Fourth Edition

Manipal Prep Manual of Medicine

As per the latest NMC Guidelines | Competency Based Medical Education (CBME) Curriculum under Graduate Medical Education Regulation

Fourth Edition

Manipal Prep Manual of Medicine

As per the latest NMC Guidelines | Competency Based Medical Education (CBME) Curriculum under Graduate Medical Education Regulation

Manthappa M MD
Professor and Unit Chief
Department of Medicine and
Vice Principal, JSS Medical College
JSS Academy of Higher Education and Research
Mysuru, Karnataka

Former Associate Professor, Department of Medicine
Kasturba Medical College, Manipal University (now MAHE)
Manipal, Karnataka
Email: manthappa74@gmail.com

CBSPD

CBS Publishers & Distributors Pvt Ltd

New Delhi • Bengaluru • Chennai • Kochi • Kolkata • Lucknow • Mumbai
Gujarat • Hyderabad • Jharkhand • Nagpur • Patna • Pune • Uttarakhand

Disclaimer

Science and technology are constantly changing fields. New research and experience broaden the scope of information and knowledge. The author has tried his best in giving information available to him while preparing the material for this edition of the book. Although all efforts have been made to ensure optimum accuracy of the material, yet it is quite possible some errors might have been left uncorrected. The publisher, the printer and the author will not be held responsible for any inadvertent errors or inaccuracies.

Fourth Edition

Manipal Prep Manual of Medicine

ISBN: 978-81-992096-7-1

Fourth Edition: 2026
First Edition: 2011
Reprint: 2015
Second Edition: 2016
Reprint: 2017, 2018, 2019, 2020
Third Edition: 2021
Reprint: 2022, 2023, 2024

Published by Satish Kumar Jain and produced by Varun Jain for

CBS Publishers & Distributors Pvt Ltd
4819/XI Prahlad Street, 24 Ansari Road, Daryaganj, New Delhi 110 002, India
Ph: 011-23289259, 23266838 Website: www.cbspd.com
e-mail: delhi@cbspd.com

Corporate Office: 204 FIE, Industrial Area, Patparganj, Delhi 110 092, India
Ph: 011-4934 4934 Fax: 011-4934 4935 e-mail: publishing@cbspd.com; publicity@cbspd.com

Branches

- **Bengaluru:** Seema House 2975, 17th Cross, K.R. Road, Banasankari 2nd Stage, Bengaluru 560 070, Karnataka, India
  Ph: +91-80-26771678/79 Fax: +91-80-26771680 e-mail: bangalore@cbspd.com
- **Chennai:** 18/8B, Subbarayan Street, Shenoy Nagar, Chennai 600 030, Tamil Nadu, India
  Ph: +91-44-42032115, 26681266 e-mail: chennai@cbspd.com
- **Kochi:** 42/1325, 1326, Power House Road, Opposite KSEB, Power House, Ernakulam 682 018, Kochi, Kerala, India
  Ph: +91-484-4059061–65, 67 Fax: +91-484-4059065 e-mail: kochi@cbspd.com
- **Kolkata:** 147, Hind Ceramics Compound, 1st Floor, Nilgunj Road, Belghoria, Kolkata 700 056, West Bengal, India
  Ph: +91-33-25633055/56 e-mail: kolkata@cbspd.com
- **Lucknow:** Basement, Khushnuma Complex, 7 Meerabai Marg (behind Jawahar Bhawan), Lucknow 226 001, UP, India
  Ph: +91-522-4000032 e-mail: tiwari.lucknow@cbspd.com
- **Mumbai:** PWD Shed, Gala No. 25/26, Ramchandra Bhatt Marg, Next JJ Hospital Gate No. 2, Opp. Union Bank of India, Noorbaug, Mumbai 400 009, Maharashtra, India
  Ph: +91-22-66661880/89 e-mail: mumbai@cbspd.com

Representatives

- **Gujarat** • **Hyderabad** • **Jharkhand** • **Nagpur** • **Patna** • **Pune** • **Uttarakhand**

For trade terms please contact customercare@cbspd.com
For general enquiries please contact info@cbspd.com

Printed at: Paras Offset Pvt. Ltd., New Delhi, India

to

My brother MK Swamy
and
my daughter Prathiksha

Foreword to the Fourth Edition

It is always a distinct pleasure and honour to write a Foreword for the exemplary work of Dr Manthappa M. The fourth edition of the *"Manipal Prep Manual of Medicine"* marks yet another significant milestone in his continuous dedication to advancing medical education and clinical practice.

In our contemporary digital era, access to information is abundant; however, the sheer volume of online resources often poses challenges in discerning accuracy and reliability. Dr Manthappa's widely acclaimed manual distinctly addresses this challenge, effectively synthesizing crucial medical knowledge into a clear, reliable, and easily comprehensible format.

Revised and updated textbooks remain essential components in effective medical education, particularly when combined with modern pedagogical approaches such as case-based learning and problem-solving techniques. The current educational landscape, shaped by the introduction of the new National Education Policy and Competency-Based Medical Education (CBME), presents unique challenges for both students and educators alike. Additionally, rapid technological advancements in diagnostics and laboratory medicine have reshaped clinical practice, occasionally overshadowing traditional bedside skills and fundamental clinical reasoning.

Acknowledging these shifts, Dr Manthappa has meticulously updated and extensively revised each chapter to incorporate the most recent advancements in medicine. The integration of the CBME framework ensures the content meets contemporary academic standards and practical requirements. Furthermore, the expanded use of clear illustrations and enhanced images significantly contributes to effective learning, aiding quicker comprehension and better retention.

This manual, with its concise yet thorough presentation, will undoubtedly serve as an invaluable resource not only for undergraduate medical students but also for students pursuing allied and paramedical health sciences.

I extend my heartfelt congratulations to Dr Manthappa for his tireless efforts and remarkable contributions to medical education. I am confident that this edition will continue to benefit countless learners and educators alike, and I wish him and the publishers enduring success.

Dr H Basavana Gowdappa MD (Medicine) FACP FICC
Professor, Department of Medicine, JSS Medical College
Vice Chancellor, JSS Academy of Higher Education and Research
Mysuru, Karnataka, India

Foreword to the First Edition

It is my pleasure to write the Foreword to this book. Medical textbooks have increased in their size due to explosion in medical knowledge over the last few decades. Advancement in technology and understanding of microbes, cellular and subcellular structures and functions have made practice of medicine highly complicated. However, for effective grooming of a basic medical doctor essential requirement is through understanding of concepts and scientific approach. This book has effectively filled the gap between the standard textbooks and actual requirement of the medical student. Narrative style is unique, very simple and easy to grasp. Each chapter has received utmost attention and the concepts are conveyed very clearly. Like other books by Dr Manthappa, this book also stands out of its objective to the point approach and clarity.

Though there are many books on medicine for undergraduates, very few of them are good to read and understand from the student's perspective. **Manipal Prep Manual of Medicine** is one of those few books which are easy to read and understand and provide actionable information in concise form to the student preparing for the exam and start his practice. Medicine is an ever-changing subject and any book is incomplete without the most recent information. Here, in this book, the author has included the most recent information to make it up-to-date.

I congratulate the author for writing this wonderful book and I am sure that medical students will benefit from this book immensely.

Dr Raviraja V Acharya MD DNB (Internal Medicine)
Professor and Head
Department of Medicine
Kasturba Medical College
Manipal Academy of Higher Education
Manipal, Karnataka, India

Special thanks to

Dr H Basavana Gowdappa, Professor of Medicine, Former Principal of JSS Medical College, and currently serving as the Vice Chancellor of JSS Academy of Higher Education and Research (JSSAHER), Mysuru, for kindly writing the foreword to the fourth edition and for his insightful and creative suggestions that significantly enhanced the quality of the book.

Dr Raviraja V Acharya, Professor and Head, Department of Medicine at Kasturba Medical College, Manipal Academy of Higher Education, Manipal. He was my mentor during my tenure as a faculty member in his unit at KMC Manipal, and his guidance and encouragement were instrumental in inspiring me to write the first edition. I am also grateful to him for writing the foreword to the first edition.

Preface to the Fourth Edition

I am delighted to place before you the fourth edition of *Manipal Prep Manual of Medicine*. There has been an overwhelming response to previous three editions of this book because medical students liked the simple, compact, and lucid presentation of the subject matter. The fourth edition has been thoroughly revised and updated to reflect current medical knowledge and evolving academic standards.

Every paragraph has been carefully reviewed, and several new illustrations and diagrams have been added to enhance understanding. Many new topics as specified in the CBME (competency based medical education) syllabus have been incorporated to align with current curricular requirements. The aim remains to present information in a manner that is clear, concise, and easy to grasp, without creating confusion.

I have noticed that getting clarity on some topics, medical students have to refer multiple textbooks or other sources of medical literature because no single book is perfect in all the aspects. For example, definition of a disease may be good in one book, clinical features in another book. It is very difficult for medical students to refer multiple books on all the occasions due to lack of time and vast medical syllabus. I have referred several standard medical textbooks and recent medical literature while writing this book so that up-to-date information with maximum clarity is available to you.

This book is not a substitute for standard medicine text books. It has been written with the intention of helping the students grasp the subject matter easily and provide for the actual requirements of students. Read this book at least twice before your exams. Higher the number of revisions, the better it is. Remember that intelligence and memory are not the same. A genius can have poor memory, and an idiot can have photographic memory. Albert Einstein was a genius but had poor memory. So even if you are very intelligent, it does not mean that you always have good memory. Good memory depends on the number of revisions, and the trick is to revise the subject matter more times, to remember better.

The purpose of the book is fulfilled if it makes you a better student and a better doctor by making you more knowledgeable. Write to me if you have any queries or suggestions to improve the book. I have provided my email address below.

Wishing you happy reading and happy learning.

Manthappa M

Preface to the First Edition

The idea of writing this book came to me because I felt the need for a book which would be simple and yet not miss out any important information. This is what I have maintained throughout this book, matter is very simple and easy to grasp without any scope for confusion.

I have referred several standard medical textbooks and other medical resources while writing this book so that the best information with maximum points is made available to you. I have also included line diagrams wherever necessary which can be easily reproduced by the reader.

This book is not a substitute for standard textbooks on medicine. It has been written with the idea of helping the students grasp the subject matter easily and provide the actual requirements of a student. Read this book at least twice before your examinations. Higher the number of revisions, the better it is. Remember that intelligence and memory are not the same. A genius can have poor memory and an idiot can have photographic memory. Albert Einstein was a genius but had poor memory. So even if you are very intelligent, it does not mean that you always have good memory. Good memory depends on the number of revisions and the trick is to revise the subject matter several times to remember the facts better.

The purpose of the book is served if it makes you a better student and a better doctor by making you more knowledgeable. If you have any queries or suggestions to improve the book, I would appreciate your writing to me at my email id. All the best and happy reading.

Manthappa M

Contents

Foreword to the Fourth Edition by Dr H Basavana Gowdappa — *vii*
Foreword to the First Edition by Dr Raviraja V Acharya — *ix*
Preface to the Fourth Edition — *xi*
Preface to the First Edition — *xii*

1. Infectious Diseases — 1
2. Diseases of Respiratory System — 115
3. Diseases of Cardiovascular System — 180
4. Diseases of Gastrointestinal System — 298
5. Diseases of Nervous System — 352
6. Diseases of Blood — 454
7. Diseases of Liver and Biliary System — 516
8. Diseases of Kidney and Urinary Tract — 560
9. Endocrinology and Diabetes Mellitus — 589
10. Diseases of Immune System, Connective Tissue and Joints — 644
11. Nutritional Disorders — 675
12. Psychiatric Disorders — 693
13. Fluid and Electrolyte Disorders — 713
14. Oncology — 724
15. Genetic Disorders — 738
16. Diseases of the Skin — 748
17. Poisoning, Venomous Bites and Environmental Diseases — 772
18. Emergency Medicine and Critical Care — 800
19. Role of Physician in the Community, Medicolegal and Ethical Issues in Health Care — 809
20. Geriatrics — 822
21. Case Scenario-based Discussions — 842

Index — *859*

Chapter 1

Infectious Diseases

Q. What are infectious diseases?

"Infectious diseases" is a broad term encompassing illnesses caused by pathogenic microorganisms. These diseases can spread directly or indirectly from person to person or via vectors, animals, or the environment.

Types of infectious agents:

1. Bacteria, e.g. *Mycobacterium tuberculosis* causing tuberculosis.
2. Viruses, e.g. influenza virus, SARS-CoV-2 (COVID-19).
3. Fungi, e.g. *Candida albicans* causing candidiasis.
4. Parasites, e.g. Plasmodium species causing malaria.
5. Prions, e.g. misfolded proteins causing diseases like Creutzfeldt-Jakob disease.

Q. Define the terms: Colonization, infestation, infection, bacteremia, sepsis and septic shock.

Colonization

- This is the simple presence of potentially pathogenic microorganisms on or within a host (like on the skin, mouth, intestines or airway) without causing disease. However, colonization may progress to infection.
- Example: Normal flora such as *Staphylococcus epidermidis* on the skin.
- Clinical relevance: Colonization does not require treatment unless there is a risk of progression to infection (e.g. in immunocompromised patients).

Infestation

- Infestation refers to presence of parasites inside or on the host. Examples: Head louse infestation, worm infestation.

Bacteremia

- Presence of viable bacteria in the bloodstream is called bacteremia which may or may not cause symptoms. It can result from day-do-day activities such as tooth brushing or dental procedures. Bacteremia usually does not cause any symptoms such as fever and often usually resolves on its own.
- Clinical relevance: Rarely it can progress to sepsis and septic shock.

Infection

- The invasion and multiplication of pathogenic microorganisms in the host, leading to tissue damage and eliciting an immune response, e.g. pharyngitis, pneumonia, viral hepatitis.

Sepsis

- A life-threatening condition that arises when the body's response to an infection causes widespread inflammation and organ dysfunction. Sepsis is usually associated with fever, weakness, tachycardia, tachypnea and multi-organ dysfunction.

Septic Shock

- Sepsis that causes dangerously low blood pressure is called septic shock (SBP <90 or MAP <70). It is a type of vasodilatory or distributive shock. It carries high morbidity and mortality.

Q. Discuss the serological (immunological) methods used in the diagnosis of infectious diseases.

- Serological (immunological) methods involve detection of antigen or antibody of a microorganism in a given sample. These are as follows:
    - Enzyme-linked immunosorbent assay (ELISA)
    - Rapid immunochromatographic test
    - Western blot (immunoblot) test
    - Immunofluorescence test
    - Complement fixation test
    - Agglutination test
    - Immunodiffusion
    - Immunoelectrophoresis

Enzyme-linked Immunosorbent Assay (ELISA)

- **ELISA** is a widely used laboratory technique for detecting and quantifying substances, typically antigens (proteins, peptides, or hormones) or antibodies, in biological samples such as blood, serum, or plasma.
- ELISA relies on the specific interaction between an antigen and an antibody, combined with an enzyme-

linked detection system that produces a measurable color change or signal when a substrate is added.
- ELISA tests are usually performed in microwell plates.

Steps in a Typical ELISA Test

- Antigen or antibody is immobilized on a 96-well microplate.
- Clinical sample is added into these microwells. If a specific antigen or antibody is present in the clinical specimen, it is captured by the coated antigen/antibodies on the ELISA plate.
- A second antibody to the target protein conjugated with an enzyme is then added which is captured by the target protein. The unbound material is washed out. A chromogenic substrate (to the enzyme) is then added. Development of color by the action of hydrolyzing enzyme on chromogenic substrate indicates the presence of the specific antigen or antibody. Color intensity is measured by the spectrophotometer.
- There are many variations of ELISA, but the basic principle remains the same as described above. In the first-generation ELISAs either crude antigen or single antigen is used for the test. In the second and third-generation ELISAs multiple antigens or recombinant antigen or/and specific peptides are used, which improves the sensitivity and specificity of the test.
- ELISA is routinely used to detect antibodies against HIV and hepatitis A virus.

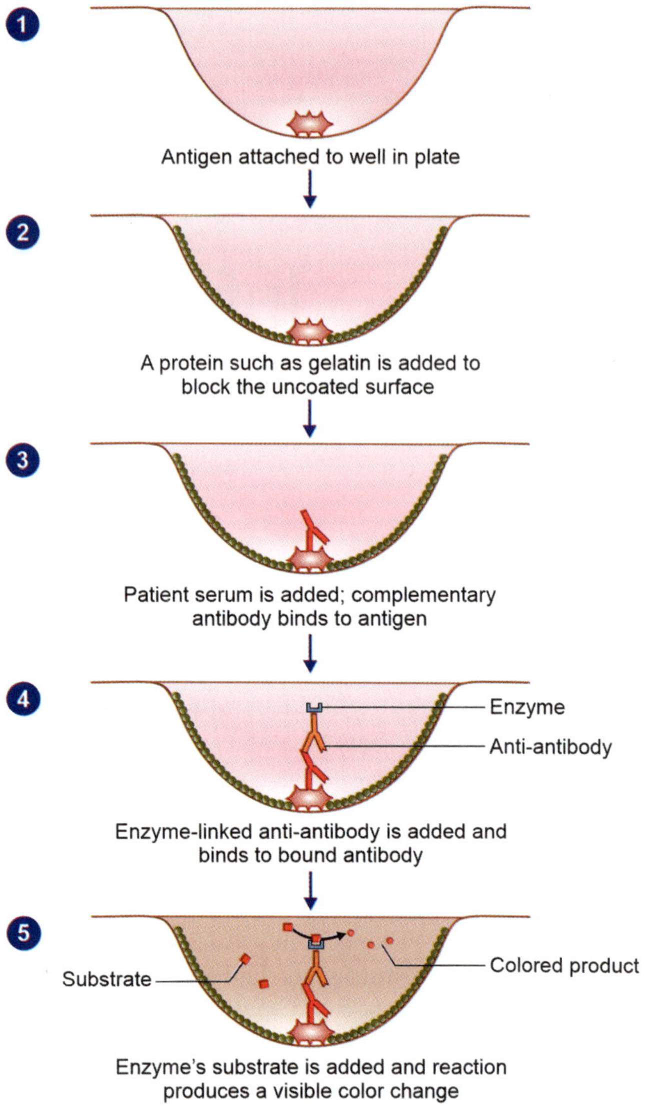

Figure 1.1: ELISA

Rapid Immunochromatographic Test

- ICT is based on the **lateral flow assay** principle, where a liquid sample flows along a nitrocellulose strip and interacts with reagents pre-applied to specific zones. Detection is achieved through visual signals, often color changes, that indicate the presence of the target analyte. This allows rapid detection of antigen or antibodies in patient's body fluids. Clinical sample (blood or urine) is added to the wells provided in the kit. The sample diffuses across the plate and the presence of specific proteins is indicated by the development of colored bands on the strip. These diagnostic strip tests are simple, rapid, cheap and reliable and can be used at home and clinics. Such kits have been developed for dengue; malaria, etc. Urine pregnancy test kit is also an example of immunochromatographic test which uses specific antibodies to selectively identify hCG in urine.

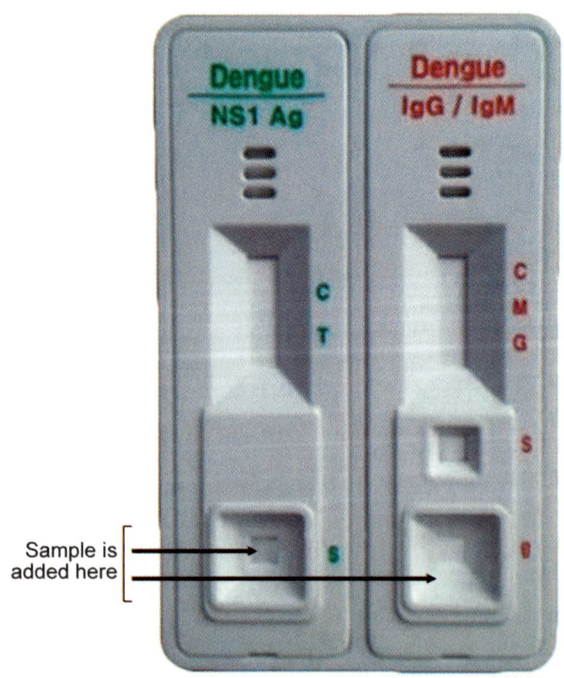

Figure 1.2: Rapid chromatographic test

Western Blot (Immunoblot) Test

- In Western blot, antibodies to multiple specific proteins are detected. Hence, it has high specificity. Microbial protein is run on gel electrophoresis to separate the ligands, which are then transferred on to a nitrocellulose membrane strip. Patient's serum is added to this nitrocellulose strip. If there are antibodies to a specific microorganism, they bind to antigens present on the strip. Enzymatically labeled anti-immunoglobulins can be added now which bind to the antibodies and visualized by the addition of an enzyme substrate to produce colored bands. This test is commonly used to confirm the diagnosis of HIV infection.

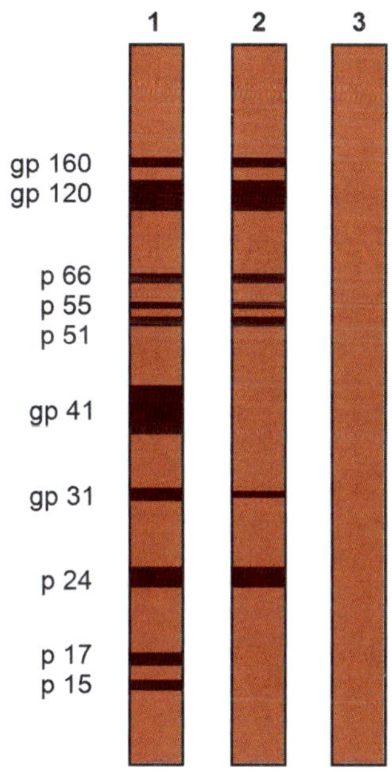

Figure 1.3: Western blot test

Test 1 is a control as it shows all the proteins tested for are present.

Test 2 is a positive result as it shows there are antibodies for 7 of the HIV proteins.

Test 3 is a negative result.

Immunofluorescence Test

- This test makes use of immunoglobulin (antibody) labeled with fluorescent dye to detect antigens or antibodies. It requires a fluorescent microscope to read the signal. It is commonly used to detect infections with herpes virus, dengue virus and rabies virus.

Direct Immunofluorescence

- Direct immunofluorescence or direct fluorescent antibody (DFA) test uses a single antibody labeled with fluorescent dye to detect the presence of a specific antigen. If a specific antigen of a microorganism is present in patient's serum, it combines with the antibody labeled with a fluorescent dye which can be detected as a fluorescent signal under a fluorescence microscope. This test is highly sensitive and specific.

Indirect Immunofluorescence

- Here two antibodies are used. The first antibody recognizes the target antigen and binds to it, and the second antibody, which is labeled with a fluorescent dye recognizes the first antibody and binds to it.
- This test is more complex than the direct immunofluorescence test and takes more time but allows more flexibility. Patient's serum is incubated with a specific microbial antigen. If specific antibodies are present in the patient serum, they combine with the antigen. Next, fluorescent-labeled antisera is added and the fluorescent signal is looked for.

Applications of Immunofluorescence

- Diagnosing autoimmune diseases (e.g. lupus with kidney biopsies).
- Detecting pathogens directly (e.g. *Treponema pallidum* in syphilis, *Plasmodium falciparum*).
- Detecting viral antigens (e.g. influenza, herpes simplex virus).

Complement Fixation Test

- Complement fixation test (CFT) is a serological method used to detect the presence of specific antigens or antibodies in a patient's serum by measuring the activity of the complement system. It is based on the principle that antigen-antibody complexes consume complement proteins, preventing them from lyzing red blood cells in a controlled test environment.
- Patient's serum is heat treated to remove any free complement. The serum is mixed with a known antigen (for antibody detection) or antibody (for antigen detection). Standardized complement proteins are added to the mixture. The mixture is incubated to allow formation of antigen-antibody complexes and complement fixation. Sensitized sheep red blood cells and hemolytic antibodies (anti-sheep antibodies) are then added.
- If antibodies are present in the patient's blood, there is formation of antigen-antibody complex and complement gets fixed to these complexes (used up), hence there is no complement left to lyse the RBCs. If there is no antibody, complement remains unused and it lyzes the sensitized sheep RBCs. Absence of hemolysis means complement fixation test is positive which means that specific antibodies are present. This test has been largely superseded by other methods such as ELISA and PCR, but still useful for the following.

Applications

- CFT is used to detect antibodies against pathogens that cause infectious diseases.
- Detection of autoimmune diseases: CFT can help detect autoimmune diseases by identifying autoantibodies (systemic lupus erythematosus (SLE) (anti-dsDNA antibodies), rheumatic fever.
- Screening for immunodeficiency: Identifying deficiencies in components of the complement system.
- Research applications: Studying complement-mediated immune mechanisms.

Agglutination Test

- An agglutination test detects the presence of antigens or antibodies in a sample through the clumping (agglutination) of particles such as red blood cells, latex beads, or bacteria.
- *Types of agglutination tests:* Direct agglutination test (DAT), indirect agglutination test (passive agglutination), hemagglutination test, coombs test (antiglobulin test), bacterial agglutination test.

Direct Agglutination Test (DAT)

- DAT is a diagnostic method that detects antigens naturally present on the surface of cells, such as red blood cells, bacteria, or other pathogens, by directly observing the agglutination caused by the binding of specific antibodies to these antigens.

- When antibodies specific to the antigens on the surface of a cell or pathogen are mixed, they bind to the antigens, forming cross-links between the cells. This interaction leads to visible clumping (agglutination) of the cells, which indicates the presence of the antigen.

Applications of DAT

- To determine ABO and Rh blood groups with specific anti-A, anti-B, and anti-D sera.
- Diagnosis of diseases like brucellosis, typhoid, and certain fungal infections by detecting antigens directly.
- Detection of Leishmania in visceral leishmaniasis.
- Identification of bacterial species by using antisera specific to bacterial antigens (e.g. serotyping Salmonella or Shigella species).

Indirect (Passive) Agglutination Test

- Unlike the direct agglutination test, this test uses artificially coated particles, such as latex beads, gelatin, or red blood cells, to which the antigens or antibodies are bound. These coated particles act as carriers to amplify the visible agglutination reaction.
- When antibodies (from the patient sample) interact with antigens (coated on the artificial particles) or *vice versa*, the particles clump together, forming visible agglutination. This method is termed "passive" because the antigens or antibodies are not naturally present on the particles but are artificially attached.
- In latex agglutination test, latex particles coated with specific antibody are mixed with patient's serum. If there are specific antigens in the patient's serum, there is agglutination of antibody coated latex particles. This test is used to detect toxins of *Vibrio cholerae* and staphylococci.
- In hemagglutination test, RBCs are coated with known antigens. If mixed with serum containing specific antibodies, there is agglutination of RBCs. This is used in the diagnosis of syphilis and herpes virus infections.

Immunodiffusion

- Immunodiffusion is a diagnostic test which involves diffusion through a substance such as agar gel. Here a specific antigen or antibody is placed in one well and patient's serum or body fluid is placed in another well and left for 48 hours. The antigen and antibody diffuse through the agarose gel towards each other and a precipitation line is formed between the two wells.

Immunoelectrophoresis

- It is a technique used to analyze and identify specific proteins in a sample, often serum or other body fluids. It combines the principles of electrophoresis and immunodiffusion to separate and characterize proteins based on their size, charge, and antigenic properties. This test is conducted on agarose gel.
- *Electrophoresis:* Proteins in the sample are separated based on their charge and size by applying an electric field to a gel.
- *Immunodiffusion:* After electrophoresis, a trough is cut into the gel, and specific antibodies are added. Proteins (antigens) and antibodies diffuse through the gel and form visible precipitin arcs where they interact.

Clinical Applications

- Detection of abnormal proteins: Useful in conditions like multiple myeloma and other plasma cell dyscrasias.
- Quantification of immunoglobulins: Identifies IgG, IgA, IgM, and their subtypes in cases of immune deficiency or overproduction.
- Identification of specific proteins: Useful for confirming the presence of specific proteins in serum or other fluids.

Q. Discuss the molecular methods used in the diagnosis of infectious diseases.

- Molecular methods have revolutionized the diagnosis of infectious diseases by providing rapid, sensitive, and specific detection of pathogens. These methods rely on the identification of nucleic acids (DNA or RNA) unique to the pathogen. These are polymerase chain reaction (PCR), southern blotting and northern blotting.

Polymerase Chain Reaction (PCR)

- This is the most specific and sensitive test of all molecular techniques. Here the nucleic acid sequence of a microorganism is amplified so that it becomes easily detectable. Since each microorganism has unique DNA/RNA sequences, it is possible to select a PCR primer that specifically identifies a particular microorganism.
- Multiple microorganisms can be identified in single clinical sample using 'multiplex' PCR.
- Fluorescent dyes can be attached to different primers and the final nucleic acid polymers examined by light spectroscopy.
- Reverse transcriptase (RT)-PCR amplifies very small amounts of any kind of RNA (mRNA, rRNA) and makes complementary DNA, which is then amplified with conventional PCR. HIV viral copies are estimated by this method.
- Real-time PCR (qPCR) is used to quantify the organisms and is used in estimation of HIV viral load.
- The disadvantages of PCR are its high cost and false-positive results. False positive results happen if there is any contamination from laboratory or other sources.

Applications

- Detecting bacterial (e.g. *Mycobacterium tuberculosis*), viral (e.g. HIV, influenza), fungal, and parasitic infections.
- Monitoring viral load in chronic infections (e.g. hepatitis B or C).

- Multiplex PCR is used to detect multiple pathogens in respiratory, gastrointestinal, or central nervous system infections (e.g. multiplex panels for meningitis/ encephalitis pathogens).
- Most widely used method for detecting COVID-19 (reverse transcription polymerase chain reaction—RT-PCR).

Southern Blotting

- Southern blot is a method for detection of a specific DNA sequence in DNA samples. Southern blot is named after biologist Edwin Southern who developed this technique.
- DNA fragments are separated by gel electrophoresis and transferred on to a blotting paper. A DNA probe (this is a piece of single stranded DNA with known sequence labeled with a radioactive isotope or a fluorescent signal) is then added to the blotting paper. DNA probe will bind to its complementary DNA if present. This is then washed to remove any unbound DNA probe.
- Even after washing if there is radioactivity or fluorescence, it means that a specific DNA complementary to DNA probe is present. Since each microorganism has specific DNA sequences, it indicates the presence of that particular microorganism in the clinical specimen.

Applications

- **Gene detection:** Identifying the presence or absence of specific genes in an organism's genome.
- **Gene mapping:** Locating genes or mutations associated with specific genetic diseases.
- **RFLP analysis:** Studying restriction fragment length polymorphisms for genetic diversity, forensic analysis, or paternity testing.
- **Diagnosis of genetic disorders:** Detecting mutations or deletions associated with diseases like sickle cell anemia or cystic fibrosis.
- **Viral genome detection:** Identifying viral DNA in infected samples (e.g. HPV, HBV).

Northern Blotting

- This is same as Southern blotting except that RNA fragments are used to detect and quantify specific RNA molecules in a sample instead of DNA.

Applications

- Detect RNA viruses like HIV or influenza in infected samples.
- **Gene expression analysis:** Measure mRNA levels to study gene activity under different conditions or during development.

Q. Define fever of unknown origin (FUO). Enumerate the causes of FUO. How do you approach a case of FUO?

- Fever of unknown origin (FUO) or pyrexia of unknown origin (PUO) is prolonged febrile illness without an established etiology despite intensive evaluation and diagnostic testing **(Table 1.1)**.

Category-based Definitions of FUO

TABLE 1.1: Category-based definitions of FUO

Category	Commonly used definition
Classic FUO	Temperature >38.3°C (100.9°F) recorded on several occasions for >3 weeks, despite 3 outpatient clinic evaluations, 1 week of intensive outpatient investigation, or 3 days of hospital-based evaluation (*remember* 3,3,1,3).
Healthcare-associated FUO	
• ICU patient	Temperature >38.3°C (100.9°F) recorded on several occasions in an ICU patient despite ≥3 days of investigations. Fever must not have been present or incubating on admission.
• Non-ICU patient	Same definition as for ICU patient, except patient is hospitalized but not critically ill.
• Postoperative patient	Same definition as for ICU patient, except fever is usually defined as ≥38.0°C (100.4°F).
FUO in immunocompromised patients	
• Neutropenic patients	Temperature ≥38.3°C (100.9°F) sustained over a one-hour period, recorded on several occasions over at least 3 days, despite appropriate antimicrobial therapy. Neutropenia is defined as <500 neutrophils/µl or impending fall to that level within 48 hours.
• Patients with HIV and CD4 count <200 cells/µl	Temperature ≥38.3°C (100.9°F) recorded on several occasions for >3 weeks for outpatient or >3 days for inpatient despite appropriate evaluation.
Travel-associated FUO	Temperature >38.3°C (100.9°F) recorded on several occasions for >3 weeks, despite 3 outpatient clinic evaluations, 1 week of intensive outpatient investigation, or 3 days of hospital-based evaluation, in a patient who traveled to another country, typically within the prior 12 months.

Causes of FUO (Table 1.2)

TABLE 1.2: Causes of FUO

Infections (most common cause of FUO)
Bacterial
• Tuberculosis (very common cause of FUO)
• Typhoid
• Brucellosis
• Infective endocarditis
• Syphilis
• Melioidosis
• Sinusitis
• Osteomyelitis
• Prostatitis
• Dental abscesses
• Cholangitis
• Intra-abdominal abscesses (subphrenic, renal, retroperitoneal, and paraspinal abscesses)

(*Contd.*)

TABLE 1.2: Causes of FUO *(Contd.)*
Viral • HIV • Chronic hepatitis (B, C, D) • Infectious mononucleosis
Parasitic • Malaria • Amebiasis • Leishmaniasis • Malaria • Strongyloidiasis • Toxocariasis • Toxoplasmosis • Trichinellosis • Babesiosis
Rickettsial infections • Q fever • Rickettsial pox • Rocky Mountain spotted fever • Scrub typhus
Fungal • Candidiasis • Histoplasmosis • Mucormycosis • Blastomycosis • Cryptococcal disease
Neoplasms (second most common cause of FUO) • Lymphoma • Leukemia and other hematologic malignancies • Liver involvement with hepatoma or metastases • Renal cell carcinoma • Colon carcinoma • Atrial myxoma
Inflammatory and connective tissue disorders • Rheumatoid arthritis • Systemic Lupus erythematosus (SLE) • Sarcoidosis • Inflammatory bowel disease (IBD) • Polyarteritis nodosa (PAN) • Giant cell arteritis (common in elderly patients) • Polymyalgia rheumatica • Crohn's disease • Granulomatous hepatitis • Kikuchi disease
Miscellaneous • Drug fever • Factitious fever • Periodic fever (familial mediterranean fever)
Undiagnosed Even after extensive workup some FUOs may remain undiagnosed. Some of them may resolve spontaneously.

APPROACH TO A CASE OF FUO

Detailed History

- Since FUO has a broad range of possible causes, the history should be thorough, structured, and tailored to uncover subtle clues that may guide the diagnostic process.

Fever Characteristics

- **Onset:** When did the fever start?
- **Pattern:** Is the fever continuous, remittent, intermittent, or relapsing? Tertian fever (occurring every third day) in malaria, step ladder type fever (typhoid), undulant fever (evening fevers resolving by morning in brucellosis), week-long fever with week-long remission (relapsing fever in borreliosis), week-long high fevers with week-long remissions (known as Pel-Ebstein fever seen in Hodgkin's disease).
- **Temperature range:** Document the highest and lowest recorded temperatures.
- **Diurnal variation:** Is the fever higher in the evening or morning?
- **Response to medications:** Does the fever respond to antipyretics?

Associated Symptoms

- Weight loss, night sweats (e.g. tuberculosis, malignancy).
- Rash or skin lesions (e.g. vasculitis, lupus).
- Joint pain/swelling (e.g. rheumatoid arthritis, Still's disease).
- Lymph node enlargement (e.g. lymphoma, sarcoidosis).
- Neurological symptoms (e.g. meningitis, encephalitis).
- Cough, chest pain, dyspnea (e.g. pneumonia, fungal infections).
- Abdominal pain, jaundice (e.g. liver abscess, hepatitis).
- Diarrhea (intestinal infections, typhoid, HIV)
- Itching after a hot bath (lymphoma)
- Painful nodules on shins (tuberculosis, fungal infections, lymphoma)
- Contact with infection (tuberculosis) or animals (cat scratch disease, brucellosis) or birds (psittacosis).
- Inquire about symptoms involving all major organ systems.

Exposure History

- High-risk sexual behavior (HIV, hepatitis-B, hepatitis-C).
- Animal contact: Pets (toxoplasmosis, cat scratch disease, leptospirosis), livestock (brucellosis, Q fever).

Travel History

- Recent or past travel to endemic regions.
- Malaria, typhoid, or arboviruses (e.g. dengue, chikungunya) in tropical regions.
- Histoplasmosis or blastomycosis in the Mississippi River Valley.
- Tuberculosis or brucellosis in high-risk areas (suspect infections endemic in places visted).
- Drug therapy (suspect drug fever).

Occupational History

- Healthcare workers (tuberculosis, viral hepatitis).
- Farmers or veterinarians (zoonoses like anthrax, brucellosis, leptospirosis).
- Recent dental treatment (possibility of endocarditis).

- History of immunosuppression such as HIV infection or steroid therapy (suspect opportunistic infections).
- History of previous abdominal surgery, trauma, endoscopy, or gynecologic procedures increase the likelihood of an occult intra-abdominal abscess.

Past History

- Chronic diseases:
  - Diabetes (predisposes to infections).
  - Autoimmune diseases (e.g. lupus, sarcoidosis).
- Surgical history:
  - Prosthetic devices or implants (infection risk).
  - Splenectomy (increased susceptibility to encapsulated organisms).

Family History

- Hereditary autoinflammatory syndromes (e.g. familial Mediterranean fever).
- Genetic predisposition to autoimmune diseases or malignancies.
- Family history of TB or HIV or other infections can predispose other family members to same infection.

Treatment History

- Recent medications: Antibiotics, anticonvulsants, or antiarrhythmics can cause drug fever.
- Immunosuppressants: Increased risk of opportunistic infections.
- Recent dental treatment can lead to infective endocarditis.
- Hospitalizations: Nosocomial infections (e.g. catheter-associated infections).
- Foreign devices: Pacemakers, prosthetics, or central lines (risk of infection).
- Recent blood transfusions: Risk of HIV, hepatitis, malaria.

Personal History

- Alcohol abuse: Risk of liver abscess, TB, pneumonia.
- Diet: Raw or undercooked foods—risk of salmonellosis or toxoplasmosis. Unpasteurized milk—brucellosis or listeriosis.

Stress or Psychogenic Factors

- Factitious fever (self-induced).

Clinical Examination

- Do a complete physical examination. A meticulous, systematic physical examination can reveal subtle signs pointing toward the underlying cause. Since FUO encompasses a broad spectrum of conditions, the examination must be comprehensive and focused on detecting infectious, inflammatory, neoplastic, or other systemic causes.

Vital Signs

- Document the height and pattern of fever. Measure body temperature more than once and in the presence of a nurse to exclude factitious fever.
- BP: BP may be low in septic shock and myocarditis.
- Pulse: Pulse rate usually increases by 10 per degree Celsius rise in temperature. Relative bradycardia (i.e. pulse rate does not correspond to the raise in temperature) may be seen in enteric fever, brucellosis and some viral infections. Relative tachycardia, i.e. pulse rate more than expected to the raise in temperature may be seen in myocarditis, sepsis, hypovolemia and thyrotoxicosis.
- Respiratory rate: High respiratory rate usually points to some respiratory pathology such as pneumonia, empyema, ARDS, etc.

General Examination

- Significant weight loss: TB, HIV, malignancy.
- Pallor: May point to hematological malignancy, or a disseminated process such as TB involving bone marrow.
- Jaundice: Points to hepatobiliary disease (hepatitis, liver abscess, etc.).
- Clubbing: TB, chronic suppurative lung disease.
- Splinter hemorrhages: Infective endocarditis.
- Look for lymphadenopathy: Tuberculosis, infectious mononucleosis, HIV, lymphoma, malignancy.
- Skin and mucosal lesions
  - Maculopapular rash (rickettsial infections, viral exanthems).
  - Skin rashes in connective tissue diseases (e.g. butterfly rash in SLE, heliotrope rash in dermatomyositis).
  - Janeway lesions, Osler's nodes (infective endocarditis).
  - Petechiae or purpura (meningococcemia, vasculitis, infective endocarditis).
  - Erythema nodosum (sarcoidosis, tuberculosis, inflammatory bowel disease).
  - Eschars (rickettsial infections).
  - Oral ulcers in Behcets disease.
- Sternal tenderness: Seen in hematological malignancy due to bone marrow proliferation.
- Spinal tenderness: Pott's spine, epidural abscess.
- Signs of meningeal irritation like neck stiffness and Kernig's sign: Meningitis.
- Always examine the fundus and retina (papilloedema in meningitis, retinal leisons in CMV infection, disseminated candidiasis, tuberculosis).

Systemic Examination

- *CVS:* Carefully examine heart for any murmurs (infective endocarditis).
- *Abdomen:* look for any tenderness (deep abdominal infections) hepatosplenomegaly (enteric fever, malaria, hepatitis, hemolytic anemia, hematological malignancies), ascites (peritoneal tuberculosis, malignancy), renal angle tenderness (pyelonephritis).
- *RS:* Inspect for respiratory distress or cyanosis. Auscultate for crackles (pneumonia, pulmonary fibrosis), wheezing, or pleural rubs. Check for signs of pulmonary infections or embolism.

- *Musculoskeletal system*: Examine for joint swelling, warmth, or pain (rheumatoid arthritis, reactive arthritis, lupus), bony tenderness (osteomyelitis, malignancies), muscle tenderness (polymyositis, trichinosis).
- *Nervous system:* Altered consciousness (meningitis, encephalitis), focal deficits (abscess, stroke), neck stiffness (meningitis, subarachnoid hemorrhage).

Investigations

- Common things are common. First rule out common diseases such as enteric fever, tuberculosis, malaria, UTI, HIV infection, etc. and then only think of rare illnesses.
- Order routine investigations like Hb, total WBC count, RBC count, differential count, platelet count, ESR and peripheral smear study. Cytopenias may suggest a pathologic process involving bone marrow such as disseminated tuberculosis, hematological malignancies, etc. A high leukocyte count is common in infections. A very high leukocyte count may suggest leukemia. Eosinophilia is seen with parasitic infections and drug reactions. A very high ESR (>100 by Westergren's method) often indicates active tuberculosis, connective tissue diseases or malignancy (myeloma, leukemia, etc.).
- Urine microscopy and culture sensitivity (to R/O UTI).
- If there is cough and sputum production send it for Gram's stain, fungus stain, AFB, malignant cells and culture/sensitivity.
- Blood culture and sensitivity for both aerobic and anaerobic organisms (infecting organism may be picked up by this).
- Complete LFT and RFT to look for any liver and renal involvement.
- Culture and examination of the stool for any ova, parasites and occult blood.
- Chest radiograph (tuberculosis, pneumonia, sarcoidosis).
- Montoux test can help in diagnosing TB.
- Lumbar puncture and CSF examination if suspecting meningitis.
- Serological investigations (WIDAL test, ASO titer, HIV-Elisa, VDRL, TPHA, Paul Bunnel test, brucella agglutination test).
- Autoimmune and inflammatory markers (to rule out connective tissue diseases): Rheumatoid factor, antinuclear antibodies.
- Tumor markers: PSA (prostate cancer). CA-125 (ovarian cancer), CA-19-9 (colorectal, pancreatic cancer), alpha-fetoprotein (HCC).
- ECG, echocardiogram (to look for signs of infective endocarditis).
- Ultrasound abdomen and pelvis to R/O any intra-abdominal pathology. Ultrasound can help in many ways. It can document any organomegaly, intra-abdominal lymphadenopathy or masses, ascites, any change in the texture of organs, any intrabdominal collections of pus.
- CT/MRI scanning (intra-abdominal lymphadenopathy, tumors, abscesses).
- Tissue diagnosis (lymph node FNAC/biopsy, liver biopsy, bone marrow examination).
- Diagnostic surgical procedures like laparoscopy, exploratory laparotomy, etc. may be required in undiagnosed cases.

Treatment

- Treatment depends on the underlying cause.
- Until a diagnosis is made, it is better to use only symptomatic treatment. Blind antibiotic therapy may make diagnosis of an occult infection more difficult, and empirical steroid therapy may mask an inflammatory response without treating the underlying cause.
- Sometimes when all the tests are negative and the cause of fever remains undiagnosed, a therapeutic trial may be indicated. For example, antituberculosis therapy (ATT) in suspected tuberculosis and steroid therapy in suspected connective tissue diseases.
- Periodic review is very important in cases of FUO as development of new signs and symptoms may help in identifying the underlying cause. In some cases, a 'second opinion' by another physician can also be very helpful as different people think from different angles.
- Many undiagnosed cases of FUO will spontaneously resolve.

Q. Chemoprophylaxis.

- Chemoprophylaxis refers to the use of drugs to prevent disease or infection in individuals who are at risk. It is widely used in both infectious diseases and non-infectious conditions and is a critical public health tool to control outbreaks, prevent complications, and protect high-risk populations.
- For example, antibiotics may be administered to immunocompromised patients to prevent opportunistic infections. Antibiotics may also be given to healthy individuals to limit the spread of an epidemic, or to patients with recurrent infections (such as urinary tract infections) to prevent recurrence.

Types of Chemoprophylaxis

Primary Prophylaxis

- Prevents the initial occurrence of a disease.
- *Example*: Using isoniazid in high-risk individuals to prevent tuberculosis.

Secondary Prophylaxis

- Prevents recurrence of a disease in previously affected individuals.
- *Example*: Sulfadiazine and pyrimethamine in HIV-positive patients to prevent recurrent toxoplasmosis.

Common Situations where Chemoprophylaxis is used

Infectious Diseases

See **Table 1.3**.

TABLE 1.3: Common situations where chemoprophylaxis is used

Situation	Goal	Chemoprophylaxis
Rheumatic fever	To prevent recurrence and further cardiac damage	Phenoxymethylpenicillin 250 mg twice daily or inj Benzathine penicillin once a month for many years as recommended
Meningitis		
• Due to meningococci	To prevent infection in close contacts	Rifampicin 600 BD for 2 days Alternatives (single dose) ciprofloxacin 500 mg orally or inj ceftriaxone 250 mg IM
• Due to *H. influenzae* type b		Rifampicin 600 mg daily for 4 days
Tuberculosis	To prevent infection in exposed tuberculin-negative individuals, infants of infected mothers and immunosuppressed patients	Oral isoniazid 300 mg daily for 6 months
Valvular heart disease **Prosthetic heart valves**	To prevent infective endocarditis in dental, oral, or upper respiratory tract procedures:	Amoxicillin, 2 g orally. If allergic to peniclin, clindamycin 600 mg or cephalexin 2 g or azithromycin 500 mg can be used. Antibiotic should be given 1 hour before the procedure orally. If patient is unable to take orally any of these can be given parenterally.
Malaria	Prevention of malaria	Chloroquine one double strength tablet per week or mefloquine 250 mg once a week.
HIV infected patient with CD4 count below 200 cells/µl	Prevention of pneumocystis jiroveci pneumonia	Trimethoprim-sulfamethoxazole, one double-strength tablet (960 mg) daily
HIV infected patient with toxoplasma IgG antibody positive and CD4+ T cell count <100/µl	Prevention of toxoplasmosis	Trimethoprim-sulfamethoxazole, one double-strength tablet (960 mg) daily
HIV infected patient with CD4 count below 50 cells/µl	Prevention of Mycobacterium avium complex infection	Azithromycin (1200 mg orally weekly) or clarithromycin (500 mg orally twice daily)

Non-infectious Diseases

- **Thromboembolism:** Low-molecular-weight heparin (LMWH) or aspirin for individuals at risk (e.g. post-surgery or immobile patients).
- **Cancer prevention:** Tamoxifen for breast cancer prevention in high-risk individuals.
- **Cardiovascular diseases:** Statins or aspirin for prevention in high-risk individuals.

Q. Opportunistic infections (Fig. 1.4 and Table 1.4).

- Opportunistic infection is an infection by a micro-organism that normally does not cause disease, but becomes pathogenic when the body's immune system is impaired. Opportunistic infections are common in following conditions:
  - Primary immune deficiency disorders
  - HIV infection
  - Steroid therapy
  - Chemotherapy for cancer
  - Immunosuppressing agents for organ transplant recipients
  - Malnutrition
  - Prolonged antibiotic therapy
- Opportunistic infections can be due to bacteria, viruses, protozoa or fungi.

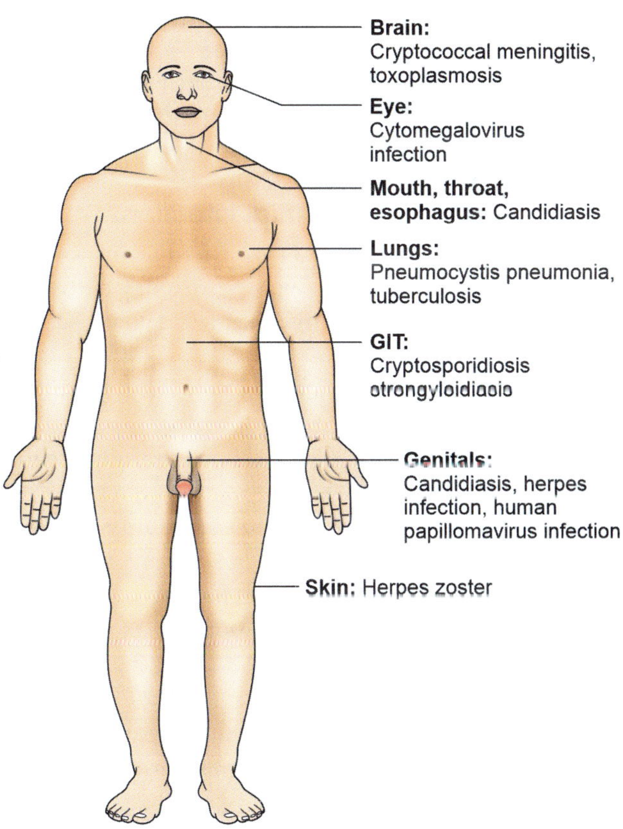

Figure 1.4: Common opportunistic infections

TABLE 1.4: Common opportunistic infections

Organism	Disease	Treatment
Viruses		
Herpes simplex virus	Encephalitis	Acyclovir
Varicella zoster virus	Disseminated herpes zoster	Acyclovir
Cytomegalovirus	Retinitis, pneumonia	Ganciclovir
Bacteria		
TB	Pulmonary or extraputlmonary involvement	Isoniazid, rifampin, pyrazinamide, ethambutol
Mycobacterium avium-intracellulare complex (MAC)	Fever, weight loss, lymphadenopathy	Clarithromycin or azithromycin + ethambutol
Fungi		
Pneumocystis jirovecii	Pneumonia	Sulphomethoxazole + trimethoprim
Candida	Mucocutaneous and esophageal candidiasis	Fluconazole, itraconazole, amphotericin-B
Cryptococcus	Meningitis	Amphotericin-B + flucytosine
Parasites		
Toxoplasma gondii	Encephalitis, pneumonia	Sulphadiazine + pyrimethamine alternative—clindamycin
Cryptosporidium	Diarrhea	Nitazoxanide
Strongyloidiasis	Diarrhea	Ivermectin, albendazole

Prevention Opportunistic Infections

- Prophylaxis in high-risk individuals
- Vaccination
- Lifestyle modifications (minimize exposure to pathogens)

Q. Nosocomial infections (hospital-acquired infections).

- Nosocomial infections (NIs), also known as hospital-acquired infections (HAIs), are infections that develop during a patient's stay in a healthcare facility and are not present or incubating at the time of admission. These infections typically appear 48 hours or more after admission or within 30 days post-discharge. The most common sites of infection are the bloodstream, lungs, urinary tract, and surgical wounds.

Common Sites of Nosocomial Infections

- *Urinary tract infections (UTIs)*: Most common HAI, often associated with indwelling urinary catheters.
- *Surgical site infections (SSIs)*: Occur at the incision site following surgery.
- *Respiratory infections*: Includes ventilator-associated pneumonia (VAP).
- *Bloodstream infections (BSIs):* Often related to central venous catheters (CVCs).
- *Gastrointestinal infections*: Most commonly caused by *Clostridioides difficile*.
- *Skin and soft tissue infections*: Can occur due to pressure ulcers or device-related infections.

Risk Factors

- *Patient-related:* Immunosuppression, comorbid conditions (e.g. diabetes, chronic lung disease), advanced age or neonatal period.
- *Procedure-related:* Indwelling devices (e.g. catheters, ventilators, IV lines), surgical procedures.
- *Environmental:* Contaminated surfaces or instruments, poor hand hygiene or infection control practices.
- *Antibiotic use:* Broad-spectrum antibiotic overuse leading to resistant organisms.

Common Pathogens in Nosocomial Infections

- Though any organism can cause a nosocomial infection, there is an increasing incidence of multidrug-resistant (MDR) pathogens causing hospital-acquired infections. Some common organisms causing nosocomial infections are as follows.
- ***Gram-positive bacteria:*** *Staphylococcus aureus* (including MRSA), Enterococcus species, gram-negative bacteria, *Escherichia coli, Klebsiella pneumoniae, Pseudomonas aeruginosa, Acinetobacter baumannii.*
- ***Fungi:*** Candida species.
- ***Viruses:*** Respiratory viruses, such as influenza or RSV.

Transmission

- Transmission usually occurs via healthcare workers, patients, hospital equipment, or interventional procedures.

Clinical Features

- Any new onset fever or any unexplained clinical deterioration in a hospitalized patient may be due to hospital acquired infection.
- Clinical features depend on the site of infection.
- Any new infiltrate on chest X-ray may due to hospital acquired pneumonia.

Investigations

- ***Complete blood count:*** usually shows leukocytosis.
- ***Blood culture and sensitivity:*** to diagnose bloodstream infection.
- ***Urine examination:*** to diagnose urinary tract infection.
- ***Chest X-ray:*** to diagnose pneumonia.
- ***Other tests*** as per clinical suspicion.

Treatment

- Treatment will be based on the type of hospital acquired infection. However, pending investigation reports, broad spectrum antibiotics can be started.
- Intravenous cannula should be removed if there is inflammation at the insertion site.
- Indwelling urinary catheter should be removed if possible.
- Surgical-site infections should be managed with a combination of surgical care and antibiotic therapy.

Prevention Strategies

- ***Hand hygiene*:** Proper handwashing or use of alcohol-based hand sanitizers.
- ***Aseptic techniques*:** During catheter insertion, IV placement, and wound care.
- ***Minimizing device use*:** Remove indwelling devices as soon as they are no longer necessary.
- ***Antibiotic stewardship*:** Avoid overuse or misuse of antibiotics.
- ***Environmental cleaning*:** Routine disinfection of surfaces and equipment.
- ***Staff training*:** Ongoing education on infection prevention practices.
- ***Isolation protocols*:** For patients with multidrug-resistant (MDR) organisms or airborne infections.

Q. Food poisoning.

- **Food poisoning** (also known as foodborne disease) refers to an acute illness caused by consuming contaminated food or beverages. It can result from the ingestion of microorganisms, their toxins, or chemical contaminants. Symptoms usually involve the gastrointestinal tract but can vary depending on the causative agent.
- Green leafy vegetables are the most common cause of food poisoning, followed by dairy items and poultry.
- Food poisoning should be suspected when many people develop the illness after ingesting the same food and the illness bears a temporal relationship to food intake.

Causes

Microorganisms

- Bacteria
  - *Staphylococcus aureus* (improperly stored meats, dairy, or cream-filled pastries).
  - *Bacillus cereus* (reheated rice, pasta, starchy foods).
  - Salmonella (e.g. in raw poultry, eggs, or dairy).
  - *Escherichia coli* (e.g. *E. coli* O157:H7 from contaminated meat or produce).
  - *Listeria monocytogenes* (e.g. in unpasteurized dairy or deli meats).
  - Vibrio species (e.g. in raw seafood).
  - *Clostridium botulinum* (improperly canned foods, honey).
- Viruses
  - Norovirus (e.g. in contaminated water, shellfish).
  - Hepatitis A (from contaminated food or water).
- Parasites
  - *Toxoplasma gondii* (from undercooked meat).
  - Cryptosporidium and *Giardia lamblia* (waterborne).
- Fungi
  - Aflatoxins produced by molds (e.g. Aspergillus on nuts and grains).

Chemical causes

- Marine toxins: Ciguatoxin, scombrotoxin fish (e.g. barracuda, tuna, mackerel)
- Plant toxins (flava beans)
- Pesticides, herbicides, or industrial chemicals.
- Heavy metals (arsenic, thallium and cadmium)
- Naturally occurring toxins (e.g. scombrotoxin in fish, mushroom toxins).

Clinical Features

- The commonest manifestation of food poisoning is a mixture of nausea, vomiting, fever, abdominal pain and diarrhea.
- Usually symptoms occur in many persons who ingest the same food.
- Symptoms usually develop within 48 hours after ingestion of food. In case of preformed toxins (staphylococcal toxin and *Bacillus cereus*) and non-infective food poisoning symptoms develop within minutes to hours.
- Specific etiologic agent can be identified by examining the suspected food, vomitus, stool or blood.

Management

- Most cases of food poisoning are self limiting.
- Intravenous fluids and electrolytes should be given to patients with severe vomiting and diarrhea.
- Antidiarrheal agents (codeine phosphate, loperamide) can be used to control diarrhea. However, they should be avoided in young children, elderly, and patients who have fever and pain abdomen suggesting infective diarrhea.
- Antibiotics are not routinely indicated unless a specific pathogen is suspected.

Prevention of Food Poisoning

Following precautions can decrease the chances of food poisoning.

- Do not drink raw (unpasteurized) milk or foods that contain unpasteurized milk.
- Wash raw fruits and vegetables thoroughly in running water before eating.
- Use precooked, perishable, or ready-to-eat food as soon as possible.
- Avoid cross contamination; keep raw meat, fish, and poultry separate from other foods.
- Thoroughly cook raw food from animal sources. Seafood and shellfish should be cooked thoroughly to minimize the risk of food poisoning.
- Refrigerate foods promptly. Never leave cooked foods at room temperature for more than two hours.

Q. Staphylococcal food poisoning.

- *Staph. aureus* is a part of the normal flora of the skin, nose, and throat. *Staph. aureus* is coagulase-positive and is the most virulent of all staphylococcal species. All other staphylococci have been collectively designated as coagulase-negative staphylococci and are less virulent.
- Food handlers may transfer the bacteria via hands to foodstuffs such as dairy products, meats, eggs, and salads.
- After the food is left at room temperature, the organisms multiply and can produce a substantial quantity of enterotoxin.

Clinical Features

- Following ingestion of contaminated food, nausea, vomiting and abdominal cramps develop within 1–6 hours. Fever and/or diarrhea may also occur in a minority of patients.
- Most cases improve rapidly. Rarely severe dehydration can occur which can be fatal.

Management

- Fluid replacement and antiemetics (domperidone, ondansetron) should be given. Antibiotics are ineffective because symptoms are caused by toxins, not active bacterial infection.
- Suspected food should be tested for the presence of enterotoxin and Staphylococcus if feasible. Public health authorities should be notified if food vending is involved.
- Prevention relies on proper food handling, hygiene, and temperature control during storage and preparation.

Q. Toxic shock syndrome (TSS).

- Toxic shock syndrome (TSS) is a toxin-mediated acute life-threatening illness, usually caused by infection with either *Staphylococcus aureus* or group A Streptococcus (GAS, also called *Streptococcus pyogenes*). The toxins produced by these bacteria act as superantigens, triggering an excessive immune response that can lead to multisystem organ failure.
- TSS was first described in a small group of children with acute febrile illness. Subsequently, it was found in young, menstruating women who were using a highly absorbent tampon that was newly introduced to the market. This was due to multiplication of vaginally colonized *S. aureus* and production of an exotoxin known as TSST-I and enterotoxin B. However, tampon associated cases of TSS have come down, and most cases are now secondary to *S. aureus* infections of skin or other sites.

Clinical Features

- TSS usually begins with nonspecific flulike symptoms such as fever and myalgia. In menstrual cases, the onset is usually 2 or 3 days after the start of menstruation.
- As the severity of illness increases, patients develop diffuse erythematous rash, hypotension, and multiple organ dysfunction. Multiple organ dysfunction manifests as vomiting and diarrhea (GIT involvement), renal failure (kidney involvement), ARDS (lung involvement), liver enzyme elevation (hepatitis), thrombocytopenia (hematological involvement), confusion, drowsiness (CNS involvement), conjunctival erythema (mucosal involvement), etc.
- Desquamation of the skin occurs during convalescence, usually 1–2 weeks after the onset of illness.

Investigations

- Investigations typically show leukocytosis, thrombocytopenia, increased urea creatinine, hypoalbuminemia and liver function abnormalities.
- Gram staining and culture sensitivity of the infected specimen.
- Blood culture may show causative organism such as Staphylococcus or Streptococcus.

Treatment

- Patient should be admitted immediately to the hospital.
- Local measures (e.g. decontamination, debridement).
- Fluid resuscitation and circulatory support.
- Empiric antibiotic therapy (e.g. clindamycin plus vancomycin) pending culture results. In addition to antibacterial effect, clindamycin also reduces the synthesis of toxin.
- For patients with group A Streptococcus infection, a combination of penicillin-G (4 million U IV q4h) and clindamycin (600–900 mg IV q8h) is used. Intravenous immune globulin can be considered for streptococcal toxic shock syndrome (specific antibody to streptococcal exotoxins).
- Duration of antibiotic treatment is 10–14 days.

Q. Enumerate the infections caused by streptococci. Write briefly on scarlet fever and erysipelas.

Streptococci are gram-positive bacteria arranged in chains. They cause a variety of infections in man which are as follows:

- Skin and soft tissue infections; cellulitis, erysipelas, necrotizing fasciitis
- Bone and joint infections
- Tonsillitis
- Scarlet fever
- Glomerulonephritis
- Rheumatic fever
- Puerperal sepsis
- Endocarditis
- Urinary tract infection
- Neonatal infections including meningitis
- Female pelvic infections
- Peritonitis
- Dental infections
- Liver abscess.

Scarlet Fever

- Scarlet fever is a bacterial illness caused by *Streptococcus pyogenes* (Group A Streptococcus, GAS). It is characterized by exudative pharyngitis, fever, and bright-red exanthema *(scarlet means bright red)*.
- Exotoxin-mediated streptococcal infections range from localized skin infection (e.g. bullous impetigo) to the widespread eruption of scarlet fever to the highly lethal streptococcal toxic shock syndrome.

Clinical Features

- Common in children aged 5–15 years.
- Scarlet fever is characterized by exudative pharyngitis, fever, and *scarlatiniform rash*. Initially patient develops fever, headache, vomiting and sore throat, followed within 24 hours by a punctate erythematous rash. Erythematous rash is caused by erythrogenic toxin.
- Initially, the exanthem is seen on the tongue which becomes bright red with prominent red papillae. This appearance is called *strawberry tongue*. The rash then appears on the neck and spreads to trunk and extremities. These rashes enlarge and join together to form a generalized erythema. Usually the rash does not affect nose, lips, palms and soles. Since the lips are not affected it remains pale and stands out against the red background of flushed cheeks. Rash is more prominent in the skin folds and is called *Pastia's lines*. Usually, the rash becomes maximum by 2 days and fades by 7 days.

Differential Diagnosis

- Includes other causes of fever with generalized rash, such as:
  - Rubella, measles, and other viral exanthems
  - Kawasaki disease
  - Toxic shock syndrome
  - Systemic allergic reactions (e.g. drug eruptions).

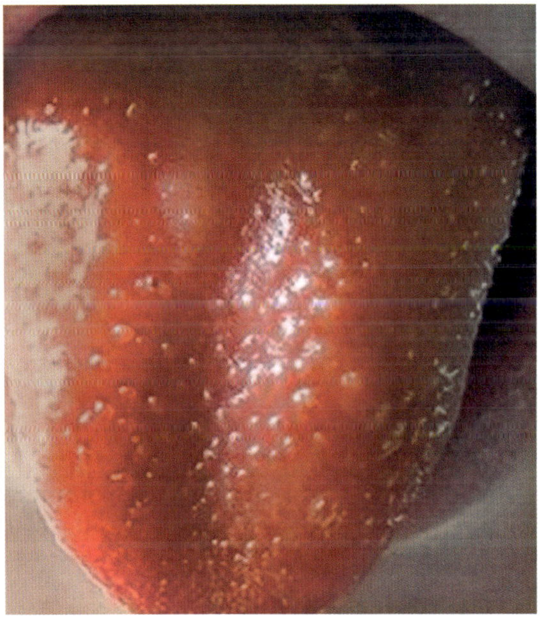

Figure 1.5: Strawberry tongue

Complications

- Otitis media, pneumonia, septicemia, osteomyelitis, toxic shock syndrome, rheumatic fever, and post-streptococcal glomerulonephritis (PSGN).

Investigations

- Complete blood count shows leukocytosis.
- Throat swab culture is the most important test to confirm the diagnosis.
- Direct antigen detecting kits allow immediate diagnosis but have less sensitivity.
- Anti-deoxyribonuclease B and antistreptolysin-O titers (antibodies to streptococcal extracellular products).

Treatment

- Penicillin is the drug of choice and is given for 7–10 days. Cephalosporins can also be used instead of penicillin. Erythromycin (or azithromycine) is an alternative for patients allergic to penicillin.

Erysipelas

- It is an infection of skin and superficial lymphatics.
- Erysipelas usually involves the face and head but other areas may also be involved.
- The skin becomes red, edematous and firm to hard in consistency due to cuticular lymphangitis. It may spread to adjacent parts and involve large areas. The margins of the erythematous areas are raised and sometimes vesicles are also seen. The patient may appear sick.
- Erysipelas of the face has to be differentiated from cellulitis. Since cellulitis is an infection of subcutaneous tissues, it does not involve the external ear which has no subcutaneous tissue, while facial erysipelas can involve external ear (Millian's sign).
- Penicillin is the drug of choice for erysipelas. Alternatives (for penicillin-allergic patients) are clindamycin, erythromycin.

Q. Listeriosis.

- Listeriosis is a serious infection caused by *Listeria monocytogenes*. *Listera monocytogenes* is an aerobic, gram-positive rod. It is an intracellular organism and is capable of invading several cell types. Listeriosis is a rare infection and primarily affects pregnant women, newborn infants, elderly, and immunocompromised patients.
- This disease is often foodborne and can result in severe systemic illness, including meningitis and sepsis.

Transmission

- The main route of acquisition of *Listeria* is through the ingestion of contaminated food products. Other modes of transmission are contact with infected animals such as rodents or ruminants. Venereal transmission occurs occasionally. Mother-to-child transmission can occur during perinatal period.

Clinical Features

- The disease is seen mainly in neonates and young children. Mother can get infected in late pregnancy which can lead to *stillbirth*. It presents as a febrile illness. The mother recovers after delivery but, occasionally, the organism persists in the genitalia to cause *habitual abortions*. If the neonate survives, the picture is one of severe infection. Neonates die in about 3 days but survivors develop suppurative meningitis.
- Listeria infection in healthy adults is uncommon but affects immunocompromised persons like AIDS patiens, diabetics, alcoholics and those with debilitating diseases. Listeria is an opportunistic infection in AIDS. *Meningitis* is often the clinical manifestation.

Investigations

- Organism can be isolated by blood culture, and culture of any infected body fluid such as CSF.

Treatment

- The *treatment of choice is intravenous ampicillin* often in combination with an aminoglycoside (synergistic effect).
- Trimethoprim-sulphamethoxazole is second-line drug and can be used if the patient is allergic to ampicillin.
- The response to treatment is slow.

Q. Discuss the etiology, pathogenesis, clinical features and complications of diphtheria. How do you investigate and manage a case of diphtheria?

Etiology

- Diphtheria is a localized infection of mucous membranes or skin that is caused by *Corynebacterium diphtheriae*. It is associated with a characteristic pseudomembrane at the site of infection.
- *C. diphtheriae* is a gram-positive bacillus and resembles *Chinese letter patterns* on *Albert's stain*.
- There are three strains of *C. diptheriae*; mitis, intermedius and gravis. Gravis causes the most severe disease.

Epidemiology

- Diphtheria affects people all over the world. But now it is uncommon due to immunization practices. It is more common during winter. It is mainly a disease of children.
- Humans are the main reservoir of *C. diphtheriae*. However, some cases have also occurred due to transmission from livestock.
- Spread occurs in close-contact settings through respiratory droplets or by direct contact with respiratory secretions or skin lesions. Fomite transmission can also occur.

Pathogenesis

- Diphtheria is initiated by entry of *C. diphtheriae* into the nose or pharynx. It multiplies locally without blood stream invasion.

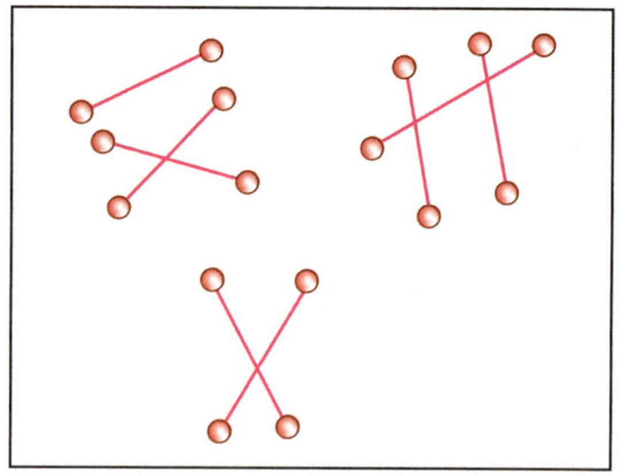

Figure 1.6: *C. diphtheriae*

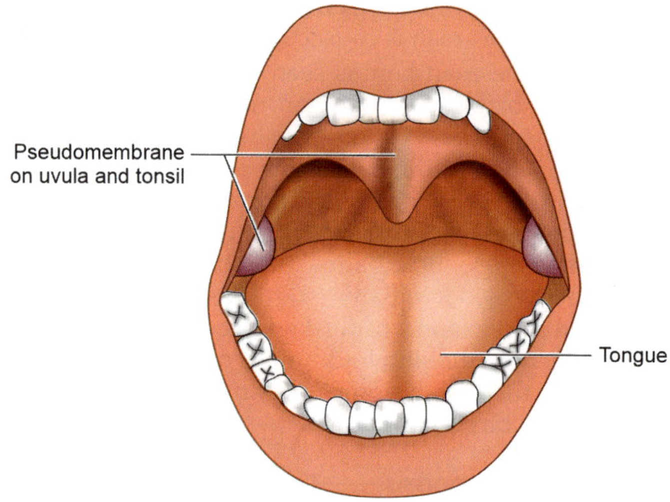

Figure 1.7: Pseudomembranes on the tonsils and uvula

- It produces a powerful exotoxin which causes local tissue necrosis and formation of a tough, adherent pseudomembrane, composed of a mixture of fibrin, dead cells, and bacteria. The membrane usually begins on the tonsils or posterior pharynx and can spread to fauces, soft palate, and into the larynx, which may result in respiratory obstruction. Toxin entering the bloodstream causes tissue damage at distant sites, particularly the heart (myocarditis), nerves (demyelination), and kidney (tubular necrosis).
- Nontoxigenic strains may cause mild local respiratory disease, sometimes including a membrane.

Clinical Features

Respiratory Diphtheria

- Nose infection presents as a chronic serosanguineous or seropurulent discharge without fever or significant toxicity. A whitish membrane may be observed on the septum.
- The **faucial (pharyngeal) form is most common**. After an incubation period of 1–7 days, the illness begins with sore throat, malaise, and mild-to-moderate fever. Grayish membrane may be present that is tightly adherent and bleeds on attempted removal. In severe cases, the patient appears toxic. Cervical

lymphadenopathy and soft tissue edema may occur, resulting in the typical *bull neck appearance* and stridor.
- Laryngeal involvement presents as hoarseness, stridor, and dyspnea.

Cutaneous Diphtheria

- Cutaneous diphtheria lesions are classically painful, deep, non-healing ulcers, which may have a grayish white membrane.

Invasive Disease

- Myocarditis presents with signs of low cardiac output and congestive failure. Conduction disturbances, ST-T wave abnormalities, arrhythmias, and heart block can occur.
- Neurologic involvement manifests as cranial nerve palsies and peripheral neuritis. Palatal and/or pharyngeal paralysis occurs during the acute phase.
- Renal failure: Due to tubular damage.

Investigations

- Gram's stain: A presumptive diagnosis of *C. diphtheriae* can be made by identifying gram-positive rods in a "Chinese letter" distribution on Gram's stain.
- Cultures from beneath the membrane, from the nasopharynx, and from suspicious skin lesions. Cultures may be negative if the patient has received antibiotics.
- Toxigenicity testing should be performed on all *C. diphtheriae* isolates.
- Polymerase chain reaction test may allow both detection of the organism and determination of toxigenicity.
- ECG may show ST-T wave changes, heart block, and dysrhythmia.

Treatment

- The goals of treatment are to neutralize the toxin by antitoxin, eliminate the infecting organism by antibiotics, provide supportive care, and prevent further transmission.

Antitoxin

- Diphtheria antitoxin is a hyperimmune antiserum produced in horses, which binds to and inactivates the diphtheria toxin.
- The antitoxin is only effective before toxin enters the cell and thus must be administered as early as possible.
- There is risk of allergic reactions to antitoxin since it contains horse serum. Hence, a test dose should be given before administration.
- The dose of antitoxin depends upon the site and severity of infection: 20,000–40,000 units for pharyngeal/laryngeal disease, 40,000–60,000 units for nasopharyngeal disease, and 80,000–120,000 units for severe disease with "bull-neck". The dose should be administered intravenously over 60 minutes.

Antibiotics

- They decrease toxin production indirectly by killing the organisms.
- Penicillin is the drug of choice. Penicillin G (25,000–50,000 units/kg IV q12 h until the patient can take orally) followed by oral penicillin V (250 mg QID) for a total of 14 days.
- Erythromycin 500 mg QID for 14 days is an alternative.

Diphtheria Toxoid Vaccine

- Patients should be given diphtheria toxoid immunization during their convalescence since natural infection does not induce immunity.

Prevention

- Isolate the patient.
- Non-immunized contacts should be given both antibiotics and diphtheria antitoxin.
- Immunized contacts are given a booster dose of diphtheria toxoid.

Q. Describe the etiology, pathogenesis, clinical features and management of tetanus. Add a note on prevention of tetanus.

- Tetanus is a serious illness caused by *Clostridium tetani* organism. It is characterized by an acute onset of hypertonia and painful muscle spasms.
- Tetanus has been described by Hippocrates and in the Indian medical writings of Sushruta.

Etiology

- *Cl. tetani* is a gram-positive, spore-forming, anaerobic bacillus. It has a drumstick appearance due to the presence of terminal spore **(Fig. 1.8)**. It is a normal commensal of human and animal gastrointestinal tracts and is widely distributed in soil. Its spores can survive for many years even in adverse conditions.
- Tetanus can occur in following situations:
  - Neonatal tetanus: Occurs when the umbilical cord is cut with an unsterile instrument or smeared with cowdung after cutting as is the practice in some areas.
  - After road traffic accidents where wounds may get contaminated easily with tetanus spores. Even a seemingly trivial injury may be able to cause tetanus.
  - People with otorrhea may develop tetanus if the ear is probed with a wire or matchstick which may carry spores on it.
  - In women after illegal abortion due to unsterile handling of the genital tract through which organisms gain entry.
  - Intramuscular injections given with contaminated needles.
  - Necrotic or gangrenous tissues due to peripheral vascular disease or any other cause.

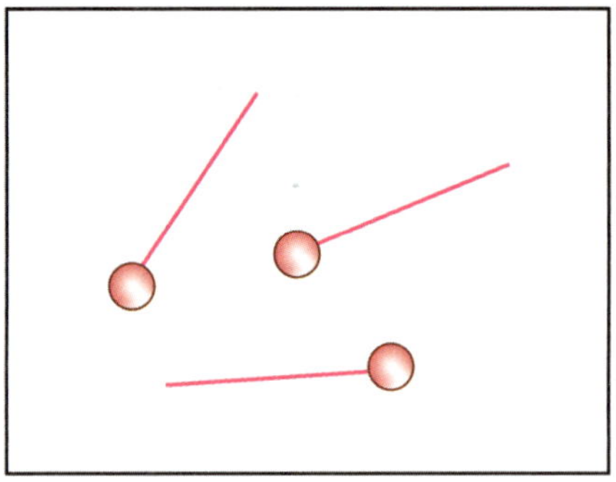

Figure 1.8: Tetanus bacilli

Pathogenesis (Fig. 1.9)

- Spores inoculated into the wound develop into bacteria. These bacteria multiply locally and produce neurotoxin tetanospasmin which is responsible for the clinical manifestations of tetanus.
- Toxin released in the wound is disseminated throughout the body and binds to motor neuron terminals in muscles, and ascends up the axon to reach nerve-cell body in the brainstem and spinal cord. The toxin then migrates across the synapse to presynaptic terminals where it blocks release of the inhibitory neurotransmitters glycine and gamma-aminobutyric acid (GABA). As a result, minor stimuli result in uncontrolled spasms, and reflexes are exaggerated.
- The time taken for the toxin to ascend from nerve endings to CNS depends on the length of nerves. Since cranial nerves are short, effect is first seen in cranial nerve territories such as face, head and neck (like lock-jaw).

Clinical Features

- The incubation period is 4–14 days (depending on the proximity of the wound to the CNS). It can be shorter or longer than this in some cases.

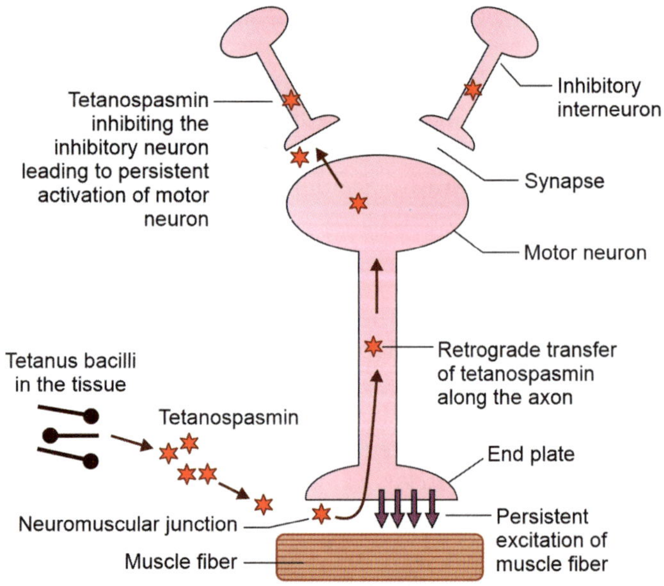

Figure 1.9: Pathogenesis of tetanus

- Tetanus can present in one of four clinical patterns:
  - Generalized
  - Localized
  - Cephalic
  - Neonatal

Generalized Tetanus

- This is the most common and most severe form.
- The classical clinical triad consists of trismus (lock jaw), muscle rigidity, and reflex spasms.
- Tetanic spasms mainly affect the muscles of the trunk, back and proximal parts of the limbs, and spare the peripheries.
- The patient first notices difficulty in opening the jaw due to increased tone in the masseter muscles (trismus, or lockjaw). Dysphagia or stiffness or pain in the neck, shoulder, and back muscles appears concurrently or soon thereafter. Abdominal and limb muscle involvement produces a rigid abdomen and stiff limbs. Sustained contraction of the facial muscles results in a grimace or sneer (risus sardonicus), and contraction of the back muscles produces an arched back (opisthotonus).
- Chest muscle spasms impair breathing. Laryngospasm may produce asphyxia.
- These spasms occur repetitively and may be spontaneous or provoked by even the slightest stimulation.
- Tetanic spasms cause contraction of both agonist and antagonist groups of muscles together.
- Patient remains fully conscious and alert throughout, even during spasms.
- Autonomic dysfunction is seen in severe cases and is characterized by labile or sustained hypertension, tachycardia, dysrhythmia, hyperpyrexia, profuse sweating, peripheral vasoconstriction, and increased plasma and urinary catecholamine levels.
- Due to repetitive muscle spasms and dysphagia, patient may develop many complications like aspiration pneumonia, fractures, muscle rupture, rhabdomyolysis, deep-vein thrombophlebitis, pulmonary embolism.
- Death can occur due to respiratory failure (most common cause) or cardiac arrest due to hypoxia.

Localized Tetanus

- Uncommon form in which manifestations are restricted to muscles near the wound. The prognosis is excellent.

Cephalic Tetanus

- Rare form of local tetanus, follows head injury or ear infection. Trismus and dysfunction of one or more cranial nerves, often the seventh nerve, are found. Cephalic tetanus may remain localized or may progress to generalized tetanus. The incubation period is a few days and the mortality is high.

Neonatal Tetanus

- Neonatal tetanus (tetanus neonatorum) is generalized tetanus that results from infection of a neonate.

Differential Diagnosis

- Inflammatory lesions inside the mouth can induce trismus (lockjaw).
- Drug induced dystonic reactions (e.g. phenothiazines, metoclopramide).
- Strychnine poisoning,
- Hypocalcemic tetany.

Treatment

- The goals of therapy are to eliminate the source of toxin, neutralize unbound toxin, prevent muscle spasms, and support the patient until recovery. Patient should be kept in a quiet room to minimize stimulation. Patient should be continuously monitored for any signs of deterioration especially respiratory compromise.

Antibiotic Therapy

- Antibiotics are given to kill tetanus bacilli so that further production of toxin is prevented.
- Penicillin is the drug of choice (10–12 million units intravenously, in divided doses daily for 10 days). Metronidazole is an alternative. Clindamycin and erythromycin can be used in those allergic to penicillin.

Antitoxin

- Antitoxin is given to neutralize the free circulating and unbound toxin. It does not have any action on the bound toxin.
- Human antitetanus globulin (ATG) is the choice and is given in a dose of 3000–6000 units intramuscularly, usually in divided doses because the volume is large. Human antitetanus immunoglobulin has a long half life; hence repeated doses are not required.
- Equine antitetanus immunoglobulin can also be used but carries risk of allergic reactions. However, it is cheaper.
- The value of injecting antitoxin proximal to the wound or infiltrating around the wound is unclear. Antitoxin does not penetrate the blood-brain barrier. The value of intrathecal administration is still not clear.

Control of Muscle Spasms

- Benzodiazepines like diazepam, lorazepam and midazolam can be used to control muscle spasms.
- Uncontrolled spasms even after giving benzodiazepines may require paralysis with a nondepolarizing neuromuscular blocking agent and mechanical ventilation.
- General anesthesia with propofol may be required for continuous spasms.
- Dantrolene and intrathecal baclofen can also be considered in severe spasms.

Supportive Measures

- Respiratory support with endotracheal intubation or tracheostomy, and mechanical ventilation, may be required.
- IV fluids should be given to maintain hydration.
- Hypertension due to autonomic dysfunction may be controlled by beta blockers, clonidine, and morphine sulfate. Intravenous magnesium sulfate also has a stabilizing effect and is useful in autonomic dysfunction.
- Hypotension or bradycardia may require volume expansion, use of vasopressors.
- Wound should be kept clean by debridement and removing any necrotic or foreign material.

Complications

Respiratory Failure

- Due to paralysis of the diaphragm and respiratory muscles.
- Mechanical ventilation is required in severe cases.

Autonomic Dysfunction

- Tachycardia, arrhythmias, fluctuations in blood pressure, and profuse sweating.

Muscle Rupture

- Due to severe, sustained muscle contractions.

Mortality

- Mortality rate is around 10–30%, particularly in older adults or those without prompt treatment.
- Prevention of tetanus

Immunization

- All partially immunized and unimmunized adults should receive vaccine, as should those recovering from tetanus. The primary series for adults consists of three doses: the first and second doses are given 4–8 weeks apart, and the third dose is given 6–12 months after the second. A booster dose is required thereafter every 10 years.
- For persons with unclean and major wounds, give tetanus immunoglobulin 250 units IM and also a dose of tetanus vaccine.

Wound care

- Wounds should be washed thoroughly and any dead tissue and slough should be excised

Q. Discuss the etiology, pathogenesis, clinical features, diagnosis and treatment of botulism.

- Botulism is a rare paralytic disease caused by botulinum toxin, which is produced by *Clostridium botulinum*.
- *C. botulinum* is an anaerobic gram-positive organism that forms terminal spores. It is found in soil and marine environments throughout the world. Botulinum toxin is the most potent bacterial toxin known.
- Has rounded ends with a characteristic "tennis racket" appearance when spores are present **(Fig. 1.10)**.

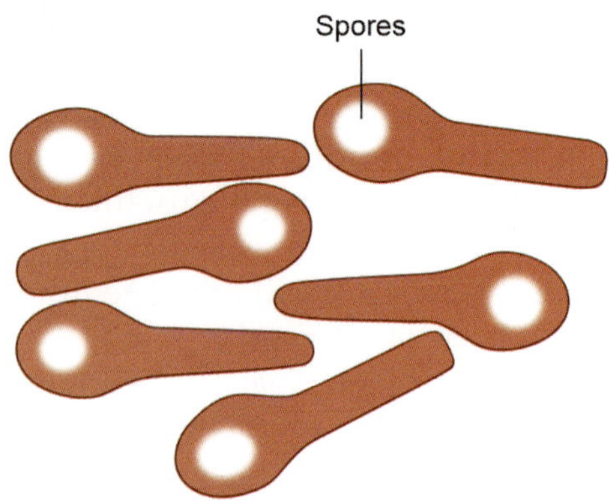

Figure 1.10: *Clostridium botulinum*

Pathogenesis (Fig. 1.11)

- Under anaerobic conditions, the spores germinate and the bacteria multiply and release the exotoxin. Botulinum toxin is absorbed through mucosal surfaces or wounds.
- Botulinum toxin inhibits release of acetylcholine at the neuromuscular junction and causes flaccid paralysis. Botulinum toxin is extremely potent and is capable of killing a person even in minute quantities. It can be used as an agent of bioterrorism.
- Naturally occurring botulism occurs in one of three forms: Food-borne botulism, infant botulism, or wound botulism. Food-borne botulism is caused by ingestion of preformed toxin present in canned foods. Infant botulism occurs due to the practice of feeding honey to infants. Honey may contain botulism organisms which may proliferate in the gut to produce toxin. Wound botulism usually occurs due to contamination of wound with organisms. Inhalational botulism is the form that would occur if aerosolized toxin was released in an act of bioterrorism.

Clinical Features

- Symptoms typically occur within 12–36 hours of exposure (foodborne botulism). Longer incubation is possible for wound botulism.
- Symmetric descending paralysis is characteristic and usually starts in the extraocular muscles, and spreads to the pharynx, larynx, and respiratory muscles before inducing a generalized flaccid paralysis. Patient may have symptoms like ptosis, blurred vision, diplopia, pooling of secretions, dysphagia and breathlessness.
- Nausea, vomiting and diarrhea may occur if the source of toxin is intestine. Paralytic ileus may develop due to intestinal muscles paralysis.
- Fever is unusual.
- Patient is conscious and alert.
- Sensory findings are absent.
- Respiratory paralysis may lead to death in untreated cases.
- A diagnosis of botulism must be considered in patients with symmetric descending flaccid paralysis without sensory deficits, who are afebrile and mentally intact.

Investigations

- Toxin can be identified in serum, stool, vomitus, gastric aspirate, and suspected foods. Mouse bioassay is the gold standard, detects toxin in serum, stool, or food. It involves injecting a suspected sample into mice and observing them for signs of botulinum toxin-induced paralysis or death.
- *C. botulinum* may be grown on selective media from samples of stool or foods.
- Wound cultures that grow *C. botulinum* suggest wound botulism.
- Electromyography (EMG) shows characteristic findings: Reduced compound muscle action potentials with incremental response to rapid repetitive stimulation.

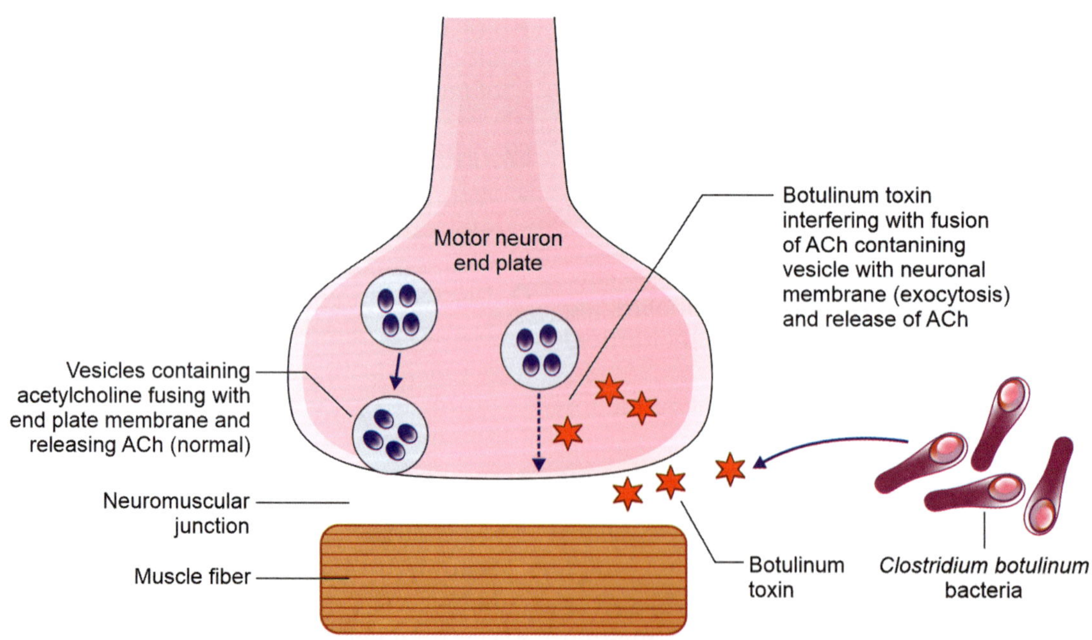

Figure 1.11: Pathogenesis of botulism

Treatment

- Botulinum antitoxin should be given intravenously as early as possible.
- Antibiotics are recommended for wound botulism along with incision and thorough debridement of the infected wound. Penicillin G or metronidazole can be used.
- The immediate threat to life is respiratory failure. Close monitoring for respiratory failure is important. If respiratory failure develops, endotracheal intubation and mechanical ventilation should be started. Tracheostomy is required if the patient needs mechanical ventilation for a long time.

Q. Gas gangrene.

- *Gas gangrene* (also known as *clostridial myonecrosis*) is a severe, life-threatening bacterial infection caused by gas-producing Clostridium species, most commonly *Clostridium perfringens*. It is characterized by rapid tissue destruction, systemic toxicity, and the production of gas within tissues.
- It usually occurs as a complication in devitalized and revascularized tissues. It is a medical emergency.

Etiology

- An 80% of cases are caused by *Clostridium perfringens*, while *C. novyi*, *C. septicum*, and *C. histolyticum* cause the remaining cases. *Clostridium perfringens* is a gram-positive, spore-forming, rod-shaped anaerobic bacterium that is widely distributed in the environment, as well as in the gastrointestinal tracts of humans and animals **(Fig. 1.12)**.
- *C. perfringens* grows in anaerobic conditions and also produces a toxin, and enzymes like collagenases and hyaluronidases which destroy the connective tissue and allow the infection to spread.

Clinical Features

- The incubation period of gas gangrene is usually short; less than 3 days.
- The first symptom is pain, along with numbness of the affected limb. There may be swelling around the wound, with pale surrounding skin. Serosanguinous foul-smelling discharge may be there from the wound. Crepitus can be elicited on palpation in and around the wound due to gas formation.
- Constitutional symptoms are severe with tachycardia and Hypotension and the patient may be stuporous. Mild-to-moderate fever may be there.
- Sometimes uterine infection can occur following criminal abortion or poor aseptic technique during labor.

Laboratory Findings

- Gas gangrene is a clinical diagnosis, and empiric therapy should be started if the diagnosis is suspected.
- X-rays may show presence of gas in the tissues.
- The smear shows the presence of gram-positive rods.
- Anaerobic culture confirms the diagnosis.

Treatment

- Wounds should be thoroughly cleansed and debrided.
- Traditionally, the antibiotic of choice for clostridial infection has been penicillin G (4 million units every 4 hours IV). Recently clindamycin has been shown to be superior to penicillin G. Combination of clindamycin and penicillin is superior to penicillin alone. Metronidazole can be used instead of clindamycin.
- Hyperbaric oxygen inhibits anaerobic bacterial growth but its effect on mortality is not clear.

Q. Describe the etiology, pathogenesis, clinical features and treatment of pseudomembranous colitis.

Etiology

- Pseudomembranous colitis is a severe inflammatory condition of the colon that occurs in some people who have taken antibiotics. This condition is characterized by the formation of pseudomembranes on the colonic mucosa.
- It is usually caused by *Clostridioides difficile (formerly called clostridium difficile)* **(Fig. 1.13)**. The name has been changed after finding out that this organism has many characteristics different from other Clostridium species.

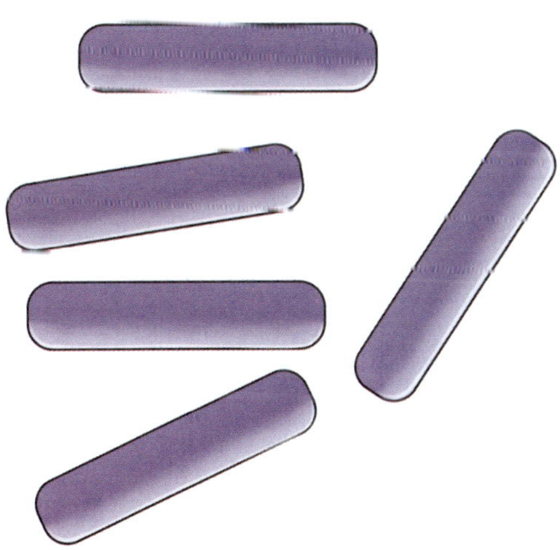

Figure 1.12: *Clostridium perfringens*

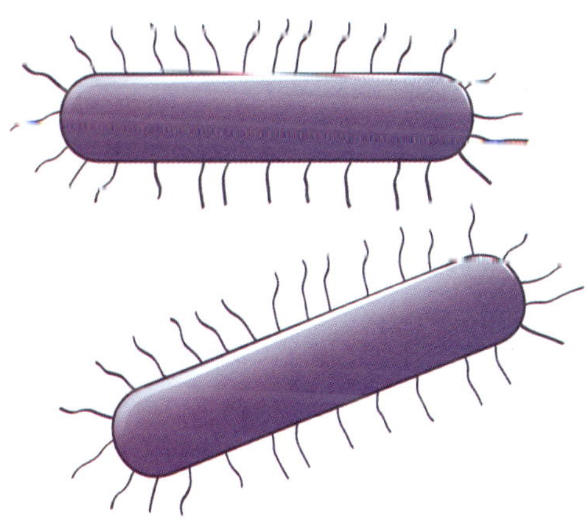

Figure 1.13: *Clostridium difficile*

- Broad spectrum antibiotics such as clindamycin and ampicillin have been implicated most often, but tetracyclines and cephalosporins are other causal agents.

Pathogenesis

- *C. difficile* colonizes the intestinal tract after the normal gut flora has been altered by antibiotic therapy.
- After colonization, *C. difficile* elaborates two large toxins: toxin A an enterotoxin, and toxin B a cytotoxin. These toxins initiate an inflammatory process in the intestinal mucosa resulting in the disruption of epithelial-cell barrier function, leading to cell death, inflammation, diarrhea, and pseudomembrane formation.
- Pseudomembranes are composed of fibrin, inflammatory cells, necrotic epithelial cells, and mucus. These plaques adhere to the colonic mucosa, giving a characteristic appearance.

Clinical Features

- Diarrhea usually begins 5–10 days after starting antibiotics. Stools may contain blood.
- Fever and abdominal pain may be present.
- Signs of dehydration may be there due to diarrhea.
- Toxic megacolon and colonic perforation (rigid abdomen and rebound tenderness) can occur in very severe cases.

Investigations

- Stool examination may show presence of WBCs and RBCs.
- Culture for *C. difficile* is slow and expensive, hence not recommended.
- Stool assay for *C. difficile* toxins (mostly toxin B). It is considered positive when cultured cells undergo cytopathic changes when exposed to stool which contains toxin.
- Enzyme-linked immunoabsorbent assay (ELISA) for toxin A and B.
- Colonoscopy/sigmoidoscopy may reveal erythematous mucosa covered by adherent pseudomembranes over the colonic mucosa.
- Abdominal X-ray or CT scan to assess for toxic megacolon or perforation if suspected.

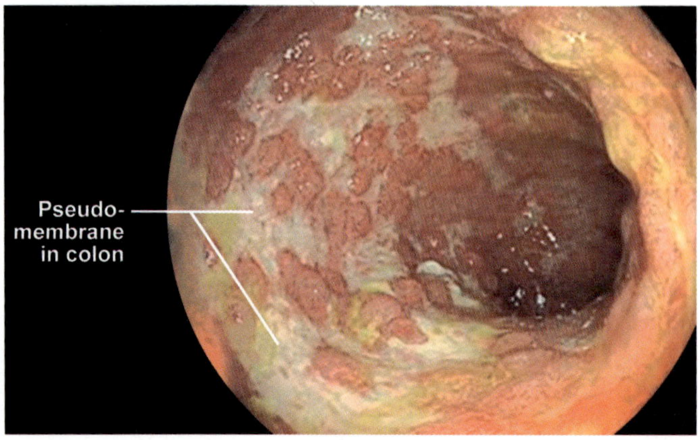

Figure 1.14: Pseudomembranes on colon

Treatment

- All antibiotics should be stopped and this alone may halt the diarrhea.
- Vancomycin (125 mg orally 4 times daily for 14 days) is the drug of choice. Fidaxomicin is an alternative (200 mg BD for 10 days). Metronidazole is no longer the drug of choice but can be used if vancomycin or fidaxomicin is not available.
- Probiotics such as Lactobacillus may be considered but benefit is doubtful.
- Surgery may be required for complications such as toxic megacolon, perforation and necrotizing colitis.

Q. Anthrax (malignant pustule, woolsorter's disease, Siberian ulcer, charbon).

- Anthrax is a zoonotic disease caused by *Bacillus anthracis*. Anthrax is also known by various names like malignant pustule, woolsorter's disease, Siberian ulcer, charbon, etc.

Etiology

- *B. anthracis* is a spore-forming gram-positive rod. Occurs singly, in pairs, or in long chains. Long chain resembles bamboo stick. It has oval, centrally located spores that do not cause swelling of the cell wall.
- Recently anthrax has attained notoriety because of its possible use in biological warfare.

Pathophysiology

- Actually, it is a zoonotic infection which affects sheep, cattle, horses and goats. Humans are affected when spores are ingested or inhaled or inoculated into broken skin. This can happen either by direct contact with these animals or contact with their products.
- After entry into the body, the spores germinate into vegetative bacteria and multiply locally.
- Spores entering the lungs are ingested by macrophages and carried via lymphatics to regional lymph nodes, where they rapidly multiply and cause hemorrhagic lymphadenitis.
- Invasion of the bloodstream leads to sepsis, killing the host.
- *B. anthracis* produces three primary toxins:
  - Protective antigen (PA): Facilitates entry of other toxins into cells.

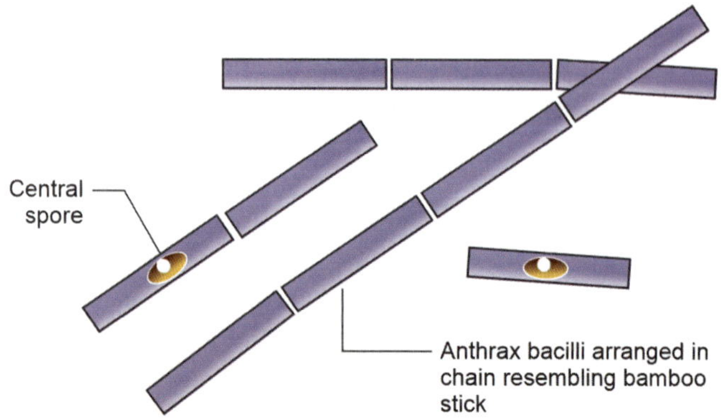

Figure 1.15: Anthrax bacilli (some have spores)

- Edema toxin (ET): Causes local swelling and fluid accumulation.
- Lethal toxin (LT): Causes tissue necrosis and systemic effects.

Clinical Features

- The incubation period is 1–5 days.
- Depending on the route of entry anthrax occurs in three forms: *cutaneous, inhalational,* and *gastrointestinal.*
- Cutaneous anthrax is the most common presentation (95%). Spores inoculate a host through skin lacerations, abrasions, or biting flies. This form most commonly affects the exposed areas of the upper extremities. Initially the cutaneous lesion appears as a small erythematous, maculopapular lesion, which subsequently undergoes vesiculation and ulceration to form a black eschar (malignant pustule). Sometimes sloughing of the eschar is associated with hematogenous spread, sepsis, and shock.
- Respiratory involvement (woolsorter's disease) is due to inhalation of spores, resulting in nonproductive cough, fever and retrosternal discomfort. Occasionally initial clinical improvement is followed by severe dyspnea, stridor, cyanosis and death. Neck and chest wall edema may develop.
- Gastrointestinal infection occurs after ingestion of spores and presents as diarrhea and vomiting, which can be bloody.
- Cutaneous anthrax may be transmitted from person to person by direct contact or fomites but gastrointestinal and inhalation anthrax are not transmitted from person to person.

Investigations

- *Chest X-ray* may show mediastinal widening in inhalational anthrax.
- *Gram's stain* shows gram-positive rods.
- *Culture* may grow B-anthracis.
- *Direct fluorescent antibody (DFA) test* and *polymerase chain reaction (PCR) assay* may identify anthrax bacillus.

Treatment

- ***Cutaneous anthrax:*** is treated with any one of the following antibiotics: ciprofloxacin, levofloxacin, doxycycline. Duration of therapy is 7–10 days.
- ***Other forms of anthrax:*** require therapy with 2 or 3 antibiotics. Antibiotic choices are ciprofloxacin, levofloxacin, meropenem, vancomycin, penicillin G, and doxycycline. Duration of therapy is 2–3 weeks.
- Monoclonal antibodies (raxibacumab or obiltoxaximab) and IV anthrax immunoglobulin can also be considered for systemic anthrax and inhalation anthrax along with antibiotics.

Postexposure Prophylaxis

- Exposed individuals should be given ciprofloxacin or levofloxacin, or doxycycline and anthrax vaccine. In addition to these, monoclonal antibodies can be considered for people exposed to inhalation anthrax.

Q. Gonorrhea, Gonococcal urethritis.

- Gonorrhea is a sexually transmitted disease (STD) caused by the bacterium *Neisseria gonorrhoeae*. It is characterized by purulent infection of the mucous membrane surfaces.
- It is one of the commonest STD world over.

Etiology

- It is caused by a gram-negative diplococcus *Neisseria gonorrhoeae* which infects the epithelium of the urogenital tract, and less frequently of the rectum and the conjunctivae. Gonococci are kidney shaped, and occur in pairs, hence the name gonococcus.

Clinical Features

- Transmission: Sexual contact (vaginal, anal, or oral). Perinatal transmission from mother to neonate during childbirth (causing ophthalmia neonatorum).
- The incubation period is 1–5 days. The common age group affected is 15–30 years.
- Asymptomatic infections can occur and more common in females. Asymptomatic individuals contribute more to transmission of infection than actual cases.

Urogenital Gonorrhea

- Gonococcal infection in males results in acute urethritis with symptoms of dysuria and purulent urethral discharge. Some patients may have mucoid urethral discharge. It may spread and cause epididymitis and prostatitis.
- In females, cervix is infected more often than the urethra. Vaginal discharge, dyspareunia (painful intercourse), and dysuria are common symptoms. Genitourinary infection can progress to pelvic inflammatory disease and lead to fever and lower abdominal pain.

Rectal Gonorrhea

- Rectal gonorrhea (proctitis) occurs in homosexual males and heterosexual females as a result of anogenital sex. The symptoms vary from mild anal

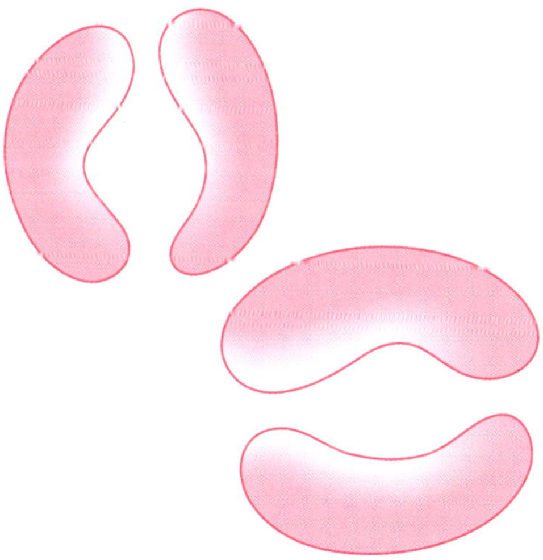

Figure 1.16: Gonococci

pruritus and mucopurulent discharge to symptoms of severe proctitis with rectal pain and tenesmus.

Pharyngeal Gonorrhea

- Pharyngeal gonorrhea (pharyngitis) may occur as a consequence of oro-genital sex and may be seen in either sex. This is generally asymptomatic.

Conjunctival Gonorrhea

- Severe conjunctivitis with purulent discharge. Risk of blindness if untreated. Ocular gonorrhea is rare in adults.

Ophthalmia Neonatorum

- It occurs in neonates as a result of contact of eyes with the infected maternal birth canal. It presents as acute purulent conjunctivitis that may affect deeper structures of the eye and may occasionally result in panophthalmitis.

Disseminated Gonococcal Infection (DGI)

- DGI can occur in both males and females leading to septic arthritis, pustular skin lesions, and meningitis. Knee is the most common site of septic arthritis.

Investigations

- Gram stain: presence of typical gram-negative intracellular diplococci establishes a diagnosis of gonorrhea.
- Nucleic acid amplification tests (NAATs) are the gold standard for detecting *Neisseria gonorrhoeae*. Common techniques include: polymerase chain reaction (PCR), transcription-mediated amplification (TMA), and strand displacement amplification (SDA).
- Culture: Grows on Thayer-Martin or chocolate agar. Useful to test antimicrobial sensitivity.

Treatment

- Ceftriaxone 500 mg intramuscular (IM) single dose is the preferred drug of choice.
- If associated *Chlamydia trachomatis* infection is also suspected, use doxycycline 100 mg orally twice daily for seven days in nonpregnant individuals or azithromycin 1 g PO single dose (in pregnant ladies).
- Disseminated gonococcal infection should be treated by parenteral antibiotics (ceftriaxone 1 g IM or IV OD) initially followed by oral therapy for a total of 7 days.
- Quinolones like ciprofloxacin (500 mg) or levofloxacin (250 mg) are alternatives but resistance is emerging.

Q. Chancroid.

- Chancroid also known as "soft chancre," is a sexually transmitted disease (STD) caused by *Haemophilus ducreyi*, a gram-negative, facultative anaerobic coccobacillus **(Fig. 1.17)**.
- It is characterized by painful genital ulcers that may be accompanied by inguinal lymphadenopathy. It is highly contagious but curable infection.

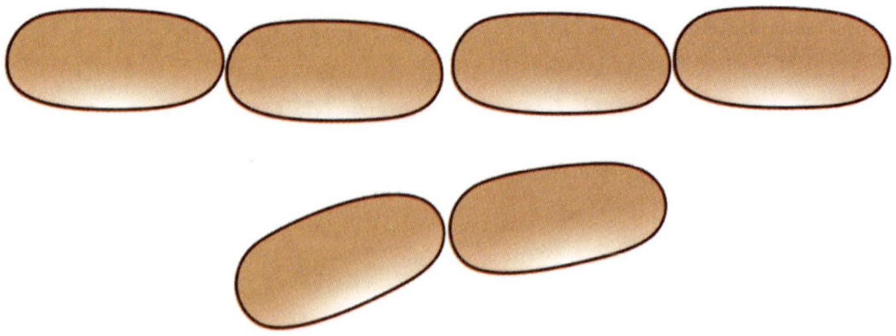

Figure 1.17: *H. ducreyi*

Etiopathogenesis

- Chancroid is caused by *Haemophilus ducreyi* which is a small gram-negative coccobacillus. A coccobacillus is a type of bacterium that has a shape intermediate between a coccus (spherical) and a bacillus (rod-shaped). This shape makes the bacterium appear oval or slightly elongated under a microscope. When examined by Gram's stain, organisms from culture often clump in long parallel strands, producing a so-called "school of fish" appearance.
- It is pathogenic only in humans, with no intermediary host. *H. ducreyi* is transmitted sexually by direct contact with purulent lesions and by autoinoculation to nonsexual sites, such as the eye and skin. *H. ducreyi* enters the skin through disrupted mucosa and causes a local inflammatory reaction. It produces a cytotoxin which plays a role in epithelial injury and development of an ulcer.

Epidemiology

- Chancroid is seen worldwide, and is associated with low socioeconomic and poor hygienic conditions. It predominantly affects young sexually active people (20–30 years of age). Chancroid is most often seen in uncircumcised men. In women it may be asymptomatic.

Clinical Features

- Incubation period is 4–10 days.
- The ulcer is seen on the prepuce in men and on the labia in women. It begins as a papule with surrounding erythema which ruptures and forms an ulcer. Ulcers are usually multiple, very painful, non-indurated and soft, have undermined edges with a base of granulation tissue and slough.
- Tender inguinal lymphadenopathy occurs in about half the patients. These lymph nodes may become fluctuant (bubo) and rupture spontaneously.

Diagnosis

- Gram's stain of material from a bubo or biopsy from ulcer reveals large numbers of gram-negative coccobacilli, arranged in a 'school of fish' pattern **(Fig. 1.18)**.
- Culture is the most definitive method of diagnosis, but the organism is fastidious.
- Immunofluorescence test and serologic assays for antibodies are newer laboratory tests.
- Polymerase chain reaction (PCR) can rapidly detect *H. ducreyi* in clinical samples and may supersede culture in future.

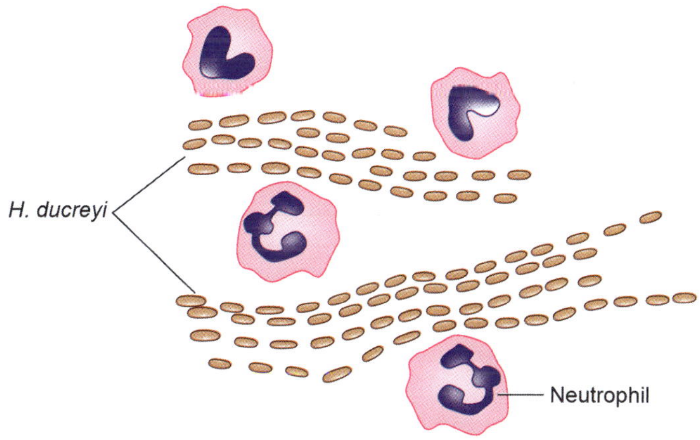

Figure 1.18: School of fish appearance of *H. ducreyi*

Differential Diagnosis

- Chancroid ulcer has to be differentiated from genital ulcer due to syphilis, lymphogranuloma venereum, herpes simplex virus-2, and granuloma inguinale.

Treatment

- A single 1 g oral dose of azithromycin will cure most people.
- Alternative regimens include ceftriaxone (250 mg intramuscularly as a single dose), or ciprofloxacin (500 mg orally twice a day for 3 days), or erythromycin (500 mg orally three times a day for 7 days).
- Fluctuant lymph nodes may require needle aspiration or incision and drainage.

Q. Pertussis (whooping cough).

- Pertussis (*per*: intensive, *tussis*: cough) is a highly contagious acute respiratory tract infection caused by *Bordetella pertussis*, a gram-negative coccobacillus.
- A severe bout of cough is followed by a deep inspiration with characteristic sound (whoop). Hence the name "whooping cough."
- The Chinese name for pertussis is "the 100-day cough," which accurately describes the course of the disease.

Epidemiology

- Pertussis occurs worldwide but the incidence has come down due to vaccination. Periodic epidemics however continue world over.
- The infection is more common and serious in infancy and early childhood. It is highly communicable.
- Even with the decline after vaccination, pertussis still continues to be a major health hazard.

Pathogenesis

- The organism is spread by respiratory droplets from patients.
- Infection is initiated by attachment of the organism to the ciliated epithelial cells of the nasopharynx. Attachment is mediated by surface adhesins. At the site of attachment, the organism multiplies, producing a variety of toxins that cause local mucosal damage and systemic effects. There is local cellular invasion, but systemic dissemination does not occur. Systemic manifestations are due to toxins.
- It is not exactly known what causes the paroxysmal cough that is the hallmark of pertussis. Pertussis toxin may be responsible for cough. Local mucosal damage may contribute.
- Bronchopneumonia can develop in some persons.
- Seizures and encephalopathy can occur and are due to hypoxia from coughing paroxysms or apnea.

Clinical Features

- The incubation period is 1–3 weeks (but mostly between 7 and 10 days).
- Classically, there are three stages: Catarrhal, paroxysmal and convalescent.

Catarrhal Stage

- Lasts 1–2 weeks. It resembles common cold and is characterized by running nose, fever and mild cough.

Paroxysmal Stage

- Begins during the second week of illness. Lasts for 2–6 weeks or longer. The cough becomes more frequent and spasmodic with repetitive bursts of 5–10 coughs, often within a single expiration. The episode may be terminated by an audible whoop, which occurs due to rapid inspiration against a closed glottis at the end of a paroxysm. Post tussive vomiting is frequent.
- During a paroxysm, there may be impressive neck-vein distension, bulging eyes, tongue protrusion, and cyanosis.
- The cough is present throughout the day and night and may be precipitated by acts such as yawning, stretching, laughing, yelling, or exercise.
- The whoop may be absent in infants, partially immune older children, and adults, which makes the diagnosis difficult in them. Most complications occur during the paroxysmal stage

Convalescent Stage

- Decrease in intensity and frequency of the cough over 1–2 weeks.

Differential Diagnosis

- Includes conditions with severe cough lasting more than 2 weeks. These are adenovirus infection, endobronchial tuberculosis, inhaled foreign body, and hyperreactive airway disease.

Complications

- Infants and young children have more complications.
- Respiratory complications: Otitis media, pneumonia due to *B. pertussis* itself or secondary bacterial infection, atelectasis, emphysema, bronchiectasis, pneumothorax and pneumomediastinum.
- Neurological complications: Seizures and encephalopathy.

- Severe cough leads to marked increase in pressure in various body compartments, which may cause epistaxis; retinal, subconjunctival and intracranial hemorrhage; inguinal hernia; rectal prolapse; rupture of the diaphragm; rib fracture.
- Malnutrition can occur due to prolonged disease.

Laboratory Findings

- Pertussis is mainly a clinical diagnosis.
- There may be lymphocytic leukocytosis.
- Confirmation of diagnosis depends on culture of *B. pertussis* (gold standard for diagnosis of pertussis) from a nasopharyngeal swab or cough plate in Bordet-Gengou medium or Regan-Lowe agar (commonly used). Cultures are often positive in the catarrhal and early paroxysmal stage.
- Polymerase chain reaction (PCR): Preferred diagnostic test. Highly sensitive and specific. Detects DNA of *Bordetella pertussis* in nasopharyngeal swab or aspirate. Results available within 24–48 hours.
- Serology: Detects antibodies against *Bordetella pertussis* antigens. Useful during the convalescent stage (after 2–4 weeks of symptoms). Limited value in the early stages of illness.
- Direct fluorescent antibody test: Uses fluorescent-labeled antibodies to detect *B. pertussis* antigens in nasopharyngeal specimens. Low sensitivity and specificity compared to PCR or culture. Rarely used in modern clinical settings.
- Chest X-ray may show lung infiltrates.

Management

- Patient should be admitted to hospital if there is respiratory distress, neurological signs and dehydration.
- *Antibiotics:* Purpose is to eradicate the infecting bacteria from the nasopharynx. Antibiotics should be given early to reduce the risk of prolonged disease. **Macrolide antibiotics (azithromycin, clarithromycin) are the drugs of choice** for treatment of pertussis. Trimethoprim-sulfamethoxazole is an alternative for individuals allergic to macrolides.
- *Supportive measures:* Include providing adequate nutrition and hydration and avoiding factors aggravating cough such as excessive crying. Complications are managed as per sytandard guidelines.

Prevention

- Isolate the patient for 4–5 days after starting antibiotics to prevent spread to others.
- *Chemoprophylaxis:* with azithromycin or erythromycin should be given to all household contacts whether they have been vaccinated or not.
- *Vaccination*: all children under 7 years of age should be vaccinated with DTaP (diphtheria, tetanus, acellular pertussis). Vaccination against pertussis is part of standard childhood vaccination. For adults, a single booster with Tdap (containing lower doses of the diphtheria and pertussis components than the childhood DTaP) is recommended after age 19 years.

Q. Discuss the etiology, pathogenesis, clinical features, diagnosis and management of typhoid fever (enteric fever).

Q. Rose spots.

Q. Complications of typhoid fever.

- Typhoid is a systemic infection caused by *Salmonella enterica* serotype Typhi (previously called Salmonella Typhi).
- Salmonella enterica serotype Paratyphi A, B, or C causes paratyphoid fever, a milder illness.
- The disease was initially called typhoid fever because of its clinical similarity to typhus. Since the primary site of infection is intestine, the term enteric fever was proposed as an alternative name. However, to this day, both names are used interchangeably.
- However, old name 'S. Typhi' remains the shorthand, ensuring simplicity and continuity.

Etiology

- *Salmonella enterica* serotype Typhi is gram-negative, facultative anaerobic, motile bacillus. It possesses a lipopolysaccharide (LPS) outer membrane and flagella. Salmonellae are present worldwide but cause disease only where poor hygiene and overcrowding exist.

Pathogenesis (Fig. 1.19)

- Humans are the only reservoir of S. Typhi. Organisms originate from patients with typhoid, or from carriers excreting organisms in their stools. Human hands, flies, or insects then transfer these organisms to food or drink. Since S. Typhi survive freezing and drying, infection can also occur through ice or canned food. Shellfish from polluted waters may transmit the disease. Decreased stomach acidity is a risk factor for infection to occur.
- Once salmonellae reach the small intestine, the bacteria penetrate and traverse through the intestinal wall through phagocytic cells that reside within Peyer's patches. After crossing the epithelial layer of the small intestine, S. Typhi and S. Paratyphi are phagocytosed by macrophages. Infected macrophages release inflammatory mediators, causing necrosis of Peyer's patches. Necrosis leads to oval or longitudinal ulcers along the antimesenteric border of the ileum.
- Once phagocytosed, salmonellae disseminate throughout the body in macrophages via the lymphatics and colonize reticuloendothelial tissues (liver, spleen, lymph nodes, and bone marrow) where they start multiplying. Patients have relatively few or no symptoms during this initial incubation stage.
- Once the number of bacteria reaches a critical stage, they invade blood stream and rest of the body. At this stage, signs and symptoms, such as fever and abdominal pain appear. Peyer's patches can get enlarged and necrosed due to mononuclear cell infiltration. Bacteria also reach gallbladder via blood stream and multiply there. From the gallbladder, bacteria reach the intestine and are excreted in the

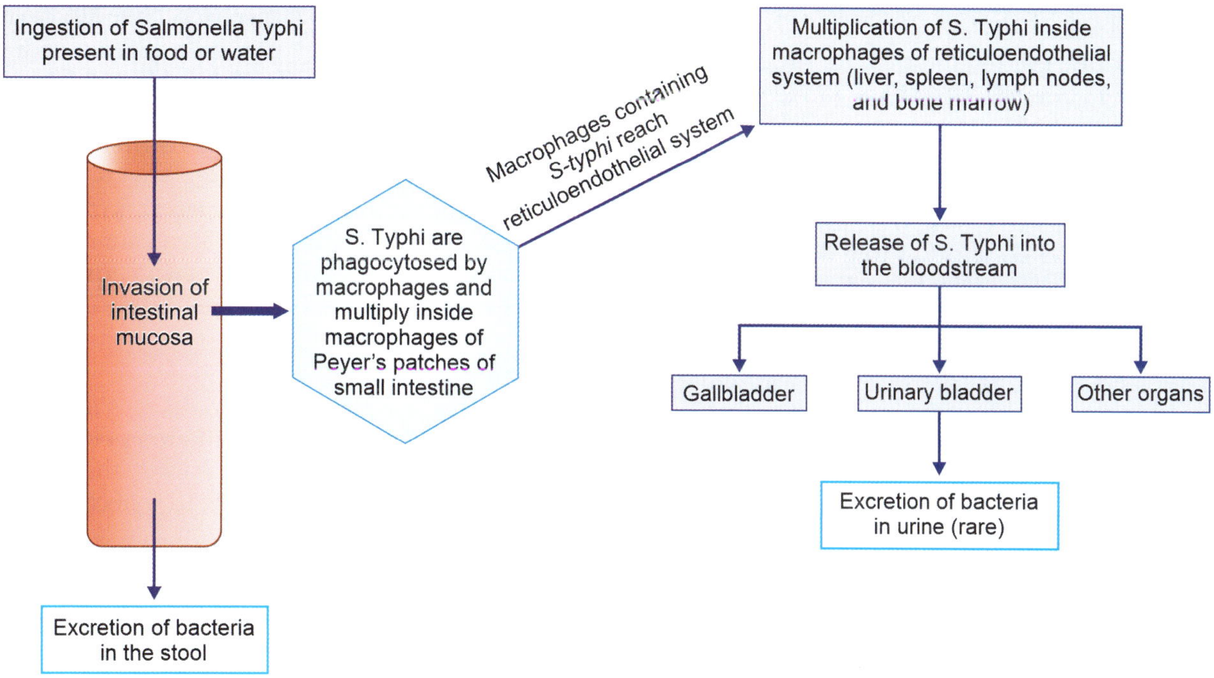

Figure 1.19: Pathogenesis of typhoid fever

stool which can spread to others via contaminated foods. Some patients become chronic carriers carrying the bacteria in their gall bladder and are responsible for much of the transmission of the organism. Carriers remain asymptomatic, but may shed bacteria in their stool for decades.

Clinical Features

- The incubation period averages 10–14 days.
- The onset of the disease is insiduous, with headache, malaise, anorexia and fever. The fever is remittent (does not touch the baseline) sometimes increasing in a step-like manner (step ladder fever) to reach a peak towards the end of the first week. Thereafter it plateaus and remains for two to three weeks. Accompanying chills are common but frank rigors are rare. Headache is present and often disabling.
- With the passing days debility sets in and in some cases progresses to mental dullness and delirium, characterized by muttering and picking at bedclothes.
- Abdominal discomfort with mild bloating and constipation usually occurs, but diarrhea can also occur. Stools may have a 'pea soup' appearance.
- Hepatosplenomegaly may develop by the end of the first week. Mild jaundice may be present.
- The typical rash of typhoid (rose spots) develops in the second week but is seldom seen in Indian patients. "Rose spots" are pink macules, 2–3 mm in size, occur in small crops on the chest and abdomen, blanch on pressure and last for 2–3 days.
- Complications may develop in the third week of illness (intestinal perforation, bleeding, delirium or altered mental status ("typhoid state").
- In the absence of complications, typhoid fever usually subsides.

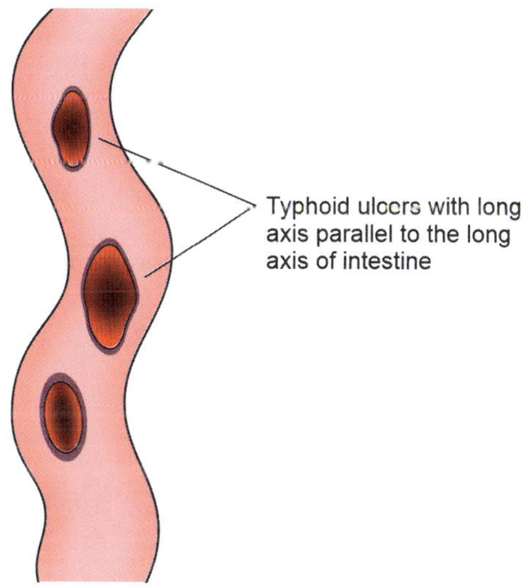

Figure 1.20: Typhoid ulcers

Complications

- Complications are uncommon now due to availability of effective antibiotics.
- *Bleeding:* Erosion of blood vessels in necrotic Peyer's patches or in the intestinal wall can initiate bleeding.
- *Intestinal perforation:* Typhoid ulcers can perforate. Usually happens in 3rd week of illness.
- Typhoid can affect almost all the organs. Hence, pneumonia, meningitis, nephritis, cholecystitis, hepatitis, myocarditis, osteomyelitis, encephalitis can occur.
- Involvement of the central nervous system can present as stupor, delirium, convulsions, encephalitis, cerebellar ataxia, extrapyramidal signs, myopathy and deafness.
- Acute renal failure and disseminated intravascular coagulation are rare complications.

Investigations

- The diagnostic "gold standard" for enteric fever is culture of S. Typhi or S. Paratyphi. Blood cultures are positive in 90% during the first week of infection but decrease to 50% by the third week. Cultures of stool and urine may also be positive. Bone marrow culture is the most sensitive test ((90% sensitive) and may remain positive even with up to 5 days of antibiotic therapy. Culture of intestinal secretions (best obtained by a noninvasive duodenal string test) can be positive despite a negative bone marrow culture. If blood, bone marrow, and intestinal secretions are all cultured, the yield of a positive culture is >90%. Stool cultures, can be positive during the third week of infection in untreated patients.
- The Widal test is very helpful in diagnosis. There can be false-positive and false-negative results. The test is positive if O antigen titer is more than 1:160. A four-fold rise in serum agglutinins against the somatic (O) antigen of the bacillus is diagnostic rather than a single test. Titers against the flagellar (H) antigen are less specific. Usually, it becomes positive after the 1st week of illness. Early antimicrobial therapy may dampen the immunologic response.
- Typhidot-M test is a new test which detects IgM antibody against typhoid bacilli. It has high sensitivity and specificity and is better than WIDAL test.
- Polymerase chain reaction: Detects S. Typhi DNA in blood or other samples. High sensitivity and specificity.
- Relative bradycardia and leukopenia may be a clue to diagnosis.
- LFT may show mild elevation of AST and ALT.

Treatment

- Third generation cephalosporins are currently the drugs of choice. Ceftriaxone (1–2 g intravenously or intramuscularly) for 10–14 days is the treatment of choice in severe typhoid. But ceftriaxone resistance is also increasing.
- Azithromycin is an alternative to cephalosporins, especially for uncomplicated typhoid fever (1 g orally once a day for 7 days or 500 mg orally for 10 days).
- Carbapenems (e.g. meropenem) are used for extensively drug-resistant (XDR) S. Typhi.
- There is widespread resistance to quinolones. Hence, they should not be used as first line therapy.
- Paracetamol can be used to control fever, headache and myalgia.
- Supportive measures include good nutrition and hydration. Soft and bland diet should be given because of inflamed bowel. Laxatives and enemas should be avoided because of the same reason.
- In cases of severe typhoid fever (fever, altered sensorium or septic shock; and a positive culture for S. Typhi or S. Paratyphi A), dexamethasone treatment should be considered. One trial showed that treatment with dexamethasone decreased the mortality rate.
- About 1–4% patients become chronic carriers of typhoid bacilli. They can be a source of infection to others (remember Typhoid Mary). Carrier state can be treated with oral amoxicillin, TMP-SMX, ciprofloxacin, or norfloxacin. Antibiotics should be given for 6 weeks. However, in cases of anatomical abnormality (e.g. gallstones or kidney stones), eradication of the infection often cannot be achieved by antibiotic therapy alone and requires surgical correction of the abnormalities.

Prognosis

- The mortality rate of typhoid fever is less than 1% in treated cases. Elderly or debilitated persons are likely to do poorly. With complications, the prognosis is poor. Relapses occur in up to 10% of cases.

Q. Paratyphoid fever.

- Paratyphoid fever is a systemic illness caused by infection with *Salmonella enterica* serotypes Paratyphi A, Paratyphi B, or Paratyphi C. These bacteria are closely related to *Salmonella enterica* serotype Typhi (S. Typhi), the cause of typhoid fever, and the clinical presentation, diagnosis, and management of paratyphoid fever is similar to that of typhoid fever, though usually less severe.

Q. Typhoid vaccines.

- Vaccination against typhoid is recommended for,
  - Persons traveling to developing countries
  - People who have intimate or household contact with a case or chronic carrier
  - Laboratory workers who frequently work with S. Typhi.
  - People living in endemic areas
- There are two main types of typhoid vaccines: inactivated (injectable) and live-attenuated (oral).
- Following typhoid vaccines are currently available. None of the typhoid vaccines protect against paratyphoid fever.

1. ViCPS

- Type: Inactivated subunit vaccine.
- It consists of purified Vi polysaccharide from the bacterial capsule.
- It is given as 0.5 ml intramuscularly (single dose) and is well tolerated. It maintains its efficacy for 2 years. Booster dose is given every 2 years in endemic areas.
- Provides about 50–80% protection.
- Safe for immunocompromised individuals.
- It should not be used below 2 years, because it is not effective in children under 2 years.

2. Typhoid Conjugate Vaccine (TCV)

- Type: Conjugate vaccine (Vi polysaccharide linked to a carrier protein like tetanus toxoid).
- Linkage of a protein moiety results in T-cell dependent differentiation of B cells. Thus, TCVs are highly

immunogenic and suitable for use in children below 2 years.

- Given as single intramuscular injection.
- Provides long-lasting immunity (**5+ years**), reducing the need for frequent boosters.
- High efficacy (>80% in preventing typhoid fever).
- Recommended by the **WHO** for routine immunization in endemic areas.

3. Ty21a (oral vaccine)

- Type: live attenuated vaccine. Contains a weakened strain of S. Typhi (Ty21a).
- The vaccine is supplied as a packet of four enteric-coated capsules that must be kept refrigerated. It should be given as one capsule every other day until all four capsules have been taken. Booster doses are given every 5 years. Vaccine-elicited immunity occurs 14 days after receipt of the last dose, with an efficacy of 50–80 percent. It maintains its efficacy for 4 years. It is well tolerated. Ty21a is commonly used vaccine because it can be given orally and has fewer side effects.
- Not recommended for pregnant women, immunocompromised individuals, and children below 6 years.

Comparative Summary of Typhoid Vaccines

(Table 1.5)

TABLE 1.5: Typhoid vaccines

Feature	ViCPS	TCV	Ty21a
Type	Inactivated subunit	Conjugate	Live-attenuated
Route	IM Injection	IM Injection	Oral
Age group	≥2 years	≥6 months	≥6 years
Doses	Single	Single	4 doses
Booster	Every 2 years	Every 5 years (optional)	Every 5 years
Protection	~50–80%	~80–90%	~60–70%
Duration	2–3 years	≥5 years	~5 years
Use in infants (<2 years)	No	Yes	No

Q. Typhoid carrier.

- A person who excretes salmonella organism in stool or urine for more than 12 months after the acute infection is called chronic carrier.
- About 1–5% of patients become chronic carriers after Salmonella Typhi infection, and the rate is higher in patients with cholelithiasis or other biliary tract abnormalities.
- Chronic urinary carriage of S. Typhi is rare and is usually associated urinary tract abnormalities such as urolithiasis, prostatic hypertrophy or *Schistosoma haematobium* infection.
- Chronic carriers do not develop recurrent symptomatic disease. They develop high level systemic immunity so that they and do not develop clinical disease but excrete large numbers of organisms in the stool.
- Chronic carriers act as source of infection to others, particularly if involved in food preparation. Hence, eradication of carrier state should be done if such individuals are identified.

Diagnosis

- Stool culture is the gold standard test to detect carrier state but has low sensitivity. At least three stool samples should be collected, separated by at least 24 hours.
- Serologic screening is not recommended (detection of antibodies against Vi antigen) for carrier diagnosis.

Treatment

- For patients with a fluoroquinolone-susceptible isolate, treatment with ciprofloxacin (500–750 mg orally twice daily) or levofloxacin (500 mg orally once daily) for 4 weeks is recommended.
- Cholecystectomy should be considered if there is any abnormality such as cholelithiasis.
- For patients with a fluoroquinolone-resistance, possible regimens include ampicillin or amoxicillin, or trimethoprim-sulfamethoxazole.

Q. Shigellosis.

- *Shigella* species are a common cause of diarrhea worldwide. Shigellosis refers to infection of the intestinal tract by Shigella species.

Etiology

- There are 4 species; *Shigella dysenteriae, S. flexneri, S. sonnei and S. boydii.*
- *S. flexneri* is the predominant species causing diarrhea followed by *S. sonnei.*
- *Shigella dysenteriae* type-1 is the most virulent of the shigellae.

Epidemiology

- Shigellosis occurs mainly in the developing countries.
- Shigella infection is associated with the 'gay bowel syndrome' of homosexuals, and travellers' diarrhea of tourists to the developing countries.
- The disease spreads by feco-oral route. Infection is transmitted by fingers and flies. Food and water contamination can cause epidemics as in refugee camps where population densities are high and hygienic standards are low.

Pathogenesis and Pathology

- Shigella first multiplies in the small intestine and initially it may cause a secretory diarrhea. Thereafter it rapidly localizes to the colon (especially rectosigmoid portion), where inflammation with hemorrhage, microabscesses, ulceration, and mucus production results.

Clinical Features

- Symptoms usually start 2–3 days after exposure.
- The onset is sudden with fever, malaise, abdominal pain and watery diarrhea. This early phase reflects small intestinal involvement.

- Later when the colon gets involved there will be dysentery characterized by loose stools mixed with blood and mucus. There may be tenesmus. Severe cramping abdominal pain may be present.
- Nausea, vomiting, headache may occur.
- In children convulsions may occur due to the effect of neurotoxin.
- Sigmoidoscopy reveals hyperemic and inflamed mucosa, with transversely distributed ulcers with ragged undermined edges, a picture which is indistinguishable at times from inflammatory bowel disease.

Differential Diagnosis

- Shigella dysentery has to be differentiated from other causes of dysentery such as:
  - Inflammatory bowel disease
  - *Entamoeba histolytica*
  - Salmonella
  - Enteroinvasive *E. coli*
  - Yersinia
  - *Campylobacter jejuni*
  - *Vibrio parahaemolyticus*
  - *Clostridium difficile*
- Clinically it is difficult to distinguish between these and laboratory tests may be needed. Viral gastroenteritis is not usually associated with fever and the stool does not usually contain blood or pus.

Differential Diagnosis between Shigella (Bacillary) and Amebic Dysentery (Table 1.6)

TABLE 1.6: Differential diagnosis between bacillary dysentery and amebic dysentery

Bacillary dysentery	Amebic dysentery
Ulcers are distributed transversely to long axis of gut. Ulcers are serpiginous with ragged undermined edges communicating with other ulcers.	Ulcers are distributed in the long axis of gut; flask shaped. Shape is oval with regular edges. Ulcers are deep and involve all layers of intestine.
Rarely perforate.	May perforate.
Mucous membrane is inflamed. Bowel wall not thickened.	Mucous membrane not inflamed. Bowel wall thickened.
Stool scanty in quantity but very frequent; bright blood red, gelatinous viscid mucus, odorless, (red currant jelly appearance)	Stools are large quantity, mixed with blood and mucus, dark brown, foul smelling.
Tenesmus common	Tenesmus uncommon
Stool microscopy: RBCs numerous and discrete. WBCs plenty. Bacteria may be visible.	RBCs numerous and in clumps. WBCs scanty. *E. histolytica* trophozoites containing ingested red cells present.

Laboratory Findings

- Stool shows many WBCs and RBCs.
- Stool culture is positive for Shigella in most cases.
- Serological tests are used mainly during epidemics.

Complications

- ***Intestinal complications:*** Proctitis, rectal prolapse, toxic megacolon, intestinal obstruction, and colonic perforation.
- ***Systemic complications:*** Fluid/electrolyte/nutrition disturbances, neurologic disease (seizures, encephalopathy), reactive arthritis. Infrequently, hemolytic uremic syndrome has been associated with *Shigella dysenteriae* type 1 infection.

Treatment

- *Fluid and electrolyte replacement:* oral rehydration salt can be used and if the patient is unable to take orally use intravenous fluids.
- *Antibiotics:* A fluoroquinolone (such as ciprofloxacin 500 mg po q 12 hours for 5 days), or azithromycin 500 mg daily for 4 days, or ceftriaxone 2 g/day IV for 5 days. Trimethoprim-sulfamethoxazole can also be used but Shigella is likely to be resistant to this antibiotic. Fluoroquinolones are contraindicated in pregnancy.
- Antimotility drugs such as loperamide may worsen the condition and are better avoided.

Q. Describe the etiology, epidemiology, clinical features, diagnosis and management of cholera. Add a note on its prevention.

- Cholera is an acute diarrheal illness caused by *Vibrio cholerae*. The hallmark of the disease is profuse secretory diarrhea. Cholera can be endemic, epidemic, or pandemic.

Etiology

- *Vibrio cholerae* is a comma-shaped, motile, gram-negative bacillus that colonizes the human small intestine. It has a single flagellum at one end. Its antigenic structure consists of flagellar H antigen and somatic O antigen. Based on the type of O antigen, *Vibrio cholerae* is divided into various serogroups **(Fig. 1.21)**.
- O1 serogroup: Responsible for the majority of cholera outbreaks and pandemics. Serotype O1 exists in two biotypes—classical and El tor, and three serotypes—Inaba, Ogawa, and Hikojima.
- O139 serogroup: Identified in 1992 in Asia. Causes cholera in specific regions but has not led to widespread pandemics like the O1 serogroup.
- Non-O1/Non-O139 serogroups: These strains typically cause sporadic cases of gastroenteritis, wound infections, or septicemia but are not associated with epidemics **(Fig. 1.22)**.
- *V. cholerae* can survive in water for up to 3 weeks and on moist linen for about a week.

Epidemiology

- Its natural habitat is salt water.
- Cholera has 2 main reservoirs, humans and water. *V. cholerae* is rarely isolated from animals, and animals do not play a role in transmission of disease.
- Transmission occurs by the feco-oral route usually through contaminated food and water.

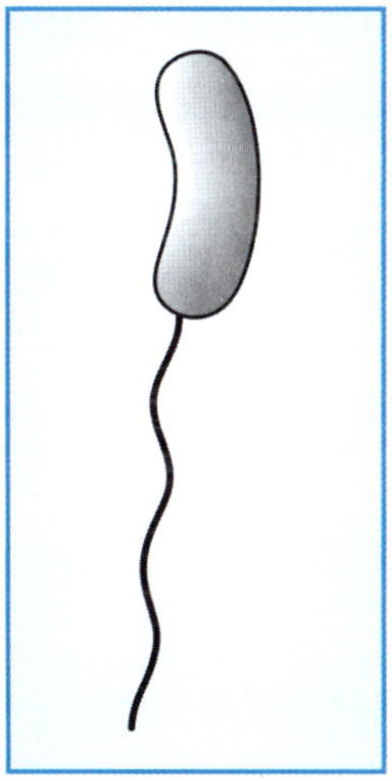

Figure 1.21: *Vibrio cholerae*

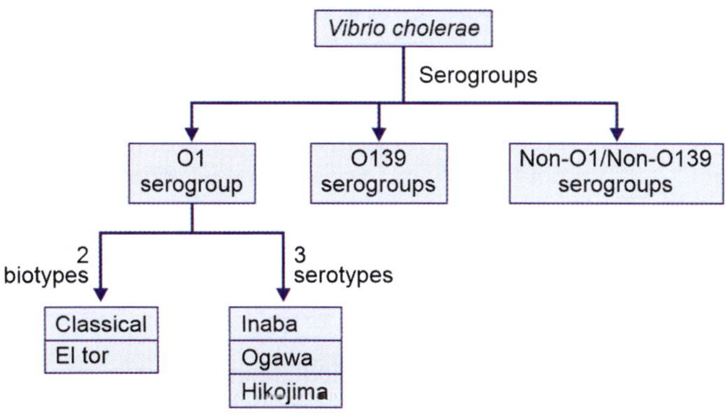

Figure 1.22: *Vibrio cholerae* classification

- *V. cholerae* belonging to O1 serogroup (classical biotype) has been so far responsible for many epidemics and first six pandemics. It has been endemic in the Ganges Delta of West Bengal and Bangladesh.
- In 1993 an outbreak of cholera occurred in India and Bangladesh for the first time with a non O1 *V. cholera.* This organism is now designated as O139 Bengal. A close watch is being kept on O139 B, as it has a potential to cause epidemics and pandemics.
- The **Seventh Cholera Pandemic** is the most recent and ongoing global cholera pandemic, caused by the El Tor biotype of *Vibrio cholerae* O1. This pandemic began in 1961 and continues to affect many parts of the world, particularly in regions with poor sanitation and limited access to clean water.

Pathogenesis (Fig. 1.23)

- Cholera is spread by feco-oral route. After ingestion, cholera bacilli colonize the small intestine, and produce an exotoxin which is responsible for the disease features.
- The exotoxin has A and B subunits. The B subunit binds to the epithelial cell wall (B–binding). The A subunit is responsible for actions (A–action). 'A' subunit activates intracellular adenylate cyclase, which causes increase in cyclic adenosine monophosphate (cAMP). cAMP in turn inhibits sodium absorption and stimulates secretion of chloride. The net effect is accumulation of sodium chloride in the intestinal lumen. Water moves passively into the intestinal lumen to maintain osmolality, and when this volume exceeds the capacity of the gut to reabsorb fluid, watery diarrhea ensues.
- Cholera causes bicarbonate loss in stools and increase in lactate because of diminished perfusion of peripheral tissues which can cause metabolic acidosis. Hypokalemia results from potassium loss in the stool.
- The organisms themselves do not damage the epithelial cells of the gut. Since the organisms do not invade the intestinal wall, stool does not contain blood.

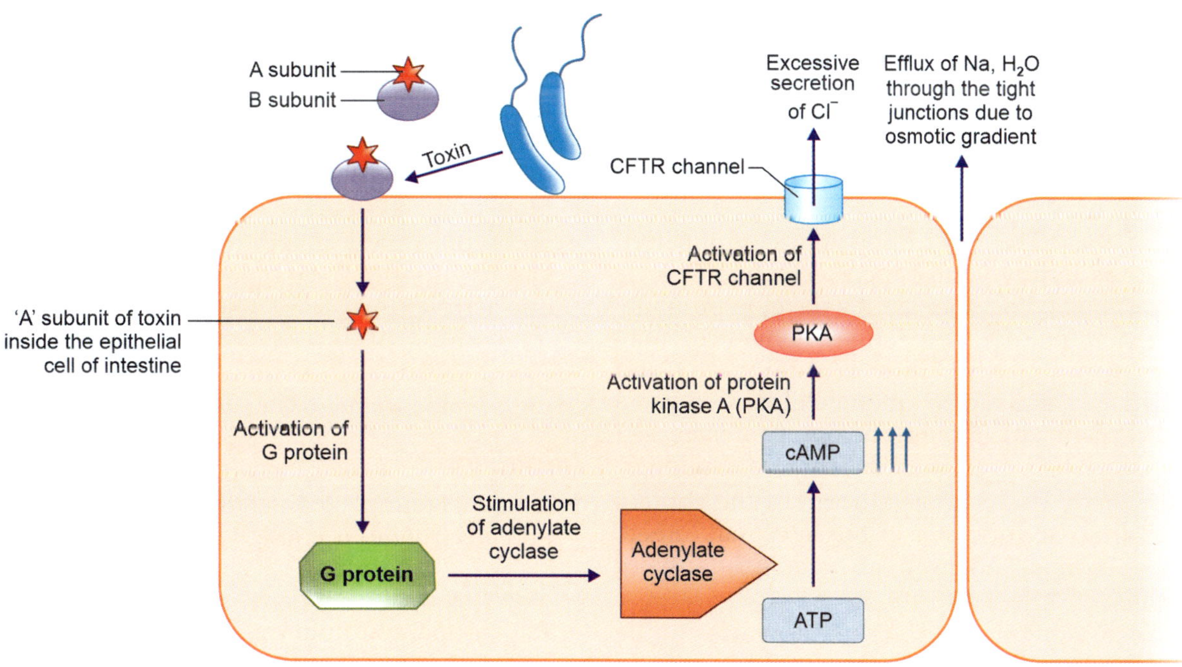

Figure 1.23: Pathogenesis of cholera

- Malnutrition increases susceptibility to cholera. Because gastric acid can quickly inactivate *V cholerae*, hypochlorhydria or achlorhydria of any cause (including *Helicobacter pylori* infection, gastric surgery, vagotomy, use of H_2 blockers and proton pump inhibitors) increases susceptibility. For unknown reasons, incidence of cholera appears to be twice as high in people with type O blood.

Clinical Features

- Cholera is predominantly a disease of children with attack rates highest in the 1–5 years age group.
- Incubation period is 1–2 days.
- Asymptomatic cases are more than symptomatic cases. Asymptomatic individuals can still shed the bacteria in their stool, contributing to the spread of the disease. Symptomatic cholera presents as follows;
- ***Gastrointestinal symptoms:*** Vomiting may begin before or after onset of diarrhea. There is sudden onset of painless, profuse, watery diarrhea. Patients may have abdominal cramping but usually do not have frank abdominal pain typically associated with dysentery. In early illness, cholera stools may contain fecal matter and bile. When cholera is severe ("cholera gravis"), stool appears like 'Rice water' because of mucus flecks floating in the watery stools (resemblance to the water in which rice has been washed). The diarrhea is usually painless, without tenesmus. Fever is uncommon; presence of fever should prompt evaluation for concurrent infection.
- ***Manifestations of hypovolemia and electrolyte loss:*** This is characterized by severe dehydration with sunken eyes, hollow cheeks, 'washerwoman's hands', and decreased urine output. Circulatory shock may develop due to dehydration, with a cold, clammy skin, tachycardia, hypotension and peripheral cyanosis. The patient usually remains alert but appears weak. Muscle cramps can occur due to loss of potassium and calcium. Children may present with convulsions due to hypoglycemia. Acute renal failure and metabolic acidosis may develop due to hypovolemic shock. If the patient survives this stage, the *recovery phase* sets in.
- ***Complications:*** The most important complication of cholera is hypovolemia and electrolyte loss, as discussed above. Pneumonia may develop probably due to aspiration of vomitus. Pneumonia itself may cause death in cholera. Chronic enteropathy and malnutrition may develop among children <5 years of age. Pregnant patients with cholera are at increased risk of miscarriage, premature delivery, and stillbirth.
- "Cholera sicca" is an unusual form of the cholera in which fluid accumulates in the intestinal lumen; circulatory collapse and death can occur in the absence of diarrhea.
- In the recovery phase, diarrhea episodes come down and there is gradual recovery of clinical and biochemical parameters.

Assessment of Dehydration (Table 1.7)

TABLE 1.7: Assessment of dehydration

	Normal (No dehydration)	*Mild-to-moderate dehydration* (if the patient has two or more of the following signs, including at least one sign marked with star*)	*Severe dehydration* (if the patient has two or more signs, including at least one sign marked with star*)
General condition	Well, alert	***Restless, irritable***	***Lethargic or unconscious; floppy***
Eyes	Normal	Sunken	Very sunken and dry
Tears	Present	Absent	Absent
Mouth and tongue	Moist	Dry	Very dry
Thirst	Drinks normally, not thirsty	***Thirsty, drinks eagerly***	***Drinks poorly or not able to drink***
Skin pinch	Goes back quickly	***Goes back slowly***	***Goes back very slowly***

Investigations

- The diagnosis is largely clinical. It should be suspected in patients with painless diarrhea without fever and abdominal pain. Stool does not contain blood.
- Antigen detection: Several rapid antigen detection-based tests are commercially available for diagnosis of cholera. Antibody-based immunochromatographic dipstick assays (for stool or rectal swab) include Crystal VC (which detects presence of O1 or O139 antigen) and Cholkit (which detects the O1 antigen only).
- Gram's stain of a stool sample may show gram-negative comma shaped organisms.
- Dark-field microscopy: Examination of stool under dark-field illumination may show motile organisms. Inhibition of their movement with type-specific antisera is diagnostic.
- Stool or rectal swabs should be taken for culture.
- Serotyping and biotyping: Once cultured, *V. cholerae* can be identified by biochemical tests; serogroup and serotype can be assigned by testing with specific antibodies. This is useful for epidemiologic studies.
- Hematocrit and serum protein are elevated in dehydrated patients because of hemoconcentration.

Treatment

- Cholera is simple to treat. Rapid replacement of fluid and electrolytes is enough in most of the cases.

Oral Rehydration Salt (ORS)

- Replacement of fluid by ORS is highly effective and has saved countless lives. ORS takes advantage of a co-transport mechanism not affected by cholera toxin wherein sodium (Na^+) moves across the gut mucosa along with actively transported glucose. Sodium loss in stool in cholera is high, so that an oral replacement solution containing 90 mmol/L Na^+ is the WHO recommendation.

- Content of WHO ORS in grams (to be added to 1 L of water)

NaCl	3.5
$NaHCO_3$	2.5
KCl	1.5
Glucose	20

- Rice-based ORS is also available. They contain rice powder instead of glucose. They have less osmolality, provide more nutritional benefits and may also reduce the amount of diarrheal stool, an effect not seen with ordinary ORS.

Intravenous Fluids

- IV fluids are required in patients who are unable to drink because of vomiting or altered mental status and in patients wo are severely dehydrated. Ringer's lactate is the best choice as it contains all the electrolytes. The total fluid deficit, which is usually estimated as 10% of body weight, can be infused within 4 hours and half of this within the first hour. Oral fluid can usually be substituted thereafter but patients with continued large-volume diarrhea require intravenous fluid until diarrhea stops. Hypokalemia may develop and can be corrected by potassium supplements. Fluid replacement is monitored by urine output.

Antibiotics

- Antibiotics are warranted for patients with cholera and moderate to severe dehydration. Although not necessary for cure, the use of an antibiotic will diminish the duration and volume of fluid loss and will hasten clearance of the organism from the stool. Single-dose tetracycline (2 g) or doxycycline (300 mg) is effective in adults but is not recommended for children <8 years of age because of possible deposition in bone and developing teeth. Antibiotics can be continued for 3–5 days, though single dose is enough for most of the cases.
- In areas where tetracycline resistance is prevalent, ciprofloxacin or erythromycin can be used for adults.

For children, furazolidone has been the recommended agent and trimethoprim-sulfamethoxazole the second choice. Azithromycin or erythromycin are also good choices for children.

Prevention

- Hygienic measures should be implemented. Avoid tap water, food from street vendors, raw or undercooked seafood, and raw vegetables. Water can be treated with chlorine or iodine, by filtration, or by boiling.

Antibiotic Prophylaxis

- Not routinely recommended. WHO recommends prophylaxis only if an average of one household member in a family of five becomes ill after the first case. Mass chemotherapy of entire communities is not effective and is not recommended.

Vaccines

- Cholera vaccination is no longer officially required for any international traveler but can be used by travelers going to endemic areas. WHO has identified 3 oral vaccines which can be used.
- These vaccines are designed to provide immunity against *Vibrio cholerae* O1 and, in some cases, O139, the serogroups responsible for cholera epidemics.
- Injectable vaccines are outdated and no longer recommended.

Here is a summarized table of cholera vaccines for easy reference **(Table 1.8)**.

Q. Describe the etiology, epidemiology, pathogenesis, Clinical Features, diagnosis and management of plague.

Etiology

- Plague is an acute febrile zoonotic disease caused by infection with *Yersinia pestis*. Yersinia is named in honor of Alexander Yersin, who first isolated this bacterium.
- *Y. pestis* is a gram-negative coccobacillus in the family Enterobacteriaceae. It has bipolar staining pattern and appears like a safety pin **(Fig. 1.24)**.
- Plague is one of the most virulent and potentially lethal bacterial diseases known.

TABLE 1.8: Cholera vaccines

Vaccine	Type	Strains covered	Doses	Protection duration	Target population
Shanchol™	Inactivated (Oral)	*V. cholerae* O1 and O139	2 doses (14 days apart)	Up to 5 years	Individuals aged 1 year and older
Euvichol-Plus™	Inactivated (Oral)	*V. cholerae* O1 and O139	2 doses (14 days apart)	Up to 5 years	Same as Shanchol™
Dukoral™	Inactivated (Oral)	*V. cholerae* O1	2 doses (adults/older children); 3 doses (ages 2–6)	Up to 2 years	Travelers to endemic areas
Vaxchora™	Live-attenuated (Oral)	*V. cholerae* O1	Single dose	3–6 months	Travelers aged 2–64 years

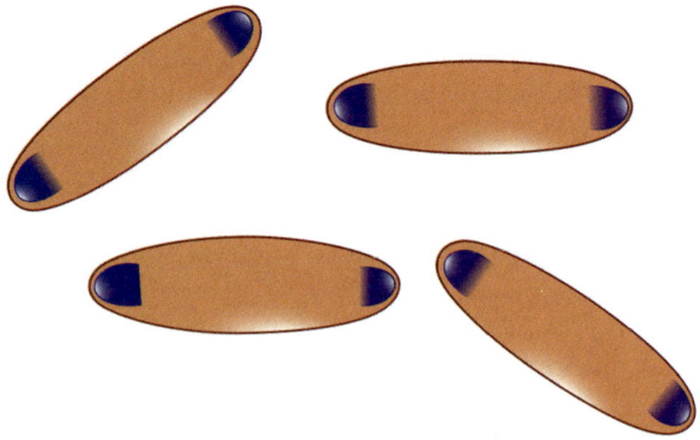

Figure 1.24: *Yersinia pestis* (bipolar staining gives safety pin appearance)

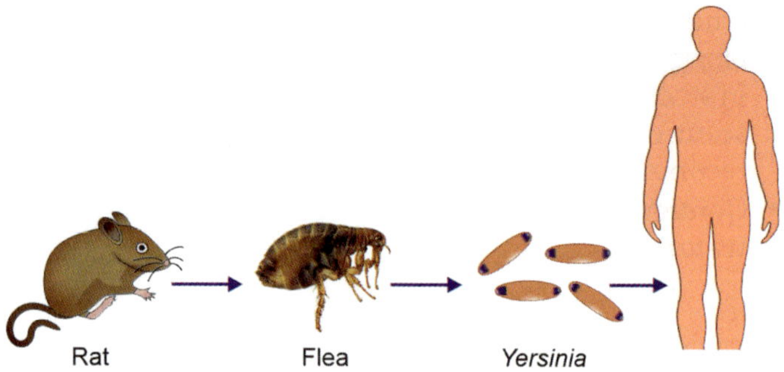

Figure 1.25: Transmission of plague

Epidemiology

- Plague is primarily a zoonotic infection of rodents and wild and domestic animals and is transmitted by fleas; humans are considered incidental hosts that do not contribute to the natural disease cycle.

Endemic Regions

- Plague is endemic in certain rural and semi-arid regions, particularly:
  - Africa: Madagascar, the Democratic Republic of Congo.
  - Asia: Parts of China, Mongolia, and Central Asia.
  - Americas: Southwestern United States, Peru, and Bolivia.
- Plague has been known for many centuries. It was described as *Mahamari* (great destroyer) in India. Since 2000, more than 95% of reported cases have been from Africa, although outbreaks involving hundreds of cases have also occurred elsewhere, including Peru and India.
- Low atmospheric temperature and humidity favor epidemics, which occur mostly from September to May.
- All the age groups and both sexes are affected.

Reservoir of Infection

- Primary reservoirs of plague are wild rodents such as rats (Rattus norwegicus in western countries, Tatera indica and Bandicota bengalensis in India), prairie dogs, and ground squirrels. Domestic rats (Rattus rattus) get infected by coming in contact with wild rats and act as secondary reservoirs. When domestic rats die or come in contact with the human population, the disease spreads.

Transmission of Infection (Fig. 1.25)

- *Vector borne:* The chief vector of the disease is the flea *Xenopsylla cheopis.* Farmers, rat catchers and those who eat rats may contract plague from the wild reservoir. When fleas feast on dead rats they ingest plague bacilli which multiply and block proventricularis. This blocked flea inoculates the host and thus spreads the disease. Dogs and cats can become infected with *Y. pestis* by eating infected rodents and possibly by being bitten by infective fleas. Both dogs and cats may transport infected fleas from rodent-infested areas to the home environment.
- *Direct contact:* Handling tissues or body fluids of infected animals can transmit the bacterium. Infection can also take place by the bite of a rat.
- *Aerosol transmission:* Inhalation of respiratory droplets from humans or animals with pneumonic plague can lead to rapid person-to-person spread.
- *Ingestion:* Consuming undercooked meat of infected animals is a less common transmission route.

Pathogenesis

- *Y. pestis* is highly invasive and pathogenic. It produces many virulence factors and also a lipopolysaccharide endotoxin which is important in sepsis, triggering the systemic inflammatory response syndrome and its complications.
- *Y. pestis* organisms inoculated through the skin or mucous membranes are carried to regional lymph nodes via lymphatic channels, although direct bloodstream inoculation and dissemination may take place. Phagocytes, which can phagocytize *Y. pestis*, may play a role in dissemination of the infection to distant sites. Plague can involve almost any organ, and untreated plague generally results in widespread and massive tissue destruction. Infected lymph nodes (buboes) contain huge numbers of *Yersinia pestis* organisms and show distorted or obliterated lymph node architecture with loss of vascular integrity, hemorrhage, necrosis, infiltration of neutrophils, and extensive serosanguineous effusion. Primary septicemic plague consists of sepsis in the absence of a bubo; secondary septicemic plague is a complication of bubonic or pneumonic plague. DIC can occur in severe cases. Vascular damage may lead to widespread ecchymoses and petechiae. Acral ischemia and gangrene may sometimes develop.
- Primary plague pneumonia is lobar or multilobar. Secondary plague pneumonia begins more diffusely. The affected lung tissue is characterized by edema, hemorrhagic necrosis, and infiltration by neutrophilic leukocytes.

Clinical Features

- Incubation period is 2–8 days.
- There is rapid onset of fever associated with headache, backache and body ache. If not treated early, plague

can follow a toxic course, resulting in shock, multiple-organ failure, and death.

- In humans, plague presents mainly as three forms; bubonic, septicemic, and pneumonic. Bubonic plague is most common type (~80% of cases) and is usually caused by the bite of an infected flea. Septicemic and pneumonic plague can be either primary or secondary to spread from other sites.

Bubonic Plague

- Results from the bite of an infected flea or contact with contaminated tissues. Initially patient experiences fever, chills, headache, myalgia and arthralgia. These symptoms are followed usually within 24 hours by pain and swelling in one or more regional lymph nodes (buboes) proximal to the site of inoculation of the plague bacillus. Since most of the flea bites are on legs, femoral and inguinal nodes are most commonly involved; axillary and cervical nodes are next most commonly affected. Within hours, the enlarging bubo becomes painful and tender. The patient usually guards against palpation, pressure, stretch and limits movements around the bubo. The surrounding tissue often becomes edematous, and the overlying skin may be erythematous, warm, and tense. At the site of flea bite, there may be a papule, pustule, or ulcer. The ulcer may be covered by an eschar.
- If treated early, bubonic plague usually responds quickly, with resolution of fever and other systemic manifestations. Without treatment, patients become increasingly toxic, and secondary plague Sepsis may result in DIC, bleeding, shock, and multi-organ failure.

Septicemic Plague

- Can arise as a primary infection or secondary to bubonic plague. Septic patients often present with gastrointestinal symptoms like nausea, vomiting, diarrhea, and abdominal pain, which may be confused with some abdominal disease. If not treated early with appropriate antibiotics, septicemic plague can be fulminant and fatal.
- Disseminated intravascular coagulation (DIC) may develop leading to: Purpura and petechiae, gangrene of extremities (blackened fingers, toes, or nose, giving rise to the term "Black Death").
- Shock may develop which manifests as refractory hypotension, renal shutdown, and obtundation. Acute respiratory distress syndrome (ARDS) can occur at any stage of septicemic plague.

Pneumonic Plague

- Pneumonic plague is often secondary to bacteremia in bubonic or septicemic plague. However, primary pneumonic plague can occur, being acquired from inhalation of *Y. pestis* from another patient or animal or laboratory specimens.
- Pneumonic plague develops more rapidly and is more fatal than other two forms. Incubation period is usually 3–5 days. The onset is often sudden, with fever, headache, bodyache, and weakness. Pulmonary signs, including tachypnea and dyspnea, cough with expectoration, and chest pain, usually start on the second day of illness. Respiratory failure may develop. Usually one lobe is involved in early stages and later on it may spread to other lobes and other lung also.

Rare Presentations

- Plague meningitis, plague pharyngitis, endophthalmitis, and lymphadenitis at multiple sites.

Diagnosis

- Plague should be suspected in any patient with fever and painful lymphadenopathy. Patient should be questioned about travel to areas of endemic disease, and potential exposure to animal or rodent vector.
- ***Gram's stain:*** Blood, aspirates from buboes, sputum and CSF can all be stained with Wright-Giemsa or Wayson's stain. Wayson's stain demonstrates the typical bipolar staining, which resembles a "closed safety pin." Gram's stain shows small gram-negative coccobacilli.
- ***Culture:*** Blood, aspirates from buboes, sputum and CSF can all be cultured. Growth of *Y. pestis* occurs on selective media (e.g. blood agar, MacConkey agar). Takes 48–72 hours; colonies appear small and non-lactose fermenting.
- ***Serology:*** demonstration of antibodies supports the diagnosis.
- ***Rapid diagnostic tests:*** Immunochromatographic tests for F1 antigen detection in field settings. Provide results within minutes.
- ***Polymerase chain reaction (PCR)****:* Rapid detection of *Y. pestis* DNA in clinical samples. Highly sensitive and specific.
- ***Chest X-ray:*** may show bronchopneumonia, consolidation, pleural effusions and hilar or mediastinal lymphadenopathy.

Treatment

- Patients should be isolated
- Streptomycin is considered the drug of choice. However, gentamicin has been shown to be equally efficacious, cheaper and easier to administer. Hence, in many places gentamicin has replaced streptomycin as the drug of choice. Other antibiotics which are effective include tetracycline, doxycycline (100 mg PO or IV twice daily), ciprofloxacin, chloramphenicol (preferred for plague meningitis due to good CNS penetration), and trimethoprim-sulfamethoxazole (160/800 mg twice daily). Antibiotics should be given for 10–14 days.
- Antibiotics are given orally but can be given parenterally in critically ill patients and to patients who cannot tolerate oral medication. In general, antimicrobial treatment should be continued for 10–14 days or for at least 3 days after the patient has become afebrile and has made a clinical recovery.

Patients initially given intravenous antibiotics may be switched to oral regimens upon clinical improvement.

- Chloramphenicol may be used to treat plague meningitis, pleuritis, endophthalmitis, and myocarditis because of its superior tissue penetration; it is used alone or in combination with streptomycin or another first-line agent.
- Complications like DIC, ARDS, and sepsis require treatment as per standard guidelines.
- Buboes may require surgical drainage.

Prognosis

- If not treated, plague is fatal in >50% of cases of bubonic disease and in nearly all cases of septicemic and pneumonic disease. Prognosis has improved now with the availability of antibiotics.

Prevention

- Avoid exposure to live or dead rodents and use insect repellents in endemic areas.
- Face-to-face contacts of patients with known or suspected pneumonic plague should be provided chemoprophylaxis with doxycycline (100 mg two times daily for 7 days). In pregnant women and children under the age of 8, trimethoprim-sulfamethoxazole has been recommended for 5–7 days. Ciprofloxacin is also effective.
- A plague vaccine exists but is not widely available and is typically reserved for high-risk laboratory personnel or populations in endemic areas.

Q. Describe the etiology, clinical features, diagnosis and treatment of melioidosis.

Etiology

- Melioidosis is an infectious disease caused by *Burkholderia pseudomallei* (previously known as *Pseudomonas pseudomallei*). It is a gram-negative organism showing bipolar staining (safety-pin appearance) like plague bacillus. It is found in the soil and stagnant waters of the tropical and subtropical regions of Asia and Australia.

Epidemiology

- Melioidosis is found predominantly in Asia, Australia, and China. It is rare in the United States.
- The routes of infection are through skin abrasions, by ingestion, and inhalation.
- Percutaneous inoculation during exposure to wet season soil or contaminated water is the predominant mode of acquiring the infection. Hence, majority of melioidosis cases occur in the monsoon wet season.

Clinical Features

- Incubation period ranges from 1 to 20 days.
- Most infections are asymptomatic.
- Immunocompromised states such as diabetes mellitus, malignancy, chronic renal failure and cirrhosis of the liver predispose to infection.
- The most common manifestation is an acute pulmonary infection (pneumonia). Localized suppurative infection can occur in almost any organ but is most common at the site of inoculation in the skin. Typical metastatic sites of infection include the liver, spleen, kidneys, prostate, bone, and skeletal muscle. Most of the patients have multiple abscesses. Septicemia may occur in some patients which may cause death. Acute or chronic fever may be present.

Pathology

- Initially lesions begin as granulomas resembling tuberculosis, with giant cells but without acid-fast bacilli. Later these lesions become microabscesses. Microabscesses enlarge to become big abscesses.

Diagnosis

- Melioidosis should be considered in patients with fever and multiple abscesses. Multiple abscesses, especially those in the liver or spleen, should alert the physician to the possibility of melioidosis.
- Confirmation of the diagnosis is by demonstration of typical safety pin-shaped organisms in smear and culture of abscesses. Pus may occasionally be sterile; hence, repeated samples should be cultured. In severe cases, blood culture may be positive.

Treatment

- The drug of choice is ceftazidime or carbapenems such as imipenem or meropenem for a minimum of 2 weeks and preferably for 4 weeks. Thereafter, combination of chloramphenicol, TMP-SMX, and doxycycline or with the single agent amoxicillin/clavulanate is recommended for 6 weeks to 6 months to eradicate infection.
- Abscesses should be drained by surgical procedures.
- Untreated, the case fatality may be 90% or more.

Q. Cat-scratch disease.

Etiology

- Cat-scratch disease is caused by *Bartonella henselae*, a gram-negative bacillus.
- It occurs throughout the world and is seen commonly in children.

Clinical Features

- Domestic cat is the animal reservoir of this microorganism. It is caused by scratch, bite, or lick of a cat and by close contact. Cats acquire the infection from flea bites but are usually asymptomatic carriers.
- Usually 3–5 days after exposure, patient develops a papule that later crusts. Still later tender regional lymphadenopathy develops. There may be mild fever and malaise. The lymphadenopathy persists for 3–5 weeks. Complications like meningitis, transverse myelitis, encephalitis, hepatitis and osteomyelitis can occur.

Investigations

- Serologic testing or PCR testing.
- Lymph node biopsy—reveals characteristic granulomatous inflammation with stellate necrosis.

Treatment

- Cat-scratch disease is generally benign and self-limiting. Antibiotics are not required except in immunocompromised patients and patients with encephalitis or other serious manifestations. It can be treated with azithromycin or doxycycline.

Q. Trench fever.

Etiology

- Trench fever, also known as *5-day fever* or *quintan fever*, is a febrile illness caused by *Bartonella quintana*, a gram-negative bacillus. It was first reported in soldiers hiding in trenches during World War I. Hence it was called trench fever.

Epidemiology

- Trench fever is seen worldwide. It is more common in United States.
- Humans are the only reservoir of this Bartonella infection. Human body louse is the carrier of *B. quintana* which is transmitted to humans when feces from infected lice are rubbed into abraded skin or the conjunctiva.

Clinical Manifestations

- Trench fever is characterized by the sudden onset of fever, headache, body ache, malaise, weight loss and aseptic meningitis.
- Some patients may have minimal symptoms.

Diagnosis

- The infection is diagnosed by finding *Bartonella quintana* in blood. In cultures it is slow to grow. The infection can also be detected serologically by demonstration of antibodies.

Treatment

- Gentamicin for 2 weeks plus doxycycline for 6 weeks.

Q. Describe the etiology, epidemiology, pathogenesis, diagnosis and treatment of brucellosis.

Etiology

- Brucellosis is a zoonotic infection transmitted to human beings from infected animals. It is also known as undulant, Mediterranean, Malta or Gibraltar fever. It is called undulant fever because of its remittent character.
- It is caused by brucella organisms which are small, non motile, gram-negative rods.
- There are many species of brucella. Out of these, *Brucella melitensis* is the commonest cause of disease in humans and is found in sheep, goats, and camels. *B. abortus* is usually acquired from cattle or buffalo. *B. suis* is usually acquired from pigs. *B. canis* is commonly acquired from dogs.

Epidemiology

- Brucellosis occurs worldwide. The disease is more common in young persons and six times more common in men than in women.
- Human brucellosis is usually associated with occupational or domestic exposure to infected animals or their products.
- The route of entry is by ingestion or inhalation or through mucosal or percutaneous exposure.
- Farmers, shepherds, goatherds, veterinarians, workers in slaughterhouses and meat-processing plants are commonly exposed to infection. Laboratory workers handling cultures or infected samples are also at risk. Others may acquire the infection through consumption of contaminated foods. The most common food items implicated are dairy products like cheese, unpasteurized milk, and ice cream. Raw meat and cosmetic products have been reported to spread the infection rarely.
- Person-to-person transmission is extremely rare, as is transfer of infection by blood or tissue donation.

Pathologenesis

- After gaining entry into human body (via ingestion, inhalation, percutaneous or mucosal exposure) organisms are taken up by macrophages and other mononuclear cells and get disseminated to local lymph nodes and different organs. Brucella then replicate in the lymph nodes and various organs. Since the organism is intracellular, it is protected from antibiotics and antibodies. Cell-mediated immunity plays an important role in clearing the infection. The host response to infection is characterized by tissue granulomas with *B. abortus* and micro-abscesses with *B. melitensis* and *B. suis*.

Clinical Features

- The incubation period varies from 1 week to several months.
- Brucellosis can present acutely, subacutely, or chronically.
- Acute or insidious onset fever which is low or high grade, remittent or intermittent, with chills and sweats, without localizing signs in most cases. Fever can be characteristically undulant, i.e. it may disappear and again appear. Fever can be associated with a relative bradycardia.
- Constitutional symptoms include anorexia, asthenia, fatigue, weakness, and malaise, and weight loss.
- Lymphadenopathy and splenomegaly is seen in 50% of the cases
- Brucellosis is a multisystem disease and affects almost all the organs. Clinical features depend on the system involved (**Table 1.9**).

TABLE 1.9: Clinical features of brucellosis

Organ system	Clinical features
Musculoskeletal system	Myalgia, arthralgia, low back pain, spine and joint pain, and, rarely osteomyelitis, suppurative arthritis
Hematologic	Hemolytic anemia, thrombocytopenia, pancytopenia
Nervous system	Depression, lethargy, dizziness, tinnitus, meningitis, encephalitis, radiculoneuritis.
Eyes	Visual disturbances, keratitis, uveitis, optic neuritis
Respiratory system	Cough, pneumonia, chronic pulmonary granuloma
CVS	Palpitations, endocarditis, myocarditis, cardiac failure
Genitourinary system	Epididymitis, orchitis
GIT	Hepatosplenomegaly, diarrhea, cholecystitis, subdiaphragmatic abscess

- Prolonged fever with a history of contact with animals or animal products and without any specific diagnosis should arouse a suspicion of brucellosis.

Investigations

- The diagnosis of brucellosis is difficult to confirm because the organism is difficult to culture and secondly, even casual contact with infected animals may induce positive serological tests in persons even without disease.
- Routine biochemical tests are usually within normal limits, although sometimes LFTs may be abnormal. WBC count is usually normal or low (relative leukopenia). Mild anemia and thrombocytopenia may be present. ESR can be elevated.
- Blood, bone marrow and lymph node culture may grow organisms.
- Serologic tests: May demonstrate antibodies to brucella. Tube agglutination test is the most common test done to detect antibodies. In endemic areas agglutinin titers of ≥1:320 to 1:640 are considered diagnostic; in nonendemic areas, a titer of ≥1:160 is considered significant. Repetition of tests after 2–4 weeks may demonstrate a rising titer.
- Polymerase chain reaction (PCR): Detects Brucella DNA in blood or tissue, providing rapid and sensitive results.
- Histopathology: Granulomas with central necrosis in tissue biopsies.
- Imaging: For complications (e.g. MRI for spondylitis, ultrasound for liver abscesses).

Treatment

- At least two antibiotics should be used. Monotherapy is not recommended. The "gold standard" for the treatment of brucellosis in adults is intramuscular streptomycin together with doxycycline. The alternative regimen (current WHO recommendation) is rifampicin plus doxycycline for 6 weeks. For patients in whom tetracyclines are contraindicated (children, pregnant women) trimethoprim-sulphomethoxazole can be used instead of tetracyclines.
- There is evidence that other aminoglycosides can be used instead of streptomycin—e.g. netilmicin or gentamicin.
- Surgery in cases of infection of prosthetic heart valves and prosthetic joints (replacement required). If abscesses develop, they need to be drained.

Prevention

- Live attenuated vaccine is available for use in animals but none is available for human beings. Using gloves and mask while handling animals, drinking pasteurized milk may protect against acquiring infection.

Q. Granuloma inguinale (donovanosis) (Granuloma venereum).

- Donovanosis is a chronic, progressively destructive bacterial infection of the genital region. It is a sexually transmitted infection.

Etiology

- It is caused by a gram-negative intracellular bacterium, *Klebsiella granulomatis*. The organism responsible for granuloma inguinale was initially described by Donovan (hence known as donovanosis) and subsequently the bacterium was classified as *Calymmatobacterium granulomatis*. Later, it was found that the molecular structure of this organism was similar to Klebsiella species and presently it is named as *Klebsiella granulomatis*. It is an intracellular bacteria and has a capsule with bipolar staining, which gives it a 'safety pin' appearance (like plague bacillus).

Clinical Features

- Incubation period is 1–12 weeks.
- Common sites of infection are genitals, and perianal region.
- The primary lesion is a painless nodule which slowly enlarges and erodes to produce bright-red ulcers with pearly rolled edges. Ulcer bleeds easily. The lesions progress slowly and heal with fibrosis. There is no lymph node involvement.
- Extragenital lesions occur in some cases and may involve oral cavity, lips, and bones. Lesions in the inguinal region may resemble lymph nodes.

Diagnosis

- *Klebsiella granulomatis* is very difficult to culture because it is extremely fastidious.
- The easiest method to visualize the organism is via smears from the base of the ulcer. The organisms are seen within the cytoplasm of macrophages. They exhibit bipolar staining with safety-pin appearance, and are referred to as Donovan bodies.
- A diagnostic PCR test has been recently developed and can be used for the detection of *C. granulomatis*.
- Serologic tests are also available

Treatment

- First-line treatment: Azithromycin 1 g orally once weekly or 500 mg daily for at least 3 weeks and until all lesions have healed.
- Alternatives: Trimethoprim/sulfamethoxazole or doxycycline or ciprofloxacin. Treatment is given for 3–5 weeks.

Q. Actinomycosis.

- Actinomycosis is a chronic suppurative granulomatous infection characterized by abscess formation and multiple draining sinuses. The main pathological feature is formation of purulent material containing granules with a yellow sulfur like appearance (termed sulfur granules).

Etiology

- The disease is caused by actinomyces bacteria. *Actinomyces israelii* is the commonest pathogen causing actinomycosis. Though actinomyces resembles fungus, actually it is a bacterium. It is gram-positive, non-acid fast, facultatively anaerobic, and branching filamentous bacteria.

Pathogenesis

- Actinomyces are normal commensals in the mouth, colon and vagina.
- Entry into tissues happens when there is a breach of the mucous membrane or from aspiration into the lung.
- Infection spreads by direct extension to contiguous tissues. Hematogenous spread to distant areas, particularly to the bone and brain, can happen.
- The organisms form visible microcolonies in the tissues called grains (sulphur granules). Sulphur granules are *in vivo* matrix of bacteria, calcium phosphate, and host material.

Clinical Features

Cervicofacial Actinomycosis ("Lumpy Jaw")

- Most common type. Painful swelling in the angle of jaw is the usual initial symptom. The swelling is purplish, firmly indurated, and feels woody or lumpy (hence, also known as lumpy jaw). There can be multiple such swellings which break to the surface, forming multiple sinus tracts discharging pus with yellowish white granules. It may spread to tongue, salivary glands, thorax, cervical spine, cranial bones and brain.

Thoracic Actinomycosis

- Results from aspiration of pharyngeal contents or dental plaques into the lungs or spread from cervicofacial actinomycosis. Patients usually c/o mild fever and cough with expectoration. Sputum can be blood-stained. Multiple abscesses may develop in the lungs which may break open into the exterior through multiple discharging sinuses. Chest X-ray shows consolidation bilaterally in the lower lung fields.

Abdominal Actinomycosis

- Results from diseased appendix. It can involve any organ in the abdomen. The disease usually presents as an abscess or mass lesion that is often fixed to underlying tissue and mistaken for a tumor. Sinus tracts may form in the abdominal wall.

Pelvic Actinomycosis

- Involves uterus and cervix. It has become common with the use of intrauterine contraceptive devices.

Rare Forms

- *CNS actinomycosis:* Can present as meningitis or multiple brain abscesses.
- *Musculoskeletal and soft-tissue actinomycosis:* Skin, subcutaneous tissue, muscle, and bone involved alone or in various combinations. Multiple cutaneous sinus tracts.
- *Disseminated disease:* Multiple organ infections. Lungs and liver most commonly involved. Presents as multiple nodules mimicking disseminated cancer.

Diagnosis

- Microscopic identification of sulfur granules in pus or tissues. Sometimes granules may be visible to the naked eye.
- Sulfur granules may also be found in mycetoma. If any doubt is there, identification of actinomyces by microscopy and culture of pus or tissue specimens will confirm the diagnosis. However, because these organisms are part of the normal flora, their identification in the absence of sulfur granules in sputum, bronchial washings, and cervicovaginal secretions is of little significance.

Differential Diagnosis

- Tuberculosis.
- Fungal infections (e.g. nocardiosis, histoplasmosis).
- Malignancies.

Treatment

- Requires prolonged antibiotic therapy (6–12 months).
- Penicillin is the drug of choice; 10–20 million units intravenously daily for 4-6 weeks followed by oral penicillin or amoxicillin for 6–12 months.
- Erythromycin, tetracycline, and clindamycin are alternatives.
- Surgical intervention: Indicated for drainage of large abscesses, debridement of necrotic tissue.

Q. Nocardiosis.

- Nocardiosis is an acute, subacute, or chronic infectious disease caused by Nocardia spp that occurs in cutaneous, pulmonary, and disseminated forms.
- Members of the genus Nocardia are ubiquitous saprophytes in soil, decaying organic matter, and fresh and salt water. Nocardia organisms are branching, beaded, filamentous, gram-positive bacteria.

- Common pathogenic species:
  - *Nocardia asteroides* (most common in pulmonary infections).
  - *Nocardia brasiliensis* (associated with cutaneous infections).
  - *Nocardia farcinica* and *Nocardia nova*.

Transmission of Infection

- Nocardia is usually transmitted to humans via one of two routes: inhalation or inoculation into the skin.
- Inhalation of contaminated dust is thought to be the most common mode of entry.
- Skin inoculation occurs via penetrating trauma from a contaminated source (e.g. puncture by a contaminated thorn) or exposure of a preexisting wound to contaminated dust, soil, or water.
- Oral ingestion via contaminated foods is another less common way of infection.

Clinical Features

- It usually causes infection in immunocompromised hosts.
- Cutaneous infection presents as ulceration, abscess, and cellulitis. Lymphocutaneous nocardiosis manifests as a nodule/ulcer at the site of injury, lymphangitis, and regional lymphadenopathy. A mycetoma is a chronic cutaneous infection that initially begins with one or more painless, slow-growing indurated nodules that eventually coalesce to form large tumors with necrotic abscesses and draining sinus tracts (Mycetomas can also be caused by fungi and other bacteria).
- Pulmonary nocardiosis is the most common clinical presentation of nocardiosis. It occurs due to inhalation of Nocardia. Pulmonary nocardiosis is usually seen as opportunistic infection in immunocompromised patients. Patients present with fever and cough with expectoration. X-ray shows lung infiltrates.
- Disseminated infection: most common site is brain. Cerebral nocardiosis presents as space-occupying lesion. Purulent meningitis may result if an abscess ruptures into the ventricles.

Diagnosis

- Microscopy
- Culture of pus and tissue specimens for nocardia.
- Molecular tests for Nocardia spp, such as polymerase chain reaction (PCR) are available in reference labs.

Treatment

Long-term antibiotic therapy is required (at least 6 months). Sulfonamides are the drugs of choice for nocardiosis. Sulfadiazine or sulfisoxazole can be used. Trimethoprim-sulfamethoxazole (TMP-SMZ) is also effective. Additional or alternative parenteral therapies include carbapenems (imipenem or meropenem), third-generation cephalosporins (cefotaxime or ceftriaxone), and amikacin alone or in combination. Combination therapy is recommended for serious infections.

Q. Mycetoma (Madura foot or Maduromycosis).

- Mycetoma is a chronic infection of the skin and subcutaneous tissue.
- It is characterized by the formation of a mass, the development of sinuses, and the discharge of grains, which are composed of the causative agent often embedded in the cement matrix.
- It is also known as Madura foot because it was first described in the Indian town of Madura region in the mid-19th century.

Etiology

- Mycetoma is caused by filamenous bacteria and true fungi.
- Mycetoma caused by filamentous bacteria is termed actinomycetoma. Most common agents of actinomycetoma are the bacteria *Nocardia brasiliensis*, *Actinomadura madurae* and *Streptomyces somaliensis*.
- Mycetoma caused by true fungi is termed eumycetoma. Eumycetoma can be caused by *Pseudallescheria boydii*, *Phialophora jeanselmei*, *Madurella mycetomi*, *Madurella grisea*, *Cephalosporium falciforme*, and *Cephalosporium recifei*.

Clinical Features

- Eumycetoma is endemic in certain tropical and subtropical regions, predominantly affecting people from rural or agricultural backgrounds who are exposed to the soil. The disease is commonly found in areas such as Africa, South Asia, and Central America, although cases have been reported worldwide.
- Mycetoma commonly affects young adults, particularly males aged between 20 and 40 years. People of low socioeconomic status and manual workers such as agriculturalists, laborers and herdsmen are commonly affected. Organisms enter the skin through minor trauma.
- Mycetoma is a chronic, deep, progressively destructive, and deforming infection of skin, subcutaneous tissues, bone, and muscle. Most of the cases involve foot but any part of the body can be involved. It manifests as a tumor-like area of localized edema or massive enlargement, with erythema and multiple draining sinus tracts. In a typical case, a triad of tumefaction, sinus tract formation, and grains (sulfur granules) is seen. The color of the grains varies depending on the pathogen.
- Note that mycetoma is different from actinomycosis. *Actinomyces israelii* can cause both actinomycosis and mycetoma.

Investigations

- Gram's stain—of secretions can show filamentous gram-positive bacteria or gram-negative fungi.
- Biopsy: shows suppurative granulomas sorrounding characteristic grains in the subcutaneous tissue. Causative filamenous bacteria or fungi can be seen in Gram's stain.
- Culture of the secretions or biopsy specimens.

Treatment

- Differentiation between actinomycetoma caused by bacteria and eumycetoma caused by fungi is important because treatment is different for both.
- For actinomycetoma (caused by bacteria), surgical debridement followed by prolonged antibiotic therapy is required. A combination of antibiotics are used including trimethroprim-sulphamethoxazole, streptomycin, dapsone and rifampicin.
- For eumycetoma (caused by fungi), surgery followed by antifungal therapy (itraconazone or voriconazole or posaconazole) is used. Duration of therapy is at least 12 months.

Q. Discuss the etiology, epidemiology, pathogenesis, clinical features, diagnosis and treatment of leprosy (Hansen's disease).

- Leprosy (Hansen's disease) is a nonfatal, chronic infectious disease caused by *Mycobacterium leprae* or *Mycobacterium lepromatosis*. To minimize the prejudice against those with leprosy, the condition is also referred to as Hansen disease, named after G.A. Hansen who discovered *M. leprae*.
- First described in ancient Indian texts from the sixth century BC.
- Mainly affects skin, peripheral nervous system, upper respiratory tract, eyes, and testes.
- Associated with social stigma.

Etiology

- *Mycobacterium leprae* and *Mycobacterium lepromatosis (a closely related species associated with diffuse lepromatous leprosy)*. The (DNA sequences of *M. leprae* and *M. lepromatosis* differ enough to distinguish them as separate species, but they share many similarities (both are obligate intracellular parasites with a tropism for nerves) and cause the same clinical disease.
- It is an acid fast and obligate intracellular organism.
- The organism grows best at 27–30°C; therefore, skin lesions tend to develop in the cooler areas of the body, with sparing of the groin, axilla, and scalp.
- Cannot be cultured *in vitro*.

Epidemiology

- 99% of leprosy cases are found in Asia, Africa and Latin America. Highest number of cases are in India.
- Affects all age groups. Peak onset is in the second and third decades of life.
- Leprosy is associated with poverty and rural residence
- Its incidence is not increased by AIDS unlike tuberculosis.
- Recently there has been a dramatic decline in leprosy cases because of effective multi-drug therapy.

Pathogenesis

- Incubation period is long, 5–10 years.
- It spreads by droplet infection when an infectious (lepromatous) patient releases the organisms by coughing and sneezing. The organism enters the body through skin, mucous membranes of the respiratory tract and possibly the gut. The infectivity of the disease is low and large percent of people exposed to the infection do not get infected.
- Leprosy has two classification schemas: the 5-category Ridley-Jopling system and the simpler 2 category WHO system.
- Ridley Jopling system divides leprosy into five clinical categories (2 polar forms and 3 borderline forms). Two polar forms are: tuberculoid (TT) and lepromatous leprosy (LL). Tuberculoid leprosy occurs in people with good immunity. Lepromatous leprosy occurs in people with low immunity. Between these forms lies a large group of patients described as the borderline group. In this group, patients showing features closer to lepromatous leprosy are designated borderline lepromatous (BL) leprosy and those with features closer to tuberculoid form are designated as borderline tuberculoid (BT) leprosy; patients with features lying midway between the two are classified as borderline (BB) leprosy.
- The World Health Organization (WHO) classification system is designed for settings with limited clinical expertise or laboratory support. It categorizes leprosy based on the number of skin lesions. Paucibacillary (PB) leprosy is defined as having five or fewer skin lesions with no detectable bacilli on skin smears. Patients with a single skin lesion are further classified as single-lesion PB. Multibacillary (MB) leprosy is characterized by six or more lesions and may include cases that test positive for bacilli on skin smears. Counting skin lesions alone may lead to misclassification of many patients with PB leprosy rather than MB leprosy, leading to undertreatment in some cases

Clinical Features

Tuberculoid (TT) Leprosy

- Occurs in people who possess a high degree of cell mediated immunity.
- More often affects brown and black people.
- The skin lesions of tuberculoid leprosy are only one or few hypopigmented macules or plaques that are sharply demarcated and hypoesthetic. Lesions usually have erythematous or raised borders, and are devoid of sweat glands and hair follicles and thus are dry, scaly, and anhidrotic.
- The regional or local nerve is thickened and may be tender. Most commonly affected nerves are ulnar, posterior auricular, peroneal, and posterior tibial nerves.
- Histology of the lesions shows granulomatous infiltrate consisting of macrophages, lymphocytes and giant cells. The infiltrate is more prominent around the nerves and the skin appendages.
- Smears from lesions show absent or very few AFB.
- Lepromin test is positive in TT leprosy.

Lepromatosus (LL) Leprosy

- Occurs in people who have less cell-mediated immunity.
- It more often affects White people.
- The skin lesions are multiple, bilaterally symmetrical, hypopigmented macules, plaques, nodules or diffuse skin infiltration. The margins are ill defined, and diffuse. Diffuse infiltration of facial skin gives rise to convoluted folds, which give the face a lion-like appearance (hence called 'leonine facies').
- Infiltration of eyebrows leads to loss of eyebrows, initially lateral third.
- Nose can get involved which can cause nasal bridge collapse and epistaxis. Nasal septum can get perforated.
- Patients with LL leprosy have late involvement of nerves which presents as distal symmetric peripheral neuropathy. Neural involvement predisposes to painless burns and trophic ulcers, deformities and resorbed digits of the hands and feet.
- Systemic involvement causes lymphadenopathy, hepatosplenomegaly, testicular involvement and gynaecomastia, and bacillemia. Smears from lesions show large number of bacilli. Lepromin test is negative in LL leprosy.
- The disease runs a slow and progressive course. Patients may die of intercurrent infections, renal failure or amyloidosis all of which are complications of leprosy.

Borderline Group

- In the BT form, the lesions show features closer to tuberculoid form of the disease. Lesions may be more or a tuberculoid lesion may have a satellite lesion close to it. In BL form, the lesions show features closer to the lepromatous form. Genuine borderline (BB) cases have features midway between tuberculoid and lepromatous leprosy.

Primary Neuritic Leprosy

- Here nerve involvement is seen without any skin lesions. Nerves are thickened and may be tender with associated loss of sensations. Facial palsy can also be a presentation.

Indeterminate Leprosy

- This is often a single hypopigmented macule which may be atrophic and may be hypoesthetic. Acid-fast bacilli may or may not be seen. At this stage it is difficult to tell which way the lesion will progress whether towards the lepromatous end or tuberculoid end.

Differenes between tuberculoid and lepromatous leprosy **(Table 1.10)**.

Diagnosis

Currently, the diagnosis of leprosy is based on clinical features. Examination of skin smears and/or biopsy can confirm the diagnosis.

Clinical Features

- In an endemic country or area, an individual should be regarded as having leprosy if he or she has one of the following features:
    - Hypopigmented or reddish skin lesion(s) with definite loss of sensation.
    - Involvement of peripheral nerves, as demonstrated by loss of sensation and weakness of the muscles of hands, feet or face.
    - Skin smear positive for acid-fast bacilli.

Skin Smears and Biopsy

- Skin smears may be taken from lesions on the ears, elbows, and/or knees. A biopsy should be taken from entirely within a lesion.

Other Diagnostic Tests

- *Measurement of anti-phenolic glycolipid-1 (PGL-1) antibodies:* This is a specific serologic test based on the detection of antibodies to phenolic glycolipid-1. This test yields a sensitivity of 95% for the detection of lepromatous leprosy but only 30% sensitive for tuberculoid leprosy.
- *Polymerase chain reaction (PCR):* This can be used to identify the Mycobacterium in biopsy samples, skin and nasal smears, and blood and tissue sections.

TABLE 1.10: Differences between tuberculoid and lepromatous leprosy

Feature	Tuberculoid leprosy (TT)	Lepromatous leprosy (LL)
Immune response	Strong cell-mediated immunity	Weak or absent cell-mediated immunity
Skin lesions	Few, well-demarcated, hypopigmented, or erythematous macules or plaques. Sensory loss over lesions.	Numerous, poorly defined macules, nodules, or plaques. Symmetrical distribution. Sensory loss late feature.
Nerve lesions	Peripheral nerves involved early. Only few nerves are involved. Nerves are thickened and may be tender.	Nerves are involved late in the disease. Symmetric involvement common
Facial changes	Slow progression, often self-limiting	Rapid progression without treatment
Bacterial load	Low or absent (paucibacillary)	High (multibacillary). Numerous bacilli present
Lepromin skin test	Positive (indicative of good immune response)	Negative (indicative of poor immune response)
Infectivity	Low, due to limited bacilli in lesions	High, as large numbers of bacilli are shed
Progression	Slow progression, often self-limiting	Rapid progression without treatment
Treatment duration	Shorter (paucibacillary regimen)	Longer (multibacillary regimen)

- *Lymphocyte migration inhibition test (LMIT):* As determined by a lymphocyte transformation and LMIT, cell-mediated immunity to *M. leprae* is absent in patients with lepromatous leprosy but present in those with tuberculoid leprosy.

Treatment of Leprosy

- There are 3 main drugs for the treatment of leprosy. These are dapsone, clofazimine, and rifampicin. Of these drugs, only rifampicin is bactericidal but dapsone is the most important.
- Other agents which are effective against leprosy are minocycline, ofloxacin and clarithromycin.
- WHO has made recommendations for the treatment of leprosy. For treatment purposes, the WHO classifies leprosy patients as paucibacillary and multibacillary. Previously, patients without demonstrable AFB in the dermis were classified as paucibacillary and those with AFB as multibacillary **(Table 1.11)**.
- Currently, most leprosy programs classify and choose the appropriate regimen for a particular patient using clinical criteria, which uses the number of skin lesions and nerves involved to classify leprosy patients into paucibacillary single-lesion leprosy (one skin lesion), paucibacillary leprosy (2–5 skin lesions) and multibacillary leprosy (more than five skin lesions).

TABLE 1.11: WHO treatment of leprosy

Form of leprosy	WHO recommended regimen (2018)	Duration of treatment
Paucibacillary (TT and BT)	Dapsone (100 mg daily) *plus* Rifampicin (600 mg/ month) *plus* Clofazimine (300 mg once monthly, and 50 mg once daily)	6 months
Multibacillary (LL, BL, BB)	Same as above	12 months

Complications of Leprosy

- **Extremities:** Distal myopathy, claw hand, loss of digits, foot drop, trophic ulcers
- **Nose:** Destruction of nasal cartilage with resultant saddle nose deformity and anosmia, epistaxis.
- **Eye:** Corneal ulcerations and development of opacities due to loss of sensation of cornea. Uveitis due to direct bacterial invasion with consequent cataracts and glaucoma.
- **Testes:** *M. leprae* can invade testes and cause aspermia or hypospermia. Erythema nodosum leprosum can also cause orchitis.
- **Amyloidosis:** Secondary amyloidosis is a complication of LL leprosy.
- **Nerve abscesses:** Seen in TT and BT forms of leprosy and can cause rapid nerve destruction which may be permanent.

Q. Write briefly about antileprosy drugs.

See **Table 1.12**.

TABLE 1.12: Antileprosy drugs

Drug	Mechanism of action	Features	Dosage	Side effects
Dapsone	Inhibition of folic acid synthesis.	Bacteriostatic. Inexpensive and relatively nontoxic	100 mg daily	Agranulocytosis Hemolytic anemia in patients with G6PD deficiency
Rifampicin	Rifampicin binds the DNA-dependent RNA polymerase complex uncoupling transcription	Most bactericidal drug available for the treatment of leprosy	600 mg monthly	Renal failure, bone marrow suppression, "flu-like" syndrome, hepatitis
Clofazimine	Binds preferentially to mycobacterial DNA and inhibits *Mycobacterium leprae* growth	Weakly bactericidal against *M. leprae*	50 mg daily	Skin pigmentation.
Ofloxacin	Interferes with bacterial DNA replication by inhibiting DNA gyrase	Bactericidal	400 mg single dose as part of ROM single dose regimen	Nausea, diarrhea and other gastrointestinal complaints CNS effects such as insomnia, headache, dizziness, nervousness, and hallucinations
Clarithromycin	Inhibits bacterial protein synthesis by binding to 50S ribosomal subunit	Bactericidal for *M. leprae*	500 mg daily	Gastrointestinal irritation, nausea, vomiting, and diarrhea
Minocycline	Inhibits protein synthesis by binding to 30S ribosomal subunit	Bactericidal for *M. leprae*	100 mg daily	Discoloration of teeth in infants or children

Q. Lepra reactions.

- Lepra reactions are immunologically mediated episodes that occur during the course of leprosy, often triggered by treatment or other factors. They occur due to abrupt change in immunological response of the body against *M. leprae*.
- They can cause acute inflammation, worsening of symptoms, and damage to nerves, leading to further disability if untreated.
- There are two main types: **Type 1 (reversal reaction)** and **type 2 (erythema nodosum leprosum)**.

Type I reaction (reversal reaction)

- Type I reactions occur in borderline forms of leprosy (BT, BB, or BL) as a result of increased activity of the body's immune system against *M. leprae*. Usually the BL form changes to BT form with treatment due to increase in immunity, hence this type of reaction is also known as reversal reaction. Cell-mediated immunity plays a major role here. It occurs both in paucibacillary and multibacillary leprosy.
- Manifestations include signs of inflammation in preexisting lesions, appearance of new skin lesions, neuritis, and rarely fever. Ulnar nerve is usually affected at elbow, which may be painful and exquisitely tender. Foot drop may result due to peroneal nerve involvement. If patients with affected nerves are not treated promptly with steroids, irreversible nerve damage may occur.

Treatment

- For mild type-1 lepra reaction, analgesics, such as acetylsalicylic acid or paracetamol are enough. For severe type 1 lepra reactions with evidence of neuritis (pain, loss of sensation or function), steroids such as oral prednisolone should be used. The usual dose of prednisolone is 40–60 mg daily (1 mg/kg) initially followed by a gradual tapering. The duration of steroid therapy is 3 months.

Type 2 Lepra Reaction (Erythema Nodosum Leprosum, ENL)

- Type 2 lepra reaction occur in patients with high load of leprosy bacilli as in multibacillary/infiltrative type of leprosy (BL and LL disease). Type 2 reaction can involve multiple organs and systems, causing generalized symptoms.
- It occurs when large number of leprosy bacilli are killed with release of their antigens. These antigens provoke an arthus type allergic reaction producing antigen antibody immune complex reaction (type III hypersensitivity) in the presence of complement system. Immune complexes are deposited in the tissues (skin, eyes, joints, lymph nodes, kidneys, liver, spleen, bone marrow, endothelium and testes) as well as in the circulation.
- Most cases of ENL follow the initiation of chemotherapy, usually within 2 years. Rarely it may occur even before the diagnosis of leprosy and may in fact point toward leprosy diagnosis.
- Patients usually present with multiple painful erythematous papules that resolve spontaneously in a few days but may recur. Patients may also have fever, arthritis, myalgia and epididymo-orchitis, iridocyclitis and lymphadenopathy. There can be anemia, leukocytosis, and abnormal liver function tests. Skin biopsy of erythematous papules reveals vasculitis or panniculitis. Rarely severe ENL can result in death.

Treatment

- Therapy for type 2 reaction includes analgesics, such as acetylsalicylic acid or paracetamol, and steroids (oral prednisolone). In patients with severe type 2 reactions, who do not respond to steroids or in whom steroids are contraindicated, *clofazimine* at high doses or *thalidomide* may be used under close medical supervision. Clofazimine often requires 4–6 weeks before an effect is seen, and therefore, initially it should be combined with steroids.

Differences between type 1 and type 2 lepra reactions **(Table 1.13)**.

TABLE 1.13: Differences between type 1 and type 2 lepra reactions

Feature	Type 1 reaction	Type 2 reaction
Immune response	Cell-mediated immunity (Th1 response)	Immune complex-mediated (Th2 response)
Occurrence	More common in borderline leprosy (BT, BB, BL)	Occurs mainly in multibacillary (lepromatous) leprosy (LL, BL)
Skin lesions	Preexisting lesions become erythematous, swollen, and tender; may ulcerate	Existing skin lesions remain unchanged and new red, painful, tender, cutaneous/subcutaneous nodules appear (ENL)
Nerve involvement	Prominent and severe, with nerve pain, swelling, and sensory/motor loss	Less common or mild nerve involvement
Systemic symptoms	Rare (primarily localized to skin and nerves)	Common; fever, malaise, arthralgia, lymphadenopathy, and more
Other organ involvement	Other organs not affected	Can involve systemic organs (e.g. iritis, orchitis, nephritis)
Histopathology	Granulomatous inflammation with increased lymphocytes in lesions	Neutrophilic infiltrates with immune complex deposition
Treatment	Corticosteroids (prednisolone) for nerve involvement; MDT continues	Corticosteroids, thalidomide (if severe), NSAIDs; MDT continues

Lucio's Phenomenon

- Lucio phenomenon is a rare complication presenting as sudden necrotizing vasculopathy in patients with longstanding, untreated lepromatous leprosy. This rare reaction is seen commonly in patients of Caribbean and Mexican origin.
- Patients develop recurrent, large, ulcerative lesions—particularly on the lower extremities. Ulcers may develop all over the body. Secondary infection and consequent sepsis can be fatal. Ulcers happen due to ischemic necrosis of skin, which in turn is due to thrombus formation in blood vessels supplying skin due to heavy parasitism of endothelial cells with AFB, and endothelial proliferation. Immune complex deposition may also play a role in thrombus formation.

Treatment

- Management requires antimicrobial therapy and corticosteroids as well as skin and wound care.

Q. Syphilis.

- Syphilis is an infectious venereal disease caused by the spirochete *Treponema pallidum*.
- It is characterized by episodes of active disease interrupted by periods of latency.

Etiology

- Syphilis is caused by *Treponema pallidum* which belongs to spirochete group.
- It is spiral in shape. Live organisms can only be seen under dark-ground illumination because of poor resolution with conventional light microscopy **(Fig. 1.26)**. Treponema organisms have characteristic to-and-fro, undulating, corkscrew-like and angulating movements.
- Syphilis is becoming a rare disease now after the discovery of penicillin. However, efforts to eradicate this disease have been unsuccessful.

Pathophysiology

- The only known natural host for *T. pallidum* is man.
- Almost all cases of syphilis are acquired by sexual contact. Less commonly, it is acquired by nonsexual personal contact, infection *in utero* (congenital syphilis), and blood transfusion. 1 in 2 persons exposed to infection gets infected.

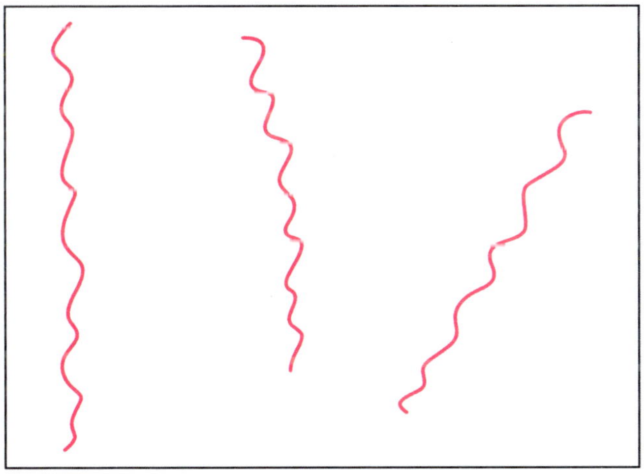

Figure 1.26: *Treponema pallidum*

- Syphilis is usually classified into 4 stages: Primary, secondary, latent, and tertiary. It can be acquired or congenital.
- *Primary syphilis:* in acquired syphilis, after exposure, *T. pallidum* penetrates intact mucous membranes or microscopic dermal abrasions and enters the lymphatics and blood to produce systemic infection. At the site of entry, a painless ulcer develops which is called chancre. Histologically, the chancre is characterized by local inflammation with infiltration by macrophages and lymphocytes. In this stage, the spirochete can be isolated from the surface of the ulceration or the overlying exudate. Whether treated or not, healing occurs with residual fibrosis.
- *Secondary syphilis* develops several weeks or months after the appearance of the primary lesion. During this stage, the spirochetes multiply and spread throughout the body. Secondary syphilis has numerous clinical manifestations. Common manifestations include malaise, fever, myalgias, arthralgias, lymphadenopathy, and rash.
- *Latent syphilis* is characterized by resolution of skin lesions and other clinical manifestations. However, serologic tests are positive for *T. pallidum*.
- *Tertiary or late syphilis* develops years after the initial infection (5–10 years later) and can involve any organ system. The most dreaded complications are neurosyphilis and involvement of the aortic valve and root. Initially syphilis mainly involves meninges and vasculature of CNS (meningovascular syphilis), later the parenchyma of brain and spinal cord is involved.
- Regardless of the stage of disease and location of lesions, histopathologic hallmarks of syphilis are endarteritis and a plasma cell–rich infiltrate. The syphilitic infiltrate is actually a delayed-type hypersensitivity response to *T. pallidum*, and can result in gummatous ulcerations and necrosis seen in tertiary syphilis. Antigens of *T. pallidum* induce treponemal antibodies and nonspecific reagin antibodies.

Clinical Features

- Acquired syphilis has predictable stages though there may not be clear cut demarcation between the stages. Four stages can usually be recognized and include (1) *primary*, (2) *secondary*, (3) *latent*, and (4) *tertiary* syphilis.

Primary Syphilis

- Primary syphilis is characterized by the development of a painless chancre at the site of entry after an incubation period of 3–6 weeks. The lesion has a punched-out base and rolled edges and is highly infectious. It has a firm consistency. In heterosexual men the chancre is usually located on the penis, whereas in homosexual men it is often found in the anal canal or rectum, in the mouth, or on the external genitalia. In women, it is usually found on the cervix and labia. Regional lymphadenopathy is usually seen. Lymph nodes are firm, nonsuppurative, and painless.

Secondary Syphilis

- Secondary syphilis has protean manifestations. These include skin and mucous membrane lesions and generalized painless lymphadenopathy. The healing primary chancre may be still present in some cases. The skin lesions are macular, papular, papulosquamous rashes, and occasionally pustules. The rahes may be very subtle and may be missed. Initial lesions are bilaterally symmetric, pale red or pink, nonpruritic, discrete, round macules that measure 5–10 mm in diameter and are distributed on the trunk and proximal extremities. After many days or weeks, red papular lesions appear. These lesions may progress to pustular lesions.
- In warm and moist areas like perianal area, vulva, scrotum, etc. papules can enlarge and become eroded to produce moist, pink or gray-white, highly infectious lesions called condylomata lata. Mucosal lesions include erosions, called mucous patches and occur on lips, oral mucosa, tongue, palate, pharynx, vulva and vagina, glans penis. The mucous patch is painless with a red periphery.
- Constitutional symptoms may accompany secondary syphilis and include fever, weight loss, malaise, anorexia and headache. Meningitis can occur rarely.
- Less commonly there can be hepatitis, nephropathy, arthritis, periostitis, iritis and uveitis.

Latent Syphilis

- In latent syphilis serologic tests for syphilis are positive but there are no clinical manifestations. In latent syphilis *T. pallidum* is present in the body. Latent syphilis can get transmitted to the fetus *in utero* and to others through blood transfusion.

Tertiary Syphilis

- Tertiary syphilis is characterized by a persistent low-level burden of pathogens, against which a potent and self-destructive immune response is mounted. It is usually very slowly progressive and noninfectious. Any organ of the body may be involved, but three main types are: *neurosyphilis, cardiovascular syphilis* and *gummatous (late) syphilis.*

Neurosyphilis

- Traditionally, neurosyphilis was considered to be a late manifestation of syphilis, but this not true and CNS can get affected anytime. CNS involvement can be asymptomatic or symptomatic. Asymptomatic neurosyphilis refers to patients without any neurological signs and symptoms but have CSF abnormalities or a positive VDRL test. Such asymptomatic patients should be treated because untreated patients may progress to symptomatic neurosyphilis.
- Neurosyphilis can be *meningeal, meningovascular, and parenchymatous syphilis*. Meningeal syphilis occurs usually within 1 year after infection, meningovascular syphilis occurs 5–10 years after infection, general paresis after 20 years, and tabes dorsalis after 25–30 years.
- *Meningeal syphilis* presents with typical signs and symptoms of meningitis like headache, nausea, vomiting, neck stiffness, and alteration of mental status.
- *Meningovascular syphilis* involves meninges and also blood vessels leading to stroke.
- *Parenchymatous syphilis* involves brain and spinal cord and manifests as general paresis and tabes dorsalis. General paresis happens due to widespread brain parenchymal damage and includes abnormalities corresponding to the mnemonic PARESIS: **P**ersonality disturbances, **A**ffect abnormalities, **R**eflex hyperactivity, **E**ye abnormality (Argyll Robertson pupils), **S**ensorium changes, **I**ntellectual impairment and **S**lurred speech. In tabes dorsalis there is demyelination of the posterior columns, dorsal roots, and dorsal root ganglia. Symptoms include ataxia, paresthesia, bladder disturbances, impotence, areflexia and loss of joint position, deep pain, and temperature sensations. Argyll Robertson pupil can be seen in both tabes dorsalis and general paresis. It reacts to accommodation but not to light. Optic atrophy also occurs frequently in tabes.

Cardiovascular Syphilis

- Cardiovascular manifestations are due to endarteritis obliterans of the vasa vasorum, which provide blood supply to large vessels. This results in weakening of tunica media and formation of aneurysm, aortitis (with linear calcification of the ascending aorta on chest X-ray), aortic regurgitation, or coronary ostial stenosis. Symptoms usually appear 10–40 years after infection. The most common finding on cardiovascular examination is a diastolic murmur with a tambour quality, secondary to aortic dilation with valvular insufficiency.

Gummatous Syphilis (late syphilis)

- Gummas are nothing but areas of granulomatous inflammation with a central area of necrosis. Gummas may be single or multiple and size varies from microscopic to many centimeters. The most commonly involved sites are skin, mucous membranes and skeletal system. Gummas of the skin produce painless and indurated nodular lesions which may break down to form punched-out ulcers with vertical edges. The ulcer heals in the middle with an atrophic tissue-paper scar and spreads peripherally. The base of the lesion is dull red and appears like 'wash-leather'. Nocturnal bone pain may occur due to bone involvement (**Fig. 1.27**).

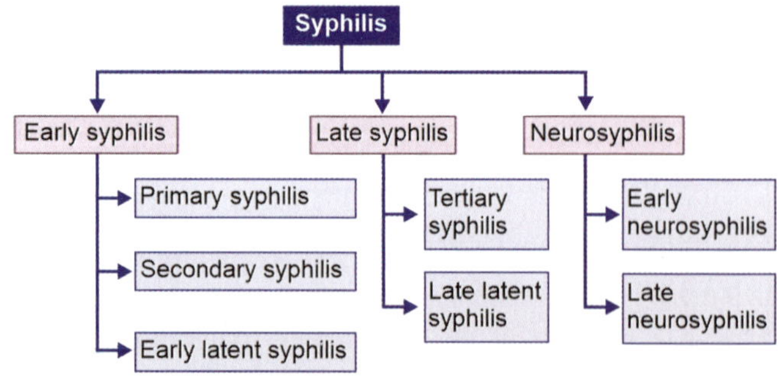

Figure 1.27: Stages of syphilis

Congenital Syphilis

- Transmission of *T. pallidum* from a syphilitic woman to her fetus across the placenta may occur at any stage of pregnancy, but the lesions in fetus develop after the fourth month of gestation.
- Treatment of the mother before 4th month of gestation can prevent fetal damage. Untreated maternal infection may lead to abortion, stillbirth, prematurity, neonatal death, or nonfatal congenital syphilis.
- Among infants born alive, congenital syphilis may or may not be clinically apparent.
- All women should be screened for syphilis in early pregnancy. In areas of high prevalence serologic screening should be repeated in the third trimester and at delivery.
- The manifestations of congenital syphilis can be divided into three types:
  - *Early manifestations:* Appear within the first 2 years of life. These are due to infection of various organs by *Treponema pallidum* and resemble secondary syphilis in the adult. These include rhinitis (snuffles), bullae (syphilitic pemphigus), vesicles, petechiae, papulosquamous lesions, mucous patches, and condylomata lata. The most common early manifestations are bone changes including osteochondritis, osteitis, and periostitis. Hepatosplenomegaly, lymphadenopathy and jaundice are also common.
  - *Late manifestations:* Appear after 2 years and are noninfectious manifestations. These include interstitial keratitis, eighth-nerve deafness, recurrent arthropathy and bilateral knee effusion known as Clutton's joints. Neurosyphilis and gummatous periostitis can also occur.
  - *Residual stigmata:* These include Hutchinson's teeth (centrally notched, widely spaced, peg-shaped upper central incisors) and "mulberry" molars (molars with multiple, poorly developed cusps). There can be abnormal facies like frontal bossing, saddle nose, and poorly developed maxillae. Saber shins, characterized by anterior tibial bowing, are rare. Rhagades are linear scars at the angles of the mouth and are caused by healing of early facial eruption.

Diagnosis

- The diagnosis of syphilis is suspected based on history and clinical features. Since the clinical features are protean, lab confirmation of diagnosis is required.

Dark-field Microscopy

- This is the most specific technique for diagnosing syphilis and can demonstrate *Treponema pallidum* in samples taken from chancre and condylomata lata. But dark-field microscopy is not widely available.

Nontreponemal Tests

- These include venereal disease research laboratory (VDRL) test, rapid plasma reagin (RPR) test and toluidine red unheated serum test (TRUST).
- Syphilis leads to the production of nonspecific antibodies that react to cardiolipin. This reaction is the basis of VDRL and rapid plasma reagin (RPR) test. Nontreponemal tests are widely used for syphilis screening.
- With nontreponemal tests, false-positive reactions can occur because of pregnancy, autoimmune disorders, and other infections. In addition, these tests may show a "prozone" phenomenon in which large amount of antibody blocks the antibody-antigen reaction, causing a false-negative test in the undiluted sample.
- These tests may be negative in early primary syphilis and late syphilis in up to one third of patients.
- After adequate treatment of syphilis, nontreponemal tests eventually become nonreactive.
- Titers are not interchangeable between different test types. Hence, the same nontreponemal test should be used for follow-up evaluations.

Treponemal Tests

- Treponemal tests detect antibodies to antigenic components of *T. pallidum*. These tests were earlier used primarily to confirm the diagnosis of syphilis in patients with a reactive nontreponemal test. However, because of widespread availability, these tests are increasingly used as an initial screening test for syphilis rather than as confirmatory tests (reverse screening).
- Specific treponemal tests include:
  - Fluorescent treponemal antibody absorption (FTA-ABS)
  - Microhemagglutination test for antibodies to *T. pallidum* (MHA-TP)
  - *T. pallidum* particle agglutination assay (TPPA)
  - *T. pallidum* enzyme immunoassay (TO-EIA) (has become the favored treponemal test in many laboratories)
  - Chemiluminescence immunoassay (CIA)
- Unlike nontreponemal tests which show a decline in titers or become nonreactive with effective treatment, treponemal-specific tests usually remain reactive for life. Therefore, treponemal-specific test titers are not useful for assessing treatment efficacy.

Treatment

- The treatment of choice in all stages of syphilis is long acting preparation of penicillin (benzathine penicillin) except in neurosyphilis where aqueous penicillin is used.
- Benzathine penicillin 2.4 million units IM (1.2 million units to each buttock) cures primary, secondary, and early (<1 year) latent syphilis. Additional doses of 2.4 million units should be given 7 and 14 days later for late (>1 year) latent syphilis.
- *Neurosyphilis* should be treated with intravenous aqueous penicillin G (3–4 million units IV Q 4h for 10–14 days) followed by benzathine penicillin 2.4 million units deep IM once a week for 3 weeks.

- For penicillin allergic patients doxycycline 100 mg BD for 1 month should be given. Doxycycline is contraindicated in pregnant women and children. In such cases penicillin should be administered after desensitization. Ceftriaxone 1 g daily IM/IV for 8 to 10 days is an alternative. At 6 and 12 months after treatment, patients with primary syphilis should be reexamined and undergo repeat serologic testing.
- *Congenital syphilis:* aqueous penicillin 50,000 units/kg IV q 12 h for the first 7 days of life and q 8 h thereafter for a total of 10 days.

Q. Venereal Disease Research Laboratory (VDRL) Test.

- VDRL is a nontreponemal antibody test to diagnose syphilis. It is quite sensitive but not very specific for syphilis. VDRL is reactive in 78% of patients with primary syphilis. It becomes positive within 4–6 weeks after infection or 1–3 weeks after the appearance of the primary lesion. Thus, these tests can be negative in early syphilis. VDRL can also be negative in some untreated patients in late syphilis. Hence, VDRL cannot be relied on for diagnosis in very early or late stage of syphilis.
- The VDRL test is based on the detection of anti-cardiolipin antibodies (nonspecific antibodies) in the patient's serum or cerebrospinal fluid (CSF). When mixed with a cardiolipin-lecithin-cholesterol antigen suspension, a positive sample produces flocculation (clumping), indicating the presence of antibodies.
- False-positive VDRL test can occur in infections (TB, HIV, Lyme disease, infectious mononucleosis, malaria), pregnancy, connective tissue diseases, liver disease, and malignancy.
- Because of frequent false-positive and false-negative VDRL test, all positive tests and all negative tests in patients in whom syphilis is strongly suspected clinically, should be verified by a specific treponemal test.
- The nontreponemal tests are quite useful for monitoring the patient's response to treatment, because the titers reflect disease activity. When these tests are used for this purpose, it is important to use the same test (either VDRL or RPR) for serial measurements because the two tests can differ significantly in their titers. When possible, it is also recommended to do the test in the same laboratory.

Q. Yaws.

- Yaws is a chronic, relapsing, nonvenereal infection caused by *Treponema pallidum pertenue*. Yaws, endemic syphilis (bejel), and pinta collectively constitute the endemic treponematoses.

Clinical Features

- The incubation period is 9–90 days (average 20 days).
- It primarily affects the skin, bones, and cartilage, and is endemic in tropical regions with poor hygiene and limited healthcare access.
- It predominantly affects children with peak incidence between 5 and 9 years of age.
- It spreads through close contact and the presence of minor skin lesions, abrasions and scratches which facilitate penetration and infection by the treponemae.
- The initial lesion may start as a painless, papillomatous nodule at the site of inoculation that may ulcerate. Initial lesion usually appears on the leg. Several weeks to months later generalized papillomatous or scaly lesions appear. Bone and joints can get affected and take the form of periostitis and osteitis. Goundou is a hypertrophic osteitis of the nasal process of the maxilla. Hyperkeratosis of soles and palms develops late. In late stages destructive gummatous lesions affecting skin, bones, and cartilage appear.
- Gangosa is the result of extensive destruction of nasal bones and cartilages. In severe cases, the whole of the palate may be destroyed, so that the nose and the mouth become one space.

Investigations

- Dark-field microscopy of the specimens from early lesions may show spirochaetes.
- Serological tests are similar to those of syphilis (VDRL, RPR, FTA-ABS, etc.) and become positive at an early stage of infection, but tend to become negative later. Serological tests cannot differentiate yaws from other treponemal infections.

Treatment

- Benzathine penicillin is the drug of choice.
- The recommended dose is 6 lakh units for those under 10 years of age, and 12 lakh units for those above 10 years of age.
- In patients allergic to penicillin, tetracycline or doxycycline can be used.

Q. Pinta.

Etiology

- Pinta is a chronic, non-venereal skin disease caused by the bacterium Treponema carateum.
- It is one of the endemic treponematoses, alongside yaws, bejel, and syphilis. Unlike syphilis, pinta primarily affects the skin without involving deeper tissues or causing systemic manifestations.
- Pinta is a Spanish word used to describe a spotted or mottled appearance. The lesions of pinta have a peculiar pigmented appearance on the skin.
- Transmission is non-venereal by contact with skin lesions. Various biting and sucking arthropods have also been implicated.

Clinical Features

- It is predominantly a disease of childhood. After infection, 2–3 weeks later, a primary lesion at the site of inoculation appears. Secondary lesions appear after a month or a year. These secondary lesions are erythematous papules which become scaly and pigmented. These lesions gradually regress and become depigmented. Lesions are found mainly on distal extremities. Trunk and face may also be involved. The lesions have to be differentiated from other depigmented lesions like leprosy, yaws, syphilis, psoriasis, tinea versicolor, and vitiligo.

Investigations

- Same as those described under yaws.

Management

- Penicillin is the drug of choice. Tetracycline or doxycycline are alternatives.

Q. Leptrospirosis.

Q. Weil's syndrome.

Etiology

- Leptospirosis is a bacterial zoonotic infection caused by Leptospira species. It is considered the most common zoonosis in the world.
- Leptospira are coiled, thin, highly motile spirochaetes **(Fig. 1.28)**.

Epidemiology

- It is a zoonosis and animals are the main reservoirs of Leptospira. Many serovars are associated with particular animals. For example, *L. pomona* and *L. interrogans* are seen in cattle and pigs; *L. grippotyphosa* is seen in cattle, sheep, goats, and voles; L. ballum and *L. icterohaemorrhagiae* are associated with rats and mice; and *L. canicola* is associated with dogs. These animals shed spirochaetes in the urine.
- Humans are accidental hosts, infected incidentally after animal or environmental exposure. Infection occurs by contact with urine-contaminated soil or water (e.g. floodwater, ponds, rivers, streams, sewage), ingestion of food or water contaminated by urine or urine-contaminated water, or direct contact with the urine or reproductive fluids from infected animals. Human-to-human transmission is rare but has been documented through sexual intercourse and breastfeeding.

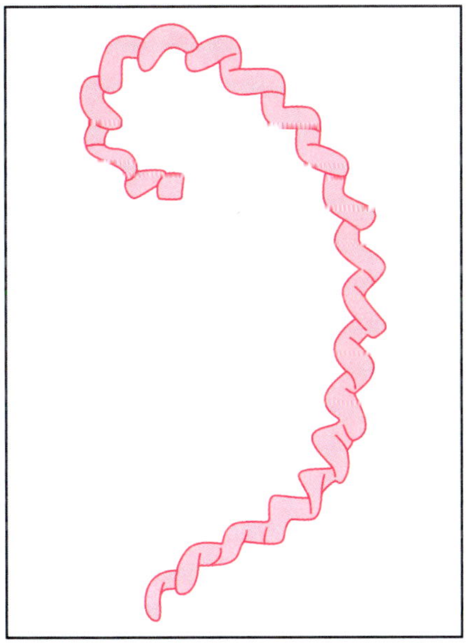

Figure 1.28: Leptospira

- The organism enters the body through cuts, abraded skin, mucous membranes, or conjunctivae.
- The disease is more common in veterinary personnel, agricultural workers, sewers, slaughter house workers and fisher men.

Pathogenesis

- The organism spreads through the blood stream to all organs. Multiplication takes place in blood and tissues.
- Leptospires damage the wall of small blood vessels leading to vasculitis. Vasculitis causes leakage of plasma, hemorrhage and volume depletion. Vasculitis is responsible for most of the manifestations of leptospirosis.
- Although any organ may be involved kidneys and liver are involved mainly. Kidney involvement leads to renal failure and oliguria. Liver involvement leads to jaundice and liver function abnormalities. Muscle involvement leads to prominent myalgia and elevated CK levels. Lung involvement can lead to ARDS and pulmonary hemorrhage.
- Meningitis can develop when there is rise in antibody titers. This association suggests that an immunologic mechanism may be responsible for meningitis.

Clinical Features

- The incubation period varies from 2 to 20 days.
- More than 90% of patients have mild and anicteric form of leptospirosis.
- Severe leptospirosis with deep jaundice (Weil's syndrome) develops in 5–10% of patients.
- Leptospirosis is characteristically biphasic and has an initial septicemic phase followed by immune phase. The distinction between the first and second phases is not always clear, and mild cases may not have the second phase.

Leptospiremic Phase (Acute Septicemic Phase)

- Lasts 2–9 days.
- Presents as an acute influenza-like illness, with fever, chills, headache, nausea, vomiting, and myalgias.
- Muscle pain is an important clinical feature.
- Headache may be intense.
- Physical examination shows fever, conjunctival suffusion, muscle tenderness, and hepatosplenomegaly. Mild jaundice may be present. Sometimes a rash also may be noted.

Immune Phase (Second Phase)

- Starts after acute phase. There is often a period of improvement between the end of the acute phase and the beginning of the immune phase. sometimes, the acute and immune phases may overlap. This second phase coincides with the development of antibodies. Fever and myalgias may be less severe in the second phase. Aseptic meningitis and uveitis may develop during second phase. Aseptic meningitis is a hallmark of the immune phase, with symptoms of headache and neck pain or stiffness occurring in approximately half of patients. Most patients become asymptomatic within a week.

- During the immune phase, leptospires are absent from the blood, and antibodies to the organism are present. The organism may be detectable in the urine during this phase.

Severe Leptospirosis (Weil's syndrome)

- Weil's syndrome, the most severe form of leptospirosis, is characterized by jaundice, renal failure, hemorrhagic tendency, and a high mortality rate.
- Initially symptoms are same as that of uncomplicated leptospirosis. However, later, jaundice, renal and vascular dysfunction develop. Jaundice is very deep and gives an orange tinge to the skin. Tender hepatomegaly is usually present. Splenomegaly may also be present.
- Dialysis may be required for renal failure. Renal function usually recovers completely with treatment.
- Pulmonary involvement occurs frequently and results in cough, dyspnea, hemoptysis and rarely respiratory failure.
- Hemorrhagic manifestations include epistaxis, petechiae, purpura, and ecchymoses. Severe GI bleeding and adrenal or subarachnoid hemorrhage occur rarely.
- Other complications of Weil's disease include rhabdomyolysis, myocarditis, pericarditis, congestive heart failure, cardiogenic shock, ARDS, necrotizing pancreatitis, septic shock and multiorgan failure.

Laboratory Features

- Microscopic agglutination test (MAT): Gold standard. It detects serovar-specific antibodies in a patient's serum by measuring their ability to agglutinate live Leptospira serovars under dark-field microscopy.
- PCR (polymerase chain reaction): Detects Leptospira DNA (useful in early infection).
- Culture (blood, CSF, urine): Rarely used in clinical practice due to its slow growth, special requirements, and low sensitivity.
- IgM ELISA: Detects IgM antibodies. It is fast, sensitive, and widely used test for early leptospirosis diagnosis.

Other Tests

- Blood examination shows anemia, increased WBCs, decreased platelet count, and high ESR.
- LFT shows elevated direct bilirubin, elevated AST and ALT and prolonged prothrombin time.
- RFT (renal function tests) show elevated blood urea and creatinine.
- CK levels are high due to muscle damage.
- Urine examination may show proteinuria, RBCs, and cellular and granular casts.
- ECG may show low voltage, prolonged QT and nonspecific ST and T wave changes.
- Chest X-ray may show patchy bronchopneumonia or ARDS.

Differential Diagnosis

- Leptospirosis should be differentiated from other febrile illnesses associated with headache, muscle pain and jaundice, such as dengue, severe malaria, enteric fever, viral hepatitis, hantavirus infections, sepsis and rickettsial diseases.

Treatment

- *Crystalline penicillin* 1.5 million units IV 6th hourly daily for 7 days OR *ceftriaxone* 1 g IV BD for 5–7 days is the drug of choice for severe cases. Mild cases can be treated with oral antibiotics such as doxycycline or azithromycin.
- Fluid and electrolyte balance should be maintained and supportive measures provided.
- Dialysis may be required for renal failure.

Q. Relapsing fever.

- Relapsing fever (RF) is a vector-borne infectious disease caused by Borrelia species. It is characterized by recurrent episodes of fever that accompany spirochetemia. Hence the name relapsing fever.
- Relapsing fever is endemic in Africa, India, Middle East and South America.

Etiology

- The infection is caused by several species of the spirochete Borrelia. There are 3 main types relapsing Fever
- *Louse-borne relapsing fever (LBRF)*: Caused by *Borrelia recurrentis* and transmitted by the human body louse (Pediculus humanus humanus).
- *Soft tick relapsing fever (STRF)*: Caused by multiple Borrelia species and transmitted by soft ticks (Ornithodoros spp.).
- *Hard tick relapsing fever (HTRF)*: Caused by *Borrelia miyamotoi* and transmitted by hard ticks (Ixodes spp.).
- The reservoirs of infection are humans (LBRF), rodents, small mammals, deer, birds (STRF, HTRF).

Pathogenesis

- Borrelia enters the bloodstream after a louse/tick bite.
- Rapid multiplication leads to high spirochetemia → fever. From the blood, spirochetes move through or between endothelial cells to invade the brain, eye, inner ear, liver, heart, testes, and other organs.
- The immune system produces antibodies against surface proteins and there is decrease in the number of oraganisms leading to afebrile period.
- Borrelia undergoes antigenic variation → new variants escape immune detection → fever relapses.

Clinical Features

- After an incubation period of 7–10 days, the illness starts with high grade fever with chills and rigors, headache, body ache and joint pain. There can be nausea, vomiting, and sleeplessness. Patients may also develop a generalized petechial or ecchymotic rash, hepatosplenomegaly, jaundice, hemorrhagic tendency and hemoptysis. Meningitis can occur rarely.

- Although patients can completely recover from the initial stage, majority will develop one or more relapses. Louse-borne fever has more chances of relapse than tick borne fever. Relapses result from antigenic variation of the spirochete's outer-surface proteins.
- Untreated, one-third of patients may die.

Diagnosis

- *Direct microscopy (blood smear) (Giemsa or Wright stain):* Detects Borrelia spirochetes during febrile episodes.
- *Direct fluorescence staining (DFA-Direct fluorescent antibody test):* Uses fluorescent-labeled antibodies that bind specifically to Borrelia antigens. Requires a fluorescence microscope for visualization.
- *PCR (Polymerase chain reaction):* Gold standard, detects Borrelia DNA in blood.
- *Serology (ELISA, Western blot):* Detects IgM/IgG antibodies against Borrelia.
- *Culture (Rarely used):* Not useful for routine diagnosis due to slow growth.

Treatment

- Treatment with doxycycline (or tetracycline), or erythromycin, or chloramphenicol is effective. For children <8 years of age and for pregnant women, erythromycin or penicillin is preferred, because of side effects of tetracyclines.
- A severe Jarish-Herxheimer reaction may occur after antibiotics are given and should be carefully watched for.
- Public health measures are needed to control the louse and tick populations.

Q. Rat-bite fever.

- Rat-bite fever (RBF) is a zoonotic bacterial infection transmitted to humans through rat bites, scratches, or by ingesting contaminated food/water. It is caused by two distinct bacteria:
  - *Streptobacillus moniliformis* (most common, North America).
  - Spirillum minus (Asia, known as Sodoku).

Clinical Features

- Streptobacillary rat-bite fever (*S. moniliformis*): Patient develops fever, migratory polyarthritis and maculo papular or petechial rash (on hands and feet).
- Spirillary rat-bite fever (Sodoku–*S. minus*): Ulceration at the bite site with regional lymphadenopathy. Relapsing fever pattern can occur for several weeks.

Diagnosis

- Blood culture: Gold standard for *S. moniliformis*. *S. minus* CANNOT be cultured *in vitro*.
- Microscopy: Gram's stain or dark-field or Giemsa stain.
- PCR (molecular testing): Detects *S. moniliformis* or *S. minus* DNA in blood, synovial fluid, or tissue samples.
- Serology: Indirect immunofluorescence or ELISA may help detect anti-Spirillum antibodies.

Treatment

- Penicillin–first choice. Doxycycline or erythromycin are alternatives.

Q. Lyme disease (Lyme borreliosis).

Q. Erythema migrans.

- Lyme disease is a **vector-borne bacterial infection** caused by *Borrelia burgdorferi* (and other Borrelia) and transmitted through the bite of **Ixodes ticks (black-legged or deer ticks)**.

Etiology

- Caused by *Borrelia burgdorferi* (and other Borrelia). These spirochetes are motile, spiral bacteria.

Epidemiology

- In nature, the reservoirs of these organisms are small mammals and birds, not deer. Deer is essential for tick life cycle but do not carry Borrelia.
- Humans acquire the infection from the bite of an infected tick of the genus Ixodes.
- The disease is seen mainly in western countries.
- Most cases occur in summer months in rural areas.
- High-risk groups: Hikers, campers, forestry workers, hunters, outdoor enthusiasts.

Clinical Features

- Lyme disease progresses through **three stages:**

Early Localized Stage (3–30 days after tick bite)

- Borrelia organisms are injected into the skin when a tick bites.
- From the injected site, the spirochaete migrates outwards, producing a red macule or papule that expands slowly to form a large annular lesion called *erythema migrans (EM)* which is the characteristic rash of Lyme disease. As the lesion increases in size, it develops a bright red outer border and central clearing or they may have a more complex target or bull's eye appearance. Without therapy, EM typically fades within 3–4 weeks. EM usually is round or

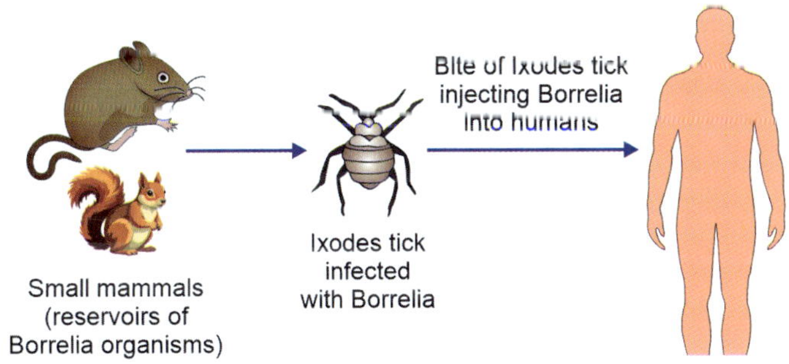

Figure 1.29: Transmission of Lyme disease

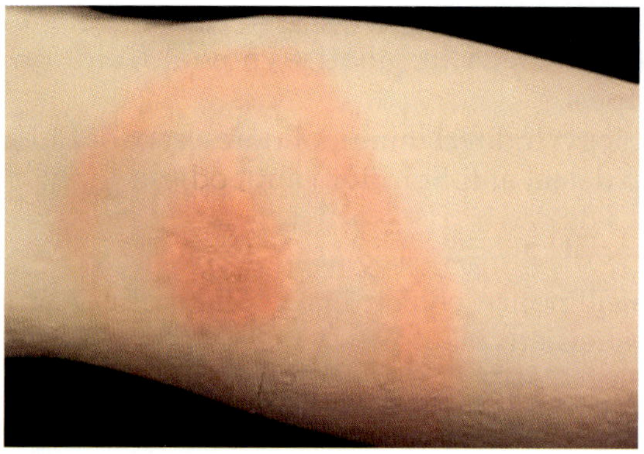

Figure 1.30: Bull's eye appearance of erythema migrans

oval, but can be triangular or linear. Often, a central punctum is present at the bite site. EM enlarges by a few centimeters per day; single lesions typically achieve a diameter of approximately 5–6 inches. Since ticks tend to bite the areas where natural barriers impede their forward motion, rash location is usually on the popliteal fossa, axillary or gluteal folds, areas near elastic bands in bra straps or underwear. In children, the scalp, face, and hairline are especially common locations. Some patients with EM may have secondary EM lesions due to hematogenous spread. These lesions generally are smaller than the primary one, lack the central punctum, and tend to be more uniform in morphology than the primary lesion. Location of secondary lesions can be anywhere.

- Fever, chills, and malaise are also present in this stage.

Early Disseminated Stage (weeks to months later)

- From the local site, organisms spread hematogenously to many sites within days or weeks after the onset of erythema migrans.
- Multiple erythema migrans lesions develop (secondary rashes).
- Patients have severe headache, neck stiffness, fever with chills, arthralgias, and fatigue.
- One or more organ systems become involved as hematologic or lymphatic spread disseminates spirochetes to distant sites. Musculoskeletal (arthritis) and neurologic symptoms are the most common. Neurologic manifestations include cranial nerve pasly especially facial nerve palsy (Bell's palsy), meningitis and encephalopathy. Cardiac involvement (Lyme carditis) presents as AV block, syncope, dyspnea, chest pain, and palpitations.

Late Stage (months to years later, if untreated)

- Chronic Lyme arthritis:
  - Intermittent or persistent large joint arthritis (especially knees).
  - Synovial fluid shows inflammatory pattern (↑ WBC, no bacteria).
- Chronic neurological symptoms:
  - Encephalopathy (memory issues, cognitive decline, depression).
  - Peripheral neuropathy (paresthesia, burning pain).

Investigations

- Lyme disease is usually diagnosed by clinical features (erythema migrans rash + tick exposure = Lyme disease).
- Lab confirmation is by testing for serum antibodies. The most frequently used test is the enzyme immunoassay (EIA) or enzyme-linked immunosorbent assay (ELISA). Positive results can be confirmed by Western blot test. However, there are many limitations to serological tests. Thirty percent of acute cases are seronegative; positive tests may reflect past rather than current infection.
- PCR testing Detects Borrelia DNA in **synovial fluid, CSF, or blood** (useful for Lyme arthritis and neuroborreliosis).
- CSF analysis (for neuroborreliosis).
- ECG (for Lyme carditis): Check for AV blocks (1st, 2nd, or 3rd degree).

Management

- *Early Lyme disease (localized stage):* Oral antibiotics are enough. Doxycycline 100 mg BID for 10–14 days. For children and pregnant patients, use Amoxicillin for 14 days.
- *Disseminated Lyme disease*: Use IV antibiotics (Ceftriaxone or or penicillin G) for 14–28 days.
- *Late Lyme arthritis*: Doxycycline (or amoxicillin) for 28 days.

Q. Epidemic typhus fever.

- Typhus refers to a group of infectious diseases that are caused by rickettsial organisms that result in acute febrile illness. Arthropod vectors transmit the rickettsial organisms to humans. The main diseases of this group are epidemic typhus, murine typhus, and scrub typhus.
- Epidemic typhus is the prototypical infection of the typhus group of diseases, and the pathophysiology of this illness is representative of all typhus fevers.
- Epidemic typhus is caused by the organism *Rickettsia prowazekii* ***(obligate intracellular gram-negative bacterium)***.

Transmission

- It is spread by the vector *Pediculus humanus corporis* (human body louse).
- Lice become infected by feeding on a human with epidemic typhus.
- *R. prowazekii* multiplies in the louse gut and is excreted in louse feces.
- Humans get infected when they scratch the bite site, introducing infected louse feces into the skin.
- No direct person-to-person transmission (except via lice).

Clinical Features

- Incubation period is ~1 week.
- The disease is characterized by high fever, severe headache, rash, and multi-organ complications, and

has historically caused devastating outbreaks during wars, famines, and poor sanitation conditions.

- Main features are high fever, severe headache, and maculopapular rash. Cough is noted frequently. There is severe generalized myalgia.
- Rash begins on the trunk, usually on the fifth day, and then spreads to extremities (centrifugal pattern) and becomes generalized. Spares the face, palms, and soles (unlike Rocky Mountain spotted fever). Initially, rash is macular, later becomes petechial or hemorrhagic.
- Photophobia and conjunctival congestion are frequently present. The tongue may be dry and coated. Neurological symptoms ("typhus meningoencephalitis"): Delirium, confusion, agitation. Seizures, coma in severe cases.
- Severe cases: Hemodynamic collapse, multi-organ failure, myocarditis, gangrene.
- Brill-Zinsser disease, a mild recrudescence of epidemic typhus, can occur years after the initial infection if host defences falter.

Investigations

- Indirect immunofluorescence assay (IFA) or enzyme immunoassay (EIA): Detects *R. prowazekii*-specific IgM and IgG antibodies.
- Weil-Felix test (low specificity)–Proteus OX-19 agglutination.
- PCR (early confirmatory test): Detects *R. prowazekii* DNA in blood, skin biopsy, or cerebrospinal fluid (CSF).
- Skin biopsy of rash lesions: Immunohistochemistry staining for Rickettsia.

Treatment

- Doxycycline is the drug of choice. It is given as 200 mg once followed by 100 mg bid for at least 7 days. Alternative is chloramphenicol 500 mg qid orally for 7–15 days. Intravenous administration of antibiotics is indicated in very sick patients. Supportive treatment is provided as needed.

Q. Scrub typhus.

Etiology

- Scrub typhus is a mite-borne infectious disease caused by *Orientia tsutsugamushi* (previously classified as Rickettsia), an intracellular gram-negative bacterium. Lacks peptidoglycan and lipopolysaccharide (LPS) (differs from classic rickettsial bacteria).

Transmission of Infection

- Scrub typhus is found in areas with heavy scrub vegetation—e.g. where the forest is regrowing after being cleared and along riverbanks. Hence, it is called scrub typhus.
- Seen in India, Asia, Australia, New Guinea, and Pacific Islands.
- *Orientia tsutsugamushi* is present in trombiculid mites. The organism is transmitted to humans through the bite of infected larval stage of mite called chiggers.
- Reservoirs of infection are rodents and small mammals (natural hosts for mites). Mites feed on animal hosts and remain infected for life. Human infection is acquired by accident.

Clinical Features

- Sudden high fever (≥39°C), headache, myalgia, and generalized body pain. Lymphadenopathy may be present. Gastrointestinal symptoms (nausea, vomiting, diarrhea, abdominal pain) may be present.
- The site of chigger bite is marked by an **eschar (pathognomonic but not always present)** which is a painless black necrotic ulcer at the mite bite site. Common locations of eschar are axilla, groin, abdomen, and neck.
- Maculopapular rash (appears after fever onset): Starts on the trunk → spreads to limbs. May progress to petechial or purpuric rash in severe cases.
- Severe cases (complications if untreated)
  - Meningoencephalitis → Delirium, seizures, coma.
  - Acute respiratory distress syndrome (ARDS) → Respiratory failure.
  - Myocarditis and shock.
  - Hepatitis, renal failure, disseminated intravascular coagulation (DIC).
  - Death may occur as a result of these complications, usually late in the second week of illness.

Investigations

- ***Serology*** (gold standard for retrospective diagnosis)***:*** Indirect immunofluorescence assay (IFA)–Detects IgM and IgG antibodies against *O. tsutsugamushi*. ELISA (IgM and IgG detection)–Alternative to IFA.
- ***PCR*** (best for early diagnosis): Detects *O. tsutsugamushi* DNA in blood, skin biopsy from eschar or rash, or CSF. Weil-Felix OX-K strain agglutination test is the oldest test available. It is inexpensive, but lacks specificity and sensitivity.
- ***Weil-Felix test*** (low sensitivity and specificity): Agglutination test using Proteus OX-K antigen (not recommended).
- ***Direct visualization*** (eschar biopsy or immunohistochemistry): Giemsa or immunofluorescence staining of eschar biopsy.

Treatment

- Drug of choice is doxycycline (100 mg bid PO for 7–15 days).
- Alternatives are azithromycin (especially for pregnant ladies and children) and chloramphenicol 500 mg qid PO for 7–15 days.

Q. Q fever.

- Q-fever is so named because when an outbreak occurred in Australia, it was unknown what type of fever it was. Hence it was named as Q (for query) fever. But later the microorganism responsible for Q fever was isolated.

- Q fever is a **zoonotic infectious disease** caused by *Coxiella burnetii*, an obligate intracellular, gram-negative bacterium. It is found in wild (mammals, birds, and ticks) and domestic animals (cattle, sheep, and goats).
- It is transmitted among animals by ticks. Infected animals shed it through their milk and conceptional products during delivery into soil.
- Human disease is acquired by inhalation of contaminated aerosols, handling infected animals, and by drinking contaminated milk. Veterinarians are at increased risk of infection. It can also be acquired through blood transfusion.

Clinical Features

- Incubation period is 2–3 weeks.

Acute Q Fever (most common form)

- Fever, chills, and severe headache.
- Pneumonia (atypical, interstitial or lobar pneumonitis): presents as dry cough, pleuritic chest pain, dyspnea. Can mimic viral pneumonia or Legionnaires' disease.
- Hepatitis: Hepatosplenomegaly, elevated liver enzymes. Granulomatous hepatitis (pathognomonic "doughnut-shaped" granulomas) **(Fig. 1.31)**.
- Myalgia, fatigue, and night sweats.

Chronic Q Fever (1–5% of infected individuals)

- Develops months to years after acute infection.
- Endocarditis (most common chronic manifestation): Affects prosthetic heart valves, immunocompromised patients. Causes culture negative endocarditis.
- Chronic hepatitis, osteomyelitis, chronic fatigue syndrome.

Q. Fever in Pregnancy

- Increased risk of miscarriage, preterm birth, intrauterine growth restriction (IUGR).

Diagnosis

- *Polymerase chain reaction (PCR)* on a blood sample, tissue, or respiratory secretions can be used for rapid diagnosis.
- *Serologic methods:* Indirect immunofluorescence assay (IFA): Method of choice. A fourfold increase in IgG antibody titer by immunofluorescent assay (IFA) of paired acute and convalescent specimens is the diagnostic gold standard to confirm the diagnosis of Q fever.
- *Immunohistochemistry or culture* of affected tissue can provide definitive confirmation of infection by *Coxiella burnetii*.
- *Blood culture (not useful): C. burnetii* is intracellular and does not grow in routine cultures.
- *Histopathology (for granulomatous hepatitis or endocarditis biopsies)*: "Doughnut granulomas". "Doughnut granulomas" are a distinctive histopathologic feature characterized by central fibrinoid necrosis surrounded by a ring of epithelioid histiocytes and an outer layer of lipid vacuoles.

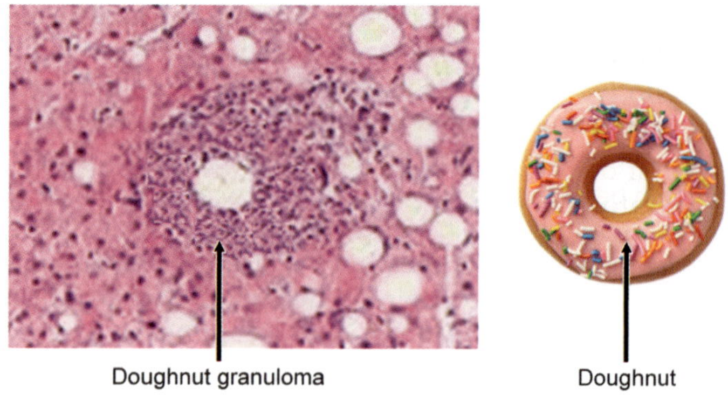

Figure 1.31: Doughnut granuloma

Treatment

- Doxycycline 100 mg BID for 14 days is the first-line treatment.
- In pregnancy, trimethoprim-sulfamethoxazole is recommended for treatment.
- Quinolones are also effective.
- Chronic Q fever (Endocarditis): Doxycycline + Hydroxychloroquine (for 18–24 months). Hydroxychloroquine alkalinizes intracellular pH, enhancing bacterial clearance.

Q. Psittacosis (parrot fever).

- Psittacosis, also known as parrot fever, is a zoonotic respiratory infection caused by *Chlamydia psittaci*, an obligate intracellular gram-negative bacterium.
- It primarily affects birds, including parrots, pigeons, and poultry.
- Organisms are transmitted to humans through contact with infected birds or their fecal materials. Organisms enter human body through inhalation. It is common among pet bird (pigeon and parrot) owners and poultry (chicken and duck) farmers.

Clinical Features

- H/o bird contact present. Incubation period is 1–2 weeks. It presents as atypical pneumonia with fever and tachypnea. Examination may show relative bradycardia. Chest examination may show crepitations and signs of consolidation. Lung lesions are more extensive than the clinical features suggest. Respiratory failure can occur.
- Rarely extrapulmonary complications can occur and include myocarditis, encephalitis, meningitis, pancreatitis, glomerulonephritis, and disseminated intravascular coagulation.

Diagnosis

- Serological methods are preferred. These include complement fixation (CF) and microimmunofluorescent antibody test (MIF).
- Molecular methods such as real-time PCR have high sensitivity and specificity and can be used for rapid diagnosis.
- Culture is difficult and hazardous to laboratory personnel.

- X-ray reveals patchy shadows, most often in the lower lobes.

Treatment

- Oral doxycycline 100 mg twice daily for 21 days is curative.
- Azithromycin is the second-line therapy when tetracyclines are contraindicated. Fluoroquinolones can be used in severe cases.

Q. Lymphogranuloma venereum (LGV).

- LGV is a sexually transmitted infection caused by *Chlamydia trachomatis* serovars L1, L2, and L3. LGV is predominantly a disease of lymphatic tissue. These serotypes can invade and reproduce in regional lymph nodes.

Clinical Features

- The peak incidence of LGV corresponds to the age of greatest sexual activity: the second and third decades of life.
- Three stages of LGV have been identified.

Primary Infection (3–12 days post-exposure)

- It is characterized by a painless genital ulcer. These lesions spontaneously heal within a few days.

Secondary Infection (2–6 weeks later)

- This stage is due to direct extension of the infection to regional lymph nodes (i.e. inguinal and/or femoral nodes).
- Painful, unilateral or bilateral inguinal lymphadenopathy ("buboes"). Buboes may break down to form multiple discharging sinuses with extensive scarring.
- Groove sign (Enlarged inguinal and femoral lymph nodes separated by the inguinal ligament).
- There is often accompanying fever, malaise, and myalgia.
- Anal intercourse may lead to hemorrhagic proctitis with regional lymphadenopathy.
- Meningoencephalitis can develop rarely.

Late LGV

- Genital elephantiasis (due to lymphatic obstruction), strictures, urethral and rectal fistulas may occur as a late complication.

Diagnosis

- NAAT (nucleic acid amplification test): Gold standard test. Detects *C. trachomatis* DNA in genital, rectal, or lymph node samples.
- Serology (less commonly used): Complement fixation test (CFT) detects high LGV-specific antibody titers.
- Direct microscopic examination of lymph node aspirates shows typical intracytoplasmic inclusions or elementary bodies.

Treatment

- Recommended treatment is doxycycline 100 mg BD for 21 days. Macrolides (erythromycin or azithromycin) are alternatives.
- Surgical drainage for suppurative bubo may be required.

Q. Influenza.

- Influenza is an acute respiratory illness caused by influenza viruses.

Etiology

- Influenza viruses are encapsulated, single-stranded RNA viruses of the family Orthomyxoviridae **(Fig. 1.32)**.
- There are 4 types of influenza viruses; A, B, C, and D.

Influenza A

- Causes seasonal epidemics and pandemics (e.g. H1N1, H3N2).
- Causes seasonal epidemics and pandemics.
- Infects humans, birds, pigs, horses, and other animals.
- Undergoes both antigenic drift and antigenic shift.
- Subtypes classified by hemagglutinin (HA) and neuraminidase (NA) proteins.
- Examples: H1N1 (swine flu), H3N2, H5N1 (avian flu), H7N9.

Influenza B

- Causes seasonal epidemics (but no pandemics).
- Infects humans only.
- Undergoes antigenic drift only (no antigenic shift).
- Two major lineages: Victoria and Yamagata.

Influenza C

- Milder illness, less common.
- Does not cause epidemics or pandemics.
- Infects humans and pigs.

Influenza D

- Primarily affects cattle, not humans.

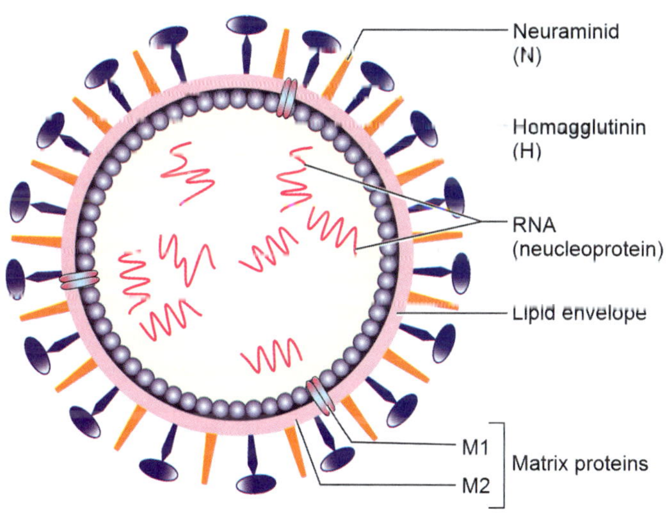

Figure 1.32: Influenza A virus

Epidemiology

- Type A is responsible for major epidemics and B for localized outbreaks. Epidemics usually occur during the winter months. Influenza-A pandemics cause considerable school and work absenteeism. Influenza-B causes less severe outbreaks mostly in schools and military camps.
- A remarkable feature of influenza virus A is it can undergo periodic antigenic variations. Major antigenic variations, called antigenic shifts, are associated with pandemics and are seen with influenza-A viruses only. Minor variations are called antigenic drifts. Antigenic shift happens due to re-assortment of gene segments between viral strains and 'antigenic drift' from point mutations.

Antigenic Drift

- Small point mutations in HA (hemagglutinin) and NA (neuraminidase) genes → leads to gradual evolution of the virus.
- Responsible for seasonal epidemics.
- Responsible for yearly flu vaccine updates.
- Seen with both influenza A and B.

Antigenic Shift

- Antigenic "shift" refers to major HA or NA gene mutations, leading to emergence of a novel influenza A virus that is antigenically and genetically distinct from viruses previously circulating in humans.
- Causes sporadic cases as well as pandemics.
- Occurs when two different influenza viruses infect the same host (e.g. swine, birds, or humans).
- Leads to novel viral subtypes with no preexisting immunity.
- Only occurs in influenza A.
- Example: 2009 H1N1 pandemic (Swine flu–Reassortment of human, avian, and swine influenza strains).

Pathogenesis

- The disease is acquired by inhalation of droplets generated by coughs and sneezes.
- It can also spread through hand-to-hand contact, personal contact, and fomites.
- The infection involves the ciliated columnar epithelial cells, but can also involve alveolar cells, mucous gland cells and macrophages. The infected cells of the tracheobronchial tree eventually become necrotic and desquamate.
- The host response to influenza involves both cell mediated and humoral immunity.
- Systemic symptoms in influenza such as fever and myalgia are due to the induction of cytokines.

Clinical Manifestations

- The incubation period varies from 18 to 72 hours.
- Both influenza A and B viruses can cause illnesses ranging from mild to severe.
- Influenza characteristically begins with the abrupt onset of fever, nonproductive cough, and myalgia. Other common symptoms include including malaise, sore throat, nausea, nasal congestion, and headache. Fever may last for as long as a week.
- Systemic examination is usually normal.
- Most patients recover in 1 week, although cough may persist for 1–2 weeks longer. In some patients weakness may persist for several weeks.
- Complications include pneumonia (influenza pneumonia or secondary bacterial pneumonia), Reye's syndrome, myocarditis, encephalitis, transverse myelitis and, rarely, Guillain-Barre syndrome.
- Critically ill patients may present with multi-organ failure, shock, and sepsis.

Diagnosis

- Influenza should be suspected in patients with abrupt onset of fever, cough, and myalgia when influenza virus is circulating.
- Common sample types for testing: Nasopharyngeal swab (most sensitive), throat swab, nasal aspirate or wash, bronchoalveolar lavage (for severe cases).
- ***Rapid influenza diagnostic tests (RIDTs):*** Detects viral antigens in respiratory samples. Results in 10–15 minutes. Low sensitivity, especially in adults. Cannot distinguish between influenza A and B subtypes.
- ***Rapid molecular assays (RT-PCR and NAATs):*** Detects viral RNA (nucleic acid). More accurate than RIDTs. Sensitivity: 90–100%. Results in 30–60 minutes. Can distinguish between influenza A and B subtypes. Disadvantages are more expensive, and require specialized equipment.
- ***Reverse transcription polymerase chain reaction (RT-PCR):*** Gold standard for influenza diagnosis. Detects and quantifies viral RNA. Can identify specific strains and subtypes. Results in 2–6 hours.
- ***Serological testing:*** Detects antibodies against influenza in blood. Not useful for early diagnosis. Used in epidemiological studies.

Treatment

- Most cases of influenza resolve spontaneously without any complications. Symptomatic therapy with paracetamol for fever and myalgia, cough suppressant syrup for dry cough are enough for such cases. Aspirin should be avoided because of the risk of Reye's syndrome. Patients should be advised to rest and maintain hydration during acute illness.
- Antiviral drugs are available to treat influenza (most effective if taken within 48 hours). Antiviral drugs are recommended for high-risk patients (elderly, those with comorbidities, immunocompromised). Choices are as follows:
    - Oseltamivir, 75 mg two times daily for 5 days.
    - Zanamivir (inhaled), two times daily for 5 days.
    - Baloxavir, 40 mg orally as a single dose.
    - Peramivir, 600 mg intravenously as a single dose.
- Antibiotics are indicated for secondary bacterial infections.

Prevention

- Influenza vaccines are the most effective way to prevent flu infection and its complications. They are updated annually to match circulating strains and are recommended for everyone aged 6 months and older. Influenza vaccine is recommended for all persons aged 6 months or older every year if there are no contraindications.
- Inactivated influenza vaccine (IIV): Contains killed virus. Given as 0.5 ml intramuscularly. Safe for all age groups, including pregnant women and immunocompromised individuals.
- Live-attenuated influenza vaccine (LAIV): Contains a weakened live virus. Given as nasal spray. Only for healthy individuals aged 2–49 years. Not recommended for pregnant women and immunocompromised individuals.
- Recombinant influenza vaccine (RIV): Produced using genetic technology (no eggs used). Available as a quadrivalent vaccine (RIV4). Does not contain live virus. Given as an IM injection. Safe for individuals with egg allergies.

Q. Discuss the etiology, clinical features, diagnosis and management of H1N1 influenza (Swine Flu).

- H1N1 influenza, commonly known as swine flu, is a respiratory illness caused by the H1N1 strain of the influenza A virus. It was responsible for the 2009 pandemic and continues to circulate as a seasonal flu strain.
- Originally detected in pigs, hence the name swine flu. Outbreaks of H1N1 influenza (swine flu) are common in pigs year-round.
- Transmission of swine influenza viruses to humans is uncommon. However, transmission can occur to humans via contact with infected pigs or environments contaminated with swine influenza viruses. Once a human becomes infected, he or she can then spread the virus to other humans.
- In 2009, cases of influenza like illness were first reported in Mexico on March 18; the outbreak was confirmed as H1N1 influenza A. During this outbreak, nearly 100,000 were hospitalized, and about 3900 died. On June 11, 2009, WHO raised the pandemic alert level to phase 6 (indicating a global pandemic) because of widespread infection beyond North America to Australia, the United Kingdom, Argentina, Chile, Spain, and Japan.

Clinical Features

- Incubation period: 1–4 days.
- Manifestations of H1N1 influenza (swine flu) are similar to those of seasonal influenza. Patients present with symptoms of acute respiratory illness, such as fever, chills, fatigue, cough, sore throat, body aches, and headache. In addition, diarrhea and vomiting may occur.
- Clinical deterioration is characterized by primary viral pneumonia and ARDS, which destroys the lung tissue and does not respond to antibiotics, and multi organ dysfunction including the heart, kidneys, and liver. Patients with severe disease have dyspnea, cyanosis, dehydration, and altered mental status.

Diagnosis

- Clinicians should consider the possibility of H1N1 infection in patients who present with febrile respiratory illness. The CDC criteria for suspected H1N1 influenza are as follows:
  - Onset of acute febrile respiratory illness within 7 days of close contact with a person who has a confirmed case of H1N1 influenza A virus infection, OR
  - Onset of acute febrile respiratory illness within 7 days of travel to a community (within the United States or internationally) where one or more H1N1 influenza A cases have been confirmed, OR
  - Acute febrile respiratory illness in a person who resides in a community where at least one H1N1 influenza case has been confirmed.
  - If H1N1 is suspected, the clinician should obtain a respiratory swab and send it for H1N1 testing.

Laboratory Confirmation of Diagnosis

- Real-time RT-PCR is the recommended test for confirmation of H1N1 cases. This is done on swab sample from the nose or throat.
- Rapid influenza diagnostic tests (RIDTs): Quick but less accurate.

Management

Supportive Therapy

- Patients should be isolated to prevent spread of infection to others. Bedrest, increased fluid intake, cough suppressants, antipyretics and analgesics (e.g, acetaminophen, nonsteroidal anti-inflammatory drugs) for fever and myalgias. Severe cases may require intravenous hydration and ventilator support.

Antiviral Agents

- Serious patients should be treated with antiviral agents. Drugs of choice are oseltamivir (TAMIFLU) or zanamivir. These two drugs inhibit neuraminidase on the surface of influenza virus that destroys an infected cell's receptor for viral hemagglutinin. By inhibiting viral neuraminidase, these agents decrease the release of viruses from infected cells and, thus, viral spread.
- Antiviral drugs reduce the risk of pneumonia a leading cause of death in H1N1 and the need for hospitalization. Oseltamivir should be started as early as possible (preferably within 48 hours) in a dose of 75 mg BD for 5 days. Where oseltamivir is unavailable or cannot be used for any reason, zanamivir may be given. Zanamivir is given by inhalation in a dose of 10 mg BD for 5 days. Peramivir (IV) and baloxavir, single-dose oral (newer option) are other options. Pregnant women and patients with underlying medical conditions are at higher risk of developing complications and should be given antivirals as soon as H1N1 is suspected even before laboratory confirmation.

Reducing the Spread of Infection

- Patients who develop flulike illness (i.e. fever with either cough or sore throat) should be strongly encouraged to self-isolate in their home for 7 days after the onset of illness or at least 24 hours after symptoms have resolved, whichever is longer.
- While in home isolation, patients and other household members should be given infection control instructions, including frequent hand washing with soap and water. Patients with H1N1 influenza should wear a face mask when within 6 feet of others at home.
- If the patient must go into the community (e.g. to seek medical care), he or she should wear a face mask.
- Patients should call the physician before meeting and should avoid mixing with other OPD patients at clinic or hospital.
- Prophylaxis with antiviral agents should be considered for close household contacts of a confirmed or suspected case who are at high risk for complications (e.g. chronic medical conditions, persons >65 years or <5 years, pregnant women), school children at high risk for complications who have been in close contact with a confirmed or suspected case, healthcare providers who were not using appropriate personal protective equipment during close contact with a confirmed or suspected case. Antivirals should not be used for postexposure chemoprophylaxis in healthy children or adults.
- School closure should be considered upon a confirmed case of H1N1.
- Public gatherings should be avoided in a place where there has been a confirmed case of H1N1.

Vaccine

- Vaccine stimulates active immunity to influenza virus infection by inducing production of specific antibodies. H1N1 vaccine is available as an IM injection and as an intranasal product.
- A quadrivalent vaccine containing four strains of influenza viruses including H1N1 is available now which can be used.
- Vaccination is recommended for all pregnant women, adults, and children over six months of age.

Prognosis

- H1N1 influenza tends to cause high morbidity but low mortality rates (1–4%). Complications are more likely in children, elderly, pregnant women and people with other comorbid illness.

Q. Varicella-zoster virus infection (chickenpox) (HHV-3).

Etiology

- The causative agent of varicella or chickenpox is varicella-zoster virus (VZV; human herpes virus-3). It is a DNA virus belonging to Herpesviridae family.
- It produces two clinical entities: Varicella (chickenpox) and herpes zoster (shingles).
- Chickenpox is the primary infection, and usually occurs in childhood. Chickenpox rarely occurs twice but the virus remains latent in the dorsal root ganglia and cranial nerve ganglia. Years later it may be reactivated to cause vesicular eruption in the relevant sensory dermatomes which is known as herpes zoster (shingles).

Transmission Routes

- Transmission occurs via contact with aerosolized droplets from nasopharyngeal secretions of an infected individual or by direct cutaneous contact with vesicle fluid from skin lesions. Airborne transmission of VZV has also been reported.

Clinical Features

- Chickenpox affects children commonly.
- Incubation period is 10–21 days.
- There may be a prodrome of low-grade fever, headache and malaise lasting 1–2 days before the onset of rash.
- Rash appears first on the face and trunk and then spreads to other parts of the body (centripetal rash). Lesions can also be found on the mucosa of the pharynx and vagina. Rashes may be pruritic and centripetal with relative sparing of the peripheries. To start with rashes are maculopapular and, in a few hours, become vesicles. Vesicles become pustules which later form crusts **(Fig. 1.33)**. New lesions continue to appear for 2–4 days so that all stages of the eruption are present simultaneously (pleomorphic rash). Rashes usually heal without scarring. Lesions can get secondarily infected with bacteria, usually *Streptococcus pyogenes* or *Staphylococcus aureus*.

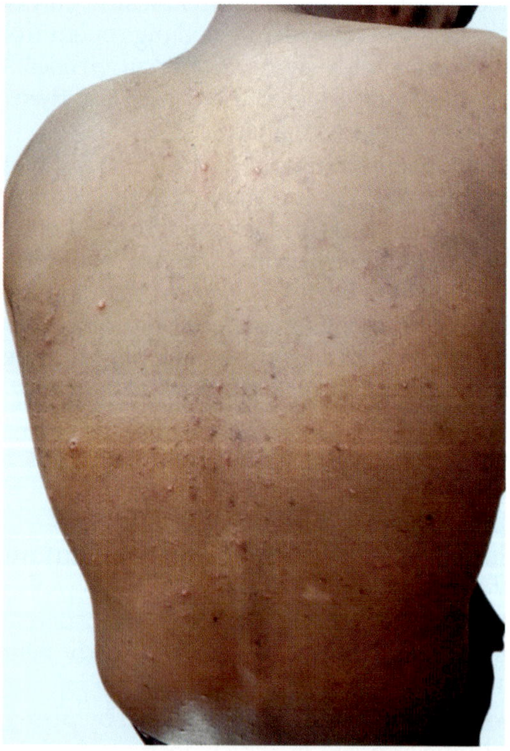

Figure 1.33: Chickenpox eruptions

Diagnosis

- Diagnosis is mainly based on clinical features.
- Diagnosis can be confirmed where necessary by:
  - PCR (polymerase chain reaction): Most sensitive test.
  - Direct fluorescent antibody (DFA) test: Detects VZV in skin lesions.
  - Serologic tests (IgM, IgG antibodies): Determines past infection or immunity.

Treatment

- Most people recover with supportive treatment.
- Antiviral agents like acyclovir, famciclovir and valacyclovir are recommended for adolescents and adults with chickenpox of ≤24 hours duration.
- Antibiotics may be used for secondary bacterial infection of skin lesions.

Complications

- CNS involvement in the form of cerebellar ataxia, meningitis, encephalitis, transverse myelitis, and Guillain-Barre syndrome.
- Involvement of other organ systems can produce varicella pneumonia, myocarditis, nephritis, hepatitis and arthritis.
- Reye's syndrome (hepatic encephalopathy), another complication, is associated with aspirin therapy.

Varicella Prevention and Vaccination

Varicella vaccine (live attenuated vaccine)

- Highly effective (90–95%) in preventing severe disease, included in childhood vaccination schedules.
- Adults who never had chickenpox should get 2 doses, 4–8 weeks apart. It is given IM (deltoid) or subcutaneously. (Note that intramuscular vaccines need to be given to deltoid in adults. Giving into gluteal region has poor immunological response).
- Pregnant women should not receive the varicella vaccine, as it is a live virus vaccine.

Q. Herpes zoster (shingles).

Etiology

- Etiologic agent is varicella-zoster virus (VZV) which is the same virus causing chickenpox. After an attack of chickenpox VZV remains latent in the dorsal root ganglia and cranial nerve ganglia. Years later it may be reactivated to cause vesicular eruption in the relevant sensory dermatomes which is known as herpes zoster (shingles).

Clinical Features

- The first symptom is severe burning or shooting pain in the affected dermatome followed by erythematous maculopapular eruption in 2–3 days. These eruptions turn into vesicles and start crusting. The skin eruption is usually unilateral **(Fig. 1.34)**.
- The total duration of disease is generally between 7 and 10 days.

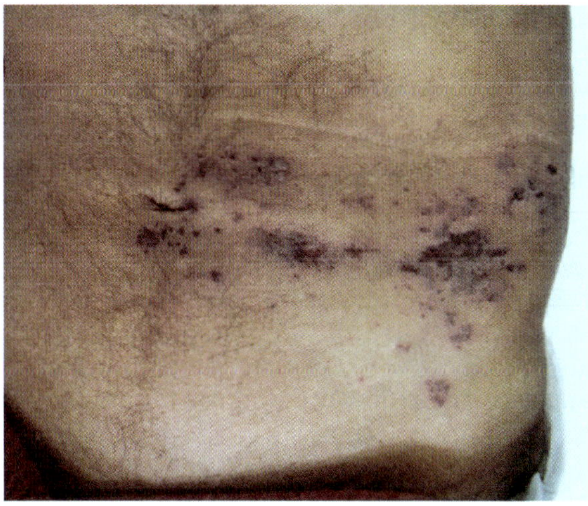

Figure 1.34: Herpes zoster affecting T-10 dermatome on left side

- Local skin hyperalgesia is a clue to the neural origin of pain.
- The dermatomes from T3 to L3 are commonly affected.
- In ophthalmic herpes the Gasserian ganglion (trigeminal ganglion) is affected and the ophthalmic branch of the trigeminal nerve is involved. Lesions develop on the nose, conjunctiva and cornea of the affected side. Corneal lesions heal leaving behind opacities causing blindness.

Treatment

- Antiviral drugs are indicated for the treatment of shingles. Drugs used are same as for varicella (acyclovir or famciclovir or valacyclovir).
- Herpes zoster causes severe pain which may be difficult to control. NSAIDs and opioid analgesics can be used along with neuron modulator drugs such as carbamazepine, gabapentin, amitriptyline and lidocaine patches to control pain.

Complications

- Postherpetic neuralgia: In postherpetic neuralgia, pain persists even after the lesions have healed. Pain of postherpetic neuralgia may be sharp and intermittent or constant and may be debilitating. It may persist for months or years or permanently. Treatments for postherpetic neuralgia include gabapentin, pregabalin, cyclic antidepressants, topical capsaicin or lidocaine ointment, and botulinum toxin injection.
- CNS: Complications include meningoencephalitis and transverse myelitis. Sometimes weakness and wasting in segments supplied by the nerve root may occur due to motor neuritis.
- Immunocompromised patients can develop severe disease with multiorgan involvement.

Prevention of Herpes Zoster

- Herpes zoster vaccination decreases the risk of developing herpes zoster and postherpetic neuralgia. A recombinant herpes zoster vaccine is available in most countries (brand name SHINGRIX). It is given AS IM injection: 0.5 ml administered as a 2-dose series. 1st dose on any day, followed by 2nd dose between 2 and 6 months after 1st dose.

Q. Infectious mononucleosis (glandular fever).

Etiology

- Infectious mononucleosis (IM) is a disease caused by Epstein-Barr virus (EBV). EBV is a DNA virus belonging to the family Herpesviridae. EBV also causes many tumors in human beings like nasopharyngeal carcinoma, Burkitt's lymphoma, and Hodgkin's lymphoma.
- Infectious mononucleosis (IM) is also known as *glandular fever* or *kissing disease*. Later it was called infectious mononucleosis because it is characterized by absolute lymphocytosis and atypical mononuclear cells in the blood.
- It is characterized by a triad of fever, pharyngitis, and lymphadenopathy.

Pathogenesis

- In humans it spreads commonly through saliva ('the kissing disease') and rarely by blood transfusion.
- After entry into the body the virus multiplies primarily in B-lymphocytes but also may replicate in the epithelial cells of the pharynx and parotid duct. Infected B cells are responsible for the dissemination of infection throughout the lymphoreticular system, i.e. liver, spleen, and peripheral lymph nodes. Infected B lymphocytes produce antibodies against the virus. Cytotoxic T cells are also produced by the body against the EBV-infected B lymphocytes.

Clinical Features

- Incubation period is 4–8 weeks. Infectious mononucleosis is a disease of childhood, adolescence and low socioeconomic groups.
- Initially there is a prodrome of fatigue, malaise, and myalgia.
- Prodrome is followed by typical features such as fever, sore throat, and lymphadenopathy.
- Fever is usually low grade. Lymphadenopathy most often affects the posterior cervical nodes but may be generalized.
- A generalized maculopapular rash is occasionally seen. Rash may develop if ampicillin is taken.
- Splenomegaly is seen in 50–60% of patients with IM. Splenic rupture is a rare but potentially life-threatening complication of IM.
- IM should be suspected in an adolescent or young adult with fever, sore throat and lymphadenopathy (especially posterior cervical lymphadenopathy).
- The illness usually lasts 2–4 weeks but weakness can persist for a long time.
- Complications include splenic rupture, thrombocytopenia, autoimmune hemolytic anemia, meningitis, encephalitis, and GB-syndrome.

Investigations

- Blood count shows absolute lymphocytosis and atypical mononuclear cells (hence the name infectious mononucleosis).
- Liver enzymes may be raised but jaundice is rare.
- Paul-Bunnel test and Monospot test (detect heterophile antibodies) are usually positive.
- Demonstration of antibodies to viral capsid antigen (i.e. VCA-IgG and VCA-IgM).

Differential Diagnosis

- Other infections which produce fever and lymphadenopathy: streptococcal pharyngitis, cytomegalovirus, acute HIV, or Toxoplasma.
- Lymphoma.

Treatment

- There is no specific treatment for infectious mononucleosis. Antiviral drugs do not have much benefit.
- Supportive measures, rest and antipyretics are given as required.
- Ampicillin should be avoided in suspected infectious mononucleosis because it causes rash.
- Corticosteroids can be helpful for complications such as impending airway obstruction, severe thrombocytopenia, and hemolytic anemia.

Q. Chronic fatigue syndrome (Myalgic encephalomyelitis).

- Chronic fatigue syndrome (CFS) also known as myalgic encephalomyelitis is a disorder characterized by unexplained, persistent, and sometimes debilitating fatigue.
- It can be difficult to diagnose because there are no objective clinical or laboratory findings associated with this disorder.
- Note that CFS is different from fibromyalgia.

Etiology

- The exact etiology of CFS is unknown and is likely to be multifactorial. Possible triggers include:
- *Viral infections*: Some cases develop after infections like:
  - Epstein-Barr virus (EBV, linked to infectious mononucleosis)
  - Human Herpesvirus-6 (HHV-6)
  - Cytomegalovirus (CMV)
  - Enteroviruses
  - COVID-19 (associated with long COVID)
- *Immune system dysfunction*: Some patients show signs of immune dysregulation.
- *Hormonal imbalances*: Abnormal levels of cortisol or thyroid hormones may play a role.
- *Genetic factors*: Family history may increase susceptibility.
- *Psychological and environmental stressors*: Trauma, stress, and environmental toxins may contribute.

Clinical Features

- CFS is more common in young and middle-aged adults, in women and in Caucasians.
- CFS/ME is more than just being tired. It involves a wide range of physical, neurological, and cognitive symptoms.

Core Symptoms (required for diagnosis)

- Severe, persistent fatigue (>6 months, unexplained, not improved by rest)
- Post-exertional malaise (PEM): Worsening of symptoms after physical or mental activity, lasting for days or weeks.
- Unrefreshing sleep: Waking up feeling exhausted despite sleeping enough.

Additional Symptoms

- Cognitive impairment ("brain fog"): Difficulty with memory, concentration, and processing information.
- Chronic pain: Muscle pain, joint pain, headaches, and nerve pain.
- Autonomic dysfunction: Dizziness, orthostatic intolerance (difficulty standing for long periods, POTS.)
- Gastrointestinal issues: IBS-like symptoms (bloating, diarrhea, constipation).
- Increased sensitivity: Sensitivity to light, noise, smells, and medications.
- Physical examination is normal, with no objective signs of muscle weakness, arthritis, neuropathy, or organomegaly.
- Many patients have underlying depression.

Treatment

- There is no specific therapy. Treatment focuses on symptom relief and lifestyle modifications.

Lifestyle Improvement

- Pacing (energy conservation strategy): Avoid pushing too hard to prevent "crashes" (PEM).
- Sleep hygiene: Regular sleep schedule, avoiding screens before bedtime.
- Diet and nutrition: Balanced diet, avoiding processed foods and excessive sugar.
- Cognitive therapy and stress management: Helps with coping mechanisms.

Medications (symptom-based)

- Pain relief: NSAIDs, low-dose antidepressants (e.g. amitriptyline for pain).
- Sleep aids: Melatonin, low-dose trazodone.
- Neuropathic pain treatments: Gabapentin, pregabalin.
- Dizziness and autonomic symptoms: Midodrine, fludrocortisone.

Q. Human papillomavirus infections.

- Human papillomavirus (HPV) is a common sexually transmitted infection (STI) caused by the HPV virus family.
- Human papilloma viruses are DNA viruses belonging to the family Papillomaviridae.
- They infect the skin and mucous membranes. Infections produce warts or may be associated with a variety of benign and malignant neoplasms. Some HPV infections (such as 16, 18, 31, 33, and 45) cause cervical cancer.
- Most of the infections are seen in children and young adults. Warts can be common warts (verruca vulgaris), plantar warts (verruca plantaris) or anogenital warts (condyloma acuminatum). Anogenital warts are sexually transmitted.
- Complications of warts include itching and bleeding with secondary infection. Warts in the respiratory tract may obstruct the airway.
- Many HPV lesions resolve spontaneously. Treatment options are cryosurgery, application of caustic agents, electrodesiccation, surgical excision, and ablation with a laser. Topical antimetabolite, such as 5-fluorouracil is also effective.
- HPV vaccination:
    - Gardasil 9 (covers HPV 6, 11, 16, 18, 31, 33, 45, 52, 58): Protects against genital warts and cancer. Recommended for:
    - Girls and boys (ages 9–14)–Best if given before sexual activity.
    - Catch-up vaccination: Recommended up to age 26, sometimes 45 (depending on risk).

Q. Measles (rubeola).

- Measles (also known as rubeola) is a highly contagious, acute, viral exanthematous disease.

Etiology

- Measles is caused by measles virus which is a RNA virus belonging to the family of paramyxoviruses.

Epidemiology

- It most commonly affects preschool children. Incidence of measles has come down after the introduction of measles vaccine.
- Measles virus is transmitted by inhalation of respiratory droplets. It can also spread through direct contact with larger droplets.
- The virus is present in nasopharyngeal secretions, blood and urine during the prodromal period and for a short time after the rash appears.
- Patients are contagious from 4 days before the onset of rash until 4 days after the onset of rash. Infectivity is maximum during the prodromal phase.

Clinical Features

- Incubation period is 10–14 days.
- Measles starts with a prodrome of malaise, cough, lacrimation, nasal discharge, and fever. At this stage it resembles influenza.
- Just before the onset of the rash, Koplik's spots appear as 1–2 mm blue-white spots on a bright red

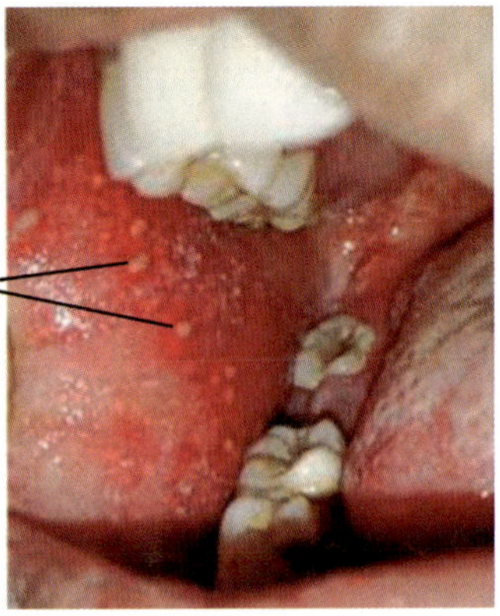

Figure 1.35: Koplik's spot

background. Koplik's spots are usually seen on the buccal mucosa alongside the upper second molars. They are pathognomonic of measles because they are not seen in any other disease. The spots disappear after the onset of rash **(Fig. 1.35)**.

- Rash appears 3–4 days after the onset of fever. Rash begins first at the hairline and behind the ears, and then spreads downward to the trunk and limbs. Rashes do not spare the palms and soles, are erythematous, nonpruritic, and maculopapular. Rash is monomorphic, i.e. all rashes have similar morphology. Rash fades in the same order in which it appeared.
- The entire illness lasts about 10 days. The disease tends to be more severe in adults than in children.

Diagnosis

- Measles is diagnosed mainly by clinical features. Fever + 3 C's (cough, coryza, conjunctivitis) + rash.
- Diagnosis can be confirmed by detecting serum anti-measles IgM antibody. IgM antibody is detectable three days after the appearance of rash. Anti-measles IgG antibody appears 7 days after the appearance of rash.
- A quick diagnosis of measles can be made by demonstration of measles antigen by immunofluorescent staining of a smear of respiratory secretions.
- Measles virus can be cultured and isolated from respiratory secretions or urine.
- PCR for measles virus RNA can also diagnose measles.

Treatment

- There is no specific treatment for measles.
- Patient should be isolated.
- Most people recover spontaneously and only supportive treatment is necessary.
- Ribavirin may be considered for use in immunocompromised individuals.
- Administration of vitamin A has been shown to prevent complications especially in malnourished children.
- Secondary bacterial complications are treated with appropriate antibiotics.

Complications

- ***Respiratory tract complications:*** Laryngitis, croup, or bronchitis, otitis media, pneumonia.
- ***CNS complications:*** Encephalitis, transverse myelitis, subacute sclerosing panencephalitis (SSPE). SSPE is a chronic, rare form of measles encephalitis. It is common in children who have measles before the age of 2 years. SSPE is now rare due to widespread vaccination against measles. Clinical features are progressive dementia which evolves over several months.
- ***Gastrointestinal complications:*** Hepatitis, appendicitis, and mesenteric adenitis.
- ***Others:*** Myocarditis, glomerulonephritis, post-infectious thrombocytopenic purpura and reactivation of tuberculosis.

Prevention

- Immediate protection can be obtained by giving immunoglobulin within 6 days of exposure to the disease. Measles vaccine given within 72 hours of exposure may also protect against disease.
- Active immunization with measles vaccine is included in the national immunization program. A single dose of vaccine is given at 8–9 months of age. **It provides lifelong immunity**. Giving MMR vaccine at 15–18 months takes care of occasional failure of measles vaccine given at 8–9 months of age. However if there is an epidemic of measles, vaccination may be given at 6 months of age followed by another dose at 15 months of age.

Q. Rubella (German measles).

- Rubella is an acute viral exanthematous disease caused by rubella virus, a RNA virus.
- It is also known as German measles because it was first recognized to be different from measles in Germany.

Epidemiology

- Humans are the only natural hosts for rubella infection.
- It spreads by respiratory droplets or is maternally transmitted to the fetus causing congenital infection.
- The peak incidence of the disease is in children of 5–12 years of age.

Clinical Manifestations

- Incubation period is usually 2–3 weeks.
- The disease is characterized by fever, rash, and lymphadenopathy.
- It is more severe in adults than children.
- There is usually a prodrome of low-grade fever, malaise, anorexia and sore throat, followed by lymphadenopathy and appearance of skin rash. Rash often begins on the face and spreads down the body. It is maculopapular, not as intense as measles rash, and does not merge. It disappears in the same order. Lymphadenopathy usually affects suboccipital,

cervical and post-auricular nodes but rarely axillary nodes can also be involved. Complications are rare and include arthritis (in women), encephalitis and thrombocytopenia.

- *Congenital rubella*: Maternal infection in early pregnancy can lead to fetal infection, leading to teratogenic effects and congenital rubella. Sensorineural hearing loss is the most common manifestation of congenital rubella syndrome. Other signs of congenital rubella are cataract, heart disease (patent ductus arteriosus), deafness, and many other defects like mental retardation, microcephaly, and thrombocytopenic purpura. Infection in the first trimester leads to more severe congenital rubella in the fetus.
- *Key features*: Mild fever + maculopapular rash + postauricular lymphadenopathy.

Investigations

- Rubella-specific IgM and IgG antibodies (serology).
- RT-PCR for rubella RNA (throat swab, blood, or urine).

Treatment

- Isolate the patient for 7 days after the onset of rash to prevent spread of infection to others.
- There is no specific treatment. Most cases recover spontaneously.
- Antipyretics like paracetamol can be used to treat fever.
- Pregnant women exposed to rubella: Serologic testing (IgM/IgG) immediately. If infected, counseling on pregnancy risks and potential termination (if early pregnancy).

Prevention

- Presently all infants are routinely immunized against rubella by giving MMR vaccine at 12–15 months of age. Live rubella virus vaccine containing RA 27/3 strain, and a recombinant DNA vaccine is now available.
- Vaccine is administered in a single dose of 0.5 ml subcutaneously. Immunity wanes after 10–15 years and hence the vaccine may have to be repeated at 10–15 years of age. Rubella vaccine may also be administered to anyone who is thought to be susceptible to the infection.
- Live rubella vaccine is contraindicated during pregnancy and it is recommended that pregnancy be avoided for at least 3 months after rubella vaccination.

Q. Mumps.

- Mumps is an acute, communicable, systemic viral infection whose most distinctive feature is swelling of parotid glands. It can involve other salivary glands, meninges, pancreas, and the gonads.

Etiology

- Mumps is caused by mumps virus which is a member of the paramyxovirus group. It is a RNA virus.

Epidemiology

- Mumps occurs worldwide but the incidence has decreased after the introduction of MMR vaccine which contains mumps component also.
- Mumps occurs mainly during winter and spring. It is mainly a disease of childhood, but nowadays adults are getting affected more commonly. Both sexes are affected equally.
- Epidemics occur in close populations, such as in schools and military services.
- Mumps is highly infectious and spreads rapidly among susceptible people living in close quarters.
- Mumps virus is transmitted by droplet nuclei, saliva, and fomites. Fomites contaminated by infected saliva and possibly also by urine transmit the infection. Transmission of infection occurs a day before the appearance of the parotid swelling and for about three days after the swelling disappears.
- One attack of mumps or vaccination confers lifelong immunity.

Clinical Features

- Incubation period is 2–3 weeks.
- Mumps starts with a prodrome of fever, malaise, myalgia, and anorexia.
- Parotitis may develop within the next 24 hours or may be delayed upto a week. Parotitis is usually bilateral, although sometimes only one side is affected. Parotid glands are involved most commonly and submaxillary and sublingual glands are involved rarely. Parotid gland becomes swollen and tender. Gland swelling increases for a few days and then gradually subsides within a week.
- Other than parotitis, orchitis is the most common manifestation. Testis becomes swollen, painful and tender. Testicular atrophy develops in half of the affected men. However, since orchitis is usually unilateral and other testes remains unaffected, sterility is rare. Oophoritis can occur in women but less common than orchitis and does not lead to sterility.
- Aseptic meningitis is a common manifestation of mumps in both children and adults. Mumps meningitis is usually self-limiting, although cranial nerve palsies are rarely seen. Rarely, encephalitis can occur, which presents as high fever with altered sensorium. Other CNS problems occasionally seen are sensorineural deafness, cerebellar ataxia, facial palsy, transverse myelitis, Guillain-Barré syndrome, and aqueductal stenosis leading to hydrocephalus.
- Other clinical manifestations are pancreatitis, myocarditis, mastitis, thyroiditis, nephritis, arthritis, and thrombocytopenic purpura.

Differential Diagnosis

- Mumps has to be differentiated from other causes of parotid gland swelling, such as,
  - Influenza, parainfluenza and Coxsackie virus infections

- Bacterial parotitis due to staphylococcal infection
- Obstruction of Stenson's duct by a calculus
- Parotid tumor
- Sarcoidosis
- Sjögren's syndrome.

Diagnosis

- Diagnosis is mainly by clinical features (parotid gland swelling + fever + fatigue).
- Serological detection of IgM antibodies.
- Virus isolation by culturing appropriate clinical specimens.
- PCR.

Treatment

- Symptomatic treatment; analgesics and antipyretics for fever and pain, cold compresses for parotid swelling.
- Patients with meningitis or pancreatitis may require hospitalization.
- Patients with orchitis are also treated symptomatically with bed rest, nonsteroidal antiinflammatory agents, support of the inflamed testis and ice packs.

Prevention

- Patients should be isolated to prevent transmission to others
- Passive immunization using immunoglobulin is not effective to prevent infection in close contacts and is not recommended.
- Active immunization is routinely given as MMR vaccine (measles, mumps, rubella) subcutaneously at 15 months of age or later; repeat dose may be necessary after 5–10 years. MMR vaccine is also recommended for susceptible older children, adolescents, and adults, particularly adolescent males who have not had mumps. Vaccine should not be given to pregnant women, immunosuppressed patients, or persons with advanced malignancies.

Q. Discuss the etiology, epidemiology, pathogenesis, clinical features, diagnosis and treatment of rabies.

Q. Prevention of rabies.

Q. Post-exposure prophylaxis of rabies.

- Rabies is an acute lethal viral infection of the central nervous system caused by rabies virus. It is a preventable zoonotic disease.
- Rabies is one of the oldest, best known, and most feared human diseases. It has the highest case fatality rate of any human infectious disease.

Etiology

- Rabies virus is a bullet-shaped virus, with a single-stranded ribonucleic acid (RNA), nucleocapsid core and lipoprotein envelope. It belongs to the family of Rhabdoviridae and genus Lyssavirus **(Fig. 1.36)**.

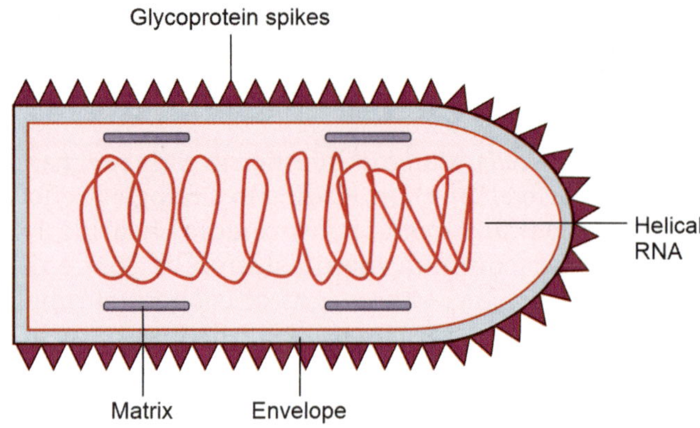

Figure 1.36: Rabies virus

Epidemiology

- Rabies has a worldwide distribution except Antarctica, New Zealand, Japan, parts of Europe, and some Caribbean Islands.
- Mammals are the main reservoir of rabies virus.
- Rabies exists in two forms: (i) urban rabies, found in unimmunized domestic dogs and cats, (ii) sylvatic rabies, found in skunks, foxes, raccoons, mongooses, wolves, and bats.
- The main reservoir of rabies throughout the world is the domestic dog. Domestic animals usually acquire infection from sylvatic reservoirs of infection.
- Human infection occurs through contact with unimmunized domestic animals or from exposure to wild animals.
- Mandatory vaccination of domestic dogs against rabies has resulted in decreased incidence of rabies.

Transmission

- Rabies is transmitted by the bite of infected animals, commonly dogs or cats or saliva contact with open wounds or mucous membranes. The saliva of these animals is the reservoir of infection. Rarely, transmission takes place through transplantation of infected tissues such as cornea or inhalation of aerosol containing virus.
- Although laboratory studies have demonstrated aerosol transmission of the rabies virus, documented cases in humans are extremely rare. To date, only four cases have been reported—two spelunkers exposed in a single cave and two laboratory workers handling live virus.

Pathogenesis (Fig. 1.37)

- Rabies is a highly neurotropic virus that evades immune surveillance by its sequestration in the nervous system.
- After the entry of live virus through saliva following a bite, viral replication starts in striated muscle cells. The virus then spreads centripetally up the nerve to the CNS, via peripheral nerve axoplasm, at a rate of ~3 mm/hour. Once the virus reaches the CNS, it multiplies there and then passes centrifugally along somatic and autonomic nerves to other tissues—the

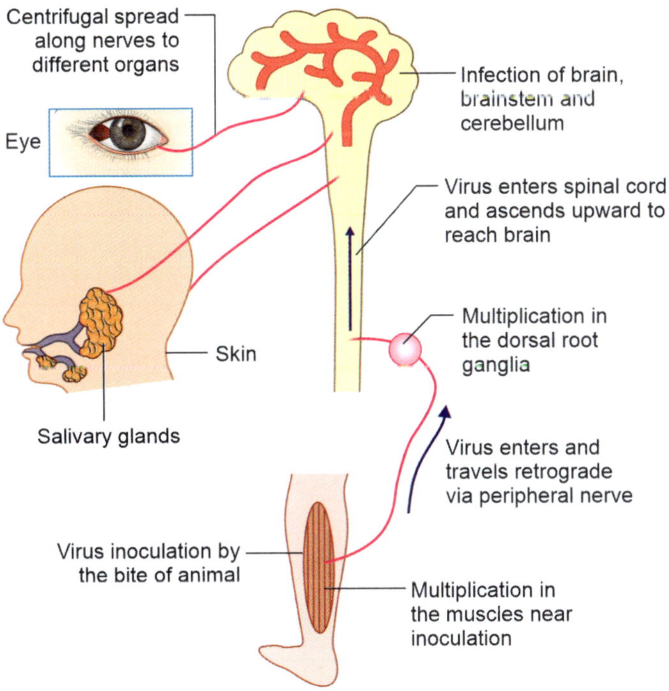

Figure 1.37: Pathogenesis of rabies

salivary glands, adrenal medulla, kidneys, lungs, liver, skeletal muscles, skin, and heart. In the salivary glands virus can multiply again and secreted into saliva which is infective to others.

- The most characteristic pathologic finding of rabies in the CNS is the formation of cytoplasmic inclusions called Negri bodies within neurons. Negri body is an eosinophilic mass of fibrillar matrix and viral particles. Negri bodies are not found in at least 20% cases of rabies, hence, their absence does not rule out the diagnosis of rabies.

Clinical Features

Incubation Period

- The incubation period of rabies ranges from 10 days to over 1 year (mean 1–3 months). Rarely, cases of human rabies with an extended incubation period (2–7 years) have been reported. The incubation period depends on the amount of virus introduced, host defense mechanisms, and the distance that the virus has to travel from the site of inoculation to the CNS.
- Incubation period is less than 50 days if the patient is bitten on the head or neck or if a heavy amount of virus is inoculated. A person with a scratch on the hand may take longer to develop symptoms of rabies than a person who receives a bite to the head.
- The rabies virus is segregated from the immune system during this period, and no antibody response is observed.

Prodromal Symptoms

- *Prodromal stage:* This stage lasts from a few days to one week and is characterized by low-grade fever, fatigue, malaise, nausea, vomiting, headache, myalgia, sore throat and dry cough. There may be complaint of paresthesia, fasciculations or intense itching at the site of virus inoculation which is pathognomonic of rabies and occurs in 50% of cases during this phase. These sensations are due to the multiplication of virus in the dorsal root ganglion of the sensory nerve supplying the area. In addition, percussion myoedema (mounding of the muscle upon percussion) may be present during the prodrome and throughout the illness. Except for these sensations/fasciculations all other symptoms resemble any other viral prodrome.

Clinical Rabies

- Infection may evolve into two major forms of disease, including encephalitic (referred to as "furious" in animals) rabies or paralytic (referred to as "dumb" in animals). Both follow the prodromal symptoms described above. In humans, encephalitic rabies is more common (80% of cases).
- Encephalitic rabies presents with fever, hydrophobia, aerophobia, pharyngeal spasms, and hyperactivity. This is the most common form. This stage is characterized by periods of excessive motor activity, excitation, agitation, hallucinations, confusion, muscle spasms, meningismus, opisthotonic posturing, seizures, and focal paralysis. Initially they are interspersed with lucid intervals, but as the disease progresses the lucid periods get shorter until the patient lapses into coma. Hyperesthesia, with excessive irritation to bright light, noise, touch, and breezes are often seen. Abnormalities of the autonomic nervous system include dilated pupils, increased sweating, lacrimation, salivation and postural hypotension. Evidence of upper motor neuron paralysis, with weakness, exaggerated deep tendon reflexes, and extensor plantar responses, is always found. Paralysis of the vocal cords may produce dysphonia. Brainstem dysfunction manifests as diplopia, facial paralysis, and dysphagia with excessive salivation. The combination of excessive salivation and difficulty in swallowing give the appearance of "foaming at the mouth." Attempt to swallow liquids produces painful, violent, involuntary contraction of the diaphragmatic, accessory respiratory, pharyngeal, and laryngeal muscles-called *hydrophobia*. Hydrophobia is the most characteristic clinical feature of rabies and is seen in only ~50% of rabies cases. Patient develops an overwhelming terror of water due to involuntary pharyngeal muscle spasms during attempts to drink. Later in the disease, even the sight or mention of water may trigger involuntary spasms. Aerophobia is also pathognomonic of rabies although it occurs less often than hydrophobia (approximately 9% in one series). Pharyngeal spasms are triggered by a draft of air and can last approximately 5–15 seconds.
- Paralytic (dumb) rabies occurs in less than 20% of patients. It presents as ascending flaccid quadriparesis with sphincter involvement, mimicking Guillain-Barré syndrome. Paralysis is usually most prominent in the bitten limb. Usually, there will be fasciculations and loss of deep tendon and plantar reflexes. As the

paralysis progresses, there is paralysis of the muscles of deglutition and respiration, leading to death. Encephalitis may occur late in the course of disease.

Stage of Coma and Death

- This begins within 10 days of onset, and the duration varies. The patient soon lapses into coma, and dies of respiratory failure. After the onset of brainstem symptoms, patient survives for only 4–5 days and rarely for 20 days maximum. If artificial supportive measures are instituted, patient may survive longer but many complications may appear like hypotension, cardiac arrhythmias, ARDS, etc. which can kill the patient.

Diagnosis

Antemortem Diagnosis (before death)

- No single test can reliably confirm rabies in a living patient. A combination of the following tests is used:

Direct fluorescent antibody test (DFA) on skin biopsy

- *Specimen*: A full thickness skin biopsy (5–6 mm in diameter) should be taken from the nape of the neck (rich in nerve endings) at the hairline. The sample should contain a minimum of 10 hair follicles.
- *Method*: Detects rabies virus antigens using fluorescent-labeled antibodies.
- *Significance*: Most reliable antemortem test for rabies.

Reverse transcription polymerase chain reaction (RT-PCR)

- *Specimen*: Saliva, cerebrospinal fluid (CSF), or skin biopsy.
- *Method*: Detects rabies virus RNA.
- *Significance*: Highly sensitive and can confirm early infection.

Rabies virus neutralizing antibodies (RVNA) in serum or CSF

- *Specimen*: Blood serum or cerebrospinal fluid (CSF).
- *Method*: Measures the presence of rabies-specific antibodies.
- *Significance*: Antibodies are usually absent in the early stage but appear later in the disease. This is not a very useful test because rabies virus–specific antibodies may be found in serum as a result of previous vaccination against rabies. However, detection of antibodies in the serum or CSF of a previously unimmunized patient is diagnostic of rabies.

Viral culture

- *Specimen*: Saliva or CSF.
- *Method*: Inoculation into cell cultures or laboratory animals.
- *Significance*: Rarely used due to time constraints and biosafety risks.

Postmortem Diagnosis (after death)

- Definitive confirmation of rabies is usually done postmortem through brain tissue examination.

Direct fluorescent antibody (DFA) test on brain tissue

- *Specimen*: Brain tissue from the hippocampus, cerebellum, or brainstem.
- *Method*: Uses fluorescent antibodies to detect rabies virus antigens.
- *Significance*: **Postmortem DFA on brain tissue** remains the **gold standard** for definitive diagnosis.

Histopathology and Negri bodies

- *Specimen*: Brain tissue.
- *Method*: Microscopic examination for *Negri bodies* (cytoplasmic inclusions in neurons).
- *Significance*: Classical finding but not always present, so additional testing is required.

RT-PCR and viral isolation

- *Specimen*: Brain tissue.
- *Method*: PCR amplification or virus isolation in cell cultures.
- *Significance*: Highly sensitive and confirms viral presence.

Treatment

- There is no specific treatment for rabies. Medical management is supportive and palliative. Death is inevitable once clinical signs develop.
- The bite wound should be cleaned, debrided and carefully examined for any foreign body (e.g. broken tooth). Generally, leave wounds to heal by secondary intention to permit drainage of wound fluids and prevent infection. The following therapy has been recommended though there is no proof that they are effective.
    - Rabies vaccination to accelerate the immune response.
    - Intramuscular human rabies immune globulin (HRIG) to promote clearance of the infection.
    - Intravenous and intraventricular ribavirin
    - Intravenous and intraventricular IFN-α
    - Intravenous infusion of ketamine, a dissociative anesthetic agent and a noncompetitive antagonist of the N-methyl-D-aspartate receptor has been shown to inhibit virus replication at high concentrations.

Prevention of Rabies

- Rabies is almost 100% fatal once symptoms appear, but it is entirely preventable through vaccination. Hence, all efforts should be made to prevent rabies. Prevention of rabies can be divided into pre-exposure prophylaxis and post-exposure prophylaxis.

Pre-exposure Prophylaxis

- It should be given to all those at risk of developing rabies like veterinarians, animal handlers and laboratory workers.
- 3 doses of vaccine (preferably HDCV–Human diploid cell vaccine) are administered intramuscularly on days 0, 7, and 21 or 28. Booster doses are required

TABLE 1.14: Post-exposure prophylaxis of rabies

Category	PEP vaccine regimen	RIG (rabies immunoglobulin)
Category I: Touching or feeding animals, animal licks on intact skin	Not required	Not required
Category II: Nibbling of uncovered skin, minor scratches or abrasions without bleeding	**Patients who have NOT been previously immunized:** Immediate vaccination with the following regimens: • 1-site IM on days 0, 3, 7, and between days 14 and 28 • 2-sites IM on day 0 and 1-site IM on days 7 and 21	Not required
	Patients who have been previously immunized: • 1-site IM on days 0 and 3	Not required
Category III: Single or multiple transdermal bites or scratches, contamination of mucous membrane or broken skin with saliva from animal licks, exposures due to direct contact with bats	**Patients who have NOT been previously immunized:** Immediate vaccination with one of the following regimens: • 1-site IM on days 0, 3, 7, and between days 14 and 28 • 2-sites IM on day 0 and 1-site IM on days 7 and 21	RIG should be administered (20 IU/kg body weight on day 0.
	Patients who have been previously immunized:* • 1-site IM on days 0 and 3	Not required

Previously immunized patients include those who have received pre-exposure prophylaxis and those who have completed a post-exposure vaccine regimen >3 months ago. Post-exposure prophylaxis (except for wound care) is not recommended for individuals who have a rabies exposure <3 months after completing a post-exposure vaccine series.
Rabies immunoglobulin (RIG) should be infiltrated into and around the wound. For small wounds, the maximal quantity that is anatomically feasible should be administered. The WHO no longer recommends injecting the remainder of the RIG IM at a site distant from the wound, which differs from ACIP (Advisory Committee on Immunization Practices) recommendations in the United States. ACIP recommends that If any RIG remains after thorough wound infiltration, it should be administered intramuscularly at a site distant from the rabies vaccine administration.
2 sites IM on day 0 means give two full doses of vaccine at each deltoid region. 1-site IM means give one dose to any one deltoid.
Do not give the vaccine into gluteal region as absorption and immunogenicity is poor.

every 1–3 years for those at continuous risk (e.g. veterinarians, wildlife handlers).
- Note that people who receive pre-exposure prophylaxis still require PEP after exposure but can skip rabies immunoglobulin (RIG).

Post-exposure Prophylaxis

- Rabies vaccination should be given as per the WHO recommendations given below.
- Tetanus toxoid should be given if not given in the last 5 years.
- Wound should be cleaned with water and antiseptic lotions. Wound should not be sutured **(Table 1.14)**.

Q. Negri bodies

- **Negri bodies** are eosinophilic (pink-staining), cytoplasmic inclusions found in neurons infected with the *rabies virus*. They are considered a **histopathological hallmark** of rabies and play an important role in postmortem diagnosis **(Fig. 1.38)**.
- Primarily found in **pyramidal cells** of the hippocampus and **Purkinje cells** of the cerebellum. Can also be seen in the thalamus, brainstem, and spinal cord.
- They are round or oval in shape. Measure **2–10 µm** in diameter.
- Made of aggregates of viral ribonucleoprotein (RNP).
- Staining: Appear eosinophilic (pink/red) in hematoxylin and eosin (H&E) stain. Best visualized with Seller's stain.
- Diagnostic significance: Presence of Negri bodies is highly suggestive of rabies but not always found,

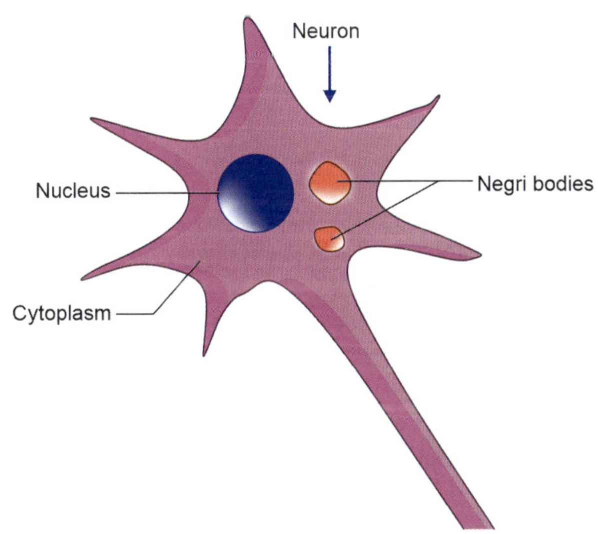

Figure 1.38: Negri bodies

especially in early cases. Found in 71–90% of human rabies cases. Absence does not rule out rabies. Definitive confirmation of rabies still requires additional tests like direct fluorescent antibody (DFA) test, RT-PCR, or virus isolation.

Q. What are arboviruses? List common arboviruses and the diseases caused by them.

- Arboviruses are a group of viruses transmitted by arthropods to vertebrate hosts like man. The word arbovirus is an acronym (arthropod-borne virus).The arthropods which transmit the infection are called vectors and include mosquito, tick, sand fly or midges.

These infections generally occur during warm weather months, when mosquitoes and ticks are active.

- Clinical manifestations of arbovirus infections include fever, rash, arthritis, encephalitis, or hemorrhagic fever.

Classification of Arboviruses

Arboviruses come from various viral families, including:

Flaviviridae (Flaviviruses)

- Dengue virus (DENV): Dengue fever
- Zika virus: Zika fever
- Yellow fever virus (YFV): Yellow fever
- Japanese encephalitis virus (JEV): Japanese encephalitis
- West Nile virus (WNV): West Nile fever

Togaviridae (Alphaviruses)

- Chikungunya virus (CHIKV): Chikungunya fever.
- Equine encephalitis viruses: Encephalitis.

Bunyaviridae (Bunyaviruses)

- Rift Valley fever virus (RVFV): Rift Valley fever.

Reoviridae

- Colorado tick fever virus: Colorado tick fever.
- Identification of infecting virus can be done by isolation of virus from blood, CSF (if there is encephalitis) or other specimens. Serological diagnosis can be made by demonstrating rising antibody titres usually by complement fixation or hemagglutination inhibition. IgM capture ELISA permits early diagnosis.

TABLE 1.15: Common arboviruses and the diseases caused by them

Arbovirus	Disease	Transmitted by (vector)	Clinical manifestations
Chikungunya virus	Chikungunya fever	Aedes mosquito	Fever, arthritis
Dengue virus	Dengue fever	Aedes mosquito	Fever, rash, hemorrhagic fever
Yellow fever virus	Yellow fever	Aedes mosquito	Fever, jaundice, hemorrhagic fever
Zika virus	Zika virus disease	Aedes mosquito	
Japanese encephalitis virus	Japanese encephalitis	Culex mosquito	Encephalitis
West Nile virus	West Nile fever, encephalitis	Culex mosquito	Fever, rash, hepatitis, encephalitis
Kyasanur forest disease virus	Kyasanur forest disease	Tick	Encephalitis, hemorrhagic fever
Colorado tick fever virus	Colorado tick fever	Tick	Fever, myalgia, encephalitis, hemorrhagic fever

Q. Yellow fever.

Etiology

- Yellow fever is a viral hemorrhagic fever caused by yellow fever virus which is a flavivirus. The disease was labeled "yellow" because of profound jaundice observed in affected individuals. It is a disease of monkeys found in Africa and South America. It has not been reported from Asia.
- The infection is transmitted by *Aedes aegypti* mosquito from monkeys to humans (urban areas). Also transmitted by Haemagogus and Sabethes (jungle transmission in South America).
- Yellow fever is an internationally notifiable disease.

Pathogenesis

The virus is transmitted via the saliva of an infected mosquito. Local replication of the virus takes place in the skin and regional lymph nodes with subsequent dissemination to all parts of the body. Liver is the most important organ affected in yellow fever. Hepatocellular damage is characterized by lobular steatosis, necrosis, and apoptosis with subsequent formation of Councilman bodies (degenerative eosinophilic hepatocytes). Other important organs affected are kidneys, lymph nodes, spleen, brain and bone marrow. The terminal phase is marked by delirium, stupor, and coma due to cerebral edema and microscopic perivascular hemorrhage.

Clinical Features

- Yellow fever is a hemorrhagic fever with hepatic necrosis. The incubation period varies from 3 to 6 days.
- Patients present with high fever, headache, retrobulbar pain, arthralgia, a flushed face and conjunctival suffusion. Relative bradycardia (Faget sign) is present from the second day onwards. The patient then makes an apparent recovery and feels well for many days. Thereafter again patient develops increasing fever, jaundice and hapatomegaly. Hemorrhages, hematemesis, melena, and encephalopathy occur due to extensive hepatic involvement.
- Disseminated intravascular coagulation (DIC), induced by liver dysfunction, leads to consumption of platelets and clotting factors.
- Tachypnea and hypoxia with impending respiratory failure may develop as a consequence of sepsis and acute respiratory distress syndrome (ARDS).
- In late stages of disease, shock and multi-organ dysfunction syndrome (MODS) dominate the clinical picture.

Diagnosis

- LFT shows raised bilirubin, AST, ALT and prolonged prothrombin time.
- Complete blood count usually shows leukopenia and thrombocytopenia.
- Serology: Enzyme-linked immunosorbent assay (ELISA) can identify IgM antibody against yellow fever virus.

- Detection of yellow fever antigen using monoclonal enzyme immunoassay in serum specimens.
- Detection of viral genome sequences in tissue or in blood or other body fluid using polymerase chain reaction (PCR) assay.
- Histopathology: Liver biopsy is contraindicated due to risk of hemorrhage. However, it can be done for postmortem confirmation of diagnosis. Findings include mid-zone necrosis, fatty degeneration and intracellular hyaline necrosis (Councilman bodies).
- Urine analysis: Usually shows severe albuminuria which is a constant feature in yellow fever and its presence helps differentiate yellow fever from other causes of viral hepatitis.

Treatment

- There is no specific treatment. Only supportive treatment is required. Bed rest, analgesics, and maintenance of fluid and electrolyte balance are important.
- Fresh frozen plasma is given to actively bleeding patients due to prolonged prothrombin time.
- A nasogastric or orogastric tube may be required to provide nutritional support.
- Patients with renal failure or refractory acidosis may require dialysis.

Prevention

- It is easily prevented by a live attenuated Yellow fever vaccine, which provides lifelong immunity with a single dose. Recommended for travelers to endemic areas. Some countries require an international certificate of vaccination for entry. The certificate is valid 10 days after vaccination and lasts for a lifetime. It is contraindicated in infants of less than 6 months, pregnant women, immunocompromised persons, and people with severe egg allergies (since the vaccine is produced in eggs).

Q. Describe the etiology, pathogenesis, clinical features, diagnosis and management of dengue fever.

Q. Dengue hemorrhagic fever.

Etiology

- Dengue fever is a viral hemorrhagic fever caused by dengue virus which belongs to Flavivirus family. There are four closely related dengue viruses (dengue 1–4).
- Dengue is the most common arthropod-borne viral (arboviral) illness in humans.

Epidemiology

- It is mainly found in Asia and Africa and is transmitted by the daytime-biting female *Aedes aegypti* mosquito.
- Occurs mostly during and shortly after the rainy season.
- Most often affects children.
- Humans are infective during the viremic stage which lasts for 3 days.
- Mosquitoes become infective about 2 weeks after feeding on an infected individual, and remain so for the rest of their lives.

Pathogenesis

- Primary infection leads to classic dengue fever. Dengue hemorrhagic fever (DHF) and dengue shock syndrome (DSS) are due to reinfection by a different serotype of dengue virus. Prior infection with a serotype leads to antibody production and sensitizes the person to reinfection. Reinfection with a different serotype leads to enhanced antibody-mediated macrophage activation. Macrophages produce vasoactive inflammatory mediators which result in vascular leak. Severe vascular leak results in shock.
- Endothelial damage also leads to hemorrhagic manifestations. Hemorrhage is often widespread and associated with pleural effusions and ascites. Focal hepatic necrosis, immune complex–mediated glomerulonephritis, and transient bone marrow suppression may be seen.

Clinical Features

- Clinical manifestations can be of 3 types (WHO 1997 classification)
    - Classic dengue fever
    - Dengue hemorrhagic fever (DHF)
    - Dengue shock syndrome (DSS)

Classic Dengue Fever

- Presents as a nonspecific biphasic (saddle back fever) febrile illness.
- Incubation period is 4–5 days.
- Disease is more severe in adults than children. About 80% of infected infants and children remain asymptomatic.
- The disease starts with sudden onset fever, chills, headache, conjunctival suffusion, myalgia, joint pain, and severe backache. Because of severe muscle, joint and bone pains, it is also called "breakbone" fever.
- A maculopapular rash may appear in over 50% of cases. Rash spares palms and soles. Petechiae may appear all over the body but more prominent on the extensor surface of the limbs.
- The fever subsides after 3–4 days for a couple of days, and returns again in a mild form and subsides.

Dengue Hemorrhagic Fever

- Severe form of dengue fever.
- Dengue hemorrhagic fever typically begins like classic dengue fever. The initial fever lasts approximately 2–7 days. However, in persons with dengue hemorrhagic fever, the fever reappears, giving a biphasic or saddleback fever curve.
- The critical feature of dengue hemorrhagic fever is plasma leakage. Plasma leakage is caused by increased capillary permeability and may manifest as hemoconcentration (≥20% rise in hematocrit above baseline), as well as pleural effusion and ascites. Bleeding is caused by capillary fragility and thrombocytopenia and may manifest in various forms, ranging from petechial skin hemorrhages to life-threatening gastrointestinal bleeding. Hypotension occurs due to hemorrhages.

Dengue Shock Syndrome

- As the term implies, dengue shock syndrome is essentially dengue hemorrhagic fever with progression into circulatory failure, with ensuing hypotension and shock. This is an even more severe form of the disease.
- Aggressive fluid replacement is required to correct the intravascular fluid deficits.

WHO 2009 Classification

- In 2009, the WHO introduced a revised classification scheme consisting of the following categories:
  - Dengue without warning signs
  - Dengue with warning signs
  - Severe dengue.

Dengue without Warning Signs

- *A presumptive diagnosis of dengue infection may be made in the setting of residence in or travel to an endemic area plus fever and two of the following:*
  - Nausea/vomiting
  - Rash
  - Headache, eye pain, muscle ache, or joint pain
  - Leukopenia
  - Positive tourniquet test

Dengue with Warning Signs

- *Dengue with warning signs of severe infection includes dengue infection as defined above in addition to any of the following:*
  - Abdominal pain or tenderness
  - Persistent vomiting
  - Clinical fluid accumulation (ascites, pleural effusion)
  - Mucosal bleeding
  - Lethargy or restlessness
  - Hepatomegaly >2 cm
  - Increase in hematocrit concurrent with rapid decrease in platelet count
  - Issues related to plasma leakage are described further above. (*See* 'Dengue hemorrhagic fever' above.)

Severe Dengue

- *Severe dengue includes infection with at least one of the following:*
  - Severe plasma leakage leading to:
    - Shock
    - Fluid accumulation with respiratory distress
  - Severe bleeding (as evaluated by clinician)
  - Severe organ involvement:
    - Aspartate aminotransferase (AST) or alanine aminotransferase (ALT) ≥1000 units/L
    - Impaired consciousness
    - Organ failure

Investigations

Direct Detection of the Virus (early phase: days 1–5)

These tests detect viral components in the blood and are most useful in the first few days of illness.

NS1 antigen test

- Detects non-structural protein 1 (NS1) of the dengue virus.
- Positive within 1–5 days of fever onset.
- Rapid test kits available, but ELISA-based tests are more reliable.

RT-PCR (reverse transcription polymerase chain reaction)

- Detects viral RNA in the blood.
- High sensitivity in the first 1–5 days of illness.
- Confirms the serotype (DENV-1, DENV-2, DENV-3, or DENV-4).

Indirect Detection (antibody tests) (late phase: days 5–10+)

- These tests detect immune response to the dengue virus.

IgM antibody test (Dengue ELISA/ICT)

- Appears around days 5–7 and stays for 2–3 months.
- Useful for diagnosing recent infection.

IgG antibody test

- Appears later (days 7–10) and can persist for years.
- High IgG levels suggest past infection or secondary dengue.
- IgM-/IgG+ in early illness suggests secondary dengue, which has a higher risk of severe disease.

Dengue duo test (Combo NS1 and IgM/IgG Rapid Test)

- Detects both NS1 antigen and antibodies in a single test.
- Helps differentiate early and late-stage infections.

Other Tests

- Low WBC counts, thrombocytopenia and altered LFT. Thrombocytopenia is an important feature. Platelet count should be monitored daily.
- Hematocrit (Hct) level: Rising hematocrit (≥20% increase) → Indicates plasma leakage (dengue hemorrhagic fever). Hematocrit drop + low platelets → Suggests internal bleeding.
- Elevated AST/ALT (>1000 U/L): Suggests liver involvement in severe dengue.
- Prolonged PT, APTT: Suggests bleeding risk in severe dengue.
- Chest X-ray may show pleural effusion.
- Ultrasound: May show pleural effusion, ascites, pericardial effusion (polyserositis), and a thickened gallbladder wall.

Treatment

- There is no specific treatment for dengue. Treatment is mainly supportive. Paracetamol is used to treat fever and body aches.
- Do not use NSAIDs (ibuprofen, aspirin, diclofenac) → Can increase bleeding risk.

- IV fluids and blood transfusions are given to replace intravascular volume loss.
- Platelet transfusions: Indications are as follows:
    - **Severe bleeding irrespective of platelet count:** Gastrointestinal bleeding, intracranial hemorrhage, massive hematuria, pulmonary hemorrhage (coughing up blood).
    - **Platelet count <20,000/mm³ with significant risk factors for bleeding:** Persistent mucosal bleeding (e.g. gums, nose**), l**iver dysfunction (elevated PT/INR, low fibrinogen), dengue with coagulopathy (disseminated intravascular coagulation—DIC), Dengue shock syndrome with worsening organ failure.
    - **Platelet count <10,000/mm³:** Even without active bleeding (risk of spontaneous hemorrhage).

Prevention

- *Mosquito control:* elimination of breeding sites, fogging.
- *Personal protection against mosquito bites*: Protective clothing, mosquito repellents, use of mosquito nets, installation of window/door screens to keep mosquitoes out.
- *Dengue vaccines*: Two different vaccines have been licensed for use and are available in some countries.
    - **CYD-TDV (Dengvaxia):** Live attenuated tetravalent vaccine. WHO-recommended, approved in multiple countries for people aged 9–45 years with previous dengue infection. Not for dengue-naïve individuals (can increase severe dengue risk on first infection). Pre-vaccination screening needs to be done to confirm past dengue infection. Requires three doses (0, 6, and 12 months).
    - **TAK-003 (Qdenga):** This is also a live-attenuated tetravalent vaccine, approved in some countries. Provides protection against all four dengue virus serotypes. Given as two doses, 3 months apart. Advantages of this vaccine are it ccan be given to dengue-naïve individuals and only two-dose are required.

Q. Ebola virus disease.

- Ebola virus disease (formerly known as Ebola hemorrhagic fever) is a severe, often fatal illness, with a case fatality rate of up to 90%. It is one of the world's most virulent diseases.

Etiology

- Ebola is a RNA virus. It is a member of the family *Filoviridae*, taken from the Latin *"filum,"* meaning thread-like, based upon their filamentous structure. Marburg virus is also a Filovirus and causes illness similar to Ebola virus **(Fig. 1.39)**.
- The genus Ebolavirus is currently classified into 6 species: Sudan, Zaire, Tai Forest, Reston, Bundibugyo and Bombali). The Zaire species of Ebola virus is among the most virulent human pathogens known. The 2014 outbreak of Ebola virus disease in West Africa is due to *Zaire ebolavirus*.

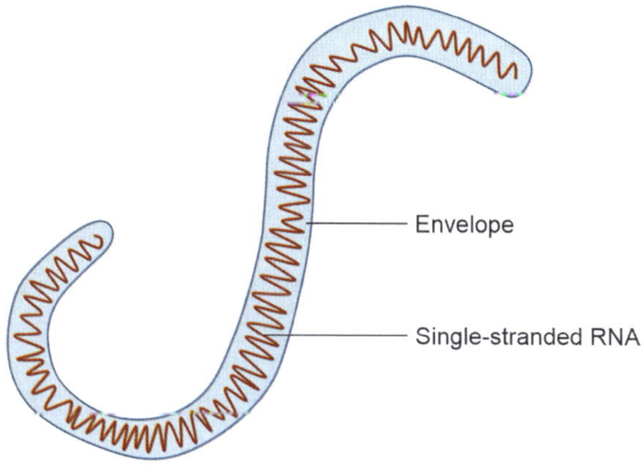

Figure 1.39: Filum shaped Ebola virus

Epidemiology

- Ebola virus disease (EVD) first appeared in 1976 in 2 simultaneous outbreaks, one in Nzara, Sudan, and the other in Yambuku, Democratic Republic of Congo. The latter occurred in a village near the Ebola River, from which the disease takes its name. In addition to causing human infections, Ebola virus has also spread to wild nonhuman primates, such as macaques, chimpanzee and gorilla in Central Africa. This has also triggered some human epidemics due to handling of and/or consumption of sick or dead animals by local villagers as a source of food.
- The 2014 outbreak of Ebola virus disease in West Africa is due to Zaire ebolavirus. Since then, there have been several outbreaks of the *Zaire* species in the Democratic Republic of the Congo, and an outbreak of the Sudan species in Uganda.

Transmission

- The reservoir host of Ebola virus is not known. It is thought that various bat species may serve as a source of infection for both humans and wild primates. Ebola is introduced into the human population through close contact with the blood, secretions, organs or other bodily fluids of infected animals such as chimpanzees, gorillas, bats, and monkeys.
- Human to human transmission occurs through direct conact (through broken skin or mucous membranes) with the blood, secretions, organs or other bodily fluids of infected people, and with fomites contaminated with these fluids.
- Burial ceremonies in which mourners have direct contact with the body of the deceased person can also play a role in the transmission of Ebola.
- People remain infectious as long as their blood and body fluids including semen and breast milk contain the virus. Men can transmit the virus through their semen for up to 7 weeks after recovery from illness.

Pathogenesis

- Ebola virus replicates well in virtually all cell types, including endothelial cells, macrophages, and parenchymal cells of multiple organs. Viral replication is associated with cellular necrosis. In addition to sustaining direct damage from viral infection, patients infected with Ebola virus have high circulating levels of proinflammatory cytokines, which contribute to the severity of the illness. The final effect of all this is widespread inflammation, DIC and tissue necrosis.

Clinical Manifestations

- Incubation period is approximately 7–10 days. Humans are not infectious until they develop symptoms.
- Initial symptoms are sudden onset of fever, fatigue, muscle pain, headache and sore throat. This is followed by vomiting, diarrhea, rash, symptoms of impaired kidney and liver function.
- Hemorrhagic phase usually starts after 7 days. This is characterized by uncontrolled internal and external bleeding (e.g. oozing from the gums, epistaxis, bruising, purpura, hematemesis, blood in the stools).
- There may be neurological symptoms (confusion, seizures, coma).
- Disease may progress to multi-organ failure (shock, kidney and liver failure).
- Death occurs due to severe fluid loss, shock, and organ failure in 50–90% of cases.
- Patients without any complications may recover 10–12 days after the onset of disease.

Investigations

- RT-PCR (reverse transcription polymerase chain reaction): Gold standard and is extremely useful for rapid diagnosis.
- ELISA (enzyme-linked immunosorbent assay): Detects Ebola antibodies.
- Virus isolation by cell culture (high-risk, rarely performed).
- Other blood tests:
  - CBC: Low WBC, low platelets.
  - Coagulation profile: Prolonged PT, APTT (DIC).
  - Liver enzymes: Elevated AST, ALT.
  - Kidney function: High creatinine, low urine output.

Treatment

- No virus-specific therapy is available, and at present treatment is mainly supportive.
- Supportive care with oral or intravenous fluids and treatment of specific symptoms improves survival.
- Management of bleeding and coagulopathy: Blood transfusion (if severe anemia), fresh frozen plasma (FFP), platelets, clotting factors if DIC develops.
- Monoclonal antibody therapies: A triple-monoclonal antibody product (atoltivimab, maftivimab, and odesivimab (REGN-EB3) has been approved for treatment of Ebola. Another one is Ansuvimab. All these monoclonal antibodies effectively neutralize the virus.
- Investigational treatments: Remdesivir (used for COVID-19)—Some activity against Ebola. Favipiravir (RNA polymerase inhibitor)—Limited evidence.

Prevention

- Ervebo (rVSV-ZEBOV): Live-attenuated Ebola vaccine (Zaire ebolavirus strain). Approved for high-risk populations (Congo, West Africa).
- Reducing the risk of human-to-human transmission from direct or close contact with people with Ebola symptoms, particularly with their bodily fluids. Barrier nursing precautions should be used while treating a patient with Ebola.
- Reducing the risk of wildlife-to-human transmission from contact with infected fruit bats or monkeys/apes and the consumption of their raw meat.
- Avoid visiting endemic areas.

Complications

- Death due to multiorgan failure and DIC or hemorrhage.
- Late hepatitis, uveitis, and orchitis have been reported, with isolation of virus from semen or detection of PCR products in vaginal secretions for several weeks.

Q. Japanese encephalitis.

Etiology

- This is encephalitis caused by Japanese encephalitis (JE) virus which is a flavivirus.
- JE virus is the most important global cause of arboviral encephalitis.
- It is found throughout Asia, including Russia, Japan, China, India, Pakistan, and Southeast Asia.
- In India it occurs in epidemics, mostly affecting children in Tamil Nadu, West Bengal, Bihar and Assam.

Transmission

- JE virus is transmitted in an enzootic cycle between mosquitoes and vertebrate hosts, primarily pigs and birds such as herons and egrets. Mosquitoes get infected when they feed on these animals and then transfer the virus to humans. It is spread by Culex mosquitoes (most often by *Culex tritaeniorhynchus*). Vaccination of these animals may reduce the transmission of the virus.
- Humans are considered accidental dead-end hosts in the JE virus transmission cycle because they do not develop a level or duration of viremia sufficient to infect mosquitoes. JE virus is not spread from person to person through direct contact. JE virus transmission through blood transfusion has been documented in a JE-endemic area.

Pathogenesis

- Mosquito bite injects JEV into human skin → Virus enters the bloodstream (viremia).
- Primary replication in lymphoid tissues (dendritic cells, macrophages).
- Spreads to the CNS through the blood-brain barrier (BBB).
- Causes neuronal infection and destruction → Direct damage to neurons in the thalamus, basal ganglia, brainstem, spinal cord.

- Cytokine storm and immune response → Causes brain edema, necrosis, and gliosis.
- Increased intracranial pressure (ICP) → Leads to seizures, paralysis, coma.

Clinical Features

- Japanese encephalitis resembles any other viral encephalitis.
- Incubation period is 5–15 days.
- All ages can be affected though children are affected more frequently.
- The encephalitis mainly involves the thalamus and the substantia nigra.
- Patient presents with a prodrome of fever, vertigo, sore throat, and respiratory symptoms. Headache, meningeal signs, photophobia, vomiting and altered mental status follow quickly. Patient may be disoriented and comatose. Cranial nerve palsies, hemiparesis, monoparesis, difficulty in swallowing, and frontal lobe signs are all common. Convulsions and focal signs may appear during the course of the disease.
- The acute encephalitis usually lasts from a few days to as long as 2 to 3 weeks. Complete recovery may take weeks to months.

Investigations

- Initial leukocytosis followed by leukopenia.
- Serological tests: Detection of JEV-specific IgM antibodies in CSF or serum by ELISA (gold standard test).
- PCR (RT-PCR for JEV RNA): Detects JEV RNA in blood or CSF. Useful for early-stage detection.
- CSF analysis: Shows a lymphocytic pleocytosis.
- MRI or CT scan: Both show abnormalities in the thalamus, basal ganglia, midbrain, pons, and medulla.
- EEG (electroencephalography) may show generalized slowing, and epileptiform activity.

Treatment

- There is no specific therapy for Japanese encephalitis. Management is mainly supportive.
- Elevated intracranial pressure, respiratory failure, and convulsions should be managed as per standard protocols.
- Nutrition should be maintained by Ryle's tube feeds. Bladder should be catheterized if the patient is in altered sensorium or comatose. Fluid and electrolyte balance should be maintained.

Prevention

- Japanese encephalitis is the most common vaccine-preventable cause of encephalitis in Asia. A vaccine is available for human use. It is given as two doses administered intramuscularly (IM) on days 0 and 28. WHO recommends JE vaccination in endemic areas and for travelers to high-risk regions.
- Pig population and mosquitoes should be controlled.

Q. Kyasanur forest disease (KFD).

- Kyasanur forest disease (KFD) is an acute febrile illness caused by KFD virus which is a flavivirus. It is named as Kyasanur forest disease because the disease was first recognized in the Kyasanur forest of Shivamogga district, Karnataka.

Epidemiology

- Endemic areas: Karnataka, Kerala, Tamil Nadu, Goa, Maharashtra. In Karnataka, it is found in Shivamogga, Mangaluru, Udupi, Uttara Kannada and Chikkamangalur districts.
- Monkeys (black faced langur and bonnet) are the main reservoirs of this virus **(Fig. 1.40)**.
- Man gets infected when the tick-*Haemophysalis spinigera* bites man after feeding on monkeys. Bites happen usually during summer when people visit the forest area to collect wood.
- Outbreaks occur every 3–5 years, often linked to monkey deaths.
- Human is the dead end in natural cycle of the virus. There is no human to human transmission of KFD.

Clinical Features

- Incubation period is 4–6 days.
- Sudden onset of fever with chills and rigors, severe headache, body ache, backache, orbital pain and weakness. Vomiting and diarrhea can also be there. There can be bleeding manifestations like epistaxis, gum bleeding, hematemesis and melaena. Encephalitis and meningitis may develop in severe cases.
- Examination usually reveals relative bradycardia, hypotension and conjunctival congestion. Lymphadenopathy may be noted in the neck and axilla.
- Fever usually subsides in 10–12 days. However, some patients can have recurrence of fever.

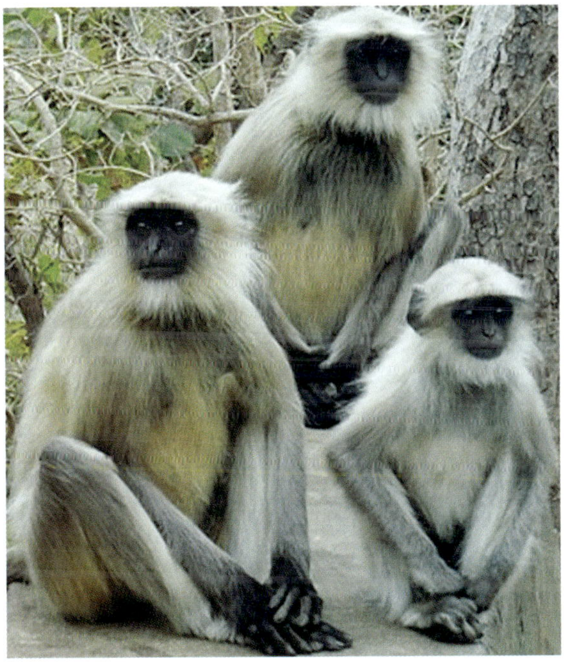

Figure 1.40: Black-faced Langur monkey

Investigations

- Leukopenia and thrombocytopenia.
- Diagnosis can be confirmed by isolation of virus from the blood during fever. Requires specialized lab.
- Detection of IgM antibodies against KFD virus by ELISA.
- RT-PCR or (reverse transcription polymerase chain reaction): Gold standard for early detection.

Treatment

- There is no specific treatment. Only symptomatic and supportive measures ae required. The condition usually resolves without any sequelae. The mortality is 5–10%.

Prevention

- KFDV vaccine (killed whole-virus vaccine) is available for use and is recommended for people in high-risk areas (forest workers, farmers, tourists).
- People should avoid visiting forests when there is death of monkeys. Those visiting the forest area ahould wear protective clothing and apply insect repellants (dimethyl phthalate) and take bath on return.

Q. Chikungunya fever.

- Chikungunya is a mosquito-borne viral disease. Chikungunya virus is a RNA virus that belongs to the family Togaviridae.
- The disease was first identified in Tanzania in 1952 and has since caused outbreaks in Africa, Asia, Europe, and the Americas. The name 'chikungunya' derives from a word in the Makonde language of Tanzania, meaning "to become contorted" and describes the stooped appearance of sufferers with joint pain (arthralgia).
- It is transmitted by the bite of an infected female *Aedes aegypti* and *Aedes albopictus* mosquitoes—the same vectors responsible for dengue and Zika viruses.
- A large epidemic occurred in southern India in 2006 due to the emergence of a new viral variant in immunologically naive population.

Pathogenesis

- Patients with chikungunya fever typically develop viremia within a few days of infection, and the virus directly invades and replicates within the joints.
- Chikungunya virus (CHIKV) causes a self-limiting febrile illness but has profound inflammatory effects on the joints, muscles, and blood vessels. The persistence of inflammatory cytokines in synovial tissue explains why some patients suffer from chronic arthritis-like symptoms long after viral clearance. While severe complications are rare, the disease can be debilitating, particularly in elderly and immunocompromised individuals.

Clinical Features

- Self-limiting illness.
- Incubation period is 3–7 days.
- Characterized by sudden onset of fever, headache, malaise, arthralgias or arthritis, myalgias, and low back pain.
- Joint symptoms can be quite painful and usually involve small and large joints. Patient may not be able to walk.
- A maculopapular skin rash is seen (often on the trunk and limbs) in approximately half of cases on the 2nd–5th day of illness.
- Fever subsides within seven days, but joint pain may persist for weeks to months.

Laboratory Features

- Leukopenia, anemia, thrombocytopenia, and elevated liver enzymes.
- Serological tests: Such as enzyme-linked immunosorbent assays (ELISA) can detect the presence of IgM and IgG anti-chikungunya antibodies.
- RT-PCR (reverse transcription polymerase chain reaction): Detects viral RNA in the blood during the acute phase (0–7 days).
- Virus isolation: Possible in specialized labs but not commonly used in routine diagnostics.

Treatment

- There is no specific antiviral treatment. Only supportive treatment is required such as NSAIDs for fever and joint pain.
- For persistent joint pain even after 2–3 weeks, steroids can be used. A typical initial dose is prednisone 10–20 mg daily for five days, depending upon severity, then tapered off over the next 10 days. More severely affected patients may require steroids for 1–2 months.

Prevention

- Mosquito control.
- Personal protection against mosquito bites.
- A vaccine is available which can be used for high risk individuals in endemic areas.

Q. Discuss the transmission, pathogenesis, clinical features, investigations and management of human immunodeficiency virus (HIV) infection.

Q. Enumerate the AIDS indicator conditions.

- Human immunodeficiency virus (HIV) is a single stranded RNA virus belonging to retroviridae family and lentivirus genus **(Fig. 1.41)**.
- There are two types of HIV virus, **HIV-1** (most common, responsible for the global pandemic), and **HIV-2** (less virulent, found mainly in West Africa).
- HIV virus is spherical in shape and has a lipid bilayer derived from host cell membrane, studded with glycoprotein **(gp)120 and gp41 spikes.** These spikes are essential for virus entry into the cells. The virus has a cone-shaped protein core made of **p24 protein** (important for diagnosis). The core contains two copies of the single-stranded RNA genome and viral enzymes. Important viral enzymes are: Reverse transcriptase (converts viral RNA into

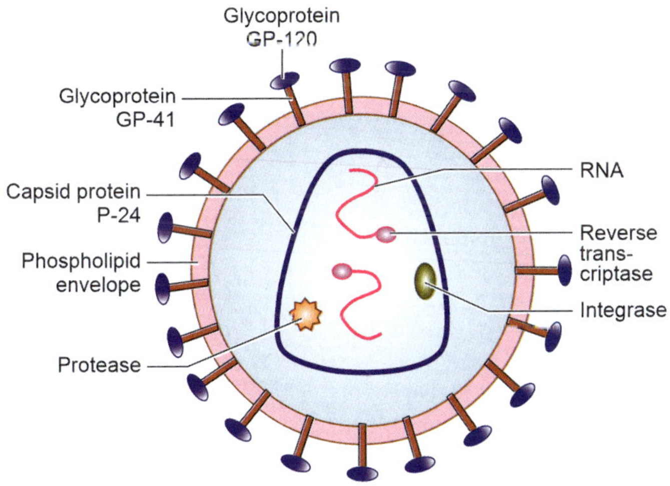

Figure 1.41: HIV virus

DNA), integrase (integrates viral DNA into host genome), and protease (cleaves viral polyproteins for maturation).

- HIV infection leads to AIDS (acquired immunodeficiency syndrome) a condition in which the immune system begins to fail, leading to life-threatening opportunistic infections. Immune deficiency is due to destruction of CD4 lymphocytes.
- AIDS was first recognized in the United States in 1981 in male homosexuals. Since then, it has grown to become a major pandemic in the world. It has become the second leading cause of disease burden world-wide and the leading cause of death in Africa. In 1983, HIV was isolated from a patient with lymphadenopathy, and by 1984 it was demonstrated clearly to be the causative agent of AIDS.
- Till now more than 25 million deaths have been attributed to AIDS. The current estimate of worldwide disease prevalence is more than 33 million HIV infections. Two thirds of these cases are in developing countries, mainly sub-Saharan Africa and Southeast Asia.
- Most AIDS cases occur in adults aged 25-49 years (70% of cases).

Transmission of HIV

- Transmission of HIV occurs through almost any body fluid such as blood, vaginal fluid, or breast milk. Within these bodily fluids, HIV is present as both free virus particles and virus within infected immune cells.
- The four major routes of transmission are unsafe sex, contaminated needles, breast milk, occupational exposure (healthcare workers via needlestick injuries), and transmission from an infected mother to her baby at birth (vertical transmission). >70% of infections occur because of unsafe sexual practices. Transmission through blood transfusion has largely been eliminated by the universal screening of blood products for HIV.

Pathogenesis

- HIV infects mainly cells of immune system such as helper T cells (CD4+ T cells), macrophages, and dendritic cells. HIV enters into these cells by binding to CD4 receptor through its gp-120 molecule. The virus replicates itself by generating a DNA copy from its RNA by reverse transcriptase. Newly generated viral DNA becomes incorporated into the host DNA. The host cell machinery produces viral proteins. New virions are assembled and released, infecting other CD4+ cells.
- HIV infection leads to fall in CD4+ T cells by three main mechanisms: Direct viral killing of infected cells; increased rates of apoptosis of infected cells; and killing of infected CD4+ T cells by CD8 cytotoxic lymphocytes that recognize infected cells. When CD4+ cell count declines below a critical level, cell-mediated immunity is lost, and the body becomes more susceptible to opportunistic infections and various neoplasms.
- Progressive failure of immune system leads to development of AIDS characterized by development of opportunistic infections and malignancies. The speed of progression of HIV infection to AIDS is variable depending on viral load, host, and environmental factors. Most will progress to AIDS within 10 years of HIV infection.

Clinical Stages and Natural History of HIV Infection

- Clinical HIV infection undergoes 3 distinct phases: Acute HIV infection, chronic HIV infection, and AIDS.

Acute HIV infection (also called primary HIV infection or acute seroconversion syndrome)

- This stage is characterized by rapid viral replication leading to an abundance of virus in the peripheral blood with levels commonly approaching several million viruses per mL. There is a marked drop in the number of circulating CD4+ T cells. It usually occurs 2–6 weeks after exposure to HIV and lasts an average of 28 days. The immune system responds to the replication of virus by activation of CD8+ T cells, and antibody production against the viral antigens. Hence, this phase is also called seroconversion phase.
- Most people develop flu-like illness during this stage. Common symptoms are fever, lymphadenopathy, pharyngitis, rash, myalgia, malaise, aphthous ulcers, hepatosplenomegaly, oral candidiasis, and weight loss. All these signs and symptoms are not specific for HIV infection and can be seen in many other infectious diseases. Hence, diagnosis may be missed at this stage
- During the acute HIV infection stage, the level of HIV in the blood is very high, which greatly increases the risk of HIV transmission.

Chronic HIV Infection (asymptomatic infection)

- Chronic HIV infection can be further subdivided into the following stages:
  - Chronic infection, without AIDS.
  - AIDS, characterized by a CD4 cell count <200 cells/µl or the presence of any AIDS-defining condition.

Chronic infection, without AIDS

- During this stage, strong immunity reduces the viral load and patient may remain asymptomatic except for the possible presence of persistent generalized lymphadenopathy (PGL, defined as enlarged glands at ≥2 extra-inguinal sites). But HIV remains active within lymphoid organs, and also as free viral particles. Patient remains infective during this stage also. CD4 count decreases usually at a rate between 50 and 150 cells/year.
- Patients may experience recurrent or persistent oropharyngeal or vulvovaginal candidiasis, as well as oral hairy leukoplakia. Additionally, seborrheic dermatitis is a common early manifestation of chronic HIV infection.
- Bacterial folliculitis, particularly caused by *Staphylococcus aureus*, is frequently observed.
- Infections caused by herpes simplex virus (HSV), varicella-zoster virus (VZV), human papillomavirus (HPV), and molluscum contagiosum tend to be more severe in HIV-positive individuals, often presenting with frequent recurrences or rapid progression.
- This stage can last from two weeks to ten years or more.

AIDS stage:

- This stage represents the most advanced stage of HIV infection, indicating AIDS (acquired immunodeficiency syndrome). At this stage, the immune system is severely compromised with CD4+ count usually <200 cells/µl. It is characterized by three types of conditions; (1) Severe opportunistic infections, (2) HIV-associated malignancies, and (3) Neurological and systemic conditions.

Severe opportunistic infections

Fungal Infections

- *Pneumocystis jirovecii* pneumonia (PCP)
- Candidiasis (esophageal, bronchial, tracheal, or pulmonary)
- Cryptococcal meningitis (*Cryptococcus neoformans*)
- Disseminated histoplasmosis and coccidioidomycosis

Bacterial Infections

- Tuberculosis (extrapulmonary or disseminated TB)
- Recurrent bacterial pneumonia (>2 episodes in 12 months)
- *Mycobacterium avium* complex (MAC) (disseminated or extra-pulmonary)
- Salmonella septicemia (recurrent non-typhoidal salmonella)

Viral Infections

- Cytomegalovirus (CMV) disease (retinitis, esophagitis, colitis, or CNS involvement)
- Herpes simplex virus (HSV) infection (chronic ulcers >1 month, esophagitis, pneumonitis)
- Progressive multifocal leukoencephalopathy (PML) (JC virus)
- Protozoal infections
- CNS toxoplasmosis (*Toxoplasma gondii*)
- Cryptosporidiosis and isosporiasis (chronic diarrhea >1 month)

HIV-associated malignancies (AIDS-defining cancers)

- Kaposi's sarcoma (KS) (caused by HHV-8).
- Non-Hodgkin's lymphoma (NHL) (including primary CNS lymphoma).
- Invasive cervical cancer (HPV-associated).

Neurological and systemic conditions

- HIV wasting syndrome (unexplained weight loss >10%, chronic diarrhea, weakness, fever).
- HIV-associated encephalopathy (HIV dementia).

Investigations

Screening tests (initial HIV tests)

Rapid HIV tests

- These tests are used for initial rapid diagnosis of HIV (point-of-care) and have high sensitivity.
- HIV rapid antibody tests: Example: TRIDOT, HIV rapid card, determine HIV-1/2. Detects: HIV-1 and HIV-2 antibodies.
  - Sample: Finger-prick blood, serum, plasma, or oral fluid.
  - Time: 5–30 minutes.
  - Limitation: Cannot detect HIV during the "window period" (first 2–8 weeks).
- HIV 4th generation rapid test
  - Detects: HIV-1/2 antibodies + p24 antigen.
  - Advantage: Detects infection earlier than antibody-only tests.

ELISA (enzyme-linked immunosorbent assay)

- 4th generation HIV ELISA (antigen-antibody test)
  - Detects: HIV-1/2 antibodies + p24 antigen.
  - Window period: Detects infection within 2–4 weeks.
  - Accuracy: Very high (sensitivity >99%).
  - Next step: If positive, confirm with a Western blot or HIV RNA test.
- 3rd generation ELISA
  - Detects: Only HIV antibodies.
  - Limitation: Misses very early HIV infections (window period: 3–8 weeks).

Confirmatory tests (to confirm HIV diagnosis)

- If an initial test (e.g. Rapid test or ELISA) is positive, confirmatory testing is done to rule out false-positives.
- Western blot (WB)
  - Detects: HIV-specific proteins (gp120, gp160, gp41, p24, etc.).
  - Used to confirm HIV-1 and HIV-2 infections.
  - Limitation: Takes longer and may be inconclusive in early infection.
- Immunofluorescence assay (IFA)
  - Confirms HIV antibodies using fluorescent-labeled HIV antigens.
  - Used as an alternative to Western Blot.

Early detection tests (for acute HIV and window period)

- These tests detect HIV before antibodies develop, useful in high-risk exposure cases.

HIV RNA PCR (Nucleic acid test, NAT)

- Detects HIV viral RNA (as early as 10–14 days post-exposure).
- Early diagnosis (before antibodies appear).
  Detecting acute HIV infection (window period cases).
  Monitoring viral load in HIV-positive patients.
- Limitation: Expensive and not used for routine screening.

HIV p24 antigen test

- Detects HIV p24 protein (viral core protein).
- Window period: Detects infection as early as 2–4 weeks.
- Often combined with HIV antibody test (4th Gen ELISA).

Monitoring tests (for HIV-positive patients)

- Once diagnosed with HIV, these tests monitor disease progression and treatment response.

CD4 count test

- Measures: CD4 T-cell count (immune function).
- Normal: 500–1500 cells/µl.
- AIDS: CD4 <200 cells/µl.
- Used to decide when to start opportunistic infection prophylaxis.

HIV viral load test (HIV RNA PCR)

- Measures: Amount of HIV RNA in blood (copies/ml).
- Used to: Monitor ART effectiveness, determine disease progression, detect hiv treatment failure.
- Goal of ART: HIV RNA <50 copies/mL (Undetectable viral load).

Other tests

- Hepatitis-B surface antibody (HBsAg).
- Hepatitis-C IgG antibody.
- Hepatitis-A IgG antibody.
- Toxoplasma antibody.
- Cytomegalovirus (CMV) IgG antibody.
- Treponema serology (VDRL and TPHA).
- Chest X-ray.

Treatment of the HIV Infection

- The treatment of HIV infection is based on antiretroviral therapy (ART), which consists of a combination of drugs that suppress the replication of the virus, prevent progression to AIDS, and improve survival.

Goals of HIV Treatment

- Suppress HIV viral load (<50 copies/ml—undetectable)
- Restore and maintain immune function (Increase CD4 count)
- Prevent progression to AIDS and opportunistic infections
- Reduce transmission (Undetectable = Untransmittable)
- Improve quality of life and longevity

When to Initiate ART (anti-retroviral therapy)

- Latest guidelines recommend that ART should be started immediately for all people with a confirmed HIV diagnosis regardless of CD4 count.

Classes of Antiretroviral Drugs

- *See* **Table 1.16**.

First-line ART Regimens

- ART consists of a **combination of three drugs** from at least **two different classes** to ensure viral suppression and prevent drug resistance.
- First-line ART (preferred regimen).

Drug class	Preferred medications
NRTI (Nucleoside reverse transcriptase inhibitor)	Tenofovir (TDF/TAF) + Lamivudine (3TC) or Emtricitabine (FTC)
INSTI (Integrase inhibitor)	Dolutegravir (DTG)

- **Preferred regimen:** Tenofovir + Lamivudine or Emtricitabine + Dolutegravir. This combination (TLD) can be given once daily.

Alternative ART Regimens (if integrase inhibitor is contraindicated)

- Tenofovir + Lamivudine or Emtricitabine + Efavirenz (NNRTI-based).
- Tenofovir + Lamivudine or Emtricitabine + Atazanavir/Ritonavir (Protease inhibitor based).

ART Monitoring (after starting treatment)

- CD4 count: Monitors immune function (every 6–12 months).
- Viral load (HIV RNA PCR): Should become undetectable (<50 copies/mL) within 6 months.

TABLE 1.16: Antiretroviral drugs

Class	Mechanism of action	Examples	Common side effects
Nucleoside/nucleotide reverse transcriptase inhibitors (NRTIs)	Block reverse transcriptase, preventing viral replication	Tenofovir (TDF, TAF), lamivudine (3TC), emtricitabine (FTC), zidovudine (AZT), abacavir (ABC), stavudine (d4T), didanosine (ddI)	Lactic acidosis, peripheral neuropathy, renal toxicity (TDF), anemia (AZT)
Non-nucleoside reverse transcriptase inhibitors (NNRTIs)	Directly inhibit reverse transcriptase	Efavirenz (EFV), nevirapine (NVP), Etravirine (ETR), rilpivirine (RPV), doravirine (DOR)	Rash, liver toxicity, CNS side effects (EFV)
Integrase strand transfer inhibitors (INSTIs)	Block viral integration into host DNA	Dolutegravir (DTG), raltegravir (RAL), elvitegravir (EVG), bictegravir (BIC), cabotegravir (CAB)	Insomnia, weight gain, headache
Protease inhibitors (PIs)	Inhibit HIV protease enzyme, preventing viral maturation	Atazanavir (ATV), darunavir (DRV), lopinavir (LPV), ritonavir (RTV), saquinavir (SQV), indinavir (IDV), tipranavir (TPV), fosamprenavir (FPV)	GI intolerance, lipid abnormalities, Insulin resistance
Entry inhibitors (Fusion and CCR5 antagonists)	Prevent virus from entering host cells	Maraviroc (MVC) (CCR5 antagonist), enfuvirtide (T-20) (Fusion inhibitor)	Injection site reactions (T-20), hepatotoxicity (MVC)
Post-attachment inhibitors	Blocks HIV from attaching to CD4 receptor	Ibalizumab (IBA)	Infusion reactions
Capsid inhibitor	Prevents proper assembly of viral capsid	Lenacapavir (LEN)	Injection site reactions

- Liver and kidney function tests: Monitors ART toxicity.
- Lipid profile and blood sugar: Needed for long-term ART effects.

Reduction of HIV Transmission (mother-to-child and person-to-person)

Prevention of Mother-to-child Transmission

- Transmission of HIV from mother to child can occur during pregnancy, labour and delivery, or breast feeding. Preventing mother-to-child transmission (MTCT) of HIV is crucial to reducing neonatal HIV infections. This can be achieved through Antiretroviral Therapy (ART) during pregnancy, safe delivery practices, and postnatal prophylaxis for the newborn.
- During antenatal period, HIV-infected women who are pregnant should start antiretroviral treatment with at least three medications. Recommended regimens are Tenofovir + Lamivudine + Dolutegravir (TLD). During labor, intravenous administration of ZDV, 2 mg/kg loading dose, followed by a continuous infusion of 1 mg/kg per hour until delivery should be given.
- Neonatal HIV prophylaxis: Neonates born to HIV-positive mothers should receive antiretroviral (ARV) prophylaxis immediately after birth to reduce the risk of perinatal HIV transmission as per the following regimens.
    - Mother on effective ART with undetectable viral load (<50 copies/ml) before delivery: Zidovudine (AZT) alone for 4 weeks (28 days).
    - Mother not on ART or viral load >50 copies/mL at delivery: 1. Zidovudine + Nevirapine or 2. Zidovudine + Lamivudine + Nevirapine (triple ARV prophylaxis) for 6 weeks (42 days).
    - Test infant for HIV at birth, 6 weeks, 3–6 months, and 18 months.
- Because HIV can be transmitted in breast milk, women with HIV should not breastfeed their babies. Baby milk formula is a safe and healthy alternative to breast milk in such situations.

Prevention of Person-to-person Transmission

- Precautions regarding sexual practices and injection drug use.
- Universal screening of donor blood and blood products for HIV.
- Occupational exposure precautions: Healthcare workers should use PPE (gloves, goggles) when handling blood or body fluid of HIV infected patient.
- Pre-Exposure Prophylaxis (PrEP) for HIV-negative individuals at high risk: Tenofovir + Emtricitabine daily reduces risk by 99% in sexual transmission. Recommended for: HIV-negative partners in relationship with HIV positive individuals, men who have sex with men (MSM), and sex workers and high-risk individuals.
- Post exposure prophylaxis (*see* below for details) if there is accidental exposure to a known source of HIV.
- Vaccines are under development. So far, no HIV vaccine has provided long-term protection in large trials.

Q. Opportunistic infections in AIDS.

- Opportunistic infections are those which usually occur in a person with weakened immune system such as patients with AIDS.
- Opportunistic infections usually occur when CD4 count is below 200. However, certain opportunistic infections in HIV infected person indicate that the person is having AIDS irrespective of the CD4 count.
- An opportunistic infection may be caused by various pathogens-bacteria, viruses, fungi, or protozoa.

Common Opportunistic Infections in HIV

Viral

- Cytomegalovirus (CMV): CMV retinitis.
- Human herpes virus 8 (HHV-8): Kaposi's sarcoma.
- Human papillomavirus (HPV): Cervical cancer.
- Epstein barr virus (EBV): Primary CNS lymphoma.

Bacterial

- Mycobacterium tubercrulosis: pulmonary or extra-pulmonary tuberculosis.
- Mycobacterium avium complex (MAC): Disseminated infection with multi-organ involvement.

Fungal

- Candida: Oropharyngeal and esophageal candidiasis.
- *Pneumocystis jirovecii*: Pneumonia.
- Cryptococcosis: Usually manifests as meningitis.
- Histoplasmosis: Disseminated infection.
- Coccidioidomycosis: Disseminated infection.
- Microsporidia: Causes diarrhea.

Protozoal

- *Toxoplasm godii*: Toxoplasmosis of brain.
- Cryptosporidiosis: Intestinal infection leading to diarrhea.
- Isosporiasis: Intestinal infection leading to diarrhea.

Prophylaxis for Common Opportunistic Infections

- Every attempt should be made to prevent opportunistic infections in HIV infected patients as they cause significant morbidity and mortality.
- Prophylaxis of opportunistic infection is usually based on the CD4 count. If the CD4 count increases above the levels that are used to initiate prophylaxis—prophylactic therapy can be discontinued **(Table 1.17)**.

Treatment of Opportunistic Infections in HIV

See **Table 1.18.**

Q. Post exposure prophylaxis (PEP) for HIV.

- Immediate decontamination: wash the area with soap and water. Small wounds and punctures may be cleansed with an antiseptic such as alcohol, iodophors, or chlorhexidine. For mucous membrane exposure, irrigate the area with water or sterile saline.

TABLE 1.17: Prophylaxis for opportunistic infections

CD4 count	Opportunistic infection against which prophylaxis is indicated	Drugs used for prophylaxis
All HIV-infected patients with positive PPD reactions (defined as >5 mm of induration for HIV-infected patients)	*Mycobacterium tuberculosis*	Isoniazid, 300 mg daily, plus pyridoxine 50 mg orally daily, for 9 months
CD4 counts ≤200 cells/µl	*Pneumocystis jiroveci* pneumonia	Trimethoprim-sulfamethoxazole, one double-strength tablet (960 mg) daily or dapsone 50–100 mg daily
CD4 counts <100 cells/µl with a positive IgG toxoplasma serology	Toxoplasmosis	Trimethoprim-sulfamethoxazole (one double-strength tablet daily)
CD4 counts <50 cells/µl	*Mycobacterium avium* complex (MAC) infection	Azithromycin (1200 mg orally weekly) or clarithromycin (500 mg orally twice daily)

TABLE 1.18: Treatment of opportunistic infections and complications of HIV

Opportunistic infection or complication	Treatment
Mycobacterium tuberculosis	Standard 4 drug antitubercular therapy for 6–9 months. ART is delayed for a period of 2–8 weeks following initiation of antitubercular therapy to prevent IRIS (Immune reconstitution inflammatory syndrome)
***Pneumocystis jiroveci* infection**	Trimethoprim-sulfamethoxazole, 15 mg/kg/d (based on trimethoprim component) orally or intravenously for 21 days. PLUS Prednisone (if PaO_2 <70 mm Hg)
***Mycobacterium avium* complex infection**	Clarithromycin + Ethambutol ± Rifabutin for ≥12 months
Toxoplasmosis	Sulfadiazine and pyrimethamine combined with leucovorin for 4–6 weeks minimum.
Cryptococcal meningitis	Amphotericin B with flucytosine intravenoulsy for 2 weeks, followed by fluconazole orally.
Cytomegalovirus retinitis	Valganciclovir or ganciclovir or foscarnet 3–6 months
Esophageal candidiasis or recurrent vaginal candidiasis	Fluconazole, 100–200 mg orally daily for 2–3 weeks.
Herpes simplex infection and herpes zoster	Acyclovir or famciclovir or valacyclovir or foscarnet.

Testing of Source of Exposure

- If the source person is available, test them as soon as possible to determine whether post-exposure prophylaxis (PEP) is needed for the exposed person. HIV rapid test (antibody test) is recommended as the results are available immediately. If HIV rapid test is negative, and the source is suspected to be in the HIV window period (with recent high-risk behavior), an HIV RNA test may be needed for confirmation.
- If the **source is HIV-negative**, PEP is **not needed**.
- If the **source is HIV-positive or unknown, start PEP immediately** while awaiting results of further tests.
- Also check source person's HBV and HCV status as there is a possibility of these infections also.

Testing of Exposed Person

- Any person exposed to potential source of HIV (e.g. needle-stick injury, sexual exposure, or blood contact) should be tested for HIV immediately and at follow-up intervals.
- Test the exposed person immediately for HIV, HCV antibody, HbsAg, and in females of childbearing age, pregnancy testing. HIV testing must be done before starting PEP.
- Immediate HIV testing (baseline): Perform 4th generation hiv antigen/antibody test. If high-risk exposure, consider HIV RNA PCR.
- If HIV positive → means, pre-existing HIV infection, start full ART instead of PEP.
- If negative → No established HIV infection, start PEP.
- Repeat HIV testing should be done at 4 and 12 weeks postexposure. If any test at 4 or 12 weeks is positive, confirm with an HIV RNA PCR and initiate full ART. Testing again at 6 months is considered if there is high-risk exposure.

Recommended PEP Regimen

- PEP should be initiated as soon as possible, ideally within 72 hours of exposure (earlier = better). First dose of PEP should be offered to the exposed worker while the evaluation is underway.
- Three-drug PEP regimens are now the recommended regimens for all exposures due to the safety and tolerability of new HIV drugs. The preferred 3-drug PEP regimen is as follows:
- **Preffered regimen: Tenofovir + Emtricitabine + Dolutegravir or Raltegravir (TED or TER)**. This combination is given once daily and is well tolerated.

- **Alternative regimen: Zidovudine + Lamivudine + Lopinavir/Ritonavir or Atazanavir/Ritonavir** (Effect of atazanavir or lopinavir can be boosted by adding ritonavir). This combination is used for pregnant women or dolutegravir contraindications.
- Duration of PEP is 28 days.

Q. Immune reconstitution inflammatory syndrome (IRIS).

- The term "immune reconstitution inflammatory syndrome" (IRIS) refers to a collection of inflammatory disorders associated with paradoxical worsening of preexisting infectious processes following the initiation of antiretroviral therapy (ART) in HIV patients. IRIS has been reported in 10–32% of patients starting ART.

Pathogenesis

- As the immune function improves following the initiation of ART, systemic or local inflammatory reactions may occur at the sites of preexisting infections. The syndrome appears to result from an unbalanced immune reconstitution of effector and regulatory T cells in patients receiving ART. Macrophages and natural killer cells are also suspected to play a role in IRIS.
- Presence of opportunistic infection at the time of initiation of ART is a clear risk factor for the development of IRIS. A variety of mycobacterial, viral, fungal and parasitic opportunistic infections are associated with IRIS. *Mycobacterium tuberculosis* (TB) is one of the commonest pathogen known to cause IRIS.
- Determining whether clinical deterioration is caused by treatment failure, IRIS, or both requires assessment of the persistence of active infections with cultures and can be difficult.

Risk Factors for IRIS

- IRIS is more likely in patients with:
  - Low baseline CD4 count (<50 cells/µl).
  - High HIV viral load at ART initiation.
  - Rapid immune recovery after starting ART.
  - Early ART initiation during opportunistic infection treatment (e.g. TB, Cryptococcus).

Clinical Features

- Patient usually presents with worsening or appearance of new clinical or radiological features. Manifestations depend on the underlying opportunistic infection.
- IRIS usually develops within 4–8 weeks after ART initiation.
- Can be fatal in severe cases (e.g. cryptococcal IRIS with brain edema).

Common Infections Associated with IRIS

- *See* **Table 1.19**.

TABLE 1.19: Common infections associated with IRIS

Infection	Symptoms of IRIS
Tuberculosis (TB)	High fever, worsening lung infiltrates, lymph node enlargement, worsening pleural effusion and pericardial effusion. Pre-existing CNS tuberculosis may worsen due to inflammation and present with worsening of headache and altered mental status
Cryptococcal meningitis	Severe headaches, fever, increased intracranial pressure
Cytomegalovirus (CMV) retinitis	Worsening eye inflammation, vision loss
Mycobacterium avium complex (MAC)	Fever, lymphadenopathy, worsening lung disease
Progressive multifocal leukoencephalopathy (PML)	New or worsening neurological symptoms
Toxoplasmosis	Worsening brain lesions, seizures

Treatment

- Opportunistic infections should be optimally treated. Non-steroidal anti-inflammatory drugs (NSAIDs) can be used for milder manifestations of IRIS and steroids for cases with severe inflammation. ART should be continued unless there is life threatening IRIS.

Prognosis

- Majority of patients with IRIS have a self-limiting disease course. However, significant morbidity and mortality may be seen with ARDS and CNS involvement.

Prevention

- ART should be initiated before the onset of severe immunodeficiency.
- Screen and treat OIs before starting ART.
- Delay ART initiation in some infections (e.g. Cryptococcus, TB meningitis). WHO recommends that TB should be treated first and after 2–4 weeks, ART to be initiated.
- Monitor patients closely in the first 2 months after starting ART.

Q. Coronavirus infection.

- Coronaviruses are RNA viruses whose name derives from their characteristic crown-like appearance in electron microsope. Coronaviruses are important human and animal pathogens. They can cause upper and lower respiratory tract infections which can be severe.
- Coronaviruses are classified into four genera: Alpha, beta, gamma, and delta coronaviruses. The human coronaviruses (HCoVs) are in two of these genera: alpha coronaviruses and beta coronaviruses. Beta coronaviruses include Middle East respiratory syndrome coronavirus (MERS-CoV), and the severe acute respiratory syndrome coronavirus (SARS-CoV).
- A novel coronavirus, designated as SARS-CoV-2 was identified as the cause of a cluster of pneumonia cases in Wuhan, a city in China, at the end of 2019.

This virus is a beta-coronavirus (same group as SARS virus). It subsequently spread throughout China and elsewhere, becoming a global health emergency. The disease caused by SARS-CoV-2 is designates as COVID-19 (which stands for coronavirus disease 2019).

Classification of Coronaviruses

- Coronaviruses belong to the family **Coronaviridae** and are classified into four genera **(Table 1.20)**:

TABLE 1.20: Classification of coronaviruses

Genus	Examples	Diseases
Alpha-coronavirus	HCoV-229E, HCoV-NL63	Mild respiratory infections (common cold)
Beta-coronavirus	SARS-CoV, MERS-CoV, SARS-CoV-2 (covid-19)	Severe respiratory diseases
Gamma-coronavirus	Infects birds	Not human pathogens
Delta-coronavirus	Infects birds and some mammals	Not human pathogens

Q. COVID-19 infection.

- COVID-19 is caused by the severe acute respiratory syndrome coronavirus-2 (SARS-CoV-2), a highly transmissible RNA virus first identified in December 2019 in Wuhan, China. It led to a global pandemic declared by the WHO on March 11, 2020.
- The exact origin of SARS-CoV-2 is unknown but it is probably of animal origin from bats. There is speculation that it has spread from bats to other mammals and then to human beings.

SARS-CoV-2

- This virus is an enveloped, single-stranded RNA virus belonging to the Coronaviridae family. The virus is spherical (~100 nm in diameter) with a lipid bilayer envelope containing key structural proteins. Spike proteins play a crucial role in binding to angiotensin-converting enzyme 2 (ACE2) receptors of host cells to enter the cell by endocytosis **(Fig. 1.42)**.

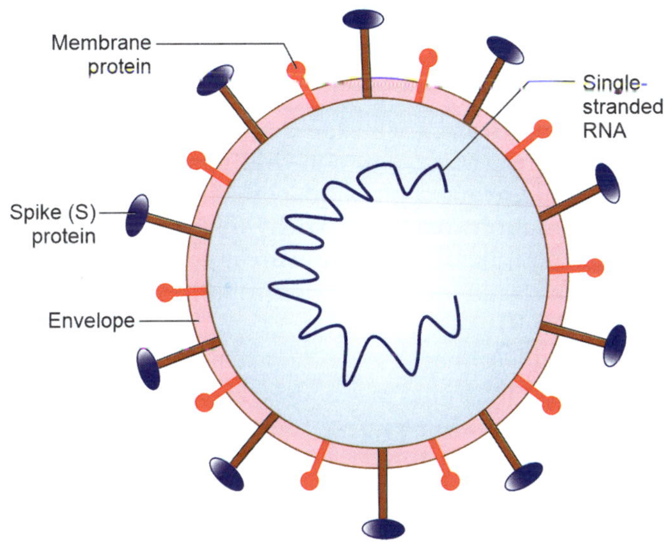

Figure 1.42: COVID-19 virus

Pathophysiology

- The route of transmission of SARS-CoV-2 is coughing and sneezing via respiratory droplets. The virus enters the lungs through the respiratory tract and attacks alveolar epithelial type 2 (AT2) cells. AT2 produces a surfactant to decrease the surface tension within alveoli. The virus binds to ACE2 receptors on alveolar epithelial cells through its spike protein. ACE2 receptors are also found in kidneys, heart, intestine, pancreas, and endothelial cells. Once inside the host cell, the virus releases its RNA. The RNA uses the host cell ribosome to produce viral proteins. It also uses RNA dependent RNA polymerases to duplicate its RNA.
- The virus then leads to an inflammatory response activating macrophages and CD4+ T helper cells which in turn release cytokines (IL-1, IL-6, and TNFα) and chemokines into the bloodstream. Excessive release of these cytokines can lead to cytokine storm. The release of these molecules causes vasodilation and increased capillary permeability. The leakage of plasma into the interstitial spaces of the alveoli cells will lead to alveolar collapse and impaired gaseous exchange. In the later stages of the disease, all these steps cause difficulty in breathing, hypoxemia, and respiratory failure. All these abnormal inflammatory responses can lead to septic shock and multi-organ failure.

Clinical Features

- Incubation period is within 14 days following exposure, with most cases occurring approximately 5 days after exposure.
- The clinical spectrum of COVID-19 varies from asymptomatic cases to severe pneumonia characterized by respiratory failure requiring mechanical ventilation, to multi-organ failure and death.
- Mild disease presents with symptoms of an upper respiratory tract viral infection, including mild fever, cough (dry), sore throat, nasal congestion, malaise, headache, and muscle pain. Loss of taste and/or smell, diarrhea, and vomiting are usually present.
- Severe disease manifests as pneumonia characterized by fever, fatigue, dry cough, dyspnea, low oxygen saturation (SpO_2 <94%), and bilateral infiltrates on chest imaging. Approximately 20% of the infected patients develop complications such as respiratory failure, septic shock, or other organ failure requiring intensive care. Mortality rate is around 3%. Most of the deaths have occurred in patients with underlying medical comorbidities.
- Children seem to be less affected than adults.
- Complications and death rate are more among elderly people and those with comorbid illness such as diabetes mellitus, hypertension, heart disease, and pre-existing lung diseases.

Diagnosis

- Bilateral infiltrates on chest X-ray.
- High-resolution CT (HRCT) of chest is one of the most important test in the diagnosis of COVID-19 pneumonia. Most common findings are multifocal bilateral "ground glass opacities" associated with consolidation areas with patchy distribution, mainly in the peripheral/subpleural areas.
- Lymphopenia or elevated neutrophil-to-lymphocyte ratio (NLR).
- Elevated D-dimer.
- Increased liver enzymes and LDH.
- RT-PCR (real-time reverse transcriptase-polymerase chain reaction) to detect viral RNA: Specimens should be collected from both the upper respiratory tract (naso- and oropharyngeal samples) and lower respiratory tract such as expectorated sputum, endotracheal aspirate, or bronchoalveolar lavage.
- *Antigen test:* Antigen tests provide rapid results but have a higher chance of missing an active infection. These tests also require a nasal swab or nasopharyngeal swab.
- Antibody test: detection of IgM or IgG antibodies against SARS-CoV-2 indicates COVID-19. But these tests take time to become positive and hence are not useful in early diagnosis.

Management

- The possibility of COVID-19 should be considered in patients with fever and/or lower respiratory tract symptoms who reside in endemic areas or who have had recent close contact with a confirmed or suspected case of COVID-19.
- Choice of treatment is based on the severity COVID-19 infection.

COVID-19 severity and treatment approach (**Table 1.21**).

Key points for outpatient treatment of COVID-19

- In mild disease, COVID-19-specific therapy is not required for immunocompetent, healthy individuals ≤64 years who do not have any risk factors for progression to severe disease. Risk factors are diabetes, cardiac disease, prior lung disease, pregnant patients, and immunocompromised patients.
- For patients who have risk factors as described above, **COVID-19-specific therapy** is given as per the following algorithm.

Key points for inpatient treatment of COVID-19

- Patients with suspected or confirmed COVID-19 who require hospitalization should be cared for in a facility that can provide an airborne infection isolation room.
- Supportive care for sepsis and acute respiratory distress syndrome is required.
- Guidelines recommend injection remdesivir only, for patients who do not require oxygen. For patients who require oxygen, injection remdesivir and dexamethasone (6 mg per day for up to 10 days) should be used. Other steroids (methylprednisolone, hydrocortisone) can be used instead of dexamethasone. Steroids are not recommended for patients who do not require oxygen. Remdesivir injection is recommended for 5 days.
- For patients who have escalating oxygen requirements despite dexamethasone, have elevated inflammatory markers, and are within 96 hours of hospitalization, baricitinib or tocilizumab should be added along with remdesivir and dexamethasone.
- *Anticoagulants:* COVID-19 patients have a higher incidence of thrombotic complications (venous thromboembolism, MI, stroke). Hence anticoagulant therapy with heparin or LMWX is recommended for all admitted patients for 5–10 days.

TABLE 1.21: COVID-19 severity and treatment approach

Severity	Symptoms	Treatment approach
Mild	Fever, cough, sore throat, loss of taste/smell, fatigue	• Home isolation and supportive care Hydration, rest, paracetamol for fever Monitor oxygen saturation (SpO_2). • Antivirals usually not required. • Antivirals required only for those at risk of progressing to severe disease (age >65, diabetes, COPD, cardiac disease, immunocompromised). For such patients Nirmatrelvir + ritonavir is given orally twice daily for 5 days.
Moderate	Shortness of breath, pneumonia (SpO_2 90–94%)	• Hospitalization if needed. • Oxygen therapy (nasal cannula). • Antivirals (Remdesivir) if within 5 days of symptoms (Injection Remdesivir, IV, 200 mg on day 1, then 100 mg daily on day 2 and day 3). • Injection dexamethasone, 6 mg per day for up to 10 days. • **Anticoagulant therapy** with heparin or LMWX is recommended for all admitted patients for 5–10 days.
Severe	ARDS, respiratory failure (SpO_2 <90%)	• ICU admission. • High-flow oxygen, ventilator support if needed. • Baricitinib or tocilizumab (for cytokine storm). • Anticoagulation (to prevent blood clots). • Dexamethasone.

- For patients with severe respiratory failure, extracorporeal membrane oxygenation (ECMO) may be considered.
- There are insufficient data to recommend drugs such as azithromycin, chloroquine, and ivermectin.
- There is limited role for monoclonal antibodies or convalescent plasma in most hospitalized patients. Most trials have not shown benefit.

Prevention

- Early recognition of suspect cases, immediate isolation, and institution of infection control measures.
- Individuals with suspected infection in the community should be advised to wear a medical mask to contain their respiratory secretions and seek medical attention.
- WHO advises general measures to reduce transmission of infection, including diligent hand washing, respiratory hygiene, and avoiding close contact with ill individuals.
- WHO also advises exit screening for international travelers from areas with ongoing transmission of COVID-19 virus to identify individuals with fever, cough, or potential high-risk exposure.
- Quarantine is meant to separate and restrict the movement of close contacts who were exposed to COVID-19 case to see, if they become sick. The recommended duration is based on the incubation period, which is up to 14 days for the SARS-CoV-2 virus. Quarantine is recommended for 14 days after their last exposure for asymptomatic close contacts either testing negative or not tested.
- Isolation is meant to separate COVID-19 patients from others. Isolation is recommended for people with COVID-19 symptoms and those who are COVID-19 positive. Isolation is usually recommended for 10 days from the day of symptom onset or from the day of positive test for asymptomatic patients.
- Strict adherence to these measures has been successful at controlling the spread of infection in select areas.

Vaccines

- COVID-19 vaccines play a crucial role in preventing severe illness, hospitalization, and death. Multiple vaccines have been developed using different technologies to combat the SARS-CoV-2 virus.

Types of COVID-19 Vaccines

See **Table 1.22**.

Q. Omicron variant of COVID-19

- Omicron variant is a highly mutated strain of the SARS-CoV-2 virus, first identified in South Africa in November 2021. It rapidly spread worldwide due to its high transmissibility and ability to partially evade immune responses. Below are key aspects of Omicron:
- Omicron has over 50 mutations, with more than 30 mutations in the spike protein.
- These changes increase binding to human ACE2 receptors, enhancing transmissibility.
- It is more immune-evasive, reducing vaccine effectiveness but not completely eliminating protection.
- Omicron evolved into multiple subvariants. Each subvariant exhibited higher transmissibility and immune escape, but vaccines continued to provide protection against severe illness.

Clinical Features

Omicron infections tend to cause milder symptoms compared to previous variants (e.g. Delta).

Common symptoms include

- Sore throat
- Runny nose
- Fatigue
- Headache
- Fever
- Cough (often dry)
- Less frequent loss of taste and smell (which was common in earlier variants).

Transmissibility

- Highly contagious, spreading faster than Delta.
- Causes shorter incubation periods (as little as 2–3 days).
- Led to major global surges in late 2021 and 2022.

Severity and Hospitalization

- Lower severity than Delta, but high case numbers overwhelmed healthcare systems.

TABLE 1.22: COVID-19 vaccines

Vaccine type	Examples	Mechanism of action
Inactivated virus vaccines	Sinovac, Covaxin	Contains killed SARS-CoV-2 virus, which triggers an immune response without causing disease.
mRNA vaccines	Pfizer-BioNTech, Moderna	Uses mRNA to instruct cells to produce the spike (S) protein, triggering an immune response.
DNA vaccines	ZyCoV-D	This vaccine uses DNA plasmids (small circles of double-stranded DNA) that encode the spike protein, which are introduced directly into the vaccine recipient's cells using an intradermal injection device. The recipient's cells then produce the spike protein against which immunity develops.
Viral vector vaccines	Sputnik V	Uses a modified adenovirus to deliver the spike protein DNA into human cells. Human cells use the DNA to produce spike protein, which induces immunity.
Protein subunit vaccines	Novavax, Corbevax	Contains purified spike protein fragments that stimulate the immune system.

- Higher reinfection rates but lower risk of severe disease, hospitalization, and death (especially in vaccinated individuals).

Vaccine and Immunity Response

- Reduced vaccine effectiveness against infection but still strong protection against severe disease and death.
- Booster doses significantly improved immunity against Omicron.
- Prior infection with other variants provided partial but incomplete protection.

Treatment

- Treatment of Omicron follows general COVID-19 management guidelines, focusing on symptom relief, antiviral medications, and supportive care.
- For mild cases, only supportive care is needed.
- Moderate to severe cases require specific antiviral treatment. Nirmatrelvir + Ritonavir) given within 5 days of symptom onset. Molnupiravir is an alternative oral antiviral for patients who cannot take Nirmatrelvir + Ritonavir, but is less effective.
- Remdesivir (IV) is used for hospitalized patients or high-risk outpatients (diabetes, heart disease, COPD, immunocompromised).
- Monoclonal antibodies (e.g. Sotrovimab, Bebtelovimab) have lost effectiveness against newer Omicron subvariants due to mutations. Not recommended for current Omicron strains.
- Corticosteroids and anti-inflammatory drugs: Dexamethasone (or prednisone) → Used in severe cases requiring oxygen support. Tocilizumab (IL-6 inhibitor) or Baricitinib (JAK inhibitor) → Used for cytokine storm in hospitalized patients.

Prevention

- Standard protocols to prevent transmission of infection (Masking, social distancing, etc.).
- Vaccines provide protection against severe illness.
- Booster vaccinations with updated formulations (bivalent vaccines targeting Omicron + original strain) have been released.
- Development of antiviral drugs (Paxlovid, Molnupiravir) to reduce hospitalization risk.

Q. Human metapneumovirus (HMPV).

- Human Metapneumovirus (HMPV) is a respiratory virus from the Paramyxoviridae family, closely related to the Respiratory Syncytial Virus (RSV). It is spherical in shape and has single-stranded RNA (**Fig. 1.43**).
- It primarily causes upper and lower respiratory tract infections, particularly in infants, elderly individuals, and immunocompromised patients.
- HMPV has four subtypes: A1, A2, B1, B2 (similar to RSV subgroups).

Epidemiology

- Worldwide distribution, peaks in winter and early spring.

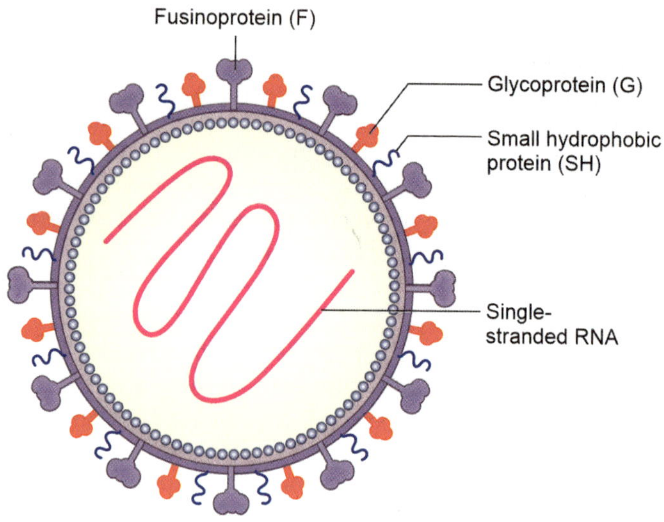

Figure 1.43: HMPV

- Most children are infected by age 5 (like RSV).
- Causes severe infections in neonates, elderly, and immunocompromised patients.

Transmission

- Droplet transmission: Coughing, sneezing, direct contact.
- Fomite transmission: Survives on surfaces for short periods.

Clinical Features

Upper respiratory tract infections (URTI)

- Common cold-like symptoms (cough, rhinorrhea, congestion), fever, sore throat, hoarseness (mild cases).

Lower respiratory tract infections (LRTI)

- Bronchiolitis: Wheezing, crackles, respiratory distress (like RSV).
- Pneumonia: Fever, hypoxia, infiltrates on chest X-ray.
- Asthma exacerbation: Infected children with asthma may have worsening symptoms.
- Severe cases: ICU admission required for respiratory failure in elderly or immunocompromised patients.

Diagnosis

- RT-PCR (Gold standard): Detects viral RNA in nasopharyngeal swabs.
- Direct immunofluorescence assay (DFA): Detects viral antigens.
- Serology (ELISA, neutralization tests): Detects past infections (not useful in acute cases).
- HMPV is often coinfected with RSV, influenza, or bacterial pneumonia, making diagnosis tricky.

Treatment

- There is no specific antiviral therapy.
- Supportive treatment: Oxygen if hypoxic, fluids and antipyretics, bronchodilators for wheezing.
- Severe cases: ICU admission, mechanical ventilation in high-risk patients.

Prevention

- Hand hygiene: Reduces spread via fomites.
- Contact precautions: Especially in hospitals and daycare centers.
- Avoid exposure: High-risk individuals should avoid sick contacts.
- No vaccine is available yet.

Q. Discuss the etiology, pathogenesis, Clinical Features, diagnosis and management of malaria.

Q. Life cycle of malarial parasite.

Q. Tests to diagnose malaria.

Q. Chemoprophylaxis for malaria.

- Malaria is a disease caused by the protozoan parasite of the genus Plasmodium.

Etiology

- Five species of Plasmodium namely, *Plasmodium vivax, P. falciparum, P. ovale, P. malariae* and *P. knowlesi* are responsible for almost all human infections. Out of these, *P. falcifarum* causes severe infection and is responsible for most of the deaths due to malaria.

Epidemiology

- Malaria is the most important of the parasitic diseases of humans. It has been eliminated from the United States, Canada, Europe, and Russia. Malaria is very common in tropical countries. *P. falcipurum* predominates in Africa, New Guinea, and Hispaniola. *P. vivax* is more common in Central America. Both falciparum and vivax are common in South America, the Indian subcontinent, eastern Asia, and Oceania. *P. malariae* and *P. ovale* is mainly confined to Africa.
- *P. knowlesi* has been identified on the island of Borneo and Southeast Asia.

Pathogenesis and life cycle of malarial parasite

- It is transmitted by the bite of infected anopheles mosquitoes (**Fig. 1.44**).
- Human infection begins when a female anopheles mosquito bites man and inoculates sporozoites into the blood. These sporozoites are motile forms of the malarial parasite and are carried via the bloodstream to the liver.
- In the liver sporozoites invade hepatic parenchymal cells and start multiplying there to produce schizonts. Schizonts contain merozoites. This initial replication in the liver is called the exoerythrocytic cycle. In *P. vivax* and *P. ovale* infections, some of these schizonts may remain dormant (hypnozoites) for upto a year or longer. These dormant forms are the cause of relapses in vivax and ovale.
- After 8–14 days, the swollen liver cell containing merozoites (schizont) bursts, releasing motile merozoites into the bloodstream. Each merozoite can invade an RBC and start multiplying there. Attachment to RBC is mediated by a receptor on the RBC. In the case of *P. vivax*, this receptor is related to the Duffy blood-group antigen. Those who have Duffy-negative blood group (West African) are resistant to *P. vivax* malaria.
- Inside the RBCs, the merozoites develop into ring-stage trophozoites. Some trophozoites mature into schizonts and some trophozoites differentiate into gametocytes. Schizonts contain many merozoites. When the RBC ruptures, these daughter merozoites are released, each capable of invading a new RBC and repeating the cycle. Gametocytes (sexual forms) are picked up by mosquitoes when they bite human beings. Inside the mosquito's midgut the male and female gametocytes join to form a zygote. This zygote becomes an ookinete which penetrates and develops

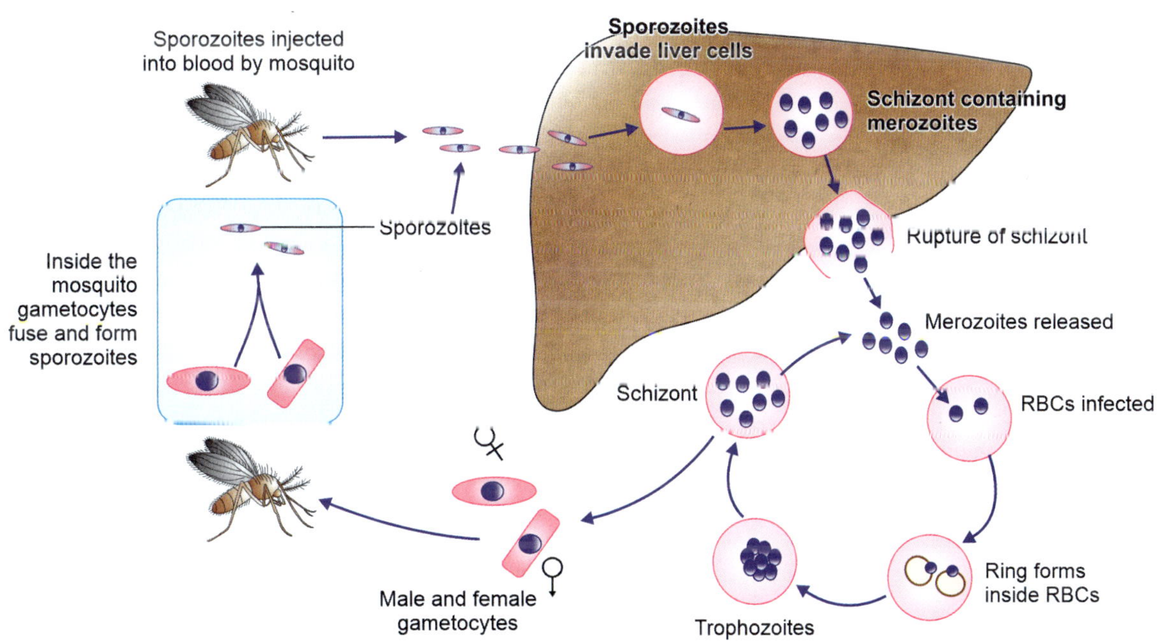

Figure 1.44: Malaria—life cycle

in the mosquito's gut wall to become oocyst. Oocyst develops by asexual division and bursts to release motile sporozoites, which migrate to the salivary gland of the mosquito to await inoculation into another human at the next feeding.

- Malaria can also develop after blood transfusion without any incubation period. The hepatic phase is absent as the erythrocytic infection is directly transmitted.

Clinical Features

- The incubation period for vivax, ovale and falciparum infections is 8–24 days. For *P. malariae* it is 15–30 days.
- The initial symptoms of malaria are nonspecific and include malaise, nausea, vomiting, headache, fatigue, body ache and fever. Some cases may also have abdominal pain, arthralgia, or diarrhea. Though myalgia may be prominent, it is not as severe as in dengue fever or leptospirosis. Muscle tenderness is absent unlike in leptospirosis or typhus fever. Classic malarial symptoms with intermittent fever, chills, and rigors are usually seen with *P. vivax* or *P. ovale* infection but not in all cases.
- Fever in vivax and ovale comes once in 3 days (tertian malaria) and once in 4 days *P. malariae* (quartan malaria). However this time pattern may not be seen in all cases of malaria. In falciparum fever comes daily and does not follow any pattern. Fever can rise above 40°C.
- Children can have febrile convulsions at the time of fever.
- Cerebral malaria should be suspected in anybody with falciparum malaria presenting with seizures.
- Physical examination is essentially normal except fever, mild anemia, mild jaundice and mild splenomegaly. Anemia and jaundice are due to destruction of RBCs (hemolysis) by the parasites. Splenomegaly is common in malaria-endemic areas and reflects repeated infections. Mild hepatomegaly may also be seen particularly in young children.
- Severe malaria especially falciparum can present with features of sepsis with multi-organ dysfunction. Patients may present with impaired consciousness or coma, renal failure, liver impairment, low platelet counts, and ARDS.
- Serious renal damage may occur due to progressive glomerulonephritis in *Plasmodium malariae* infection due to deposition of immune complexes. The glomerulonephritis does not respond to antimalarial drugs or corticosteroids.

Differences in Malaria caused by different Plasmodium *species*

See **Table 1.23**.

Causes of Anemia in Malaria

- Destruction of RBCs by parasites.
- Enlarged spleen causing sequestration of RBCs and hemolysis.
- Dys-erythropoiesis.
- Folate deficiency due to depletion of stores.
- Drug-induced (chloroquine, primaquine) hemolysis in patients with G6PD deficiency.

Investigations

- It is difficult to diagnose malaria clinically with accuracy; hence treatment should be started on clinical grounds in endemic areas pending laboratory confirmation.

Peripheral Smear

- The diagnosis of malaria can be easily made by demonstration of asexual forms of parasites in the peripheral blood smear. If initial smears are negative, repeat smears should be made preferably at the time of fever. Thick and thin smears are made and stained

TABLE 1.23: Differences in malaria caused by different *Plasmodium* species

	P. vivax	*P. ovale*	*P. falciparum*	*P. malariae*	*P. knowlesi*
Incubation period	8–24 days	8–24 days	8–24 days	15–30 days	7–14 days
Fever pattern	Tertian	Tertian	No periodicity	Quartan	Quotidian (every 24 hours)
Exo-erythrocytic cycle	Yes	Yes	No	No	Yes
Relapses	Yes	Yes	No	No	No
Red cell preference	Young RBCs	Reticulocytes	Young RBCs (but can invade cells of all ages)	Older cells	All RBCs
RBC morphology	Enlarged RBCs with large sing ring form. Schüffner's dots present	Infected RBCs oval-shaped with fimbriated ends. Large single ring form. Schüffner's dots present	Normal RBC size. Multiple rings per RBC Small ring forms. Schüffner's dots absent	Normal RBC size. Band form trophozoies seen. Schüffner's dots absent	Normal-sized and shaped RBCs. Single ring Schüffner's dots absent
Gametocyte shape	Round/oval	Round/oval	Crescent/banana	Round	Round

with Giemsa stain. Thick smear detects parasites (higher sensitivity). Thin smear is useful to identify species and life cycle stages. Gametocytes may persist for days or weeks after clearance of asexual parasites. Presence of gametocytes without asexual forms does not indicate active infection.

Rapid Diagnostic Tests (RDT)

- *Rapid diagnostic tests* for malaria are based on the presence of certain Plasmodium antigens or enzymatic activities. Assays may involve detection of a histidine-rich protein 2 (HRP-2) associated with malaria parasites (especially *P. falciparum*) and detection of Plasmodium-associated lactate dehydrogenase (pLDH). These tests are rapid and almost as sensitive as thick smear but do not quantify the severity of infection and remain positive for weeks after infection. These tests are quick and do not need microscope. Useful in rural areas.
- *HRP-2 based tests*: Histidine-rich protein-2 (HRP-2) based serologic assays can detect parasite antigens in blood from a fingerprick sample. PfHRP2 dipstick or card test can detect only falciparum.
- *Plasmodium LDH based tests*: The pLDH-based assays specifically detect the parasite lactate dehydrogenase enzyme using a panel of monoclonal antibodies. Different species can be identified. Example is OptiMAL test.

Flouroscent Technique (MP-QBC)

- Malaria parasite by quantitative buffy coat (MP-QBC) is a technique that is as sensitive as thick smear.
- Blood is collected in a glass micro tube containing acridine orange stain, anticoagulant, and a float. This is centrifuged to concentrate the parasitized cells around the float. Malarial parasites take up fluorescent stain and can be easily detected under fluorescence microscopy. This test is ideal for processing large numbers of samples rapidly. But this test cannot identify the species of malaria.

Other Tests

- In addition to the tests listed above, new molecular techniques, such as PCR assay testing and nucleic acid sequence-based amplification (NASBA) are also available for diagnosis. They are more sensitive than thick smears but are expensive and are mainly used in research labs.

Other Laboratory Findings

- There may be normochromic normocytic anemia, increased WBC count, neutrophilia, and increased ESR. In severe falciparum malaria there may be metabolic acidosis, increased bilirubin, elevated liver enzymes, thrombocytopenia, increased urea creatinine, and hypoglycemia.

Treatment

See **Table 1.24**.

Criteria for Severe Malaria

Malaria is considered to be severe when patients have ≥ 1 of the following. Severe malaria is most often due to *P. falciparum*.

- Impaired consciousness/coma.
- Repeated generalized convulsions.
- Renal failure (Serum creatinine >3 mg/dl).
- Jaundice (Serum bilirubin >3 mg/dl).
- Severe anemia (Hb <5 g/dl).
- Pulmonary edema/acute respiratory distress syndrome.

TABLE 1.24: Regimens for the treatment of malaria

Chloroquine-sensitive strains of all species of malaria (*P. vivax, P. falciparum, P. malariae, P. ovale, P. knowlesi*	Chloroquine (10 mg of base/kg stat followed by 5 mg/kg at 12, 24, and 36 hours) OR Amodiaquine OD 3 days) In addition to above, primaquine (0.5 mg of base/kg per day) should be given for 14 days to prevent relapses in vivax and ovale. Primaquine kills the hypnozoites present in liver and prevents relapses. Tafenoquine 300 mg single dose is an alternative to primaquine in adults ≥16 years. Primaquine should not be given in severe G6PD deficiency
Chloroquine-resistant uncomplicated *Plasmodium vivax and Falciparum* (suspect this in areas known to harbor resistant strains. Ovale and malariae are usually sensitive)	Quinine sulfate (10 mg/kg 3 times a day for 3 or 7 days) plus Doxycycline 100 mg twice a day for 7 days OR Artemether-lumefantrine (BD for 3 days with food) OR Atovaquone/proguanil 4 adult tablets once a day for 3 days *Primaquine or Tafenoquine should be given to prevent relapses as mentioned above.*
Severe malaria, all Plasmodium species including falciparum	Severe malaria is an emergency and parenteral artemisinin derivatives or quinine should be used irrespective of chloroquine sensitivity. IV artesunate 2.4 mg/kg body weight at 0, 12, 24, and 48 hours followed by one of the following (a) Artemether-lumefantrine (BD for 3 days with food) OR (b) Atovaquone/proguanil 4 adult tablets once a day for 3 days OR (c) Doxycycline100 mg twice a day for 7 days *Primaquine or tafenoquine should be used to prevent relapses if P. vivax or P. ovale is likely or confirmed*

- Hypoglycemia (plasma glucose <40 mg/dl).
- Metabolic acidosis.
- Circulatory collapse/shock (systolic BP <80 mm Hg).
- Abnormal bleeding and DIC.
- Hemoglobinuria.
- Hyperthermia (temperature >104°F).
- Hyperparasitemia (>5% parasitized RBCs in low endemic and >10% in hyperendemic areas).

Supportive Measures

- Include IV fluids, antipyretics, blood transfusion to correct severe anemia, and bed rest.

Relapses

- Relapses occur in vivax and ovale malaria due to hepatic hypnozoites. Since hepatic hypnozoites are absent in falciparum malaria, relapses do not occur in falciparum malaria.

Prevention of Malaria

Decreasing the Mosquito Population

- Spraying of insecticides
- Biological methods such as use of mosquito larva eating fish in water reservoirs.

Personal Protection

- Use of clothes extending up to the wrists and ankles when outdoors and mosquito nets when indoors to avoid mosquito bites. Application of insect-repellant creams on the exposed body surfaces like legs and hands.

Chemoprophylaxis

- Recommended for nonimmune visitors to endemic areas and to pregnant women living in endemic areas.
- Travelers should start taking antimalarial drugs at least 1 week before visiting the area and continue for 4 weeks after returning from the endemic area.
- Chloroquine 500 mg per week or mefloquine 250 mg orally per week or doxycycline 100 mg orally once daily can be used for prophylaxis. Doxycycline is contraindicated in pregnant women and children less than 8 years.

Malaria Vaccine

- The development of malaria vaccines has made significant progress, particularly with the **RTS,S (Mosquirix)** vaccine, and the newer **R21/Matrix-M** vaccine showing promising results.

Complications of Malaria

- Complications usually happen in severe falciparum malaria.

- Cerebral malaria
- Severe anemia
- Renal failure
- Pulmonary edema
- Acute respiratory distress syndrome (ARDS), and respiratory failure
- Hypoglycemia
- Circulatory collapse
- DIC
- Acidosis
- Hemoglobinuria
- Jaundice

Q. Cerebral malaria.

- Cerebral malaria is the most severe complication of falciparum malaria with high mortality rate. It is more common in children, pregnant women, splenectomised and in non-immune individuals.

Pathophysiology of Cerebral Malaria

- The main pathology in cerebral malaria is sequestration of parasitized red cells in brain microvasculature. This process is known as **rosetting** and **sequestration**. This leads to:
  - **Reduced blood flow** and **hypoxia** (lack of oxygen) in brain tissue.
  - **Inflammatory responses** that can cause swelling and damage to brain cells.
  - **Clotting abnormalities**, leading to the formation of microclots and contributing to further brain damage.

Clinical Features

- Cerebral malaria manifests as diffuse encephalopathy and presents as impaired state of consciousness and/or seizures, and can result in coma and death. Focal neurologic signs are unusual. Although some passive resistance to head flexion may be detected, frank neck rigidity is absent. This feature can differentiate cerebral malaria from meningitis. The corneal reflexes are preserved except in deep coma. Flexor or extensor posturing may be seen. Some patients have retinal hemorrhages, papilledema, and cotton wool spots. Convulsions can occur and are usually generalized.
- Cerebral malaria is universally fatal if untreated, and even with treatment mortality is high. About 10 percent of patients who survive cerebral malaria have persistent neurologic abnormalities even after recovery.

Diagnosis

- Diagnosis is typically based on the presence of **Plasmodium falciparum** infection (confirmed by a **blood smear** or **rapid diagnostic test**) along with symptoms suggestive of **neurological involvement** (e.g. coma, seizures).
- **CT/MRI scans:** These may be done to rule out other causes of altered consciousness (such as strokes or infections) and to assess the extent of cerebral damage.

Treatment

Antimalarial Treatment

- **Intravenous artesunate:** Artesunate is the preferred treatment for severe malaria, including cerebral malaria. It is an artemisinin-based therapy that rapidly reduces parasitemia and is associated with better outcomes compared to older drugs like quinine.
- **Intravenous quinine:** If artesunate is not available, quinine can be used as an alternative. However, artesunate is generally preferred because of its superior efficacy and safety profile.
- After the patient improves, treatment can be switched to oral artemisinin-based combination therapies to complete the course.

Supportive Care

- *Anticonvulsants*: Seizures are common in cerebral malaria, and anticonvulsant medications (e.g. phenytoin or benzodiazepines) may be administered to control them.
- *Management of raised intracranial pressure*: This may include mannitol or hyperventilation to reduce brain swelling.
- *Fluid and electrolyte management*: Careful monitoring of fluid balance is essential to avoid both dehydration and cerebral edema (swelling of the brain).
- *Blood glucose control*: Hypoglycemia can be a common complication in malaria, especially in children, so maintaining normal blood glucose levels is important.
- *Oxygen therapy*: To manage hypoxia and support breathing in severe cases.

Q. Blackwater fever.

- Blackwater fever is a serious and potentially fatal complication of ***Plasmodium falciparum*** malaria. It is characterized by **hemolysis** (destruction of red blood cells), **hemoglobinuria** (presence of hemoglobin in urine which makes the urine appear **dark or "black")** and **acute renal failure.**
- This condition is rare but can be seen in individuals who have had **recurrent malaria infections** or are exposed to **malaria** in areas where the disease is highly endemic.

Pathophysiology of Blackwater Fever

- *Severe hemolysis:* The infection with *Plasmodium falciparum* leads to the rupture of red blood cells, releasing hemoglobin into the bloodstream. The immune system may respond by attacking both the infected and uninfected red blood cells.
- *Hemoglobinuria:* The free hemoglobin released from the lysed red blood cells is filtered by the kidneys and excreted in the urine, causing it to turn dark or reddish-brown (resembling "blackwater"). Hemoglobin in the urine is toxic to the kidneys and can lead to renal failure if not managed promptly.
- *Renal failure:* The kidneys may become overwhelmed by the large amounts of hemoglobin, which can clog kidney tubules and cause acute kidney injury (AKI). The hemoglobin and other cellular debris can lead to tubular necrosis.
- *Immune response:* The phenomenon is often associated with immune sensitization due to repeated or chronic malaria infections. It is also linked to drug-induced hemolysis when taking antimalarial drugs like quinine or sulfadoxine-pyrimethamine.

Clinical Features

- Dark or "black" urine (the hallmark of the condition).
- *Fever*: Often high and persistent, associated with malaria.
- *Jaundice*: Due to liver dysfunction from massive red blood cell destruction.
- *Abdominal pain*: Particularly in the right upper quadrant, where the liver is located.
- *Hemolytic anemia*: Manifested by pallor (paleness), fatigue, and weakness.
- *Acute renal failure*: Decreased urine output, swelling (edema), and signs of kidney damage.
- *Rapid pulse and hypotension*: Due to fluid loss from hemolysis and kidney dysfunction.

Diagnosis of Blackwater Fever

- Blackwater fever is diagnosed based on clinical presentation and laboratory tests.
- *Urine examination*: The dark, "black" urine is a key sign. Laboratory analysis of urine may reveal free hemoglobin, indicating hemolysis.
- *Blood smear:* A thick and thin blood smear can confirm the presence of *Plasmodium falciparum* in the blood.
- *Hemoglobin levels*: A low hemoglobin level is consistent with hemolytic anemia.
- *Renal function tests*: Blood tests, including serum creatinine, blood urea nitrogen (BUN), and electrolyte levels, will assess kidney function and the degree of renal impairment.
- *Liver function tests*: Elevated liver enzymes may be present due to the liver's involvement in the disease process.

Treatment of Blackwater Fever

Antimalarial Treatment

- Artesunate is the preferred treatment for severe malaria caused by *Plasmodium falciparum*, including cases of blackwater fever. Artesunate is more effective than quinine and is associated with lower mortality and fewer side effects.
- If artesunate is unavailable, quinine can be used, though it may worsen hemolysis in some patients, especially in those with quinine-induced blackwater fever.
- ACTs (artemisinin-based combination therapies) are effective in treating the malaria infection once the patient stabilizes.

Management of Hemolysis and Anemia

- Blood transfusions may be necessary to manage severe anemia resulting from massive red blood cell destruction.
- Fluids and electrolyte management: Adequate hydration is essential, but care must be taken to avoid fluid overload, especially in patients with renal failure.

Supportive Care for Renal Failure

- Dialysis: In cases of acute kidney injury (AKI) or renal failure, hemodialysis or peritoneal dialysis may be needed to support kidney function until recovery.
- Monitoring renal function: Regular monitoring of renal parameters (e.g. serum creatinine, BUN, and urine output) is crucial.

Prognosis of blackwater fever

- Blackwater fever can be fatal, especially in uncontrolled cases or if renal failure is severe and not managed properly. Mortality is higher in individuals who develop severe anemia, acute renal failure, or shock.
- With early recognition, prompt treatment of malaria, and supportive care, many patients can recover from blackwater fever. However, renal damage may be permanent in some cases, especially if the kidney failure is prolonged or severe.

Q. Tropical splenomegaly (hyperreactive malarial splenomegaly).

- Tropical splenomegaly, also known as hyperreactive malarial splenomegaly (HMS) or tropical splenomegaly syndrome (TSS), is a condition characterized by enlargement of the spleen (splenomegaly) that occurs as a result of chronic or repeated malaria infections, particularly in areas with high transmission rates of malaria.
- It is prevalent in areas where malaria is endemic.

Pathogenesis

- The exact mechanism behind hyperreactive malarial splenomegaly is not fully understood, but it is believed to be due to a chronic, exaggerated immune response to repeated malaria infections. The primary features of this syndrome include:
  - *Chronic malaria infections*: the spleen acts as a primary site for filtering out infected red blood cells during malaria infection. In individuals living in areas with high malaria transmission, repeated exposure to Plasmodium parasites leads to immune stimulation over time.
  - *Excessive splenic response*: Spleen becomes hypertrophied (enlarged) as it works to filter out the increasing number of infected red blood cells. This results in splenomegaly. The hyperreactive immune response can lead to the excessive production of antibodies, which further contributes to splenic enlargement.
  - *Immunological overreaction*: Individuals with hyperreactive malarial splenomegaly often have a heightened immune response that leads to excessive immune complex formation, activation of T cells, and B cells. This response can be particularly pronounced in people with genetic predispositions to such an overreaction, such as those with certain MHC haplotypes (major histocompatibility complex).
  - *Parasitic load and immune clearance*: A high parasitic load over time can overwhelm the spleen's filtering capacity, causing it to enlarge significantly. This enlargement is often disproportionate to the severity of the malaria infection.

Clinical Features

- Most commonly observed in children, but it can occur in adults with frequent malaria exposure.
- Patients with tropical splenomegaly present with an abdominal mass or a dragging sensation in the abdomen. Occasionally sharp abdominal pain may be noted due to perisplenitis.
- Anemia and pancytopenia are usually present.
- These patients are prone for respiratory and skin infections and many die due to infection and secondary sepsis.
- In rare, severe cases, a ruptured spleen can occur due to its extreme enlargement, leading to hemorrhagic shock. This is a medical emergency.

Treatment

- The first-line treatment for malaria is artemisinin-based combination therapies (ACTs), which are highly effective in reducing the parasitic load.
- If the patient has chronic or repeated malaria infections, long-term antimalarial prophylaxis may be recommended to prevent future episodes.
- Splenectomy: In some cases, where the splenomegaly is severe and associated with complications such as splenic rupture or severe anemia, splenectomy (removal of the spleen) may be considered. However, this is not a routine procedure and is only used in severe cases

Q. Describe the etiology, life cycle, pathogenesis, Clinical Features and treatment of amebiasis.

- Amebiasis is an infection caused by the intestinal protozoan *Entamoeba histolytica*. The diseases produced by ameba include dysentery and abscesses in the liver and other organs.

Epidemiology

- Amebiasis is found all over the world.
- Amebiasis is more common in the developing world, where overcrowding, poor sanitation and economic backwardness are common. In developed countries, it is an important infection among male homosexuals, intravenous drug users and patients with AIDS.
- 90% of infections are asymptomatic and only 10% produce clinical symptoms.

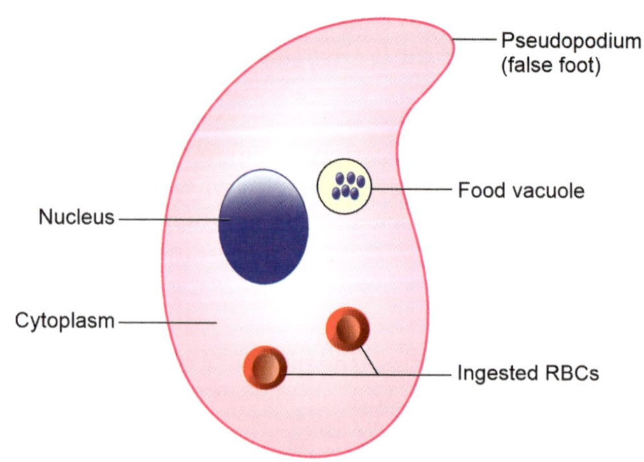

Figure 1.45: *Entamoeba histolytica*

Life cycle of ameba and pathogenesis (Fig. 1.46)

- The infection is transmitted through the feco-oral route.
- Man is the only reservoir of infection and excretes the cystic form of the organism in the feces, which can survive in the environment for several weeks. Man acquires infection by ingestion of viable cysts from fecally contaminated water, food, or hands. Less commonly it is acquired through oral and anal sexual practices. Once ingested, cysts are able to resist the acidic gastric juice, and reach small intestine, where the cysts develop into motile trophozoites. Trophozoites remain as harmless commensals in the colon in most patients. However in some patients, the trophozoites invade the bowel mucosa, and cause colitis which presents clinically as dysentery.
- There are usually mucosal ulcers which typically have the shape of a flask in cross-section (wide base and narrow neck) **(Fig. 1.47)**. Amebic ulcers occur most commonly in the rectum but may occur anywhere in the colon.
- Trophozoites can also enter the bloodstream and get carried to different organs like liver, lungs, or brain where they may produce abscesses. The necrotic contents of a liver abscess appear like "anchovy sauce". Some trophozoites undergo encystation and produce infectious cysts which are shed in the stool and the life cycle can get repeated again.
- Trophozoites if ingested cannot cause infection because they are rapidly killed by exposure to air or stomach acid.

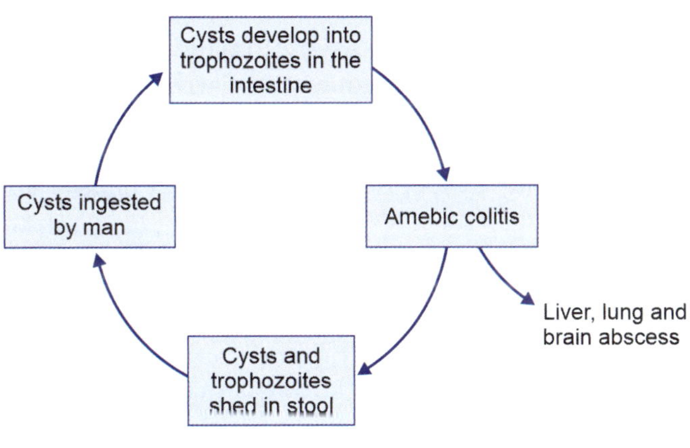

Figure 1.46: Life cycle of ameba

Clinical Features

- Amebic infections are clinically classified as intestinal and extraintestinal.

Intestinal Amebiasis

- Most patients with Intestinal amebiasis are asymptomatic. Those who become symptomatic present with dysentery. Lower abdominal pain, malaise and mild diarrhea develop gradually. Abdominal pain is usually colicky. Patients may pass up to 10–12 stools per day. The stools appear dark brown, contain little fecal material and consist mainly of blood and mucus. Fever is uncommon unlike bacterial diarrhea. Almost all patients have blood in the stools.
- Severe intestinal infection may present with severe abdominal pain and high fever. Some patients may develop toxic megacolon where there is severe gaseous dilation of colon. Rarely patients develop chronic amebic colitis, which can be confused with inflammatory bowel disease.

Extraintestinal amebiasis

- Extraintestinal infection by *E. histolytica* most often involves the liver. Other sites include the brain, spleen, lungs and pelvic organs.
- Patients present with fever and right-upper-quadrant pain. Pain is dull or pleuritic in nature and may radiate to the right shoulder. Point tenderness over the liver and right-sided pleural effusion is common. Hepatomegaly is usually seen, but jaundice is rare. Although the initial site of infection is the colon, most patients do not give a history of dysentery. Most abscesses occur in the right lobe of liver. Amebic liver abscess can present as FUO and should be considered in the differential diagnosis of fever of unknown origin.

Complications

- Perforation of amebic ulcers and toxic megacolon.
- Liver abscesses may become big and rupture into adjacent structures such as the pleural cavity, lungs, pericardium and peritoneum which can be fatal.

Investigations

- ***Stool examination:*** This is the best test to diagnose amebic dysentery. A saline preparation of freshly

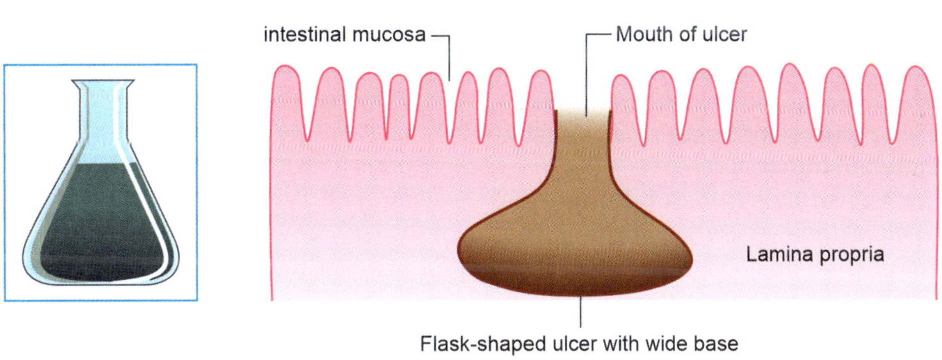

Figure 1.47: Flask-shaped amebic ulcer

passed stool is examined for motile trophozoites. Cysts also may be seen. Stool can be cultured for *Entamoeba histolytica* and other bacteria.

- ***Colonoscopy or sigmoidoscopy:*** The test is useful to see the typical ulcers and also to distinguish it from other ulcerative and inflammatory lesions like acute bacillary dysentery and ulcerative colitis, and to obtain swabs and biopsies for appropriate examinations.
- ***Ultrasound or CT scan of abdomen:*** It is useful to identify amebic liver abscess and also the size and location of the abscess.
- ***Serological tests:*** Demonstration of presence of anti-amebic antibodies in the serum is an important way of diagnosing amebic infections. Especially useful for extraintestinal amebiasis such as liver abscesses.

Treatment

- Metronidazole 400 mg thrice a day for 7 days is effective. Tinidazole can also be used.
- Newer agents like tinidazole, secnidazole or ornidazole are equally effective and allow less frequent dosing.
- Along with above agents, it is useful to give luminal amebicides like diloxanide furoate or iodoquinol or Paromomycin which act in the gut lumen and have minimal systemic absorption. Asymptomatic cyst passers do not require treatment.
- Liver abscess requires the above drugs at a higher dosage. If liver abscess does not respond to medical therapy, it can be aspirated under ultrasound guidance by introducing a pig-tailed catheter. Chloroquine has also been used for patients with hepatic amebiasis.
- Complications such as perforation, toxic megacolon and stricture require appropriate surgical treatment.

Q. Describe the etiology, clinical features, diagnosis and treatment of giardiasis.

- Giardiasis is one of the most common parasitic diseases worldwide and is due to *Giardia lamblia* which is a protozoan. It causes intestinal disease and diarrhea.
- *Giardia lamblia* (also known as *Giardia intestinalis* or *Giardia duodenalis*) is a flagellated protozoan and has a pair of nuclei which give it an owl-eyed appearance. Flagellae are responsible for its motility **(Fig. 1.48)**.

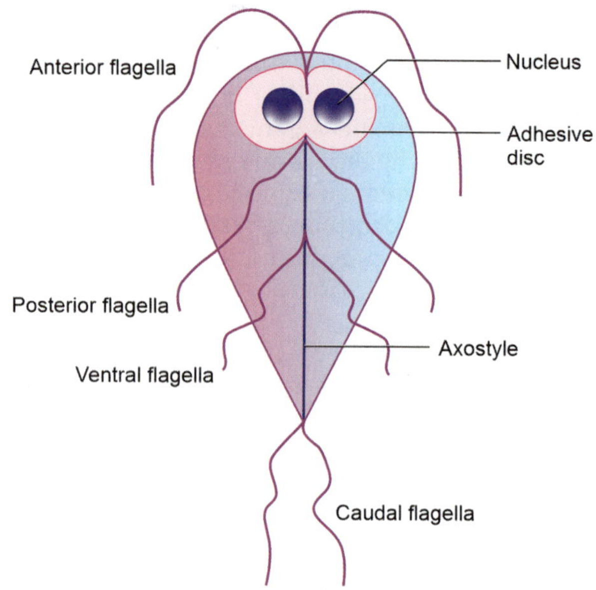

Figure. 1.48: *Giardia lamblia*

Pathogenesis

- Infection spreads through feco-oral route and is acquired by ingestion of cysts present in food or water. The cysts excyst in the intestine and become trophozoites which have owl eyed appearance. Giardia colonizes the mucosa of upper small intestine but does not invade the mucosa.
- Giardia attach to the mucosa of duodenum and jejunum with the help of their ventral suction disc. They interfere with gut function by mechanical covering of the mucosa by a large number of parasites and causing villous atrophy in the jejunal mucosa leading to a reduced absorptive surface. In most infections the gut morphology is normal, but in a few cases there may be changes resembling tropical sprue and gluten-sensitive enteropathy on histopathology. The pathogenesis of diarrhea in giardiasis is not known.
- Both trophozoites and cystic forms are excreted in the stool, but only cysts are infective to others. High levels of secretory IgA in breast milk are believed to protect suckling infants from infection. Giardiasis is an important cause of traveler's diarrhea and is also an important cause of diarrhea in immunosuppressed individuals.

Clinical Features

- *Giardia* infection can be asymptomatic.
- Acute giardiasis may manifest as diarrhea, abdominal pain, bloating, belching, flatus, nausea, and vomiting. This illness is usually self-limiting. Patients may also present with dyspeptic symptoms with nausea and anorexia.
- Chronic giardiasis may present with malabsorption, steatorrhea and weight loss. Such patients usually have villous atrophy, with malabsorption of fat, carbohydrates, vitamin B_{12} and lactose intolerance. Children with chronic giardiasis may have growth impairment.
- Giardiasis can be life-threatening in patients with hypogammaglobulinemia.

Diagnosis

- Stool examination: Detection of cysts or trophozoites in the feces by microscopy.
- Stool antigen tests (ELISA or immunofluorescence Assay-IFA): Highly sensitive and specific for detecting Giardia antigens in stool. More reliable than microscopic examination.
- PCR testing (molecular diagnosis): Detects Giardia DNA with high accuracy.
- Endoscopic sampling of duodenal fluid and biopsy of the mucosa may be required to detect the parasite. This is rarely done.

Treatment

- Metronidazole is the drug of choice and is given either as 200 mg thrice daily for 7 days or as a single dose of 2.4 g. Tinidazole or secnidazole are alternatives. All infected symptomatic persons should be treated.

Q. *Trichomonas vaginalis* (Trichomoniasis).

- Trichomoniasis is a sexually transmitted infection (STI) caused by the protozoan parasite *Trichomonas vaginalis*. It is one of the most common non-viral STIs worldwide and primarily affects the urogenital tract.
- *Trichomonas vaginalis* is a pear-shaped protozoan and causes infection of the vagina, urethra and prostate **(Fig. 1.49)**.

Clinical Features

- In women, it causes vaginitis which presents as yellow and frothy vaginal discharge with burning and itching. They may also complain of dysuria, increased urinary frequency and dyspareunia.
- In men, trichomoniasis presents with urethritis and prostatitis, but may be asymptomatic.

Diagnosis

- The diagnosis is made by detection of motile Trichomonads in wet smears prepared from vaginal, urethral or prostatic secretions.
- Nucleic acid amplification test (NAAT): Most sensitive and specific test. Detects *T. vaginalis* DNA in vaginal, cervical, or urine samples.
- Rapid antigen tests: Point-of-care antigen tests available but less sensitive than NAAT.

Treatment

- Metronidazole is the drug of choice and is given as 200 mg thrice a day for 7 days or as a single 2 g dose. Tinidazole also can be used. Both partners should be treated to prevent reinfection.

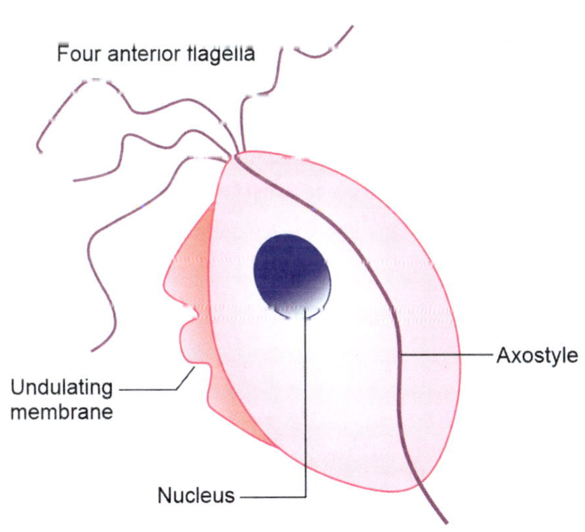

Figure 1.49: *Trichomonas vaginalis*

Q. Describe the etiology, clinical features, diagnosis and treatment of leishmaniasis.

- The term leishmaniasis refers collectively to various clinical syndromes caused by intracellular protozoa of the genus Leishmania. The name leishmaniasis comes from the scientist Sir William Leishman who first discovered the organisms in a patient who died of leishmaniasis. It is a vector-borne (sandfly) zoonosis, with rodents and canids as reservoir hosts and humans as incidental hosts.
- The clinical spectrum of leishmaniasis ranges from self-healing cutaneous ulcers to fatal visceral disease. These syndromes fall into three broad categories:
  - Visceral leishmaniasis (VL): This is also known as kala-azar and is the most serious form of the disease.
  - Cutaneous leishmaniasis (CL): This is the most common type.
  - Mucocutaneous leishmaniasis (ML).

Etiology

The various species of leishmania causing human disease are as follows:

- *Visceral leishmaniasis*: *Leishmania donovani*, *L. infantum*.
- *Cutaneous leishmaniasis*: *L. major*, *L. tropica*, *L. mexicana*, *L. braziliensis*.
- *Mucocutaneous leishmaniasis*: *L braziliensis*.

Epidemiology

- Leishmaniasis mainly occurs in tropical regions. India and neighboring Nepal, Bangladesh, Sudan, and Brazil are the four largest foci of visceral leishmaniasis.
- Cutaneous leishmaniasis occurs mainly in Afghanistan, Pakistan, Ethiopia, Kenya, and Uganda.

Life Cycle and Pathogenesis (Fig. 1.50)

- Leishmania parasites are transmitted to man by the bite of sandflies (Phlebotomus and Lutzomyia). Visceral leishmaniasis can also be transmitted by blood transfusion or needle sharing.
- Leishmania exists in the sandfly as a motile, spindle-shaped promastigote with an anterior flagellum. As the flies feed on hosts including man, they regurgitate the promastigote stage into the skin. Promastigotes are phagocytized by macrophages and inside the macrophages develop into the nonflagellated amastigote stage. This amastigote multiplies by binary fission and are released after rupture of macrophages. Released amastigotes are phagocytized by other macrophages and start multiplying there. Some amastigotes can be ingested by sandflies where they transform back into promastigotes and ready to infect other hosts.
- There is inflammatory response against leishmania organisms with increased production of gamma interferon (IFN), tumor necrosis factor alpha (TNF), and other proinflammatory cytokines. In addition to these proinflammatory cytokines and chemokines, patients with active disease also have markedly

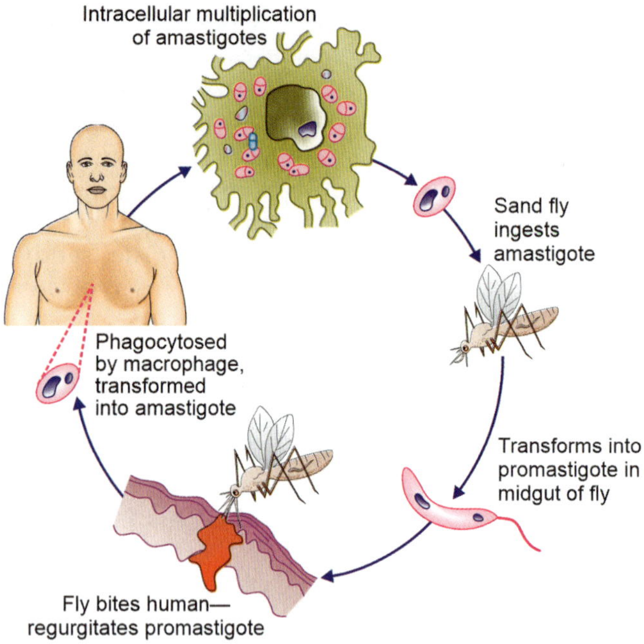

Figure 1.50: Life cycle of leishmaniasis

elevated levels of IL-10 in serum as well as in lesions. IL-10 inhibits the killing of amastigotes by inhibiting macrophages. This inflammation along with inhibition of killing of amastigotes causes nodules, necrosis, ulceration and destruction of tissues seen in leishmaniasis.

Clinical Features

Visceral Leishmaniasis (kala-azar)

- It is a potentially lethal widespread systemic disease characterized by darkening of the skin as well as the pentad of fever, weight loss, hepatosplenomegaly, pancytopenia, and hypergammaglobulinemia.

Cutaneous Leishmaniasis (CL)

- A few days or weeks after the bite of a sandfly, a papule develops and grows into a nodule that ulcerates. The base of the ulcer, which is usually painless, consists of necrotic tissue and crusted serum. Satellite lesions and local lymphadenopathy may be present.
- In diffuse cutaneous leishmaniasis, multiple, widespread non-ulcerating cutaneous papules, nodules and infiltration is seen.
- Post kala-azar dermal leishmaniasis (PKDL): Develops months to years after the patient's recovery from visceral leishmaniasis. Cutaneous lesions include hypopigmented macules, erythematous papules, nodules and plaques.

Mucocutaneous Leishmaniasis (ML)

- Lesions in or around the nose or mouth are the typical presentation of ML. Patients usually give history of self-healed CL preceding ML by 1–5 years. Typically, ML presents as nasal stuffiness and bleeding followed by destruction of nasal cartilage, perforation of the nasal septum, and collapse of the nasal bridge. Subsequent involvement of the pharynx and larynx leads to difficulty in swallowing and phonation. The lips, cheeks, and soft palate may also be affected. Secondary bacterial infection is common, and aspiration pneumonia may be fatal.

Diagnosis

- The diagnosis is established by demonstration of parasites. Amastigotes can be demonstrated by light-microscopic examination of a specimen (smear, biopsy) obtained from the infected site.
- Culture can be done in Novy-MacNeal-Nicolle (NNN) blood agar.
- Immunologic methods for diagnosis include serologic assays and skin testing for delayed-type hypersensitivity reactions. Traditional serologic methods like indirect fluorescent testing do not reliably distinguish past from current infection.
- Other methods of parasitological confirmation include animal inoculation, and polymerase chain reaction (PCR).

Treatment

- Three groups of drugs are commonly used in the treatment of leishmaniasis.
  - *Pentavalent antimonials*—sodium stibogluconate and meglumine antimoniate
  - *Pentamidine* isetheonate and pentamidine methanosulphonate
  - *Amphotericin B*
- All these drugs have to be given parenterally (IM or IV) for effective cure.
- *Miltefosine*: This is the first oral compound approved for the treatment of leishmaniasis. It has a long half-life (150–200 hours) and its mechanism of action is not clearly understood.

Q. Visceral leishmaniasis (kala-azar, Dumdum fever).

Etiology

- Visceral leishmaniasis (Kala-azar) is caused by *Leishmania donovani* and *L. infantum*. Kala-azar means 'black fever' in Hindi which refers to characteristic darkening of the skin seen in this condition.

Epidemiology

- Most cases of visceral leishmaniasis occur in Bangladesh, northeastern India (particularly Bihar state), Nepal, Sudan, and northeastern Brazil.
- Visceral leishmaniasis is transmitted by sandflies.
- It can also spread by blood transfusion or needle sharing.

Pathogenesis

- Infection begins in macrophages at the inoculation site as described above and disseminates throughout the reticuloendothelial system. Reticuloendothelial cells undergo hyperplasia which leads to enlargement of the spleen, liver, lymph nodes, and bone marrow. Bone-marrow infiltration, hypersplenism, autoimmune hemolysis, and bleeding all lead to pancytopenia.

Clinical Features

- The incubation period varies from weeks to months but can be as long as years.
- Males are affected more than females and children are affected more than adults.
- Onset of symptoms is usually insidious or subacute, with slow progression of malaise, fever, weight loss, and splenomegaly (with or without hepatomegaly) over a period of weeks to months.
- Patients usually present with daily fever. Some patients have 2 fever spikes per day (double quotidian fever) with rigors. Occasionally continuous fever can occur.
- Skin manifestations in VL are frequent. Kala-azar means "black sickness" and refers to characteristic darkening of the skin seen in this condition.
- Hepato-splenomegaly is often present and splenomegaly can be massive. Lymphadenopathy is also present.
- Anemia is present in most patients due to hemolysis, hypersplenism, and bone marrow suppression.
- Jaundice, hypoalbuminemia, edema and ascites can be there due to liver involvement.
- Death occurs due to secondary infections.

Diagnosis

- *Microscopy (gold standard):* Kala-azar can be diagnosed by demonstration of the parasite in smears or cultures of a tissue aspirate or a biopsy specimen (e.g. of spleen, liver, bone marrow, or lymph node).
- *Antibody detection* by direct agglutination test (DAT) and ELISA are the tests of choice for field diagnosis.
- *PCR* is a sensitive test and can also identify the species. It can be performed on almost any tissue. It is not widely available.
- *Culture:* Leishmania can be grown in NNN (Novy-MacNeal-Nicolle) medium. Takes several weeks.
- *Montenegro skin test:* Similar to TB skin test, detects delayed hypersensitivity reaction. Positive in cutaneous and mucocutaneous leishmaniasis, but negative in active visceral leishmaniasis.

Treatment

First-line Treatment

- Liposomal amphotericin B (IV, 3–5 mg/kg for 5 days)
- Miltefosine (oral, 28 days): Teratogenic, avoid in pregnancy.

Alternative Treatments

- Pentavalent antimonials (Sodium stibogluconate or Meglumine antimoniate)
- Combination therapy (Paromomycin + Miltefosine).

Prevention

- *Vector control*: Sandflies should be controlled by spraying insecticides such as pyrethroids.
- *Avoid sandfly bites*: Insecticide-impregnated mosquito net and repellants can be used for personal protection against sandfly bites.
- *Early detection and treatment*: Prevents complications and transmission.
- *Vaccine:* Currently, no widely available vaccine.

Q. Trypanosomiasis.

Q. American trypanosomiasis (Chagas' disease).

Q. African trypanosomiasis (sleeping sickness).

- Trypanosomiasis is caused by protozoans belonging to the genus Trypanosoma.
- There are mainly two types of trypanosomiasis, American trypanosomiasis and African trypanosomiasis.
- American trypanosomiasis (Chagas disease) is caused by *Trypanosoma cruzi*. African trypanosomiasis (sleeping sickness) is caused by *Trypanosoma brucei*.

American Trypanosomiasis (Chagas' disease)

- Chagas' disease is caused by the hemoflagellate protozoan *Trypanosoma cruzi* (flagellated protozoan). *T. cruzi* is found only in the Americas. It is the leading cause of congestive heart failure in areas of Latin America where it is endemic.

Pathogenesis

- It is transmitted to man by the bite of triatomine bug (also known as kissing bug). These bugs ingest organisms while sucking blood from infected animals or humans. Ingested organisms multiply in the gut of the bugs, and infective forms (trypomastigotes) are passed in the feces at the time of bite. Transmission occurs when breaks in the skin, mucous membranes, or conjunctivae become contaminated with bug feces.
- *T. cruzi* can also be transmitted by blood transfusion, organ transplantation and from mother to fetus.
- A nodular swelling or chagoma develops at the site of entry. Lymphatic spread then carries the organism to regional lymph nodes. When the histiocytes or other inflammatory cells ingest the parasites, they transform into amastigotes. After local multiplication, the organisms can assume the trypomastigote form and invade the bloodstream, carrying the infection to all parts of the body. Cells of the reticuloendothelial system; cardiac, skeletal, and smooth muscles; and neural cells are preferentially parasitized.
- During the acute phase of illness, the parasite is believed to directly destroy host cells. The pathogenesis of the cardiac and GI alterations typical of the chronic phase is not well understood. Loss of ganglionic neurons and nerve fibers along with inflammatory reaction are important pathological findings.

Clinical Features

- An indurated inflammatory lesion called "chagoma" often appears at the site of parasite entry.
- If the bite occurs near the eye, unilateral painless edema of palpebrae and periocular tissues associated with preauricular lymphadenopathy (Romana's sign) occurs. These initial local signs are followed by malaise, fever, and anorexia.

- Cardiac abnormalities are the most frequent manifestations of chronic Chagas' disease. Congestive heart failure is the first sign of chagas heart disease. Other features are arrhythmias and heart blocks (commonly RBBB-right bundle branch block). Death usually occurs due to heart failure.
- Involvement of GI tract produces dysphagia, regurgitation, hiccups, constipation, and abdominal pain.
- Muscle involvement leads to myositis and myalgia.
- Nervous system involvement leads to meningoencephalitis.

Diagnosis

- Microscopic examination of anticoagulated blood or of the buffy coat can show the motile trypanosomes (trypomastigotes).
- PCR: Detects parasite DNA in blood/tissues.
- Serology (ELISA, IFA) detects *T. cruzi* antibodies.
- ECG, echocardiography, barium swallow–Assess organ involvement.

Treatment

- There is no satisfactory treatment for Chagas' disease. Only two drugs—nifurtimox and benznidazole are available for treatment and these drugs cause severe side effects. Nifurtimox, a nitrofurantoin derivative, is given for 3 or 4 months. New drugs are being developed.

African Trypanosomiasis (Sleeping Sickness)

Etiology

- *Trypanosoma brucei gambiense* → West African Sleeping Sickness (chronic, 97% of cases). *Trypanosoma brucei rhodesiense* → East African Sleeping Sickness (acute, more severe).

Life Cycle

- Tsetse fly becomes infected when it bites infected mammalian hosts. After multiplication in the midgut of the tsetse fly, the parasites migrate to the salivary glands. Parasites are transmitted to another mammalian host when the tsetse fly bites. The injected trypanosomes multiply in the blood of new host and invade all the organs causing illness.

Clinical Features

- A painful chancre may appear in some patients at the site of bite associated with enlargement of the regional lymph nodes.
- Enlargement of the nodes of the posterior cervical triangle is known as 'Winterbottom's sign' and is characteristic of *T. brucei gambiense* infection.
- Hematogenous and lymphatic dissemination is marked by the onset of fever, headache, arthralgia, lymphadenopathy and hepatosplenomegaly.
- If untreated, CNS gets involved, producing sleepiness during the day (hence called sleeping sickness), nighttime insomnia, mental confusion, coma and death. CNS involvement occurs weeks to months after the initial infection.
- In rhodesience infection, death from myocarditis and intercurrent infection can occur before sleeping sickness.

Diagnosis

- Microscopy (gold standard): Trypomastigotes are found in blood, lymph, or CSF (thick and thin smears).
- Serological tests have not become popular because of variable sensitivity and specificity.
- PCR techniques are not yet commercially available.

Treatment

- Drugs used in the treatment of African trypanosomiasis include pentamidine, suramin, eflornithine, and melarsoprol.

Prevention

- Avoid areas which harbor tsetse flies, wear protective clothing and use insect repellents. Chemoprophylaxis is not recommended, and no vaccine is available at present.

Q. Babesiosis.

- Babesiosis is a tick-borne infectious disease caused by protozoan parasites of the genus Babesia. These protozoans are obligate intracellular parasites of red blood cells (RBCs).
- Wild and domestic animals are the natural reservoirs of Babesia. Transmission to humans is incidental.
- There are many species, but *Babesia microti* is responsible for most of the infections.

Epidemiology

- Most of the cases occur in the United States. Sporadic cases are reported in Europe and the rest of the world including India. The number of cases of *B. microti* illness has increased steadily over the last decade.

Life Cycle and Pathogenesis

- The nymphal stage of the deer tick *Ixodes scapularis* is the primary vector (it also carries Lyme disease) for transmission of *B. microti*. Transmission occurs from May through September with three-fourths of cases presenting in June and July. The incubation period is 1–6 weeks. Babesiosis can also be acquired through blood transfusion. There are case reports of congenital babesiosis also.

Clinical Features

- Babesiosis causes malaria-like illness with fever and hemolytic anemia. Patients present with fever

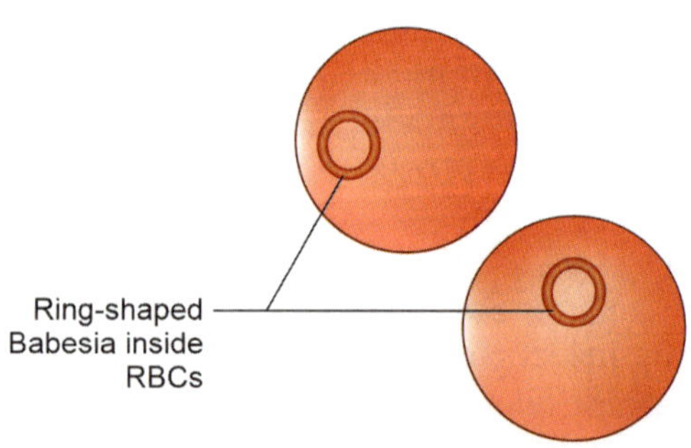

Figure 1.51: Babesia inside RBCs

associated with chills, sweats, headache, myalgia, anorexia, dry cough, arthralgia, and nausea.

- Physical examination is usually normal except for fever. Occasionally, hepatosplenomegaly may be seen. Rarely jaundice, pharyngeal erythema, retinal infarcts, and retinopathy with splinter hemorrhages is seen.
- Severe babesiosis can occur in immunocmpromised states such as asplenia, HIV/AIDS, malignancy, and immunosuppression. Complications such as severe hemolytic anemia, hemoglobinuria (due to RBC destruction) ARDS, disseminated intravascular coagulation, congestive heart failure, and renal failure can occur in severe babesiosis. Splenic infarcts and rupture have also been reported.

Diagnosis

- Babesiosis should be considered in patients who presents with flu-like symptoms and has recently resided in or traveled to an endemic area.
- Babesiosis is diagnosed by identification of Babesia in a peripheral blood smear. Babesia species appear as ring forms (similar to malaria but no pigment) inside RBCs.
- Polymerase chain reaction (PCR) can be used to identify DNA of babesia.
- Serological tests detect IgG and IgM antibodies against babesia. Used in chronic or past infections. Not useful for early detection.
- Complete blood count (CBC): Hemolytic anemia → ↓ Hemoglobin, ↑ Reticulocytes, ↓ Platelets
- Elevated lactate dehydrogenase (LDH) and bilirubin (due to RBC destruction)

Treatment

- Treatment is indicated in symptomatic patients with positive Babesia tests.
- Mild *B. microti* illness: oral atovaquone plus azithromycin for 7–10 days. Clindamycin plus quinine is the second choice.
- Severe *B. microti* illness: IV clindamycin plus oral quinine is given for 7–10 days.

Q. Toxoplasmosis.

- Toxoplasmosis is a disease caused by an intracellular protozoan parasite *Toxoplasma gondii*. Toxoplasmosis can be congenital or acquired.
- Congenital toxoplasmosis is transmitted from the mother to the fetus during pregnancy.
- Acquired infection is due to ingestion of cysts excreted in the feces of infected cats or from eating undercooked meat (especially lamb and pork).
- Infection can also be acquired through blood transfusion and organ transplantation.

Life Cycle and Pathogenesis

- The cat is the definitive host in which the sexual phase of the cycle takes place. Asexual cycle occurs in humans, mammals, birds (intermediate hosts).
- *T. gondii* exists in three forms: **oocysts** (infectious stage in the environment), **tachyzoites** (rapidly multiplying form during active infection), **bradyzoites (tissue cysts)** (latent infection form in muscle, brain).
- Cats ingest infected animals (rodents, birds) containing bradyzoite tissue cysts. The parasite undergoes sexual reproduction in the cat's intestines. Oocysts are formed in the cat and shed in feces. Vegetables or grass contaminated by cat feces can be ingested by animals, birds, and humans. Ingested oocysts become cysts (bradyzoites) in the muscle of animals.
- Human infection occurs by ingestion of oocysts in food or water contaminated with cat feces (most common mode of infection) or by eating raw or undercooked meat containing bradyzoite cysts, most commonly lamb, pork, or rarely beef. Toxoplasmosis can be transmitted transplacentally if the mother becomes infected during pregnancy.
- After ingestion of oocysts or bradyzoite cysts, tachyzoites are released and spread throughout the body. Tachyzoites later form bradyzoite cysts in many organs especially in CNS, eyes, heart, lungs, and adrenals. The cysts can reactivate later in immunocompromised patients such as AIDS patients.

Clinical Features

- Infections may manifest in several ways as follows:

Asymptomatic Infection

- Immunocompetent individuals often have no symptoms or mild flu-like illness.

Acute Toxoplasmosis (symptomatic cases)

- Fever, muscle aches, headache
- Lymphadenopathy (swollen lymph nodes)
- Fatigue

Ocular Toxoplasmosis

- Presents with retinitis and choroiditis. Symptoms are photophobia, ocular pain, and blurred vision. Can lead to blindness if untreated.

Congenital Toxoplasmosis (severe in infants)

- Occurs when the mother is infected during pregnancy. Clinical features are as follows;
- Hydrocephalus (fluid accumulation in the brain)
- Intracranial calcifications (seen on imaging)
- Chorioretinitis (eye inflammation leading to blindness)
- Seizures, intellectual disability

Toxoplasmosis in Immunocompromised Patients (HIV/AIDS, organ transplants)

- Reactivation of latent infection
- Severe brain infection (toxoplasmic encephalitis)
    - Clinical features are headache, altered mental status, seizures, coma, fever, and sometimes focal neurologic deficits.
    - Ring-enhancing brain lesions on MRI/CT scan

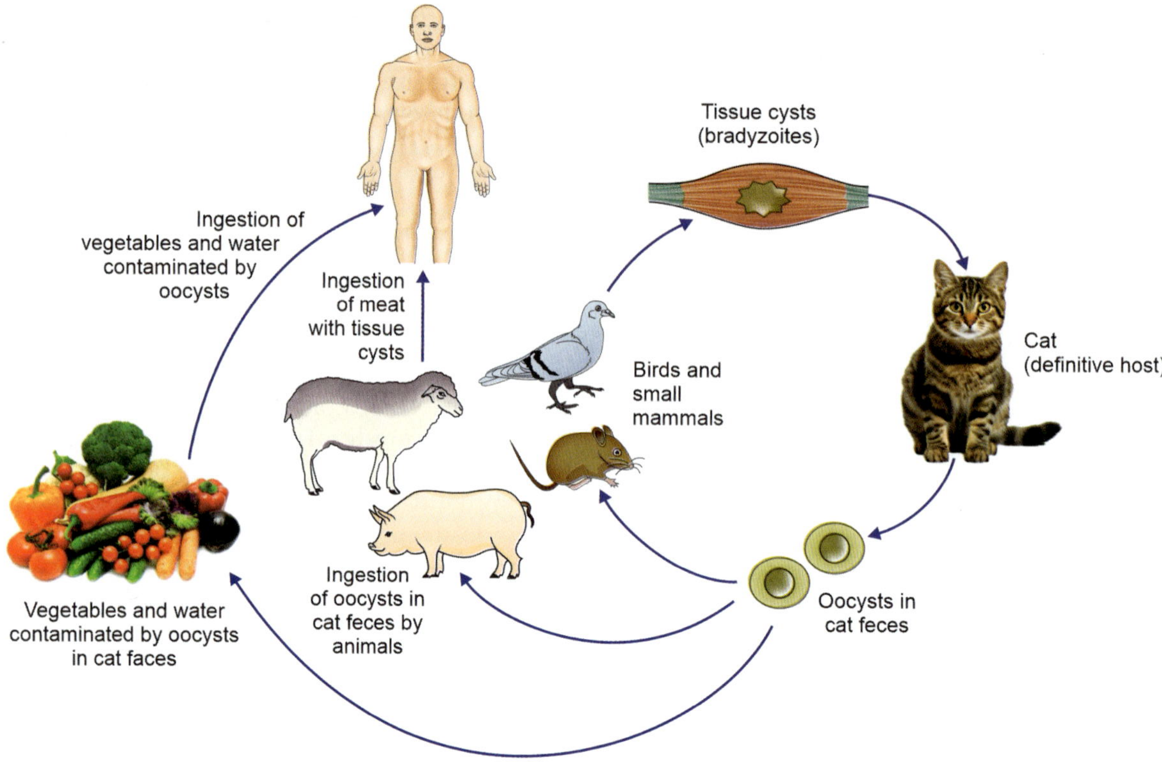

Figure 1.52: Life cycle of toxoplasmosis

- Disseminated disease: May present with pneumonitis, myocarditis, polymyositis, diffuse maculopapular rash, and high fevers. This may occur with or without CNS disease.

Investigations

- *Serological tests* like detection of antibodies are helpful in the diagnosis. A rise in the titer of IgM antibodies indicates acute infection. IgG antibodies indicate past infection (lifelong immunity). Antibodies persisting in an infant beyond 6 months of age imply congenital toxoplasmosis.
- *Biopsy* of a lymph node may show tachyzoites or histological changes.
- *Contrast CT or MRI of brain* should be done in suspected CNS toxoplosmosis which will show multiple ring enhancing lesions.
- *PCR:* Detects parasite DNA in blood, amniotic fluid, or cerebrospinal fluid.

Management

- Immunocompetent persons do not require specific treatment as the infection usually resolves spontaneously. But infants, immunosuppressed patients and those with eye involvement require treatment.
- *First-line therapy* (6 weeks minimum): Pyrimethamine + Sulfadiazine + Leucovorin (Folinic acid).
  - Pyrimethamine → Antiprotozoal drug.
  - Sulfadiazine → Kills Toxoplasma.
  - Leucovorin → Protects against pyrimethamine toxicity
- *Alternative if sulfa allergy:*
  - Pyrimethamine + Clindamycin + Leucovorin.

Toxoplasmosis and Pregnancy

- If a seronegative woman acquires toxoplasmosis in first trimester of pregnancy, there is a high risk of fetal damage. Hence, termination of pregnancy should be considered in such women.
- If a woman is already seropositive before becoming pregnant, then there is no risk of fetal damage.
- Spiramycin is used for pregnant women to prevent fetal transmission.

Prevention

- Avoid undercooked meat → Cook meat to ≥65°C (149°F).
- Wash hands and vegetables thoroughly.
- Pregnant women should avoid cat litter, raw meat, and unpasteurized dairy.
- HIV patients who are seropositive for *T. gondii* and who have a CD4+ T lymphocyte count of <100/µl should receive trimethoprim-sulfamethoxazole (TMP-SMX) as prophylaxis against toxoplasmosis.

Q. Describe the pathogenesis, clinical features, investigations and treatment of Pneumocystis infection.

Q. *Pneumocystis jiroveci* pneumonia (*Pneumocystis carinii*).

- *Pneumocystis jiroveci* (formerly known as *Pneumocystis carinii*) is an opportunistic fungal pulmonary pathogen and is an important cause of pneumonia in the immunocompromised individuals.
- Pnemocystis is now classified as a fungus. However, unlike fungi, Pneumocystis lacks ergosterol and is not susceptible to antifungal drugs.

- Pneumocystis has worldwide distribution and most people are exposed to the organism in childhood itself.

Pathogenesis

- Pneumocystis infection develops usually in immunocompromised individuals. HIV patients who have CD4+ counts below 200/μl have high chances of developing *Pneumocystis jiroveci* infection. Other persons at risk are patients on immunosuppressive therapy (particularly glucocorticoids) for cancer, organ transplantation, and other disorders; children with primary immunodeficiency diseases; and premature malnourished infants.
- After being inhaled, Pneumocystis reaches the alveoli, and attaches to type-I alveolar cells. The main defence against Pneumocystis is alveolar macrophages, which ingest and kill the organism. If the immune system of the host is compromised, Pneumocystis multiplies and damages the type I alveolar cells, alters surfactant, and increases alveolar capillary permeability. Lung sections stained with hematoxylin and eosin, show the alveoli filled with a foamy exudate. In severe disease, there is interstitial edema, fibrosis, and hyaline membrane formation.

Clinical Features

- The incubation period is 1–2 months.
- Patients with pneumocystis pneumonia present with fever, dyspnea, and dry cough. Physical findings include tachypnea, tachycardia, and cyanosis, but there are few lung findings (i.e. symptoms are more than signs). Pneumothorax may occur sometimes and management is difficult.
- Although Pneumocystis usually remains confined to the lungs, disseminated infection can occur and involves lymph nodes, spleen, liver, and bone marrow. Eye lesions (choroiditis) also occur and may be confused with CMV retinitis.

Investigations

- *Chest X-ray* shows bilateral diffuse infiltrates mainly in the perihilar regions.
- *High-resolution CT* (HRCT) scan: Ground-glass opacities, worse in perihilar areas.
- *ABG (arterial blood gas)* analysis shows reduced arterial oxygen pressure (PaO_2), and respiratory alkalosis (alkalosis is due to tachypnea). There is increased alveolar-arterial oxygen gradient (PAO_2–PaO_2). PAO_2–PaO_2 of >35 mm Hg indicates poor prognosis.
- *Pulmonary function tests* show reduced diffusing capacity of the lung (DLCO) and an increased uptake of tracer with nuclear imaging (gallium-67 citrate scan).
- *Serum lactate dehydrogenase (LDH)* levels are usually elevated due to lung parenchymal damage.
- Beta-D-glucan (Fungal marker)—often elevated.
- Since there is little sputum production, sputum can be induced by inhalation of 3% saline and stained with *Methenamine silver and toluidine blue* which selectively stain the wall of *P. jiroveci* cysts. Fiber-optic bronchoscopy with bronchoalveolar lavage (BAL) is more sensitive (>90%) than induced sputum.
- *Transbronchial biopsy and open lung biopsy* are performed only when the diagnosis remains in doubt.

Treatment

- Treatment should be started as soon as the diagnosis is suspected.
- Trimethoprim-sulphamethoxazole (TMP–SMX) is the drug of choice for all types of pneumocystis infections and is given for 21 days. Alternative for sulfa allergic patients is atovaquone (oral) or dapsone + trimethoprim.
- Other effective drugs include clindamycin + primaquine. Pentamidine IV.
- Steroids (prednisone 40 mg BID, for 5 days, then taper) improve the prognosis in HIV infected patients with pneumocystis. However, one should be cautious about associated tuberculosis.

Prevention

- Primary prophylaxis is indicated for HIV-infected patients with CD4 counts less than 200 cells/cumm. Secondary prophylaxis is indicated for patients with prior pneumocystis. Prophylaxis can be stopped if CD4 >200 cells/μl for ≥3 months on ART.
- TMP-SMX (one double strength tablet once daily) is the drug of choice.
- Alternatives if there is sulfa allergy are as follows;
  - Dapsone (Check for G6PD deficiency before use)
  - Atovaquone (Less effective but well-tolerated)
  - Aerosolized Pentamidine (For those unable to take oral meds).

Q. Name the different tape worms which infest human beings.

- Tapeworms are parasitic flatworms (Cestodes) that infect the intestines of humans and animals.
- Adult worms reside in the gastrointestinal tract, but the larvae can be found in any organ.
- Humans are either the definitive hosts where the adult worms reside in GIT (*Taenia saginata*,

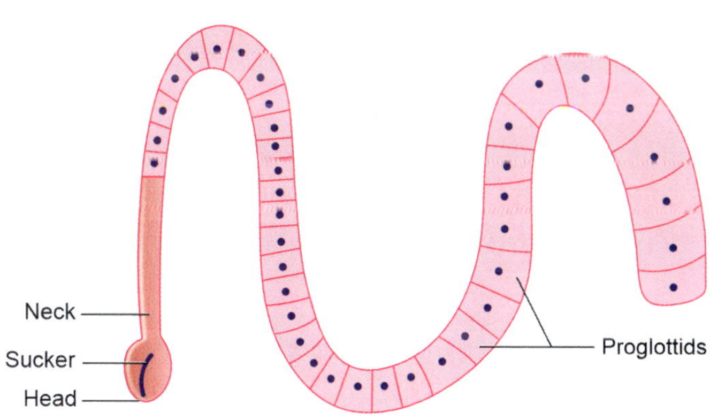

Figure 1.53: Tape worm

Infectious Diseases 1

Diphyllobothrium, Hymenolepis, and *Dipylidium caninum*) or the humans are intermediate hosts where larval-stage parasites are present in the tissues (echinococcosis, sparganosis, and coenurosis).

- For *Taenia solium*, humans can be both definitive and intermediate hosts.
- An adult tapeworm consits of a head (scolex), a neck, and a chain of individual segments (proglottids). The scolex is the attachment organ through which tapeworm attaches to the intestinal mucosa. Neck is the narrow part behind scolex from which proglottids (segments) form. Mature proglottids produce eggs. Proglottids are hermophrodites and cross-fertilization between proglottids occurs. Big worms can be several metres in length. The entire worm is covered with an elastic cuticle. Tapeworms absorb nutrients directly through the cuticle since they do not have any GI tract.
- Tapeworms infecting humans are as follows.

Types of Tapeworms and their Transmission

See **Table 1.25**.

Q. Taenia saginata (beef tapeworm).

- *T. saginata* (also called the cattle or beef tapeworm) occurs in all countries where raw or undercooked beef is eaten. This worm can reach 4–12 meters in length.

Life Cycle

- Humans are the only definitive host for the adult stage of *T. saginata* and cattle are intermediate hosts. It lives in the upper jejunum. It attaches to jejunal mucosa through a scolex which has four suckers. Eggs are passed in the feaces and can live for months to years on vegetation. Cattle may ingest these eggs while grazing. Inside the cattle intestine, the eggs hatch and release larvae. Larvae invade the intestinal wall, and are carried to striated muscle, where they becomes cysticerci. When raw or undercooked beef is eaten by humans, this cysticerci can grow into adult worm in the intestine.
- Unlike *T. solium* (pork tapeworm), *T. saginata* does not cause neurocysticercosis because its larvae do not infect human tissues.

Clinical Features

- Patients may notice worm segments (proglottids) in their feces. The proglottids are often motile.
- Abdominal pain or discomfort, nausea, decreased appetite, weakness, and weight loss (rare) can occur.
- Severe infestation may produce vitamin B_{12} deficiency (similar to *Diphyllobothrium latum*), intestinal obstruction, and appendicitis or pancreatitis (if proglottids block ducts).

Diagnosis

- Stool microscopy: Detection of eggs or proglottids in the stool. Eggs may also be present in the perianal area; thus, if proglottids or eggs are not found in the stool, the perianal region should be examined with use of a cellophane-tape swab.
- Eosinophilia and elevated serum IgE levels may be present.

Treatment

- Praziquantel, given as a single dose (10 mg/kg) is effective against this tape worm. Niclosamide (2 g) is an alternative.

Prevention

- Proper cooking of beef and pork, inspection of beef before cooking, and proper disposal of human feces are measures which can prevent *T. saginata* infestation.

Q. *Taenia solium* and cysticercosis (pork tapeworm).

Q. Neurocysticercosis (NCC).

- *T. solium* is the pork tapeworm.
- It can cause two forms of infection. In humans, infection can be with adult tapeworm in the intestine or with larval forms in the tissues (cysticercosis).
- It has worldwide distribution.

Life Cycle (Fig. 1.54)

- Humans are the only definitive hosts for *T. solium*; pigs are the usual intermediate hosts. The adult tapeworm usually stays in the upper jejunum. It has a scolex with two sucking disks through which it attaches to the mucosa. The adult worm is about 3 meters in length and may live for years. Proglottids (segments) contain eggs and are passed in the feces. Eggs can survive in the environment for many months. These eggs are infective to humans and animals. If eggs are ingested by animals and man (through contaminated food, hands, water), the larvae are released in the intestine, penetrate the intestinal wall, and are carried to many tissues. In the tissues, larvas become encysted in 2–3 months (cysticerci). These cysticerci can survive for

TABLE 1.25: Types of tapeworms and their transmission

Tapeworm species	Intermediate host	Infection source	Disease
Taenia solium	Pigs	Undercooked pork	Taeniasis, Neurocysticercosis
Taenia saginata	Cattle	Undercooked beef	Taeniasis
Diphyllobothrium latum	Fish (freshwater)	Raw/undercooked fish	Diphyllobothriasis (Vitamin B_{12} deficiency)
Echinococcus granulosus	Dogs, sheep	Dog feces	Hydatid disease (Cystic echinococcosis)
Echinococcus multilocularis	Foxes, rodents	Fox/dog feces	Alveolar echinococcosis
Hymenolepis nana	Humans, rodents	Contaminated food/water	Hymenolepiasis (common in children)

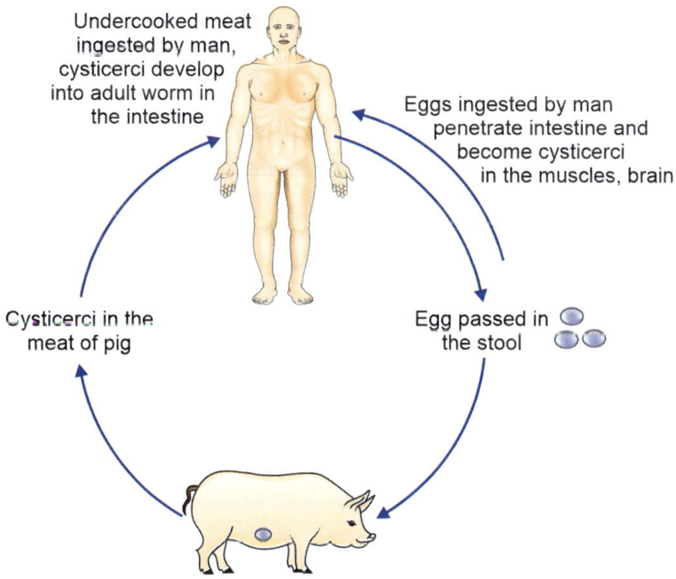

Figure 1.54: Life cycle of *Taenia solium*

months to years. Humans also acquire infection by ingesting undercooked pork containing cysticerci. In this case ingested cysticerci develop into adult tapeworms in the intestine. Autoinfection may occur if an individual ingests eggs from his own feces.

- Note that NCC does not occur by eating pork. Pork meat containing cysticerci when ingested by man develop into adult tape worm in the intestine (cysticercosis will not develop). Cysticercosis in humans develops only when the eggs of *T. solium* are ingested. Hence, food or water, especially raw vegetables contaminated with *T. solium* eggs can cause cysticercosis including neurocysticercosis.

Clinical Manifestations

- Intestinal infection with *T. solium* is usually asymptomatic or produces epigastric discomfort, nausea, weight loss, and diarrhea. Worm segments (proglottids) may be noted in feces.
- In cysticercosis, the clinical manifestations depend on the location of cysticerci. Cysticerci are commonly found in the brain, subarachnoid space, spinal cord, skeletal muscle, subcutaneous tissue, and eye.
- Cysticerci in the brain (neurocysticercosis-NCC) act like space occupying lesions. Seizures (most common clinical manifestation of NCC), hydrocephalus (due to obstruction of CSF flow by cysticerci), signs of raised intracranial pressure including headache, nausea, vomiting, changes in vision, dizziness, ataxia, or confusion, may be present. Patients with hydrocephalus may develop papilledema or display altered mental status. Chronic meningitis and strokes can also occur.
- In the eye they may cause blindness.

Diagnosis

- Stool examination may show eggs or worm segments.
- Definitive diagnosis of cysticercosis is difficult because it requires biopsy and histopatholgical studies which are sometimes difficult to obtain as in brain infection. However, a clinical diagnosis can be made based on Clinical Features, imaging studies, serologic tests, and exposure history.
- MRI/CT scan of brain shows ring enhancing lesions. Demonstration of a scolex within a cystic lesion is considered diagnostic of neurocysticercosis.
- Serology (ELISA, Western Blot): Detects antibodies against *T. solium*.

Treatment

Intestinal infection

- Praziquantel (10 mg/kg) as a single dose is effective. Niclosamide (2 g) is an alternative.

Neurocysticercosis

- Praziquantel 50–60 mg/kg daily in three divided doses for 15 days or albendazole (15 mg/kg per day for 10–14 days hasten the resolution of cysticercosis.
- Both drugs can exacerbate the inflammatory response due to dying parasites which may be prevented by addition of steroids.
- Antiepileptics for seizures.
- Obstructive hydrocephalus is treated by the removal of the cysticercus via endoscopic surgery or by ventriculoperitoneal shunting.

Prevention of *T. solium* infection

- Properly cook pork (≥63°C/145°F for 3 minutes).
- Handwashing and sanitation (prevents fecal-oral transmission).
- Deworm pigs and prevent pigs from consuming human feces.
- Mass deworming campaigns in endemic areas.
- Improved meat inspection and food hygiene.

Q. Diphyllobothriasis.

- *Diphyllobothrium latum* (fish tapeworm) is a parasite of freshwater fish. *D. latum* is the largest tapeworm of humans (up to 10 meters in length).

Life Cycle

- It occurs when humans eat raw or undercooked freshwater fish containing infectious larvae. The adult tapeworm lives usually in the ileum and occasionally in the jejunum. The adult worm has 3000–4000 proglottids (segments) which release eggs daily into the feces. If an egg reaches water, it hatches and releases a free-swimming larva which is eaten by crustaceans (Cyclops). Inside the crustacean the larva develops into a procercoid. When the crustacean is swallowed by a fish, the larva migrates into the fish's flesh and grows into a sparganum larva. Humans acquire the infection by ingesting undercooked infected freshwater fish. Inside the human intestine, the larva matures into an adult worm. Diphyllobothriasis occurs worldwide, especially where lakes are contaminated by sewage.

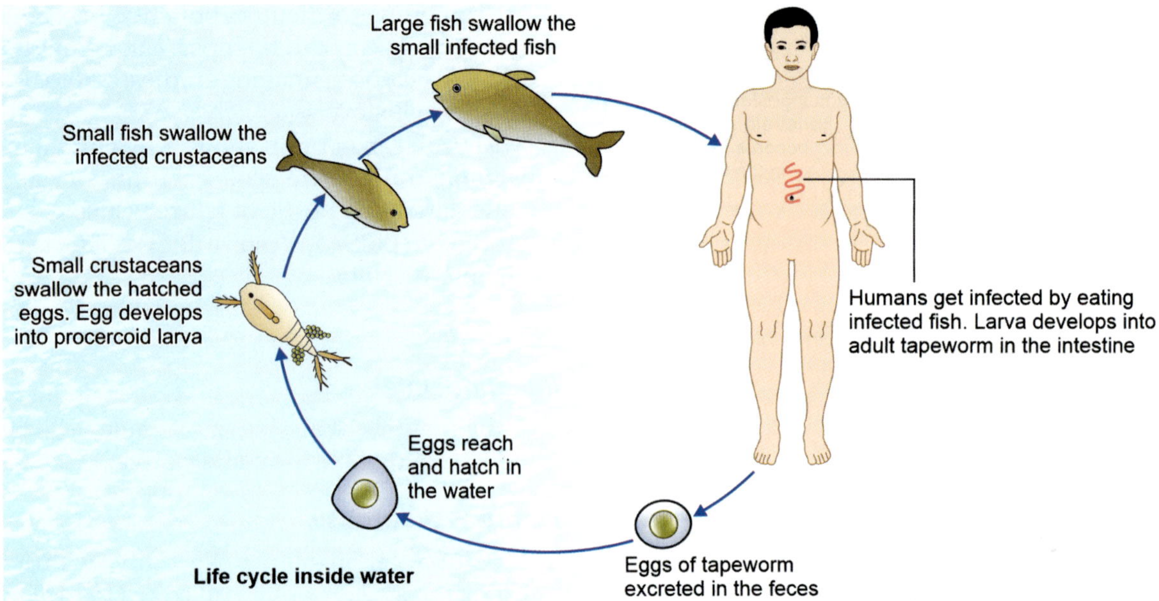

Figure 1.55: Life cycle of fish tapeworm

Clinical Manifestations

- Most *D. latum* infections are asymptomatic. Some may have abdominal discomfort, diarrhea, vomiting, weakness, and weight loss.
- Rarely worm can cause intestinal obstruction, cholangitis or cholecystitis by mechanically blocking the lumen.
- Because the tapeworm absorbs vitamin B_{12}, vitamin B_{12} deficiency can develop which manifests as megaloblastic anemia.

Diagnosis

- Stool microscopy (gold standard test): May show eggs or worm segments (proglottids) in the stool.
- Megaloblastic anemia in severe cases. Eosinophilia may be present.
- PCR and serology (for species identification): Used in research or outbreaks.

Treatment

- Praziquantel, 5–10 mg/kg as a single dose is highly effective. Niclosamide (2 g) is an alternative.

Prevention and control

- Properly cook fish.
- Avoid raw freshwater fish (sushi, ceviche, sashimi, smoked fish).
- Proper sewage disposal (prevents egg contamination in lakes/rivers).

Q. Hymenolepis nana (dwarf tapeworm).

- This is the most common human tapeworm worldwide.
- This is the smallest tapeworm (2–4 cm in length) infesting human beings.
- Only tapeworm which does not require an intermediate host. Hence the only tapeworm capable of direct human-to-human transmission.
- *H. nana* is endemic all over the world. Infection is spread by feco-oral contamination.

Life Cycle

- *H. nana* is the only tapeworm which does not require an intermediate host. Both the larval and adult phases take place in the humans. The adult worm resides in the proximal ileum. The eggs are released into the feces and when ingested by a new host, the oncosphere is freed and penetrates the intestinal villi, becoming a cysticercoid larva. Larva migrates back into the intestinal lumen, attaches to the mucosa, and matures into adult worm. Eggs may also hatch before passing into the stool, causing internal autoinfection.

Clinical Manifestations

- Infection is usually asymptomatic. Occasionally anorexia, abdominal pain, and diarrhea may be seen.

Diagnosis

- Detection of eggs in the stool.

Treatment

- Praziquantel (25 mg/kg once) is the drug of choice. It is effective against both the adult worms and the cysticercoids. Niclosamide (2 g) is an alternative.

Q. Echinococcosis (dog tape worm) (hydatid cyst).

- Echinococcosis, also known as hydatid disease, is a zoonotic infection caused by the larval stage of the *Echinococcus* tapeworm. The most common species affecting humans are:
    - *Echinococcus granulosus*—cystic echinococcosis (hydatid cyst disease).
    - *Echinococcus multilocularis*—alveolar echinococcosis (more severe).
    - *Echinococcus vogeli* and *Echinococcus oligarthrus*—rare, cause polycystic echinococcosis.

- Humans are accidental intermediate hosts: They become infected by ingesting tapeworm eggs from dog feces or contaminated food/water.

Life Cycle (Fig. 1.56)

- Like other cestodes, echinococcal species have both intermediate and definitive hosts. The definitive hosts are dogs that pass eggs in their feces. These eggs are ingested by intermediate hosts—sheep, cattle, humans, goats, camels, and horses either through contaminated food/water or while grazing. Eggs develop into cysts in the muscles of intermediate hosts. When a dog ingests beef or lamb containing cysts, they develop into adult worms in dogs and life cycle is completed.
- When humans ingest the eggs, embryos escape from the eggs, penetrate the intestinal mucosa, enter the portal circulation, and are carried to various organs, most commonly the liver and lungs where they develop into fluid-filled unilocular hydatid cysts. These cysts consist of an external membrane and an inner germinal layer. Daughter cysts and brood capsules develop from the inner germinal layer. New larvae, called protoscolices, develop within the brood capsule. The cysts expand slowly over a period of years.
- The life cycle of *E. multilocularis* is same except that the intermediate hosts are rodents.

Clinical Manifestations

- Echinococcal cysts remain asymptomatic until their expanding size elicits symptoms in the involved organ. Liver and lungs are involved commonly.
- Patients with liver cysts often present with abdominal pain or a palpable mass in the right upper quadrant. Compression of a bile duct can cause biliary obstruction and jaundice.,
- Lung involvement presents with cough, chest pain, dyspnea, and hemoptysis. Right lung is involved more commonly.
- CNS involvement leads to seizure, neurological deficits and raised ICT.
- Involvement of the heart leads to conduction defects and pericarditis.
- Cysts in the kidney can cause hematuria or flank pain.
- Involvement of bone leads to pathologic fractures.
- Ocular and subcutaneous cysts has also been described.
- Rupture or leakage of hydatid cyst fluid may produce fever, pruritus, urticaria, eosinophilia, or anaphylaxis. Rupture of hydatid cysts may also lead to dissemination of protoscolices, which can develop into additional cysts. Rupture can occur spontaneously or at surgery.
- The larval forms of *E. multilocularis* present as slowly growing mass in the liver with destruction of hepatic parenchyma. These cysts may lead to obstruction of biliary tree leading to obstructive jaundice, or invade adjacent structures like diaphragm, kidneys and lungs.

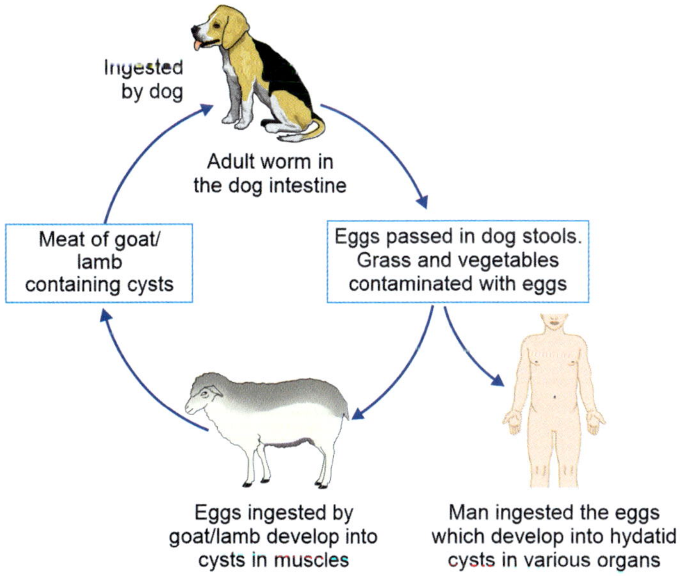

Figure 1.56: Life cycle of dog tape worm (hydatid cyst)

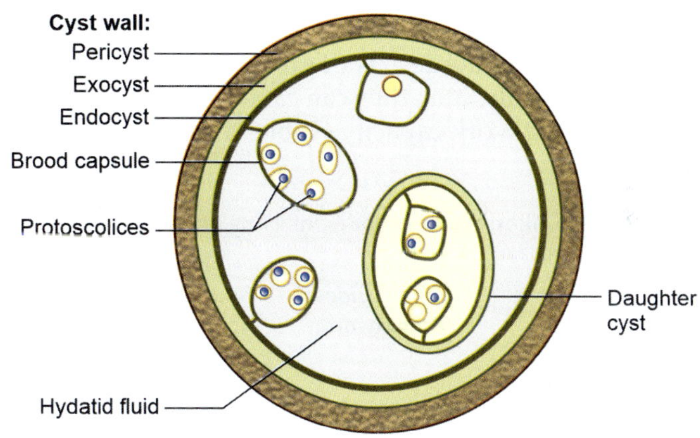

Figure 1.57: Hydatid cyst

Diagnosis

- MRI, CT, and ultrasound can define the site and size of echinococcal cysts.
- Examination of aspirated fluid from cyst for protoscolices or hooklets can make a definite diagnosis of *E. granulosus* infection, but is not usually recommended because of the risk of fluid leakage resulting in either dissemination of infection or anaphylactic reactions.
- Serologic studies for antibodies can be useful, but negative result does not rule out the diagnosis.

Treatment

- For uncomplicated *E. granulosus* cysts, PAIR (percutaneous aspiration, infusion of scolicidal agents, and reaspiration) is now the treatment of choice. PAIR is contraindicated for superficially located cysts (because of the risk of rupture), for cysts with multiple internal septae, and for cysts communicating with the biliary tree. Albendazole (15 mg/kg daily in two divided doses) should be given for at least 4 days before the procedure and continued for at least 4 weeks afterward.

- For complicated *E. granulosus* cysts (e.g. those communicating with the biliary tree), surgery is the treatment of choice. Pericystectomy is the procedure of choice, where the entire cyst and the surrounding fibrous tissue are removed. There is a risk of spillage of cyst contents during surgery. Albendazole should be given for several days before resection and for several weeks after resection. Praziquantel (50 mg/kg daily for 2 weeks), may hasten the death of the protoscolices.
- Medical therapy with albendazole alone for 12 weeks to 6 months results in cure in ~30% of cases and improvement in another 50%.
- Surgical resection remains the treatment of choice for *E. multilocularis* infection.

Q. Name the different intestinal nematodes that infest man.

Intestinal Nematodes

- Intestinal nematodes are roundworms. Their length varies from 1 mm to many centimeters. There are more than a billion people worldwide who are infected with intestinal nematodes. Though nematode infections are not usually fatal, they can cause malnutrition and diminished work capacity **(Table 1.26)**.

Q. Describe the, lifecycle, clinical features, diagnosis and treatment of *Ascaris lumbricoides* (Ascariasis).

- Ascaris is a nematode seen worldwide.
- It is transmitted through feco-oral route and is common in areas of poor sanitation.

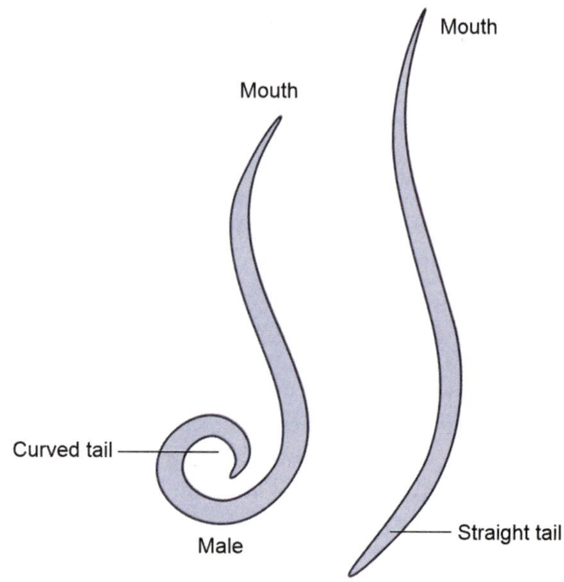

Figure 1.58: Ascaris worms

TABLE 1.26: Intestinal nematodes infesting man

	Ascaris lumbricoides **(Roundworm)**	**Hookworm (*Necator americanus, Ancylostoma duodenale*)**	***Strongyloides stercoralis***	***Trichuris trichiura*** **(Whipworm)**	***Enterobius vermicularis*** **(Pinworm)**
Endemic areas	Worldwide	Hot, humid regions	Hot, humid regions	Worldwide	Worldwide
Infective stage	Egg	Filariform larva	Filariform larva	Egg	Egg
Transmission	Feco-oral	Skin penetration (walking barefoot on contaminated soil)	Skin penetration, autoinfection	Feco-oral	Feco-oral
Gastrointestinal location of worms	Jejunum	Jejunum	Small intestine	Cecum, colon	Cecum, appendix
Adult worm size	15–35 cm	0.7–1.2 cm	2 mm	3–5 cm	0.8–1.3 cm
Pulmonary passage of larvae	Yes	Yes	Yes	No	No
Life span	1–2 years	2–8 years	Decades (owing to autoinfection)	5 years	2 months
Main symptoms	Usually asymptomatic. Rarely gastrointestinal or biliary obstruction	Iron-deficiency anemia	Gastrointestinal symptoms, malabsorption	Gastrointestinal symptoms, anemia	Perianal pruritus
Diagnosis	Detection of eggs in stool	Detection of eggs in fresh stool, larvae in old stool	Detection of larvae in stool or duodenal aspirate	Detection of eggs in stool	Detection of eggs from perianal skin on cellulose acetate tape
Treatment	Mebendazole, albendazole, pyrantel pamoate	Mebendazole, albendazole, pyrantel pamoate	Ivermectin, albendazole, thiabendazole	Mebendazole, albendazole	Mebendazole, albendazole, pyrantel pamoate

- The length of adult ascaris is 15–35 cm. Female worm is bigger with a straight posterior end. Male worm is smaller with a curved posterior end **(Fig. 1.58)**.

Life Cycle (Fig. 1.59)

- Adult worms live in the small intestine for 1–2 years. Female Ascaris worms produce eggs which are passed in the stools. These eggs mature in the soil and become infective after several weeks. Eggs can remain infective for many years. When a person swallows these eggs, eggs hatch in the intestine and produce larvae. These larvae invade the intestinal mucosa, reach lungs through circulation, break into the alveoli, ascend the bronchial tree, and are swallowed. They reach small intestine and develop into adult worms. About 2 and 3 months are required from swallowing of eggs to development of adult worms.

Clinical Features

- Most infected individuals are asymptomatic. Symptoms arise due to larval migration through the lungs or adult worms in the intestines.
- When the larvae migrate through the lungs, patients may develop a dry cough and burning substernal discomfort worsened by coughing or deep inspiration. Sometimes dyspnea and blood-tinged sputum may be seen. Low-grade fever and weight loss may be present. All these features may be mistaken for pulmonary tuberculosis. Eosinophilia develops during this symptomatic phase and subsides slowly over weeks. Chest X-ray may show eosinophilic pneumonitis (Löffler's syndrome) with round or oval infiltrates.
- In heavy infections, a large number of worms can get entangled and cause intestinal obstruction. Single worm may migrate into and occlude the biliary tree, causing biliary colic, cholecystitis, cholangitis, and pancreatitis. Sometimes worms may come out of mouth or nose.

Diagnosis

- Stool examination: Detection of ascaris eggs in the stool sample.
- Detection of larvae in sputum or gastric aspirates when they migrate through the lungs.
- Eosinophilia may be found in the blood in early stages.
- Imaging (Ultrasound, X-ray, CT scan): Large adult worm shadows may be visualized occasionally.

Treatment

- Albendazole (400 mg single dose), or mebendazole (500 mg single dose) is effective against ascariasis. These drugs are contraindicated in pregnancy and instead pyrantel pamoate (11 mg/kg once; maximum, 1 g) can be used in pregnancy.
- Intestinal obstruction requires surgery.

Prevention

- Improved sanitation and hygiene (proper disposal of feces).
- Washing hands and vegetables thoroughly.
- Health education on avoiding contaminated food and water.

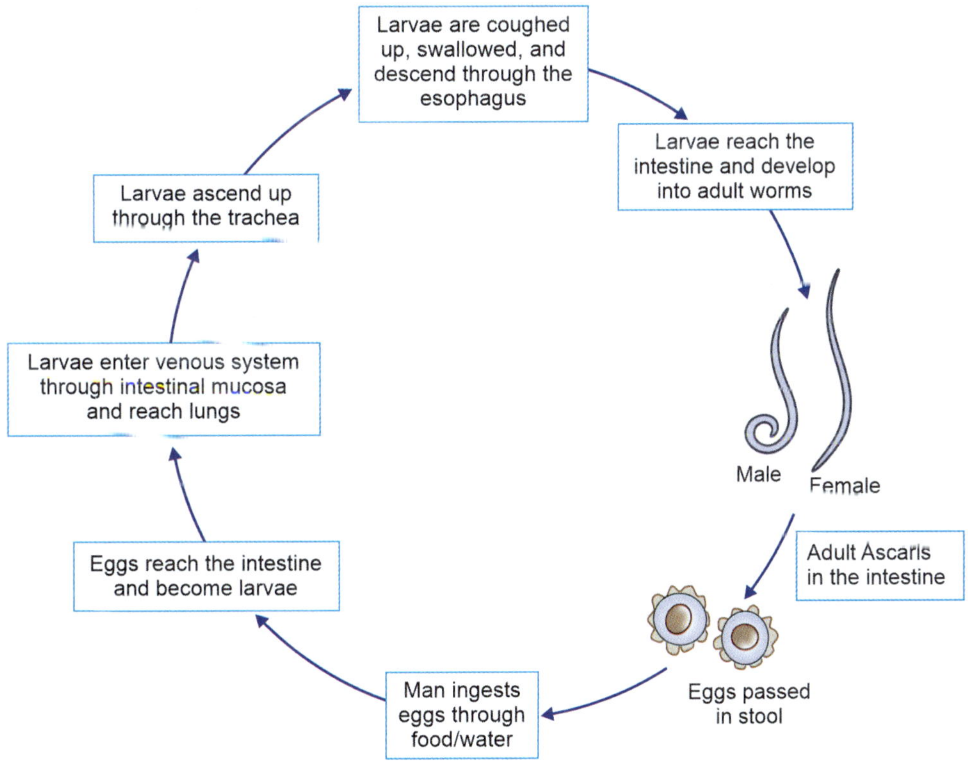

Figure 1.59: Life cycle of ascariasis

Infectious Diseases

1

Q. Describe the epidemiology, life cycle, clinical features, diagnosis and treatment of hook worm infestation.

Epidemiology

- Human hookworm disease is predominantly caused by the nematode parasites *Necator americanus* and *Ancylostoma duodenale*; and rarely by *Ancylostoma ceylonicum*, *Ancylostoma braziliense*, and *Ancylostoma caninum*.
- Ancylostoma duodenale is found in Mediterranean countries, Iran, India, Pakistan, and the Far East. Necator Americanus is found in North and South America, Central Africa, Indonesia, and parts of India. Both are found in many tropical regions, particularly Southeast Asia.
- It is common in rural areas where defecating in open fields is common. Barefoot walking is a risk factor for infection.
- Older children are affected commonly.
- *Ancylostoma caninum* and *Ancylostoma braziliense* are animal hookworms and can cause cutaneous larva migrans ("creeping eruption").

Life Cycle

- Adult hookworms are about 1 cm long. They attach to the intestinal mucosa through buccal teeth (Ancylostoma) or cutting plates (Necator) and suck blood (0.5 ml/day per Ancylostoma and 0.03 ml/day per each *N. americanus*) and interstitial fluid. The adult hookworms produce thousands of eggs daily. The eggs are passed with feces into the soil, where rhabditiform larvae hatch and develop over a 1-week period into filariform larvae. These filariform larvae penetrate the skin and reach the lungs through bloodstream. In the lungs, they invade alveoli and ascend the airways, get swallowed and reach the small intestine. In the small intestine they develop into adult worms. It takes about 6–8 weeks from skin invasion to appearance of eggs in the feces. A. duodenale lives for about 6–8 years and N. americanus for 2–5 years.

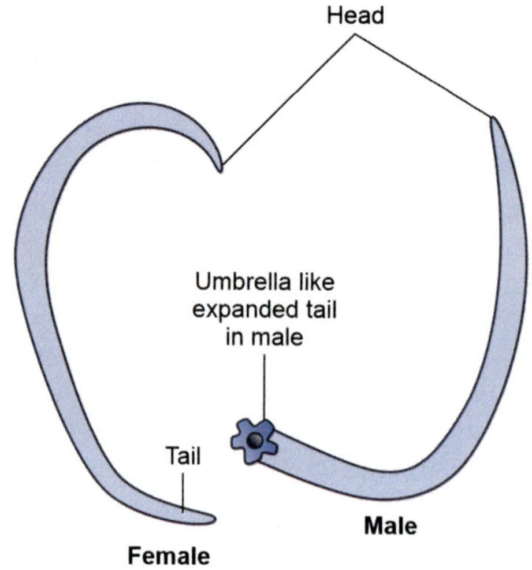

Figure 1.60: Adult hook worms (around 1 cm long)

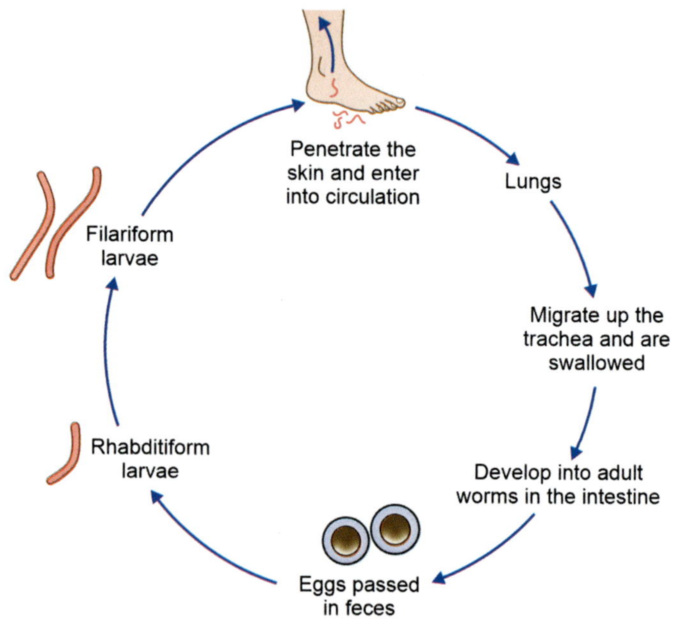

Figure 1.61: Life cycle of hookworm

Clinical Features

- Most hookworm infections are asymptomatic.
- Filariform larvae may cause pruritic maculopapular dermatitis ("ground itch") at the site of skin penetration as well as serpiginous tracks when they migrate through subcutaneous tissue (similar to cutaneous larva migrans).
- Larvae migrating through the lungs may cause transient pneumonitis.
- Mild epigastric pain or diarrhea may be seen sometimes.
- Chronic hookworm infection leads to iron deficiency anemia.

Diagnosis

- *Stool microscopy*: Detection of oval hookworm eggs in the feces. In light infections, stool-concentration procedures may be required to detect eggs. Eggs of the two species cannot be differentiated by light microscopy.
- Eosinophilia may be present.
- Microcytic hypochromic anemia, occasionally with eosinophilia is characteristic of chronic hookworm infestation.

Treatment

- Albendazole (400 mg single dose), or mebendazole (500 mg single dose), or pyrantel pamoate (11 mg/kg for 3 days) are highly effective.

Q. Strongyloidiasis.

- Strongyloidiasis is due to *Strongyloides stercoralis* which is a helminth.
- In contrast to other helminthic parasites, *S. stercoralis* can complete its entire life cycle within the human host. This unique capacity leads to repeated cycles of autoinfection and thus strongyloidiasis can persist for decades in the host.

Epidemiology

- *S. stercoralis* is found in tropical areas and is particularly common in Southeast Asia, sub-Saharan Africa, and Brazil. It is also found in some parts of United States.

Life Cycle

- Adult female worms of *S. stercoralis* are about 2-mm-long. **Parasitic adult males do not exist** and female worms produce eggs by parthenogenesis. Eggs hatch in the intestine itself, releasing rhabditiform larvae which are passed with the feces into soil. These rhabditiform larvae transform into infectious filariform larvae either directly or after a free-living phase of development in the soil. Humans acquire strongyloidiasis when filariform larvae penetrate the skin or mucous membranes and enter the body. These filariform larvae reach the lungs through bloodstream. In the lungs, they invade alveoli and ascend the airways, get swallowed and reach the small intestine. In the small intestine, larvae mature into adult worms that penetrate the mucosa of the small intestine. Alternatively, rhabditiform larvae in the intestine can develop directly into filariform larvae that penetrate the colonic wall or perianal skin and enter the blood stream to repeat the migration that establishes ongoing internal reinfection (autoinfection).

Clinical Features

- Most patients are asymptomatic or have mild cutaneous and/or abdominal symptoms.
- Recurrent urticaria is the most common cutaneous manifestation.
- Migrating larvae can elicit a pathognomonic serpiginous eruption, larva currens ("running larva"), a pruritic, raised, erythematous lesion that advances as rapidly as 10 cm/hours along the course of larval migration.
- Pulmonary phase: Can cause dry cough, wheezing, mild fever, and eosinophilia.
- Intestinal phase: Adult worms burrow into the duodenojejunal mucosa and can cause abdominal (usually epigastric) pain, which resembles peptic ulcer pain. Nausea, diarrhea, gastrointestinal bleeding, and weight loss can occur.
- Immunosuppressed states can lead to disseminated infection where larvae may invade the central nervous system, peritoneum, liver, and kidney.

Diagnosis

- Stool microscopy: Finding rhabditiform larvae in feces is diagnostic. Since the eggs hatch in the intestine, eggs are not usually found in the feces. Repeated stool examinations can improve the sensitivity of stool diagnosis.
- If stool examinations are negative, Strongyloides can be detected by sampling of the duodenojejunal contents by aspiration or biopsy.
- Detection of antibodies against Strongyloides is a sensitive method of diagnosing uncomplicated infections.
- Eosinophilia is common.

Treatment

- **Ivermectin** (200 μg/kg daily for 1 or 2 days) is the drug of choice and is more effective than albendazole (400 mg daily for 3 days, repeated at 2 weeks). Ivermectin should be given for at least 5–7 days in disseminated strongyloidiasis.
- **Albendazole** (400 mg twice daily for 7 days) is alternative if ivermectin is unavailable or contraindicated.

Q. Trichuriasis (whipworm).

- Trichuriasis is a **soil-transmitted helminthic infection** caused by ***Trichuris trichiura*** (whipworm).
- It is about 4 cm long and has a thin anterior end and a broad posterior end which gives it a characteristic whiplike appearance (hence called whipworm) **(Fig. 1.62)**.

Epidemiology

- It is found all over the world both in the tropics and subtropics.
- It most commonly affects children.

Life Cycle

- The adult worms live for many years in the colon and cecum. Their anterior ends are embedded into the mucosa. Adult female worms produce thousands of eggs per day which are passed with the feces, mature in the soil and become infective. After ingestion, infective eggs hatch in the duodenum, releasing larvae which mature and migrate to the colon. The full cycle takes about 3 months.

Clinical Features

- Most infected persons are asymptomatic.
- Heavy infections can cause abdominal pain, anorexia, and diarrhea.
- Malnutrition and growth retardation can happen in children.
- In severe cases, rectal prolapse (due to severe colonic inflammation), and dysentery-like symptoms (Trichuris dysentery syndrome) can occur.

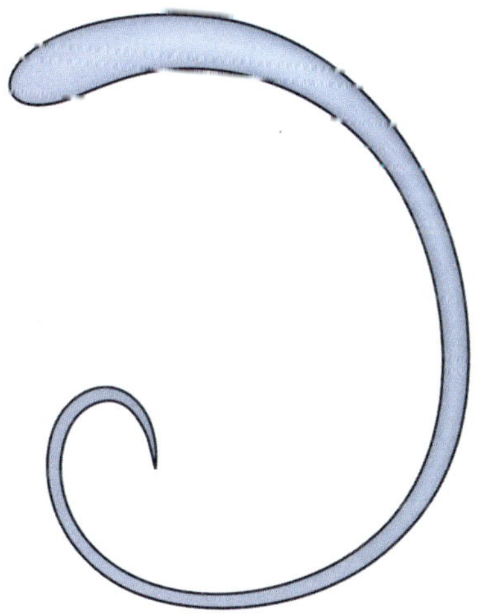

Figure 1.62: Whipworm

Diagnosis

- The characteristic lemon-shaped (or barrel shaped) whipworm eggs may be detected on stool examination. Adult worms can occasionally be seen on proctoscopy.

Treatment

- Mebendazole (500 mg once for mass treatment or 100 mg BD for 3 days for individual patient) or albendazole (400 mg daily for 3 doses) or ivermectin 200 μg/kg orally once a day for 3 days are effective against whipworm.

Q. Pinworm infestation (Enterobiasis, Oxyuriasis).

Pinworm (*Enterobius vermicularis*) is a small nematode about 1 cm long. It is more common in temperate countries than in the tropics. School children are affected commonly.

Life Cycle

- Humans are the only natural host for Enterobius. Adult worms live in the terminal ileum and colon. The female worm migrates out at night into the perianal region and lays up to 10,000 eggs. Self-infection results from perianal scratching and transport of eggs by the hands to the mouth. The larvae hatch and mature within the intestine. This life cycle takes ~1 month, and adult worms live for ~2 months. It can spread easily from one person to another.

Clinical Features

- Most pinworm infections are asymptomatic. Perianal itching is the cardinal symptom. The itching is worse at night and is due to the nocturnal migration of the female worms.
- Heavy infections can cause abdominal pain and weight loss.
- Rarely, pinworms invade the female genital tract and cause vulvovaginitis.

Diagnosis

- Since the eggs are deposited in the perianal region, they can be detected by the application of clear cellophane tape to the perianal region in the morning. Eggs get attached to the sticky cellophane tape which is then transferred to a slide and examined under microscope for characteristic pinworm eggs, which are oval and flattened along one side.
- Direct visualization: Parents may see small, white, thread-like worms in the perianal area at night.

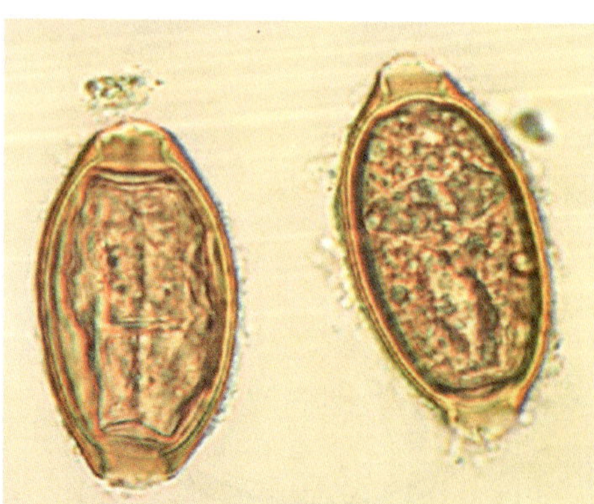

Figure 1.63: Barrel- or lemon-shaped eggs of *Trichuris trichiura*

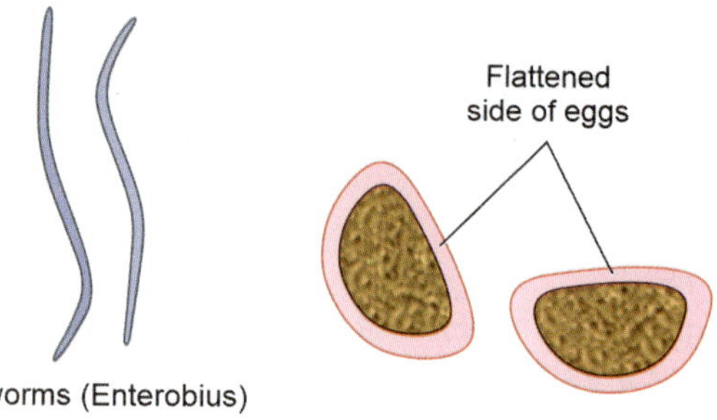

Figure 1.64: Pinworms and their eggs

Treatment

A single dose of mebendazole (100 mg), or albendazole (400 mg), or pyrantel pamoate (11 mg/kg base), is effective against pinworms. Treatment should be repeated after 2 weeks. All family members should be treated to eliminate asymptomatic reservoirs of infection.

Q. Enumerate the different filarial species which cause infection in man.

- Filariasis is a group of parasitic infections due to filarial worms (nematodes) **(Table 1.27)**. Filariasis is transmitted by mosquitoes or other arthropods.
- Eight filarial species infect humans. Out of these, four—(1) *Wuchereria bancrofti*, (2) *Brugia malayi*, (3) *Onchocerca volvulus*, and (4) *Loa loa*—are responsible for most infections.
- Adult filarial worms reside in either lymphatic or subcutaneous tissues of humans. Adult worms live for many years and produce offsprings called microfilariae, which either circulate in the blood or migrate through the skin.
- Microfilariae are ingested by the arthropod vector and there develop into new infective larvae.
- All filarial worms have similar life cycles but differ in: (1) their vector, (2) the final dwelling place of the adult worms, (3) the circadian periodicity of the microfilariae, and (4) the pathological syndromes they cause.

Q. Describe the etiology, epidemiology, pathogenesis, clinical features, diagnosis and treatment of lymphatic filariasis.

Q. *Wuchereria bancrofti.*

- Lymphatic filariasis is caused by *Wuchereria bancrofti*, *Brugia malayi*, and *Brugia timori*. The threadlike adult worms live in lymphatic channels or lymph nodes for many years. World Health Organization (WHO) has identified lymphatic filariasis as one of the major cause of permanent and long-term disability in the world.

Epidemiology

- *W. bancrofti* is the most common human filarial infection seen all over the world (90% of cases).

TABLE 1.27: Filarial species causing disease in humans

Worm species	Periodicity	Vector	Dwelling place of adult worm	Dwelling place of microfilariae
Wuchereria bancrofti	Nocturnal	Mosquitoes	Lymphatic vessels	Blood
Brugia malayi	Nocturnal	Mosquitoes	Lymphatic vessels	Blood
B. timori	Nocturnal	Mosquitoes	Lymphatic tissue	Blood
Oncocercus valvulus	None	Simulium (blackflies)	Subcutaneous	Skin
Loa loa	Diurnal	Chrysops (deerflies)	Subcutaneous	Blood
Mansonella ozzardi	None	Midges	Retroperitoneal	Blood and skin
Mansonella perstans	None	Midges	Retroperitoneal	Blood
Mansonella streptocerca	None	Midges	Skin	Skin

Humans are the only definitive host for this parasite. W. bancrofti is nocturnally periodic (microfilariae are found in peripheral blood mainly at night). Vectors for W. bancrofti are Culex fatigans mosquitoes in urban settings and anopheles or aedes mosquitoes in rural areas.

- *B. malayi* occurs mainly in China, India, Indonesia, Korea, Japan, Malaysia, and the Philippines.
- *B. timori* is seen only on islands of the Indonesian archipelago.

Life Cycle of Filariasis (Fig. 1.65)

- Adult female worms inside lymphatics release microfilariae into the bloodstream. Microfilariae are found in blood at night (nocturnal periodicity, depending on the filarial species).
- A mosquito (Culex, Anopheles, Aedes) bites an infected person and ingests microfilariae with the blood.
- In the mosquito microfilariae develop into L1 larval stage → L2 Larvae → L3 Larvae (infective stage)
- During a mosquito bite, the L3 larvae enter the human skin, migrate to the lymphatic system, and mature into adult worms over 6–12 months. Adult male and female worms mate and adult female worm releases microfilariae and the cycle repeats again.

Pathology

- Female adult worms are 8–10 cm long; males are about 4 cm long. Gravid adult females produce microfilariae that circulate in blood. Adult worms live in afferent lymphatics or sinuses of lymph nodes and cause dilatation and thickening of lymphatics. An inflammatory reaction develops in the lymphatics due to the presence of worms which further damages lymphatics and their valves leading to tortuous and blocked lymphatics. Blocked and damaged lymphatics lead to lymphedema with hard or brawny edema in the overlying skin. Death of the adult worm leads to increased inflammatory reaction and fibrosis of lymphatics which may be permanent.
- Microfilariae do not have much role in the development of lymphedema.

Clinical Features

- Patients with lymphatic filariasis usually present with subclinical microfilaremia, acute adenolymphangitis (ADL), and chronic lymphatic disease.

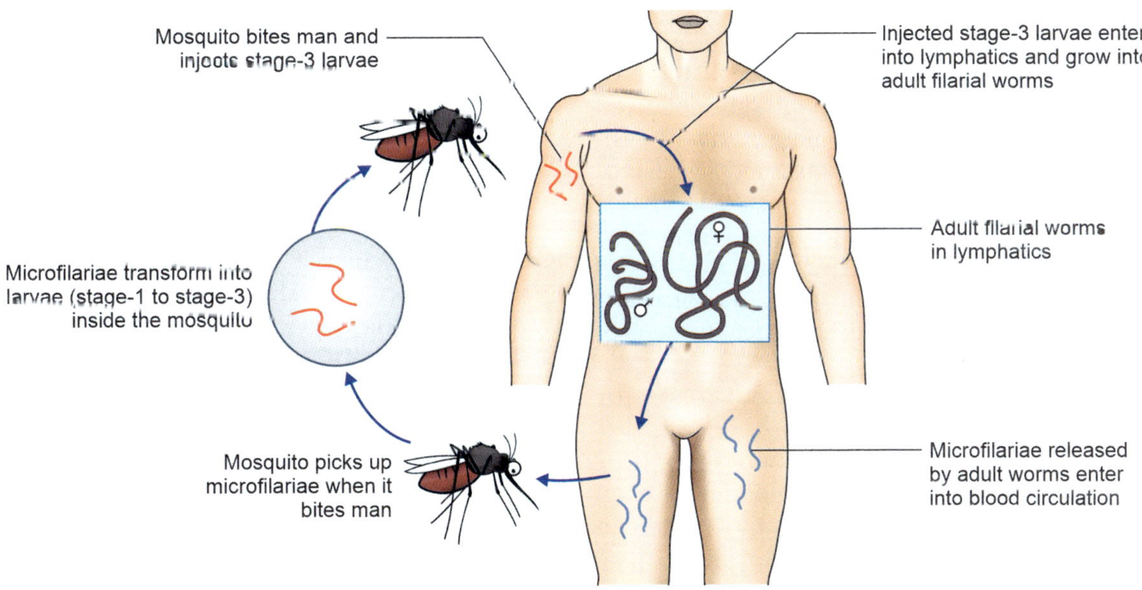

Figure 1.65: Life cycle of filariasis

- In areas where *W. bancrofti* or *B. malayi* is endemic, most infected individuals are clinically asymptomatic.
- Only very few of these asymptomatic individuals develop acute and chronic phases of infection.
- *Acute phase of infection:* leads to acute adenolymphangitis (ADL) which is characterized by fever, lymphangitis, lymphadenitis, and transient local edema. Lymphangitis is inflammation of lymphatic vessels and is retrograde extending from the lymph node to periphery. In bacterial lymphangitis ascending lymphangitis is seen. Lymphadenitis is inflammation of lymph nodes which become enlarged and painful. The lymphangitis and lymphadenitis can involve both the upper and lower limbs. Genital lymphatics involvement occurs almost exclusively with *W. bancrofti* infection and manifests as funiculitis, epididymitis, and scrotal pain and tenderness.
- *Chronic phase of infection:* Chronic filarial disease develops insidiously after many years and is due to severe lymphatic damage. This leads to lymphadema (elephantiasis) characterized by non-pitting edema due to thickening of the subcutaneous tissues and hyperkeratosis involving legs, arms, breasts, and scrotum). Recurrent infections of these edematous tissues lead to further swelling. Hydrocele and scrotal elephantiasis may develop. Renal lymphatic involvement leads to rupture of the renal lymphatics and chyluria.
- Tropical pulmonary eosinophilia (TPE) is another rare manifestation which causes low-grade fever and wheezing. Blood eosinophil count is usually high. It is most likely due to hypersensitivity reactions to microfilariae.

Diagnosis

- Definitive diagnosis can be made by detection of adult filarial worms. But this is difficult. Imaging techniques like ultrasound and Doppler can sometimes identify motile adult worms in the dilated lymphatics ("Filarial dance sign"-adult worms moving inside lymphatic vessels).
- *Microscopic examination of blood samples*: Microfilariae can be demonstrated in the blood, hydrocele fluid, or rarely in other body fluids. Blood should be collected based on the periodicity of the microfilariae. Night time blood sample should be examined in case of nocturnal periodicity.
- *Antigen test for W. bancrofti:* Antigens of *W. bancrofti* can be detected by enzyme-linked immunosorbent assay (ELISA) and immunochromatographic card test. There are currently no tests to detect antigens of brugian filariasis.
- *Antibody tests:* Enzyme immunoassay tests for antifilarial antibodies.
- *Polymerase chain reaction (PCR)* based assays for DNA of *W. bancrofti* and *B. malayi* in blood have been developed. PCR tests have high sensitivity and can detect infection in almost all infected subjects.
- In cases of kidney involvement, urine examination may show hematuria and/or proteinuria.
- Elevated eosinophils and serum IgE support the diagnosis of lymphatic filariasis.

Differential Diagnosis

- Acute filarial lymphangitis and lymphadenitis has to be differentiated from bacterial lymphangitis.
- Chronic filarial lymphedema must be distinguished from the lymphedema of malignancy, postoperative scarring, trauma, chronic edematous states, and congenital lymphatic abnormalities.

Treatment

- Diethylcarbamazine (DEC) is the drug of choice for filariasis. It has action on adult worms as well as microfilariae. It is given in a dose of 6 mg/kg/day in three divided doses for 12 days. A single dose of 6 mg/kg also has equivalent efficacy in reducing levels of microfilariae. For tropical pulmonary eosinophilia (TPE), a longer DEC treatment course of 14–21 days is generally recommended.
- Ivermectin: A single oral dose of 150 μg/kg is useful to clear microfilaria. Ivermectin does not kill adult worms.
- A single dose of albendazole plus either DEC or ivermectin has been found to be more effective than single drug. Recently single dose of a 3-drug regimen of ivermectin plus diethylcarbamazine and albendazole has been shown to be more effective than the 2-drug combination.
- Early treatment of asymptomatic persons is recommended to prevent permanent lymphatic damage. For adenolymphangitis (ADL), supportive treatment with antipyretics and analgesics is given and antibiotics are also indicated if secondary bacterial infection is suspected. In persons who have chronic lymphadema, good local hygiene should be maintained, and secondary bacterial infections should be prevented. Hydroceles are managed by repeated aspiration or surgical intervention.

Prevention and Control

- Mosquito control: Use of insecticide-treated nets, indoor residual spraying, elimination of mosquito breeding sites.
- Mass treatment with annual single-dose of Albendazole + DEC/Ivermectin in endemic regions suppress microfilaremia and interrupts transmission.
- Community use of DEC-fortified salt dramatically reduces microfilarial density (used in some regions).

Q. Tropical pulmonary eosinophilia.

- Tropical pulmonary eosinophilia (TPE) is a hypersensitivity reaction to microfilariae of *Wuchereria bancrofti* or *Brugia malayi* trapped in the lungs. It is a rare, occult form of lymphatic filariasis seen mainly in endemic tropical and subtropical regions.
- Males are affected commonly often during the third decade of life. Most cases occur in India, Pakistan, Sri Lanka, Brazil, and Southeast Asia.

Etiology

- *Wuchereria bancrofti* and *Brugia malayi* are the main causes of TPE. It is due to an exaggerated immune response to microfilariae trapped in the lungs.

Clinical Features

- Patients are usually from filaria-endemic areas.
- They usually present with nocturnal dry cough and wheezing (probably due to the nocturnal periodicity of microfilariae), low-grade fever, and high blood eosinophil counts (usually >3000 eosinophils/µl).
- The clinical symptoms are due to allergic and inflammatory reactions elicited by the microfilariae in the lungs.
- Interstitial fibrosis and lung damage can happen if this condition is not treated properly.

Investigations

- Eosinophil count is high (usually >3000 eosinophils/µl).
- Elevated IgE levels (>1,000 IU/ml).
- Filarial antibody and antigen tests (serology positive in 50% of cases).
- Chest X-ray may show increased bronchovascular markings, diffuse miliary lesions or reticulonodular infiltrates.
- Pulmonary function tests show both restrictive and obstructive defects, and decreased DLCO (diffusing capacity of lungs for carbon monoxide).

Differential Diagnosis

- Asthma.
- Allergic bronchopulmonary aspergillosis.
- Löffler's syndrome.
- Allergic granulomatosis with angiitis (Churg-Strauss syndrome).
- Systemic vasculitis (Wegener's granulomatosis).
- Chronic eosinophilic pneumonia.
- Idiopathic hypereosinophilic syndrome.

H/o of filarial exposure, nocturnal cough and wheezing, high levels of antifilarial antibodies, and a rapid response to DEC help in differentiating TPE from other conditions.

Treatment

- DEC should be given at a dosage of 4–6 mg/kg of body weight divided into 2 or 3 doses per day for 3 weeks. DEC plus albendazole is more effective than DEC alone.

Q. Onchocerciasis (river blindness).

- Onchocerciasis (river blindness) is caused by the filarial nematode *Onchocerca volvulus*. Humans acquire onchocerciasis through the bite of *Simulium* blackflies. Because the fly develops and breeds in flowing water, onchocerciasis is commonly found along rivers and is sometimes referred to as river blindness.
- This disease is seen mainly in Africa.
- It affects mainly the skin and eyes. Onchocerciasis is the second leading cause of **infectious blindness** worldwide (trachoma, caused by *Chlamydia trachomatis* is the most common infectious cause of blindness).

Life Cycle and Pathogenesis

- Man acquires infection by the bite of an infected blackfly. Infective larvae of *O. volvulus* are deposited into the skin during bite. The larvae develop into adults worms, which live in subcutaneous nodules (onchocercomas). The adult female worm releases microfilariae that migrate to all tissues including skin and eyes causing severe inflammation. Infection is transmitted to other persons when a female blackfly ingests microfilariae from the host and these microfilariae then develop into infective larvae. Adult female worms are about 40–60 cm in length and males 3–6 cm in length. These worms can live up to 18 years.

Clinical Features

- In onchocerciasis, tissue damage occurs due to microfilariae and not due to adult worms.
- Skin disease ("Onchodermatitis"): In the skin, pruritus and papular rash are the most frequent manifestations. Subcutaneous nodules form around the adult worms and are seen commonly over bony prominences. Chronic inflammatory changes in skin result in loss of elasticity, atrophy, fibrosis and premature wrinkling. All these changes may make the skin appear like Leopard skin (due to patchy depigmentation, common on shins), lizard skin (due to thickened, wrinkled skin due to chronic inflammation), and hanging groin (due to loss of skin elasticity in the groin area).
- Eye disease: In the eye, the most common early finding is conjunctivitis with photophobia. Corneal inflammation (keratitis) occurs due to microfilaria which leads to neovascularization, corneal scarring and formation of opacities. This leads to blindness. Inflammation in the anterior and posterior chambers frequently results in anterior uveitis, chorioretinitis, and optic atrophy.
- Lymphadenopathy is usually present.

Diagnosis

- Diagnosis can be confirmed by the detection of an adult worm in an excised nodule or microfilariae in a skin snip.
- Ultrasound can also visualize worm in the subcutaneous nodules.
- Antibody detection: Serology (ELISA, rapid tests). Detects IgG4 antibodies against O. volvulus (for exposure detection).
- PCR to detect onchocercal DNA in skin snips are highly sensitive and specific but not available everywhere.
- Slit lamp examination (eye involvement): Detects microfilariae in the cornea and anterior chamber.

- Mazzotti test (historical): Diethylcarbamazine (DEC) 50 mg orally → causes severe itching and rash if microfilariae are present. No longer widely used due to severe inflammatory reactions.
- Eosinophils and serum IgE levels are elevated.

Treatment

- Ivermectin is the drug of choice for onchocerciasis. It is given as a single oral dose of 150 μg/kg, repeated at 6–12 month intervals for at least 10–12 years. Ivermectin kills microfilaria and does not kill the adult worms. Ivermectin is contraindicated in pregnant or breastfeeding women.
- Doxycycline can kill the adult worms by killing **Wolbachia bacteria,** a symbiotic bacteria required for worm survival and embryogenesis.
- **Moxidectin** is a new drug that has been approved for use in onchocerciasis. It has been shown to be superior to ivermectin.
- Subcutaneous nodules near the head should be excised (because the adult worms are nearer to the eye).

Prevention

- Vector control.
- Community-based administration of ivermectin every 6–12 months to interrupt transmission.

Q. Dracunculiasis (guinea worm disease).

Etiology

- Dracunculiasis is a parasitic infection caused by Dracunculus medinensis.
- It primarily affects impoverished, rural areas with limited access to clean drinking water.
- Its incidence has declined dramatically due to global eradication efforts. But cases still occur in Sudan.

Life Cycle

- Humans are the definitive hosts (harbor adult worm) and copepods (a small crustacean, commonly known as water fleas) are intermediate hosts (harbor infective larvae).
- Humans acquire infection by drinking water containing infected copepods which harbor infective larvae. The copepods die in the stomach and release the infective larvae. The released larvae penetrate the intestinal wall, and mature in the abdominal cavity into adult worms. After mating, adult male worm dies, but gravid female worm migrates through the subcutaneous tissue, usually to lower limb. Female Dracunculus worm is very thin but length is up to 1 meter.
- A blister forms in the skin and breaks down to form an ulcer through which the worm can come out and release motile, rhabditiform larvae into water. Patients often immerse the affected region in water to relieve pain. This contact enables the worm to expel thousands of larvae into the water.
- These rhabditiform larvae are ingested by copepods where they develop into infective larvae, thus completing the cycle.

Clinical Features

Initial Stage (asymptomatic phase)

- The infection remains asymptomatic for about a year while the worm matures.

Emergence of the Worm

- Painful blister formation, often on the feet or lower legs.
- Just before blister formation, there is fever and allergic symptoms like periorbital edema, wheezing, and urticaria. The emergence of the worm is associated with local burning sensation and swelling. Intense burning sensation makes the patient to immerse the limb into water for relief, facilitating larval release.
- Sometimes the worm is visible to the naked eye when it comes out. Fever and local symptoms subside when the blister ruptures releasing larva-rich fluid. The ulcer slowly heals but can become secondarily infected. Occasionally, the adult worm does not emerge but becomes encapsulated and calcified.
- Secondary bacterial infections and cellulitis may occur.
- Arthritis or joint complications can result from worm migration.

Diagnosis

- Clinical diagnosis based on worm emergence and characteristic skin lesions.
- Microscopic examination of fluid from blisters may reveal larvae.

Treatment

- Mechanical extraction: Emerging adult worm can be gradually extracted by winding a few centimetres on a stick every day.
- Niridazole was previously tested for Guinea worm but abandoned due to severe neurotoxic effects (hallucinations, seizures). Currently there is no effective drug to kill guinea worm.
- Surgery: Rarely necessary for deeply embedded worms.

Prevention

- Guineaworm infestation can be prevented by the provision of safe drinking water.
- Vector control: Treating water sources with temephos (larvicide) kills water fleas.

Q. Describe the etiology, life cycle, clinical features, investigations and management of schistosomiasis (bilharziasis).

Etiology

- Schistosomiasis is also known as bilharziasis after Theodor Bilharz who first identified the parasite. It is caused by infection with parasitic blood flukes known as schistosomes. Schistosomes are trematodes (flat worms) which belong to the phylum Platyhelminthes.

- The organisms infect the vasculature of the gastrointestinal or genitourinary system. Human schistosomiasis is caused by following species.
  - *Schistosoma haematobium* (urogenital schistosomiasis)
  - *Schistosoma mansoni* (intestinal schistosomiasis)
  - *Schistosoma japonicum* (intestinal schistosomiasis)
  - *Schistosoma intercalatum* and *Schistosoma mekongi* (intestinal schistosomiasis, less common)

Epidemiology

- Schistosomiasis is found in South America, the Caribbean, Africa, the Middle East, and Southeast Asia. People between 15 and 20-year age group are affected commonly. It is less common in older age groups probably due to less water exposure.

Life Cycle (Fig. 1.66)

- Human infection is acquired when infective cercariae in fresh water penetrate the skin and reach the subcutaneous tissue. In the subcutaneous tissue, cercariae transform into schistosomula which travel through the bloodstream to the liver, where they mature into adults worms.
- The mature adult worms then migrate through the veins to their ultimate home in the intestinal veins (typically S. japonicum and *S. mansoni*) or the venous plexus of urinary bladder (typically *S. haematobium*). Adult worms measure 1–2 cm in length. In these organs worms mate and gravid female worms produces eggs. Eggs can penetrate the venous wall by enzyme secretion and reach the lumen of the intestine or urinary bladder from where they are passed with stools or urine. Some eggs are carried by venous blood flow to the liver and other organs (e.g. lungs, central nervous system, spinal cord). Excreted eggs hatch in freshwater, releasing miracidia (first larval stage) which enter snails. After multiplication in snail, thousands of free-swimming cercariae are released which are ready to infect humans.

Pathogenesis

- The clinical manifestations seen in schistosomiasis are due to inflammatory reaction to eggs in the tissues. Chronic inflammation leads to granuloma formation and irreversible fibrosis.

Clinical Features

- Most people with intestinal schistosomiasis are asymptomatic. In contrast, most people with urinary schistosomiasis are symptomatic.
- In general, disease manifestations of schistosomiasis occur in 2 stages: Acute and chronic stages.

Acute Infection

- During the phase of cercarial invasion, a form of dermatitis called swimmers' itch may be seen. It is seen 2 or 3 days after invasion as an itchy maculopapular rash.
- Acute shistosomiasis syndrome (also called Katayama fever) is seen during worm maturation and is characterized by a serum sickness–like syndrome with fever, generalized lymphadenopathy, hepatosplenomegaly and increased eosinophil counts.

Chronic Infection

- The clinical manifestations of chronic schistosomiasis are species-dependent. Egg deposition in the intestinal wall (*S. mansoni*, *S. japonicum*, *S. mekongi*, and *S. intercalatum*) causes colicky abdominal pain and bloody diarrhea. Eggs can penetrate the bowel adjacent to mesenteric vessels where adult worms are residing. Unshed eggs, which are swept back to the portal circulation induce granulomatous reaction in the portal tracts leading to presinusoidal blockage and portal hypertension. Portal hypertension can lead to esophageal varices and splenomegaly. Right and left upper-quadrant "dragging" pain may be experienced due to hepatomegaly and splenomegaly respectively. Bleeding from esophageal varices may

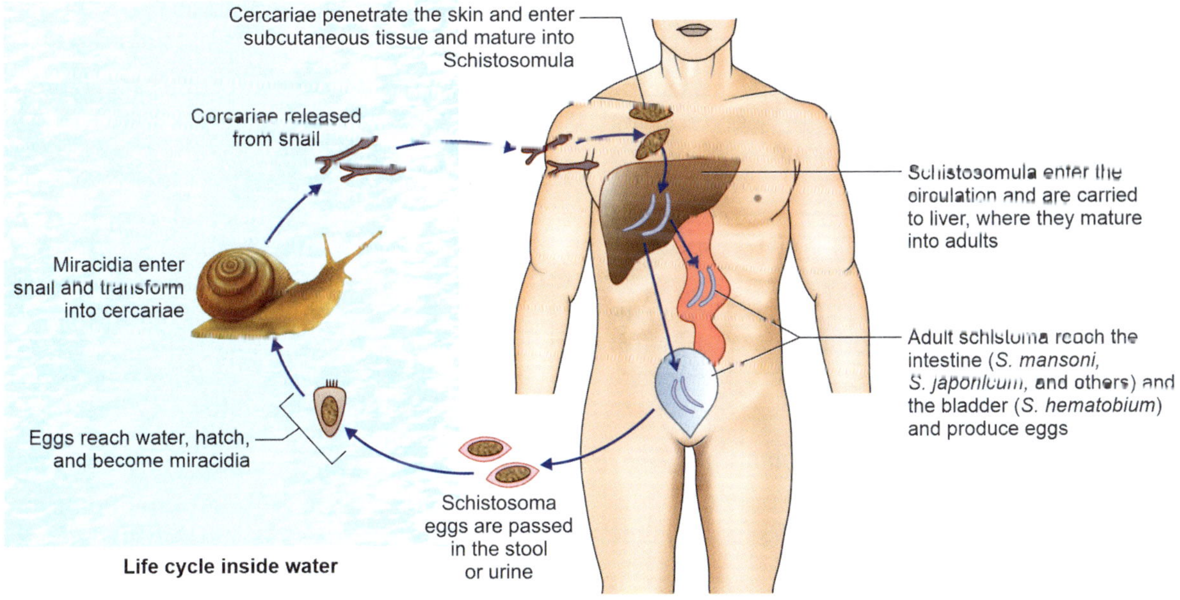

Figure 1.66: Life cycle of schistosomiasis

cause hematemesis and malena and may be the first manifestation of the disease. In late-stage disease, cirrhosis and liver failure may develop.

- Deposition of eggs in the urinary blader (*S. haematobium*) causes inflammation and granuloma formation in the urinary bladder leading to dysuria, increased frequency, and hematuria. Obstruction of the lower end of the ureters results in hydroureter and hydronephrosis. Bladder granulomas undergo fibrosis and result in typical sandy patches visible on cystoscopy. Squamous cell carcinoma has been observed to develop in damaged bladder; hence, *S. haematobium* has now been classified as a human carcinogen.
- Lungs can also get affected in schistosomiasis. Embolized eggs lodge in small lung arterioles, and produce acute necrotizing arteriolitis and granuloma formation. Later, fibrosis leads to endarteritis obliterans, pulmonary hypertension, and cor pulmonale.
- CNS schistosomiasis occurs when eggs which are carried to the brain induce a granulomatous response and fibrosis. Patients may present with epilepsy. Transverse myelitis may also be seen due to eggs traveling to the venous plexus around the spinal cord. Patients with transverse myelitis present with lower limb weakness accompanied by bladder dysfunction.

Diagnosis

- H/o travel to endemic areas and exposure to freshwater bodies is central to diagnosis.
- High blood eosinophil count and presence of schistosomal antibodies is highly suggestive of infection. Schistosomal antibodies can be detected by indirect fluorescent antibody test and ELISA.
- Examination of stool or urine may show eggs of schistosoma.
- Plain X-ray of the abdomen or CT scan may reveal intramural calcification in the wall of the bladder or colon.
- Schistosome infection can also be diagnosed by examination of tissue samples, usually rectal biopsies and rarely liver biopsy.

Treatment

- Infections with all major Schistosoma species can be treated with praziquantel. Steroids can be given along with praziquantel to suppress inflammation.

Prevention and Control

- Travelers should avoid freshwater contact especially in endemic areas.
- Application of molluscicides, provision of safe water and disposal of sewage, chemotherapy, and health education are all effective in reducing the prevalence of schistosomiasis.

Q. List the important fungi affecting human beings.

- Fungi are universally present in nature but only a few fungi belonging to Eumycetes group are pathogenic to man.
- Fungal infections, or mycoses, range from superficial to life-threatening systemic diseases. They are caused by opportunistic or primary fungal pathogens, affecting the skin, mucosa, and internal organs.

Classification of Fungal Infections

Superficial mycoses (Affect skin, hair, nails, and mucosa)

- **Tinea (Dermatophytosis)** → Caused by Trichophyton, Microsporum, Epidermophyton. These include
  - *Tinea capitis* (scalp)
  - *Tinea corporis* (body)
  - *Tinea pedis* (athlete's foot)
  - *Tinea unguium* (onychomycosis, nail infection)
  - *Tinea cruris* (jock itch)
- **Pityriasis (Tinea) Versicolor** → *Malassezia furfur* (hypo/hyper-pigmented skin patches)
- **Candidiasis** → *Candida albicans* (affects skin, oral mucosa, and genital areas)
- **Sporotrichosis** → *Sporothrix schenckii* (rose gardener's disease; subcutaneous nodules)

Systemic (deep) mycoses (affect internal organs, often in immunocompromised hosts)

- **Histoplasmosis** → *Histoplasma capsulatum* (lung infection, linked to bat/bird droppings)
- **Blastomycosis** → *Blastomyces dermatitidis* (pulmonary and skin granulomas)
- **Coccidioidomycosis** → *Coccidioides immitis* (Valley fever, flu-like symptoms)
- **Paracoccidioidomycosis** → *Paracoccidioides brasiliensis* (South American blastomycosis)

Opportunistic Mycoses (Severe infections in immunocompromised individuals)

- **Aspergillosis** → *Aspergillus fumigatus* (lung infections, allergic bronchopulmonary aspergillosis)
- **Cryptococcosis** → *Cryptococcus neoformans* (meningitis, common in AIDS patients)
- **Mucormycosis** (Zygomycosis) → Rhizopus, Mucor species (aggressive necrotizing infections, seen in diabetics and immunosuppressed patients)
- ***Pneumocystis pneumonia* (PCP)** → *Pneumocystis jirovecii* (severe pneumonia in AIDS patients)

Q. Describe the etiology, clinical features, diagnosis and treatment of candidiasis.

Etiology

- Candidiasis is a fungal infection caused by yeasts that belong to the genus Candida. Out of many species of candida, *Candida albicans* is the most common yeast causing human disease.
- *Candida albicans* is a normal oropharyngeal and gastrointestinal commensal.
- Candida species reproduce asexually by budding.

Clinical Features

- *Oropharyngeal candidiasis (thrush)* is common in neonates, patients with diabetes mellitus, HIV infection, dentures, patients treated with antibiotics, chemotherapy, or radiation therapy, patients with xerostomia and those treated with inhaled corticosteroids. Oral candidiasis (thrush) presents as well defined, painless adherent white patches in the mouth, tongue and pharyngeal mucosa. HIV infection should be ruled out in unexplained oropharyngeal candidiasis.

- *Cutaneous candidiasis* usually occurs in macerated skin, such as diapered area of infants, under pendulous breasts. It presents as red macerated areas, paronychia, balanitis, or pruritus ani. Partial alopecia can occur in scalp infections.
- *Vulvovaginal candidiasis* is especially common in the third trimester of pregnancy. It causes pruritus, white discharge, and sometimes pain on intercourse.
- Esophageal candidiasis can cause substernal pain or dysphagia. Most lesions occur in the distal third of the esophagus.
- *Systemic candidiasis* and septic shock can occur especially in immunocompromised persons. It can invade almost any organ. Hematogenous seeding is particularly common in the retina, kidney, spleen, and liver. Kidney involvement causes cystitis, pyelitis, or papillary necrosis. Retinal infection appears as unilateral or bilateral small white retinal exudates. The vitreous humor becomes cloudy, and the patient notices blurring, ocular pain, or a scotoma. Retinal detachment can occur. Infection of liver and spleen can occur in patients with acute leukemia recovering from profound neutropenia. Candida pneumonia is very rare. Candida endocarditis can occur in previously damaged or prosthetic heart valves. The source is often an intravascular catheter or illicit drug injection. Other manifestations include arthritis, subacute peritonitis, brain abscess and chronic meningitis.

Diagnosis

- Pseudohyphae are seen on a wet KOH smear prepared from the scrapings of lesion. Diagnosis can be confirmed by culture.
- Since Candida is a normal commensal, positive cultures of urine, sputum, abdominal drains, endotracheal aspirates, or the vagina is not diagnostic.
- Blood cultures are useful in the diagnosis of Candida endocarditis. Serologic tests for antibody or antigen are not useful.

Treatment

- For cutaneous candidiasis, topical antifungals are effective. Nystatin powder or ciclopirox cream or an azole is useful. Clotrimazole, miconazole, econazole, and tolnafate are available as creams or lotions.
- For vulvovaginal candidiasis, azoles are better than nystatin preparations. All azoles are equally efficacious. A single dose of 150-mg fluconazole is more convenient to use for vulvovaginitis than topical treatment but is contraindicated in pregnancy.
- For oral candidiasis clotrimazole troches can be used five times a day. Oral fluconazole (150 mg daily) can also be used.
- For esophageal candidiasis, oral fluconazole (150 mg once daily for 2–3 weeks) is the treatment of choice. Itraconazole is an alternative. For azole-resistant oropharyngeal or esophageal candidiasis a 2-week course of intravenous amphotericin B or caspofungin is effective.
- For invasive candidiasis, intravenous amphotericin B is the drug of choice. Candida endocarditis requires valve replacement along with long-term fluconazole administration.

Q. Describe the etiology, clinical features, diagnosis and treatment of Aspergillosis.

- Aspergillosis is a fungal infection caused by Aspergillus species. Aspergillus species are A. fumigatus (most common), *A. flavus*, *A. niger*, *A. nidulans*, *A. terreus*, and many other species.
- It primarily affects the lungs, sinuses, and immunocompromised patients, leading to a spectrum of diseases ranging from allergic reactions to invasive infections.
- Aspergillus is ubiquitous in the environment, and is present on dead leaves, stored grain, compost piles, hay, and other decaying vegetation.
- Infection is seen most often in immunocompromised and diabetic persons. Aspergillus can colonize the damaged bronchial tree, pulmonary cysts, or cavities. Balls of hyphae within cysts or cavities (aspergillomas) may form and can reach several centimeters in diameter.

Clinical Manifestations

- *Allergic bronchopulmonary aspergillosis (ABPA):* Can occur in patients with asthma and cystic fibrosis and lead to chronic cough, wheezing and breathlessness.
- *Chronic pulmonary aspergillosis*: This is a slowly progressing lung infection in patients with preexisting lung disease (e.g. tuberculosis, COPD). It can present as aspergilloma (fungal ball) in a cavity or chronic cavitary pulmonary aspergillosis. Patient may present with cough, hemoptysis, weight loss, and fatigue.
- *Invasive aspergillosis:* Pneumonia can occur in immunosuppressed individuals and is difficult to treat. Aspergillus may invade immunosuppressed patients through the skin at a site of minor trauma or through the upper airway mucosa. Rapid extension into the adjacent paranasal sinus, orbit, or face is common. Patients usually have a history of chronic allergic rhinitis, and present with painless proptosis, nasal obstruction, or dull aching pain. CT or MRI scan shows a solid mass pushing out the lateral wall of the ethmoid sinus or the medial wall of the maxillary sinus.
- Aspergillus can grow on cerumen and detritus within the external auditory canal and is called otomycosis.
- Other manifestations include aspergillus keratitis, endophthalmitis, and infection of intracardiac or intravascular prostheses.

Diagnosis

- Detection of hyphae in clinical specimens suggests infection.
- A fungal ball within a lung cavity can be detected using a chest X-ray or CT scan. In cavitary lesions, it appears as a mass surrounded by an air crescent (**Fig. 1.67**).
- IgG antibody to Aspergillus antigens is found in many colonized patients and almost all patients with fungus ball. Serum IgE antibody is raised in allergic bronchopulmonary aspergillosis.
- Biopsy is required for the diagnosis of invasive aspergillosis of the lungs, nose, and paranasal sinuses, etc.
- Blood cultures rarely yield positive results.

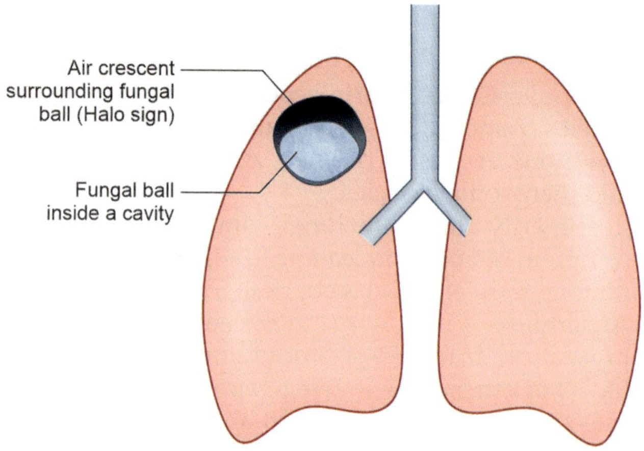

Figure 1.67: Aspergilloma inside a cavity

Treatment

- Fungus ball of the lung usually requires lobectomy.
- Allergic bronchopulmonary aspergillosis responds to short courses of steroids.
- Invasive aspergillosis is treated with voriconazole, or itraconazole or liposomal or conventional amphotericin B.

Q. Mucormycosis: zygomycosis.

Q. Rhino-orbital-cerebral mucormycosis.

- Mucormycosis is a severe fungal infection caused by fungi in the order **Mucorales**, most commonly *Rhizopus*, *Mucor*, and *Lichtheimia* species. It primarily affects immunocompromised individuals, leading to rapidly progressive and life-threatening infections.
- Predisposing factors are
  - Diabetic ketoacidosis
  - Chronic renal failure
  - Desferoxamine therapy
  - AIDS
  - Corticosteroids or cytotoxic drugs
- Infection commonly involves sinuses, orbits, and the lungs. Disseminated infection can occur in immunoccompromised and those receiving chemotherapy.

Clinical Features

Rhino-orbital-cerebral mucormycosis (ROCM)

- Most common form, often seen in diabetic ketoacidosis (DKA) and immunosuppressed patients.
- Symptoms: Facial pain, nasal congestion, black necrotic eschar, vision loss, proptosis (eye bulging), cranial nerve involvement
- Complications: Brain invasion → Meningitis, cavernous sinus thrombosis.
- It should be suspected in patients with black necrotic lesions of the nose or sinuses with cranial nerve palsies. Prognosis is poor.

Pulmonary Mucormycosis

- Seen in prolonged neutropenia, organ transplant, or cancer patients.
- Symptoms: Fever, cough, hemoptysis (coughing blood), pleuritic chest pain.

Cutaneous Mucormycosis

- Results from trauma, burns, or surgery in immunocompromised patients.
- Symptoms: Painful necrotic ulcers, black eschars
- Complications: Deep tissue invasion → Sepsis, gangrene.

Disseminated Mucormycosis

- Occurs when the infection spreads to multiple organs (brain, heart, skin, kidney, spleen). Assoiated with altered mental status and multi-organ failure. Carries high mortality.

Diagnosis

- Diagnosis is by demonstrating characteristic fungal hyphae in secretions and biopsy specimens. Cultures are frequently negative.

Treatment

- Treatment is by intravenous liposomal amphotericin B. Posaconazole is also effective. Control of diabetes and other underlying conditions is important. Extensive surgical removal of necrotic involved tissue is essential for cure.

Q. Sporotrichosis (rose gardener's disease).

- Sporotrichosis is a chronic fungal infection caused by *Sporothrix schenckii.*
- It is seen worldwide but most cases occur in Americas and Japan. It is found in soil, sphagnum moss, and decaying wood.

Clinical Features

- Infection takes place when the organism is inoculated into the skin—usually on the hand, arm, or foot, especially during gardening. Pulmonary infection develops after inhalation. Invasive infection can occur in immunocompromised persons.
- Lymphocutaneous sporotrichosis is the most common form seen. A nodule develops at the site of inoculation. This later becomes adherent to the overlying skin and ulcerates. Within a few days to weeks, similar nodules develop along the lymphatics draining this area, and these may ulcerate as well. The lymphatic vessels become indurated and are easily palpable.
- Pulmonary and disseminated sporotrichosis can occur rarely.

Diagnosis

- Microscopy and culture → Yeast form on Sabouraud agar.
- Histopathology → Cigar-shaped yeast on tissue biopsy.
- Detection of antibody is useful for diagnosis of disseminated disease, especially meningitis.
- Chest X-ray/CT → If pulmonary involvement is suspected.

Treatment

- Itraconazole orally daily for 3–6 months. Terbinafine, 500 mg twice daily, is also effective. Systemic infection is treated by intravenous amphotericin-B.
- Prognosis is good in lymphocutaneous sporotrichosis, and bad in systemic disease.

Chapter 2

Diseases of Respiratory System

- Respiratory system starts from the nose and ends at alveoli. It can be broadly divided into upper respiratory tract and lower respiratory tract.
- **Upper respiratory tract** includes nose, pharynx, and larynx.
- **Lower respiratory tract** includes trachea, right and left main bronchi, all the subsequent branches of airways, and alveoli.

Functions of Respiratory System

- *Gas exchange*: The main function of respiratory system is gas exchange.
- *Speech*: the movement of air through the vocal cords in the larynx produces speech.
- *Filtration of microthrombi* arriving from systemic veins.
- *Metabolic function*: Conversion of angiotensin I to angiotensin II. Removal or deactivation of serotonin, bradykinin, norepinephrine, acetylcholine and drugs such as propranolol and chlorpromazine.
- *Regulation of blood pH*: Respiratory system plays a crucial role in maintaining the acid-base balance of the body by regulating the levels of carbon dioxide in the blood. Too much CO_2 can make the blood more acidic, while too little can make it too alkaline. Through changes in breathing rate, the respiratory system can quickly adjust blood pH.
- *Thermoregulation*: Respiratory system helps regulate body temperature by exhaling warm air. This process aids in cooling the body, especially during intense physical activities.
- *Olfaction*: Nasal passages, which are part of the respiratory system, contain receptors for the sense of smell.

Q. Lung defense mechanisms.

- The air that we breathe contains potentially harmful particles, gases, and infectious agents. Particles, such as dust and soot, mold, fungi, bacteria, and viruses deposit on airway and alveolar surfaces. Fortunately, there are many defense mechanisms in the respiratory tract which protect us from these potentially harmful agents. Pulmonary disease often results from a failure of many of these defense mechanisms.
- These mechanisms can be categorized into mechanical, cellular, and immunological defenses.

MECHANICAL DEFENSE MECHANISMS

Nasal Hairs and Turbinates

Over 90% of particles greater than 10 microns are trapped by nasal hair and turbinates.

Coughing, Sneezing or Gagging

These physiological mechanisms expel any particles or foreign bodies that are inhaled.

Mucociliary Layer of Respiratory Tract

- The epithelium of respiratory tract is covered by a layer of mucus secreted by goblet cells and mucous glands. The respiratory epithelium is also covered by cilia which are in contact with the under surface of the mucus layer. Mucus traps dust, microbes, and debris. The cilia push the mucus blanket upwards along with the trapped particles. Cigarette smoking reduces ciliary action. In the *'immotile cilia'* syndrome and *cystic fibrosis* there is reduced ciliary function, leading to stagnation of secretions and recurrent infections.
- Lysozyme, lactoferrin or peroxide are present within the mucus. These substances provide nonspecific first-line of defense to invasion by microorganisms.

CELLULAR DEFENSE MECHANISMS

- *Alveolar macrophages:* They phagocytize foreign particles and bacteria which reach the alveoli.
- *Neutrophils:* Recruited in response to infections. Release enzymes and reactive oxygen species (ROS) to kill pathogens. Excessive activation can cause lung damage (e.g. in chronic infections or diseases like COPD).
- *Dendritic cells:* Present antigens to T-cells, linking innate and adaptive immunity. Initiate immune responses against harmful pathogens.
- *Lymphoid tissue:* The lung contains large numbers of lymphocytes which are scattered throughout the airways. These lymphocytes contribute to local immunity through differentiation into IgA-secreting plasma cells.

IMMUNOLOGICAL DEFENSE MECHANISMS

Secretary IgA

- This is present in mucus secretion which provides local immunity within the lumen of airways.

Surfactant Proteins

- Produced by alveolar type II cells.
- Enhance macrophage function and help clear bacteria and viruses.

Antimicrobial Peptides (Defensins and Cathelicidins)

Disrupt microbial membranes and kill bacteria, fungi, and viruses.

OTHER DEFENSE FACTORS

- **Alpha 1 antitrypsin:** This is present in lung secretions. It inhibits chymotrypsin and trypsin and neutralizes proteases and elastase which cause damage to lung tissue.
- **Normal microbiota:** Beneficial bacteria in the respiratory tract help prevent colonization by harmful microbes.
- **Antioxidants (Glutathione, superoxide dismutase):** Protect lung tissue from oxidative damage caused by pollution and smoking.

Clinical Implications

- Impaired defenses (e.g. smoking, chronic diseases, immunosuppression) increase susceptibility to respiratory infections like pneumonia, tuberculosis, and COVID-19.
- Overactive immune responses (e.g. asthma, hypersensitivity pneumonitis) can cause inflammation and airway damage.

Q. Pulmonary function tests (PFT).

- Pulmonary function tests (PFTs) are a group of tests used to assess lung function by measuring airflow, lung volume, and gas exchange. These tests help diagnose, monitor, and guide treatment for respiratory diseases such as asthma, COPD, and restrictive lung disorders.
- Many test results depend on the effort of patient, and suboptimal effort is a common cause of misinterpretation of results. All pulmonary function tests are measured against predicted values derived from large studies of healthy subjects. These predictions depend on age, sex, height and weight of the patient.

Indications for Pulmonary Function Testing

- Assessment of the type and severity of lung dysfunction
- Diagnosis of causes of dyspnea and cough
- Monitoring lung function in certain occupations at high risk of lung damage (e.g. mine workers)
- Monitoring response to treatment
- Preoperative assessment
- Disability evaluation.

Contraindications to Pulmonary Function Testing

- Acute severe asthma
- Respiratory distress
- Angina
- Pneumothorax
- Hemoptysis
- Active tuberculosis.

TYPES OF PULMONARY FUNCTION TESTS

Spirometry

- **Spirometry** is the measurement of lung volumes and airflow rates using an instrument called a **spirometer**.
- A **spirogram** visually represents your breathing patterns during the test. The shape of the curve on the graph plays a crucial role in diagnosing specific lung conditions:
    - **Normal spirometry pattern:** A healthy graph shows a rapid rise in airflow, reaching peak flow quickly before gradually declining. This indicates efficient lung function, where air is expelled swiftly and completely.
    - **Obstructive pattern:** This is characterized by a **'coved' or scooped-out** shape on the flow-volume loop. It presents with a reduced peak flow and a concave curve after the peak, suggesting airway obstruction that restricts airflow. If the **FEV_1/FVC ratio falls below 70%**, it indicates an obstructive respiratory condition, such as **asthma or COPD**, where airways are partially blocked.
    - **Restrictive pattern:** In contrast, a restrictive spirometry graph displays a **sharper but lower peak**, indicating **reduced lung volume**. The steep descent to baseline suggests difficulty filling the lungs with air, though air expulsion remains relatively unaffected. A **below-normal FVC** value supports this finding, pointing to restrictive conditions like **pulmonary fibrosis or scoliosis**, where lung expansion is limited.
- When taking a spirometry test, ask the patient to breathe into the spirometer mouthpiece and perform three types of breathing. First, ask him to breathe normally, also called quiet breathing, which corresponds to the tidal volume (TV). After that, ask him to take a deep breath, which will be represented in the diagram as a big increase in volume. A big inhale like this, in addition to the amount of air that was already inhaled during quiet breathing, is referred to as the Inspiratory reserve volume (IRV). Finally, ask him to perform a forced exhalation, which is the maximum amount of air possible to exhale from the lungs at once. This deep expiration will be recorded as a large decrease in volume which corresponds to the Expiratory Reserve Volume (ERV) **(Figs 2.1 to 2.3)**.
- The FVC is calculated by adding up the TV, the IRV, and the ERV. Among people with obstructive lung diseases like asthma, the FVC is lower than people with no obstructive disease.

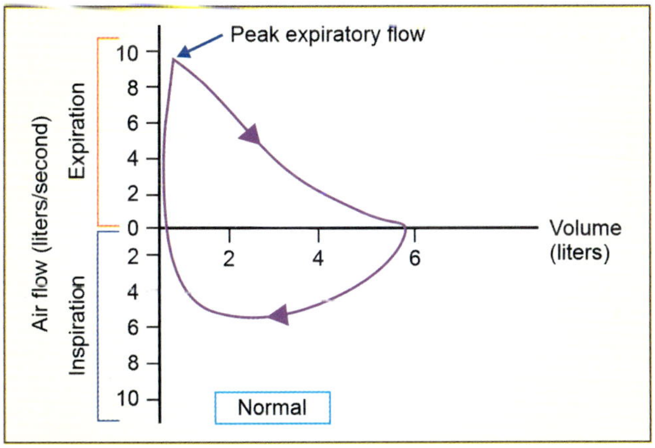

Figure 2.1: Normal spirometry

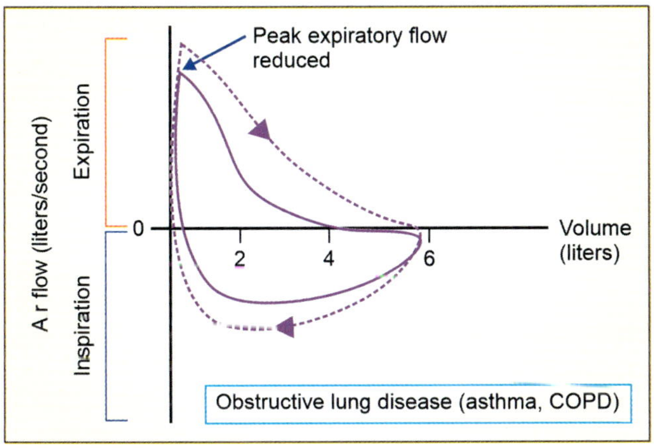

Figure 2.2: Spirometry in obstructive lung disease

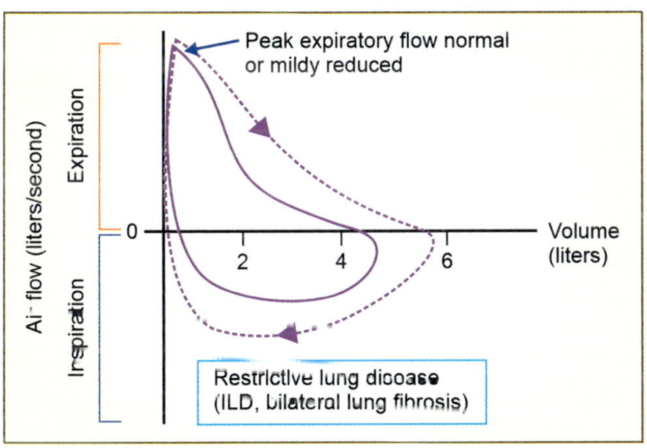

Figure 2.3: Spirometry in restrictive lung disease

Peak Expiratory Flow Rate (PEFR)

- **Peak expiratory flow fate (PEFR)** is the **maximum speed** at which air can be forcefully exhaled after a full inspiration. It is measured in **liters per minute (L/min)** and is an important parameter in monitoring **airway obstruction**. It is measured by a peak flow meter. The patient takes a deep breath and blows as hard as possible into the instrument. A pointer on the calibrated dial of the instrument moves indicating PEFR. The normal PEFR for men is 450–700 L/min and 300–500 L/min for women.
- PEFR is reduced in asthma (especially during exacerbations), COPD (due to airflow limitation), upper airway obstruction, and expiratory muscle weakness. PEF values less than 200 L/min indicate severe airflow obstruction. PEFR monitoring can quantify asthma severity, and provide an objective measurement for monitoring response to therapy in asthma. Predicted values for PEFR vary with age, sex, and height. PEFR shows diurnal variation. It is lowest on first awakening and highest many hours later. PEFR should be measured in the morning before taking bronchodilator and in the afternoon after taking a bronchodilator.

Diffusing Capacity of Lungs for Carbon Monoxide (DLCO)

- This reflects the diffusibility of gas across the alveolar/capillary membrane. It is helpful in evaluation of patients with diffuse infiltrative lung disease or emphysema. DLCO is low in emphysema and interstitial lung diseases whereas it is normal or high in asthma. DLCO is a useful screening test for patients with AIDS who are suspected to have *Pneumocystis pneumonia*. A normal DLCO is strong evidence against *Pneumocystis pneumonia*.

Arterial Blood Gas (ABG)

- ABG measurement is indicated whenever acid-base disturbance, hypoxemia, or hypercapnia is suspected.

Pulse Oximetry

- This is a noninvasive method of monitoring oxygen saturation of blood.

Cardiopulmonary Exercise Stress Testing

- This is done in patients with unexplained dyspnea. A bicycle ergometer or treadmill is used. Minute ventilation, expired oxygen and carbon dioxide tension, heart rate, blood pressure, and respiratory rate are monitored.

Q. Briefly discuss about different lung volume measurements.

Q. Difference between vital capacity (VC) and forced vital capacity (FVC).

Q. Difference between FVC and FEV_1.

Q. Differences between PEFR and FEV_1.

- The volume of gas in the lungs is divided into volumes and capacities. Tidal volume (VT) is the amount of gas inhaled and exhaled during a normal breath. Residual volume (RV) is the amount of gas remaining in the lungs at the end of a maximal exhalation. Vital capacity (VC) is the total amount of gas that can be exhaled following a maximal inhalation. FVC is the maximum amount of air exhaled forcefully after a deep breath, i.e. vital capacity performed with a maximally forced expiratory effort. The vital capacity and the residual volume together constitute the total lung capacity (TLC). The functional residual capacity (FRC) is the amount of gas in the lungs at the end of normal expiration.

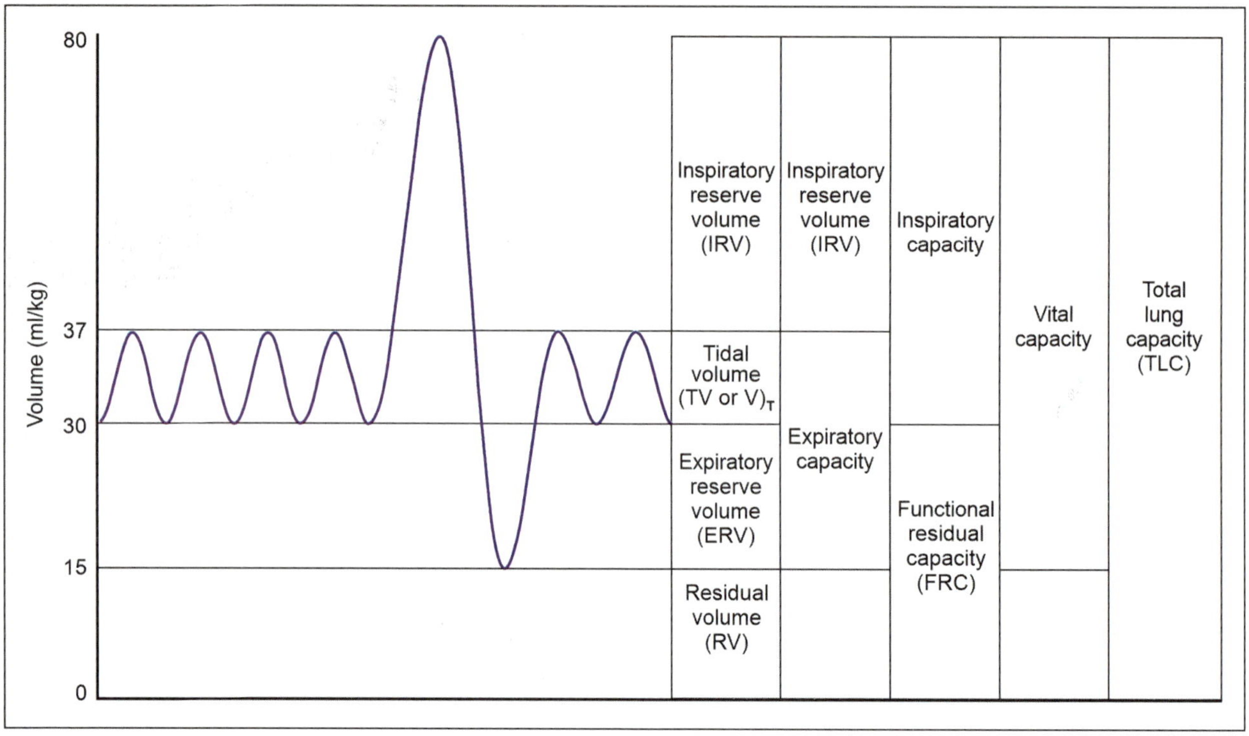

Figure 2.4: Various lung volumes

- Forced expiratory volume in the first second (FEV_1) is the amount of gas exhaled during the first second after inhaling to maximum capacity. Normal FEV_1 is about 80%. The ratio of the FEV_1 to the FVC (often referred to as the FEV_1%) is diminished in patients with obstructive lung diseases such as asthma and COPD.
- All lung volumes can be measured by spirometry except residual volume (RV), functional residual capacity (FRC), and total lung capacity (TLC). These are measured by helium dilution and body plethysmography.
- Measurement of lung volumes gives an idea about the presence and severity of obstructive and restrictive pulmonary dysfunction. Obstructive dysfunction is characterized by a fall in the ratio of FEV_1 to FVC. Causes of obstructive dysfunction include asthma, COPD, bronchiectasis, bronchiolitis, and upper airway obstruction. Restrictive dysfunction is characterized a reduction in lung volumes with a normal to increased FEV_1/FVC ratio. Causes include interstitial lung diseases, weak respiratory muscles, pleural disease, and prior lung resection.

Differences between FVC and VC

See **Table 2.1**.

Differences between PEFR and FEV_1

See **Table 2.2**.

Q. Enumerate the common signs and symptoms of respiratory disease.

Following are the common signs and symptoms of respiratory disease.

- Cough
- Hemoptysis
- Dyspnea
- Wheezing
- Chest pain (pleuritic, musculoskeletal)
- Cyanosis
- Clubbing
- Pedal edema (due to cor pulmonale)

Q. Enumerate the causes and differential diagnosis of cough.

TABLE 2.1: Differences between forced vital capacity (FVC) and vital capacity (VC)

Parameter	FVC (forced vital capacity)	VC (vital capacity)
Definition	Maximum amount of air exhaled forcefully after a maximal inspiration. It is a more dynamic test.	Maximum amount of air exhaled slowly and completely after a deep breath. It is a gentler measurement
Effort level	Measures overall lung capacity and function.	Requires **slow and steady** exhalation.
Clinical use	Assesses **both obstructive and restrictive** lung diseases.	Mainly used for assessing **restrictive** lung diseases.
Typical value	Often slightly **lower** than VC due to airway collapse in forced exhalation.	Slightly **higher** than FVC because slow exhalation prevents airway collapse.

TABLE 2.2: Differences between peak expiratory flow rate (PEFR) and forced expiratory volume in 1 second (FEV_1)

Parameter	Forced vital capacity (FVC)	Peak expiratory flow rate (PEFR)	Forced expiratory volume in 1 second (FEV_1)
Definition	Maximum **amount of air** exhaled forcefully after a maximal inspiration	Maximum **airflow speed** during forced expiration	**Volume of air** exhaled in the first second of a forced breath.
How to measure	Patient takes a deep breath and then forcefully exhales as hard and fast as possible until they cannot exhale any further.	Patient takes a deep breath and then forcefully exhales **as forcefully and quickly as possible** in a single blow.	Patient takes a deep breath and then forcefully exhales **as forcefully and quickly as possible** into a spirometer. The first second of exhalation is measured as FEV_1.
Measurement unit	Liters	Liters per minute (L/min) when measured by peak flow meter Expressed in L/sec when measured as part of spirometry	Liters
Purpose	Measures overall lung capacity and function.	**PEFR** is a quick and easy test for detecting **bronchospasm**, mainly in **asthma**. Useful for daily monitoring	Assesses how quickly air can be expelled, indicating airway resistance. Useful in **COPD and asthma** diagnosis
Measurement tool	Spirometer	Peak flow meter (handheld, easy to use at home) or spirometer.	Spirometer
Clinical use	Helps diagnose **restrictive** lung diseases.	Key indicator for **obstructive** lung diseases. used to monitor the response to treatment in asthma/COPD at home/bedside	Key indicator for **obstructive** lung diseases

Q. Discuss the approach to a case of cough.

- Cough is a reflex act of sudden, forceful expulsion of air from the lungs. It generates positive intrathoracic pressure as high as 300 mm Hg. Cough serves as a protective reflex to clear the respiratory tract of foreign particles, irritants, mucus, or pathogens.
- Cough is a frequent symptom of many respiratory diseases. Cough can occur in otherwise healthy people and is often a self-limiting symptom.
- Persistent coughing can be a socially disabling and distressing symptom, for which help is often sought.

Mechanism of Cough Production

- Cough reflex is initiated by stimulation of cough receptors (also known as mechanoreceptors and chemoreceptors) by chemical/mechanical stimuli. Cough receptors are present in in the airways (larynx, trachea, bronchi, lung parenchyma) and other parts of the body, including the pharynx, pleura, and diaphragm.
- When the cough receptors are stimulated, the signal is transmitted via afferent (sensory) fibers of the vagus nerve (cranial nerve X) to the brainstem, particularly the cough center (nucleus tractus solitarius) located in the medulla.
- The cough center in the medulla processes the sensory information from the airways. The medullary center integrates this input and generates a response that coordinates various muscles involved in coughing.
- Once the cough reflex is activated, efferent (motor) signals are sent from the cough center to various muscles involved in the cough mechanism via: vagus nerve (controls airways), phrenic nerve (controls the diaphragm), and spinal nerves (control the intercostal and abdominal muscles).
- The cough involves three distinct phases which are as follows:
    - *Inspiratory phase:* A deep inhalation occurs to fill the lungs with air (2.5–3 liters). This increases the volume of air that will be expelled during the cough.
    - *Compression phase*: The vocal cords in the larynx close, and there is a brief contraction of the expiratory muscles (diaphragm, intercostal, and abdominal muscles), creating increased pressure in the lungs. During this phase, the intrathoracic pressure rises significantly (up to 300 mm Hg), while the glottis remains closed.
    - *Expiratory phase:* The vocal cords and glottis suddenly open, and the high intrathoracic pressure rapidly releases air from the lungs through the mouth and nose. This explosive release of air helps to expel irritants or mucus from the respiratory tract. The air travels at high velocity (up to 480 km/hour or 300 mile/hour) during the cough, which is necessary to dislodge secretions or foreign bodies.

Causes of Cough

- Based on the duration, cough can be classified as.
    - ***Acute cough:*** Present for less than *three weeks*.
    - ***Subacute cough:*** Lasts *three to eight weeks* (pneumonia).
    - ***Chronic cough:*** Lasts *more than eight weeks*.
- Causes of cough based on duration are depicted in **Table 2.3**.

Differential Diagnosis of Cough

See **Table 2.4**.

TABLE 2.3: Causes of cough

Acute cough (<3 weeks)	Subacute cough (3–8 weeks)	Chronic cough (>8 weeks)
• Upper respiratory tract infections (common cold, pharyngitis) • Acute bronchitis • Pneumonia • Pulmonary embolism • Congestive cardiac failure • Inhalation of noxious chemicals or smoke • Aspiration event	• Prolonged viral infections • Tracheobronchitis • Post nasal drip • GERD	• Pulmonary tuberculosis • Bronchial asthma • COPD • Bronchiectasis • Bronchogenic carcinoma • Interstitial lung diseases (ILD) • Eosinophilic bronchitis • Tropical pulmonary eosinophilia • Post nasal drip due to perennial or allergic rhinitis, vasomotor rhinitis, or chronic sinusitis • GERD • Drugs like ACE inhibitors • Congestive cardiac failure

TABLE 2.4: Differential diagnosis of cough

Site of origin	Causes	Clinical features
Nose	Post-nasal drip due to sinusitis, rhinitis	History of rhinitis
Pharynx	Pharyngitis	Sore throat, fever
Larynx	Laryngitis, tumor, Whooping cough, croup	H/o hoarseness of voice, painful cough, fever. Stridor may be present in severe laryngitis
Trachea	Tracheitis	Retrosternal pain with cough
Bronchi	Acute bronchitis	Dry or productive cough. Worse in mornings. Wheezing present.
	Asthma	Usually dry, worse at night. Associated wheezing is usually present. Asthma-related cough may be seasonal and may worsen upon exposure to cold, dry air, or certain fumes or fragrances.
	COPD	Most patients are smokers. Sputum is usually scanty and mucoid. Associated wheezing is usually present
	Bronchogenic Ca	Persistent cough often with hemoptysis. Patient is usually a chronic smoker. Weight loss may be present.
Lung parenchyma	Tuberculosis	Productive, often with hemoptysis. Low-grade fever may be present along with weight loss.
	Pneumonia	Initially dry, later associated with sputum production
	Bronchiectasis	Sputum is mucopurulent and large quantity. Changes in posture induces sputum production
	Pulmonary edema	Often at night. Pink, frothy sputum may be produced. Signs and symptoms of cardiac failure present.
	Interstitial lung disease	Dry, irritant and distressing cough. Associated exertional dyspnea is usually present initially on exertion and later at rest also.
Pleural diseases	Pleural Effusion Pleurisy (Pleuritis) Pneumothorax Pleural Tumors (Mesothelioma, Metastases) Pleural Tuberculosis	Pleural diseases present with dry cough, and sometimes with pleuritic chest pain. There may be breathlessness in cases of pleural effusion and pneumothorax. Weight loss may be there with TB and pleural tumors.
Miscellaneous (extrapulmonary causes)	GERD	Cough is usually nocturnal. Heartburn may be present.
	ACE inhibitors	Dry cough. It follows initiation of ACE inhibitors.
	Irritation of the external auditory canal by impacted foreign bodies or cerumen	Dry cough. Ear pain and discharge may be present.

History

Age and Sex

- Bronchogenic ca and COPD are more common in elderly males. Asthma is more common in females.

Onset

- Cough of sudden onset may be associated with foreign body aspiration, allergic reactions and pulmonary edema due to left ventricular failure. Insidious onset cough occurs in COPD, interstitial lung diseases, chronic lung infections such as TB, etc.

Is the cough dry/productive?

- Significant sputum production suggests primary pulmonary pathology (such as pneumonia, lung abscess, bronchiectasis). Dry cough is more likely to be associated with upper airway infections (such as rhinitis, pharyngitis), interstitial lung disease, pleural diseases, and drug induced cough due to ACE inhibitors.

Associated Symptoms

- Presence of wheezing along with cough suggests bronchial asthma, acute bronchitis, COPD, eosinophilic pneumonia, tropical pulmonary eosinophilia, etc. Presence of breathlessness can occur in pneumonia, acute exacerbation of asthma and COPD, or significant pleural pathology. Presence of fever usually suggests an infectious etiology for cough.

Diurnal variation in cough

- Asthma has early morning cough. Cough due to gastroesophageal reflux may increase after food intake and at night due to recumbent position. Pulmonary edema due to heart failure can cause coughing at night which wakes patients (PND).

Intake of any medications

- ACE inhibitors can cause cough.

Smoking

- One of the most common causes of persistent cough is smoking. Smoking also leads to COPD and lung cancer which can present as cough.

Occupation

- Dust/chemical exposure in certain occupations can cause cough. For example, coal mine workers may develop chronic cough.

Physical Examination

General Examination

- Fever (infection), weight loss (TB, cancer), clubbing (ILD, lung cancer).

Respiratory Examination

- **Wheezing:** Asthma, COPD.
- **Crackles (Crepitations):** Pneumonia, ILD, bronchietasis.
- **Decreased breath sounds:** Pleural effusion, pneumothorax.

Cardiovascular Examination

- **Raised JVP, peripheral edema, presence of S3:** Heart failure-related cough.

Investigations

- Acute cough usually does not require any investigations. It should be treated symptomatically (with antitussives for dry cough and expectorants for productive cough). Indications for investigation in acute cough include hemoptysis, prominent systemic illness, suspicion of inhaled foreign body and suspicion of lung cancer. However, chronic chough requires many of the following investigations.

Complete Blood Count (CBC)

- Infection (↑ WBCs), eosinophilia (asthma, allergy).

Sputum Analysis and Culture

- Done in cases of productive cough. Helpful to rule out pneumonia, TB.

Chest X-ray

- It can show any pleural or parenchymal pathology such as effusion, pneumonia, mass lesions, etc.

Sinus Imaging (X-ray or sinus CT scan)

- To rule out sinusitis.

Spirometry

- Spirometry should be performed in all patients with chronic cough. It is helpful in differentiating obstructive (COPD, asthma) *vs* restrictive lung diseases (fibrosis).

High resolution computed tomographic (HRCT) scanning of chest

- HRCT scanning may be of useful for diagnosing bronchiectasis, interstitial lung diseases or detailed evaluation of any lung pathology.

Bronchial provocation testing

- Should be done in patients without a clinically obvious etiology for cough.

Bronchoscopy

- Bronchoscopy should be done if inhalation of a foreign body or endobronchial pathology is suspected.

Echocardiography

- Helpful to rule out cardiac causes of cough (heart failure, pulmonary hypertension).

24-hour esophageal pH monitoring

- To rule out gastroesophageal reflux disease as a cause of cough.

Treatment of Cough

Symptomatic Management

- Use of cough suppressants (such as codeine, dextromethorphan, levocloperastine) for dry cough and expectorants for productive cough. Do not suppress a productive cough.

Management based on cause

Condition	Management
Infectious (pneumonia, TB, bronchitis)	Antibiotics (if bacterial), supportive care
Asthma/COPD	Bronchodilators, inhaled corticosteroids
GERD-related cough	PPIs, lifestyle modifications
Postnasal drip	Antihistamines, nasal steroids
ACE inhibitor cough	Stop/change medication
Pleural causes (effusion, pneumothorax, malignancy)	Thoracentesis, pleural drainage, cancer treatment

Complications of Cough

- Cough syncope, rib fracture, pneumothorax, development of hernias.

Q. Define clubbing. Enumerate the causes and mechanism of clubbing.

Q. Hypertrophic osteoarthropathy.

- Clubbing is a physical sign characterized by bulbous enlargement of distal ends of digits. This results in "club-like" appearance of the fingers.
- Clubbed fingers are also known as watch-glass nails, drumstick fingers, and Hippocratic fingers/nails. It was first described by Hippocrates in a patient with empyema. Hence, the name Hippocratic fingers. Acropachy is another term used for clubbing.
- Clubbing itself is not a disease, but is a sign of underlying disease. Hence, it is important to look for clubbing, because if the underlying disorder is diagnosed and treated early it may be curable.
- Clubbing usually develops in the thumb and forefinger first, and later in the other fingers. Clubbing may be missed in the initial stages, unless the examiner observes the hands (and feet) carefully.
- Clubbing can be acquired or hereditary: Acquired bilateral clubbing is the most common form.

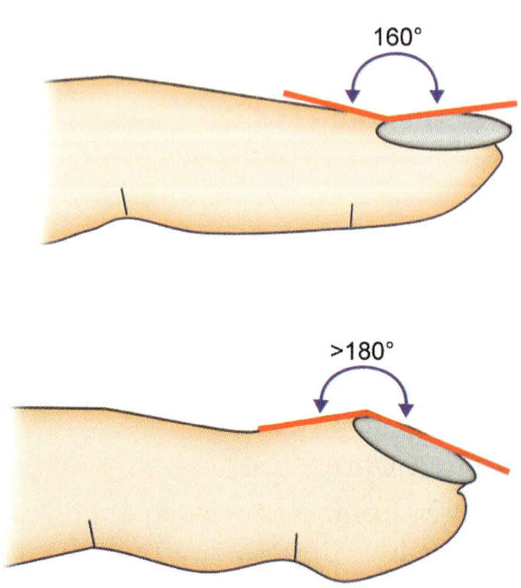

Figure 2.5: Clubbing

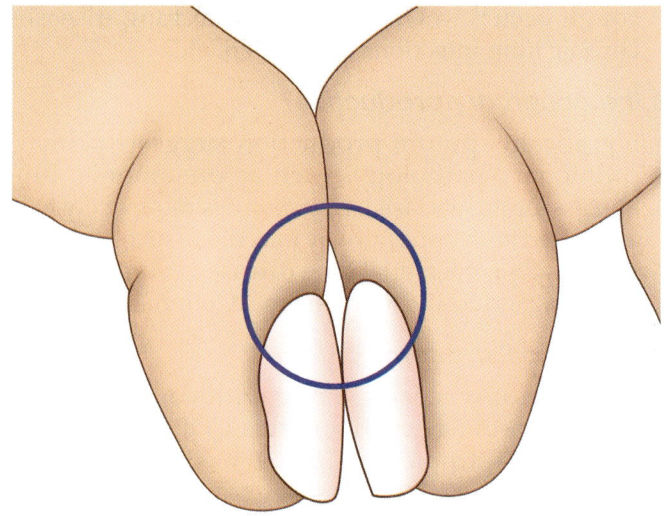

Figure 2.6: Diamond shaped Shamroth window between normal fingers

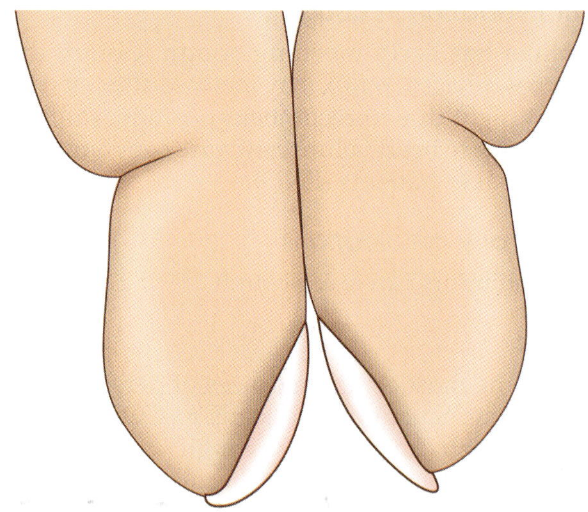

Figure 2.7: Absent Shamroth window in clubbing

Causes of Clubbing (Table 2.5)

TABLE 2.5: Causes of clubbing

Pulmonary diseases (most common cause of clubbing; account for 75% of clubbing)
- Bronchogenic carcinoma
- Pleural mesothelioma
- Metastatic carcinoma
- Lung abscess
- Chronic empyema
- Interstitial lung disease (ILD)
- Pneumoconiosis
- Cystic fibrosis
- Emphysema
- Bronchiectasis

Cardiovascular disease (2nd most common cause)
- Cyanotic congenital heart disease
- Subacute bacterial endocarditis
- Cor pulmonale
- Chronic congestive heart failure
- Atrial myxoma

(Contd.)

TABLE 2.5: Causes of clubbing *(Contd.)*

Gastrointestinal disease
• Cirrhosis (all types, especially biliary cirrhosis)
• Hepatocellular carcinoma
• Amebic liver abscess
• IBD—Crohn's, ulcerative colitis
• Sprue
Miscellaneous
• Hyperthyroidism
• Pregnancy
• Chronic osteomyelitis with amyloidosis
• Hemoglobinopathies
• Toxin exposure (Arsenic, mercury)
• Familial
Unilateral clubbing
• Aortic or subclavian artery aneurysm
• Pulmonary hypertension with patent ductus arteriosus
• Pancoast tumors
Unidigital clubbing
• Local trauma
• Median nerve injury
• Sarcoidosis
Clubbing of toes without fingers
• Coarctation of aorta

Grades of Clubbing

Grades of clubbing

Grade 1: Increased fluctuation of nailbed

Grade 2: Obliteration of nailbed angle more than or equal to 180 degree

Grade 3: Parrot beaking—Biconvexity of nail

Grade 4: Hypertrophic osteoarthropathy-with the above mentioned features plus thickening of periosteum, distal arthropathy, periosteal tenderness and heaviness of hands

Pathophysiology

- Clubbing is characterized by an increase in the pulp tissue due to proliferation of subungual connective tissue, interstitial edema, and dilation of arterioles and capillaries. This results in loss of the normal angle between the proximal nail fold and nail plate and excessive sponginess of the nail base. Normally, the angle between the nail plate and the proximal nail fold (known as Lovibond angle) is 160° in normal nails. When clubbing occurs, this angle becomes >180°.
- The exact mechanism of proliferation of subungual connective tissue resulting in clubbing remains unknown. Many theories have been proposed. Some theories are as follows.
- One proposed theory is that clubbing results from distal digital vasodilation, which in turn results in subungual tissue proliferation and edema. Many factors are thought to produce this distal vasodilation including a circulating or local vasodilator, neural mechanism, response to hypoxemia, genetic predisposition, or a combination of these factors. Many vasodilator substances are thought to be inactivated by lungs normally. In case of diseases where the blood bypasses lungs (e.g. cyanotic congenital heart diseases with right to left shunt), vasodilator substances reach the distal ends of digits and cause vasodilatation. Proposed vasodilatory factors include ferritin, prostaglandins, bradykinin, adenine nucleotides, and 5-hydroxytryptamine.
- A neural mechanism has been proposed with particular consideration of the vagal system. Increased vagal stimulation with resultant vasodilation in digits has been proposed but is not widely accepted.
- Hypoxia has been proposed as a cause of clubbing in many cardiac and lung diseases. An increase in hypoxia may activate local vasodilators, consequently increasing blood flow to the distal portion of the digits; however, many diseases with hypoxia are not associated with clubbing.
- Genetic inheritance and predisposition also may play a role in digital clubbing especially in hereditary clubbing and clubbing associated with pachydermoperiostosis.
- Currently, the most accepted theory is "Platelet hypothesis". Normally, megakaryocytes (precursors of platelets) break up into smaller platelets when they pass through pulmonary capillaries. If megakaryocytes bypass pulmonary circulation due to right to left shunt, then they preferentially lodge in the vascular beds of the fingertips and release platelet-derived growth factor (PDGF), VEGF, and other mediators. These mediators have growth-promoting activity and causes increased capillary permeability and connective tissue hypertrophy, ultimately leading to clubbing.
- A simple maneuver (described by Schamroth) readily differentiates true clubbing from these pseudo-clubbing conditions. The examiner asks the patient to hold the two thumbs back to back with the two fingertips and interphalangeal joints aligned. Because the base angle is unaltered in these conditions, an elongated, diamond-shaped area of empty space is apparent. In true clubbing, this empty space is lost. (Schamroth, while himself ill with subacute bacterial endocarditis, noted this finding as one of the earliest signs of clubbing; he also reported that the window of empty space reappeared 2 months after his endocarditis had been treated successfully.)

How to look for clubbing?

- Inspect the periungual skin. In clubbing it is stretched and shiny.
- Very early clubbing can be detected by increase in fluctuation of the nail-bed ("floating nail" sign) which is due to softening of the nail-bed. To elicit 'fluctuation', the patient's finger (pulp of index finger) is placed on the pulp of examiner's two thumbs and held in place by gentle pressure from the examiner's middle fingers on the patient's proximal interphalangeal joint. The patient's finger is now palpated over the base of the nail by the tips of examiner's index fingers. There is always some amount of fluctuation present even in normal fingers. Clubbing is diagnosed when the fluctuation becomes pronounced, creating a sensation as if the nail is floating above its bed.

- Next, bring the patient's fingers at examiners eye level and look tangentially from side. Look at the angle between the nailplate and proximal skin fold (onychodermal angle). Normally, the angle between the nail plate and the proximal nail fold (known as Lovibond angle) is 160°. When clubbing occurs, this angle becomes >180°. This is also known as"profile" sign. Obliteration of the angle between the nail and the nailbed is one of the first sign of clubbing and its most constant feature; indeed, many require it for the diagnosis.
- Schamroth sign: This sign is elicited by placing the dorsal surfaces of terminal phalanges of corresponding right and left fingers together. Normal fingers create a diamond-shaped window. In patients with clubbing, this diamond-shaped window gets obliterated and is known as Schamroth sign. Schamroth, while himself ill with subacute bacterial endocarditis, noted this finding as one of the earliest signs of clubbing; he also reported that the window of empty space reappeared 2 months after his endocarditis had been treated successfully.
- Also note the width of terminal portion and compare with the proximal part. Normally the size of terminal portion is same or less than the proximal portion of the terminal phalanx. In clubbing, there is widening of the AP and lateral diameter of terminal portion of fingers and toes giving the appearance of clubbing.

Hypertrophic Osteoarthropathy

- Hypertrophic osteoarthropathy is an advanced stage of clubbing where there is painful periosteal proliferation of long bones such as the radius, ulna, or tibia. The periostitis is often associated with mild fever and arthralgia or joint effusion.
- Hypertrophic osteoarthropathy should always be sought when clubbing is found. The symptomatic patient with hypertrophic osteoarthropathy will complain of severe burning, deep pain over the distal extremities, especially of the legs, that is worsened at night and on dependency. There may be tenderness of the distal parts of the limbs (legs, feet, forearms, hands). Distal joints may be swollen with tenderness, The examiner may elicit tenderness over bony prominences by simply pressing or by encircling the limb (e.g. the wrist) with his own fingers like a bracelet and gently squeezing it. Later, autonomic changes such as flushing, sweating, or blanching (Raynaud's phenomenon) may be noted in the affected hands and feet.

Pseudo-clubbing

- Psuedo-clubbing is seen in conditions associated with subperiosteal bone resorption of terminal phalanges. Here there is absence of soft tissue proliferation but increased curvature is present. The angle between nail and nailbed (Lovibond angle) remains normal.
- It is seen in
  - Scleroderma
  - Acromegaly
  - Hyperparathyroidism
  - Leprosy

Q. Define dyspnea. What are the mechanisms of dyspnea?

Q. Enumerate the causes of dyspnea.

Q. Discuss the differential diagnosis of acute onset dyspnea.

- Dyspnea (or breathlessness) refers to the abnormal and uncomfortable awareness of breathing.
- Dyspnea is a subjective symptom reported by patients. It is always a sensation expressed by the patient and should not be confused with rapid breathing (tachypnea) or hyperventilation. tachypnea is an increased rate of breathing (>20/min), whereas dyspnea is the sensation or feeling of difficulty or discomfort in breathing. While dyspnea can be associated with tachypnea, tachypnea need not always cause dyspnea. For example, in fever, tachypnea can be there, but no dyspnea. Dyspnea is most frequently described as shortness of breath, inability to take a deep breath, or chest tightness.

Causes of Dyspnea (Table 2.6)

- Dyspnea can be acute, subacute, or chronic. Acute dyspnea develops over minutes to hours. Chronic dyspnea develops over weeks to months.
- 90% of dyspnea cases are due to respiratory or cardiac problems.

Causes of Episodic/Intermittent Breathlessness

- Here breathlessness episode are intermittent and resolve completely between episodes. Causes are as follows:
  - Asthma
  - Pulmonary edema
  - Angina
  - Pulmonary embolism
  - Work-related dyspnea (occupational asthma)

Mechanisms of Dyspnea

See **Table 2.7**.

Grading of Breathlessness

- Severity of breathlessness can be assessed by using Modified Medical Research Council (mMRC) dyspnea scale which is as follows. It has 5 grades (0–4) and the descriptions are more focused on specific activities to make it easier for patients to self-report their level of dyspnea.

Modified Medical Research Council (mMRC) dyspnea scale
Grade 0: I only get breathless with strenuous exercise
Grade 1: I get short of breath when hurrying on level ground or walking up a slight hill
Grade 2: On level ground, I walk slower than people of the same age because of breathlessness, or have to stop for breath when walking at my own pace
Grade 3: I stop for breath after walking about 100 yards [91 meters] or after a few minutes on level ground
Grade 4: I am too breathless to leave the house or I am breathless when dressing

TABLE 2.6: Causes of dyspnea

	Acute dyspnea (minutes to hours)	Subacute dyspnea (days to weeks)	Chronic dyspnea (months to years)
Cardiovascular	• Acute pulmonary edema • Acute myocardial ischemia • Cardiac tamponade		• Chronic heart failure • IHD
Respiratory	• Acute severe asthma • Acute exacerbation of COPD • Pneumothorax • Pneumonia • Pulmonary embolism • ARDS • Foreign body aspiration • Laryngeal edema (e.g. anaphylaxis)	• Pneumonia • Pleural effusion • Lobar collapse	• COPD • Chronic asthma • Bronchial carcinoma • Interstitial lung disease • Chronic pulmonary thromboembolism • Lymphangitis carcinomatosis • Pleural effusion
Others	• Metabolic acidosis (e.g. diabetic ketoacidosis, lactic acidosis, uremia, overdose of salicylates, ethylene glycol poisoning) • Psychogenic hyperventilation (anxiety or panic-related)		• Severe anemia • Obesity

TABLE 2.7: Mechanisms of dyspnea

Mechanisms of dyspnea	Causes
Stimulation of intrapulmonary sensory nerves	• Interstitial inflammation • Pulmonary embolism
Increase in the mechanical load on the respiratory muscles	• Airflow obstruction • Pulmonary fibrosis
Stimulation of chemoreceptors	• Hypoxia • Hypercapnia • Acidosis
Reduction of lung compliance	• Pulmonary edema • Severe kyphoscoliosis • Pleural effusion • Pneumothorax

Investigations

- SpO_2 (Pulse oximetry): Assess oxygenation.
- Arterial blood gas (ABG): Evaluate hypoxia, hypercapnia, acid-base balance.
- Complete blood count (CBC): To rule out anemia (↓ Hb), infection (↑ WBC).
- D-dimer: To rule out pulmonary embolism in low-risk cases.
- BNP: Elevated in heart failure.
- Troponins: Rule out acute coronary syndrome.
- Chest X-ray (CXR). First-line investigation for pulmonary and cardiac causes.
    - Cardiomegaly, pulmonary edema → Heart failure
    - Hyperinflated lungs, flat diaphragm → COPD
    - Consolidation, opacities → Pneumonia, ARDS
    - Air/fluid collection → Pneumothorax, pleural effusion
- High-resolution CT (HRCT) → Interstitial lung disease, pulmonary fibrosis.
- CT pulmonary angiography (CTPA) → Pulmonary embolism.
- ECG, Echocardiography (ECHO) → If cardiac cause suspected.
- Pulmonary function tests (PFTs) → in cases of chronic dyspnea.

Treatment of Dyspnea

- General supportive measures.

Airway Support

- Ensure airway patency (suction if needed).

Breathing Support

- Oxygen supplementation if needed.
- Monitor respiratory rate (RR) and ABG
- Bronchodilators (nebulized salbutamol + ipratropium); if bronchospasm (e.g. asthma, COPD).
- IV steroids (hydrocortisone/methylprednisolone); if airway inflammation.
- Diuretics (furosemide IV); if pulmonary edema (e.g. heart failure).
- BiPAP if needed.
- Endotracheal intubation and mechanical ventilation (if impending respiratory failure).

Circulatory Support

- IV Fluids–If dehydration or sepsis is present.
- Vasopressors (Noradrenaline, Dobutamine)–If in shock.

Treatment Based on Underlying Cause

See **Table 2.9**.

Q. Solitary pulmonary nodule (SPN).

- Solitary pulmonary nodule (SPN) or "coin lesion" is a single round lesion, that is less than 3 cm and surrounded by normal lung parenchyma.
- A "nodule" is called a "mass" when the size is more than 3 cm. SPN is a common clinical problem and is detected incidentally on a chest X-ray or CT scan.
- The differential diagnosis of SPN is broad. The main question that has to be answered is whether it is malignant or benign.

TABLE 2.8: Differential diagnosis of acute dyspnea

Condition	Clinical features	Investigations
Pulmonary edema (due to LVF)	*History:* Chest pain, orthopnea, palpitations. Previous h/o cardiac problems. Expectoration of pink frothy sputum. *Examination:* Central cyanosis, raised JVP, sweating, cool extremities, B/L basal lung crepitations. S3 and S4 may be present.	Chest X-ray: Cardiomegaly. Prominent pulmonary vasculature. Pleural effusion may be present.
Acute pulmonary embolism	*History:* Risk factors for DVT present (recent major surgery, immobilization, stroke). Sudden onset pleuritic chest pain, hemoptysis, syncope. *Examination:* central cyanosis, elevated JVP, hypotension. Signs of DVT in the lower limbs. Breath sounds normal.	Chest X-ray: Prominent hilar vessels, oligemic lung fields, prominent pulmonary artery. ECG may show signs of pulmonary embolism such as, S1Q3T3 pattern and right bundle-branch block. Echo shows dilated pulmonary artery, dilated right ventricle.
Acute severe asthma	*History:* h/o dyspnea associated with wheezing, previous h/o asthma. Response to bronchodilators. *Examination:* Bilateral polyphonic rhonchi present over the lungs. Usually no crepitations. Prolonged expiration. Tachycardia, pulsus paradoxus and cyanosis may be present.	Chest X-ray shows hyperinflation. ECG normal. PEFR reduced.
Acute exacerbation of COPD	*History:* Smoking history present. H/o of similar episodes in the past. H/o wheezing present. *Examination:* Cyanosis, signs of COPD such as increased AP diameter of chest, pushed down diaphragm. Signs of CO_2 retention (warm periphery, flapping tremor, bounding pulses).	Chest X-ray: Hyperinflation, increased bronchovascular markings, signs of emphysema. ECG usually normal, but may show signs of pulmonary HTN.
Pneumonia	*History:* Fever with chills and rigors. Cough with purulent sputum. Pleuritic chest pain in lobar pneumonia. *Examination:* Signs of consolidation present. Crepitations present. Pleural rub may be present if there is associated pleurisy. Signs of pleural effusion may be present if there is syn-pneumonic effusion.	Chest X-ray: Pneumonic shadow. Total leukocyte count high. ECG normal
Metabolic acidosis	*History* of diabetes/renal failure present. Oliguria or anuria in renal failure. H/o ingestion of ethylene glycol, methanol, etc. which can produce metabolic acidosis. *Examination:* Smell of acetone in diabetic ketoacidosis. Anemia present in CRF. Pedal edema in renal failure	Chest-ray and ECG normal ABG shows metabolic acidosis. Ketone bodies present in urine in diabetic ketoacidosis. Urea and creatinine high in renal failure
Psychogenic hyperventilation	*History:* Previous similar episodes. H/o stressful event preceding the attack. Common in young women. *Examination:* No cyanosis. CVS and RS normal. Carpopedal spasm present due to hyperventilation induced respiratory alkalosis leading to low calcium.	All investigations are normal.
Pneumothorax	*History:* Sudden onset unilateral chest pain. H/o wheezing absent. *Examination:* Signs of pneumothorax present (trachea deviated to opposite side, hyperresonant percussion note, absent breath sounds)	Chest X-ray: Shows pneumothorax. ECG normal
Upper airway obstruction (foreign body aspiration, laryngeal edema)	*History:* Stridor present. Hoarseness of voice may be present. Patient may be unable to speak. *Examination*: Inspiratory sound localized to trachea or larynx. Lungs and heart normal.	Chest X-ray may be normal or may show foreign body if it is radiopaque. Direct laryngoscopy or bronchoscopy may show laryngeal edema or foreign body. ECG normal

TABLE 2.9: Treatment of dyspnea based on underlying cause

Cause	Treatment
Obstructive lung disease (Asthma, COPD)	Bronchodilators (salbutamol + ipratropium) IV/systemic steroids (prednisolone/hydrocortisone) Oxygen therapy/BiPAP Antibiotics (if infection present)
Pulmonary edema (heart failure, cardiogenic shock)	Diuretics (furosemide IV) Oxygen/BiPAP Vasodilators (nitroglycerin if BP is stable).
Pulmonary embolism (PE)	Anticoagulation (Heparin/LMWH) Thrombolysis (If massive PE + unstable BP) Oxygen/Mechanical ventilation (If severe hypoxia)
Pneumonia (bacterial, viral, aspiration)	Antibiotics (Empirical therapy based on severity) Bronchodilators (If wheezing present)
Pneumothorax	Needle decompression (if tension pneumothorax) Chest tube drainage (if large pneumothorax)
Anemia (severe, Hb <7 g/dl)	Blood transfusion (PRBCs) Treatment of underlying cause of anemia.
Neuromuscular disorders (myasthenia gravis, Guillain-Barré syndrome)	IV Immunoglobulin (IVIG) or plasmapheresis Ventilatory support (If respiratory muscle weakness)

Causes of Solitary Pulmonary Nodule

TABLE 2.10: Causes of solitary pulmonary nodule

Benign causes	*Malignant causes*
• **Infectious causes:** Tuberculoma, Histoplasmosis, Coccidioidomycosis Blastomycosis, Localized pneumonia, lung abscess, hydatid cyst, aspergilloma (usually surrounded by air 'halo' • **Benign neoplasms:** Hamartoma (most common benign tumor), fibroma, lipoma, chondroma • **Inflammatory/autoimmune:** Wegener's granuloma, rheumatoid nodule, sarcoidosis • **Vascular causes:** Arteriovenous malformations (AVMs), pulmonary infarct, pulmonary hematoma • **Structural causes:** Bronchogenic cyst, pulmonary sequestration	• Primary lung cancer • Carcinoid tumor • Single metastasis • Lymphoma

Diagnosis

- The main task is to distinguish between malignant and benign nodules. Malignant nodules should be excised whereas benign nodules may be left behind.
- It is not always possible to distinguish between malignant and benign lesions noninvasively. However certain clinical and radiological features may help in this aspect.
- Clinical features suggesting more chances of malignancy are:
  - Advanced age: More than 50% nodules are malignant at the age of 60 or above.
  - H/o hemoptysis, weight loss, chest pain).
  - H/o of chronic smoking.
  - H/o Exposure to carcinogens (asbestos, radon, silica, coal, etc.).
  - Previous h/o of malignancy.
- Radiographic features suggestive of benign lesions are:
  - Small size (<8 mm).
  - Smooth, well-defined borders.
  - Central, laminated, or popcorn calcification (suggests granuloma or hamartoma).
  - Slow growth (no significant change in >2 years).
- Radiographic features suggestive of malignancy are:
  - Size: Larger lesions (>8 mm) are more likely to be malignant than smaller lesions.
  - Irregular, lobulated or spiculated border.
  - Growth: Fast growing nodules are likely to be malignant.
  - Eccentric or stippled calcification.
  - Doubling time of 1–12 months.

Investigations

- Chest X-ray
- CT-scan chest
- PET scan can noninvasively distinguish between benign and malignant lesions.
- FNAC or biopsy is the gold standard to confirm or rule out malignancy.

Management

- If the probability of nodule being malignant is high, it should be resected.
- If the probability of nodule being malignant is low, it should be followed with serial CT scan. PET scan or sampling of the nodule may be alternatives for patients who are uncomfortable with a strategy of observation.

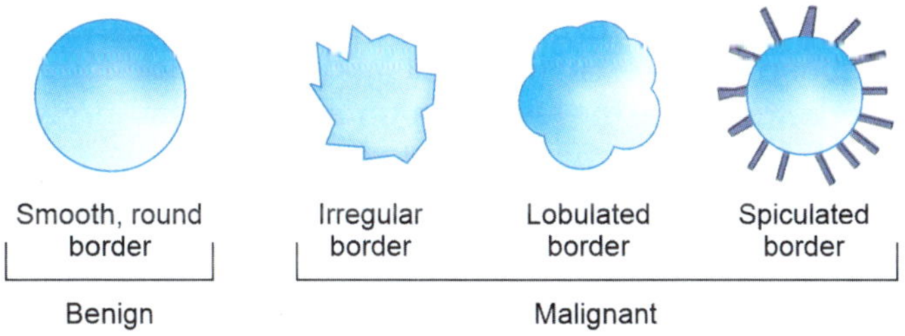

Figure 2.8: Solitary pulmonary nodule border types

Q. Define hemoptysis. Discuss the causes, clinical features, investigations and management of hemoptysis.

- The term hemoptysis refers to coughing out of blood from the lower respiratory tract (i.e. from below the vocal cords).
- Hemoptysis is often a sign of serious disease.
- True hemoptysis should be differentiated from pseudo-hemoptysis (spurious hemoptysis). Clear history of blood being coughed up or mixed with sputum reliably indicates hemoptysis.
- In pseudo-hemoptysis, there is bleeding from the upper respiratory tract which is spit or coughed out. Rarely pseudo-hemoptysis may be due to infection with organism like *Serratia marcescens* producing a red pigment. Blood that suddenly appears in the mouth without coughing suggests a nasopharyngeal origin; ask about nosebleeds and look for epistaxis or a bleeding source within the mouth.

Differentiating true hemoptysis from pseudo-hemoptysis (Table 2.11)

TABLE 2.11: Differences between true hemoptysis from pseudo-hemoptysis

	True hemoptysis	Pseudo-hemoptysis
Origin of the blood:	Blood typically originates from the lower respiratory tract (lungs or bronchi)	Blood comes from areas like the upper respiratory tract or GI tract.
Associated symptoms	Respiratory symptoms such as cough, shortness of breath, and sometimes chest pain	There may be nasal congestion, throat pain, or GI symptoms like heartburn or vomiting.
Blood color	Often produces bright red, frothy blood	Fresh or clotted, non-frothy blood
Mixed with sputum	May be	No
Chest X-ray	May be abnormal	Normal

- It is classified as trivial, mild, or massive.
- Massive hemoptysis usually refers to the expectoration of a large amount of blood and/or to a rapid rate of bleeding. There is no universally accepted volume of blood that defines massive hemoptysis but generally more than 200–600 ml in 24 hours indicates massive hemoptysis.
- A useful clinical definition of massive hemoptysis is hemoptysis that results in a life-threatening event including significant airway obstruction, significant abnormal gas exchange, or hemodynamic instability. It is better to use the term "life-threatening hemoptysis" rather than massive hemoptysis.
- Lungs have two sources of blood supply. The pulmonary arteries which arise from the right ventricle and bronchial arteries which arise from the aorta or intercostal arteries both supply the lungs. The bronchial arterial circulation is a high-pressure circuit. Though it contributes to only 1–2% of total pulmonary blood flow, bronchial circulation is frequently the source of hemoptysis.

Causes of Hemoptysis

Common causes of hemoptysis

Respiratory causes
- Tuberculosis
- Necrotizing pneumonia/lung abscess
- Bronchogenic carcinoma
- Acute bronchitis
- Bronchiectasis
- Pulmonary embolism
- Aspergilloma
- Bronchial adenoma
- Foreign body
- Diseases affecting pulmonary vasculature (Goodpasture's syndrome, polyarteritis nodosa)
- Trauma
- Catamenial hemoptysis (recurrent hemoptysis that is coincident with menses due to endometriosis in the lungs.)
- Pulmonary arteriovenous malformation (PAVM)
- Iatrogenic, e.g. post-lung biopsy, bronchoscopy

Cardiac causes
- Mitral stenosis
- Acute left ventricular failure
  (in both the above causes, hemoptysis occurs due to rupture of engorged pulmonary veins and capillaries)
- Aortic aneurysm rupturing into lungs

Bleeding and clotting disorders
- Thrombocytopenia
- Hemophilia
- Use of anticoagulants

Severity of Hemoptysis

- ***Non-life-threatening hemoptysis:*** Small amounts of blood, often streaking the sputum. This can be investigated safely as an outpatient.
- ***Life-threatening hemoptysis (formerly massive hemoptysis):*** Greater than 100–200 ml of blood in 24 hours, posing an immediate threat to airway patency and oxygenation. Massive hemoptysis requires careful monitoring of patient and immediate resuscitative measures.
- The pulmonary artery circulation supply is a low-pressure system mostly supplying the lung parenchyma; most episodes of hymoptysis are non-life-threatening and originate from the pulmonary artery circulation. In contrast, the bronchial artery circulation is relatively high-pressure from the systemic circulation mostly supplying the endobronchial tree. Although the bronchial artery circulation is responsible for only 2% of the total vascular supply to the lung, bleeding from a bronchial artery is the cause of life-threatening hemoptysis in 90% of cases.
- The pulmonary artery circulation, which supplies the lung parenchyma, is a low-pressure system, and most

episodes of hemoptysis originate from this circulation and are generally non-life-threatening. In contrast, the bronchial artery circulation, which arises from the high-pressure systemic circulation, primarily supplies the endobronchial tree. Despite accounting for only 2% of the lung's total blood supply, bleeding from the bronchial arteries is responsible for 90% of life-threatening cases of hemoptysis because this is a high pressure circulation.

Clinical Features

- Patient gives h/o of blood-streaking of sputum or frank hemoptysis.
- Patient is usually anxious.
- Massive hemoptysis may have signs of hemodynamic compromise such as tachycardia, hypotension and cold peripheries.
- Symptoms and signs of underlying disease causing hemoptysis may be present.

Differential Diagnosis of Hemoptysis based on Associated Signs/Symptoms

See **Table 2.12**.

Investigations

- Chest X-ray should be done in all cases and may show underlying pathology.
- Hemoglobin, PCV, complete blood count, including platelet count, renal function tests, urinalysis, and coagulation studies should be done.
- Sputum culture, acid-fast bacilli (AFB) stain → If infection or TB is suspected.
- High-resolution CT can diagnose unsuspected bronchiectasis and arteriovenous malformations and can also show central endobronchial lesions in many cases.
- Bronchoscopy can be done if the cause of hemoptysis is not evident from noninvasive tests.
- D-dimer, CT pulmonary angiography → If pulmonary embolism is suspected.

Management

- The cause of hemoptysis needs to be identified and treated.
- Life-threatening hemoptysis is a medical emergency. Attention should be given to airway, breathing, and circulation (ABCs). Patient should be placed in the lateral decubitus position with the involved lung dependent so that the blood does not enter the other lung.
- Volume expansion by using IV fluids or blood transfusion is required to maintain blood circulation.
- Cough suppressants such as codeine syrup and mild sedation (with benzodiazepines) are helpful.
- Nebulized adrenaline can cause pulmonary vasoconstriction and reduce hemoptysis.
- Oral tranexamic acid (500 mg tds).
- Uncontrollable hemoptysis needs rigid bronchoscopy and specific intervention. Angiography and embolization of the involved bronchial arteries is another option.
- Lung resection should be considered if the bleeding site is localized and not responding to any of the above measures.

TABLE 2.12: Differential diagnosis of hemoptysis based on associated signs/symptoms

Associated signs/symptoms (Clinical clues)	Possibility
Chronic cough, evening rise of temperature, wight loss, night sweats	TB
Massive hemoptysis without severe coughing	Pulmonary cavity and tumors
Repeated expectoration of 2–3 ml of blood in a chronic smoker with weight loss and clubbing	Bronchogenic carcinoma
Recent onset of cough, wheeze and purulent blood-streaked hemoptysis	Acute bronchitis
Recurrent episodes of hemoptysis over many years with purulent sputum, clubbing, coarse leathery crepitations	Bronchiectasis
High-grade fever, chills, rigors and sputum with hemoptysis	Pneumonia
Acute onset of dyspnea with chest pain and hemoptysis especially with predisposing factors such as recent immobilization, major surgery, or long travel	Pulmonary embolism Acute heart failure may also have such a presentation
Anticoagulant use	Coagulopathy causing hemoptysis
Ho orthopnea, PND, heart disease (RHD, MI), fine bibasal crepitations	Mitral valve disease or LVF causing hemoptysis
Recurrent hemoptysis during menses (catamenial hemoptysis)	Endometriosis of lungs
Skin lesions (purpura, ulcers)	Conditions like granulomatosis with polyangiitis (Wegener's) or Goodpasture's syndrome can cause hemoptysis, often associated with systemic vasculitic findings like purpura or ulcers

Q. How do you differentiate hemoptysis from hematemesis?

See **Table 2.13**.

Q. Describe the etiology, clinical features and treatment of acute rhinitis (common cold, acute coryza).

- Acute rhinitis is the inflammation of the nasal mucosa, most commonly caused by viral infections. It is a self-limiting condition characterized by nasal congestion, sneezing, rhinorrhea (runny nose), and mild systemic symptoms.

Etiology

- Rhinoviruses, coronaviruses, influenza and para-influenza viruses, respiratory syncytial virus (RSV), etc.
- Rhinoviruses are the most common cause.

Epidemiology

- It is more common in children and incidence decreases with advancing age.
- Common cold is a major cause of absenteeism from school and the workplace. There is no evidence that exposure to cold temperatures, fatigue, or sleep deprivation causes increased incidence of common cold.

Transmission

- Common cold viruses spread by direct contact and through respiratory droplets.

Clinical Features

- The incubation period for most common cold viruses is 24–72 hours.
- Sneezing, nasal congestion with rhinorrhea, mild malaise, photophobia and watering of eyes. Secondary infection causes the discharge to turn mucopurulent. Nasal obstruction which usually alternates. Dry cough may be noted due to post nasal discharge.
- Examination shows congested nasal mucosa with secretions.

Treatment

- Treatment is mainly symptomatic.
- Antihistamines like cetirizine, loratidine, etc. can be used to decrease nasal discharge.
- Topical decongestants (oxymetazoline, pseudo-ephedrine) may be useful to decrease nasal blockage.
- Antipyretics (paracetamol) can be used for headache and bodyache.
- Vitamin C supplementation may help in decreasing the severity of attack.

Complications

- Sinusitis
- Lower respiratory tract disease—pneumonia, acute bronchitis.
- Exacerbation of congestive heart failure, COPD, and asthma attacks.
- Otitis media.

Q. Acute bronchitis.

- Acute bronchitis is inflammation of medium sized airways.
- It is typically caused by viral infections, leading to cough, mucus production, and transient airway inflammation. It is a self-limiting condition that usually lasts 1–3 weeks.

Etiology

- *Viral causes:* It is usually due to viral infections, such as adenovirus, coronavirus, rhinovirus, influenza virus, respiratory syncytial virus, and parainfluenza viruses.
- *Bacterial causes*: Atypical infections with *Mycoplasma pneumonia, Chlamydia pneumonia* and *Chlamydia psittaci*

TABLE 2.13: Differences between hemoptysis and hematemesis

	Hemoptysis	Hematemesis
What it means	Coughing out of blood	Vomiting of blood
Source of blood	Lower respiratory tract (trachea, bronchi, or alveoli)	GI tract (esophagus, stomach, or upper small intestine)
Appearance of blood	Bright red in color, frothy due to mixing with air and surfactant and mixed with sputum or mucus	Dark brown (coffee ground appearance due to acid hematin formation). Not frothy. May be mixed with food particles or gastric contents
Associated symptoms	Coughing is the predominant symptom, along with shortness of breath, chest pain, or other respiratory symptoms	Nausea and vomiting are the key symptoms. Other symptoms are abdominal pain, epigastric pain, and melena
pH	Alkaline	Acidic
Presence of hemosiderin-laden macrophages	Yes. Macrophages come from alveoli	No
H/o melena	Absent	May be present
H/o preexisting disease	Cardiopulmonary disease	Gastrointestinal disease
Diagnosis	Chest X-ray, CT, bronchoscopy	Endoscopy, abdominal imaging

can rarely present as acute bronchitis. Secondary bacterial infection with *Strep. pneumoniae* and *H. influenzae* can occur in viral bronchitis.

- *Environmental and irritant causes*: Tobacco smoke exposure, pollution, dust, chemicals, or occupational irritants.

Clinical Features

- Patient c/o fever, malaise and dry cough. There can be scanty mucoid sputum which may later become mucopurulent. Dyspnea with wheezing is usually present.
- Examination shows diffuse B/L wheeze on auscultation. There may be signs of upper respiratory tract infection.

Investigations

- Chest X-ray is usually normal.
- Total leukocyte count may be high.
- Sputum Gram's stain and culture can give an idea about the infecting organism.
- COVID-19 or influenza testing, if symptoms are suggestive of these infections.

Treatment

- Antibiotics are prescribed if bacterial infection is suspected.
- Cough syrups give symptomatic relief.
- Bronchodilators may be needed if there are wheezes on auscultation.

Q. Describe the etiopathogenesis, types, clinical features, differential diagnosis and management of bronchial asthma.

- Asthma is a chronic inflammatory disease of airways characterized by increased responsiveness of the tracheobronchial tree to multiple stimuli.
- It is characterized by episodic airflow obstruction, which is reversible.
- Clinically, asthma presents as episodes of dyspnea, wheezing, and cough. In-between the episodes the person is usually normal.
- An attack of asthma may last a few minutes or hours or days. When the attack is severe lasting days or weeks, it is known as status asthmaticus.

Incidence and Prevalence

- About 10% of the world's population is affected by asthma. It can occur at any age, but commonly starts before the age of 10 years. In childhood, there is 2:1 male/female preponderance, but the sex ratio equalizes by the age of 30.

Etiology

- Asthma is a heterogeneous disease with both endogenous and environmental factors playing a role. Several risk factors have been implicated.

Risk factors involved in asthma

Endogenous factors	Environmental factors
Genetic predisposition	Indoor and outdoor allergens
Atopy	Diet
Airway hyperresponsiveness	Air pollution
Gender	Occupational sensitizers
Ethnicity (common in Europeans)	Respiratory infections
Obesity	
Early viral infections	

Endogenous Factors

- *Genetic predisposition:* The familial association of asthma and a high degree of concordance for asthma in identical twins indicate a genetic predisposition to the disease. More than 100 asthma susceptibility genes have been reported. Some of the chromosomes implicated are 5, 13, 14, and 17.
- *Atopy:* Atopy refers to genetic predisposition to develop an allergic reaction (as allergic rhinitis, asthma, or atopic dermatitis) and produce elevated levels of IgE upon exposure to an environmental antigen. Atopy is the major risk factor for asthma, and non-atopic individuals have a very low risk of developing asthma.
- *Airway hyperresponsiveness:* Airway hyperresponsiveness is due to chronic inflammation of the airways, which leads to bronchospasm and typical symptoms of wheezing, shortness of breath, and coughing after exposure to allergens, environmental irritants, viruses, cold air, or exercise.
- *Gender:* Asthma predominantly occurs in boys in childhood, with a male-to-female ratio of 2:1 until puberty. After puberty there is equal incidence.
- *Ethnicity:* Asthma is more common in industrialized western countries.
- *Obesity:* Obese individuals seem to be at higher risk of developing asthma.

Environmental Factors

- *Allergens:* Inhaled allergens are common triggers of asthma symptoms and have also been implicated in allergic sensitization. Exposure to house dust mites in early childhood is a risk factor for allergic sensitization and asthma. Domestic pets, particularly cats, have also been associated with allergic sensitization.
- *Diet:* The role of dietary factors is controversial. Observational studies have shown that diets low in antioxidants such as vitamin C and vitamin A, magnesium, selenium, and omega-3 polyunsaturated fats (fish oil) or high in sodium and omega 6 polyunsaturated fats are associated with an increased risk of asthma. Vitamin D deficiency may also predispose to the development of asthma.
- *Air pollution:* Air pollutants such as sulfur dioxide, ozone, and diesel particulates, may trigger asthma symptoms, but the role of different air pollutants in the etiology of the disease is less certain.
- *Occupational sensitizers:* Exposure to chemicals such as toluene diisocyanate and trimellitic anhydride,

may lead to sensitization independent of atopy. Individuals may also be exposed to allergens in the workplace such as small animal allergens in laboratory workers and fungal amylase in wheat flour in bakers.

- *Respiratory infections:* Though many vial illnesses (rhinovirus, respiratory syncytial virus) have been known to trigger asthma attack, their role in etiology is uncertain. Many patients with asthma have coexistent sinusitis.

Pathogenesis (Fig. 2.9)

- Basically, asthmatics have bronchial hyperresponsiveness compared to normal people. Hence, stimuli that normally produce no clinical response can produce clinical symptoms in asthmatics.
- Bronchial hyperresponsiveness is due to persistent subacute inflammation of the airways. The airways are edematous and infiltrated with eosinophils, neutrophils, and lymphocytes. Glandular hypertrophy and denudation of the epithelium is usually present. The inflammatory cells present in airways release mediators on provocation which produce bronchoconstriction, vascular congestion, edema formation, increased mucus production, and impaired mucociliary transport.
- Triggers include allergens like pollen, house-dust, mite, drugs like NSAIDs, exercise, inhalation of cold air, infections of the respiratory tract, air pollution, cigarette smoke, strong scents and perfumes, etc.
- Inhalation of allergens by atopic asthmatic individuals leads to the development of two types of responses. Early response, where bronchoconstriction occurs within 10–15 minutes of exposure to an allergen. This type of response usually subsides in one hour. This response is mediated by mast cells in the lumen of the airways, where they interact with inhaled allergens through surface-bound IgE molecules. Histamine and leukotriens released from mast cells mediate bronchoconstriction. The early response is reversed by bronchodilator therapy and can be prevented by prior treatment with a mast cell stabilizer such as sodium cromoglycate.
- In some individuals, the early response is followed by a later phase of bronchoconstriction which begins 4–6 hours after exposure to the allergen and can persist for 8–12 hours or longer. The late reaction responds poorly to bronchodilators, but responds to steroids. This late response is mediated by neutrophils, eosinophils and macrophages. These cells contain large quantities of powerful mediators like leukotrienes, platelet activating factor and eosinophilic major basic protein. All these mediators cause an inflammatory reaction responsible for late-phase asthmatic reaction and airway hyper-responsiveness.

Types

- Asthma can be classified into two types, extrinsic and intrinsic asthma **(Table 2.14)**.

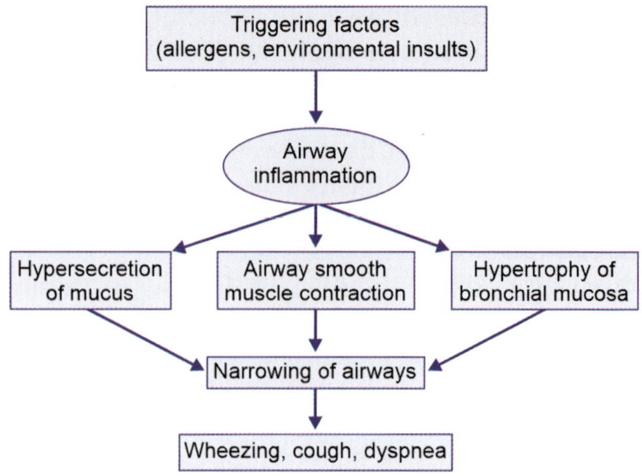

Figure 2.9: Pathogenesis of asthma

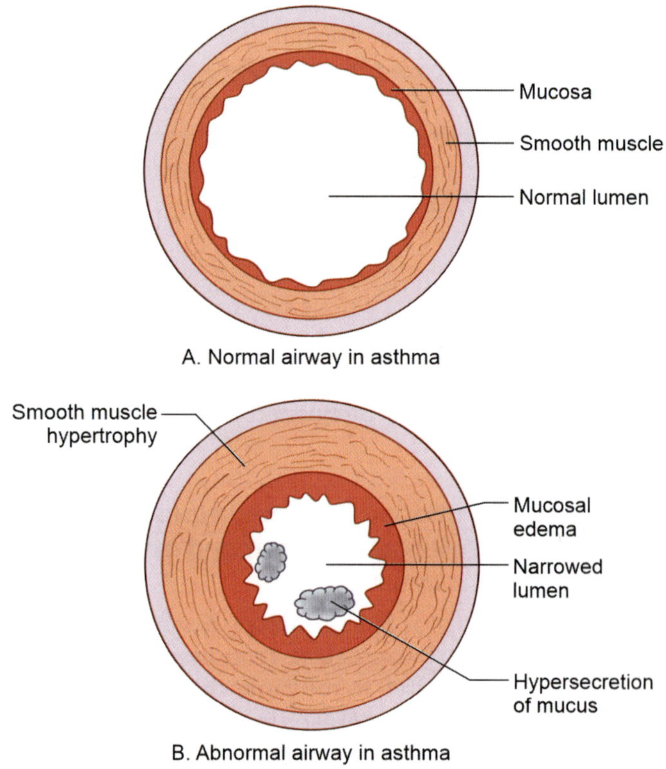

Figure 2.10: Pathology in asthma

TABLE 2.14: Classification of asthma

	Extrinsic (atopic)	Intrinsic
Etiology	Allergic	Idiopathic
Hereditary predisposition	Yes	No
Onset	Early in life	Late in life
Serum IgE levels	Elevated	Normal
Symptoms	Usually seasonal	perennial
History of allergy	Yes	No

Clinical Features

- The symptoms of asthma consist of a triad of intermittent and reversible attacks of dyspnea, cough, and wheezing. All three symptoms coexist in a typical attack of asthma. Initially patient experiences a sense of constriction in the chest, often with dry cough. Respiration becomes harsh, expiration becomes prolonged and wheezing is heard usually in expiratory phase but can be heard in both phases of respiration.

- Asthma usually worsens at night especially early morning. The end of an attack is usually marked by cough that produces thick, stringy mucus, which often takes the form of casts of the distal airways (Curschmann's spirals). Some patients may just present with intermittent dry cough or exertional dyspnea without any h/o wheezing. In these patients a bronchoprovocation test may be required to make the diagnosis of asthma.
- Examination shows tachypnea, tachycardia, mild systolic hypertension, hyperinflated lungs, with increase in AP diameter of the thorax. High pitched polyphonic rhonchi are heard all over the lungs bilaterally. The presence of cyanosis, severe tachypnea, pulse rate more than 120 per minute, widened pulse pressure, pulsus paradoxus and completely silent chest on auscultation are indicative of a severe airway obstruction.
- Extrapulmonary features sometimes seen are nasal polyps, pale nasal mucosa, cobblestone appearance to the posterior pharyngeal wall (due to associated rhinitis), and atopic dermatitis.

Differential Diagnosis

See **Table 2.15**.

Investigations

- Blood examination may show increased eosinophils.
- Total serum immunoglobulin E levels are frequently elevated.
- *Chest X-ray* may show hyperinflation.
- Pulmonary functions tests show a decrease in the forced vital capacity (FVC), peak expiratory flow rate (PEFR) and forced expiratory volume in one second (FEV_1). The FEV_1/FVC ratio is usually less than 70%. The diagnosis of asthma is established

TABLE 2.15: Differential diagnosis of asthma

Upper airway diseases ***Vocal cord paralysis, vocal cord dysfunction syndrome, laryngeal edema, tracheal narrowing***	• Typically present with stridor • Respiratory sound is more over the trachea. • Absence of diffuse rhonchi over both lung fields • Indirect laryngoscopy or bronchoscopy is diagnostic.
Allergic bronchopulmonary aspergillosis (ABPA)	• ABPA occurs in patients with asthma or with cystic fibrosis. • Immediate skin test reactivity to *Aspergillus antigens* • Serum antibodies to *A. fumigatus* positive • Peripheral blood eosinophilia • Lung infiltrates on chest X-ray
Cystic fibrosis	• Onset in childhood • Multisystem involvement • Sweat chloride test diagnostic
Endobronchial disease such as foreign-body aspiration, neoplasm, or bronchial stenosis	All these conditions usually produce localized rhonchi unlike asthma which produces bilateral diffuse rhonchi.
Acute left ventricular failure (cardiac asthma)	• There is usually S3 and S4. • Bilateral basal lung crepitations may be heard.
Carcinoid tumors	• Usually associated with stridor • Recurrent episodes of bronchospasm can occur.
Recurrent pulmonary emboli	• Risk factors for embolism present such as DVT • Pulmonary HTN may be present. • Definitive diagnosis requires chest CT or pulmonary angiography.
COPD	• Patient is usually a chronic smoker. • No true symptom-free periods • History of chronic cough and sputum production present • Progressive worsening of dyspnea
Eosinophilic pneumonias	• Fever and cough present • High eosinophil count in the blood • Chest X-ray shows bilateral diffuse opacities
Systemic vasculitis *(Churg-Strauss syndrome)*	• Multisystem involvement • Hemoptysis may be present.
Psychiatric disorders *(conversion reactions and laryngeal spasm)*	• Wheezing more on inspiration. Sound localized to trachea. Lung fields clear • Stressors present before the attack • Usually young women

by demonstrating reversible airway obstruction. Reversibility is traditionally defined as a ≥15% increase in FEV_1 after two puffs of a β_2-adrenergic agonist. Serial recordings of FEV_1 or peak expiratory flow rate (PEFR) can give an idea about the response to treatment.

- Methacholine/histamine challenge test: assesses the airway hyperresponsiveness. It is useful when spirometry findings are normal or near normal, especially in patients with intermittent or exercise-induced asthma symptoms. The patient breathes in nebulized methacholine or histamine. Both drugs provoke bronchoconstriction and the level of airflow obstruction is documented by spirometry. However, this test is not routinely done in clinical practice.
- Arterial blood gas analysis shows respiratory alkalosis and in severe attacks hypoxia. However in respiratory failure CO_2 retention causes respiratory acidosis. A rising CO_2 even in the normal range is a bad prognostic sign and indicates impending respiratory failure.
- Skin prick tests are done to identify the allergen in case of allergic or atopic asthma.

Treatment

Goals of Asthma Treatment

- Achieve and maintain control of asthma symptoms.
- Maintain normal activity levels, including exercise.
- Maintain pulmonary function as close to normal as possible.
- Prevent asthma exacerbations.
- Avoid adverse effects from asthma medications.
- Prevent asthma mortality.

Controlling Trigger Factors

- Avoidance of asthma "triggers" is important in successful asthma management. It will prevent frequent attacks and also the requirement of medications. Common asthma triggers include: allergens, respiratory infections, inhaled irritants such as tobacco smoke and air pollutants, exposure to cold air, emotional stress and gastroesophageal reflux disease. Drugs such as betablockers and NSAIDs can precipitate an attack and should be avoided.

Drug Treatment

- Drugs used in the treatment of asthma can be divided into two categories.
- First category is drugs that relax the smooth-muscle (called "quick relief medications"). Quick relief medicines are used to treat an acute attack. They can be used as and when required basis. These include β-adrenergic agonists, methylxanthines, and anticholinergics.
- Second category is drugs that prevent and/or reverse inflammation (called "long-term control medications"). These medicines prevent or decrease the attacks of asthma. Usually they are used on a regular basis. These include inhaled glucocorticoids, long-acting β_2-agonists, mast cell–stabilizers, and leukotriene modifiers.

Quick Relief Medications

See **Table 2.16.**

Long-term Control Medications

- These medicines prevent or decrease the number of attacks by preventing or reversing airway inflammation **(Table 2.17)**.

TABLE 2.16: Quick relief medications

Drug category	Mechanism of action	Side effects
Adrenergic stimulants Salbutamol, levosalbutamol, terbutaline, adrenaline, salmeterol, formoterol	They are first line therapy in acute attack. They act through adrenergic β_2 receptors which mediate smooth muscle relaxation. They can be given orally or by inhalation or by nebulization. Adrenaline and terbutaline can be given parenterally also. Salmeterol is long acting and should not be used to treat acute attacks. It is particularly helpful in nocturnal and exercise-induced asthma.	Tremors, tachycardia, and hypokalemia
Methylxanthines Theophylline, doxofylline, acebrophylline	They are considered second-line therapy. They act by inhibiting phosphodiesterase enzyme. They are usually used along with β_2 agonists in acute attacks. However, there is minimal evidence for additional benefit when used with optimal doses of β-agonists.	Nervousness, nausea, vomiting, anorexia, and headache. High levels can cause seizures and cardiac arrhythmias.
Anticholinergics Ipratropium bromide Tiotropium bromide	They have only modest efficacy. They are slow to act (60–90 minutes may be required for peak effect). They are particularly helpful in patients with heart disease, in whom the use of methylxanthines and β-adrenergic stimulants may be dangerous.	Blurred vision, urinary retention and cardiac arrhythmias

TABLE 2.17: Long-term control medications

Drug category	Mechanism of action	Side effects
Inhaled glucocorticoids Beclomethasone Budesonide Flunisolide Fluticasone Triamcinolone	Decrease airway inflammation. Since the drug is directly delivered to lungs, they have less systemic side effects and less pituitary adrenal suppression.	Oral thrush and dysphonia, cataract formation, decreased growth in children, interference with bone metabolism. Rarely pituitary adrenal suppression
Systemic glucocorticoids Hydrocortisone Prednisolone Dexamethasone	Decrease airway inflammation. Especially useful in acute severe attack of asthma but remember that they are not quick relief medications.	Pituitary adrenal suppression. May predispose to infections, cataract formation, decreased growth in children, interference with bone metabolism, and purpura
Long-acting β_2-agonists Salmeterol Formoterol	Relaxation of bronchial smooth muscle for a long time	Major side effect is tremors, tachycardia, and hypokalemia.
Mast cell stabilizers Cromolyn Nedocromil	They inhibit the degranulation of mast cells thus preventing the release of mediators	
Leukotriene modifiers Montelukast Zafirlukast Zileuton	Inhibit the synthesis of leukotrienes which mediate airway inflammation	Zileuton can cause elevations in aminotransferase levels. May predispose to the development of Churg-Strauss syndrome
Anti-IgE antibody Omalizumab	Omalizumab is a blocking antibody that neutralizes circulating IgE and inhibits IgE-mediated reactions. It reduces the number of exacerbations in patients with severe asthma. It should be used when all other medications fail to control asthma. However, it is very expensive and has to be injected subcutaneously.	Headache, upper respiratory tract infections, injection site pain, anaphylaxis
Thromboxane A_2/prostaglandin receptor antagonist Seratrodast	Seratrodast blocks the broncho-constrictor effects of prostaglandins and also decreases the inflammation by antagonising the thromboxane A_2 receptor	Drowsiness, headache, palpitations, and hepatitis

Stepwise Treatment of Asthma

- Asthma management follows a stepwise approach, adjusting treatment intensity based on the severity of symptoms and the level of control achieved. This method ensures personalized care, aiming to maintain optimal asthma control with the least amount of medication necessary **(Fig. 2.11 and Table 2.18)**.

Key Principles

- *Regular assessment*: Monitor symptoms and lung function to determine the current level of asthma control.
- *Step up/step down therapy*: Increase treatment ("step up") when asthma is not well-controlled; decrease treatment ("step down") when control is sustained for at least three months to minimize medication use.

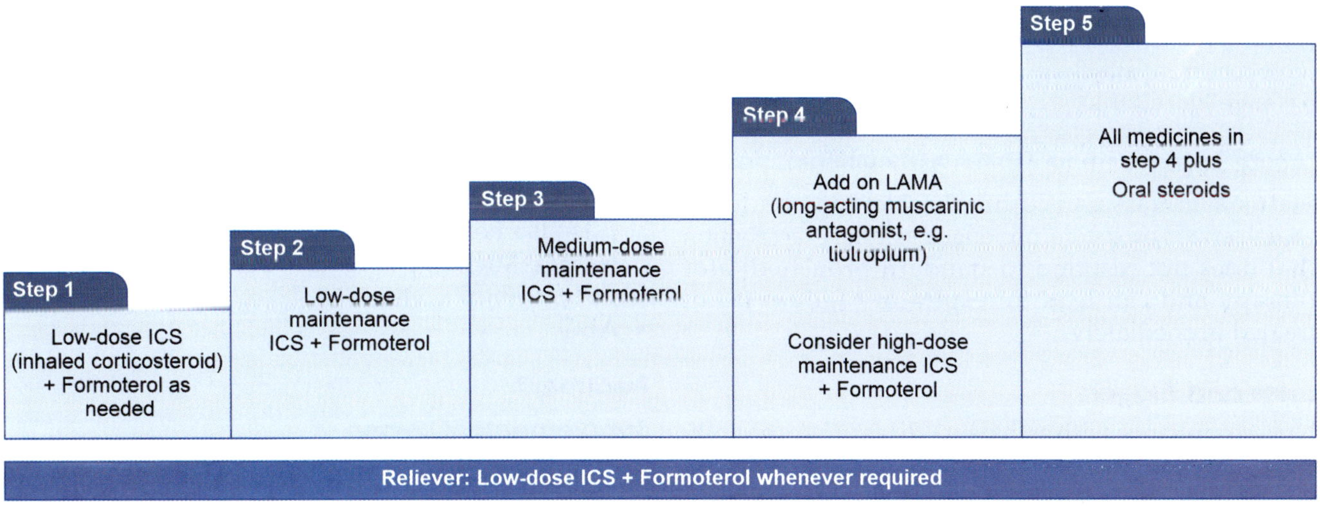

Figure 2.11: Stepwise treatment of asthma

TABLE 2.18: Stepwise treatment of asthma

Severity of asthma	Stepwise treatment
Infrequent asthma symptoms (for example, 1–2 days/week or less)	Step 1: The recommended treatment is low-dose inhaled corticosteroid (ICS) plus long-acting beta-2 agonist (LABA). Example, ICS (budesonide) plus formoterol taken whenever needed to relieve asthma. Symptoms: Studies have shown that ICS plus LABA is better than SABA alone (short-acting beta-2 agonist, example salbutamol) and also better than ICS plus SABA.
Asthma symptoms less than 3–5 days/week, with normal or mildly reduced lung function	Step 2: Patients take combination ICS-formoterol as daily maintenance treatment, and also take extra doses of the same medication whenever they have asthma symptoms. This is called "maintenance-and-reliever therapy".
Asthma symptoms most days, waking due to asthma once a week or more, or low lung function	Step 3: Patients take medium dose combination ICS-formoterol as daily maintenance treatment, and also take extra doses of the same medication whenever they have asthma symptoms.
Daily asthma symptoms, waking at night with asthma once a week or more, with low lung function, or current smokers	Step 4: High dose combination ICS-formoterol as daily maintenance treatment, and also take extra doses of the same medication whenever they have asthma symptoms. Additionally, LAMA (long-acting muscarinic antagonist, e.g. tiotropium) is added.
During acute asthma exacerbation	Treat acute exacerbations PLUS Step 5: In addition to all the medicines in step 5, addition of oral steroids are considered.

- Good control of asthma is indicated by all of the following:
  - Daytime symptoms ≤2 days per week
  - No limitation of activities
  - No symptoms during night or on waking
- Poor control of asthma is indicated by three or more of following:
  - Daytime symptoms >2 days per week
  - Any limitation of activities
  - Any symptoms during night or on waking.

Prevention of Asthma Attacks

- Avoid triggers (allergens, smoke, cold air, strong odors, pollution).
- Regular use of controller medications (ICS/LABA for persistent asthma).
- Annual influenza and pneumococcal vaccinations.
- Peak flow monitoring (for early detection of worsening asthma).

Prognosis

- Asthma is a chronic relapsing disorder. Most patients have recurrent attacks but there is no progressive lung damage like COPD.

Q. Acute severe asthma (status asthmaticus).

- Status asthmaticus is a life-threatening condition characterized by severe, prolonged asthma exacerbation that does not respond to standard bronchodilator therapy and can lead to respiratory failure if not treated immediately.

Causes and Triggers

- Non-compliance with asthma medications (especially ICS).
- Severe allergen exposure (dust, pollen, pet dander).
- Respiratory infections (viral/bacterial).
- Cold air, exercise, stress, strong odors.
- Medications (NSAIDs, β-blockers).
- Smoking, air pollution.

Clinical Features

- Patient appears severely breathless and unable to speak full sentences.
- Patient may be restless or drowsy due to hypoxia and hypercarbia.
- Use of accessory muscles (sternocleidomastoid, intercostals).
- There may be cyanosis and paradoxical pulse (>20 mm Hg drop in BP during inspiration).
- Respiratory rate is usually >30 per minute, and pulse is usually >120 beats/min.
- Wheezing is prominent. A silent chest on auscultation suggests that there is no air movement in and out of lungs due to severe airway obstruction and is a sign of impending respiratory failure.

Investigations

- Peak expiratory flow rate (PEFR): <50% predicted (severe obstruction).
- Pulse oximetry: SpO_2 <92% (suggests hypoxia).
- ECG to rule out MI with pulmonary edema which can also present with dyspnea and wheezing.
- Chest X-ray is usually normal except hyperinflation. It is also helpful to rule out other causes of breathlessness such as pulmonary edema, pneumonia, and pneumothorax, etc.
- ABG.

Treatment

Supplemental Oxygen

- Should be given to maintain a SPO_2 >90% or a PaO_2 >60 mm Hg. Venturi masks can deliver oxygen better than nasal prongs.

Bronchodilators

- Frequent administration of a short acting β_2-agonist (SABA) through nebulization is the most important measure. Nebulizations are repeated as necessary till the patient feels better. Inhalers also can be used if the patient can take it. At least three nebulizer treatments should be given in the first hour. Thereafter, the frequency of nebulization can be based on patient response and improvement.
- Administration of anticholinergic bronchodilators such as ipratropium bromide is also helpful.
- IV aminophylline infusion is rarely used now because of side effects.

Systemic Corticosteroids

- Corticosteroids should be given by intravenous route.
- Methyl prednisolone should be given at a dose of 40–60 mg every 6 hours for 2 days or until the FEV_1 (or PEFR) returns to 50% of predicted (or 50% of baseline) and then slowly tapered off.
- An equivalent dose of any other steroid (e.g. hydrocortisone 200 mg IV stat and 8th hourly or dexamethasone) can also be used.

Magnesium Sulfate

- Intravenous magnesium sulphate (2 g infused over 20 min) may be considered in patients not responding to above therapies. It relaxes bronchial smooth muscle by inhibiting calcium influx.

Mechanical Ventilation

- May be required in respiratory failure or impending respiratory failure. Signs of respiratory failure are as follows:
  - Rising $PaCO_2$, decreasing pH (respiratory acidosis).
  - Severe hypoxia despite O_2 therapy.
  - Altered mental status, exhaustion.
  - Silent chest, bradycardia, hypotension.

Antibiotics

- Are indicated if there is evidence of infection.
- Sedatives are contraindicated during an acute attack unless the patient is intubated.

Q. Chronic obstructive pulmonary disease (COPD).

- Chronic obstructive pulmonary disease (COPD) is a progressive lung disease characterized by persistent respiratory symptoms and airflow limitation due to airway and/or alveolar abnormalities.
- It is usually caused by significant exposure to noxious particles or gases most commonly cigarette smoke.
- COPD includes:
  - ***Chronic bronchitis:*** is a condition characterized by chronic cough, sputum production and airway narrowing. It is defined as a chronic productive cough for at least three months in each of two successive years, in a patient in whom other causes of chronic cough (e.g. bronchiectasis) have been excluded.
  - ***Emphysema:*** is a condition characterized by destruction of alveolar walls and enlargement of the alveoli.
- Chronic bronchitis is a clinical diagnosis whereas emphysema is a pathological diagnosis which requires biopsy to confirm the diagnosis which is not routinely done.

Epidemiology

- COPD occurs all over the world and is a public health problem. Its incidence is expected to increase further.
- In India COPD is the commonest lung disorder following pulmonary tuberculosis.
- It affects men more commonly than women probably due to smoking habits. But the prevalence is also increasing in women due to increasing smoking habits among them also.
- There is higher prevalence with increasing age probably due to cumulative lung injury

Risk Factors

- ***Smoking:*** Cigarette smoking is a major risk factor. 95% of cases are smoking-related, typically >20 pack years (1 pack year is 20 cigarettes smoked per day for 1 year). There is less evidence for cigar and pipe smoking probably due to lower dose of inhaled tobacco by-products. Passive (secondhand) smoking is also a risk factor for COPD.
- ***Airway hyperresponsiveness:*** patients with increased airway responsiveness are more likely to develop COPD.
- ***Occupational exposures:*** Several occupational exposures, like coal mining, gold mining, cotton textile dust, etc. are all risk factors for development of COPD. But their effect is less than cigarette smoking.
- ***Air pollution:*** is thought to increase the risk of developing COPD.
- ***Genetic factors:*** also play an important role, e.g. α_1 antitrypsin (α_1AT) deficiency predisposes to the development of COPD.

Pathology

- In COPD, all three components of lungs are affected, i.e. airways, lung parenchyma, and lung vasculature.

Changes in Airways

- **Chronic inflammation:** Increased neutrophils, macrophages, and CD8+ T lymphocytes release inflammatory mediators (e.g. IL-8, TNF-α, leukotrienes). Leads to airway inflammation and airway obstruction.
- **Increased number of goblet cells and submucosal gland hypertrophy:** Lead to mucus hypersecretion → mucus plugging and airway obstruction. Excessive mucus production also contributes to chronic cough and sputum. The Reid index, which indicates the ratio of thickness of the submucosal glands to that of the bronchial wall, is thus increased.

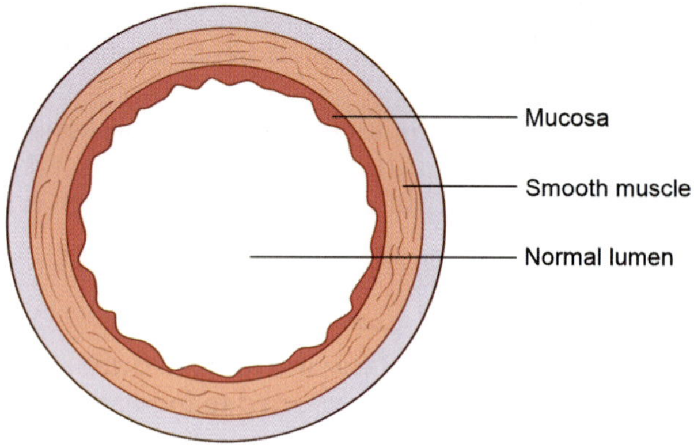

Figure 2.12: Normal airway

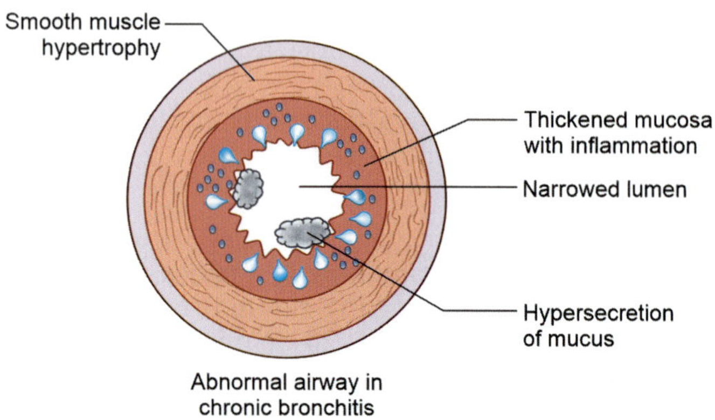

Figure 2.13: Airway changes in chronic bronchitis

- **Airway remodeling:** Fibrosis and thickening of the bronchial walls. Smooth muscle hypertrophy leading to increased airway resistance. There may be squamous metaplasia of mucous membrane which predisposes to cancer development and also impairs mucociliary clearance.
- All these changes produce airway obstruction and also predispose to recurrent infections which in turn may perpetuate airway inflammation.

Changes in Lung Parenchyma

- There is destruction of gas-exchanging air spaces distal to terminal bronchiole, i.e. the respiratory bronchioles, alveolar ducts, alveolar sacs, and alveoli (all these are together called acinus) leading to emphysema. Emphysema is classified into three pathologic types, **proximal acinar** (also known as centriacinar), **panacinar, and distal acinar**. Centrilobular emphysema is associated with cigarette smoking. It is characterized by abnormal dilation or destruction of the respiratory bronchiole, the central portion of the acinus (remember "C" for cigarettes). Panacinar emphysema is characterized by enlargement or destruction of all parts of the acinus. Panacinar emphysema is usually seen in patients with alpha-1 antitrypsin deficiency, and often affects lower lobes. In distal acinar (also known as paraseptal) emphysema, the alveolar ducts are predominantly affected. Distal acinar emphysema may occur alone or in combination with proximal acinar and panacinar emphysema **(Figs 2.14 and 2.15)**.

Changes in the Pulmonary Vasculature

- Include intimal hyperplasia and smooth muscle hypertrophy/hyperplasia due to hypoxic vasoconstriction of the small pulmonary arteries. Destruction of alveoli due to emphysema can lead to loss of the associated areas of the pulmonary capillary. All these changes lead to pulmonary hypertension. Pulmonary hypertension can lead to cor-pulmonale.

Clinical Features

- Three most common symptoms of COPD are chronic cough, sputum production, and dyspnea. The duration of these symptoms is usually months to years. The most common early symptom is exertional dyspnea. Less common symptoms include wheezing and chest tightness. Onset of these symptoms is gradual. As COPD advances, dyspnea worsens and

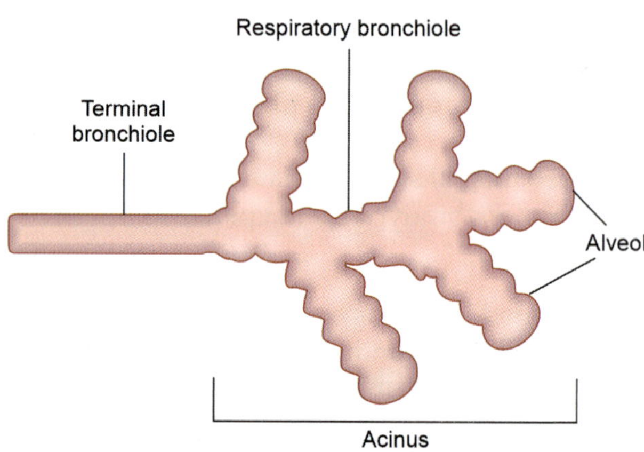

Figure 2.14: Normal acinus

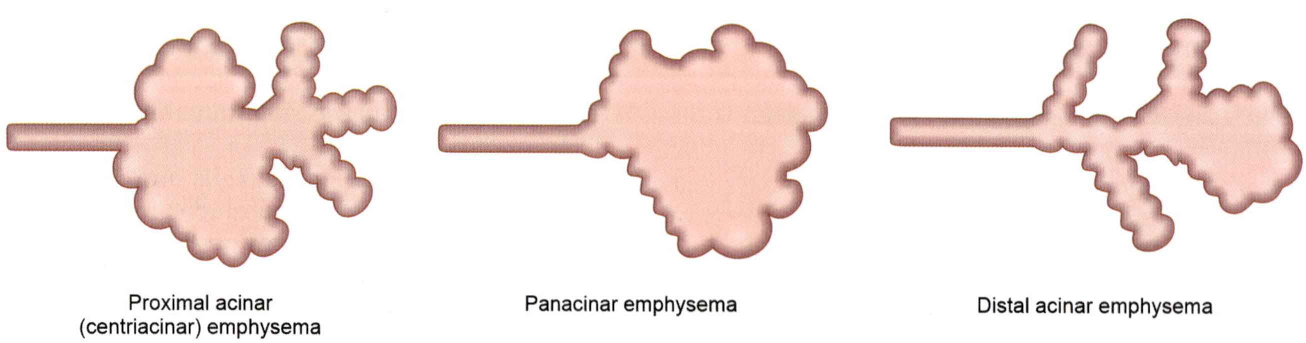

Figure 2.15: Various types of emphysema

in the most advanced stage, patients are breathless doing routine activities or even at rest.

- Episodes of exacerbations occur precipitated usually by upper or lower respiratory tract infections.
- Examination may be normal in early stages of COPD. There may be signs of smoking, like odor of smoke, tobacco staining of teeth or nicotine staining of fingernails. Clubbing is usually not seen in COPD, and if it is present other causes should be searched. Development of lung cancer is the most likely cause of newly developed clubbing in COPD patients.
- Patients with severe COPD may have cyanosis. Accessory muscles of respiration may be active, and patient sits in a characteristic "tripod" position to facilitate the actions of accessory muscles. In patients with severe COPD, expiration is prolonged and there is usually expiratory wheezing. Signs of hyperinflation of lungs are present and include a barrel shaped chest, pushed down diaphragm, and obliteration of cardiac dullness. Tidal percussion reveals decreased movement of diaphragm as it is already pushed down.
- Patients with predominant emphysema are referred to as "pink puffers," due to lack of cyanosis and pursed-lip breathing. Patients with chronic bronchitis are called "blue bloaters," due to presence of cyanosis and fluid retention. Usually, patients have features of both and cannot be simply classified.
- Patients with advanced COPD have wasting and loss of subcutaneous fat. Such wasting is a poor prognostic sign in COPD.
- In advanced COPD patient may develop pulmonary HTN and right heart failure, called cor-pulmonale. Such patients present with peripheral edema, raised JVP, congestive hepatomegaly, and ascites.

Differences between Chronic Bronchitis and Emphysema (Table 2.19)

TABLE 2.19: Differences between chronic bronchitis and emphysema

Feature	Chronic bronchitis	Emphysema
Main pathology	Airway inflammation	Destruction of alveolar walls
Main symptom	Cough	Breathlessness
Clinical appearance	Blue bloater	Pink puffer
Sputum production	Copious	Scanty
Cor pulmonale	Common	Only in advanced stage
Respiratory insufficiency	Repeated episodes	Only in advanced stage
Arterial blood gases	Abnormality early in the course of disease	Abnormality only in advanced stage

Investigations

- Spirometry (gold standard for diagnosis): The hallmark of COPD is airflow obstruction. Pulmonary function testing shows reduction in FEV_1, FVC, and FEV_1/FVC (a decreased ratio <0.70) s diagnostic of airflow obstruction. Post-bronchodilator spirometry shows lack of significant improvement in FEV_1 after administering a bronchodilator suggestive of irreversible or only partially reversible airflow obstruction.
- DLCO (diffusibility of carbon monoxide across alveolar membrane) may be reduced in emphysema reflecting destruction of alveolar walls.
- Arterial blood gas analysis (ABG) or SpO_2 may show resting or exertional hypoxemia and hypercapnia (elevated CO_2 levels).
- ECG may show evidence of right ventricular hypertrophy.
- Echocardiography: To assess for pulmonary hypertension and cor pulmonale.
- Chest X-ray may show bullae, flattening of the diaphragm and hyperlucency in emphysema. On lateral film, large retrosternal air space and localized emphysematous bullae may also be seen in emphysema. Increased bronchovascular markings may be seen in chronic bronchitis.
- High-resolution computed tomography (HRCT): Provides detailed visualization of emphysema and airway changes. Helps in distinguishing between different types of emphysema (e.g. centrilobular *vs.* panacinar).
- Hematocrit may be high due polycythemia due to chronic hypoxemia.
- If the patient is less than ≤50 years, with a strong family history, and with a minimal smoking history, serum level of alpha-1 antitrypsin (α_1AT) should be checked.

Treatment

- The treatment of COPD focuses on relieving symptoms, slowing disease progression, preventing exacerbations, and improving quality of life.
- Only smoking cessation and oxygen therapy have been shown to alter the course of COPD. All other treatments are aimed at improving symptoms and decreasing the frequency of exacerbations.

Smoking Cessation

- All patients with COPD should be strongly urged to quit smoking. Combining pharmacotherapy with traditional supportive approaches increases the chances of smoking cessation. Two drugs, bupropion, and nicotine are helpful in this regard. Nicotine is available as gum, transdermal patches, inhaler, and nasal spray. All patients should be offered pharmacotherapy, in the absence of any contraindication to treatment.

Bronchodilators

- These drugs provide symptomatic relief. These include β_2 agonists (such as salbutamol, formoterol, salmeterol), theophylline, ipratopium bromide, etc. Inhaled route is preferred as the incidence of side effects are less. In acute exacerbations these are given through nebulization **(Table 2.20)**.
- LABA + LAMA combination therapy is preferred for moderate to severe COPD.

TABLE 2.20: Bronchodilators

Class	Example	Mechanism	Use
Short-acting beta$_2$ agonists (SABA)	**Salbutamol (albuterol), terbutaline**	Bronchodilation via β_2 receptor activation	Rescue therapy
Short-acting muscarinic antagonists (SAMA)	**Ipratropium bromide**	Blocks M_3 receptors, reducing bronchoconstriction	Rescue therapy
Long-acting beta$_2$ agonists (LABA)	**Salmeterol, formoterol, indacaterol**	Long-term bronchodilation	Maintenance
Long-acting muscarinic antagonists (LAMA)	**Tiotropium, aclidinium, umeclidinium**	Prolonged M_3 receptor blockade	Maintenance

Glucocorticoids

- Inhaled glucocorticoids reduce the frequency of exacerbations. Side effects are oropharyngeal candidiasis and osteoporosis. A trial of inhaled glucocorticoids should be considered in patients with frequent exacerbations defined as two or more per year. Examples: Budesonide, fluticasone. Inhaled corticosteroids are best used in combination with LABA (e.g. Budesonide + Formoterol).
- Oral glucocorticoids can be used during exacerbations but long-term use of oral glucocorticoids is not recommended because of more side effects than benefits.

Phosphodiesterase 4 inhibitor

- Roflumilast has been shown to reduce exacerbation frequency in patients who have moderate or severe COPD in spite of taking all the above medications.

Oxygen Therapy

- Supplemental oxygen for patients with resting hypoxemia is the only therapy which decreases mortality and improves quality of life in patients with COPD. Oxygen can be given during day or at night at home (home oxygen therapy). Using it for 12 hours or more has been shown to provide significant benefit.

Mechanical Ventilatory Support

- This is required in COPD with respiratory failure as happens during exacerbations and advanced stages. Noninvasive positive pressure ventilation (NIPPV) can be given through a tight-fitting mask without tracheal intubation. Contraindications to NIPPV include hypotension, altered mental status or inability to cooperate, copious secretions or the inability to clear secretions, craniofacial abnormalities or trauma, extreme obesity, and significant burns in the head and neck region. Invasive mechanical ventilation via an endotracheal tube is indicated for patients in respiratory failure who are not candidates for NIPPV.

Surgery for COPD

- Lung volume reduction surgery can produce symptomatic and functional improvements in patients with advanced diffuse emphysema and lung hyperinflation.
- Bullectomy can be considered when a single large emphysematous bulla occupies at least 30–50% of the hemithorax.
- Lung transplantation can be an option for advanced COPD in younger patients with severe disability.

Other Measures

- Intravenous α-1 antitrypsin can be used in patients with deficiency.
- All COPD patients should receive the **influenza and pneumococcal vaccine** since *H. influenza* and Pneomococcus are the causes of frequent infective exacerbations.
- Pulmonary rehabilitation: Graded aerobic physical exercise programs improve patients' ability to carry out daily activities. Training of inspiratory muscles by inspiring against progressively larger resistive loads reduces dyspnea and improves exercise tolerance and quality of life.

Differential Diagnosis

- The most difficult disease to differentiate from COPD is asthma. Asthma typically begins early in life with episodes of dyspnea and wheezing which reverse rapidly and completely after bronchodilator therapy.
- Other differential diagnoses include cystic fibrosis, bronchiectasis, eosinophilic granuloma, lymphangioleiomyomatosis and bronchiolitis obliterans.

Prognosis

- COPD is a progressive disease. Poor prognostic factors include weight loss, presence of resting hypoxemia and the need for hospital admission for an exacerbation, especially to intensive care unit.

Q. How do you differentiate between asthma and COPD?

- Asthma and chronic obstructive pulmonary disease (COPD) are both chronic airway diseases that cause breathlessness and airflow limitation, but they have different causes, pathophysiology, clinical features, and treatment approaches **(Table 2.21)**.

Q. Asthma-COPD Overlap (ACO).

- Asthma-COPD overlap (ACO) is a clinical condition where patients exhibit features of both asthma and COPD, leading to persistent airflow limitation with both reversible (asthma-like) and irreversible (COPD-like) components. It is not a separate disease but rather a syndrome that requires a combined approach to diagnosis and treatment.

TABLE 2.21: Differences between asthma and COPD

Feature	Asthma	COPD
Age of onset	Typically childhood or young adulthood	Usually >40 years
Cause	Allergens, environmental triggers, genetic predisposition	Smoking (main cause), air pollution, occupational exposure
Pathophysiology	Reversible bronchoconstriction, eosinophilic inflammation, increased mucus production	Irreversible airway narrowing, neutrophilic inflammation, alveolar destruction (emphysema)
Airflow limitation	Reversible with bronchodilators	Partially reversible or irreversible
Symptoms	Intermittent dyspnea, wheezing, cough, nocturnal or early morning symptoms	Chronic and progressive dyspnea, cough, sputum production
Exacerbations	Triggered by allergens, cold air, exercise, respiratory infections	Triggered by infections, air pollution, smoking
Smoking history	May be absent	Almost always present
Sputum production	Less common (except in severe cases)	Common (chronic productive cough)
Spirometry (FEV_1/FVC ratio)	Reversible airflow obstruction (improves with bronchodilator)	Irreversible airflow obstruction (FEV_1/FVC <0.70, minimal response to bronchodilator)
Peak expiratory flow variability	Significant variability (diurnal variation)	Minimal variability
Response to corticosteroids	Good response to inhaled corticosteroids (ICS)	Limited response to ICS, mainly used in severe cases
Complications	Rare, if well controlled	Pulmonary hypertension, cor pulmonale, respiratory failure
Diffusion capacity of the lung for CO_2 (DLCO)	Normal or increased (hyperinflation may increase DLCO)	Reduced, especially in emphysema due to alveolar destruction
Chest X-ray/CT scan	Usually normal	Signs of hyperinflation, flattened diaphragm, and emphysematous changes
Treatment approach	ICS (inhaled corticosteroid) + LABA (long acting beta-2 agonist) as main therapy, SABA (short acting beta-2 agonist) for quick relief	LAMA (long acting muscarinic antagonist)/ LABA as main therapy, ICS used in severe cases or frequent exacerbations

Causes and Shared Risk Factors

- Smoking (main cause of COPD, but some asthmatics also smoke).
- Environmental pollutants (e.g. biomass exposure, occupational irritants).
- Airway infections (recurrent early-life infections can lead to both diseases).
- Genetics (e.g. family history of asthma or COPD).

Clinical Features

- ACO shares symptoms of both asthma and COPD, making diagnosis challenging.
- Age of onset is midlife.
- Smoking history is often present.
- Symptoms are partial reversible with bronchodilators.
- Responds moderately to inhaled corticosteroids.

Diagnosis of ACO

- ACO should be suspected when a patient has persistent airflow limitation (FEV_1/FVC <0.70) but also shows features of both asthma and COPD.

Treatment of ACO

- ACO requires a combination of asthma and COPD treatment strategies, balancing airway inflammation control (asthma) and bronchodilation (COPD).

Prognosis of ACO

- Worse than asthma alone but better than COPD alone.

Q. Define pneumonia. How do you classify pneumonia?

Definition

- Pneumonia is an acute infection of the lung parenchyma that causes inflammation and consolidation of the alveoli, leading to cough, fever, dyspnea, and sputum production.

Classification

Based on the Setting in which Pneumonia Develops

- Community acquired pneumonia (CAP)
- Hospital-acquired (nosocomial) pneumonia (HAP).
  - Ventilator-associated pneumonia (VAP)
  - Non-ventilator-associated pneumonia
- Aspiration pneumonia

Based on the Anatomical Distribution of Pneumonia

- Lobar pneumonia
- Bronchopneumonia
- Interstitial pneumonia
- Miliary pneumonia

Q. Discuss the etiology, pathology, clinical features, investigations and management of community-acquired pneumonia.

Definition

- Community-acquired pneumonia (CAP) is defined as an acute infection of the pulmonary parenchyma in a patient who has acquired the infection in the community.
- Community-acquired pneumonia (CAP) is a common and serious illness with considerable morbidity and mortality.

Etiology

- ***Bacteria:*** Most of the cases are due to bacteria
  - *Typical bacteria: Streptococcus pneumoniae, H. influenzae, Moraxella catarrhalis*, gram-negative bacilli, anaerobes, *Mycobacterium tuberculosis, Coxiella burnetiid*, etc. Out of these, the first three bacteria (*Streptococcus pneumoniae, H. influenzae, Moraxella catarrhalis*) account for almost 85% of CAP, and *Streptococcus pneumonia* (pneumococcal pneumonia) accounts for most of the cases.
  - *Atypical bacteria: Mycoplasma pneumoniae, Chlamydia pneumoniae, Legionella pneumophila.*
- ***Viruses:*** Influenza virus, parainfluenza virus, SARS-CoV-2, H1N1, respiratory syncytial virus.
- ***Fungi:*** *Pneumocystis jirovecii* (in HIV), *Histoplasma capsulatum*.

Risk Factors for Pneumonia

- ***Age***: Elderly (>65 years).
- ***Immunocompromised state***: HIV, chemotherapy, steroid therapy. Splenectomy is an important risk factor for pneumonia with *S. pneumoniae*.
- ***Chronic diseases***: Uncontrolled diabetes mellitus, COPD, heart failure.
- ***Anatomical defects***: Obstructed bronchus, bronchiectasis, or fibrosis lead to recurrent pneumonia.
- ***Lifestyle factors***: Smoking, alcohol abuse. Alcohol abuse is a risk factor for both community acquired and aspiration pneumonia.

Pathogenesis

Entry of Microorganisms into the Lung

- Microbial agents reach lungs by inhalation, aspiration, hematogenous spread from a distant site, or direct spread from a contiguous site.
- Inhalation: Droplet transmission of airborne pathogens (e.g. *Streptococcus pneumoniae*, Mycoplasma, influenza virus, TB, H1N1, SARS-CoV-2).
- Aspiration: Inhalation of oropharyngeal or gastric contents (e.g. anaerobes in aspiration pneumonia). Aspiration can occur during sleep (microaspiration), postoperatively and also during seizures and strokes.
- Hematogenous spread: Dissemination from bloodstream (e.g. *Staphylococcus aureus* in endocarditis, *E. coli* from UTI).
- Direct extension: From nearby infections (e.g. pleural infection, trauma).
- *Mycobacterium tuberculosis*, fungi, Legionella, *Coxiella burnetii*, and viruses reach the lungs through inhalation of aerosols.

Host Defense and Inflammatory Reaction in Lung

- Once microorganisms reach the alveoli, there is inflammatory response against them. This inflammatory response, rather than the proliferation of microorganisms, triggers the clinical syndrome of pneumonia. Alveolar macrophages recognize the microorganisms and release inflammatory mediators, such as interleukin (IL)-1, IL-6, and tumor necrosis factor (TNF-alpha), which results in fever. Neutrophils are recruited → Release reactive oxygen species (ROS) and proteases to kill bacteria. Inflammatory mediators released by macrophages and neutrophils create an alveolar capillary leak. RBCs can also leak into the alveoli causing hemoptysis. The capillary leak results in a radiographic infiltrate and crepitations heard on auscultation. Alveolar filling also results in consolidation of lung and impaired gas exchange.
- All patients with pneumonia have reduced vital capacity, lung compliance, functional residual capacity, and total lung capacity. Decreased compliance, hypoxemia, increased respiratory drive, increased secretions, and occasionally infection-related bronchospasm all lead to dyspnea.
- Associated pleural inflammation leads to pleuritic type chest pain.
- Pathologically pneumonia manifests as four general anatomical patterns: Lobar pneumonia, bronchopneumonia, interstitial pneumonia, and miliary pneumonia.

Lobar pneumonia

- In lobar pneumonia an entire lobe of lung is involved. Inflammation can involve pleura causing pleuritic chest pain, pleural effusion and pleural rub. There are four stages in the course of lobar pneumonia.
- Stage of congestion—occurs during the first 24 hours and is characterized grossly by redness and a doughy consistency and microscopically by vascular congestion and alveolar edema.
- Stage of red hepatization–so called because in this stage, the affected part of lung resembles liver in color and consistency. Microscopically this stage is characterized by the presence of erythrocytes, neutrophils, desquamated epithelial cells, and fibrin in the alveolar spaces. Erythrocytes give the appearance of red color.
- Stage of gray hepatization: Here the affected part of lung is dry, friable, and gray-brown due to fibrinopurulent exudate, disintegration of red blood cells, and presence of hemosiderin. The second and third stages last for 2–3 days each.
- Stage of resolution: This is characterized by resolution of above changes by enzymatic digestion of exudates, phagocytosis, and coughing out of debris.

- Atypical pneumonia (e.g. Mycoplasma, viral pneumonia) presents with diffuse interstitial inflammation rather than lobar consolidation.

Bronchopneumonia

- This pattern of pneumonia involves one or many lobes, and has patchy distribution. Causes of bronchopneumonia include *Staphylococcus aureus*, *Klebsiella pneumoniae*, viruses (H1N1, SARS-COV-2), and aspiration of oropharyngeal secretions.
- The consolidated areas are poorly demarcated. The neutrophilic exudate is more in bronchi and bronchioles, with centrifugal spread to the adjacent alveoli.

Interstitial pneumonia

- This pattern of pneumonia involves the interstitium. Inflammation may be patchy or diffuse. There is infiltration of lymphocytes, macrophages, and plasma cells into the alveolar septa. The alveoli may contain a protein-rich hyaline membrane similar to those found in adult respiratory distress syndrome (ARDS). Examples of pathogens causing interstitial pneumonia are *Mycoplasma pneumoniae*, and influenza virus.

Miliary pneumonia

- The pattern is so called because of resemblance of lesions to millet seeds. These lesions are numerous, 2–3 mm in size and diffusely distributed. They result from the spread of the pathogen to the lungs via the bloodstream. The lesions consist of granulomas or foci of necrosis.
- Miliary pneumonia occurs in miliary tuberculosis, histoplasmosis, and coccidioidomycosis. Viruses like herpesvirus, cytomegalovirus, or varicella-zoster virus can cause miliary pattern pneumonia in immunocompromised patients.

Clinical Features

The onset may be sudden or insidious.

General Symptoms

- Fever, tachycardia. Cyanosis in severe cases.
- There may be other symptoms like headache, nausea, vomiting, diarrhea, myalgia, arthralgia, and fatigue. Confusion may occur in elderly persons.

Respiratory Symptoms/Signs

- Cough (with or without sputum). Sputum is common with bacterial infections. Dry cough may be seen with viral or atypical pneumonia.
- Breathlessness.
- Pleuritic type chest pain (in lobar pneumonia).
- Hemoptysis in severe cases (especially necrotizing pneumonia due to Staphylococcus, Klebsiella)
- RS examination shows dull percussion over the area of consolidation, increased tactile and vocal fremitus, egophony, whispering pectoriloquy, bronchial breath sounds, crepitations and sometimes pleural rub. Crepitations are heard in the stage of congestion and resolution. Bronchial breath sounds are heard in the stage of consolidation. The single most useful sign of the severity of pneumonia is a respiratory rate of >30/min.

Investigations

Imaging Studies

- The most important investigation is chest X-ray. It shows pneumonic patch with or without pleural effusion. However, chest X-ray can be normal in early stages of pneumonia. Hence, it is useful to repeat chest X-ray after 1or 2 days.
- High-resolution computed tomography (HRCT) can pick up opacities even if chest X-ray is normal.
- Lung ultrasound: Identifies consolidation, pleural effusion, B-lines (alveolar flooding).

Sputum Analysis

- Gram's stain can tell whether the infecting organism is gram-positive or negative.
- AFB staining and CB-NAAT: If tuberculosis (TB) is suspected.

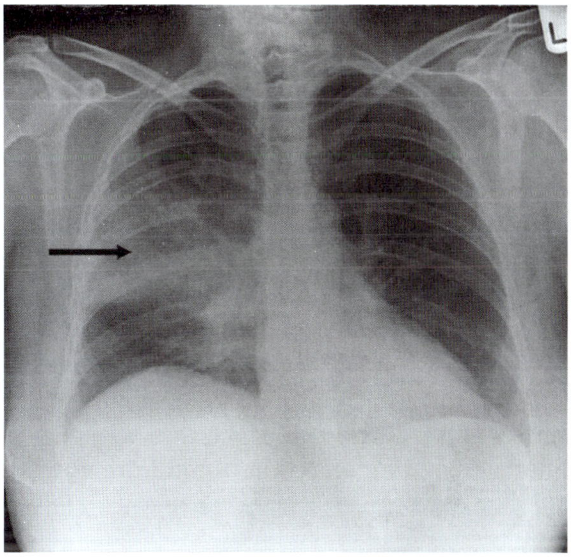

Figure 2.16: Lobar pneumonia

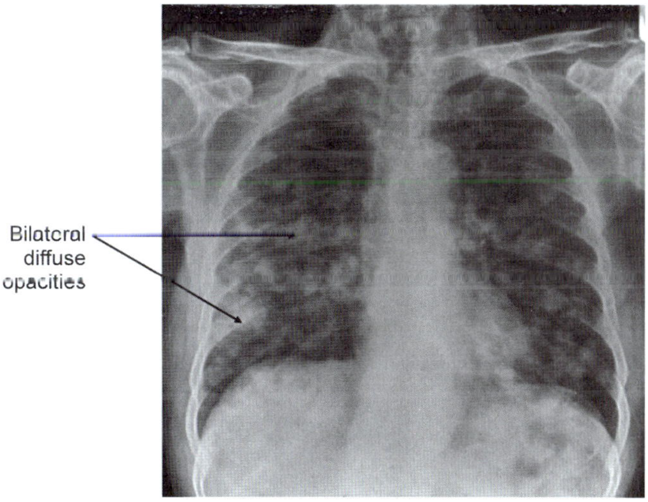

Figure 2.17: Bronchopneumonia

- Viral PCR panel *(for suspected viral pneumonia):* Detects Influenza, SARS-CoV-2, RSV, adenovirus, etc.
- Culture and sensitivity of sputum can clearly identify the organism and also antibiotic susceptibility. Culture results should always be correlated with those of Gram's staining. If an organism is cultured from sputum which was not seen on Gram's staining, the isolate may be a contaminant from upper airway.
- Some organisms should always be considered as pathogens if isolated from sputum. These include *M. tuberculosis*, Legionella, *Histoplasma capsulatum*, and *Coccidioides immitis*.

Blood Culture

- Blood should be drawn before starting antibiotics for culture and sensitivity. The organism causing pneumonia is sometimes picked up by blood culture due to bacteremia. Two sets of blood cultures should be drawn.

Serological Tests

- The detection of IgM antibody or a fourfold rise in the titer of antibody to a particular organism is a good evidence for infection by that organism. *Mycoplasma pneumoniae, Chlamydia pneumoniae, Chlamydia psittaci,* Legionella and *Coxiella burnetii*, are often diagnosed serologically.
- Serologic testing is not recommended for routine use.

Pleural Fluid Analysis

- Aspiration and analysis if pleural effusion present.

Bronchoscopy with Bronchoalveolar Lavage (BAL)

- For immunocompromised or non-resolving pneumonia.
- Collects deep lung secretions for culture, fungal, TB, viral PCR tests.

Detection of Antigens in Urine

- *Legionella pneumophila* serogroup 1 antigen can be detected in the urine of patients with Legionnaires' disease by ELISA. The urine antigen test is now the most frequently used diagnostic method for Legionnaires' disease. Antigen of *Streptococcus pneumoniae* can also be detected in the urine.

Differential Diagnosis

- Pleural effusion
- Pulmonary tuberculosis
- Pulmonary infarction
- Pulmonary edema
- Pulmonary eosinophilia
- Malignancy
- Alveolitis/cryptogenic pneumonitis/drug-induced pneumonitis
- Systemic necrotizing vasculitis
- Interstitial lung diseases.

Treatment of Pneumonia

Admit the patient if any one of the following features is there

- Respiratory rate >28/min.
- Systolic blood pressure <90 mm Hg or 30 mm Hg below baseline.
- New-onset confusion or impaired level of consciousness.
- Hypoxemia: PaO_2 <60 mm Hg while breathing room air or SPO_2 <90%.
- Unstable comorbid illness (e.g. decompensated congestive heart failure, uncontrolled diabetes mellitus, immunosuppression).
- Multilobar pneumonia, if hypoxemia is present.
- Significant pleural effusion.
- **CURB-65 scoring:** CURB-65 score is used to predict the severity and prognosis of pneumonia. It is very useful to decide whether the patient is to be admitted or not. Each risk factor scores one point, for a maximum score of 5

	Clinical parameter	Points
C	Confusion	1
U	Urea ≥20 mg/dl	1
R	Respiratory rate ≥30 breaths/min	1
B	BP systolic <90 mm Hg or Diastolic ≤60 mm Hg	1
65	Age ≥65 years	1

- If the cumulative score is 0 or 1, the risk of mortality is low and patient can be treated as an outpatient.
- If the score is 2 the risk is moderate and ideally should be treated as inpatient.
- If the score is ≥3, risk of mortality is high and the patient should be treated as inpatient preferably in ICU.

Antibiotic Therapy

- Initially empirical antibiotic therapy is started based on clinical judgment till the organism is identified. Macrolides have excellent activity against *Streptococcus pneumoniae* and atypical pathogens like *Mycoplasma pneumoniae, Chlamydia pneumoniae,* and Legionella spp and can be used as first-line therapy. Doxycycline, also has activity against *S. pneumoniae* and atypical pathogens and can be used for outpatient therapy.
- IV antibiotics can be changed to oral therapy when (1) the white blood cell count is returning toward normal, (2) there are two normal temperature readings (<37.5°C) 16 hours apart, and (3) there is improvement in cough and shortness of breath.
- Antibiotics should be given for minimum 2 weeks. Azithromycin has a long half life and needs to be given for only 5 days. Patients with severe Legionnaires' disease, pneumonia due to pseudomonas aeruginosa or other aerobic gram-negative bacilli require 21 days of therapy.
- Patients can be discharged if afebrile for 24 hours, heart rate is <100/min, respiratory rate is <24/min, systolic blood pressure is >90 mm Hg, and oxygen saturation is >90%.

TABLE 2.22: Initial antibiotic choice for community-acquired pneumonia

Clinical setting	Antibiotic choice
Out patients Previously healthy patients with no risk factors for MRSA or *Pseudomonas*: Comorbidities or antibiotics in past 3 months	Oral amoxicillin *or* doxycycline *or* macrolide antibiotic (clarithromycin or azithromycin). Oral macrolide *or* doxycycline (as above) *plus* an oral beta-lactam (amoxicillin/clavulanate or cefpodoxime, or cefuroxime). OR Monotherapy with an oral fluoroquinolone (moxifloxacin, gemifloxacin, levofloxacin) *Duration of treatment is 7 days*
Inpatients (non-severe pneumonia, usually not requiring ICU)	A respiratory fluoroquinolone. Oral/IV: moxifloxacin, or levofloxacin *or* A macrolide *plus* a beta-lactam. For intravenous therapy: ampicillin/sulbactam, or cefotaxime or ceftriaxone or ceftaroline. For patients with prior respiratory isolation of MRSA, strongly consider adding coverage for MRSA (IV vancomycin or linezolid). For patients with prior respiratory isolation of *Pseudomonas aeruginosa*, strongly consider adding coverage for *P. aeruginosa*: IV piperacillin-tazobactam, or cefepime, or imipenem, or meropenem, or aztreonam. *Duration of treatment is 7–10 days*
Inpatients with severe pneumonia (typically requiring ICU admission)	Azithromycin or a respiratory fluoroquinolone (as above) plus an intravenous anti-pneumococcal beta-lactam (as above). For patients at risk for *P. aeruginosa*, add coverage for *P. aeruginosa* (as above). If drug resistance to pseudomonas is high, consider adding either an anti-pseudomonal fluoroquinolone (ciprofloxacin or levofloxacin) or an aminoglycoside (gentamicin, tobramycin, amikacin). For patients at risk for MRSA infection, add coverage for MRSA (vancomycin, or linezolid). *Duration of treatment is 10–14 days*

General Measures

- IV fluids
- Oxygen
- Addition of bronchodilators and mucolytics may enhance sputum clearance.
- Physiotherapy to teach effective coughing techniques.
- Mechanical ventilation may be required in patients with respiratory failure.

Causes of Unresolving Pneumonia

- *Wrong diagnosis:* Other diseases may be mistaken for community acquired pneumonia. These are collagen vascular disease, tuberculosis, pneumocystis, or fungal pneumonia.
- *Improper antibiotics:* For example, amoxicillin or azithromycin to treat MRSA will lead to poor response to treatment.
- *Obstructed bronchus:* due to carcinoma or sequestration of a segment of lung.
- *Undrained or metastatic pyogenic focus,* e.g. empyema, endocarditis, splenic abscess, osteomyelitis.
- *Immunosuppressed states.*

Causes of Recurrent Pneumonia

- *Bronchopulmonary disease:* Foreign body, obstruction of bronchus due to enlarged lymph nodes or bronchogenic Ca, COPD, bronchiectasis, lung fibrosis, cystic fibrosis.
- *Cardiac diseases:* ASD, heart failure.
- *Immunodeficiency states:* HIV infection, immunosuppressant drugs, congenital immunoglobulin deficiencies.
- *Conditions leading to recurrent aspiration*: Gastroesophageal reflux disease, esophageal stricture.

Complications of Pneumonia

- Pleural effusion (common)
- Empyema
- Pneumothorax-particularly with *Staph. aureus*
- Lung abscess
- ARDS
- Sepsis with multiorgan failure
- Ectopic abscess formation (*Staph. aureus*).

Vaccination

- Pneumococcal vaccine for high-risk patients.
- Influenza vaccine to prevent secondary bacterial pneumonia.

Q. Atypical Pneumonia.

- Atypical pneumonia refers to a type of pneumonia caused by pathogens other than the most common bacteria responsible for typical pneumonia (e.g. *Streptococcus pneumoniae*). It often presents with milder symptoms and is sometimes called "walking pneumonia" because affected individuals may not feel sick enough to stay in bed.

- The origin of the term "atypical" is a matter of debate. The term may refer to the fact that these organisms are not "typical" bacteria that can be identified by standard microbiologic techniques. Others suggest that atypical refers to the mild nature of the pneumonia caused by some of these organisms compared with pneumonia caused by *Streptococcus pneumoniae.* Sometimes, some viral pneumonias have also been included as atypical pneumonia (e.g. respiratory syncytial virus).
- Atypical organisms are an inclusive term for organisms difficult to culture and not apparent on gram stain. Given their intracellular nature, they are difficult to isolate and often challenging to treat because antibiotics must be able to penetrate intracellularly to reach their intended target.

Etiology

- Atypical pneumonia is caused by following atypical organisms. Atypical organisms are an inclusive term for organisms difficult to culture and not apparent on gram stain due to their intracellular nature. The most common causative agents include:
- ***Bacteria***
  - *Mycoplasma pneumoniae* (most common cause of atypical pneumonia).
  - *Chlamydia pneumoniae.*
  - *Legionella pneumophila* (Legionnaires' disease, often linked to contaminated water sources).
  - *Coxiella burnetii.*

Clinical Features

Unlike typical pneumonia, atypical pneumonia often presents with:

- Gradual onset of symptoms
- Low-grade fever
- Non-productive (dry) cough
- Headache, myalgia (muscle pain), and fatigue
- Pharyngitis (sore throat) and hoarseness (common with *Chlamydia pneumoniae*)
- Gastrointestinal symptoms (common with *Legionella pneumophila*)
- Mild respiratory distress (rarely severe unless in immunocompromised individuals)

Diagnosis

- Chest X-ray: Often shows diffuse, patchy infiltrates rather than lobar consolidation.
- PCR or serology for *Mycoplasma* and *Chlamydia pneumoniae*
- Urinary antigen test for *Legionella pneumophila*
- Sputum Gram's stain and culture (less reliable for these pathogens)

Treatment

Atypical pneumonia does not respond to beta-lactam antibiotics (e.g. penicillins, cephalosporins) because pathogens like *Mycoplasma* lack a cell wall. Instead, treatment involves:

- Macrolides (e.g. azithromycin, clarithromycin)—first-line for *Mycoplasma* and *Chlamydia.*
- Tetracyclines (e.g. doxycycline)—alternative option
- Fluoroquinolones (e.g. levofloxacin)—used for *Legionella pneumophila.*
- Antivirals or antifungals if a viral or fungal cause is suspected.

Prognosis and Prevention

- Most cases are mild and self-limiting, but can be severe in immunocompromised individuals.

Q. Differences between typical and atypical pneumonia.

See **Table 2.23.**

TABLE 2.23: Differences between typical and atypical pneumonia

Feature	Typical pneumonia	Atypical pneumonia
Causative agents	*Streptococcus pneumoniae* (most common), *Haemophilus influenzae, Staphylococcus aureus, Klebsiella pneumoniae, Pseudomonas aeruginosa*	*Mycoplasma pneumoniae, Chlamydia pneumoniae, Legionella pneumophila, Chlamydia psittaci, Coxiella burnetii*
Fever	High fever with chills	Low-grade fever
Cough	Productive cough with purulent or rusty sputum	Nonproductive (dry) cough or scanty sputum
Chest pain	Pleuritic chest pain (sharp, worsens with breathing)	Less common, may be vague or mild
Respiratory symptoms	Significant dyspnea, tachypnea, and respiratory distress	Mild dyspnea, less severe respiratory distress. Usually not bedbound, hence called "walking pneumonia"
Extrapulmonary symptoms	Rare	More common: headache, myalgia, sore throat, gastrointestinal symptoms (esp. *Legionella*)
Chest X-ray findings	Lobar consolidation (affecting one lung segment or lobe)	Diffuse, patchy infiltrates, often interstitial
Response to beta-lactams (penicillins, cephalosporins)	Good response to beta-lactam antibiotics	Poor response (since many atypical pathogens lack a cell wall)
First-Line treatment	Beta-lactams (e.g. amoxicillin, ceftriaxone)	Macrolides (azithromycin), tetracyclines (doxycycline), fluoroquinolones (levofloxacin)

Q. Hospital-acquired pneumonia (HAP).

Q. Ventilator associated pneumonia (VAP).

- Hospital-acquired or nosocomial pneumonia refers to pneumonia that occurs at least 48 hours after admission to hospital and not incubating at the time of admission.
- It can be further divided into ventilator associated and non-ventilator associated pneumonia. Ventilator-associated pneumonia (VAP) is pneumonia that develops after 48 hours of mechanical ventilation and not incubating at the time of intubation. Non-ventilator associated pneumonia includes all other types of HAP such as postoperative pneumonia, aspiration pneumonia, etc.
- Both HAP and VAP have similar features and the following description applies to both.

Epidemiology

- 5–20 cases per 1,000 hospital admissions.
- Accounts for up to 30% of all nosocomial infections.
- Highest rates among intensive care unit (ICU) patients undergoing mechanical ventilation.
- About 1.5% of patients develop pneumonia post-operatively.
- HAP lengthens hospital stay by an average of 7–9 days per affected patient.

Risk Factors

Colonization with Potential Pathogens

- Decreased gastric acidity due to use of H_2 blockers and proton pump inhibitors.
- Antimicrobial therapy.
- Contaminated ventilator circuits or equipment.

Aspiration of Oropharyngeal Contents into Lower Respiratory Tract

- Intubation/mechanical ventilation.
- Decreased level of consciousness.
- Nasogastric intubation.
- Reduced cough (general anesthesia, thoracic and abdominal surgery).

Reduced Host Defenses

- Corticosteroid treatment, diabetes, malignancy.

Bacteremia

- Infected emboli
- Intravenous cannula infection
- Sepsis.

Organisms Causing HAP

- HAP is typically caused by multi-drug resistant (MDR) pathogens due to hospital environments and prior antibiotic exposure. Majority of HAP are caused by gram-negative bacteria. These are as follows:

Gram-negative Bacteria (most common)

- *Pseudomonas aeruginosa*
- *Klebsiella pneumoniae*
- *Escherichia coli*
- *Acinetobacter baumannii*
- Enterobacter species.

Gram-positive Bacteria

- *Staphylococcus aureus* (especially MRSA).

Fungi

- Candida species, Aspergillus in immunocompromised patients.

Clinical Features

- New or worsening cough with purulent sputum
- Fever and chills
- Dyspnea (shortness of breath), tachypnea
- Pleuritic chest pain
- Increased oxygen requirements or respiratory distress
- Leukocytosis or leukopenia
- New infiltrates on chest X-ray or CT scan.

Differential Diagnosis

- Pulmonary edema due to fluid overload or heart failure
- Pulmonary embolism
- Atelectasis
- ARDS
- Pulmonary hemorrhage.

Laboratory Tests

- Complete blood count shows increase in leukocyte count.
- Blood cultures.
- Sputum culture and Gram's staining. Endotracheal aspirate can yield good uncontaminated sample for Gram's stain and culture.
- Chest X-ray shows a new or changing pulmonary infiltrate.
- CT of the chest if necessary.
- Bronchoscopy may be required sometimes.

Management

- Since Organisms causing HAP are likely to be due to Gram-negative bacteria such as Pseudomonas, one of the following antibiotics active against Pseudomonas and other gram-negative organisms should be chosen
  - Piperacillin/tazobactam
  - Cefepime
  - Levofloxacin
  - Imipenem
  - Meropenem
- If MRSA is highly prevalent in the institution and the patient is at risk for MRSA infection, add vancomycin or linezolid.
- Aspiration pneumonia can be treated with amoxicillin clavulanic acid 1.2 g 8-hourly plus metronidazole 500 mg 8-hourly.
- Physiotherapy for immobile and elderly, and to teach coughing techniques.

Complications

- Increased mortality.
- Prolongation of mechanical ventilation.
- Pulmonary hemorrhage (especially with Pseudomonas).
- Long-term complications such as bronchiectasis and parenchymal scarring leading to recurrent pneumonias.

Prevention

- Health care providers must adhere strict hand hygiene and infection control measures.
- In patients undergoing mechanical ventilation,
  - *Extubate as early as possible*
  - *Ensure careful periodic drainage of tubing condensate.*
  - *Avoid paralytic agents and heavy sedation that can depress cough.*
  - *Continuous suctioning of secretions*
- Use small-bore enteral feeding tubes.
- Elevate the head of the bed by > 30 degrees to prevent aspiration.
- Judicious use of antibiotics to prevent MDR strains.
- Incentive spirometry is recommended to prevent postoperative pneumonia.
- Use of kinetic beds.

Q. Suppurative or necrotizing pneumonia.

Q. Staphylococcal pneumonia.

Q. *Klebsiella pneumonia.*

- Suppurative pneumonia and necrotizing pneumonia are severe forms of bacterial pneumonia characterized by lung tissue destruction, abscess formation, and extensive necrosis.

Etiology

- *Staphylococcus aureus* (including MRSA)
- *Klebsiella pneumoniae*
- *Pseudomonas aeruginosa*
- *Streptococcus pneumoniae*
- Anaerobic bacteria (e.g. Bacteroides, *Fusobacterium*, *prevotella*)—often in aspiration pneumonia.

Clinical Features

- High fever with rigors and chills
- Productive cough with foul-smelling, purulent sputum (suggestive of anaerobic infection)
- Hemoptysis due to lung tissue necrosis
- Pleuritic chest pain
- Dyspnea
- Signs of sepsis (hypotension, tachycardia) in severe cases.

Radiologic Features

- Lung abscess (cavity with air-fluid level on chest X-ray or CT).
- Patchy consolidation with central necrosis.

Complications

- Pulmonary hemorrhage (especially when there is necrosis)
- Lung abscess formation
- Empyema (pus in the pleural space)
- Bronchopleural fistula.
- Sepsis.

Treatment

- Empiric broad-spectrum antibiotics, covering both aerobic and anaerobic bacteria:
  - Beta-lactam + beta-lactamase inhibitor (e.g. piperacillin-tazobactam, ampicillin-sulbactam)
  - Or Carbapenems (e.g. meropenem for MDR pathogens)
  - Or Clindamycin or metronidazole (for anaerobic coverage)
- Drainage of abscesses or empyema if necessary
- Supportive care (oxygen, IV fluids)

Staphylococcal Pneumonia

Clinical Features

- Are same as described above.

Investigations

- Chest X-ray: Homogeneous lobar or segmental opacity. Abscess may be present with an air fluid level. Additional radiographic features include multilobar shadowing, cavitation, and pneumatoceles.
- Sputum Gram's stain and culture sensitivity.

Management

Same as described above.

Klebsiella pneumonia

Clinical Features

- More common in men, alcoholics and diabetics. It can be either community acquired or hospital acquired. It is one of the most common causes of hospital-acquired pneumonia. Upper lobe involvement common. The sputum in *Klebsiella pneumonia* is described as "red currant jelly." This is because *K. pneumoniae* causes significant inflammation and necrosis of the surrounding tissue. Complications include lung abscess, cavitation, empyema, and pleural adhesions.

Investigations

- Chest X-ray-upper lobe involvement is common. Sometimes bulging fissure sign is seen in the affected area because of severe inflammation.
- Other investigations are same as above.

Treatment

- Preferred: Third-generation cephalosporin. For severe infections, add an aminoglycoside.
- Alternatives: Aztreonam, imipenem, meropenem, aminoglycoside, or a fluoroquinolone

Q. Legionnaires' disease.

- Legionnaires' disease is a severe form of atypical pneumonia caused by *Legionella pneumophila* and related Legionella species.
- Legionnaires' disease was first recognized in 1976, when an outbreak of pneumonia took place during the annual convention of the American Legion at a Philadelphia hotel.

Etiology

- The causative agent is *Legionella pneumophila* which is a gram-negative aerobic bacillus. *Legionella pneumophila* causes 2 distinct disease entities; Legionnaires' disease (LD) and Pontiac fever. Legionnaires' disease (LD) is characterized by pneumonia. Pontiac fever is a short-term illness manifesting as fever and myalgias without pneumonia.
- Its natural habitat is water. It is ubiquitous, and is found in rivers and lakes where it can survive for years at very low temperatures.
- Human infection is acquired via inhalation aerosols from contaminated water or soil. Sources of infection are water distribution system colonized by Legionella, contaminated shower heads and faucets in patient rooms and air conditioning systems. Legionella infection is not transmitted from person to person.

Clinical Features

- The incubation period is 2–10 days.
- Males are affected more often. Smokers and the immunocompromised are also more at risk.
- It causes pneumonia which begins with high fever, cough and dyspnea.
- Extrapulmonary manifestations can occur due to bacteremia. Gastrointestinal symptoms include nausea, vomiting, diarrhea (watery, not bloody), abdominal pain, and anorexia.
- Neurologic symptoms include headache, lethargy, encephalopathy, and altered mental status.
- There may be relative bradycardia.
- Failure to respond to beta-lactam antibiotics is a clue to diagnosis.
- Key point to remember: Legionnaires' disease = severe pneumonia + GI and neurological symptoms.

Investigations

- Chest X-ray usually shows lobar or multilobar pneumonia, sometimes with a small pleural effusion.
- Sputum Gram's stain shows numerous neutrophils and gram negative rods.
- Hyponatremia, elevated creatinine and liver enzymes can occur.
- Serology: Paired serologic testing. Serum IgM antibody showing a fourfold rise in titer between paired sera or a single value of >1:256 is diagnostic.
- PCR (polymerase chain reaction): Detects Legionella DNA in respiratory secretions. Fast and reliable.
- Urinary antigen testing: Legionella lipopolysaccharide antigen is excreted in the urine and can be detected by ELISA, radioimmunoassay (RIA), or latex agglutination test. Urine antigen testing is very useful to confirm the diagnosis as this test is not affected by antibiotics and urine sample is easy to obtain than sputum.
- Sputum culture (gold standard): Legionella grows on buffered charcoal yeast extract (BCYE) agar. Takes several days but confirms species and antibiotic sensitivity.

Treatment

- Azithromycin (for 5–10 days) or levofloxacin (for 1–2 weeks) are the antibiotics of choice and are effective as monotherapy.
- Avoid beta-lactams (penicillins, cephalosporins): *Legionella* lacks a cell wall, making them ineffective.

Prevention

- Proper water system maintenance.

Q. Discuss the etiology, pathology, clinical features and management of bronchiectasis.

- Bronchiectasis is an abnormal and permanent dilatation of bronchi.
- It can be congenital or acquired and localized or diffuse.
- It leads to chronic or recurrent infection in the dilated bronchi, copious sputum production and hemoptysis.

Etiopathogenesis

- Development of bronchiectasis is mainly due to two factors; infection and obstruction or both. Infection leads to inflammation and destruction of the bronchial wall, damages respiratory epithelium and impairs mucociliary clearance. This leads to pooling of secretions, and dilatation of bronchi. Dilated bronchi become more susceptible to infection and thus, a vicious cycle results. Pulmonary tuberculosis leads to fibrosis, distorted and dilated bronchi.
- Bronchial obstruction due to any reason can lead to recurrent infections and development of bronchiectasis.
- Some congenital disorders like dyskinetic cilia or mucoviscidosis can also predispose to bronchiectasis.
- A congenital condition, Kartagener's syndrome is characterized by a combination of situs inversus, bilateral bronchiectasis and abnormal cilia lining the respiratory epithelium. This condition leads to stagnant secretions and repeated bronchial infections which lead to bronchiectasis.
- Bronchiectasis usually affects lower lobe bronchi. Upper lobe bronchiectasis is usually due to tuberculosis.
- Three forms of bronchiectasis have been recognized, namely; cylindrical, fusiform, and saccular (cystic).
    - In the cylindrical type, there is uniform dilatation of bronchi.
    - In the fusiform type, dilatation is irregular with tapering at both ends.

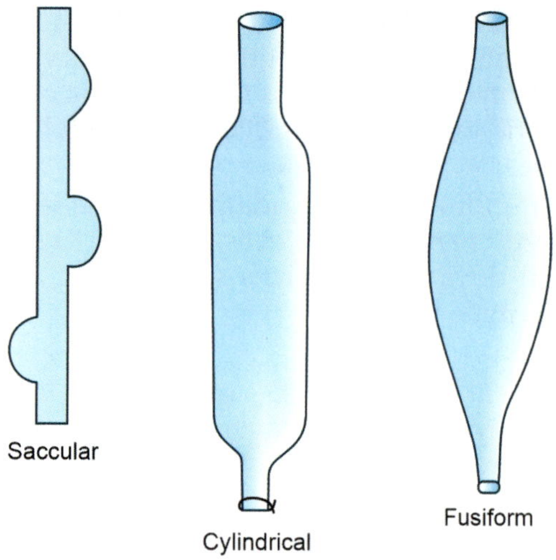

Figure 2.18: Types of bronchiectasis

- In saccular type, there are multiple bulgings from side wall of bronchi **(Fig. 2.18)**.
- The bronchial epithelium may be ulcerated with exposure of thin-walled capillaries in the submucosa which are responsible for hemoptysis.

Causes of Bronchiectasis

Bronchial Obstruction

- Foreign body
- Tumor
- Stenosis
- Enlarged lymph nodes
- Impacted secretions

Infections

- Childhood pneumonias in measles, whooping cough
- Pulmonary tuberculosis
- Bronchopulmonary aspergillosis
- Repeated chest infections due to immunodeficient states

Congenital and Genetic Disorders

- Cystic fibrosis
- Kartagener's syndrome
- Alpha-1 antitrypsin deficiency
- Immotile cilia syndrome

Clinical Features

- Persistent or recurrent cough with copious sputum for several years. There is postural variation to cough and sputum quantity depending on which area of the lung is involved. Some patients may have no sputum with cough. This entity is called bronchiectasis sicca.
- Sputum is often blood-stained, and occasionally foul-smelling. Hemoptysis can be massive due to erosion of a hypertrophied bronchial artery.
- Patients may have dyspnea and wheezing when underlying COPD is also present.
- When there is secondary infection, quantity of sputum increases, becomes more purulent and foul smelling. Patients may also have fever and other constitutional symptoms.
- Patients are usually malnourished and, in a child, there may be growth retardation.
- Physical examination may reveal coarse, leathery crepitations, wheezes, and bronchial breath sounds over the area of bronchiectasis reflecting damaged airways containing secretions and consolidation. Clubbing is usually present. Patients with severe B/L bronchiectasis may have cor pulmonale and right ventricular failure.

Investigations

- Chest X-ray may show cystic lesions in cystic bronchiectasis. B/L honeycombing (ring shadows) can occur reflecting end on view of dilated bronchi. When seen longitudinally, the dilated and thickened bronchi appear as "tram tracks". Chest X-ray may be normal in patients with limited disease.
- High-resolution computed tomography (HRCT) of the chest (gold standard test) is now the preferred method for diagnosis because it is noninvasive. It can pick up even slight abnormalities missed by chest X-ray. Sometimes the 'signet ring sign' is seen in bronchiectasis when the dilated bronchus and accompanying pulmonary artery branch are seen in cross section **(Fig. 2.19)**. The bronchus and artery should be the same size, whereas in bronchiectasis, the bronchus is markedly dilated.
- Bronchography is instillation of a radiopaque dye into airways and then taking X-ray images. This can provide excellent visualization of bronchiectatic airways and was once gold standard for the diagnosis of bronchiectasis. But now this technique has been replaced by HRCT.
- Bronchoscopy may be done if a foreign body or adenoma is suspected to be the cause of bronchiectasis.

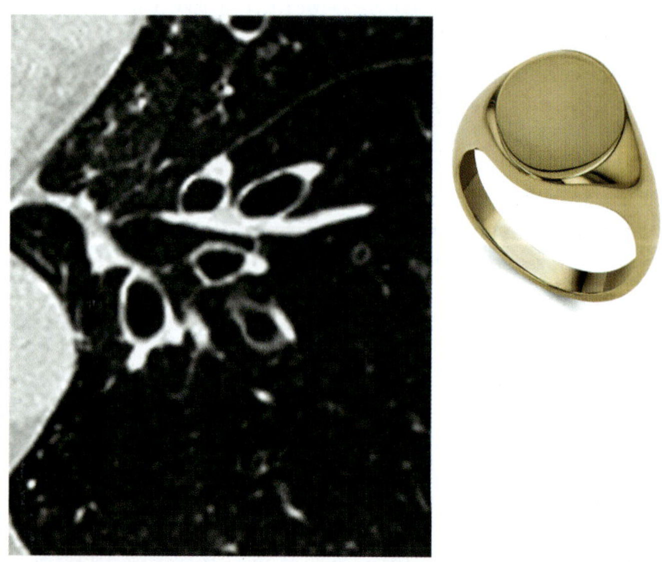

Figure 2.19: Signet ring appearance of bronchiectasis

- In diffuse bilateral bronchiectasis with early age of onset, measurement of sweat chloride levels to rule out cystic fibrosis and assessment of nasal or bronchial cilia or sperm for primary ciliary dyskinesia may be required.
- Pulmonary function tests show both restrictive and obstructive ventilatory dysfunction. Airway obstruction is due to retention of secretions and bronchial inflammation, whereas the restrictive changes are due to atelectasis and scarring of the lung parenchyma.

Management

- Medical management consists of postural drainage of the secretions, expectorants, bronchodilators and antibiotics.
- Regular physiotherapy and postural drainage prevents accumulation of secretions and repeated infections.
- Use of mucolytics like N-acetylcysteine and bromhexine may help in clearing the secretions.
- If secondary infection is suspected, broad spectrum antibiotics such as amoxicillin-clavulanate, macrolides are given. If *Pseudomonas aeruginosa* is suspected a quinolone or aminoglycoside or third-generation cephalosporin is used. Metronidazole can be added if anaerobic infection is suspected.
- Bronchodilators relieve airflow obstruction and aid clearance of secretions.
- Surgical resection is considered when bronchiectasis is localized and the morbidity is substantial despite adequate medical therapy.
- Bronchial artery embolization can be considered in patients with recurrent large hemoptysis.
- Influenza vaccination (yearly) and pneumococcal vaccination is recommended for all patients with bronchiectasis.
- Underlying conditions should be treated to slow the progression of lung disease. For example, replacement therapy in alpha-1 antitrypsin deficiency.

Complications

- Massive hemoptysis, empyema, respiratory failure, cor pulmonale, pericarditis, metastatic abscesses, and secondary amyloidosis.

Q. Cystic fibrosis.

- The first known reference to cystic fibrosis (CF) is an adage from northern European folklore: "Woe to that child which when kissed on the forehead tastes salty. He is bewitched and soon must die." This saying describes the salty sweat that is the basis of an important diagnostic test and early mortality of cystic fibrosis.
- Cystic fibrosis (CF) is a genetic (monogenic) disorder that presents as a multisystem disease. It is characterized by recurrent airway infection (which leads to bronchiectasis), exocrine pancreatic insufficiency and intestinal dysfunction, abnormal sweat gland function, and urogenital dysfunction.
- It usually presents in childhood but some patients may present in adulthood.
- Earlier, patients used to die in childhood but now because of improvement in therapy patients reach more than 30 years of age. Pulmonary involvement occurs in 90% of patients surviving the neonatal period. End-stage lung disease is the principal cause of death.

Pathogenesis

- Cystic fibrosis (CF) is an autosomal recessive disease resulting from mutation in a gene located on chromosome 7. Mutation in this gene leads to absent or defective CF transmembrane conductance regulator (CFTR). The CFTR protein functions as Cl-channel and as regulator of other ion channels. CFTR is located in the apical (lumen-facing) membrane of epithelium in the airways, pancreatic ducts, intestine, biliary ducts, and in the apical and basolateral membranes of the sweat gland duct.
- The function of CFTR channel in sweat gland is different from its function in airways, pancreatic ducts, intestine, and biliary ducts.

CFTR in Airways vs Sweat Glands

Feature	Airways (lungs, pancreas, intestines)	Sweat glands
Normal CFTR function	Secretes Cl^- and HCO_3^- into airway → Keeps mucus hydrated	Reabsorbs Cl^- and Na^+ → Makes sweat less salty
Cystic fibrosis effect	↓Cl^- secretion → Thick, dehydrated mucus	↓Cl^- reabsorption → Salty sweat
Main clinical consequence	Airway obstruction, infections, bronchiectasis	High salt loss, dehydration risk

- In the sweat duct, normally, the CFTR reabsorbs Cl^-, and Na^+ follows it, making sweat hypotonic. Abnormal or loss of CFTR prevents absorption of Cl^- which in turn prevents absorption of Na^+ to maintain electroneutrality. As a result, sweat contains high Na^+ and Cl^- concentrations making the sweat taste salty.
- In other exocrine glands (airway, pancreas, intestine, bile duct, reproductive system), normally the CFTR channel excretes Cl^- and bicarbonate into the lumen. Na^+ follows Cl^- and stays back in the lumen. Water accompanies Na^+ and Cl^- stays in the lumen thus maintaining the hydration and liquidity of mucus and secretions in the ducts. The defective CFTR in all these organs due to cystic fibrosis causes ↓ Cl^- secretion and ↓ HCO_3^- secretion into the lumen of ducts. As a result, Cl^- accumulates inside the cells. Increased Cl^- in the cells causes increased Na^+ reabsorption into the cells → water accompanies Na^+ and enters into the cell from lumen of ducts → less water in the lumen of ducts → dehydrated, thick, sticky mucus → airway obstruction, chronic infections, bronchiectasis **(Figs 2.20 and 2.21)**.

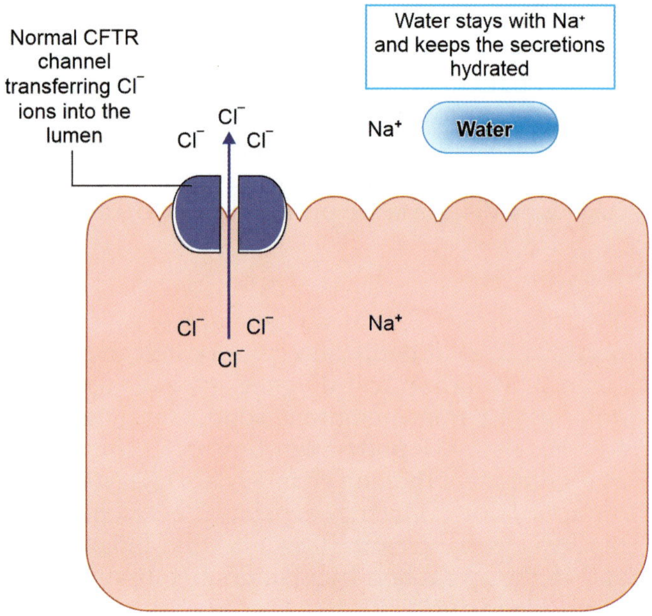

Figure 2.20: Normal CFTR channel in the airway

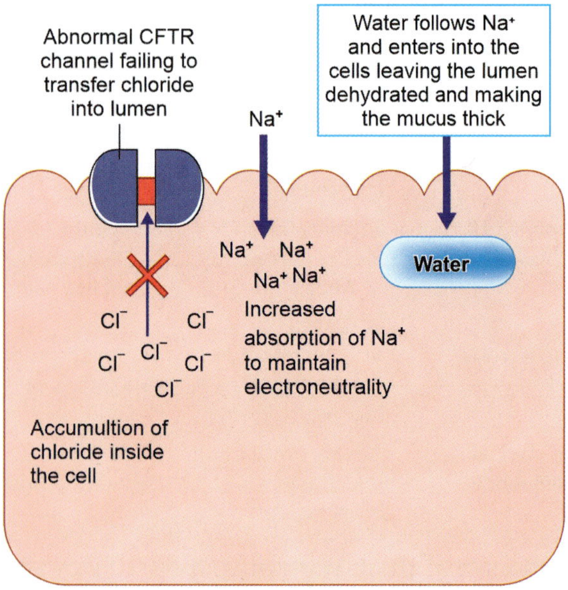

Figure 2.21: Abnormal CFTR channel in the airway

- Obstruction of the small ducts in the male genital tract also leads to the atrophy, fibrosis, or absence of the vas deferens, tail and body of the epididymis, and seminal vesicles.
- In the ileum, disruption of salt and water secretion produces thick, dehydrated intestinal contents that obstruct the ileum in the newborn, causing meconium ileus and producing meconium ileus-equivalent later in life.

Clinical Manifestations

- Patients with CF can present at several ages with a variety of clinical manifestations.
- Newborns may present with meconium ileus, infants and children may present with failure to thrive, and older children and adults may present with any of the following features.
- ***Sweat gland manifestations:*** Salty skin (excess Na^+ and Cl^- in sweat), heat intolerance and dehydration (due to excessive salt loss), electrolyte imbalances (hyponatremia, hypochloremia).
- ***Respiratory system manifestations:*** Cough is the common manifestation of respiratory system involvement due to thick mucus and recurrent infections. Episodes of cough tend to persist longer than expected for an acute respiratory illness and, with time, occur more and more frequently. Sputum is thick, purulent, and often green colored due to pseudomonas infection. With recurrent infections patient develops symptoms of bronchiectasis. Recurrent sinusitis can occur as a result of thick mucus blocking the sinus openings.
- ***Gastrointestinal system manifestations:*** Pancreas involvement leads to fat and protein malabsorption and also diabetes due to pancreas damage. Patients have steatorrhea due to malabsorption. Children may present with failure to thrive due to malabsorption. Generalized edema can occur due to hypoproteinemia. Intestinal involvement can present as distal intestinal obstruction syndrome due to thick mucus blocking the intestines, constipation and rectal prolapse.
- ***Hepatobiliary manifestations:*** Include biliary cirrhosis, portal hypertension, cholestasis and gall-stones.
- ***Reproductive system manifestations:*** Male infertility due to congenital bilateral absence of the vas deferens (CBAVD). In females, thick cervical mucus leads to reduced fertility by blocking the entry of sperm (but pregnancy is possible).

Investigations

- Newborn screening: Immunoreactive trypsinogen (IRT) test (elevated in CF), followed by genetic testing (CFTR mutations).
- Sweat chloride test (gold standard): ↑ Sweat chloride (>60 mmol/L in children, >80 mmol/L in adults). Performed twice for confirmation.
- Pancreatic function tests: ↓ Fecal elastase (exocrine pancreatic insufficiency).
- Genetic testing: For the presence of CFTR gene mutation (e.g. ΔF508).
- Other useful tests include chest X-ray, CT chest, pulmonary function tests, etc.

Treatment

Airway Clearance and Pulmonary Care

- Chest physiotherapy (chest percussion and postural drainage) are helpful in clearing purulent secretions.
- High-frequency chest wall oscillation (HFCWO)–"Vest therapy". Loosens and clears mucus.
- Use of positive expiratory pressure (PEP) devices.
- Hypertonic saline nebulization (3–7%) → Helps loosen mucus.
- Dornase alfa (pulmozyme) → Breaks down mucus DNA, improves clearance

Antibiotics

- Lung infections require an intensive course of parenteral antibiotics for 2–3 weeks. The choice of antibiotics is based on sputum cultures and sensitivity. Since *Pseudomonas aeruginosa* is a particularly common pathogen, a combination of an aminoglycoside and a beta-lactam antibiotic are commonly used.

Bronchodilators

- Bronchodilator therapy should be considered during exacerbations and in hospitalized patients.

Pancreatic Enzyme Replacement

- Since pancreatic enzymes are deficient in cystic fibrosis, pancreatic enzyme supplementation (lipase, trypsin) at mealtimes is recommended. The fat-soluble vitamins A, D, and E are also given daily since they also require pancreatic enzymes for absorption. Vitamin K may be given as required based on prothrombin time.

CFTR Modulator Therapy

- Corrects defective CFTR function to improve chloride transport and reduce mucus thickness.
- **Ivacaftor:** The cystic fibrosis transmembrane conductance regulator (CFTR), ivacaftor, has been shown to improve lung function, reduce the risk of pulmonary exacerbations, and reduce the concentration of sweat chloride.
- **Elexacaftor + Tezacaftor + Ivacaftor (Trikafta):** This triple combination is very effective and improves CFTR function in 90% of CF patients.

Gene Therapy

- The best approach to treat this disease would be to transfer a normal CFTR gene or cDNA into the affected cells. Progress in this area of research has been substantial and it is hoped that successful gene therapy will become a reality.

Other Supportive Measures

- Adequate salt should be taken during hot weather since excess salt is lost in the sweat.
- Adequate immunizations, including influenza, and Pneumococcus are mandatory.
- Smoking should be avoided.
- Laxatives (PEG, lactulose) for constipation.
- Ursodeoxycholic acid (UDCA) for liver disease prevention.

Lung Transplantation

- Should be considered for patients with an FEV_1 less than 30% predicted.

Q. Etiology, clinical features and management of lung abscess.

- A lung abscess is a localized collection of pus within lung tissue due to necrotizing infection, often caused by bacteria.

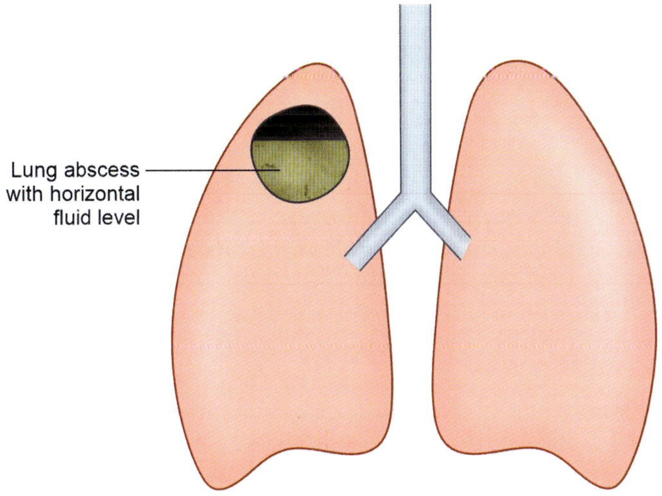

Figure 2.22: Lung abscess (schematic view)

- It is usually single and measures >2 cm in diameter. The formation of multiple small (<2 cm) abscesses is occasionally referred to as necrotizing pneumonia.
- Lung abscess may be acute or chronic, single or multiple.

Etiology

- Lung abscess is caused most frequently by bacteria, usually anaerobes.
- The routes of infection include *aspiration of oral secretions, endobronchial obstruction, and hematogenous seeding of the lung*. Lung abscess can also occur due to secondary infection of a pre-existent cavity, cyst or bulla. A lung neoplasm may cavitate and mimic lung abscess.
- Aspiration of the oropharyngeal secretions is the most common way of abscess formation. It usually occurs in patients with altered consciousness, anesthesia, alcohol intoxication, sedative drugs, head injury, cerebrovascular accidents, esophageal stricture, and during seizures. Poor oral hygiene and dental caries is a risk factor for development of abscess.
- Bronchial obstruction due to tumor or foreign body and bronchiectasis may predispose to secondary infection and abscess formation. Immunodeficient state is also a predisposing factor.
- Hematogenous seeding of the lungs occur due to suppurative thromboembolism (e.g. septic embolism due to IV drug use) or right-sided endocarditis. Typically, multiple lung abscesses occur in such cases.

Organisms Causing Lung Abscess

- Anaerobic bacteria (most common)
  - *Peptostreptococcus, Fusobacterium, Prevotella, Bacteroides.*
- Aerobic bacteria
  - *Staphylococcus aureus, Klebsiella pneumoniae, Streptococcus species.*
- Gram-negative bacteria
  - *Pseudomonas aeruginosa, Enterobacteriaceae.*

- Fungal (rare)
  - Aspergillus, Nocardia.
- Parasitic (rare)
  - *Entamoeba histolytica.*

Pathology

- By definition a lung abscess is more than 2 cm in diameter and has a wall of variable thickness. The abscess cavity is usually filled with purulent secretions.
- Posterior segments of the right upper lobe and apical segments of the lower lobe of both lungs are affected commonly after aspiration. Abscesses due to other mechanisms may involve any segment. An abscess usually communicates with a bronchus.

Clinical Features

- Patients usually present with high-grade fever with chills and rigors. Cough with purulent sputum, dyspnea and chest pain are usually present. Hemoptysis may also be present.
- Physical examination may show clubbing in chronic lung abscess. There may be amphoric or cavernous bronchial breath sounds over the cavity. Crepitations and pleural rub may be heard.

Investigations

- Blood count shows polymorphonuclear leukocytosis.
- X-ray chest shows the abscess cavity with fluid level.
- CT scan (gold standard): Defines abscess size, location, and rule out malignancy. Also differentiates lung abscess from loculated empyema.
- Gram's stain and culture of sputum or bronchial aspirate can identify the causative organism.
- Blood cultures (if sepsis is suspected).
- Bronchoscopy is indicated if foreign body or tumor is suspected.

Complications

- Bronchopleural fistula and empyema formation.
- Pericarditis.

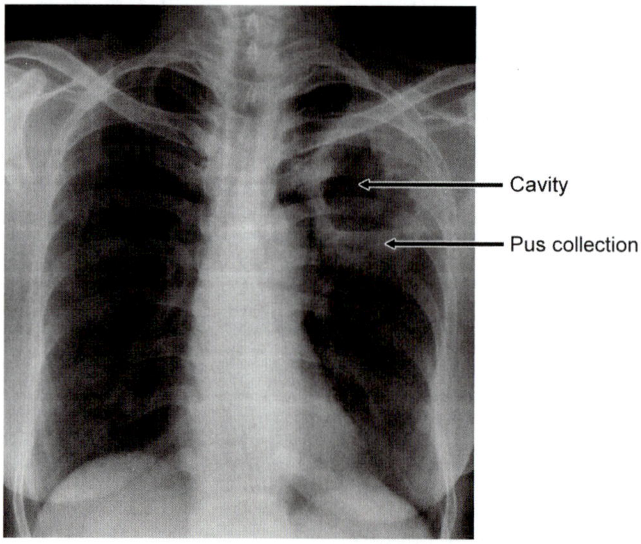

Figure 2.23: Lung abscess (X-ray view)

- Massive hemoptysis.
- Metastatic infection (brain abscess, purulent meningitis).
- Secondary amyloidosis may develop in chronic lung abscess.

Treatment

- Intravenous clindamycin or amoxicillin-clavulanate can be used as initial therapy pending organism identification. Penicillin plus metronidazole is another option especially if aspiration is suspected.
- Lung abscess which develops in hospital are usually caused by *Klebsiella pneumoniae*, *Pseudomonas aeruginosa*, *S. aureus* and anaerobes, and require treatment with a combination of a third-generation cephalosporin, aminoglycoside and metronidazole.
- Antibiotic therapy should be continued until radiographic resolution of the abscess cavity is demonstrated. Usually, 4–6 weeks of therapy is required.
- Physiotherapy in the form of postural drainage can help clear the secretions.
- Chronic abscesses not responding to medical therapy require surgical resection.

Q. Describe the etiology, pathogenesis, clinical features, diagnosis and management of pulmonary tuberculosis.

Q. Describe the etiology, pathogenesis, clinical features, diagnosis and management of post primary (reactivation) pulmonary tuberculosis.

Q. Antituberculous drugs.

Q. Newer methods of diagnosis of tuberculosis.

Q. Sequelae of tuberculosis.

- Tuberculosis is a chronic infectious disease caused by *Mycobacterium tuberculosis*. It is one of the oldest infections known. It usually affects the lungs, although in up to one-third of cases other organs are involved. Tuberculosis is curable if properly treated. Untreated disease can be fatal within 5 years in more than half of cases.

Etiology

- *M. tuberculosis* is a rod-shaped, non-spore-forming, aerobic bacterium. Robert Koch discovered this bacillus.
- They do not take up Gram's stain because of the high lipid content, but can be stained by the Ziehl-Neelsen stain. After staining with Z-N stain they resist decolorization with acid. That is why they are also known as acid fast bacilli.
- Acid fastness is mainly due to the organism's high content of mycolic acids, long-chain cross-linked fatty acids, and other cell-wall lipids. Other microorganisms which are acid fast are Nocardia, Rhodococcus, *Legionella micdadei*, Isospora, and Cryptosporidium.
- Mycobacteria are rapidly destroyed by sunlight and ultraviolet light. But if protected from sunlight they can survive for weeks to months. Tubercle bacilli in milk are killed by pasteurization.

Epidemiology

- According to the WHO, there were 10.6 million new cases of tuberculosis worldwide in 2022 and 1.3 million deaths. India is the highest TB burden country with an estimated 2.7 million tuberculosis (TB) cases, as of 2023. It is estimated that about 40% of the Indian population is infected with TB bacteria, the vast majority of whom have latent rather than active TB. Recent data on global trends indicate that incidence is falling in most regions.
- The incidence of tuberculosis is highest among adult men than women. The risk increases in the elderly, due to waning immunity and comorbidity.
- Genetic factors also play a role in innate non-immune resistance to infection with *M. tuberculosis*. Hence, susceptibility to tuberculosis differs in different populations.

Pathogenesis (Fig. 2.24)

- TB spreads via airborne droplets containing *M. tuberculosis* bacilli, expelled when an infected person coughs, sneezes, or speaks.
- The risk of infection is directly related to the duration and intensity of exposure to air contaminated with infected droplets. Patients whose sputum is smear-positive can have up to 1 lakh organisms per ml of sputum and are highly infectious. Respiratory secretions aerosolized by coughing, sneezing or talking are sufficiently small (1–10 μ) and can remain suspended for long periods. A cough can produce 3000 infectious droplet nuclei. Talking for 5 minutes can also produce similar number of droplets, and sneezing produces more droplets. A single droplet is sufficient to infect a person if prolonged exposure is there. In hospital wards, six air changes per hour eliminate infectiousness; hence, good ventilation is important to prevent infection.
- Majority of inhaled droplet nuclei containing bacilli are trapped in the upper airways and expelled by ciliated mucosal cells. Some bacilli reach the alveoli. There, alveolar macrophages phagocytose the bacilli. Now two things can happen. Either macrophages kill the bacilli and clear the infection or the bacilli multiply within macrophages and kill the macrophages. There are many mechanisms by which the bacilli can survive inside macrophages without getting killed. Other cells residing in alveoli such as dendritic cells and monocytes also put up resistance against bacilli. Dendritic cells in the alveoli migrate to local lymph nodes to activate T-helper cells.
- If bacilli multiply within macrophages, then, macrophages produce cytokines (TNF-α, IL-12, IFN-γ) to recruit more immune cells such natural killer (NK) cells, dendritic cells (DC), neutrophils, and macrophages to the site of infection. TNF alpha released by macrophages also induces differentiation of monocytes into epithelioid histiocyte cells. Some of these epithelioid histiocyte cells fuse to form giant cells. All these cells (NK cells, B cells, giant cells, dendritic cells, neutrophils, macrophage, foam cells, and epithelioid macrophages) surround the bacilli and form a nodular granulomatous structure called the granuloma (tuberculoma) with caseating center made of necrotic cells. The granuloma is a prison to wall off the bacteria from spreading systemically. This initial granuloma is usually located in the subpleural regions of the lower part of the upper lobe or upper part of the lower lobe of the lung, and is called **Ghon focus**. M. tuberculosis spreads via lymphatics to the hilar and paratracheal lymph nodes where it also induces granuloma formation and lymph node enlargement. **Ghon focus** (the primary site of infection in the lung parenchyma) **plus involvement of regional lymph nodes** (hilar and paratracheal lymph nodes) together **is called Ghon complex**. *M. tuberculosis* also induces the macrophage to express and secrete vascular endothelial growth factor (VEGF) into the extracellular spaces. VEGF induces growth of new blood vessels into the granuloma so that immune cells can reach the granuloma and kill the bacilli.
- The granuloma may remain like this for years or may progress further within few days. If the granuloma remains without any clinical manifestation, it is called latent TB infection since the bacilli may remain dormant within the granulomas. However, it has been suggested to use the term 'persister' instead of 'latent TB' since the bacilli may remain active during this "latent" stage.
- While all these things are going on in the lung tissue at the intial site of infection (phagocytosis of bacilli, granuloma formation, etc.), the dendritic cells which have migrated to local lymph nodes activate T-cells (CD4 cells) residing at lymph nodes. Now the T cells start differentiating and become ready to attack the bacilli which is called cell mediated immunity which is very important in containing and controlling bacilli. But this second line of defense from T-cells may take 3 weeks or more. Within these 3 weeks, bacilli would have extensively multiplied and potentially spread to other organs. In HIV patients, due to reduced CD4 count, TB is a common infection.
- If the granuloma progresses further manifesting with clinical illness without becoming latent TB, it is called as **primary TB** and is common among children in the first few years of life and among immunocompromised persons.
- If the latent TB persists for many years and then reactivates to produce clinical features, it is called **secondary or post-primary TB**, which, because of frequent cavitation, is more often infectious than is primary disease. This reactivation can occur due to waning immunity in old age, HIV infection, or use of immunosuppressive drugs.

Risk Factors for Developing Reactivation (also known secondary or post-primary TB)

- HIV infection
- Silicosis
- Chronic renal failure/hemodialysis
- Diabetes

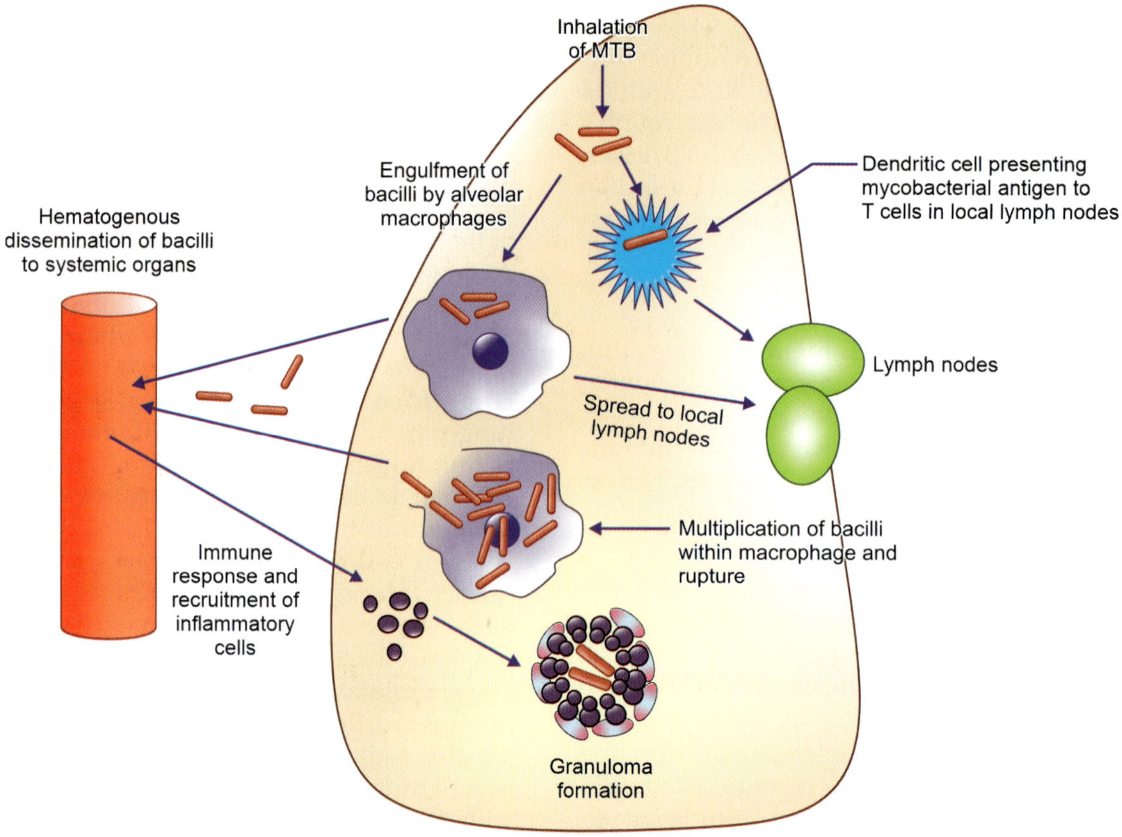

Figure 2.24: Pathogenesis of TB

- IV drug use
- Immunosuppressive treatment
- Tobacco smoking
- Malnutrition

Clinical Features

- Manifestations of pulmonary tuberculosis (TB) can be divided into three stages; primary tuberculosis, latent tuberculosis, and reactivated (secondary) tuberculosis.

Primary Tuberculosis

- Fever is the most common symptom. It is usually low grade, often worse in the evening. and can last for weeks to months.
- Night sweats: Profuse sweating, especially during sleep.
- Weight loss: Due to chronic inflammation and increased catabolism.
- Dry cough initially which may become productive later.
- Fatigue and malaise: Weakness due to prolonged illness.
- Loss of appetite: Contributes to weight loss. Pleuritic chest pain and pleural effusion can be present.
- The physical examination is usually normal but signs of pleural effusion may be present.

Latent TB (immune control of infection)

- Asymptomatic (no active disease).
- No transmission risk.
- Can reactivate if immunity weakens (HIV, diabetes, malnutrition, corticosteroid use).

Secondary (reactivation or post primary) TB

- Secondary TB accounts for most of the adult cases. It results from reactivation of a previously dormant focus acquired at the time of the initial infection. It affects apical posterior segments commonly.
- Symptoms begin insidiously and include cough, weight loss and fatigue, fever and night sweats. Patients may present with only fever and night sweats without cough. Pleuritic chest pain, dyspnea and hemoptysis are also reported by some patients. Pleuritic chest pain signifies inflammation abutting or invading the pleura. Cavity formation is more common with secondary TB. Dyspnea occurs when there is extensive parenchymal involvement, pleural effusion, or a pneumothorax. Pleural effusion can progress to frank empyema.
- Initially cough may be dry. But as the disease progresses, cough becomes productive with yellow or yellow-green sputum. Frank hemoptysis, due to caseous sloughing or endobronchial erosion, typically is present later in the disease and is rarely massive.
- Physical findings include weight loss, signs of pleural effusion, crepitations and signs of consolidation if large areas are involved. Amphoric breath sounds may be heard over cavities. Clubbing may be present.

Endobronchial Tuberculosis

- Endobronchial tuberculosis may develop by direct extension to the bronchi from an adjacent parenchymal focus such as cavity, or spread of organisms to the bronchi through infected sputum.

- Endobronchial TB can cause obstruction, atelectasis, bronchiectasis, and tracheal or bronchial stenosis.
- Symptoms of endobronchial TB include cough with sputum and hemoptysis.
- Physical findings include diminished breath sounds, rhonchi or wheezing due to narrowing of bronchus.

Summary of Clinical Features

Feature	Primary TB	Latent TB	Secondary TB
Fever	Mild, low-grade	None	High, persistent
Cough	Dry or mild	None	Chronic, productive
Hemoptysis	Rare	None	Common
Weight loss	Mild	None	Severe
Night sweats	Occasional	None	Frequent
Chest pain	Sometimes	None	Common (pleuritic)
Hilar lymphadenopathy	Common	None	Rare
Cavitary lesions	Absent	None	Common
Contagious	Yes	No	Yes

Diagnosis

- ***Chest X-ray:*** in primary tuberculosis it may show pleural effusion, pulmonary infiltrates usually on right side and perihilar region, and hilar lymphadenopathy (Ghon complex). In post primary tuberculosis it may show cavities, hilar adenopathy and fibrosis. In miliary TB, numerous small, millet-seed-like nodules are seen.
- ***CT scan chest:*** Provides more detailed visualization of cavitary lesions, fibrosis, and pleural involvement.
- ***Microscopy:*** Sputum is stained by **Ziehl-Neelsen (ZN) stain**. At least three sputum samples should be tested. *Mycobacterium tuberculosis* are visible as red bacilli. Demonstration of acid-fast bacilli on sputum smear does not confirm the diagnosis of tuberculosis, since non tuberculous mycobacteria may colonize the airways or cause pulmonary disease. Cultures of sputum for *M. tuberculosis* is diagnostic. **Fluorescent Auramine-Rhodamine stain** is more sensitive than Ziehl-Neelsen. In patients who do not produce sputum or those whose sputum is negative for AFB but still TB is suspected, fiberoptic bronchoscopy can be used to obtain specimens. Through fiberoptic bronchoscopy, bronchial washings are obtained and tested for AFB. Fiberoptic bronchoscopy can also diagnose endobronchial TB and biopsies also can be obtained. Early morning aspiration of gastric contents after an overnight fast is an alternative to bronchoscopy. Gastric aspirates are suitable only for culture and not for stained smear, because non tuberculous mycobacteria may be present in the stomach in the absence of tuberculous infection.
- ***Culture (gold standard test):*** Tubercle bacilli grow slowly in culture. Hence it may take 6–8 weeks to grow them in solid media (Löwenstein-Jensen (LJ) medium). Liquid culture media (*BACTEC*) may allow detection of mycobacterial growth in as little as several days. Once *M. tuberculosis* is grown in culture drug sensitivity tests also can be done to rule out MDR TB. Sensitivity testing is done when a treatment regimen is failing, and when sputum cultures remain positive even after 3 months of therapy. *M. tuberculosis* may sometimes be cultured in blood of 15% of patients with tuberculosis. Pleural fluid cultures for *M. tuberculosis* are positive only rarely.
- ***Histopathology:*** In patients with TB pleural effusion, needle biopsy of the pleura reveals granulomas in 50% of patients.
- ***Serologic tests:*** demonstration of IgG antibody against mycobacterial antigens by ELISA. This test is not done routinely.
- ***Adenosine deaminase (ADA):*** ADA level of >50 U/L in pleural fluid is highly suggestive of tuberculous pleural effusion.
- ***PPD skin testing (Montoux test):*** In the absence of a history of BCG vaccination, a positive skin test provides additional support for the diagnosis of tuberculosis.
- ***Drug susceptibility testing:*** Universal DST is considered by the WHO as the current standard of care for all TB patients and should consist of DST to at least rifampin for all initial isolates of *M. tuberculosis*, as rifampin resistance is an excellent proxy for MDR-TB diagnosis.

Newer Methods of Diagnosis of Tuberculosis

- **IFN-gamma release assays (IGRA):** These assays measure T cell release of IFN-gamma in response to stimulation with TB-specific antigens. A positive test result suggests that *M. tuberculosis* infection is likely; a negative result suggests that infection is unlikely. An indeterminate result indicates an uncertain likelihood of *M. tuberculosis* infection. There are two commercially available kits T-SPOT.TB and QuantiFERON-TB Gold. IGRAs are more specific than tuberculin test because of less cross reactivity due to BCG vaccination and infection by nontuberculous mycobacteria. IGRA does not help differentiate latent tuberculosis infection from active tuberculosis.
- **Nucleic acid-based tests:** These are based on the detection of DNA of mycobacterium TB. The available tests in this category are: Line probe Assay (LPA), CB-NAAT (cartridge based nucleic acid amplification test, and TrueNat.
- ***Line probe Assay (LPA):*** LPA is a rapid technique based on polymerase chain reaction (PCR) that is used to detect *Mycobacterium tuberculosis* and its sensitivity to rifampicin and isoniazid. LPA can be used for testing culture isolates as well as AFB smears.
- ***CB-NAAT (cartridge based nucleic acid amplification test):*** this test is marketed as GeneXpert and the kits are manufactured by a California based company. CB-NAAT is an automated cartridge-based molecular

technique which not only detects *Mycobacterium tuberculosis* but also rifampicin resistance within two hours and has been endorsed by WHO for rapid diagnosis of tuberculosis.

- ***TrueNat:*** This is **real-time PCR-based molecular test** for the rapid diagnosis of **tuberculosis (TB)** and **rifampicin (RIF) resistance**. It is similar to CB-NAAT. It is developed by a Bengaluru based Indian company and can diagnose TB within 3 hours as well as test for resistance to Rifampicin. It is a portable, battery-operated device–suitable for decentralized testing (district and primary healthcare centers). The sensitivity and specificity of TrueNAT test is equal to CB-NAAT. Due to the portability of its battery-powered testing platform, test can be done even at remote places. ICMR has recommended the use of TrueNat for diagnosis of TB and for detecting resistance to Rifampicin. In view of the recommendations of ICMR and the ease of use of TrueNat in peripheral settings, it has been planned to use this test across the country.
- ***TB-LAMP (Loop-mediated isothermal amplification):*** This is a rapid, molecular-based test for tuberculosis (TB) detection. It is endorsed by the World Health Organization (WHO) as an alternative to sputum smear microscopy, particularly in resource-limited settings. Detects *Mycobacterium tuberculosis* complex (MTBC) DNA. Faster than culture and smear microscopy—results available in <1 hour. Highly sensitive—detects both smear-positive and smear-negative TB cases. Does not require sophisticated lab equipment—works at a constant temperature (isothermal). Can be performed by non-specialist staff. Disadvantages of TB-LAMP is that it cannot detect drug resistance, and false positives may occur in some cases.

Treatment of Tuberculosis (TB)

- The two main aims of TB treatment are (1) to prevent morbidity and death by curing TB while preventing recurrences and emergence of drug resistance, and (2) to interrupt transmission by rendering patients noninfectious to others.

Antituberculous Drugs

- There are five main first-line drugs for the treatment of tuberculosis: Isoniazid, rifampin, pyrazinamide, ethambutol, and streptomycin (HRZES). Note that streptomycin is put under first line drugs by WHO whereas it is put under second line drugs by CDC (centre for disease control).
- Rifampicin, Isoniazid, and streptomycin are bactericidal. Pyrazinamide and ethambutol are bacteriostatic.
- The treatment regimen usually consists of initial intensive treatment for 2 months followed by 4–6 months of continuation phase. Initial phase includes 4 or more drugs and continuation phase 2 or more drugs.

First-line Drugs

See **Table 2.24**.

Second-line Drugs Used in MDR TB

See **Table 2.25**.

- Three new TB drugs, bedaquiline, delamanid, and pretomanid have become available. These are recommended by the World Health Organization (WHO) for the treatment of drug-resistant TB along with other drugs.

TABLE 2.24: First-line drugs

Drug	Mechanism of action	Dose/day	Side effects
Isoniazid	Inhibition of mycolic acid synthesis. It also disrupts DNA, lipid, carbohydrate synthesis and metabolism	5 mg/kg	Hepatitis, peripheral neuropathy, drug fever
Rifampicin	Inhibits bacterial DNA-dependent RNA polymerase	10 mg/kg	Hepatitis, flu-like syndrome, thrombocytopenia (rare)
Ethambutol	Exact mechanism unknown. Thought to inhibit the synthesis of arabinogalactan, a mycobacterial cell wall constituent	15 mg/kg	Optic neuritis
Pyrazinamide	Inhibits fatty acid synthetase-I (FASI) of *M. tuberculosis*	25 mg/kg	Hepatitis, hyperuricemia

TABLE 2.25: Second-line drugs used in MDR TB

Group	Drugs
Group A: Drugs to be prioritized and included in all regimens, unless they cannot be used.	Levofloxacin or moxifloxacin Bedaquiline Linezolid
Group B: Drugs to be added in all regimens, unless they cannot be used.	Clofazimine Cycloserine or terizidone
Group C: Drugs to be used to complete the regimen and when drugs from groups A and B cannot be used.	Delamanid Imipenem-cilastatin or meropenem Amikacin or streptomycin Ethionamide or prothionamide p-Aminosalicylic acid

Treatment of Tuberculosis

The treatment of tuberculosis (TB) depends on whether the infection is:

- ***Drug-susceptible TB (DS-TB):*** Treated with first-line anti-TB drugs.
- ***Multidrug-resistant TB (MDR-TB)*** and extensively drug-resistant TB (XDR-TB): Requires second-line drugs and longer treatment.
- ***Latent TB infection (LTBI):*** Requires preventive therapy to stop progression to active TB.

Treatment of drug-susceptible TB (DS-TB)

- The WHO-recommended treatment for drug-sensitive pulmonary TB includes:

Standard first-line treatment (6 months regimen)

- **Intensive phase (first 2 months): HRZE daily**
  - H–Isoniazid (INH)
  - R–Rifampicin (RIF)
  - Z–Pyrazinamide (PZA)
  - E–Ethambutol (EMB)
- **Continuation phase (next 4 months): HR daily**
  - H–Isoniazid
  - R–Rifampicin

Shorter regimen (4 months)

WHO has approved a shorter 4-month TB regimen using rifapentine (RPT) and moxifloxacin (MFX) in some cases.

- **Intensive phase:** 2 months of daily administration of:
  - Isoniazid (H)
  - Rifapentine (P)
  - Moxifloxacin (M)
  - Pyrazinamide (Z)
- **Continuation phase:** 2 months of daily administration of:
  - Isoniazid (H)
  - Rifapentine (P)

DOTS (Directly Observed Treatment-short Course)

- Treatment default is a major problem in TB treatment. To improve this DOTS has been designed. DOTS is defined as "observation of the patient by a health care provider or other responsible person as the patient ingests anti-TB medications." Drugs can be given only two or three times per week.
- Standard 6 months regimen consisting of 2 months intensive phase and 4 months of continuation phase is given.
- Although DOTS programs require significant resources, they are very effective. DOTS programs have been found to improve cure rate while decreasing the incidence of drug resistance and treatment failure.
- The Center for Disease Control and Prevention (CDC) and the American Thoracic Society (ATS) recommend that DOTS be considered for all patients.

DOTS-Plus

- DOTS-Plus is an extension of the DOTS strategy designed to treat multidrug-resistant TB (MDR-TB) using second-line anti-TB drugs. It ensures proper drug administration, adherence monitoring, and drug resistance management.
- Duration of treatment is typically 9–24 months, depending on drug resistance.

Monitoring Treatment

- Monitoring tuberculosis (TB) treatment is essential to assess treatment response, detect drug resistance early, and prevent relapse or failure. The WHO recommends a structured monitoring approach that includes clinical, microbiological, and radiological assessments.

Clinical Monitoring

Symptom improvement

- Fever, cough, weight loss, and night sweats should gradually improve within the first 2 months. Persistent or worsening symptoms may indicate treatment failure or drug resistance.

Weight gain

- A steady increase in weight suggests good response to treatment. Failure to gain weight may indicate malabsorption, poor adherence, or treatment failure.

Drug side effect monitoring:

- Rifampicin → hepatitis, flu-like syndrome
- Isoniazid → Peripheral neuropathy, hepatitis
- Pyrazinamide → hepatitis, joint pain
- Ethambutol → Optic neuritis (blurred vision, color blindness)
- The most important side effect of ATT is hepatitis. Baseline LFT should be done for all patients before starting ATT. LFT should be monitored monthly thereafter. Up to 20% of patients have small increases in AST (aspartate aminotransferase) up to three times the upper limit of normal without any symptoms. This is of no consequence. For patients with symptomatic hepatitis and those with marked (five to six-fold) elevations in serum levels of AST, treatment should be stopped and drugs reintroduced one at a time after liver function tests have returned to normal.
- Pyrazinamide should be stopped if the patient develops gouty arthritis. Individuals who develop autoimmune thrombocytopenia secondary to rifampicin should not receive the drug thereafter. Similarly, the occurrence of optic neuritis with ethambutol is an indication for permanent discontinuation of this drug

Sputum Testing

Sputum microscopy

- Performed at month 2, 5, and 6 (or end of treatment).
- Persistent AFB positivity at month 2 may indicate poor treatment response. AFB smear becomes negative little later than culture due to the presence of dead bacilli in the sputum.
- Smear-positive at month 5 → Treatment failure (switch to MDR-TB regimen).
- AFB smear and culture is difficult in patients with extrapulmonary tuberculosis. In these cases, the response to treatment should be assessed clinically or radiologically.

Sputum culture (for drug-resistant TB monitoring)

- More sensitive than smear microscopy.
- Should be negative by month 2–3. Persistent positivity suggests treatment failure.

CB-NAAT (GeneXpert)/Line probe assay (LPA)

- Detects drug resistance early (e.g. rifampicin/Isoniazid resistance).
- WHO recommends using CB-NAAT if sputum remains positive at month 2 or 5.

Chest X-ray

- Can be done at end of treatment (month 6 or 9, depending on the regimen) to assess resolution of lung lesions. Serial chest radiographs are not recommended to monitor response to treatment, as radiographic changes may lag behind bacteriologic response

Treatment Failure and Relapse

- As mentioned above, MDR TB should be suspected when a patient's sputum smear and cultures remain positive after 2 months (i.e. at the end of intensive phase).
- When sputum smear and cultures remain positive even at the end of 5 months, it indicates treatment failure. In such cases approach should be as for MDR TB.

Special Considerations in TB Treatment

- TB-HIV Co-Infection: Antiretroviral therapy (ART) should be started within 2 weeks of TB treatment if CD4 <50 or within 8 weeks if CD4 >50. Rifampicin interacts with ART (alternative drugs like Rifabutin may be used).
- TB in pregnancy: HRZE regimen is safe in pregnancy. Avoid Streptomycin (SM) due to ototoxicity in the fetus.
- Extrapulmonary TB (EPTB) treatment: Same regimen as pulmonary TB, but duration may be extended to 9–12 months for TB meningitis, bone TB, and disseminated TB.

Sequelae of Pulmonary Tuberculosis

- Fibrosis and destruction of the lung
- Bronchiectasis
- Lung abscess
- Aspergilloma (fungal ball)
- Scar carcinoma
- Chronic respiratory failure and cor pulmonale
- Chronic tuberculous empyema and fibrothorax
- Amyloidosis

Prevention

- *Early diagnosis and treatment:* TB should be diagnosed and treated early in order to prevent deterioration of the disease and spread of the infection.
- *Examination of close contacts:* The close contacts of TB patients, usually the household contacts, should be examined. Tuberculin skin testing and/or chest x-ray examination is done for close contacts.
- *Leading a healthy life style:* Smoking and alcohol intake should be stopped. Balanced diet should be taken. Adequate exercise, enough rest and sleep should be encouraged.
- *Chemoprophylaxis:* For household contacts of TB patients and those with AIDS infection and Hodgkin's lymphoma, Isoniazid, 300 mg/day for 1 year, can reduce the incidence of tuberculosis.
- *BCG (Bacille Calmette-Guerin) vaccination:* All newborn babies should be vaccinated to protect them against tuberculosis.

Q. MDR tuberculosis.

- Multidrug-resistant tuberculosis (MDR-TB) refers to tuberculosis resistant to both isoniazid and rifampicin.
- Primary drug-resistance occurs in a patient who has never received antituberculosis therapy. Secondary resistance refers to the development of resistance during or following chemotherapy, for what had previously been drug-susceptible tuberculosis.

Diagnosis

- Sputum should be sent for culture and sensitivity. Nowadays WHO recommends universal drug susceptibility testing for all patients in the beginning of treatment so that we can know whether a patient has drug resistant TB from the beginning itself. If a patient cannot produce sputum, sputum induction should be done by hypertonic saline nebulization. If an adequate sample is still not produced, bronchoscopy may be used to obtain sputum samples or other specimens. In extrapulmonary tuberculosis, samples of involved tissue (e.g. lymph nodes, bone, blood) should be obtained for culture and sensitivity testing as well as pathology.
- Susceptibility testing for first-and second-line agents should be performed at a reliable reference laboratory.
- Features which suggest drug-resistant tuberculosis are:
  - Previous treatment for active tuberculosis
  - Tuberculosis treatment failure or relapse in a patient with advanced HIV infection
  - Contact with a case of drug-resistant tuberculosis
  - Failure to respond to empiric therapy

Treatment of TB Resistant only to Isoniazid

- Rifampicin + pyrazinamide+ ethambutol + levofloxacin (RZEL) for 6-months. If fluoroquinolone is contraindicated use only first three drugs (RZE) for 6 months.

Treatment of Rifampicin Resistant TB (RR-TB) and MDR-TB

- MDR TB should be managed by medical personnel with expertise and experience in treating such cases. Laboratory facilities to document drug susceptibility and monitor response should be available.

- When MDR TB is suspected, sputum for culture and drug susceptibility testing (DST) should be sent and patient should be started on empirical MDR regimen till the DST results are available.
- Usually longer regimens are used in the treatment of RRTB and MDR TB.

Regimens for Rifampicin Resistant TB (RRTB) and MDR-TB

Longer MDR-TB Regimen (duration of 18–20 months)

- All three group A agents and at least one group B agent should be included to ensure that treatment starts with at least four effective drugs and at least three drugs are included for the rest of the treatment after bedaquiline is stopped.
- If only one or two group A agents are used, both group B agents are to be included.
- If the regimen cannot be composed with agents from groups A and B alone, group C agents are added to complete it.

Regimen composition

- Bedaquiline (BDQ)
- Levofloxacin (LFX) or Moxifloxacin (MFX) (Fluoroquinolone)
- Linezolid (LZD)
- Clofazimine (CFZ)
- Cycloserine (Cs) or terizidone (Trd)

Alternative drugs (if needed)

- Delamanid (DLM)–If BDQ is unavailable.
- Ethambutol (E), pyrazinamide (Z), or amikacin (Am)–If necessary.

Shorter MDR-TB Regimen (9–11 months)

- This is all-oral, bedaquiline-containing regimen.
- Preferred if there is no resistance to fluoroquinolones.
- Regimen composition

Intensive phase (4–6 months duration, 7 drugs)

- Bedaquiline (BDQ) (first 6 months)
- Levofloxacin (LFX) or Moxifloxacin (MFX) (fluoroquinolone)
- Linezolid (LZD)
- Clofazimine (CFZ)
- Pyrazinamide (Z)
- Ethambutol (E)
- Isoniazid (high-dose) (Hh) or ethionamide (Eto)

Continuation phase (5 months duration)

- All the above drugs without bedaquiline (BDQ)

Monitoring of Patients on MDR Regimen

- Close monitoring is essential during treatment of MDR-TB patients. To assess treatment response, sputum smears and cultures should be done monthly until smear and culture conversion. (Conversion is defined as two consecutive negative smears and cultures taken 30 days apart.) After conversion, monitoring is at least monthly for smears and quarterly for cultures.

Surgery

- Surgery can be considered in patients with sputum cultures positive for longer than three months despite appropriate therapy or with isolates resistant to all of the first-line oral agents. Patients with localized pulmonary disease, which can be completely removed at operation, are most likely to benefit from surgery. However drugs should be continued for at least 18 months after surgery.

Q. XDR tuberculosis.

Q. Pre-XDR TB.

- Extensively drug-resistant tuberculosis (XDR-TB) refers to tuberculosis resistant to at least isoniazid, rifampicin, fluoroquinolones, and one of the second line injectable drugs.
- Pre-XDR TB is MDR-TB + resistance to fluoroquinolones (but sensitive to injectables).
- XDR-TB is harder to treat and requires specialized regimens with newer drugs.
- WHO now recommends all-oral regimens (BPaL for XDR-TB) to avoid toxic injectables.

WHO-recommended Treatment for XDR-TB

Regimen	Drugs used	Duration
BPaL (new preferred regimen)	Bedaquiline (Bdq) + Pretomanid (Pa) + Linezolid (Lzd)	6–9 months
Longer individualized regimen	Based on drug susceptibility	18–24 months

Prevention of XDR-TB

- Strict DOTS therapy: Ensure correct TB treatment from the start.
- Rapid testing (GeneXpert, LPA): Detect resistance early.
- Infection control in hospitals and prisons.
- Avoid unnecessary use of second-line drugs to prevent resistance.

Q. Latent TB infection (LTBI)

- Latent TB is a condition where a person is infected with *Mycobacterium tuberculosis* (*M. tb*) but does not have active disease. The bacteria remain dormant (inactive) in the body, and the person does not show symptoms or spread TB to others.
- Can become active TB if the immune system weakens (HIV, diabetes, immunosuppressive drugs).

Diagnosis of Latent TB

- Absence of clinical symptoms.
- Lab tests: There are two main tests to detect latent TB: tuberculin skin test (Mantoux test), and interferon-gamma release assay (IGRA)
  - Mantoux test: Involves injection of purified protein derivative (PPD) intradermally. If the reaction (induration of skin) is ≥10–15 mm after 48–72 hours, it is considered as positive for latent TB. However, this test cannot distinguish between latent and active TB.
  - Interferon-gamma release assay (IGRA): IGRA is a blood test used to detect latent tuberculosis infection (LTBI) by measuring the release of interferon gamma by immune system's response to *Mycobacterium tuberculosis* antigens. It is an alternative to the Tuberculin Skin Test (TST) and is more specific, especially in BCG-vaccinated

individuals. Types of IGRA tests available are QuantiFERON-TB Gold Plus (QFT-Plus) and T-SPOT.TB Test

- Chest X-ray (Done if Montoux or IGRA is positive): Normal in latent TB (used to rule out active TB).

Treatment of LTBI

Treatment is given to prevent development of active TB. It is recommended for: close contacts of TB patients, HIV-positive individuals, and immunocompromised patients (e.g. diabetes, cancer, transplant recipients).

WHO-recommended LTBI Treatment Regimens

Regimen	Drugs	Duration	Dosing frequency
1HP	Rifapentine + Isoniazid	**1 month**	Once weekly
3HP	Rifapentine + Isoniazid	**3 months**	Once weekly
3HR	Rifampicin + Isoniazid	**3 months**	Daily
4R	Rifampicin	**4 months**	Daily

Q. DOTS (directly observed therapy-short course).

- DOTS is an internationally recommended strategy by WHO to treat TB. DOTS plus is to treat MDR-TB. The WHO-recommended DOTS strategy was launched formally as Revised National TB Control Programme (RNTCP) in India in 1997. Since then, it has played an important role in controlling the incidence and prevalence of TB in India.
- The five key components of DOTS are
  - Political commitment to control TB;
  - Case detection by sputum smear microscopy examination among symptomatic patients;
  - Patients are given anti-TB drugs under the direct observation of the health care provider/community DOT provider;
  - Regular, uninterrupted supply of anti-TB drugs; and
  - Systematic recording and reporting system that allows assessment of treatment results of each and every patient and of whole TB control program.
- In DOTS, the responsibility of ensuring regular and complete treatment of the patient lies with the health system.
- WHO recommends that daily treatment should be used throughout the course of treatment and this has been implemented in India and other countries.
- Recently the effectiveness of DOTS strategy has been questioned because it requires lot of manpower to implement DOTS and also requires multiple visits by the patient to a health care facility. Hence nowadays self-administration of anti TB drugs by the patient is preferred and this is tracked by using latest technologies such as printing a code number on the drug packet which the patient has to send to the healthcare facility.
- National Tuberculosis Elimination Programme (NTEP) (earlier called RNTCP program 0 has now introduced daily regimen for treating TB. For newly diagnosed TB cases, treatment in intensive phase will consist of 2 months of INH, rifampicin, pyrazinamide and ethambutol in daily dosage. This is followed by continuation phase of 4 months where 3 drugs (INH, rifampicin, and ethambutol) are given daily. In the previously treated TB cases, intensive phase will be of 3 months. For the initial 2 months, 5 drugs are used (INH, rifampicin, pyrazinamide and ethambutol plus injection streptomycin). After 2 months, injection streptomycin is stopped and the remaining 4 drugs are given daily for another 1 month. Continuation phase will be for 5 months consisting of 3 drugs daily (INH, rifampicin, and ethambutol).

Q. Classification of TB based on treatment history (WHO/NTEP Classification) (Table 2.26).

TABLE 2.26: Classification of TB based on treatment history

Type	Definition
New TB case	Patient **never treated for TB** or received treatment for **less than 1 month.**
Previously treated TB case	Patient who has received TB treatment for **more than 1 month.**
Relapse TB	Patient previously **declared cured** but develops TB again!
Treatment after failure	Patient whose TB treatment **failed (positive sputum after treatment completion).**
Treatment after lost to follow-up (TALF)	Patient who **stopped TB treatment for at least 2 months** and returns with TB.
Other previously treated cases	Patients who **do not fit the above categories** (e.g. patients transferred from another center).

- New and relapse TB cases are started on first-line drugs unless resistance is detected.

Q. Tuberculin skin test (Montoux test).

- The Mantoux tuberculin skin test (TST) is a diagnostic tool used to detect latent TB infection (LTBI) or active TB disease in some cases. It measures the immune response to purified protein derivative (PPD) injected into the skin.

Principle of the Test

- The test works by detecting a delayed-type hypersensitivity (DTH) reaction to *Mycobacterium tuberculosis* antigens in previously exposed individuals. If the immune system has encountered TB before, T-cells respond to PPD by releasing cytokines, causing a localized skin reaction.

Doing the Test

- The Mantoux test is done by intradermal injection of 0.1 ml of PPD (purified protein derivative) into the volar aspect of the forearm using a 27-gauge needle.

Interpretation of Test

- Test is read after 48–72 hours. If the test is positive an induration surrounded by erythema is formed. The maximum diameter of the induration (not redness) is recorded and interpreted as follows:

> 15 mm or ulceration-strongly positive
> 10 mm-positive
5 to 9 mm-indeterminate
< 5 mm-negative

- Induration of 5 mm or more is considered positive in HIV infected and other immunosuppressed patients.
- Its negative predictive value is higher than positive predictive value. Hence, tuberculin test is more useful to exclude the diagnosis of tuberculosis rather than to diagnose it.
- A positive reaction indicates that the individual has been exposed to Mycobacterium (*M. tuberculosis*) but the individual may or may not be suffering from active disease. A strongly positive test may indicate recent infection. The test is positive in 85% of infected individuals.
- Ten per cent of recent tuberculin converters may develop active disease in their lifetime and 5% do so within the first two years of infection.
- The test is of limited value in the diagnosis of active TB because of its relatively low sensitivity and specificity and its inability to discriminate between latent infection and active disease.
- False-negative results can occur in miliary TB, sarcoidosis, HIV/AIDS, malnutrition, recent viral infections, or immunosuppression.
- False-positive results can occur due to BCG vaccination or exposure to non-TB mycobacteria.

Key Points

- The Mantoux test is a simple, cost-effective screening tool for TB exposure.
- It is useful for detecting latent TB (LTBI) but not reliable for active TB diagnosis.
- IGRA is preferred over Mantoux in BCG-vaccinated individuals.

Q. Miliary tuberculosis.

OR

Q. Disseminated tuberculosis.

- Miliary TB is a severe and disseminated form of tuberculosis where *Mycobacterium tuberculosis* spreads hematogenously (through the bloodstream) to multiple organs, forming tiny, millet-seed-like granulomas throughout the body.
- Miliary TB occurs when TB bacilli escape from a primary lung lesion and spread via the bloodstream.

Risk Factors for Miliary TB

- Immunocompromised patients (HIV/AIDS, malnutrition, diabetes, chemotherapy).
- Children and elderly individuals (weaker immune response).
- Untreated or poorly managed TB cases.
- Chronic diseases (renal failure, organ transplantation).

Clinical Features

General Symptoms

- Fever, night sweats, anorexia, weakness, and weight loss.

Pulmonary Symptoms

- Dry cough or productive cough.
- Breathlessness, respiratory distress.

Extrapulmonary Symptoms (other organs involved)

- Liver involvement: Hepatomegaly, jaundice
- Spleen involvement: Splenomegaly
- CNS involvement (Tuberculous meningitis): Headache, neck stiffness, confusion
- Bone marrow suppression: Anemia, pancytopenia
- Adrenal TB: Addison's disease (adrenal insufficiency).
- Severe cases can present with multiorgan dysfunction.
- Eye examination may show choroidal tubercles.

Diagnosis of Miliary TB

- ***Chest X-ray:*** Often shows "miliary" (diffuse, small, 1–2 mm nodules throughout both lungs.
- ***HRCT chest:*** It has higher sensitivity and specificity than chest radiography in displaying randomly distributed millet seed like lesions.
- ***Ultrasound abdomen:*** May reveal diffuse liver disease, hepatomegaly, splenomegaly, or para-aortic lymph nodes.
- ***Tuberculin test:*** Is frequently negative.
- ***Sputum microscopy:*** Is negative for AFB in most cases.
- ***Bronchoalveolar lavage and transbronchial biopsy:*** May be required in some cases to establish diagnosis.
- ***Liver or bone-marrow biopsy:*** May show tuberculous granulomas.

Treatment

- Military tuberculosis is treated with standard anti-tuberculous therapy.
  - Intensive phase (2 months): HRZE (Isoniazid + Rifampicin + Pyrazinamide + Ethambutol).
  - Continuation phase (4–7 months): HR (Isoniazid + Rifampicin).

Q. Causes of hemoptysis in pulmonary tuberculosis.

- Active tuberculosis.
- Rupture of Rasmussen's aneurysm (arises from bronchial arteries when TB extends into the adventitia and media causing thinning of the vessel wall).
- Post-tubercular bronchiectasis,
- Aspergilloma invading an old healed cavity,
- Scar carcinoma arising from the healed scar of TB.

Q. Fall and rise phenomenon in tuberculosis (TB).

- It is seen in patients who are treated with ineffective antituberculous therapy.
- Initially after the commencement of treatment there is fall in bacterial load and clinical symptoms. Sputum becomes negative on microscopy. Later as the treatment is continued there is again a rise bacterial load and worsening of clinical symptoms. This is called the fall and rise phenomenon.

Causes of the Fall and Rise Phenomenon

- Drug resistance (MDR-TB or XDR-TB): Initial symptom relief due to partial response, but later the patient worsens as ineffective drugs fail to eliminate resistant bacilli.
- Non-adherence to TB treatment: This results in partial bacterial killing, selection of drug-resistant TB strains.
- Paradoxical reaction (immune response to TB killing): TB treatment triggers an exaggerated immune response leading to worsening symptoms (e.g. enlarging lymph nodes, worsening lung lesions).
- Immune reconstitution inflammatory syndrome (IRIS) in HIV-TB: Worsening TB symptoms despite proper treatment (fever, lymph node enlargement, worsening lung lesions).

Management of the Fall and Rise Phenomenon

- For drug resistance: Shift to MDR/XDR-TB regimen (Bedaquiline, Linezolid-based).
- For poor adherence: Enforce DOTS therapy and patient education.
- For paradoxical reactions/IRIS: Continue TB drugs, add steroids if severe.
- Regular follow-up and microbiological monitoring are essential to detect treatment failure early.

Q. Extrapulmonary tuberculosis (EPTB).

- Extrapulmonary tuberculosis (EPTB) is defined as disease outside the lung parenchyma.
- During the initial seeding of infection with *M. tuberculosis*, hematogenous dissemination of bacilli to a number of organs can occur. These localized infections can progress to primary tuberculosis or remain dormant and get activated later. Extrapulmonary tuberculosis, therefore, can either be a presentation of primary or reactivation tuberculosis.
- Extrapulmonary tuberculosis may be generalized or confined to a single organ. Extrapulmonary tuberculosis is found in 15–20% of all tuberculosis cases. The incidence is higher in young children and immunocompromised patients.
- Extrapulmonary sites most commonly involved, in descending order of frequency are
  - Lymph nodes (most common type of EPTB)
  - Pleura
  - Upper airways
  - Genitourinary tract
  - Bones/joints

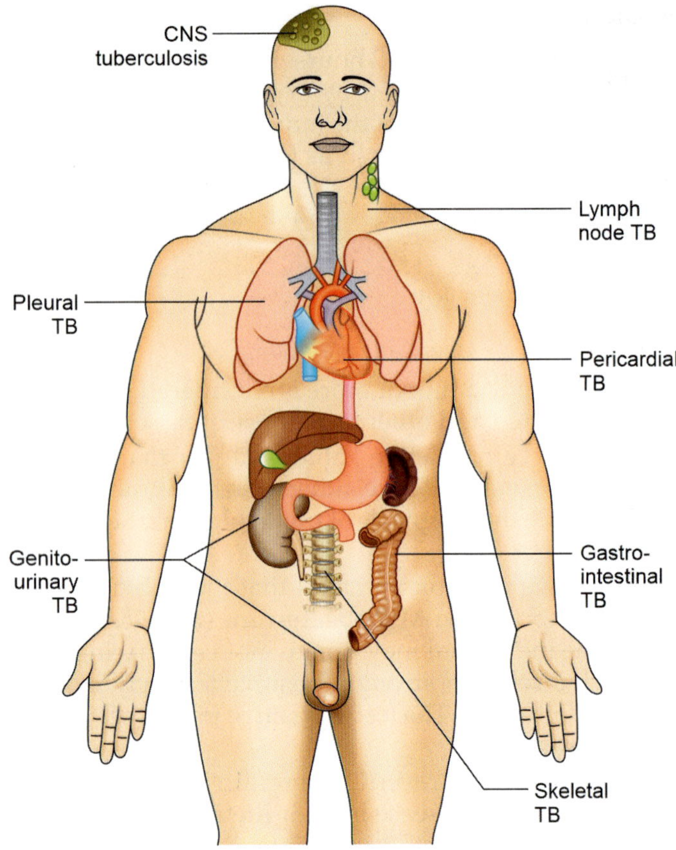

Figure 2.25: Sites of extrapulmonary TB

  - Meninges
  - Peritoneum
  - Pericardium
  - Skin
  - Eyes

Lymph Node TB (Tuberculous Lymphadenitis; Scrofula)

- This is the most common form of EPTB.
- Painless swelling of lymph nodes, usually at cervical and supraclavicular sites. Lymph nodes may be inflamed and tender and may have a fistulous tract to skin draining caseous material. Multiple lymph nodes may get matted together. Systemic symptoms are usually absent except in immunocompromised patients.
- Other lymph nodes which can get involved are axillary, inguinal, mesenteric, and mediastinal lymph nodes.
- Tuberculous mediastinal lymphadenopathy can present with dysphagia, esophageal perforation and vocal cord paralysis due to recurrent laryngeal nerve involvement.

TB Infection in the Pleural Space

- This is the second most common EPTB form.
- Patients usually present with unilateral pleural effusion
- Symptoms include pleuritic chest pain, breathlessness, dry cough, fever, and night sweats.

- Diagnosis is by pleural fluid analysis: Exudative, high protein, lymphocyte-predominant, low glucose, ADA (adenosine deaminase) >40.

TB of Upper Airways (Epiglottis, Pharynx, Larynx)

- It usually occurs as a complication of advanced cavitary pulmonary TB, Clinical features include hoarseness, dysphagia and chronic productive cough.

Genitourinary Tract TB

- Clinical features include increased urinary frequency, dysuria, hematuria, flank pain. In the initial stages patients may be asymptomatic.
- In men, epididymo-orchitis and prostatitis may develop. Sinus tracts may form draining pus externally.
- In women, it may present as pelvic pain, infertility, and menstrual abnormalities.

Skeletal TB

- Weight-bearing joints (spine, hips, and knees—in that order) are involved often.
- Spinal TB (Pott's disease, tuberculous spondylitis) often involves ≥ 2 adjacent vertebral bodies. Upper thoracic spine is affected commonly in children. Lower thoracic and upper lumbar vertebrae are usually affected in adults. Clinical features include back pain, low grade fever and night sweats. Spinal cord compression produces paraplegia. Kyphosis develops in advanced disease due to vertebral body collapse.
- Joint involvement leads to pain and swelling, difficulty in walking.

CNS Tuberculosis

- *Tuberculous meningitis:* It presents as subacute febrile illness which evolves over 1–2 weeks but may present acutely. Clinical features include headache, altered mental status (confusion/lethargy), and neck rigidity. Cranial nerve palsies may be present particularly ocular nerve palsies producing diplopia. Involvement of cerebral arteries (vasculitis) leads to occlusion and focal neurological signs including stroke. Obstructive hydrocephalus can develop due to fibrin deposition in the subarachnoid space.
- *Tuberculoma:* tuberculomas are caseous foci within the substance of the brain that develop from deep-seated tubercles acquired during hematogenous dissemination. They act like intracranial space-occupying lesions (ICSOL) and present with seizures and focal neurological deficits
- *Spinal tuberculous arachnoiditis:* it is characterized by focal inflammatory disease at single or multiple levels in the subarachnoid space producing gradual encasement of the spinal cord by a gelatinous or fibrous exudate. Patients present with signs and symptoms of nerve root and cord compression such as radicular pain, hyperesthesia or paresthesias; lower motor neuron paralysis; and bladder or rectal sphincter dysfunction. Vasculitis may lead to thrombosis of the anterior spinal artery and infarction of the spinal cord.

Gastrointestinal TB

- It can involve bowel or peritoneum.
- Bowel involvement (ileocecal region involved commonly) produces abdominal pain often mimicking appendicitis. Other features are diarrhea, obstruction, hematochezia and palpable abdominal mass. Constitutional symptoms such as fever, weight loss, and night sweats are common. Bowel wall involvement produces ulcerations/fistulae simulating Crohn's disease. Anal fistulae can develop due to rectal involvement.
- Tuberculous peritonitis produces abdominal pain, fever and ascites. The classic doughy abdomen on palpation is rarely observed in tuberculous peritonitis.

Pericardial TB (Tuberculous Pericarditis)

- Onset is usually subacute. Clinical features include fever, retrosternal pain and pericardial friction rub. Pericardial effusion may develop and lead to cardiac tamponade. Constrictive pericarditis may ultimately appear.

Less Common Sites

- Eyes: Chorioretinitis, uveitis, phlyctenular conjunctivitis.
- Tuberculous otitis: Hearing loss, otorrhea, tympanic membrane perforation.
- Skin: Abscesses, chronic ulcers, scrofuloderma, lupus vulgaris, erythema nodosum.
- Adrenal glands: Signs of adrenal insufficiency such as weight loss, weakness, hypotension, hyperpigmentation.

Treatment of Extrapulmonary Tuberculosis

- Treatment of extrapulmonary TB is same as that of pulmonary tuberculosis.

Q. Indications for corticosteroids in tuberculosis treatment.

- There are some situations where steroids are given along with antituberculous therapy (ATT) to improve the final outcome.

Indications

- *Allergic reactions to antituberculosis drugs.*
- *Pericardial tuberculosis*: Reduces inflammation, scarring, amount of effusion and development of constrictive tuberculosis.
- *Tuberculosis of the eye, larynx and ureteric involvement in genitourinary TB*: Reduces inflammation, tissue destruction and scarring.
- *Tuberculous meningitis:* Reduces adhesions, obstructive hydrocephalus and improves final outcome.
- *Adrenal tuberculosis*: Need to replace steroids.
- *Severe Miliary TB:* Reduces systemic inflammation and multi-organ involvement.

Dosage

- TB meningitis requires a dose of 40–60 mg prednisolone per day for 4–6 weeks and then gradually tapered off.
- Adrenal TB requires replacement dose of steroids: Hydrocortisone 20–30 mg/day OR prednisolone 5–7.5 mg/day lifelong.
- For other indications 40–60 mg of prednisolone daily is given for 4–6 weeks and then gradually tapered off.

Q. Discuss the etiology, clinical features, investigations and treatment of interstitial lung disease (ILD).

Q. Idiopathic pulmonary fibrosis (cryptogenic fibrosing alveolitis).

- The interstitial lung diseases (ILDs) also known as diffuse parenchymal lung diseases are a group of disorders characterized by diffuse parenchymal lung involvement.
- Even though the pathology begins in the interstitium (hence the name ILD), ILD is not restricted to interstitium, but also involves other structures such as alveoli and airways.
- Interstitial lung diseases (ILD) produce a restrictive ventilatory defect without airway obstruction, decreased pulmonary diffusing capacity, and hypoxemia.
- Two histopathological patterns of ILDs are recognized (1) those with predominant inflammation and fibrosis, and (2) those with predominant granulomatous reaction in interstitium.

Causes of ILD

- There are numerous causes of ILD. But only a few causes account for majority of ILDs. When the cause is unknown it is called idiopathic pulmonary fibrosis (cryptogenic fibrosing alveolitis).

Classification of interstitial lung diseases (ILDs) *See* **Table 2.27.**

TABLE 2.27: Classification of interstitial lung diseases (ILDs)

Category	Subtypes/examples
Idiopathic interstitial pneumonias (IIP)	• Idiopathic pulmonary fibrosis (IPF) • Non-specific interstitial pneumonia (NSIP) • Desquamative interstitial pneumonia (DIP) • Respiratory bronchiolitis-ILD (RB-ILD) • Cryptogenic organizing pneumonia (COP) • Acute interstitial pneumonia (AIP)
ILD associated with connective tissue diseases (CTD-ILD)	• Rheumatoid arthritis-ILD • Systemic sclerosis-ILD • Systemic lupus erythematosus (SLE-ILD) • Polymyositis/dermatomyositis-ILD • Sjögren's syndrome-ILD
Granulomatous ILDs	• Sarcoidosis • Hypersensitivity pneumonitis (HP)
Occupational and environmental ILDs (Pneumoconioses)	• Asbestosis • Silicosis • Coal workers' pneumoconiosis (CWP) • Berylliosis
Drug-induced ILDs	• Amiodarone • Methotrexate • Bleomycin • Nitrofurantoin
Radiation-induced ILD	• Radiation pneumonitis • Radiation fibrosis
Other ILDs	• Lymphangioleiomyomatosis (LAM) • Pulmonary Langerhans cell histiocytosis (PLCH)

Clinical Features

- Chronic dyspnea (most common complaint). Dyspnea is progressive and worsened by exertion. Sudden worsening of dyspnea, especially if associated with acute chest pain, may indicate spontaneous pneumothorax.
- Chronic dry cough.
- Wheezing and chest pain are rarely seen.
- There may be h/o occupational exposure to organic or inorganic dust.
- General examination may show clubbing, cyanosis, tachypnea, and use of accessory respiratory muscles.
- Examination of the chest may show decreased expansion bilaterally and fine end inspiratory crepitations bilaterally usually at the base of the lungs. Advanced disease may show findings of pulmonary hypertension and cor pulmonale.
- In addition to the above findings patients may have features of underlying disease causing ILD. For example, patients with systemic sclerosis may have Raynaud's phenomenon; those with rheumatoid arthritis may have joint involvement. Those with SLE may have malar rash.

Investigations

Chest X-ray

- Reticulonodular shadows, ground glass opacities and honeycombing may be seen diffusely and bilaterally more in basal areas.
- Chest X-ray may also show features of underlying disease. For example, bilateral hilar lymphadenopathy may be seen in sarcoidosis and egg-shell calcification of hilar lymph may be seen in silicosis.

High-resolution Computed Tomography (HRCT) Chest

- HRCT is superior to chest X-ray for early detection and confirmation of ILD. It shows the reticulonodular pattern and honeycombing. It can also identify any underlying disease like sarcoidosis better than chest X-ray. HRCT allows better assessment of the extent and distribution of disease. If lung biopsy is planned HRCT is useful to know from which area biopsy should be taken.

Lung Biopsy

- Lung biopsy is the most definitive method for diagnosing ILD. Biopsy should be done before starting treatment. Fiberoptic bronchoscopy with multiple transbronchial lung biopsies (four to eight samples) is the procedure of choice. If a specific diagnosis is not possible by transbronchial biopsy, then surgical lung biopsy by video-assisted thoracic surgery or open thoracotomy is indicated.

Pulmonary Function Tests

- Spirometry shows a restrictive defect with reduced total lung capacity (TLC), functional residual capacity, and residual volume. FEV_1 and forced vital capacity (FVC) are reduced due to decreased TLC. The FEV_1/FVC ratio is usually normal or increased.
- Diffusing capacity of the lung for carbon monoxide (DLCO) is decreased.
- Arterial blood gas analysis may reveal hypoxemia and respiratory alkalosis (due to hyperventilation). CO_2 retention occurs in end-stage disease.

Other Investigations

- Investigations to find out the cause for ILD should be done based on clinical features of the patient.
- ANA should be done if SLE or other connective tissue disease is suspected. RA factor and anti-CCP antibody may be positive in rheumatoid arthritis. Antineutrophilic cytoplasmic antibodies (ANCA) may be positive in Wegener's granulomatosis. Patients with extrinsic allergic alveolitis have precipitable antibodies against the offending antigen.
- Lymph node biopsies are helpful in diagnosing tuberculosis, sarcoidosis or histiocytosis-X.

Treatment

- ILD progresses slowly and results in respiratory failure. Treatable causes should be identified and treated. Treatment is mainly directed at suppressing inflammatory process, thereby reducing further lung damage. Existing fibrosis cannot be reversed by treatment.
- For idiopathic pulmonary fibrosis, antifibrotic agents pirfenidone or nintedanib can be tried. These drugs do not reverse fibrosis, but they slow disease progression.
- For inflammatory ILDs (e.g. connective tissue associated ILD, hypersensitivity pneumonitis), steroids are the mainstay of therapy, but the success rate is low. A common starting dose is, prednisolone 0.5–1 mg/kg once-daily orally. This dose is continued for 1–3 months, and the patient is reassessed. If the patient is stable or improved, the dose is tapered to 0.25–0.5 mg/kg and is maintained at this level for an additional 1–3 months. If the patient's condition continues to worsen even on glucocorticoids, another drug (cyclophosphamide or azathioprine or mycophenolate mofetil) is added. Rituximab can be considered in severe connective tissue associated ILD.
- Hypoxemia (SpO_2 <88%) should be managed by supplemental oxygen.
- If all these therapies fail, lung transplantation may be considered.

Q. Farmer's lung (Hypersensitivity pneumonitis).

- Farmer's lung is a type of hypersensitivity pneumonitis induced by the inhalation of organic dust, mold, and bacteria from hay, straw, grain, or silage. It leads to immune-mediated lung inflammation.

Pathophysiology

- The growth of mold spores occurs when hay is not dried properly. Incidence of Farmer's lung peaks during late winter and early spring and is mostly seen after the harvest season. It is most prevalent in damp climates. When the farmer inhales the mold spores and other particles they induce an allergic reaction in the alveoli which leads to accumulation of fluid, protein, and inflammatory cells in the alveoli. This leads to impaired gas exchange and compromise in lung function. Chronic exposure leads to fibrotic changes in the lungs and permanent damage.

Clinical Features

- Farmer's lung can present as acute, subacute, or chronic disease. It should be suspected when there is history of symptoms such as cough, fever, and shortness of breath when exposed to mold in work environment.

Acute Stage

- This occurs after 4–8 hours after exposure. Symptoms includes headache, irritating cough, and shortness of breath upon physical exertion.

Subacute Stage

- This occurs after repeated exposure. Symptoms persist without further exposure, and increase in severity. Symptoms include: shortness of breath upon exertion, chronic cough, fatigue, occasional fever and sweating, decrease in appetite, aches and pains.

Chronic Stage

- Symptoms persist for long time. There is fibrosis, irreversible damage, and respiratory failure. Bibasilar inspiratory crackles ("Velcro crackles") are often heard.

Investigations

- HRCT chest: Ground-glass opacities, centrilobular nodules, fibrosis.
- Pulmonary function tests (PFTs): Restrictive pattern (↓FVC, ↓TLC), ↓DLCO.
- Bronchoalveolar Lavage (BAL): ↑ Lymphocytes (>20%).
- Serology: Precipitating IgG antibodies to organic antigens.

Prevention

- Chronic farmer's lung disease is permanent and cannot be reversed; hence appropriate measures should be taken to prevent it.
- Provision of good ventilation at work areas.
- Proper drying of agricultural products.
- Use of a mask while working with moldy hay or crops.

Treatment

- Adequate rest and reducing the exposure to the antigens through masks and increased ventilation.
- Corticosteroids (prednisolone 0.5–1 mg/kg/day, taper over 4–8 weeks).

Q. Pneumoconioses.

- Pneumoconioses (dusty lungs) are a group of chronic interstitial lung diseases caused by inhalation of inorganic dust. After inhalation, dust particles get deposited in the alveoli and cause inflammation and fibrosis (interstitial fibrosis).
- The principal cause of the pneumoconioses is workplace exposure; environmental exposures have rarely given rise to these diseases.
- Pneumoconioses take many years to develop and manifest, although in some cases (e.g. silicosis) rapidly progressive forms can occur after short periods of intense exposure. When severe, these diseases lead to respiratory failure, disability, and premature death. From a public health perspective, these conditions are entirely man-made, and can be avoided through appropriate dust control.
- Overall, most physicians do not encounter these diseases very frequently.

Common Causes of Pneumoconiosis (Table 2.28)

TABLE 2.28: Common causes of pneumoconiosis

Pneumoconiosis	Caused by	High-risk occupations
Silicosis	Silica dust	Mining, quarrying, construction, sandblasting
Asbestosis	Asbestos	Shipbuilding, insulation work, construction
Coal workers pneumoconiosis	Coal dust	Coal miners, power plant workers
Berylliosis	Beryllium	Aerospace, electronics, nuclear industries
Siderosis	Iron oxide	Welding, iron foundries
Stannosis	Tin oxide	Mining, tin smelting, welding, tin plating, manufacturing of tin-based products
Byssinosis ("Brown lung")	Cotton, flax, hemp dust	Textile industry workers

Clinical Features

- Progressive shortness of breath
- Chronic cough, may be dry or productive
- Crackles (bibasilar), present in fibrotic pneumoconioses
- Clubbing and cyanosis, cor pulmonale in advanced cases.

Investigations

- Chest X-ray/HRCT chest: Nodules and fibrosis seen in both the lungs.
- Pulmonary function tests: usually show restrictive pattern.

Treatment

- Exposure prevention: Use masks, ventilation, protective gear.
- Steroids and immunosuppressants to slow down fibrosis.
- Supportive care: Oxygen therapy, pulmonary rehab, bronchodilators (if obstruction present).

Q. Silicosis.

- Silicosis is a progressive fibrotic lung disease caused by chronic inhalation of crystalline silica dust. Less commonly, it can be caused by inhalation of silicates, minerals containing silicon dioxide bound to talc. It leads to inflammation, fibrosis, and respiratory impairment.
- Silicosis is the most common occupational lung disease. Workers at greatest risk are those who move or blast rock and sand (miners, quarry workers, stonecutters) or who use silica-containing rock or sand abrasives (sand blasters; glass makers; foundry, gemstone, and ceramic workers; potters).

Pathogenesis

- After inhalation, silica particles are deposited in the alveoli. Alveolar macrophages ingest the silica particles and enter lymphatics and interstitial tissue. The macrophages cause release of cytokines (tumor necrosis factor-alpha, interleukins), growth factors (tumor growth factor), and oxidants, stimulating parenchymal inflammation, collagen synthesis, and, ultimately, fibrosis.
- Over time, silica-laden macrophages, fibroblasts, and collagen aggregate to form silicotic nodules. As nodules coalesce, they form progressive massive fibrosis (PMF), causing severe respiratory dysfunction.
- Silicosis can present in following forms:

Acute Silicosis

- Occurs after exposure to high concentrations of crystalline silica. Symptoms develop within a few weeks or months after massive exposure.

Accelerated Silicosis

- Develops over 5–10 years of moderate exposure, leading to quicker fibrosis progression.

Chronic Silicosis

- It develops slowly, usually appearing 10–20 years after first exposure.

Clinical Presentation

- Silicosis is a progressive disease, often beginning asymptomatically before advancing to severe respiratory distress. The primary symptoms include:
- Progressive dyspnea on exertion
- Chronic dry cough
- Fatigue and weight loss (seen in advanced cases)
- Pleuritic chest pain (sometimes).
- Auscultation often reveals bibasilar crackles, especially in late-stage disease.
- Severe lung disease may lead to cor pulmonale with associated right ventricular heave, raised JVP, hepatomegaly, and peripheral edema.
- Patients usually die of respiratory failure.

Investigations

- *Chest X-ray:* Most commonly silicosis is diagnosed by a routine chest radiograph. Chest X-ray shows multiple nodule (opacities) ranging from 1 to 10 mm size seen predominantly in the upper lung zones initially and in advanced disease all over the lungs. Progressive massive fibrosis (PMF) manifests as bilateral upper lobe masses, which are formed by the coalescence of nodules. The hilar lymph nodes may show 'egg shell calcification'.
- *CT/HRCT chest:* This is more sensitive than chest X-ray in picking up nodules, fibrosis, honeycombing and pleural thickening.
- *Pulmonary function tests:* Show restrictive lung disease pattern and decreased diffusing capacity of the lungs for carbon monoxide (DLCO).
- Echocardiogram may show pulmonary HTN, and features of cor pulmonale (dilated RA, RV).
- *Lung biopsy:* This is usually not necessary because diagnosis can be made by clinical features and above investigations. However, if the diagnosis is in doubt, lung biopsy may be considered.
- *Tuberculin skin test:* Using purified protein derivative (PPD) is indicated in all persons with silicosis as they are prone to develop tuberculosis.

Complications

Silicosis is associated with several severe complications, including:

- *Progressive massive fibrosis (PMF):* Large fibrotic masses in the lungs, causing severe lung impairment.
- *Silico-tuberculosis (Silico-TB):* Silica exposure weakens lung immunity, increasing susceptibility to tuberculosis (TB).
- *Lung cancer:* Chronic silica exposure is a recognized risk factor for lung malignancies, especially in smokers.
- *Cor pulmonale*: Right heart failure due to pulmonary hypertension caused by chronic lung fibrosis.

Treatment

- Currently, there is no cure for silicosis, and treatment primarily focuses on symptom management and disease progression control.
- Patient should be advised to avoid further exposure to silica dust and quit smoking.
- Bronchodilators may be helpful to relieve bronchial obstruction.
- Corticosteroid therapy (prednisolone) has been shown to produce significant improvements in lung volumes, carbon monoxide diffusing capacity, and partial pressure of arterial oxygen.
- Lung transplantation should be considered in end-stage silicosis with respiratory failure.
- Antifibrotic agents such as pirfenidone and nintedanib are being studied.
- Experimental approaches to treatment include whole-lung lavage and aluminum inhalation.

Prevention

- Use of respiratory masks, dust control systems, and proper ventilation in high-risk workplaces.
- Regular workplace monitoring to limit silica exposure levels.

Q. Coal worker's pneumoconiosis (CWP).

Etiology

- Coal workers' pneumoconiosis (CWP) also known as black lung disease is a chronic occupational lung disease caused by prolonged inhalation of coal dust.
- It is caused by inhaling high-carbon coal mine dust (anthracite and bituminous). Anthracosis is the asymptomatic accumulation of carbon without a consequent cellular reaction. Such accumulation can be found in most urban dwellers and tobacco smokers. Inhaled coal dust becomes a problem when body reacts to it with consequent fibrosis in the lungs. The risk of CWP increases with dust level in the mine and cumulative exposure to coal mine dust.
- CWP is called "simple" if all radiographic opacities are less than 1 cm in diameter. If any opacity is 1cm or more on chest X-ray, it is termed complicated CWP or progressive massive fibrosis (PMF). Exposure to coal mine dust is also associated with bronchitis.

Pathology

- The inhaled coal dust causes an inflammatory reaction in the lungs leading to accumulation of macrophages and other inflammatory cells. Chronic inflammation leads to fibrosis. The characteristic lesion of CWP is coal macule, which is focal collection of coal dust and pigment-laden macrophages. As these macules extend, they join other macules in the vicinity, forming discrete areas of interstitial fibrosis. This growing collagen network causes distention of the respiratory bronchioles, forming focal areas of emphysema (commonly centrilobular emphysema).
- Macules may arrest or may enlarge and form nodules which may join together to produce progressive massive fibrosis. Progressive massive fibrosis (PMF) is diagnosed pathologically if nodules reach at least 2 cm, (or X-ray wise 1 cm or more). These lesions are

rich in collagen and disrupt the lung's architecture. PMF leads to severe lung restriction, respiratory failure, and pulmonary hypertension.

Clinical Manifestations

- Many patients are asymptomatic in early stages of disease and incidentally diagnosed by chest X-ray.
- Patients may present with cough and black sputum production.
- Progressive dyspnea may occur in advanced disease.
- Severe lung disease may lead to cor pulmonale with associated right ventricular heave, raised JVP, hepatomegaly, and peripheral edema.

Investigations

- *Chest X-ray:* In simple disease, the chest radiograph typically shows small nodules that tend to predominate in the upper lung zones. Reticular opacities may also be present, more often in cigarette smokers. X-ray findings and clinical symptoms do not correlate with each other because there can be significant symptoms with little or no radiographic abnormality. Progressive massive fibrosis is associated with progressive dyspnea, pulmonary hypertension, cor pulmonale and respiratory failure.
- *High-resolution CT (HRCT) scan*: More sensitive than X-ray for detecting early nodules and fibrosis.
- *Pulmonary function tests* (PFTs): Restrictive pattern in advanced disease (↓ TLC, ↓ FVC).
- *Other tests:* are same as those done for silicosis.

Treatment

- Same as that of silicosis.

Prognosis

- Simple pneumoconiosis alone does not increase mortality. Progressive massive fibrosis is associated with more severe morbidity and increased mortality.

Q. Beryllium disease.

- Beryllium disease, also known as berylliosis, is a chronic granulomatous lung disease caused by exposure to beryllium dust or fumes. It primarily affects workers in industries such as aerospace, nuclear, electronics, and metal refining. The disease occurs in two forms: *See* pathogenesis.

Pathogenesis

- Acute beryllium disease (ABD): A rare, severe chemical pneumonitis due to high-dose exposure.
- Chronic beryllium disease (CBD): A delayed hypersensitivity reaction leading to granulomatous lung inflammation and fibrosis, similar to sarcoidosis. Beryllium is transported to extrapulmonary sites such as the liver, spleen, skin and lymph nodes where granulomas are formed.

Clinical Features

- Acute beryllium disease occurs from exposure to a high concentration of dust or fumes. Patient presents with pharyngitis, tracheobronchitis and chemical pneumonitis.
- Chronic beryllium disease resembles sarcoidosis and is characterized by formation of granulomas in the lung and other organs. It differs from most pneumoconioses in that it is a cell-mediated hypersensitivity disease. Patients present with exertional dyspnea, dry cough, weight loss, fatigue, and chest pain. Physical examination shows crepitations in the lungs, lymphadenopathy, hepatosplenomegaly, and skin rash.

Investigations

- ***Chest X-ray:*** In acute berylliosis, chest X-ray shows diffuse or localized infiltrate. In chronic cases, chest X-ray or CT scan may show reticulonodular opacities and hilar adenopathy. In advanced disease there is honeycomb appearance of lung.
- ***Pulmonary function tests:*** Show a restrictive ventilatory defect and decrease in diffusion capacity.
- ***Beryllium lymphocyte proliferation test (BeLPT):*** Gold standard for diagnosing beryllium sensitization.

Treatment

- Consists of removal from exposure, oxygen and corticosteroids for both acute and chronic beryllium disease.

Q. Asbestosis.

Definition

- Asbestosis is a **chronic, progressive interstitial lung disease** caused by **long-term inhalation of asbestos fibers**. The disease is characterized by slowly progressive, diffuse pulmonary fibrosis.

Etiology

- Asbestos refers to a group of naturally occurring, heat-resistant fibrous silicates. Because of its heat-resistant and structural properties asbestos is used in construction and shipbuilding materials, automobile brakes, and some textiles. Chrysotile (a serpentine fiber), crocidolite, and amosite (amphibole, or straight fibers) are the 3 main types of asbestos that cause disease. All types of asbestos fibers cause asbestosis, pleural disease, and lung cancer.

Epidemiology

- People working in asbestos mines, textiles and brake lining factories, construction trades and workers using insulators are exposed to asbestos. Since a large number of buildings now have asbestos-containing materials, maintenance and demolition workers also get exposed to asbestos. However, exposure of building occupants to asbestos is quite low. The risk of asbestosis increases with cumulative exposure to asbestos fibers and manifestations usually appear after 15–20 years of exposure.

Pathology

- After inhalation asbestos fibers get deposited at respiratory bronchiole and alveolar duct bifurcations. Macrophages are attracted to these sites and an inflammatory reaction begins which results in fibrosis. Initially this fibrotic reaction is found at the site of deposition of asbestos fibers, but later involves the whole lung. Amphibole fibers may be more toxic than chrysotile because their structure allows them to deposit more efficiently in the distal lung parenchyma and reduces their rate of clearance. In advanced cases, extensive fibrosis destroys the normal architecture of the lung and causes honeycombing (cystic spaces bounded by fibrosis). Lungs become small and stiff with macroscopically visible fibrosis and honeycombing. Asbestos bodies are visible under microscopy.

Clinical Manifestations

- Patients present with dry cough and exertional dyspnea. Fine crepitations are heard on auscultation of the chest in basal areas bilaterally. Cyanosis and clubbing may be present in advanced cases.
- In advanced cases, features of cor pulmonale such as right ventricular heave, raised JVP, hepatomegaly, and peripheral edema may be present.

Investigations

- Chest X-ray shows irregular opacities most prominent in the basal areas. Pleural thickening and calcified pleural plaques may also be present.
- High-resolution CT is more sensitive to detect the pleural and pulmonary disease.
- Spirometry typically shows a reduced forced vital capacity (FVC) with absence of airflow obstruction, and reduced DLCO.
- Lung biopsy is usually not required but can help in definitive diagnosis. Both fibrosis and asbestos bodies can be visualized through microscopy.

Treatment

- There is no specific treatment for asbestosis. Further exposure should be avoided. Oxygen supplementation is needed if there is hypoxemia. Smoking should be stopped. Lung transplantation may be considered for advanced disease.

Complications

- Lung cancer → Most common cause of death in asbestosis patients.
- Malignant mesothelioma → Associated with pleural plaques, highly aggressive.
- Pulmonary hypertension and cor pulmonale → Due to chronic hypoxia.

Q. Byssinosis (Monday fever).

- Byssinosis as "Monday fever" or "brown lung disease," is is an occupational lung disease caused by exposure to cotton, flax, or hemp dust in textile industries.
- It is a chronic obstructive airway disease that primarily affects workers in cotton mills, textile factories, and flax processing plants.

Pathogenesis

- Cotton, flax, or hemp fibers contain bacterial endotoxins from gram-negative bacteria.
- When cotton dust is inhaled, these endotoxins trigger airway inflammation and bronchoconstriction.
- This leads to cytokine release (TNF-α, IL-1, IL-6), neutrophilic inflammation, and airway hyperreactivity. Repeated exposure over time causes chronic bronchitis and irreversible airflow limitation.

Clinical Features

- Patient presents with asthma-like symptoms on the first day of work (Monday) after a weekend off (hence called "Monday fever"). Patient c/o chest tightness, wheezing, dyspnea, and cough (worsens at the start of the workweek).
- Symptoms improve over weekends or vacations but return with re-exposure.
- With repeated exposure over a period of years, symptoms may continue till midweek or end of the week.

Diagnosis

- Diagnosis should be suspected in any patient with asthma-like symptoms (chest tightness, dyspnea, wheezing) and history of exposure to raw cotton.
- Pulmonary function tests show airflow obstruction and a reduction in ventilatory capacity.

Treatment

- Avoidance or reduction of exposure to raw cotton dust.
- Bronchodilators and inhaled steroids

Q. Eosinophilic lung diseases (ELD)

- Eosinophilic lung diseases (ELD) are a group of pulmonary disorders characterized by lung infiltration with eosinophils. They can be primary (idiopathic) or secondary (due to infections, drugs, autoimmune conditions, or malignancies) **(Table 2.29)**.
- Hallmark feature is increased eosinophils in the lungs, bronchoalveolar lavage (BAL), or peripheral blood.

TABLE 2.29: Classification of eosinophilic lung diseases

Category	Disease examples
Primary (Idiopathic) No known external cause	• Acute eosinophilic pneumonia (AEP) • Chronic eosinophilic pneumonia (CEP) • Eosinophilic granulomatosis with polyangiitis (EGPA, Churg Strauss)
Secondary	• Parasitic infections (Löffler's syndrome) • Drug-induced eosinophilic pneumonia • Hypereosinophilic syndrome (HES)

General Clinical Features of ELD

Respiratory symptoms

- Progressive dyspnea (shortness of breath)
- Cough (dry or productive)

- Wheezing (especially in EGPA)
- Chest pain (pleuritic in some cases)

Systemic symptoms

- Fever, night sweats, malaise (CEP, AEP)
- Weight loss (CEP, EGPA, parasitic infections)
- Fatigue and myalgias (EGPA, HES)

Investigations

- Peripheral eosinophilia: >500 cells/µl suggests eosinophilic disorder. >1500 cells/µl in hypereosinophilic syndrome (HES).
- IgE levels (elevated in parasitic infections, atopic diseases).
- ANCA (for EGPA).
- Parasitic serologies (if suspected).
- CXR and CT scan: Bilateral opacities, ground-glass infiltrates, peripheral consolidation.
- Bronchoscopy with BAL: BAL eosinophilia. Lavage fluid can be analysed to rule out infections (fungal, parasitic, mycobacterial).
- Lung biopsy (if uncertain): Vasculitis (EGPA), granulomas, fibrosis, eosinophilic infiltration.

Treatment of Eosinophilic Lung Diseases

- First-line therapy: Corticosteroids (prednisone 0.5–1 mg/kg/day, taper over weeks–months).
- Immunosuppressive therapy (severe/refractory cases): Cyclophosphamide, azathioprine, methotrexate (for EGPA, HES).
- Biologics: Mepolizumab, benralizumab (anti-IL-5) for EGPA and HES.
- Infectious Causes: Anti-parasitics (albendazole, ivermectin for Löffler's syndrome).
- Drug cessation (if drug-induced).

Q. Write a brief note on obesity hypoventilation syndrome (Pickwickian syndrome).

- Obesity hypoventilation syndrome (OHS) is defined as the presence of awake alveolar hypoventilation in an obese individual which cannot be attributed to other conditions associated with alveolar hypoventilation.
- Obesity hypoventilation syndrome (OHS) exists when an obese individual (body mass index >30 kg/m^2) develops awake alveolar hypoventilation ($PaCO_2$ >45 mm Hg). Other conditions which cause alveolar hypoventilation such as pulmonary disease, skeletal restriction, neuromuscular weakness, hypothyroidism, or pleural pathology should be ruled out before diagnosing OHS.
- Obesity is the hallmark of OHS (BMI >30 kg/m^2) and the prevalence of this disorder increases with increasing BMI. About 90% of OHS individuals will have coexisting obstructive sleep apnea (OSA). Note that OHS and OSA are different entities.

Pathophysiology

- Obesity puts extramechanical load on rib cage and abdomen and reduces the compliance of the chest wall. As a result the FRC (functional residual capacity) is reduced, particularly on lying down.
- Most patients have a defect in the central respiratory control system. These patients have been shown to have a decreased responsiveness to carbon dioxide rebreathing, hypoxia, or both.
- Chronic hypercapnia and hypoxemia leads to polycythemia, pulmonary hypertension and cor pulmonale.

Clinical Features

- Patients are usually middle-aged and very obese (BMI ≥30 kg/m^2).
- Both sexes are equally affected.
- Daytime hypersomnolence (excessive sleepiness).
- Morning headaches (due to hypercapnia).
- Fatigue, poor concentration, and memory impairment.
- Dyspnea on exertion.
- There may be cyanosis, secondary polycythemia, and cor pulmonale.

Investigations

- Chest X-ray reveals cardiomegaly.
- ECG/Echocardiography shows evidence of pulmonary HTN and right ventricular hypertrophy.
- ABG may show hypoxemia and hypercapnia (type-II respiratory failure).
- Elevated serum bicarbonate (>27 mEq/L): Almost all patients with OHS have an elevated serum bicarbonate, which is a compensatory mechanism for respiratory acidosis due to chronic hypercapnia.
- Thyroid function tests to rule out hypothyroidism which can be contribute to hypoventilation and obesity.
- Pulmonary function tests: usually restrictive pattern is seen.
- Sleep study (polysomnography) shows coexisting obstructive sleep apnea (OSA) in most of these patients.

Treatment

- Noninvasive positive airway pressure (PAP) therapy: First-line treatment. Reduces hypercapnia, improves oxygenation, and decreases respiratory workload
  - BiPAP (bilevel positive airway pressure) → Preferred in severe hypercapnia.
  - CPAP (continuous positive airway pressure) → Used if OSA is predominant.
- The definitive treatment is to make the patient lose weight. Sometimes surgery is needed (e.g. gastric bypass surgery) to help with weight loss.
- Oxygen therapy: Low-flow supplemental oxygen if persistent hypoxia (PaO_2 <55 mm Hg) despite positive airway pressure therapy. Avoid excessive O_2 → Can worsen CO_2 retention by reducing respiratory drive.
- Use of sedatives, and alcohol should be avoided because they worsen hypoventilation.
- Respiratory stimulants: Oral medroxyprogesterone acetate and acetazolamide can be used as last resort

for patients who continue to have serious alveolar hypoventilation despite PAP therapy and weight loss to increase respiratory drive.

Q. Sleep apnea.

Q. Obstructive sleep apnea.

Q. Central sleep apnea.

- Sleep apnea is defined as intermittent cessation of the airflow at the nose and mouth during sleep for at least 10 seconds. Most patients have apnea for 20–30 seconds, and it may even last as long as 2–3 minutes.
- Sleep apnea has been classified into 3 types:
  1. Obstructive sleep apnea (OSA)
  2. Central sleep apnea (CSA)
  3. Mixed sleep apnea

Obstructive Sleep Apnea (OSA)

- Obstructive sleep apnea (OSA) is a sleep disorder that involves cessation or significant decrease in airflow in the presence of breathing effort. In this disorder airflow ceases because of occlusion of the upper airway, usually at the level of the oropharynx. The respiratory drive is normal.
- The obstruction results in progressive asphyxia until there is a brief arousal from sleep, whereupon the airway patency is restored and airflow resumes. The patient again returns to sleep. This sequence of events may occur many times in the night causing fragmentation of sleep which causes daytime somnolence.
- The upper airway collapses because the negative pressure during inspiration exceeds the ability of airway dilator and abductor muscles to keep the airway open. During deep sleep there is reduced activity of muscles of the upper airway resulting in airway collapse. In many patients, upper airway may be structurally narrow due to enlarged adenoids, and obesity. Thus obesity is an important cause of obstructive sleep apnea.

Causes of OSA

- OSA occurs when the muscles at the back of the throat relax excessively during sleep, leading to airway collapse. Key risk factors include:
- Obesity (most common cause)
- Enlarged tonsils/adenoids (especially in children)
- Narrow airway (due to genetics or structural abnormalities)
- Smoking and alcohol use
- Aging (muscle tone decreases with age)
- Neuromuscular disorders (e.g. stroke, myasthenia gravis)

Clinical Features

- Patients are usually obese and are between 30 and 60 years of age.
- Loud snoring is the most common symptom. Many patients have snoring which precedes the onset of OSA by many years. Snoring is due to narrowing of the upper airways during sleep. However, snoring alone does not warrant an investigation for OSA.
- Gasping, choking, or pauses in breathing while sleeping.
- Excessive daytime sleepiness and fatigue.
- Morning headaches.
- Difficulty concentrating (brain fog), memory loss.
- Mood changes (depression, irritability).
- High blood pressure (OSA is linked to cardiovascular diseases).
- Asystole or dangerous arrhythmias can occur during the apnea, hypoapnea episodes.
- Some patients develop pulmonary hypertension, right ventricular failure, and secondary polycythemia.

Investigations

- Sleep study (polysomnography) is the definitive investigation of choice. It is a detailed overnight sleep study that includes recording of multiple parameters simultaneously. These include ECG to detect arrhythmias, electroencephalogram (EEG) to know sleep stages, the chin electromyogram (activity decreases in REM), and the electro-oculogram (EOG) to detect REM sleep. Pulse oximetry is used to know oxygen saturation during apnea episodes.

Treatment

- *General:* Weight reduction if obese, avoidance of alcohol and CNS depressant drugs, and avoidance of sleeping in the supine position.
- *Oral appliance therapy:* Oral appliances act by moving (pulling) the tongue forward or by moving the mandible and soft palate anteriorly, enlarging the posterior airspace. They open or dilate the upper airway.
- *Specific:* CPAP (continuous positive airway pressure) ventilation is the definitive treatment for OSA. It prevents upper airway occlusion by splinting the pharyngeal airway with a positive pressure delivered through tight fitting face mask.
- *Surgical options:* If patients cannot tolerate CPAP, surgical procedures aimed at increasing the upper airway dimensions (uvulopalatopharyngoplasty, linguaplasty, mandibular advancement) etc can be considered. Tracheostomy should be considered in patients with severe OSA.

Central Sleep Apnea (CSA)

- Central sleep apnea is due to transient abolition of central drive to the ventilatory muscles. The brain fails to send proper signals to the respiratory muscles, leading to pauses in breathing during sleep.
- This usually happens due to fall of PCO_2 during sleep below the critical level required for respiratory stimulation. As a result, apnea develops until PCO_2 rises and again stimulates respiration.

Causes of CSA

- CNS diseases: Central respiratory drive can be abnormal in CNS diseases like brainstem tumor, infarction, or infection, Parkinson's disease, encephalitis and high cervical cord compression.

- Primary central sleep apnea—no identifiable cause.
- CSA due to high-altitude periodic breathing—seen at high elevations (>8,000 ft).
- Heart failure—Cheyne-Stokes breathing (CSB).
- Use of opiates and other CNS depressants—suppress brainstem respiratory control.

Clinical Features

- Patients complain of sleeping poorly, nocturnal awakenings, morning headache, daytime fatigue and sleepiness.
- Patients may also present with history of recurrent respiratory failure, polycythemia, pulmonary hypertension and right-sided heart failure.

Investigations

- Polysomnography is the investigation of choice and shows recurrent apnea with absent respiratory effort (whereas respiratory effort is present in obstructive sleep apnea).
- Echocardiography (if heart failure is suspected).
- Brain imaging (MRI/CT scan) for stroke or neurological disorders.

Treatment

- Patients with hypoxemia benefit from nocturnal supplemental oxygen.
- Positive airway pressure (PAP) therapy: BiPAP or CPAP (as for OSA) can be effective, although the treatment is less well tolerated than in patients with OSA.
- Respiratory stimulants such as acetazolamide (used for high-altitude CSA) or theophylline may help but results are variable.

Q. Enumerate the causes of pleural effusion. Give the differential diagnosis, clinical features, investigations and management of pleural effusion.

- A pleural effusion is an abnormal collection of fluid in the pleural space.

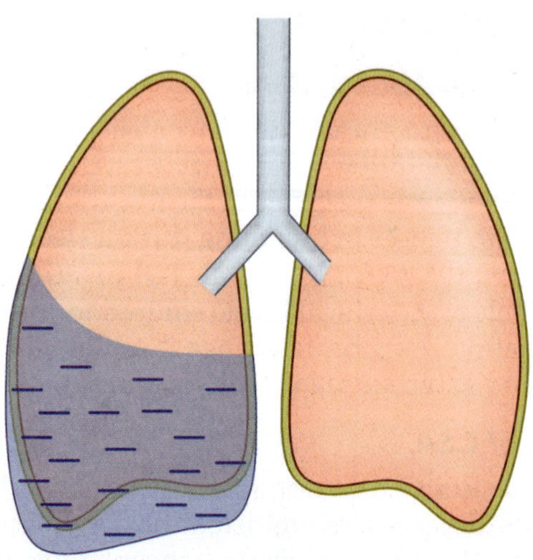

Figure 2.26: Pleural effusion

- It results from excess fluid production or decreased absorption or both.
- Normally about 10–20 ml of fluid is present in the pleural space which is similar in composition to plasma except low protein (<1.5 gm/dl). Pleural fluid accumulates as a result of
    1. Increase in vascular permeability (e.g. pneumonia).
    2. Increase in hydrostatic pressure (e.g. cardiac failure).
    3. Decrease in pleural pressure (e.g. atelectasis).
    4. Decrease in plasma osmotic pressure (e.g. nephrotic syndrome).
- Pleural effusion can be exudative or transudative based on lights criteria.

Light's Criteria to Distinguish Pleural Transudate from Exudate

Pleural fluid is an exudate if one or more of the following criteria are met:

- Pleural fluid protein: Serum protein ratio >0.5
- Pleural fluid LDH: Serum LDH ratio >0.6
- Pleural fluid LDH > two-thirds of the upper limit of normal serum LDH

Causes of Pleural Effusion

Transudative Pleural Effusion

- Congestive heart failure
- Cirrhosis with portal HTN
- Nephrotic syndrome
- Peritoneal dialysis
- Hypoalbuminemia
- Atelectasis
- Constrictive pericarditis
- Superior vena cava (SVC) obstruction

Exudative Pleural Effusion

- Pneumonia
- Tuberculosis
- Subphrenic abscess
- Hepatic abscess
- Esophageal perforation
- Malignancy
- Pancreatitis (acute, chronic)
- Pulmonary embolism
- Sarcoidosis
- Connective tissue diseases (SLE, rheumatoid arthritis)
- Ovarian hyperstimulation syndrome
- Chylothorax
- Meigs' syndrome

Clinical Features

- Patients may be asymptomatic in mild pleural effusion.
- *Dyspnea:* This is the most common symptom associated with effusion.
- *Cough:* Cough is often mild and dry. More severe cough with sputum suggests an underlying pneumonia or endobronchial lesion causing effusion.

- *Pleuritic chest pain:* Chest pain indicates pleural irritation, and occurs in pleural infection, mesothelioma, or pulmonary infarction. Pain is pleuritic in nature and is typically described as sharp or stabbing and is exacerbated with deep inspiration. Pain may be localized to the chest wall or referred to the ipsilateral shoulder or upper abdomen because of diaphragmatic irritation. Pain may diminish as the pleural effusion increases which separates inflamed pleural surfaces from each other.
- *Other symptoms:* Symptoms of underlying disease may be present. Lower limb edema, orthopnea, and paroxysmal nocturnal dyspnea may suggest congestive cardiac failure as the cause of pleural effusion. Night sweats, fever, hemoptysis, and weight loss should suggest TB. Hemoptysis also suggests the possibility of malignancy or endobronchial pathology, or pulmonary infarction. An acute febrile episode, purulent sputum production, and pleuritic chest pain may suggest effusion associated with pneumonia (syn: pneumonic effusion).
- Examination shows decreased chest movements, stony dull percussion note, and absent breath sound on the affected side. Vocal fremitus and vocal resonance are decreased. Pleural rub may be heard sometimes. Mediastinal shift may be seen in massive pleural effusion. There may be signs and symptoms of underlying disease causing pleural effusion. Peripheral edema, distended neck veins, and S3 gallop suggest congestive cardiac failure. Presence of jaundice and ascites suggest liver disease (cirrhosis with portal HTN). Lymphadenopathy or a palpable mass suggests malignancy.

Investigations

Chest X-ray

- Pleural effusion appears as a curved shadow at the lung base, blunting the costophrenic angle and ascending towards the axilla on the erect chest X-ray. Minimum 200 ml of fluid is required to produce a shadow on chest X-ray, but smaller effusions can be identified by ultrasound or CT scanning.

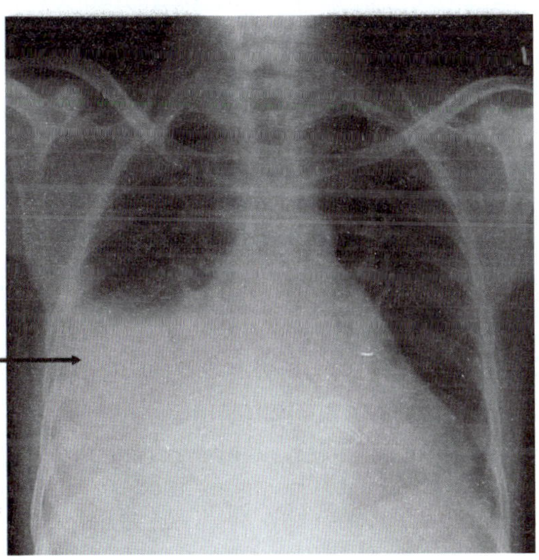

Figure 2.27: Pleural effusion on right side

Ultrasound Chest

- This is more accurate than chest X-ray to detect pleural effusion. It can also be used to guide pleural aspiration and pleural biopsy. It can also distinguish pleural fluid from pleural thickening.

CT Scan

- CT is better than both X-ray and ultrasound in showing pleural abnormalities and underlying disease.

Pleural Fluid Aspiration and Analysis

- If the cause of effusion is obvious (e.g. heart failure) it may not be necessary to do diagnostic pleural aspiration. Most bilateral pleural effusions are transudates and do not require aspiration for analysis. However, if the cause is not obvious and effusion is unilateral, aspiration is necessary to establish a diagnosis.
- Color and texture of fluid can give clue about the possible diagnosis. It is straw colored in transudates, turbid and purulent in empyema and hemorrhagic in pulmonary infarction or malignancy. A milky, opalescent fluid suggests a chylothorax. Black pleural fluid is seen in infection with *Aspergillus niger* or *Rizopus oryzae*, malignant melanoma, and charcoal-containing empyema.
- Biochemical analysis allows classification into transudate and exudates (*see* Light's criteria). Measurement of adenosine deaminase level (ADA) in pleural fluid is very helpful in the diagnosis of tuberculosis. ADA level of >50 U/L is highly suggestive of TB. Increased interferon-gamma concentrations (>140 pg/ml) also support the diagnosis of tuberculous pleuritis. Increased triglyceride and cholesterol levels are seen in chylothorax. Increased amylase level is seen in effusion due to pancreatitis. A low pH <7.2 suggests empyema or complicated syn-pneumonic effusion. Glucose <60 mg/dl suggests infection, malignancy, or rheumatoid effusion.
- Microbiological investigations should be done such as Gram's stain, culture sensitivity and AFB stain. PCR for tuberculosis should be done in most cases of pleural effusion.
- Cell count, cell type and malignant cytology should also be requested.

Pleural Biopsy

- Combining pleural aspiration with biopsy increases the diagnostic yield. An Abrams needle is used for pleural biopsy. Pleural biopsy is better obtained under ultrasound or CT guidance. Video-assisted thoracoscopy allows the operator to directly visualize the pleura and obtain biopsy.

Management

- Asymptomatic transudative effusions need not be drained.
- *Therapeutic aspiration* should be considered in symptomatic patients (e.g. dyspnea).

- *Chest tube drainage*: Insertion of intercostal drainage tube (ICD) is required in complicated parapneumonic effusions and empyema.
- *Pleurodesis:* involves instilling an irritant (such as talc, doxycycline) into the pleural space to cause inflammatory changes that result in bridging fibrosis between the visceral and parietal pleural surfaces, obliterating the pleural space. Pleurodesis is used for recurrent malignant effusions.
- *Surgery:* Pleurectomy, or decortication is considered in refractory or recurrent cases (e.g. malignant effusion).
- *Treatment of the underlying cause:* for example, heart failure, nephritic syndrome, pneumonia, etc. will often be followed by resolution of the effusion.

Complications if Untreated

- Empyema (infected pleural fluid leading to sepsis).
- Fibrosis and pleural thickening (restrictive lung disease).
- Respiratory failure in large or rapidly accumulating effusions.

Q. Empyema.

- Empyema is collection of pus in the pleural space.

Etiology

- Empyema develops when pyogenic bacteria, fungi, parasites, or mycobacteria invade the pleural space, either from an adjacent pneumonia or from direct inoculation (e.g. penetrating chest injuries) or other source.
- Following are the causes of empyema:

Traumatic	Penetrating chest injuries
Iatrogenic	Thoracic surgery
	Following pleural aspiration, and intercostal tube drainage
Infections	Pneumonia (most common cause)
	Tuberculosis
	Bronchiectasis
	Lung abscess
	Mediastinitis
	Osteomyelitis of ribs, vertebrae
Spread from other sites	Rupture of subphrenic abscess and liver abscess

Clinical Features

- Patient usually presents with fever, pleuritic chest pain, and dyspnea. Cough with purulent sputum may be seen in bronchopleural fistula.
- Examination reveals decreased chest movement, stony dull percussion note, absent breath sounds, tenderness and bulging of intercostal spaces on the side of empyema. Clubbing is usually present.
- Rarely, empyema can penetrate the pleura and collect in the subcutaneous tissue forming a swelling on the chest wall which increases on coughing (cough impulse). This is called "empyema necessitans", and is seen in actinomycotic infection.
- Patient may be toxic with signs of sepsis. Chronic empyema leads to pleural thickening, chest deformity and scoliosis. Extensive pleural calcification may occur.

Diagnosis

- Empyema should be suspected in any case of pneumonia with pleural effusion.
- Chest X-ray appearance of empyema is the same as that of pleural effusion, but loculations may be present more often.
- Chest CT scan (gold standard): Shows loculated fluid collection with septations, and thickened pleura.
- Ultrasound of chest can show fibrin strands suggesting empyema.
- Aspiration of pleural fluid can confirm the diagnosis of empyema. Gram's stain, AFB stain and culture should be done from the pleural aspirate. The pleural fluid appears turbid, pus like, pH is usually less than 7.2, LDH level is more than 1000 IU/L and glucose content is less than 60 mg/dl, and WBC count is >50,000 cells/µl.

Complications

- Sepsis with septic shock
- Pleural thickening with calcification and fibrosis
- Bronchopleural fistula
- Deformities of the thoracic cage
- Chronic discharging sinus
- Secondary amyloidosis
- Metastatic infection.

Management

- Antibiotics are given based on culture and sensitivity. Pending culture sensitivity results, combination of penicillin (Gram's positive cover), an aminoglycoside (gram negative cover) and metronidazole (anaerobic cover) may be used. The duration of treatment is usually 6 weeks.
- Empyema due to tuberculosis or other organisms such as *Entamoeba histolytica* and Actinomyces should be treated with appropriate antibiotics.
- Empyema should be drained either by closed or open methods. Closed drainage is done by needle aspiration or intercostal tube drainage under a water seal. ICD can be removed when the drainage is less than 25–50 ml in 24 hours for two consecutive days. Open drainage by thoracotomy is required if there is bronchopleural fistula or multiple loculations, or the fluid is too thick.
- Video-assisted thoracoscopic surgery (VATS) (for loculated/organizing empyema): For patients not responding to antibiotics and chest tube drainage.

Q. Bronchogenic carcinoma (lung cancer).

Q. Paraneoplastic syndrome.

- Bronchogenic carcinoma refers to lung cancer that originates from the bronchi or bronchioles. Bronchogenic carcinoma can be divided into following types.
  - ***Non-small cell lung cancer (NSCLC)***
    - Adenocarcinoma

- ✦ Squamous cell carcinoma
- ✦ Large cell carcinoma
- ❑ ***Small cell lung cancer (SCLC)***
  - ✦ *Oat cell carcinoma*
- NSCLC accounts for approximately 85% of all lung cancers. Identifying the type of cancer is important, because SCLC has a high response rate to chemotherapy and radiation whereas NSCLC can be cured by surgery in certain stages and is not curable by chemotherapy alone.
- ***Adenocarcinoma:*** Most common type (40–50%). Occurs often in non-smokers. Located peripherally in the lungs.
- ***Squamous cell carcinoma*** (25–30%): Strongly linked to smoking. Located centrally in the lung. May cause cavitary lesions and hypercalcemia (via PTHrP production).
- ***Large cell carcinoma*** (5–10%): Poorly differentiated and aggressive. Peripheral lung location. Poor prognosis due to rapid progression.
- ***Small cell lung cancer*** (SCLC): 15% of cases. Highly aggressive, rapid growth, early metastasis. Strongly associated with smoking. Located centrally in the lung. Often associated with paraneoplastic syndromes (SIADH, Cushing's syndrome, Lambert-Eaton myasthenic syndrome).

Incidence and Prevalence

- Bronchogenic Ca is the most common cancer in men. It is one of the leading causes of cancer death in both men and women. The incidence of lung cancer peaks between ages 55 and 65 years.
- Males are affected more often than females probably due to smoking habits. However, incidence in females is also increasing because of increased smoking habits in women also.
- Incidence is higher in urban than in rural areas, probably due to air pollution.
- Adenocarcinoma, arising from the bronchial mucosal glands, is the most common NSCLC cancer. Squamous cell carcinoma is the next common ca.

Etiology

- Smoking is the main cause of bronchogenic carcinoma. Ninety percent of patients with lung cancer are current or former cigarette smokers. The relative risk of developing lung cancer is increased by about 13-fold in smokers. There is a significant dose-response relationship between the risk of lung cancer and the number of cigarettes smoked per day. The risk is increased 60–70-fold for a man smoking two packs a day for 20 years as compared with a nonsmoker. Besides the dose, the form of tobacco smoked is also believed to be important. Those who smoke only pipes or cigars have a lower risk. Bidi smoking is equally harmful. The risk of lung cancer is lower among users of filter than non-filter cigarettes. The risk decreases after stopping smoking. Passive smoking can also increase the risk of lung cancer. The risk may be about twice as compared to non-smokers without such exposure.
- Cigarette smoke contains many carcinogenic polycyclic hydrocarbons like 3, 4 benzopyrine. Squamous cell carcinoma and oat cell carcinoma are common in smokers, whereas adenocarcinoma is common in nonsmokers.
- Other risk factors for developing lung cancer include air pollution, ionizing radiation, chromates, metallic iron and iron oxides, arsenic, nickel, beryllium, asbestos, petrochemicals, hematite and mustard gas. Adenocarcinoma can develop in areas of chronic scarring (scar carcinoma).
- Genetic factors like mutations in oncogenes may play an important role in the development of Ca. All other risk factors may work by inducing tumor oncogenes.

Pathology

- Adenocarcinomas commonly present as mid-zone or peripheral mass lesions. Poorly differentiated adenocarcinomas tend to metastasize early and have a poor prognosis. Large cell carcinomas are made up of large malignant cells with abundant cytoplasm.
- Squamous cell Ca grows relatively slowly and often presents with local symptoms. Small cell carcinoma grows faster and proves rapidly fatal due to early metastasis. Small cell Ca is more often central than peripheral. The classical oat cell type is characterized by round or oval nuclei with scanty cytoplasm.

Clinical Features

- The signs and symptoms of lung cancer are due to local tumor growth, invasion or obstruction of adjacent structures, regional lymph node involvement, metastases and remote effects of tumor products (paraneoplastic syndromes). The patient may be asymptomatic and may be diagnosed incidentally by a chest X-ray.

Symptoms due to Local Growth

- Central or endobronchial tumor may cause cough, hemoptysis, wheeze and stridor, dyspnea, and obstructive pneumonia. Obstruction of airways can produce wheezing, and unilateral wheezing suggests a localized obstruction.
- Peripheral tumor may cause pain from pleural or chest wall involvement, cough, and dyspnea.
- Bronchogenic carcinomas may cavitate and lead to lung abscess formation.

Symptoms due to Local Invasion

- Local spread of tumor into the mediastinum or involvement of mediastinal lymph nodes may cause tracheal compression, dysphagia due to esophageal compression, hoarseness due to recurrent laryngeal nerve paralysis, elevation of the hemidiaphragm and dyspnea due to phrenic nerve paralysis and Horner's syndrome (enophthalmos, ptosis, miosis, and ipsilateral loss of sweating) due to sympathetic chain compression. Pleural effusion can occur.

- Pancoast syndrome results due to a tumor in the apex or in the superior sulcus of the lung with involvement of the C8 and T1 nerves, cervical sympathetic chain with consequent pain radiating to medial side of arm and forearm, shoulder pain and Horner's syndrome.
- Other problems of local spread include superior vena cava compression, cardiac involvement with resultant malignant pericardial effusion and tamponade, arrhythmia, or cardiac failure.

Symptoms due to Metastases

- Common sites of metastases of lung carcinoma include brain, bone, adrenals, and liver.
- Symptoms are referable to the organ system involved. Brain metastases produce neurologic deficits; bone metastases produce pain and pathologic fractures; bone marrow invasion presents with pancytopenia; liver metastases produce jaundice; and biliary obstruction; spine metastases produces cord compression.

Paraneoplastic Syndromes

- Paraneoplastic syndromes are clinical syndromes due to nonmetastatic systemic effects of a cancer. They are not due to the local effect of tumor and not due to its metastases. These syndromes result from substances produced by the tumor, and they occur remotely from the tumor itself.
- Paraneoplastic syndromes occur in approximately 10% of patients with bronchogenic carcinoma and occasionally are the presenting symptom. Paraneoplastic manifestations of lung cancer include cachexia, weight loss, hypercalcemia, SIADH, Eaton-Lambert syndrome, etc.

Physical Signs

- Physical examination may reveal clubbing, osteoarthropathy of the wrists and ankles, and lymphadenopathy especially in the supraclavicular regions. RS examination may be normal or show collapse, or consolidation. Pleural effusion may be present. Monophonic wheeze may be heard in localized airway obstruction.

Investigations

Imaging Studies

- Chest X-ray may show an isolated solitary mass lesion. Cavitation or abscess formation may be seen. Doubling time of more than 18 months and presence of calcification strongly suggest a benign diagnosis. Segmental, lobar or massive collapse of the lung may be present. Associated hilar and mediastinal lymphadenopathy may be present. Pleural and pericardial effusion may be present due to invasion of the pleura and pericardium. An elevated diaphragm suggests phrenic nerve involvement. Secondary deposits in the ribs and other bones may be present.
- CT scan of the chest is very useful and helps in differentiating malignant lesions from benign ones. It can also pick up mediastinal lymphadenopathy and metastatic disease in the brain, liver, adrenal, kidney and lymph nodes of the abdomen.
- MRI is particularly useful to detect vertebral, spinal cord, and mediastinal invasion.
- PET-CT scan detects metastases (brain, liver, bones, adrenal glands).

CT-guided Needle Biopsy

- Best for peripheral tumors (adenocarcinoma, large cell carcinoma).

Bronchoscopy

- Bronchoscopy is useful to diagnose and obtain biopsy in case of centrally located and endobronchial tumors. When the lesion is endoscopically visualized, diagnosis can be established in more than 90% of cases. Bronchoscopy can also reveal paralysed vocal cords and bronchial aspirate and bronchial washings can be obtained to test for malignant cells.

Sputum Cytology

- Cytological examination of sputum may show malignant cells. If pleural effusion is present, it should be aspirated and examined for malignant cells. CT-guided FNAC or biopsy from the mass is also helpful for cytological examination.

Mediastinoscopy and Thoracoscopy

- These are sometimes used to take biopsy from lesions and lymph nodes.

Other Diagnostic Techniques

- Biopsy of involved lymph nodes or of a metastatic nodule in the skin, liver, bone or pleura can help in diagnosis.

Management

Non-small Cell Lung Cancer (NSCLC) Treatment

- Surgical resection of the primary tumor and regional lymph nodes is the treatment of choice for stage I and II NSCLC (tumor is localized without distant metastases). It is not useful in SCLC.
- Chemotherapy + Radiation for stage III and unresectable cases.
- For stage IV (distant metastases) → Chemotherapy + Targeted therapy + Immunotherapy (PD-L1 inhibitors) + Palliative care.
- Commonly used chemotherapy drugs are cisplatin, etoposide, docetaxel, gemcitabine, carboplatin in various combinations.

Small Cell Lung Cancer (SCLC) Treatment

- Limited stage → Chemotherapy (Cisplatin + Etoposide) + Radiation.
- Extensive stage → Chemotherapy ± Immunotherapy (atezolizumab, durvalumab).
- Prophylactic cranial irradiation (PCI) → Recommended to reduce brain metastases.

Key Points

- Most common type of lung cancer: NSCLC (Adenocarcinoma most frequent).
- Strongest risk factor: Smoking (>85% of cases)
- Symptoms: Persistent cough, hemoptysis, weight loss, dyspnea
- Best diagnostic tool: CT scan + Biopsy (bronchoscopy for central tumors, needle biopsy for peripheral tumors)
- Treatment: Surgery for early NSCLC; chemotherapy + immunotherapy for advanced cases
- SCLC is highly aggressive, with early metastasis and poor prognosis.

Q. Tumors of the mediastinum.

- Mediastinal tumors are abnormal growths that develop in the mediastinum, the central compartment of the thoracic cavity located between the lungs.
- Mediastinum can be divided into four major compartments: Superior, anterior, middle and posterior **(Fig. 2.28)**.
- The location of each compartment and the tumors that can occur within them are given in **Table 2.30**.

TABLE 2.30: Tumors of mediastinum

Divisions of mediastinum	Tumors
Superior mediastinum Above a line joining the lower border of the 4th thoracic vertebra and the upper end of the sternum	• Retrosternal goiter • Persistent left superior vena cava • Enlarged lymph nodes due to TB • Prominent left subclavian artery • Tumors of thymus • Dermoid cyst • Lymphoma • Aortic aneurysm
Anterior mediastinum In front of the heart	• Retrosternal goiter • Dermoid cyst • Tumors of thymus • Lymphoma • Enlarged lymph nodes due to TB • Hiatus hernia
Middle mediastinum Between the anterior and posterior compartments	• Pericardial cyst • Bronchogenic cyst • Aortic aneurysm • Bronchial carcinoma • Lymphoma • Sarcoidosis
Posterior mediastinum Behind the heart	• Neurogenic tumors • Meningocele • Paravertebral abscess • Esophageal lesion • Diaphragmatic hernia • Aortic aneurysm • Foregut duplication

Clinical Features of Mediastinal Tumors

- Benign tumors can cause pressure effect on trachea or superior vena cava. But most of the time benign tumors are asymptomatic and are diagnosed when chest X-ray is taken for some other reason.
- Malignant tumors can invade and compress adjacent structures. Symptoms and signs depend on the structure compressed which are as follows.

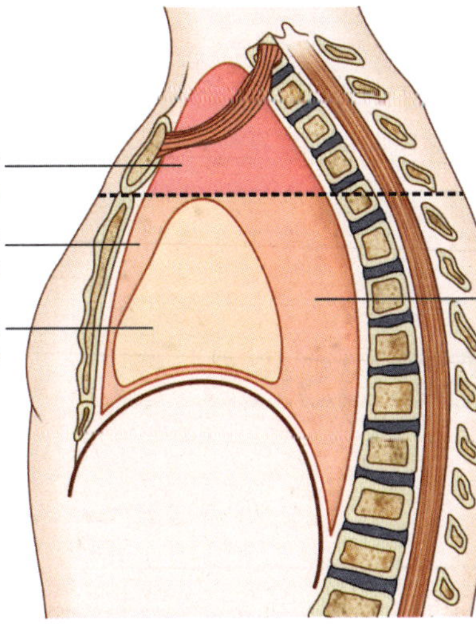

Figure 2.28: Divisions of mediastinum

- *Trachea and bronchi*: Stridor, breathlessness, cough, pulmonary collapse.
- *Esophagus:* Dysphagia.
- *Phrenic nerve:* Diaphragmatic paralysis, paradoxical chest movement.
- *Recurrent laryngeal nerve:* Hoarseness of voice and 'bovine' cough.
- *Sympathetic trunk:* Horner's syndrome.
- *Superior vena cava:* Elevation of JVP, edema of the head and neck and upper limbs. Dilated veins seen on chest wall.
- *Pericardium:* Pericarditis and/or pericardial effusion.

Investigations

- *Chest X-ray:* Tumor may be visualized. Mediastinal widening may be present.
- *CT chest:* This can easily pick up mediastinal growths, the extent of spread and enlarged lymph nodes.
- *Bronchoscopy:* May show intrabronchial lesion which has spread to mediastinum.
- *Mediastinoscopy:* This can directly visualize the tumors and take biopsy also.

Management

- Treatment depends on the nature of mediastinal pathology. Benign tumors should be removed surgically because they may cause symptoms later.

Q. Miliary mottling in chest X-ray.

- The term miliary mottling refers to innumerable, small 1–2 mm nodules (resembling millet seeds) scattered throughout the lungs. Causes of miliary mottling can be remembered by the mpnemonic "Hi STOP MAC"

Hi: Histoplasmosis, Histicytosis X, Hemosiderosis
S: Sarcoidosis
T: TB
O: Oil embolism
P: Pneumoconiosis
M: Metastasis
A: Alveolar microlithiasis
C: Coccidioidomycosis

Chapter 3

Diseases of Cardiovascular System

- The cardiovascular system comprises the heart, arteries, veins, and capillaries. Its primary function is to transport nutrients and oxygen-rich blood to all parts of the body and to carry deoxygenated blood back to the lungs.
- The cardiovascular system consists of 2 main loops: systemic circulation and pulmonary circulation. Pulmonary circulation allows for the oxygenation of the blood, and systemic circulation allows oxygenated blood and nutrients to reach the rest of the body.

Q. Describe the blood supply and venous drainage of the heart.

- Heart is supplied by mainly by two coronary arteries (left main and right coronary arteries) which arise from the aorta just distal to the aortic valve **(Fig. 3.1)**.

Left main Coronary Artery (LCA)

- Left main coronary artery arises from the left aortic sinus of ascending aorta.
- Its main branches are left anterior descending artery (LAD) and left circumflex artery (LCx).
- LAD runs in the anterior interventricular groove, and supplies anterior wall of both ventricles and anterior 2/3 of interventricular septum.

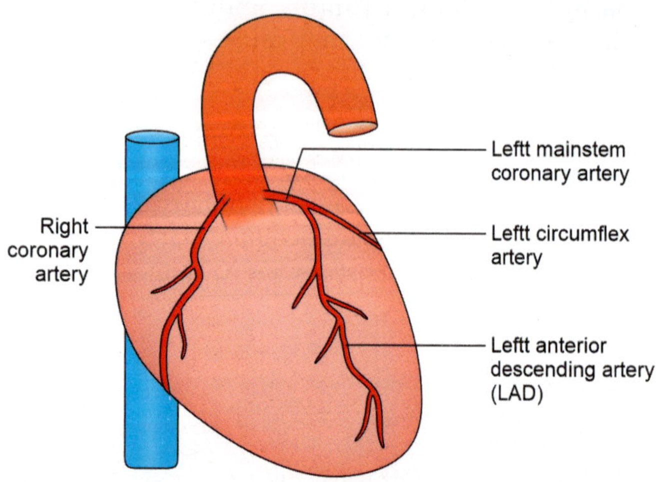

Figure 3.1: Blood supply of heart

- Left circumflex artery (LCx) runs in the left atrioventricular groove and supplies left atrium, lateral and posterior walls of the left ventricle.
- LAD gives diagonal branches and septal perforation branches which supply the anterior part of the septum, anterior wall and apex of the left ventricle. LCx artery supplies the lateral, posterior and inferior segments of the LV.
- Occlusion of the LAD or LCx causes infarction of the left ventricular areas supplied by them. Occlusion of the left main coronary artery is usually fatal.

Right Coronary Artery (RCA)

- The right coronary artery (RCA) arises from the right aortic sinus of the ascending aorta.
- It runs in the right atrioventricular groove and gives off branches.
- It supplies right atrium and right ventricle, SA node (in 60%), AV node (in 80%), inferior part of the left ventricle, and posterior part of the interventricular septum.
- Since the RCA supplies SA and AV node in most people, occlusion of the RCA can cause sinus bradycardia and AV nodal block. Occlusion of RCA also causes infarction of the right ventricle and inferior part of the left ventricle.

Venous System of the Heart

- Mainly consists of coronary sinus with its draining veins, the anterior right ventricular veins and the Thebesian veins. The coronary sinus lies in the posterior AV groove and drains into the right atrium. Thebesian veins are small veins which drain directly into the cardiac chambers.

Lymphatic Drainage

- Lymphatics from the heart travel with the coronary vessels and then drain into the thoracic duct.

Q. Nerve supply of the heart.

- The heart is supplied by both sympathetic and parasympathetic fibers.

Sympathfetic Supply (Cardio-accelerator)

- Sympathetic fibers arise from the first five thoracic segments (T1–T5) of the spinal cord and pass through cervical and upper thoracic symphathetic ganglia. Sympathetic system supplies muscle fibers in the atria and ventricles and the electrical conducting system.
- Effects of sympathetic stimulation:
  - Increases heart rate (positive chronotropic effect).
  - Increases force of contraction (positive inotropic effect).
  - Enhances conduction velocity (positive dromotropic effect).
  - Increases myocardial oxygen demand.

Parasympathetic Supply (Cardio-inhibitory)

- The parasympathetic fibers start in the medulla and pass through the right and left vagus nerves. They supply the AV and SA nodes via muscarinic (M_2) receptors and have an inhibitory effect.
- Effects of parasympathetic stimulation:
  - Decreases heart rate (negative chronotropic effect).
  - Reduces force of contraction (negative inotropic effect).
  - Slows conduction velocity (negative dromotropic effect).
- Afferent impulses from the heart pass via the spinal cord and the spinothalamic tract into the posteroventral nucleus of the thalamus.

Q. Describe briefly the conduction system of the heart (Fig. 3.2).

- The cardiac conduction system is made of specialized conduction tissue and consists of the sinotrial (SA) node, internodal atrial pathway, AV node, the bundle of His, bundle branches and terminal Purkinje fibers.
- The SA node is oval in structure, about 1–2 cm long and 0.5 cm thick. It is located at the junction of the right atrium and superior vena cava. SA node is made of special cells and it generates the impulses normally.
- The AV node is situated in the lower right atrium above the insertion of the medial leaflet of the tricuspid valve. It is also ovoid in shape and measures 1 × 3 × 5 mm. It continues as the bundle of His which passes into the ventricular tissue.

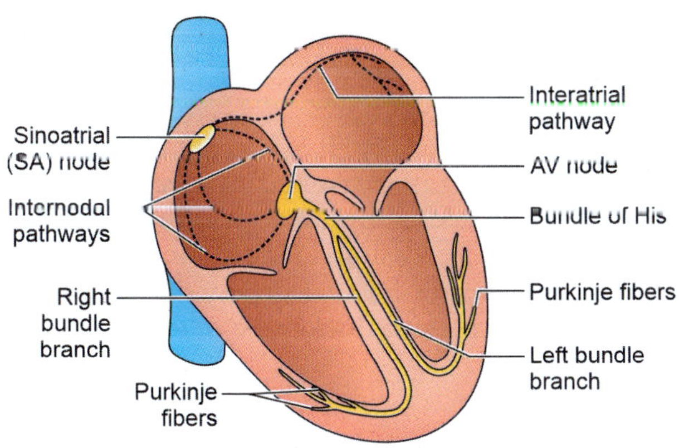

Figure 3.2: Conducting system of heart

- The bundle of His is about 2 cm in length. It divides into right and left bundle branches. The left bundle branch passes down the left side of the interventricular septum. Left bundle branch gives rise to two fascicles known as anterosuperior and posteroinferior fascicles. Right bundle branch is a continuation of bundle of His and runs on the right side of the interventricular septum. Both left and right bundle branches give rise to Purkinje fibers which ultimately supply the ventricles.
- The normal cardiac impulse is generated by SA node. This impulse passes to the AV node through atria. There is a delay in the AV node followed by transmission of the impulse to ventricles through the bundle of His and its branches. The delay in the AV node is responsible for the PR interval on ECG.

Q. Emumerate the symptoms of cardiac disease.

- The major symptoms associated with cardiac disease are:
  - Chest pain (discomfort)
  - Dyspnea
  - Fatigue
  - Edema
  - Palpitations
  - Syncope
  - Cough
  - Cyanosis

Q. What are the causes of chest pain? Discuss the differential diagnosis of chest pain.

Causes of Chest Pain

Cardiac

- Angina
- Myocardial infarction
- Pericarditis

Noncardiac

- Aortic dissection
- Pulmonary hypertension
- Pulmonary embolism
- Gastroesophageal reflux
- Esophageal spasm
- Peptic ulcer
- Gallbladder disease
- Musculoskeletal disease (costochondritis, rib fracture, muscle pain)
- Pleuritis
- Herpes zoster
- Pneumothorax

Differential Diagnosis of Chest Pain

Angina

- Felt in the retrosternal region. Usually radiates to left side of neck, jaw, epigastrium, shoulder, and arms. Felt as pressure, burning, squeezing, or heaviness. Usually lasts <20 min. Precipitated by exercise, cold weather, or emotional stress; relieved by rest or nitroglycerin. Prinzmetal's angina may come even at rest. Associated symptoms include sweating, palpitations, dizziness and dyspnea.

- *Main investigations:* ECG will show ST depression and T wave inversion. Cardiac enzymes (CK-MB, troponins) and echocardiogram will be usually normal.

Myocardial Infarction

- Pain is same as angina but more severe and lasts 30 min or longer. It is not relieved by rest or nitroglycerin. Associated symptoms include dyspnea, sweating, weakness, nausea, and vomiting.
- *Main investigations:* ECG will show ST elevation and pathological Q waves. Cardiac enzymes (CK-MB, troponins) will be elevated. Echocardiogram shows regional wall motion abnormality.

Pericarditis

- Pain is sharp, stabbing and knifelike and lasts for many hours to days. Usually felt over the precordium and may radiate to neck or left shoulder. It is more localized than the pain of myocardial ischemia. It is aggravated by deep breathing and supine position; relieved by sitting up and leaning forward. Auscultation shows pericardial friction rub.
- *Main investigations:* ECG will show ST elevation (with concavity upward). Echocardiogram may show pericardial effusion or constriction.

Aortic Dissection

- Pain is felt in the anterior chest. It is sudden onset, excruciating, tearing, knifelike and may radiate to back. It usually occurs in people with uncontrolled hypertension or Marfan's syndrome. There may be murmur of aortic insufficiency and pulse or blood pressure asymmetry between the limbs.
- *Main investigations:* Echocardiogram may show the dissection. CT or MR angiography can confirm the diagnosis.

Pulmonary Embolism

- Chest pain is felt in the substernal or over the region of pulmonary infarction. It is of sudden onset and pleuritic (with pulmonary infarction) or angina-like. It lasts minutes to <1 hour and aggravated by breathing. Associated symptoms include dyspnea, tachypnea, tachycardia, hypotension, signs of acute right-sided heart failure, pleural rub, and hemoptysis.
- *Main investigations:* Chest X-ray may show wedge shaped opacity. ECG may show S1Q3T3 pattern. Echocardiogram may show signs of pulmonary hypertension with dilated right atrium and right ventricle.

Pulmonary Hypertension

- Pain is felt like pressure in the substernal region. Pain is aggravated by exertion. Associated findings include dyspnea and signs of pulmonary hypertension.
- *Main investigations:* Echocardiogram may show signs of pulmonary hypertension with dilated right atrium and right ventricle.

Gastroesophageal Reflux

- Pain is burning type, felt in epigastric and retrosternal region and lasts 10–60 min. It is worsened by postprandial recumbency and relieved by antacids.
- *Main investigations:* Upper GI scopy (gastrointestinal scopy) may show reflux esophagitis, regurgitation of stomach contents into the esophagus.

Esophageal Spasm

- Pain is felt as pressure, tightness, or burning sensation in the retrosternal area. It lasts for 2–30 min and closely mimics angina. Esophageal spasm can be relieved by nitrates adding on to its confusion with angina.
- *Main investigations:* Esophageal manometry can record the increased pressure in the lower part of esophagus due to spasm. Endoscopy is also useful to visualize the inside of esophagus.

Peptic Ulcer

- Pain is burning type, felt in epigastric region and lasts for a long time. It is relieved by food or antacids and aggravated by spices and alcohol. Associated nausea, vomiting and melena may be present.
- *Main investigations:* Endoscopy will show the ulcer in the stomach or duodenum.

Gallbladder Disease

- Cholesystitis and cholelithiasis can cause epigastric, right upper quadrant, or substernal pain. Pain is felt as burning or pressure sensation and lasts for a long time. It often increases after a meal.
- *Main investigations:* Ultrasound abdomen may show gallstones or features of cholecystitis.

Musculoskeletal Disease

- Like costochondritis can cause chest pain. Pain is aching type and lasts for a variable duration. Pain is aggravated by movement. Localized tenderness may be present.
- *Main investigations:* ECG and other routine investigations will be normal.

Pleuritis

- Pain is felt superficially. It is usually unilateral, and well localized. It is worsened by deep breath and cough. Associated symptoms include cough, fever, crepitations and occasional rub.
- *Main investigations:* Chest X-ray may show underlying pneumonia or pleural thickening or effusion.

Herpes Zoster

Pain is sharp or burning with dermatomal distribution. Vesicular rash may appear in the dermatomal area.

Pneumothorax

- Pain is sudden onset and lasts for many hours. Pain is usually unilateral on the side of pneumothorax. Associated features include tracheal shift to opposite side, dyspnea, absent or diminished breath sounds on the side of pneumothorax.
- *Main investigations:* Chest X-ray will show the pneumothorax (air in the pleural space).

Q. Define syncope. Enumerate the causes of syncope. Dicuss the approach to a case of syncope.

- Syncope is a sudden, transient loss of consciousness with loss of postural tone followed by spontaneous recovery due to global cerebral hypoperfusion. This definition excludes seizures, coma, shock, or other states of altered consciousness. Near-syncope is light-headedness and a sense of an impending faint without loss of consciousness.
- Loss of consciousness happens due to global cerebral hypoperfusion. It is typically associated with a BP <60 mmHg for ≥6 seconds. It is characterized by rapid onset, short duration and spontaneous complete recovery.
- Though most cases of syncope are benign, there can be serious underlying problems such as cardiac disorders.

Causes of Syncope (Table 3.1)

- Syncope is classified as neurally mediated, cardiac, and orthostatic hypotension.

TABLE 3.1: Causes of syncope
Reflex mediated (most common type)
• Vasovagal syncope
• Situational syncope (cough, sneeze, swallow, micturition, defecation)
• Carotid sinus syncope
Cardiac
• Valvular heart diseases (AS, MS)
• Aortic dissection
• Atrial myxoma
• Cardiac tamponade
• Hypertrophic obstructive cardiomyopathy
• Myocardial ischemia, infarction
• Pulmonary embolism
• Pulmonary hypertension
• Arrhythmias
Orthostatic hypotension
• Autonomic neuropathy
• Volume depletion
• Drugs (alpha blockers, beta-blockers, nitrates)
Miscellaneous
• Psychogenic syncope
• Hyperventilation
• Transient ischemic attack
• Vascular steal syndromes (subclavian steal syndrome)

Approach to a Case of Syncope

History

- Elicit a detailed history of the event from the patient or bystanders.
- Ask whether there was definite loss of consciousness. In the absence of a clear witness account this may be difficult to establish—encourage the patient to describe the events in detail.
- Assume transient loss of consciousness if any following features are there:
    - A witness confirms a period of unresponsiveness.
    - The patient describes 'waking up'on the ground, especially if there is no recollection of falling.
    - There are facial injuries (most conscious patients can protect their face as they fall).
- Transient loss of consciousness is unlikely if:
    - There was no loss of postural tone
    - Patient recalls landing on the ground
    - Witness account suggests interaction with or awareness of the environment throughout the episode.
- ***Precipitating factors:*** include fatigue, sleep or food deprivation, hot weather, alcohol consumption, pain, and strong emotions such as fear or apprehension. If present, likely reflex syncope.
- ***Details of patient activity before the event:*** Activity prior to syncope may give a clue to the etiology of symptoms. Syncope may occur at rest; with change of posture; on exertion; after exertion; or with specific situations such as shaving, coughing, voiding, or prolonged standing. Syncope occurring within 2 minutes of standing suggests orthostatic hypotension.
- ***Position of the patient immediately before the syncope occurred:*** Syncope while standing indicates orthostatic hypotension. Syncope while seated or lying is more likely to be cardiac.
- ***Symptoms prior to the onset of syncope:*** Faintness, dizziness, or light-headedness occurs prior to true syncope. Other symptoms, such as vertigo, weakness, diaphoresis, epigastric discomfort, nausea, blurred or faded vision, pallor, or paresthesias, may also occur prior to true syncope. An aura prior to loss of consciousness may suggest seizure. Syncope on exertion, presence of chest pain, dyspnea, and palpitations may suggest cardiac cause. Severe headache, focal neurologic deficits, diplopia, ataxia, or dysarthria prior to the syncopal event suggest neurological cause such as intracranial bleed or vertebrobasilar insufficiency.
- ***Duration of loss of consciousness*** (LOC) can indicate the cause. True syncope is associated with LOC lasting for few seconds to few minutes. In neurological problems, LOC usually lasts longer, few minutes to hours.
- Confusion after syncope, tongue bite, urinary and fecal incontinence, convulsive activity, and myalgias indicate siezure as the cause of LOC.
- Obtain drug history, because many drugs cause postural hypotension and syncope. These are calcium channel blockers, alpha-blockers, diuretics, etc.

- Past history of cardiac disease, sizure disorder, diabetes (hypoglycemia), etc. should be asked. H/o pregnancy should be asked because ectopic rupture can cause syncope.

Physical Examination

- Look for the presence of following and consider appropriate possibilities **(Table 3.2)**.

TABLE 3.2: Clinical findings and possible cause of syncope

Clinical finding	Possible cause of syncope
Vary rapid or very slow pulse during syncope	Think of tachyarrhthmia or bradyarrhythmia
Irregularly irregular pulse	Think of atrial fibrillation with or without cardioembolic TIA
Weak thready pulse	Think of dehydration, hemorrhage or cardiac failure
Pallor	Consider anemia or hemorrhage as cause of syncope
Raised JVP, peripheral edema	Heart failure
Unilateral lower limb edema	Suspect DVT with pulmonary embolism
Drop in BP after standing by more than 20 mm Hg systolic or 10 mm Hg diastolic	Orthostatic hypotension
Ejection systolic murmur in aortic area	Aortic stenosis
Hyperpigmentation of skin, weight loss	Adrenal insufficiency
Rashes over the body	Allergic reaction

- CVS: Look for murmurs, signs of cardiac failure such as basal crepitations of lung, presence of S3 and presence of arrhythmias.
- CNS: Look for any signs of head injury, pupilary abnormalities, cranial nerve deficits, motor deficits, abnormal deep tendon reflexes, and sensory deficits. Severe neuropathies may correlate with vasodepressor syncope.
- RS/Abdomen: Look for any abnormalities.

Investigations

- Check blood glucose immediately using glucometer to rule out hypoglycemia. Other tests include complete blood count, serum electrolytes, cardiac enzymes, LFT and renal function tests.
- ECG: to rule out acute myocardial infarction or myocardial ischemia, arrhythmias, conduction defects.
- Stool for occult blood to rule out any GI bleed.
- Urine pregnancy test in women to rule out ectopic rupture.
- Chest radiography: May show evidence of diseases such as pneumonia, heart failure, pulmonary embolism, etc.
- Computed tomography (CT) of the head: To rule out any intracranial pathology such as hemorrhage or infarction in patients with neurologic deficits or in patients with head trauma secondary to syncope.
- CT of the chest and abdomen: Indicated only in select cases (e.g. suspected aortic dissection, ruptured abdominal aortic aneurysm, or pulmonary embolism [PE]).
- Echocardiography: Test of choice for evaluating cardiac causes of syncope such as heart failure, valvular heart diseases, etc.
- Tilt-table test: Useful for confirming autonomic dysfunction and postural hypotension causing syncope. Here patient is put on a table which is then tilted to an angle of 70° for up to 45 minutes while the ECG and blood pressure are monitored.
- Electroencephalography (EEG): Indicated if seizure is a likely diagnosis.
- Stress test: A cardiac stress test is appropriate for patients in whom cardiac syncope is suspected and who have risk factors for coronary atherosclerosis.

Management

- Treatment depends on the cause or precipitant of the syncope.
- Situational syncope: Patient education regarding the condition.
- Orthostatic syncope: Patient education; wearing elastic compression stocking to lower limbs, mineralocorticoids, and other drugs (e.g. midodrine); elimination of drugs associated with hypotension; increasing oral fluid intake.
- Cardiac syncope: Antiarrhythmic for arrhythmia induced syncope or pacemaker insertion. Surgical correction if any valvular heart disease is present.

Q. Write briefly about vasovagal syncope.

- Vasovagal syncope (earlier called neurocardiogenic syncope) (also known as the "common faint") is the most common cause of syncope. Majority of patients are young women between 15 and 45 years old. Vasovagal syncope is likely if there is history of specific triggers, such as emotional stress, pain, prolonged standing, hot weather, etc.

Pathophysiology

- Regardless of the trigger, the mechanism of syncope is similar in the various vasovagal syncope syndromes. There is an exaggerated autonomic reflex, resulting in enhancement of parasympathetic nervous system tone (vagal) and withdrawal of sympathetic nervous system tone.
- Increased parasymphathetic tone results in cardioinhibitory response, characterized by decreased heart rate (negative chronotropic effect) and decreased contractility (negative inotropic effect) leading to a decrease in cardiac output resulting in a loss of consciousness.
- Decreased sympathetic tone results in drop in blood pressure (to as low as 80/20) without much change in heart rate. This occurs due to dilation of the blood vessels, due to withdrawal of sympathetic tone.

- Though any of the above mechanisms can lead to syncope, majority of people with vasovagal syncope have both of the above mechanisms playing a role.

Causes and Triggers

Emotional Triggers ("classic vasovagal syncope")

- Fear (e.g. sight of blood, pain, injury)
- Emotional distress (e.g. anxiety, bad news)

Orthostatic Triggers ("situational syncope")

- Prolonged standing (e.g. in crowded places)
- Dehydration or heat exposure
- Sudden postural change (standing up quickly)

Reflex Triggers

- Coughing (Cough syncope)
- Swallowing (Swallow syncope)
- Micturition (Micturition syncope)
- Defecation (Straining during bowel movements)

Clinical Features

Prodromal Phase (before fainting)

- Lightheadedness or dizziness.
- Feeling sweaty or clammy.
- Nausea.
- Blurry vision.
- Looking pale or gray.
- Weakness.

Syncope (loss of consciousness)

- Brief (few seconds to minutes).
- Loss of muscle tone (may fall suddenly).
- No postictal confusion (unlike seizures).
- Feeble pulse, hypotension.

Recovery Phase

- Rapid recovery upon lying down.
- Fatigue, weakness, nausea may persist for a few minutes.

Investigations

- *Tilt table test*: Reproduces symptoms in orthostatic hypotension by tilting the patient upright while monitoring vitals.
- *ECG and Holter Monitor*: Rule out arrhythmias.
- *Echocardiogram*: Rule out structural heart disease.
- *Blood tests*: Rule out anemia, electrolyte imbalances, hypoglycemia.

Treatment

Acute Management

- Lay the patient flat, elevate legs (improves venous return).
- Ensure airway patency if unconscious.

Preventive Strategies

- Try to avoid situations that trigger fainting.
- Maintain good hydration and salt intake: Increases blood volume.
- If there are frequent attacks affecting the quality of life, following medications can be used.

Pharmacological Treatment (for frequent attacks affecting the quality of life)

- Alpha-1-adrenergic agonists (such as midodrine), which raise blood pressure.
- Corticosteroids (fludrocortisone) help raise sodium and fluid levels.
- Selective serotonin reuptake inhibitors (SSRIs such as paroxetine) help to regulate the nervous system response.

Q. Define cyanosis. Describe the mechanism and causes of cyanosis.

Q. Describe the mechanism of central and peripheral cyanosis. How do you differentiate central from peripheral cyanosis?

Q. Differential cyanosis.

- Cyanosis refers to a bluish discoloration of the skin and mucous membranes due to an increased quantity of deoxygenated hemoglobin or abnormal hemoglobin in the blood.
- Cyanosis is seen when deoxygenated hemoglobin (reduced hemoglobin) concentration in arterial blood is more than 5 g/dl. Cyanosis is also seen when methemoglobin (>1.5%) or sulfhemoglobin (>0.5%) is present in blood.
- It is easily detected on the lips, nail beds, ears, and malar eminences. The degree of cyanosis is modified by the color and thickness of the skin.
- Cyanosis can be divided into two types, central and peripheral.

Mechanism of Cyanosis

- It is the *absolute quantity* rather than the *relative quantity* of reduced hemoglobin which is important in producing cyanosis. Thus in severe anemia even if the reduced hemoglobin percentage is more; still the absolute quantity is less and hence, may not produce cyanosis. The opposite is true in polycythemia where hemoglobin is increased and can produce cyanosis even with lesser percentages of reduced hemoglobin.
- In central cyanosis PaO_2 is reduced or an abnormal hemoglobin is present, and it affects both skin and mucous membranes. Peripheral cyanosis is due to slowing of peripheral circulation which leads to greater extraction of O_2 from the blood and causes cyanosis. It results from vasoconstriction and diminished peripheral blood flow which occur in cold exposure, shock, congestive failure, and peripheral vascular disease. Peripheral cyanosis usually spares mucous membranes of oral cavity and tongue. In congestive heart failure both peripheral and central cyanosis may coexist.

Causes of Cyanosis (Table 3.3)

TABLE 3.3: Causes of cyanosis
Central cyanosis
Decreased FIO_2
• High altitude
Respiratoy causes
• Pneumonia
• ARDS
• COPD
• Interstitial lung disease
• Pulmonary embolism
• Respiratory failure due to any cause
• Ventilation perfusion mismatching (pulmonary arteriovenous fistulas)
Cardiac causes
• Cyanotic congenital heart diseases.
• Congestive heart failure with pulmonary edema
Hemoglobin abnormalities
• Methemoglobin
• Sulfhemoglobin
Peripheral cyanosis
• Cardiac failure
• Cold exposure
• Peripheral vascular disease
• Venous obstruction
• Raynaud's phenomenon

Differentiation between Central and Peripheral Cyanosis (Table 3.4)

TABLE 3.4: Differentiation between central and peripheral cyanosis

Feature	Central cyanosis	Peripheral cyanosis
Mechanism	Decreased arterial saturation	Decreased blood flow in the affected areas
Affected sites	Generalized involving both skin and mucous membranes	Affects only skin. Mucous membranes spared
Evidence of respiratory or cardiovascular disease	Present	Absent
Temperature of peripheries	Warm	Cold
Clubbing of fingers	Usually present and may suggest congenital cyanotic heart disease or pulmonary disease	Absent
Massage or warming of a cyanotic extremity	Cyanosis persists	Cyanosis disappears or decreases
Breathing 100% oxygen	Cyanosis may disappear	Persists
PaO_2	Decreased	Normal

Differential Cyanosis

- Here, cyanosis is present only in lower half of the body. Upper half of the body remains pink. It can be seen in patent ductus arteriosus with reversed shunt due to pulmonary hypertension. The deoxygenated blood in the pulmonary artery goes through the PDA, empties into the descending aorta, after the origin of left subclavian artery **(Fig. 3.3)**. Hence deoxygenated blood flows through the descending aorta into trunk and lower limbs. Hence cyanosis is seen lower half of the body (lower half of trunk and both lower limbs. Upper half of the body including both upper limbs, head and neck remain pink as they continue to receive oxygenated blood **(Fig. 3.4)**.
- It is usually seen in neonates with patent ductus arteriosus (PDA) and pulmonary arterial hypertension.
- In adults, differential cyanosis is pathognomonic for a large untreated patent ductus arteriosus (PDA) associated with Eisenmenger syndrome (right to left shunt due to pulmonary hypertension).

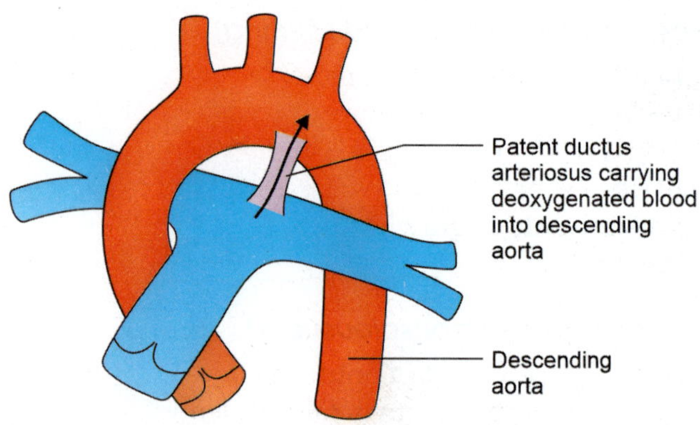

Figure 3.3: Mechanism of differential cyanosis

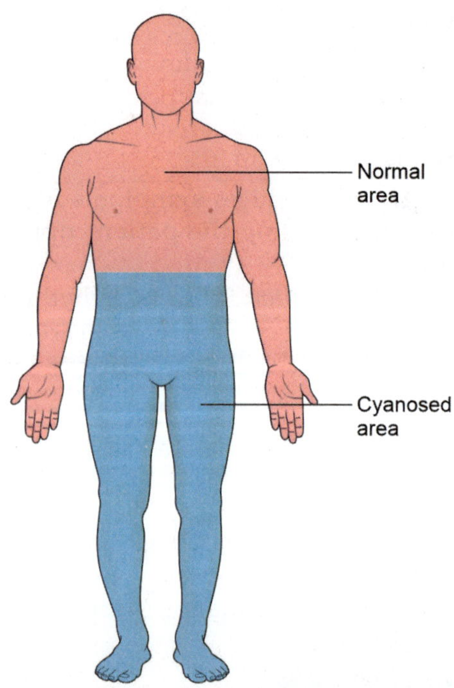

Figure 3.4: Differential cyanosis: Normal and cyanosed area

Reverse Differential Cyanosis (cyanotic upper limbs and normal lower limbs)

- This is seen in infants with transposition of the great arteries (TGA) with coarctation of the aorta or interrupted aortic arch and TGA with suprasystemic pulmonary vascular resistance. In this setting, the descending aorta is filled with oxygenated blood from the pulmonary circulation, and hence lower half of the body remains pink whereas upper half of the body is cyanosed.

Pseudocyanosis

- Several drugs and heavy metals can result in a bluish or slate-gray pigmentation of the skin that can be confused with cyanosis. This drug-induced skin discoloration is called sometimes as pseudocyanosis. Note that oxygen saturation is normal in pseudocyanosis.
- It occurs on exposure to drugs such as amiodarone, gold or silver salts.

Clinical Features

- Onset of cyanosis in the early perinatal period is highly suggestive of a congenital cause whereas a more recent onset suggests an acquired cause.
- General examination shows bluish hue in the skin and mucus membranes.
- History of exposure or physical contact with substances like dapsone and sulfur-containing drugs suggests hemoglobinopathies like methemoglobinemia.
- Current or frequent exposure to cold suggests peripheral cyanosis.
- Breathlessness (in central cyanosis)
- Clubbing (in chronic cyanotic heart disease)
- Cold extremities (in peripheral cyanosis).
- Detailed physical examination should be done to look for any cardiac or lung abnormality.

Investigations

- *Pulse oximetry (SpO_2)*: Measures oxygen saturation. Reduced in central cyanosis, normal in peripheral cyanosis.
- *Arterial blood gas (ABG):* Decreased arterial oxygen saturation (SaO_2) is seen in central cyanosis whereas ABG is normal in peripheral cyanosis.
- *Complete hemogram*: To know the presence of anemia, polycythemia, etc. which can influence the degree of cyanosis.
- *Methemoglobin and carboxyhemoglobin levels:* To rule out methemoglobinemia.
- *Chest X-ray*: To rule out lung diseases such as pneumonia, ILD.
- *Hyperoxia test*: High flow oxygen is given and patient is observed for the disappearance of cyanosis. In some cases of central cyanosis disappears. There will not be any change in peripheral cyanosis.
- *Echocardiography:* This can identify cyanotic heart diseases, heart failure, etc.

Treatment

- Oxygen support can be provided to resolve the hypoxia (especially in central cyanosis). Oxygen can be provided through nasal cannula, oxygen mask, and assisted ventilation.
- Warming of extremities (for peripheral cyanosis due to cold exposure).
- Treatment of underlying cause:
  - For methemoglobinemia-induced cyanosis, the standard treatment is with methylene blue.
  - Diuretics and inotropes for heart failure.
  - Surgical intervention is for the correction of congenital heart disease causing cyanosis.
  - Antibiotics for pneumonia, anticoagulants for DVT.

Q. Define palpitation. Enumerate the causes of palpitation. How do you approach a case of palpitation?

- Palpitations are defined as the abnormal awareness of one's own heartbeat.
- Palpitations occur whenever there is a change in heart rate, rhythm, and stroke volume.
- Patients may describe the sensation as skipping, fluttering, racing, pounding, thudding, or jumping. While episodes can be distressing and scary, the majority are benign, with less than half stemming from a heart rhythm abnormality.
- Palpitation is a very common and sometimes frightening symptom. It may be due to cardiac or noncardiac problems. Differentiating cardiac from noncardiac cause is important because there is a risk of sudden death in those with an underlying cardiac etiology.

Causes of Palpitation (Table 3.5)

TABLE 3.5: Causes of palpitation

Cardiac conditions
• *Change in heart rate:* Bradyarrhythmias, tachyarrhthmias, sinus tachycardia
• *Change in rhythm:* Atrial fibrillation, ectopic beats
• *Change in stroke volume:* Aortic regurgitation, mitral regurgitation, congestive cardiac failure
• *Mitral valve prolapse*
Noncardiac
• *High output states*: Thyrotoxicosis, anemia, Paget's disease, AV fistulas, pregnancy
• *Psychological*: Panic attack, anxiety
• *Metabolic disorders:* Hypoglycemia, pheochromocytoma
• *Physiological:* Stress, fear, exercise
• *Drugs:* Sympathomimetic agents, anticholinergic drugs, cocaine, amphetamines, caffeine nicotine, alcohol

Approach to a Patient with Palpitations

- Evaluation of the patient presenting with palpitations begins with a history, physical examination, and 12-lead ECG. Additional testing should be guided by clinical clues.

History

- Detailed history and physical examination are important for finding out the cause of palpitations.
- The key components of a detailed history include, age of onset, description of the symptoms including rhythm, situations that commonly result in the symptoms, mode of onset (rapid or gradual), duration of symptoms, factors that relieve symptoms (rest, Valsalva), other associated symptoms such as chest pain, dyspnea, light-headedness or syncope.
- Age of onset of palpitation: The age of onset might sometimes provide clues to potential causes, although it's essential to consider various factors for an accurate diagnosis. Here are some age-related considerations for palpitations: Infancy and childhood onset – think of congenital heart diseases, and emotional factors. Onset later in life, think of late presentation of congenital heart disease or other structural heart disease.
- Ask the patient to describe and tap out the rhythm. A rapid regular rhythm is more likely to be secondary to paroxysmal supraventricular tachycardia or ventricular tachycardia, and an irregular rhythm is more likely to be atrial fibrillation, or tachycardia with variable block.
- Onset and termination of palpitation: Abrupt onset and abrupt termination of palpitation is seen in supraventricular (PSVT) and ventricular tachycardia. H/o of termination of palpitations with a Valsalva maneuver suggests supraventricular tachycardia. Gradual onset and gradual termination suggests sinus tachycardia especially when is brought on by exertion.
- Nature of the palpitation: Is it rapid, forceful, or irregular? ask patient to tap out the rhythm.
- If the patient says palpitation is regular and normal speed during symptom (described as 'forceful' or 'strong), it may be due to increased stroke volume (e.g. aortic regurgitation, anemia, vasodilators, or simply awareness of the normal heartbeat). This type of regular palpitation with normal speed is against an arrhythmia. Try to look for evidence of causes described above.
- A clear history of an occasional 'jolt' or 'jump' in the chest or isolated 'dropped' or 'skipped' beats is highly suggestive of ectopic beats– such patients can usually be reassured without further investigation.
- Timing of palpitations: how quickly do they come on and subside? How often do these episodes occur, and how long do they typically last.
- Associated symptoms: Presyncope, syncope or chest pain: Palpitations associated with chest pain may suggest myocardial ischemia. When light-headedness or syncope accompanies the palpitations, ventricular tachycardia, supraventricular tachycardia, or other arrhythmias should be considered.
- H/o taking any medicines including over the counter medications should be asked. Sympathomimetic agents used as nasal decongestants, cough syrups containing terbutaline and salbutamol can cause palpitations. Excess caffeine consumption, alcohol, and illicit drug use (cocaine, methamphetamines) can also cause palpitations.
- Past medical history: Ask about previous episodes of arrhythmias, heart or thyroid disorders, history of underlying cardiac disease such as rheumatic heart disease, ischemic heart disease.
- Family history should note occurrences of syncope or sudden death at an early age (suggest significant arrhythmias).

Some Arrhythmias which Cause Palpitations

- Ectopic beats (extra-systoles) are a benign cause of palpitation at rest and are abolished by exercise. The premature ectopic beat produces a small stroke volume and an impalpable impulse due to incomplete left ventricular filling. The subsequent compensatory pause leads to ventricular overfilling and a forceful contraction with the next beat. Accordingly, patients often describe 'missed beats', sometimes followed by a particularly strong heart beat ('jolt' or 'thump').
- Atrial fibrillation (AF): Sudden onset rapid, irregular neat. Can be associated with breathlessness if very rapid. Can be followed by diuresis. While exercise or alcohol may trigger AF; it is often of spontaneous onset.
- Supraventricular tachycardia produces sudden paroxysms of rapid, regular palpitation that can sometimes be terminated with vagal stimulation using Valsalva breathing maneuvers or carotid sinus pressure (abrupt onset and abrupt termination). It is often followed by diuresis due to secretion of BNP. It often affects young patients with no other underlying cardiac disease.
- Ventricular tachycardia can produce similar symptoms (regular rapid beat) but is more commonly associated with presyncope or syncope, and tends to affect patients with cardiomyopathy or previous myocardial infarction.

Review of Systems

- Should cover symptoms of causative disorders, including heat intolerance, weight loss, and tremor (hyperthyroidism); chest pain and dyspnea on exertion (myocardial ischemia); and fatigue, weakness, heavy vaginal bleeding, and/or dark tar-like stools (anemia).

Examination

- Note the general status of the patient: whether anxious or agitated because these can produce palpitation.
- Look for any abnormality in vital signs such as fever, hypertension, hypotension, tachycardia, bradycardia, tachypnea, and low oxygen saturation. Note the pulse volume and rhythm. Irregular rhythm is seen in atrial fibrillation.
- Look for pallor (anemia can cause palpitation) any thyroid abnormality (thyromegaly) or exophthalmos (thyrotoxicosis can cause palpitation).

- CVS: Look for murmurs (suggests valvular heart disease), cardiomegaly and presence of S3 (suggests cardiac failure). Also note the rate and regularity of the heart beats.

Investigations

- ECG to rule out any arrhythmias. Normal resting ECG does not exclude cardiac arrhythmia. Hence ambulatory ECG monitoring should be considered if arrhythmia is strongly suspected inspite of normal ECG.
- Echocardiogram to rule out any structural heart disease.
- Exercise stress testing (treadmill testing) is indicated in patients who experience palpitations with exertion.
- Other tests such as hemoglobin, thyroid function tests, 24-hour urinary catecholamine levels (pheochromocytoma), etc. depending on suspicion.

Management

- Treatment depends on the underlying cause.
- Most cases of palpitations are due to an awareness of the normal heart beat, a sinus tachycardia or benign extrasystoles that have been triggered by stress, an intercurrent illness, or the effects of caffeine, alcohol and nicotine. In these situations, patient should be reassured.
- Beta-blockers may be tried for persistent benign palpitations.

Q. Describe the different types of radial pulse and their clinical importance.

Q. Clinical importance of radial pulse examination.

- Examination of radial pulse can indicate the underlying diagnosis.
- Examination of the pulse involves assessment of the following: Rate, rhythm, volume, character, condition of the vessel wall, radioradial and radiofemoral delay.
- Other peripheral pulses such as femorals, dorsalis pedis, posterior tibials, subclavians and temporals should be palpated and assessed for any delay or difference in volume. In coarctation of the aorta, the volume of the femoral pulse is lower than radial pulse and also delayed.
- Pulse volume and character are better assessed in the carotid artery. All other parameters can be assessed in the radial pulse.
- The normal carotid and aortic pulse consist of an early percussion wave due to left ventricular ejection, and a second smaller peak tidal wave representing the reflected wave from periphery. However, normally, peripheral pulses such as radial and femoral are felt as single waveform.

Rate

- The normal pulse rate for adults at rest typically falls within the range of 60–100 beats per minute (bpm).
- Pulse rate of more than 100 per minute is called as tachycardia.
- Pulse rate of less than 60 per minute is called as bradycardia.
- In healthy young individuals who breathe at a normal rate, the heart rate undergoes rhythmic variations in response to the phases of respiration. Heart rate increases during inspiration and decreases during expiration, especially while breathing deeply. This phenomenon, known as sinus arrhythmia, is considered a normal occurrence and is attributed to fluctuations in parasympathetic nerve signals affecting the heart.
- During inspiration, there is inhibition of vagal tone, which increases heart rate. This effect is often more pronounced in children and adolescents and tends to become less prominent after the age of 30.

Causes of Tachycardia (Table 3.6)

TABLE 3.6: Causes of tachycardia

Physiological
• Infancy: In newly born infant, pulse rate is about 130/min
• Childhood: In children PR is higher than adults, it comes to adult level at around 20 years of age
• After exercise
• After eating
• During emotions like fear, anger, excitement
• In pregnancy
• In high ambient temperature
• During inspiration (heart rate slightly increases)
Pathological
• Fever: Pulse rate increases by approximately 10 beats per minute per degree centigrade rise in body temperature.
• Anemia: Tachycardia occurs as a compensatory mechanism to improve oxygen supply to tissues.
• Thyrotoxicosis: Thyroxin increases the number of β receptors in heart and also increases sensitivity of these receptors to catecholamines.
• Tachyarrhthmias (supraventricular tachycardia, atrial flutter, atrial fibrillation, ventricular tachycardia).
• Hypovolemia (dehydration, blood loss)
• Heart failure
• Certain drugs (phenylephrine, adrenaline, noradrenaline, atropine, terbutaline, amphetamines)

Causes of Low Pulse Rate (bradycardia) (Table 3.7)

TABLE 3.7: Causes of bradycardia

Physiological
• Old age
• During deep expiration
• In athletes; because of their increased vagal tone
• During sleep and meditation.
Pathological
• Hypothyroidism: decrease in thyroxin levels will decrease the number of β receptors and their sensitivity to catecholamines.
• Raised intracranial pressure: increased intracranial pressure will lead to Cushing's reflex.
• Heart block: Decrease in pulse rate depends on degree of heart block. In complete heart block, rate may be 30–40/minute.
• Certain drugs, e.g. beta blockers, digoxin.
• Obstructive jaundice.

Rhythm

- Normally the pulse is regular except for a slight increase in rate on inspiration and slowing on expiration (sinus arrhythmia).

Irregularly Irregular

- Atrial fibrillation
- Atrial flutter with a varying AV block
- Multifocal atrial tachycardia (MAT)
- Frequent extrasystoles

Completely Regular (loss of normal sinus arrhythmia)

- Autonomic neuropathy.

Regularly Irregular

- Sinus arrhythmia
- Pulsus bigeminus, trigeminus
- Partial AV blocks

Volume

- This is the amplitude of pulse wave as judged by the palpating finger. It depends on pulse pressure and is graded as high volume, normal volume, and low volume.

High-volume Pulse (water hammer, collapsing or Corrigan's pulse)

- Aortic regurgitation
- Patent ductus arteriosus
- Mitral regurgitation
- Ventricular septal defect
- High output states (anemia, hyperthyroidism, beriberi, Paget's disease, arteriovenous fistula)
- Increased stroke volume (complete heart block).

Low-volume Pulse

- Hypovolemia
- Cardiogenic shock
- Tachycardias
- Dilated cardiomyopathy
- Heart failure
- Mitral stenosis
- Aortic stenosis

Varying Volume Pulse (alternate high and low volume pulses)

- Left ventricular failure.

Character of the Pulse

Pulsus Paradoxus

- This is an exaggeration of the normal phenomenon of low-volume pulse during inspiration and better volume during expiration (normal fall by <10 mm Hg on inspiration). Hence, the name "paradoxus" is a misnomer.
- *Mechanism of pulsus paradoxus:* In normal people, there is reduction of itrathoracic pressure during inspiration, which causes pooling of blood in the right ventricle and pulmonary vasculature, which in turn results in decreased venous return to left ventricle and low stroke volume. Exaggeration of this normal response can be caused by,
- Restriction of diastolic filling of ventricles (constrictive pericarditis, massive pericardial effusion). Limitation in the diastolic filling of the right atrium and right ventricle during inspiration results in lowering of left ventricular stroke volume.
- Right ventricular failure. This leads to decreased venous return to left ventricle and low left ventricular stroke volume.
- Increased respiratory effort (severe asthma). During inspiration, owing to enhanced intrathoracic negative pressure, there is pooling of blood in pulmonary veins resulting in lowered left ventricular stroke volume.

Causes of pulsus paradoxus

- Constrictive pericarditis
- Cardiac tamponade
- Restrictive cardiomyopathy
- COPD
- Severe asthma
- Tension pneumothorax.

How to look for pulsus paradoxus

- Pulsus paradoxus is better appreciated in the peripheral pulses (radial). During inspiration there is decrease in the volume of radial pulse.
- An even better way of measuring pulsus paradoxus is by using sphygmomanometer and stethoscope. BP cuff is tied around the arm and inflated until all Korotkoff sounds are absent, then pressure is released very slowly from the cuff. The first sounds auscultated will be heard only during expiration, and this pressure should be noted. Next, as cuff pressure is dropped further, the pressure should be noted when Korotkoff sounds are heard during both inspiration and expiration. The difference between these two systolic pressures quantifies pulsus paradoxus.

Reverse Pulsus Paradoxus

- This refers to inspiratory rise in arterial pressure.
- It is seen in hypertrophic cardiomyopathy, positive pressure ventilation and AV dissociation.

Water Hammer or Collapsing Pulse or Corrigan's Pulse

- This is characterized by a rapid upstroke, a rapid down stroke and a high volume.
- The rapid upstroke is due to increased stroke volume. Rapid downstroke is due to either diastolic leak back into left ventricle (e.g. aortic regurgitation) or rapid run off to the periphery due to low systemic vascular resistance (e.g. AV fistula).

Causes of water hammer pulse

- Aortic regurgitation
- Ruptured sinus of Valsalva
- Patent ductus arteriosus
- Mitral regurgitation
- Hyperkinetic circulatory states (anemia, hyperthyroidism, beriberi, Paget's disease, arteriovenous fistula).

How to check for collapsing pulse

The fundamental principle of eliciting the water hammer pulse is to elevate the patient's arm above the heart and to palpate the patient's wrist (radial pulse) with the examiner's palm. Place the patient in supine position at a slight recline. Wrap around the patient's wrist with your palm and feel for the radial pulse with your palm. Now increase the grasp so that radial pulse is slightly occluded. The patient's arm is then raised above the patient's head. The water hammer pulse will feel like a tapping impulse with the palm of examiner's hand.

Pulsus Alternans

- This is alternate large volume and low volume pulse. There is a difference of 10–40 mm Hg in systolic pressure between beats.
- It is due to the alternate strong and weak contraction of the left ventricle. When the ventricle contracts poorly there is less stroke stroke volume producing weak pulse. Less stroke volume also leads to increased end diastolic volume in left ventricle which leads to strong contraction and high volume pulse in the next beat according to Starling's law.
- The pulse must be absolutely regular to diagnose pulsus alternans and distinguish it from pulsus bigemini which also has beats of alternating strength, although the rhythm is irregular.
- It is seen in cardiac failure.

Pulsus Parvus et Tardus

- This is a slow rising, low volume, well sustained pulse, seen in aortic stenosis.
- Anacrotic pulse is a variant of pulsus parvus in which a notch is palpable between the slowly rising percussion and tidal waves.

Pulsus Bisferiens

- A double pulse noticed during systole in the peripheral pulse is called pulsus bisferiens. This is derived from the Latin word, which means strike twice (bis = twice, ferio = strike). It is also called a biphasic wave. Pulsus bisferiens manifests as a single central pulse wave featuring two prominent peaks, separated by a noticeable mid-systolic dip. The initial component, known as the percussion wave, results from the rapid ejection of blood from the left ventricle. The subsequent component, referred to as the tidal wave, represents a reflected wave originating from the periphery, resulting from the recoil effect of an artery.
- Pulsus bisferiens is often confused with the dicrotic pulse. The main difference is that both peaks of pulsus bisferiens occur in systole, whereas in dicrotic pulse, one peak occurs in systole and the other in diastole.
- Pulsus bisferiens is a combination of slow raising pulse (anacrotic) and collapsing pulse. This is typically seen in AS with AR. Hypertrophic cardiomyopathy with obstruction (HOCM). Other causes are: severe aortic regurgitation, large PDA (patent ductus arteriosus) or arteriovenous fistula.
- The precise mechanism of pulsus bisferiens is not understood. A normal central pulse has two waves; a percussion wave (larger) and a tidal wave (smaller), which are not easy to distinguish clinically. But in the above conditions, these are exaggerated by a wider mid-systolic gap leading to two distinct waves.

Dicrotic Pulse/Twice Beating Pulse

- Dicrotic pulse also has two peaks, but one peak occurs in systole and the other in diastole (in bisferiens pulse both peaks occur in systole). It is called 'Twice beating pulse because the dicrotic wave is prominent and gives impression of 2 beats. It is better appreciated during inspiration.
- It is almost impossible to distinguish between pulsus bisferiens and dicrotic pulse clinically, without a pulse recording.
- The exact mechanism is not fully understood.

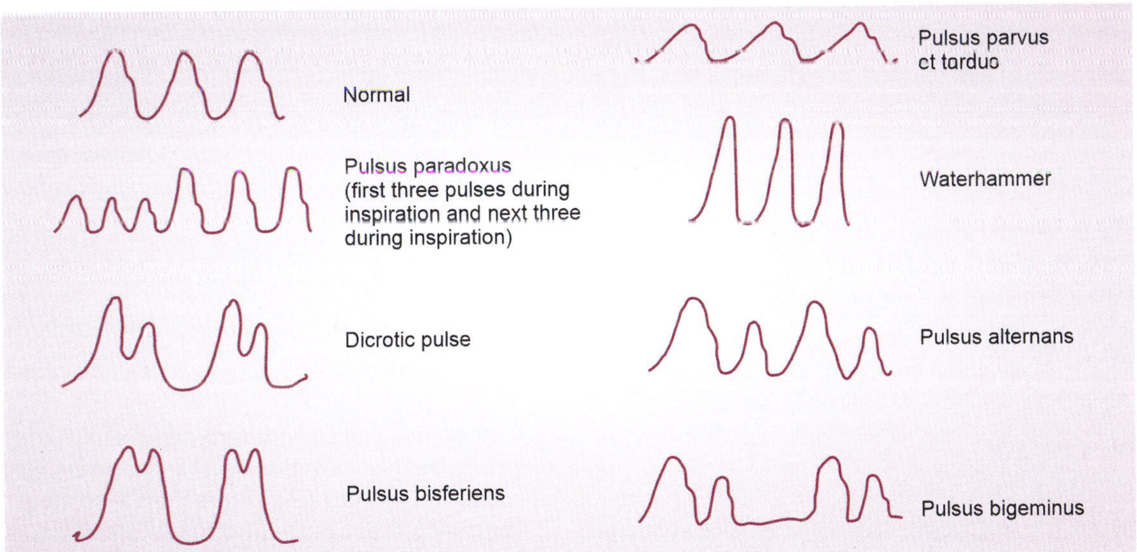

Figure 3.5: Different types of pulses

Causes

- Fever
- Cardiac failure
- Sepsis
- Cardiac tamponade
- Occasionally seen in normal individuals after exercise.

Pulsus Bigemini or Trigemini or Quadrigemini

Here the pulse is regularly irregular and is due to fixed unifocal extrasystoles coming after every normal beat (bigemini) or after every two (trigemini) or three normal beats (quadrigemini), with a pause after the extrasystole.

Condition of Arterial Wall

This can be assessed by rolling the radial artery with fingers against the underlying bone. Normally it feels soft and elastic. If the wall is thickened, it feels hard and tortuous.

Radiofemoral and Radioradial Delay

- Delayed femoral pulse compared to the radial pulse is seen in coarctation of aorta (post-subclavian), aorto-arteritis, or saddle embolus. Radiofemoral delay can be assessed by simultaneous palpation of these two arteries.
- Unequal radial pulses and radioradial delay may be seen in coarctation of aorta (pre-subclavian).
- Unequal carotid pulses could be due to atherosclerotic stenosis in one of the arteries.

Q. Discuss the mechanism of jugular venous pulse.

Q. Describe the importance of examination of JVP. What are the normal wave patterns of JVP and their variations? How do you differentiate JVP from carotid pulse?

- Examination of jugular veins can give valuable clues regarding volume status, central venous pressure, and right heart events. Since there are no valves between the right atrium and internal jugular veins, right atrial pressure is reflected in these veins.

Why is JVP Important?

Assessment of Right Heart Function

- Elevated JVP → Suggests right heart failure, pulmonary hypertension, tricuspid valve disease, or pericardial tamponade.
- Decreased JVP → Seen in hypovolemia, dehydration, or hemorrhage.

Diagnosing Heart and Lung Diseases

- Raised JVP + Bilateral pedal edema → Right heart failure.
- Raised JVP + Pulmonary symptoms → Cor pulmonale (pulmonary hypertension).
- Raised JVP + Hypotension → Cardiac tamponade or constrictive pericarditis (Kussmaul's sign).

How to Measure JVP

- The patient should be in supine position, torso elevated to 45 degrees, and the head extended backward and turned slightly to the left (around 30 degrees to left). Normally the neck veins should not be visible and collapse in this position. The height of JVP is measured as the vertical distance between the top of the venous pulsation and the angle of Louis (sternal angle, where the manubrium meets the sternum). This measurement is normally ≤3 cm. Anything above 3 cm is considered abnormal.
- The centre point of right atrium is about 5 cm below the sternal angle. Hence, if 5 cm is added to the height of JVP measured, we get a rough estimate of central venous pressure (CVP) which is normally ≤8 cm H_2O. Elevated JVP is >8 cm.
- Some clinicians choose to use the clavicle as a reference point with the patient in seated position. Clavicle is easily located and venous pulsations above that level are clearly abnormal.

Causes of Elevated JVP (Table 3.8)

TABLE 3.8: Causes of elevated JVP
• Right heart failure (cor pulmonale)
• Volume overload
• Tricuspid regurgitation
• Tricuspid stenosis
• Pulmonary HTN
• Pulmonary embolism
• Constrictive pericarditis
• Cardiac tamponade
• Sup vena cava obstruction (non-pulsatile elevation)
• Massive ascites or right sided pleural effusion

Distinguishing JVP from Carotid Pulse (Table 3.9)

Jugular venous pulse should be differentiated from carotid pulse as the later can sometimes be mistaken for the jugular venous pulsation.

TABLE 3.9: Differences between JVP and carotid pulse

JVP	Carotid pulse
Visible but not palpable	Visible and palpable
Obliterated by pressure at root of neck	Not obliterated
Multiple wave forms	Single wave form
Hepatojugular reflux present	Absent
Definite upper level	No definite upper level
On sitting up upper level of column decreases	No change
Upper level falls on inspiration	No change

Wave forms of JVP and their Mechanism

- JVP has 3 positive (a, c, v) and 2 negative waves (x and y).
- *The 'a' wave occurs due to right atrial contraction.* A prominent '*a*' wave is seen in patients with reduced right ventricular (RV) compliance from any cause. A cannon '*a*' wave occurs with A-V dissociation (complete heart block) and RA contraction against a closed tricuspid valve. '*a*' wave is absent in atrial fibrillation

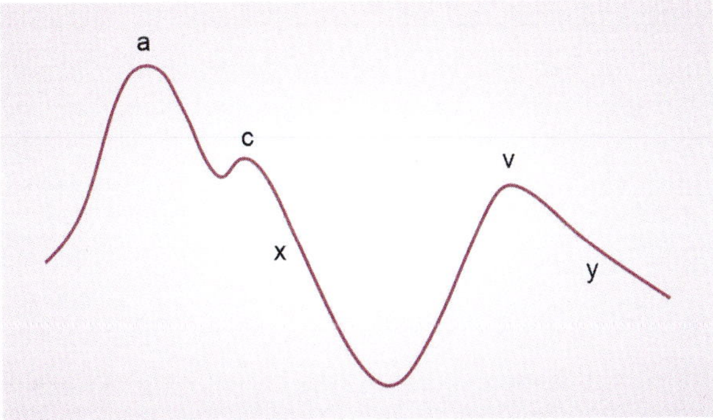

Figure 3.6: Waveforms of JVP

because there is no coordinated atrial contraction. Cannon A waves need to be distinguished from giant A waves that occur in right heart structural changes such as tricuspid valvulopathies, right ventricular hypertrophy, and pulmonary hypertension. To the observer of the jugular, venous-pressure giant A waves and Cannon A waves may appear similar. From physical exam alone it might be difficult to differentiate between the two.

- *Next 'x' descent follows and is due to the fall in pressure in the atrium during atrial diastole.* In normal individuals, the x' descent is the predominant waveform in the jugular venous pulse.
- The *'x'* descent is interrupted by a *positive 'c' wave which is due to the ventricular systole* pushing the closed tricuspid valve into the right atrium, elevating its pressure.
- *The 'v' wave is due to venous filling of right atrium,* and occurs at the end of ventricular systole. Its height depends on RA compliance and the amount of blood in the RA. Normally *v* wave is smaller than the *'a'* wave. In patients with atrial septal defect (ASD), the *'a'* and *'v'* waves may be of equal height.
- *The 'y' descent follows the 'v' wave peak and reflects the fall in RA pressure after tricuspid valve opening.* If there is resistance to ventricular filling in early diastole, the *'y'* descent will be blunted (e.g. pericardial tamponade, tricuspid stenosis). A steep *'y'* descent occurs when the ventricular diastolic filling occurs early and rapidly, as with pericardial constriction. The corresponding auscultatory phenomenon is the pericardial knock.

Key Timing Features of JVP Waves (Table 3.10)

TABLE 3.10: Key timing features of JVP waves

JVP Wave	Phase of cardiac cycle	Relation to carotid pulse
a wave	Atrial contraction (late diastole)	Just before carotid pulse
c wave	Tricuspid valve bulging (early systole)	Occurs with carotid pulse
x descent	Atrial relaxation (mid-systole)	Follows the carotid upstroke
v wave	Venous filling of RA (late systole)	Peaks just after the carotid pulse
y descent	Tricuspid valve opening (early diastole)	Occurs after the carotid pulse

Q. Kussmaul sign.

- Normally, the JVP falls with inspiration and increases with expiration. This is because of decrease in intrathoracic pressure and pulmonary vascular resistance during inspiration inspite of increased venous return to the right side of the heart during inspiration. As a result, pulmonary artery, right ventricle and right atrial pressures fall leading to decrease in JVP inspite of increased venous return. During expiration, due to increased positive intrathoracic pressure, pulmonary circulation is compressed by the thoracic cage resulting in increased pulmonary resistance and pressure.
- However, in some patients, there is a lack of a decrease or even an increase in JVP during inspiration, and this abnormal finding is called Kussmaul sign.
- Kussmaul sign is seen in the following conditions:
    - Constrictive pericarditis
    - Restrictive cardiomyopathy
    - Acute severe asthma or COPD
    - Pulmonary embolism
    - RV infarction
    - Right-sided volume overload
    - Advanced systolic failure
- In all these conditions, increased venous return in inspiration cannot be accommodated in the right side of the heart and pulmonary vasculature leading to inspiratory increase in JVP.

Q. Hepatojugular reflux (abdominaojugular reflux).

- Abdominojugular reflux is performed using firm and consistent pressure over the upper abdomen, preferably the right upper quadrant, for 10–30 seconds.
- Normally there is either no rise or only a transient (2–3 seconds) rise in JVP which falls down even if the pressure on the abdomen is continued.
- A sustained rise in JVP until abdominal pressure is released indicates impaired right heart function. This abnormal response is called hepatojugular reflux.
- Patient should not hold his or her breath or perform a Valsalva-like maneuver during the procedure because these can falsely elevate the venous pressure.

Significance

- This can help to confirm that the pulsation is caused by the JVP.
- Abdominojugular reflux indicates a volume-overloaded state and limited compliance of an overdistended or constricted venous system. It is positive in right heart failure. But the normal response is lost in SVC obstruction and Budd-Chiari syndrome.

Q. Discuss the mechanism and variations of first heart sound.

- The first heart sound is mainly due to closure of the mitral and tricuspid valves. It coincides with the R wave on the ECG.
- Normally S1 is louder than S2 at the apex (mitral area). The loudness of the mitral valve closure depends upon 3 things: the degree of valve opening, the force

of ventricular contraction shutting the valve, and the integrity of the valve. Think of a slamming door. The amount of its noise will depend on how far open the door is, how hard you slam it, and the integrity of the door.

- S1 has two components: mitral component (M1) due to mitral valve closure and tricuspid component (T1) due to tricuspid valve closure. Normally these two components are not heard separately as the tricuspid valve closure sound is too faint to hear. However splitting of first heart sound can be heard sometimes.

Variations of First Heart Sound

Causes of Loud S1

- *Thin chest wall* (sound is better conducted through the thin chest wall to stethoscope).
- *Tachycardia:* The faster the heart rate and the faster the rise in ventricular pressure, the louder the S1, because mitral leaflets close rapidly from a widely open position.
- *Mitral stenosis*: In mitral stenosis, the increased left atrial pressure causes the mitral valve leaflets to be more widely separated, and as they close from widely separated position, produce loud S1.
- *Tricusipid stenosis*: Reason for loud S1 is same as MS.
- *Hyperkinetic states (anemia, thyrotoxicosis, fever):* All these produce tachycardia and loud S1 as described above. Additionally, increased force of contraction of left ventricle also contributes to loud S1.

Causes of Quiet (Muffled) S1

- *Thick chest wall (obesity), emphysema, pericardial effusion:* sound transmission to stethoscope becomes less.
- *Bradycardia:* Due to prolonged diastole, the mitral and tricuspid valves would have already drifted towards closure position, hence close from a less widely open position leading to muffled S1.
- *Calcified anterior mitral leaflet:* In severe to critical mitral stenosis the valve leaflets are so calcified and immobile that M1 sound is diminished or absent.
- *Heart failure:* Decreased LV pressure during systole results in less forceful closure of mitral valve and hence muffled S1.
- *Mitral regurgitation*: Mitral valves will not close and hence soft or absent S1 (however, tricuspid component of S1 may still be heard in tricuspid area).
- *Long P–R interval (first-degree heart block):* Longer PR results in longer diastolic filling time, which in turn results in gradual filling of LV and gradual increase in LV pressure. This gradual increase in pressure causes the mitral valve leaflets to slowly drift together towards the closing position. Therefore, when ventricular systole occurs in the setting of a long PR interval, the leaflets will be separated by a smaller distance, and the S1 sound will be softer due to less excursion of leaflets (imagine a door closing from a smaller distance *vs* closing from a widely open position. Door closing from a smaller distance produces less sound and door closing from a widely open position produces loud sound).

Varying Intensity of S1

- Varying intensity of S1 refers to an inconsistent loudness of the first heart sound between beats. Varying intensity of S1 occurs in atrial fibrillation (AF). This occurs when there are fluctuations in ventricular contraction strength, mitral/tricuspid valve position, or AV conduction time.

Causes of varyining intensity of S1 and its mechanism

TABLE 3.11: Causes of varyining intensity of S1 and its mechanism

Causes	Mechanism
Atrial fibrillation	In AF, there is an absence of organized atrial contraction, leading to variable ventricular filling times. The PR interval is constantly changing, causing different degrees of mitral valve opening at systole. When mitral valve closes from widely open position (due to short PR interval), there will be loud S1. When mitral valve closes from less open position (due to drifting of valvfe towards closed position due tyo long diastole due to long PR interval), there will be soft S1. This results in beat-to-beat variability in S1 intensity.
Atrioventricular (AV) dissociation (e.g., complete heart block)	In third-degree (complete) heart block, the atria and ventricles beat independently. The PR interval varies, and hence the position of mitral and tricuspid valves varies before final closure. This will lead to varying S1.
PVCs (premature ventricular contractions)	Early ventricular beats → inconsistent ventricular filling → different valve closure positions → varying S1.

Splitting of S1

- Not heard normally because both mitral and tricuspid valves close simultaneously.
- Splitting can be seen in following conditions
  - Complete RBBB. RBBB causes the electrical impulse to reach the right ventricle late and hence delayed contraction of right ventricle, hence split becomes obvious.
  - Pacing of left ventricle. Left ventricle is activated first and contracts first leading to early production of mitral component of S1 leading to split S1.
- A split S1 heart sound is best heard at the tricuspid area as tricuspid component of S1 is soft and may not be heard in other areas. In tricuspid area, you can appreciate both mitral and tricuspid components of S1 if there is a split. Inspiration delays the closure of the tricuspid valve in a normal person, due to increased venous return, thereby enhancing the splitting of the S1 sound.

Q. Discuss the mechanism and variations of second heart sound.

- The second heart sound (S2) is produced by closure of the aortic and pulmonary valves. It has two components; aortic component (A2) due to closure of aortic valve and pulmonary component (P2) due to closure of pulmonary valve.
- Normally A2 comes first and then P2.

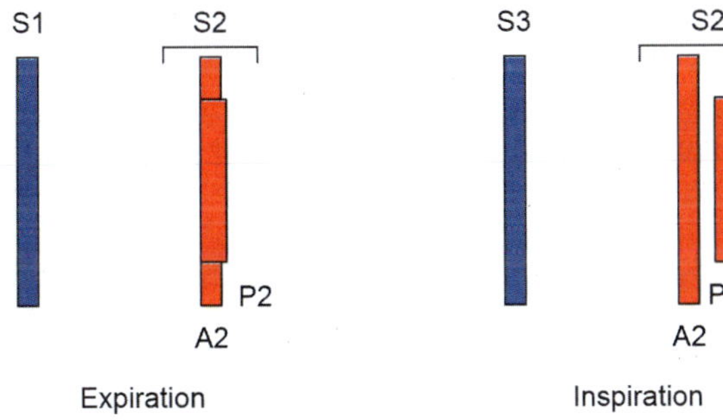

Figure 3.7: Normal single S2 in expiration and split S2 during inspiration

- Normally, during inspiration, there is increased venous return to right ventricle and hence pulmonary valve closes late. At the same time due to decreased venous return to left ventricle, aortic valve closes early. This causes physiological splitting of second heart sound during inspiration. During expiration the sound is heard as single. A split S2 is best heard at the pulmonary area since P2 is much softer than A2 and is better heard at the pulmonary area **(Fig. 3.7)**.

Variations of Second Heart Sound

- Loud A2 (loud aortic component of S2)
- Soft A2 (soft aortic component of S2)
- Loud P2 (loud P2 component of S2)
- Soft P2 (soft P2 component of S2)
- Wide fixed split S2
- Wide mobile split S2
- Reversed (paradoxical) splitting of S2
- Single S2

Loud A2 (loud aortic component of S2) (Table 3.12)

TABLE 3.12: Loud A2

Causes	Mechanism
Hypertension	High aortic pressure → Aortic valve snaps shut forcefully → Loud A2
Aortic root dilatation (aortic aneurysm, syphilitic Aortitis, Marfan syndrome)	Increased aortic tension → Stronger recoil force on valve → Louder closure sound

Soft A2 (soft aortic component of S2) (Table 3.13)

TABLE 3.13: Soft A2

Causes	Mechanism
Severe aortic stenosis	Calcified, immobile aortic valve → Reduced valve closure force → Soft or absent A2
Severe aortic regurgitation	Aortic valve fails to close properly → Reduced closing intensity → Soft A2 (may also be absent if regurgitation is severe).
Tetralogy of Fallot (post-surgical correction)	Aortic valve is more anteriorly placed → Increased transmission of A2 sound.
(Contd.)	
Hyperdynamic circulation (e.g. fever, anemia, hyperthyroidism)	Increased stroke volume → More forceful closure of aortic valve → Loud A2.

Loud P2 (loud P2 component of S2) (Table 3.14)

TABLE 3.14: Loud P2

Causes	Mechanism
Pulmonary hypertension	Increased pulmonary artery pressure → Pulmonary valve closes forcefully → Loud P2
ASD	
	Left-to-right shunt → Increased pulmonary blood flow → Pulmonary hypertension over time → Loud P2

Soft P2 (soft P2 component of S2) (Table 3.15)

TABLE 3.15: Soft P2

Causes	Mechanism
Pulmonary stenosis	Thickened, immobile pulmonary valve → Weak closure → Soft or absent P2.
Tetralogy of Fallot	Severe RV outflow obstruction → Less blood flow across pulmonary valve → Soft or absent P2.
Severe fight ventricular failure (e.g. RV infarction, dilated cardiomyopathy)	Weak RV contraction → Low pulmonary artery pressure → Reduced P2 intensity.

Wide Fixed Split S2

- Normally during inspiration, A2 and P2 components of S2 are separated, because inspiration increases venous return to the right heart, delaying pulmonary valve (P2) closure. Inspiration also reduces left ventricular (LV) return, causing earlier aortic valve (A2) closure. This creates a physiologic split of S2. But during expiration, they are close together or single.
- **In wide fixed split S2,** A2 and P2 are separated more than normal during both inspiration and expiration. The split does not change with respiration (unlike normal S2 splitting) **(Fig. 3.8)**.

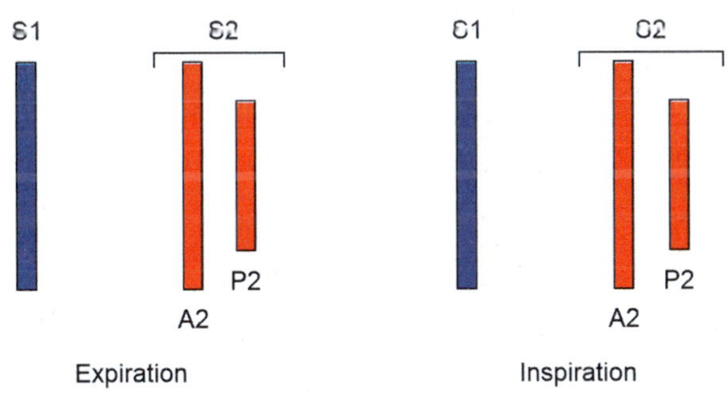

Figure 3.8: Wide fixed split S2

Causes of wide fixed split S2 (Table 3.16)

TABLE 3.16: Causes of wide fixed split S2	
Causes	**Mechanism**
Atrial septal defect ASD)	Left-to-right shunt → Increased RV volume → Prolonged RV systole → Delayed P2. Venous return does not change significantly with respiration, making the split fixed.
Severe right ventricular failure	RV is unable to vary its stroke volume during respiration

Wide Mobile Split S2 (Fig. 3.9)

- A2 and P2 are separated both during inspiration and expiration, but the split increases further during inspiration.

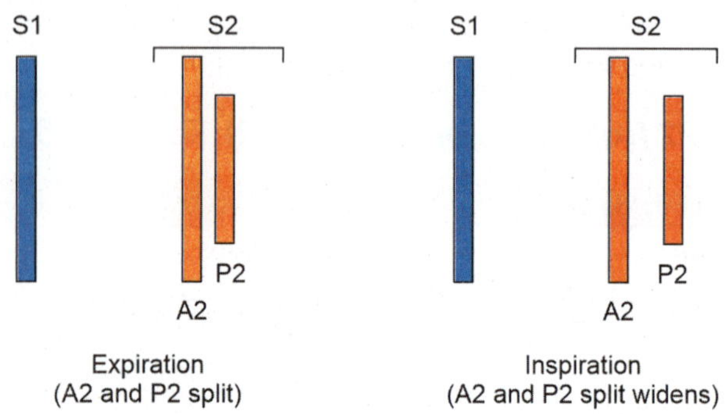

Figure 3.9: Wide mobile split S2

TABLE 3.17: Causes of wide mobile split S2	
Causes	**Mechanism**
Right bundle branch block (RBBB) – most common	Delayed RV depolarization → Delayed RV contraction → Delayed P2 closure → Split S2
Pulmonary stenosis	Obstruction of RV outflow → Prolonged RV systole → Delayed P2
Severe mitral regurgitation	Decreased left ventricular ejection time (early A2)
Ventricular septal defect (VSD) with left-to-right shunt	Decreased left ventricular ejection time (early A2)
Pulmonary hypertension with right heart failure	Prolonged right ventricular ejection time → delayed P2

Reversed (paradoxical) Splitting of S2

- A2 follows P2 instead of preceding it (i.e. the normal order is reversed) **(Fig. 3.10 and Table 3.18)**.

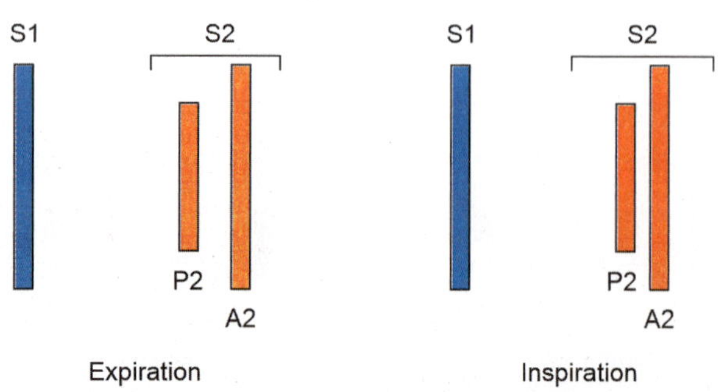

Figure 3.10: Reversed spliting of S2

TABLE 3.18: Reversed (paradoxical) splitting of S2	
Causes	**Mechanism**
Left bundle branch block (LBBB)	Delayed left ventricular (LV) depolarization → Delayed LV contraction → Delayed A2
Severe aortic stenosis or HOCM	Obstruction at aortic valve → Prolonged LV systole → Delayed A2
Severe systemic hypertension	Increased LV afterload → Prolonged LV systole → Delayed A2
Artificial right ventricular pacing	Right ventricle contracts first, hence P2 comes first
Left bundle branch block (LBBB)	Delayed left ventricular (LV) depolarization → Delayed LV contraction → Delayed A2

Single S2

- A single S2 occurs when either A2 or P2 is absent or both sounds fuse together, making only one audible heart sound instead of two **(Table 3.19)**.

TABLE 3.19: Single S2	
Causes	**Mechanism**
Severe aortic stenosis, severe aortic regurgitation	Absent A2 → Single S2
Absent pulmonary valve, pulmonary atresia, tetralogy of Fallot, truncus arteriosus	Absent P2 → Single S2
Eisenmenger ventricular septal defect, common ventricle	Fusion of A2 and P2 → Single S2

Q. Discuss the mechanism and significance of S3 (ventricular gallop) and S4 (atrial gallop).

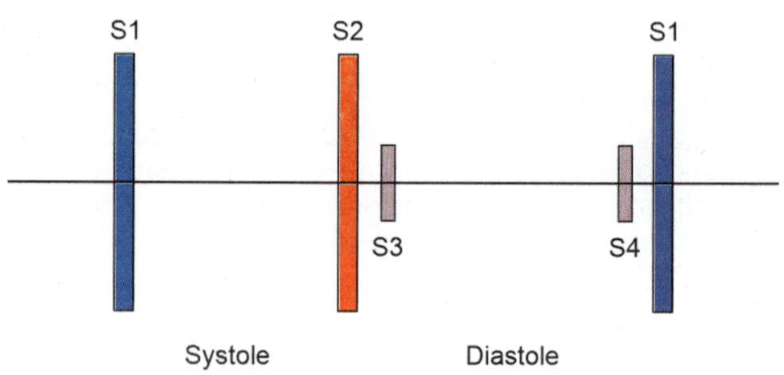

Figure 3.11: 3rd and 4th heart sounds

Third Heart Sound (S3)

- Third heart sound (S3 also known as ventricular gallop) occurs during the rapid filling phase of ventricular diastole (early part of diastole). It is a benign finding in children and young adults. When heard in elderly it usually indicates underlying cardiac disease.
- S_3 occurs when the ventricle suddenly reaches its elastic limits and abruptly decelerates the onrushing column of blood. Thus, an S3 can be produced by excessive rapid filling into a ventricle with normal compliance, as with high-output states and MR, or

by a normal or less than normal rate of filling into a ventricle with decreased compliance, as in patients with HCM. Likewise, decreased rates of filling into overfilled ventricles with large end-systolic volumes, as seen in patients with LV systolic dysfunction, will also produce this sound.

Causes of S3 (Table 3.20)

TABLE 3.20: Causes of S3

Physiological	Pathological
• Children and young adults • Pregnancy • Well trained athletes	• Cardiac failure • Hyperkinetic circulatory states (anemia, thyrotoxicosis, beriberi) • Mitral or tricuspid regurgitation • Aortic or pulmonary regurgitation • Right sided S3 is always pathological (seen in ASD, TR, right heart failure)

- S3 can be left or right sided. A left-sided S3 is a low-pitched sound best heard over the LV apex in the left lateral decubitus position with the bell of stethoscope and with the breath held in expiration. Right-sided S3 (seen in right heart failure) is best heard at the left lower sternal border with the patient supine and on inspiration.
- S3 has to be differentiated from split S2, opening snap of mitral stenosis, and a diastolic click related to mitral valve prolapse.

Fourth Heart Sound (S4)

- S4 occurs in late-diastole, immediately before S1 due to forceful atrial contraction against a poorly compliant ventricle and is therefore heard just before S1. S4 is also known as atrial gallop. It is also low pitch like S3 except for its timing, sounds much like an S3, but is more difficult to hear than S3. It can arise from left or right-side of the heart. S4 occurs in conditions causing diastolic dysfunction and poor ventricular compliance. Presence of S4 is always abnormal.

Causes of S4

- *Left sided S4*: Severe aortic stenosis, systemic hypertension, hypertrophic obstructive cardiomyopathy, IHD. All these conditions are diastolic dysfunction and poor ventricular compliance.
- *Right sided S4*: RVH, pulmonary hypertension, pulmonary stenosis, right ventricular infarction (compliance becomes less).

Comparing the 3rd and 4th Heart Sounds

S3 (ventricular gallop)	S4 (atrial gallop)
Occurs in early diastole during passive LV filling	Occurs in late diastole during active LV filling
May be normal at times	Almost always abnormal
Requires a very compliant LV	Requires a noncompliant LV
Can be a sign of systolic CHF	Can be a sign of diastolic CHF

Q. List the investigations used in the evaluation of cardiac disorders.

Investigations usually Done in Cardiac Disorders are as follows

- Cardiac biomarkers
  - Troponins (Troponin I, Troponin T): Gold standard for diagnosing myocardial infarction.
  - Creatine Kinase-MB (CK-MB): Used to assess myocardial damage.
  - Brain Natriuretic Peptide (BNP) and NT-proBNP: Markers for heart failure.
  - Myoglobin: Early marker of myocardial injury.
- Electrocardiography (ECG)
  - *Resting ECG*
  - *Exercise (stress) ECG*
  - *Ambulatory ECG (holter monitoring)*
- Echocardiography (ECHO)
  - *Two-dimensional echocardiography*
  - *Doppler echocardiography*
  - *Transesophageal echocardiography*
- Chest X-ray
- Cardiac catheterisation
- Computed tomographic (CT) imaging
- Magnetic resonance imaging (MRI)
- Radionuclide imaging
  - *Blood pool imaging to assess ventricular function*
  - *Myocardial perfusion imaging*
- Intravascular ultrasound (IVUS)
- Endomyocardial biopsy.

Q. Cardiac biomarkers.

- Cardiac biomarkers are substances released into the bloodstream when the heart is damaged or under stress.
- They are crucial in diagnosing, assessing prognosis, and guiding the management of various cardiac disorders, particularly myocardial infarction (MI), heart failure, and myocarditis.

Important Cardiac Biomarkers

Troponins (Troponin I and Troponin T)

- Troponins are regulatory proteins involved in cardiac muscle contraction. They are released into the bloodstream when cardiac myocytes are damaged.

Uses of troponins

- They are highly sensitive and specific for myocardial damage and have replaced older markers like CK-MB and myoglobin for MI diagnosis.
- Gold standard for diagnosing acute myocardial infarction (STEMI & NSTEMI).
- Serial testing (at 0, 3, and 6 hours) is recommended to confirm a rise/fall pattern.
- Differentiates unstable angina (normal troponins) from NSTEMI (elevated troponins).
- High-sensitivity troponin (hs-Tn) is more sensitive and detects even minor myocardial injury.

- Higher troponin levels correlate with worse outcomes in MI, heart failure, and sepsis.
- Persistently high troponin levels suggest ongoing myocardial injury.

Troponin kinetics in myocardial infarction (MI)

- Elevates: Within 3–6 hours after myocardial injury.
- Peaks: At 12–24 hours.
- Returns to normal: Over 7–14 days.

Limitations of troponins

- Delay in elevation (3–6 hours) means very early MI may not be detected.
- Noncardiac conditions can cause mild elevations (epsis, pulmonary embolism, stroke, renal failure) requiring clinical correlation.

Creatine Kinase-MB (CK-MB)

- Specific to myocardial cells, though also found in skeletal muscle. Although less specific than troponins, CK-MB is useful in detecting reinfarction and distinguishing cardiac from skeletal muscle injury.
- Elevates: Within 4–6 hours after myocardial infarction
- Peaks: At 12–24 hours.
- Returns to normal Within 48–72 hours. This is faster than troponins because of short half life. Hence, useful to detect reinfarction.
- Noncardiac causes of CK-MB elevation: Skeletal muscle injury (trauma, intense exercise, rhabdomyolysis, chronic kidney disease (due to delayed clearance), and hypothyroidism.

Myoglobin

- A very early marker of muscle injury (cardiac and skeletal).
- Elevates: Within 1–2 hours after myocardial infarction.
- Peaks: At 6–12 hours.
- Returns to normal: Within 24 hours.
- High sensitivity, but low specificity—not used alone for MI diagnosis.

Brain Natriuretic Peptide (BNP) and N-Terminal proBNP (NT-proBNP)

- NP and NT-proBNP are natriuretic peptides released by the ventricles in response to ventricular wall stretch due to volume overload or pressure overload.
- Markers of heart failure (HF), reflecting ventricular wall stress.
- BNP >100 pg/ml or NT-proBNP >300 pg/ml suggests HF.
- Elevated in congestive heart failure (CHF), acute coronary syndrome (ACS), and pulmonary hypertension.
- NT-proBNP is more stable and has a longer half-life, making it a more reliable marker in chronic heart failure.
- Used for: Diagnosing and prognosticating heart failure. They help differentiate cardiac vs. non-cardiac causes of dyspnea and assess disease severity.
- Other causes of elevated BNP:

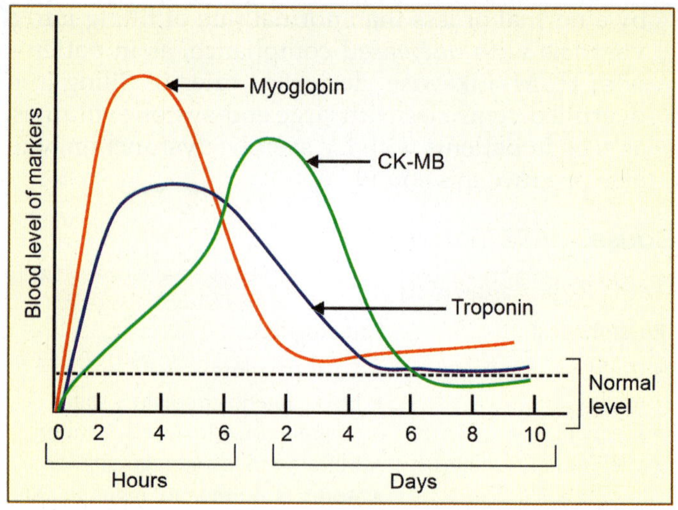

Figure 3.12: Elevation and fall of cardiac biomarkers after MI

  - Acute coronary syndrome (MI, unstable angina).
  - Atrial fibrillation.
  - Pulmonary hypertension.
  - Valvular heart disease.
  - Renal failure (reduced BNP/NT-proBNP clearance).
  - Sepsis (inflammatory cytokine activation).
  - Chronic lung diseases (e.g. COPD, pulmonary embolism).
  - Liver cirrhosis (fluid overload).

Q. Electrocardiography (ECG).

- ECG is a recording of electrical activity of the heart.
- Normally, cardiac activation starts in the sinoatrial node, goes to atrium, AV node, and then to ventricles through bundle of His and its branches. Each of this stage gives rise to electrical current, which is recorded by the electrodes placed on the chest wall creating the ECG. Though SA node generates impulses, this is not recorded on ECG. Similarly, atrial repolarization produces little electrical activity and cannot be recorded on ECG. Except these two events, all other events are recorded on the ECG.
- ECG consists of the following waves and segments.

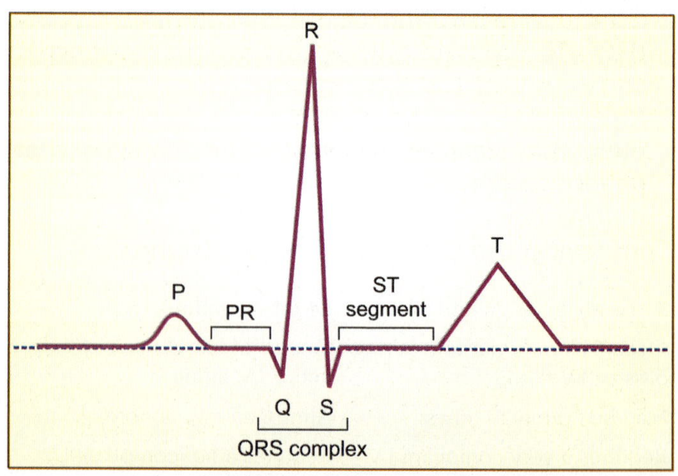

Figure 3.13: Normal ECG

P wave	Due to atrial depolarization
PR interval	Beginning of P wave to start of QRS. It represents the delay in conducting the sinus impulse to ventricles in AV node
QRS complex	Due to ventricular depolarization
ST segment	Flat segment after QRS
T wave	Ventricular repolarization
QT interval	Start of QRS to end of T wave. Represents the total duration of ventricular depolarisation and repolarisation

Uses of ECG

- To determine the cardiac rhythm and the condition of the conducting tissues
- To diagnose myocardial ischemia and infarction
- To know the effects of some drugs on the heart
- To know the chamber size
- Electrolyte imbalance.

Q. Treadmill test (TMT) or exercise stress test or stress ECG.

- Many patients complain of symptoms suggestive of angina on exertion but their resting ECG is normal. Such patients can be made to exercise (walk on a treadmill) and the ECG is recorded continuously during exertion. Such ECG may show ST, T changes proving ischemia or other changes.

Indications for Exercise (stress) ECG

- Evaluation of patients with suspected angina.
- Silent ischemia detection—identifies ischemia in patients without symptoms.
- Evaluation of atypical symptoms—helps assess unexplained dyspnea, fatigue, or dizziness.
- Evaluation of functional capacity.
- Assessment of prognosis and functional capacity after myocardial infarction.
- Assessment of outcome after coronary revascularisation, e.g. coronary angioplasty.
- To diagnose and evaluate the treatment of exercise-induced arrhythmias.

Procedure

- Different exercise protocols are used to gradually increase heart workload. The commonly used exercise protocol is Bruce Protocol. Patient is made to walk on treadmill and 12-lead ECG is continuously recorded during exercise. The speed of treadmill and incline is increased every 3 minutes. Blood pressure, heart rate and symptoms are monitored regularly throughout the test. Test continues till until target heart rate (85% of max HR, Max HR = 220–age in years) is reached or symptoms occur.
- Both false positive and false negative tests can occur with stress test. However, in patients with symptoms suggestive of angina, exercise testing has much better sensitivity and specificity, and is clinically very useful.

Positive Stress Test

- Anginal pain occurs.
- ST, T changes s/o ischemia (ST segment shifts of >1 mm).
- Fall in BP (SBP drop >10 mm Hg from baseline).
- Exercise-induced arrhythmia (ventricular tachycardia, frequent PVCs, atrial fibrillation).
- A positive stress test requires further evaluation (e.g. coronary angiography, stress imaging).

Contraindications for Stress Test

- Unstable angina
- Decompensated heart failure
- Severe hypertension (>180/110 mm Hg at rest)
- Uncontrolled cardiac arrhythmias
- Advanced atrioventricular block
- Acute myocarditis or pericarditis
- Severe aortic stenosis
- Severe hypertrophic obstructive cardiomyopathy
- Significant tachyarrhythmias or bradyarrhythmias
- Acute systemic illness (pulmonary embolism, aortic dissection).

Q. Ambulatory ECG (Holter monitoring)

- A standard electrocardiograph (ECG) records the heart's electrical activity for only a few seconds. This can detect abnormalities that are constant; however, sometimes abnormal heart rhythms and ischemic events may occur only briefly or unpredictably. To detect such problems, continuous ambulatory ECG, in which the ECG is recorded continuously for 24–48 hours or longer while the person engages in normal daily activities is used. These records are then analyzed for rhythm and ST-T alterations.

Indications

- To evaluate unexplained palpitations (these can be due to transient arrhythmias).
- To diagnose the cause of recurrent syncope or near syncope (could be due to transient arrhythmias or cardiac ischemic events).
- To detect transient episodes of arrhythmias or silent myocardial ischemia.
- To detect pacemaker malfunctions and monitor implantable cardioverter-defibrillator (ICD) activity.

Technique

- There are many portable devices for ambulatory ECG recording. These devices are compact, battery-operable, can be worn by the patient and permit continuous data recording during daily activities of the patient. Holter monitor is one such small instrument which can be worn by the patient for 24–48 hours. Event recorders record only the abnormal rhythm whenever they occur. Many of these devices have the facility to transmit ECG recordings to a cardiac centre through the telephone.

Q. Echocardiography (Echo).

- Echocardiography is nothing but ultrasound of the heart. Images of the heart are obtained by placing the ultrasound transducer on the chest wall.
- It is commonly used because it is noninvasive.

Common Indications for Echocardiography

- Assessment of ventricular function
- Evaluation of valvular heart diseases
- Identification of vegetations in endocarditis
- Identification of structural heart disease
- Detection of pericardial effusion
- Identification of cardiac masses such as myxoma, clots, mural thrombus, etc.

2D Echocardiography

- 2D echocardiography (2D Echo) provides real-time, cross-sectional images of the heart. It allows visualization of cardiac chambers, valves, great vessels, and pericardium to assess heart structure and function.
- However, 2D echo does not provide any hemodynamic information (velocity, direction of blood flow, etc.). These parameters can be detecetd by Doppler echocardiography. Combined 2D and color Doppler echocardiography can assess flow and hemodynamic information also. Modern echocardiography systems integrate both 2D imaging and Doppler capabilities, allowing for a comprehensive assessment of cardiac structure and function in a single examination.

Doppler Echocardiography

- Doppler echocardiography is based on the *Doppler effect* described by Christian Doppler. When an ultrasound beam with known frequency is transmitted to the heart, it is reflected by red blood cells. The frequency of the reflected ultrasound waves increases when the red blood cells are moving toward the source of ultrasound and decreases when the red blood cells are moving away.
- The speed and direction of movement of blood across the valves and arteries can be detected by this technique.
- Advanced techniques include three-dimensional echocardiography and intravascular ultrasound.

Uses of Doppler echocardiography

- It is very useful to evaluate valvular heart diseases. It can detect the severity and direction of blood flow in valvular heart disease such as aortic regurgitation or mitral regurgitation, etc.
- To estimate pressure gradients, e.g. across stenosed aortic valve.

3D Echocardiography

- Provides real-time 3D images. Advanced transducers capture 3D heart anatomy.
- Advantages over 2D echo include enhanced depth and spatial accuracy, more accurate for detailed cardiac anatomy, valve disease, congenital defects, and surgical planning.

Transesophageal Echocardiography

- Here an ultrasound probe is passed into the esophagus and placed behind the left atrium. It can obtain clear images of cardiac structures especially valves and left atrium.

Uses

- It is useful to pick up vegetations in infective endocarditis which may not be detected by surface echocardiography.
- It is also useful for investigating patients with prosthetic (especially mitral) valve dysfunction, congenital abnormalities (e.g. atrial septal defect), aortic dissection, and systemic embolism.

Q. Uses of computed tomographic (CT) and MRI imaging in the evaluation of cardiovascular disease.

- Computed tomography (CT) and magnetic resonance imaging (MRI) are advanced imaging modalities used for detailed structural and functional assessment of cardiovascular diseases (CVD). They complement echocardiography when more precise anatomical, perfusion, or tissue characterization is needed.

CT Imaging

- CT imaging is most useful for imaging the aorta in suspected aortic dissection. It is also useful to image the chambers of the heart, great vessels, pericardium and surrounding structures.
- CT angiogram: Noninvasive imaging of the coronary arteries is possible by using CT angiogram. CT images of the proximal coronary arteries are comparable to conventional coronary angiography. The patency of coronary artery bypass grafts can also be assessed by using CT angiogram.
- CT pulmonary angiography (CTPA): Gold standard for pulmonary embolism diagnosis.

Magnetic Resonance Imaging (MRI)

- MRI is now considered the gold standard for the assessment of regional and global systolic function, myocardial infarction (MI) and viability, and the assessment of congenital heart disease.
- It is particularly useful in detecting infiltrative conditions (such as amyloidosis, sarcoidosis) affecting the heart. The right ventricular wall which is difficult to see on echocardiogram is readily visualized on MRI.
- Aortic dissection and aneurysms: Alternative to CT in patients with renal impairment (no contrast required in some cases).

Q. Cardiac catheterization.

Q. Coronary angiography (CAG).

Cardiac Catheterization

- Cardiac catheterization is an invasive procedure where a specially designed thin catheter is introduced into the heart through an artery or vein under fluoroscopic guidance to evaluate and treat cardiovascular conditions. Introducing the catheter into the left side

of the heart is called left heart catheterization and into the right side is called right heart catheterization.
- Gold standard for diagnosing and treating coronary artery disease.

Technique

- Cardiac catheterisation is performed under light sedation and local anesthesia.
- Left heart catheterization is performed through radial, brachial and femoral artery routes. Right heart catheterization is performed through basilic or femoral vein route.

Indications

- To assess coronary artery disease by coronary angiogram (CAG).
- Revascularisation procedures such as balloon angioplasty and stenting.
- To assess the size and function of the ventricles by ventriculography.
- To assess pulmonary artery pressure.
- To detect intracardiac shunts by measuring oxygen saturation in different chambers.
- To measure intracardiac/intravascular pressures and flow.
- Measurement of hemodynamic data in critically sick patients.
- For nonsurgical closure of atrial septal defect, ventricular septal defect or patent ductus arteriosus in carefully selected cases.
- For temporary/permanent cardiac pacing.
- To perform endomyocardial biopsy.

Contraindications

- Marked untreated ventricular irritability (risk of ventricular tachycardia/ventricular fibrillation).
- Electrolyte abnormalities and digitalis toxicity.
- Marked untreated congestive heart failure.
- Uncontrolled hypertension.
- Concurrent febrile illness.
- Renal impairement: Risk of worsening of reanal impairement due to contrast-induced nephropathy.
- Severe liver disease: Risk of bleeding.
- Severe anemia.

Coronary Angiography (CAG)

Definition

- Coronary angiography is obtaining anatomical details of coronary arteries by injection of radioopaque contrast material into the coronary arteries and their radiological filming.

Technique

- A thin, flexible catheter is inserted into an artery, typically via the femoral artery (groin) or radial artery (wrist).
- The catheter is carefully guided toward the heart using fluoroscopy (X-ray guidance).
- A contrast dye (iodine-based) is injected through the catheter into the coronary arteries.
- Real-time X-ray images (angiograms) are captured to assess blood flow and detect blockages.
- If a significant blockage is found, additional procedures like angioplasty or stent placement may be performed during the same session.

Indications

- For evaluation of unexplained chest pain with high suspicion of angina.
- To establish the site and severity of coronary artery disease in patients with definite angina.
- Prior to coronary artery bypass surgery.
- To perform balloon angioplasty and stenting.
- To perform intracoronary thrombolytic therapy.
- To assess the patency of coronary bypass grafts after surgery.

Contraindications

- See above under cardiac catheterization.

Complications

- While generally safe, coronary angiography carries some risks, including:
- Bleeding or hematoma at the catheter insertion site.
- Allergic reaction to the contrast dye.
- Arrhythmias.
- MI or stroke (rare but possible).
- Kidney damage (especially in patients with pre-existing kidney disease).
- Death may occur in cases with advanced coronary disease. However, its incidence is very low (0.1% or less).

Q. Role of radionuclide imaging in the evaluation of cardiac disorders.

- Injecting gamma-emitting radionuclides and picking up the gamma rays emitted by the heart by gamma camera can be used to assess the ventricular function and myocardial perfusion.
- *Radionuclide ventriculography*: Left ventricular function can be assessed by injecting the isotope intravenously (Tc-99m-labeled RBCs). Isotope mixes with blood and enters ventricles. Using the gamma camera, the amount of isotope-emitting blood in the heart can be measured in systole and diastole which gives information about ventricular function.
- *Myocardial perfusion Imaging (SPECT and PET):* Myocardial perfusion imaging involves obtaining scintiscans of the myocardium at rest and during stress after the administration of an intravenous radioactive isotope (such as Technetium-99m sestamibi, Thallium-201, Rubidium-82). It can give information about myocardial perfusion and identify areas of ischemia or infarction. Positron emission tomography (PET) scan can give more accurate quantitative information regarding myocardial perfusion.

Q. Intravascular ultrasound (IVUS).

- IVUS is an advanced intravascular imaging technique, performed along with cardiac catheterization. Here, a miniature ultrasound probe (transducer) on the tip of a coronary catheter is passed into the coronary arteries and detailed images of the interior walls of the arteries are obtained. IVUS shows a cross section of both the interior, and the arterial wall. Visualization of arterial wall is not possible by conventional angiogram, which shows only the luminal narrowing **(Fig. 3.14)**.

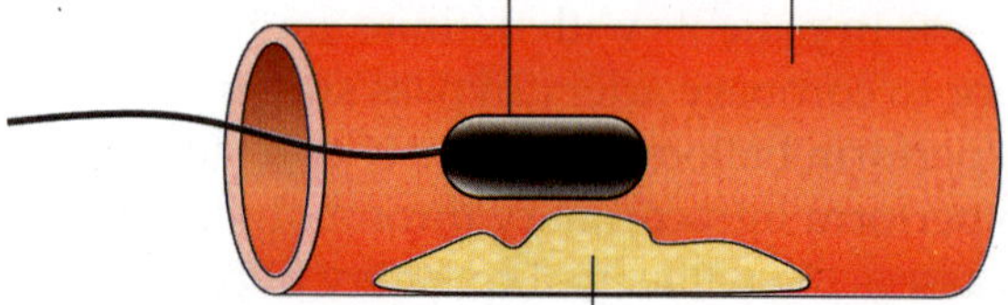

Figure 3.14: IVUS

Uses of IVUS

- Evaluation of coronary artery disease (CAD): IVUS can give a cross sectional view of coronary artery—from the inside out. This helps in assessment of plaque burden and morphology. It helps to differentiate between soft, fibrous, and calcified plaques.
- Helps in the selection of correct size stents and balloons for angioplasty.
- To confirm accurate stent placement and optimal stent deployment.
- IVUS can also be used to view the aorta and structure of the artery walls (which can show plaque buildup), find which blood vessel is involved in aortic dissection.

Advantages of IVUS over Angiography

Feature	IVUS	Angiography
Plaque characterization	Yes	No
Assessment of vessel wall	Yes	No
3D cross-sectional imaging	Yes	No
Guidance for stent placement	Yes	Limited
Detects early atherosclerosis	Yes	No

Q. Define heart failure. Describe the etiology, classification, clinical features, investigations and management of heart failure (congestive cardiac failure).

Q. Precipitating causes of heart failure.

Q. Role of ACE inhibitors in the management of heart failure.

Q. Role of beta-blockers in the management of heart failure.

Definition

- HF as a complex clinical syndrome that results from any structural or functional impairment of ventricular filling or ejection of blood leading to cardinal manifestations of dyspnea, fatigue, and fluid retention.
- It is a common health problem especially in industrialized countries.

Causes of Heart Failure

- Heart failure can result from structural, functional, or metabolic abnormalities affecting the heart. The causes can be broadly categorized into cardiac (primary) and noncardiac (secondary) conditions. All these causes lead to heart failure by one of the following mecahnisms, either singly or in combination: (1) intrinsic pump failure, (2) increased workload on heart, (3) impaired filling of cardiac chambers **(Table 3.21)**.

Precipitating Causes of Heart Failure

- Precipitating causes make the previously compromised heart fail. These include,
- ***Infection:*** Any infection may precipitate HF. Fever, tachycardia, hypoxemia, and the increased metabolic demands due to infection may place additional burden on a compromised heart and lead to heart failure.
- ***Arrhythmias:*** Tachyarrhythmias reduce the time available for ventricular filling, and cause ischemic myocardial dysfunction in patients with ischemic heart disease. Atrioventricular dissociation as happens in many brady- and tachyarrhythmias results in the loss of the atrial booster pump mechanism, thereby raising atrial pressure and reduce cardiac output.
- ***Physical, dietary, fluid, environmental, and emotional excesses:*** sudden increase in sodium intake, physical overexertion, excessive environmental heat or humidity, and emotional crises all may precipitate HF.
- ***Discontinuation of drugs:*** Such as antihypertensives, diuretics, etc. given for heart failure may precipitate heart failure.
- ***Ingestion of drugs:*** Such as NSAIDs can precipitate heart failure.
- ***Myocardial infarction:*** a new infarction on a previously compromised heart may precipitate heart failure.
- ***Pulmonary embolism:*** may result in right heart failure.
- ***Anemia:*** In the presence of anemia, the oxygen needs of the metabolizing tissues can be met only by an increase in the cardiac output. An already compromised heart may not be able to tolerate such an increased demand and may fail.
- ***Thyrotoxicosis and pregnancy:*** Thyrotoxicosis and pregnancy are high cardiac output states which place increased demand on heart.
- ***Uncontrolled hypertension:*** Uncontrolled BP either due to renal problems or discontinuation of antihypertensives may result in cardiac decompensation.
- ***Myocarditis:*** Rheumatic, viral, and other forms of myocarditis may precipitate HF in patients with or without preexisting heart disease.

TABLE 3.21: Causes of heart failure

Cardiac causes of heart failure

Coronary artery disease (CAD) (most common cause):
- Myocardial infarction (heart attack): Leads to permanent myocardial damage and reduced contractility (HFrEF).
- Chronic ischemia: Causes myocardial stunning or hibernation, leading to progressive HF.

Cardiomyopathies
- Dilated cardiomyopathy (DCM): Weak, enlarged heart with reduced pumping ability (HFrEF). Causes include genetic mutations, viral infections, toxins, and alcohol.
- Hypertrophic cardiomyopathy (HCM): Thickened heart muscle reduces ventricular filling, leading to diastolic dysfunction (HFpEF).
- Restrictive cardiomyopathy (RCM): Stiff ventricles impair relaxation and filling (HFpEF). Common causes: Amyloidosis, sarcoidosis, hemochromatosis.

Valvular heart diseases
- Aortic Stenosis (AS): Increased afterload leads to LV failure.
- Mitral Regurgitation (MR) and Aortic Regurgitation (AR): Chronic volume overload leads to dilated LV and HF.
- Mitral Stenosis (MS): Causes left atrial hypertrophy and pulmonary congestion, leading to right heart failure.

Arrhythmias
- Atrial fibrillation (AF): Reduces cardiac output and worsens HF.
- Tachyarrhythmias: Cause tachycardia-induced cardiomyopathy.
- Bradyarrhythmias and heart Block: Cause low cardiac output leading to HF.

Pericardial diseases
- Constrictive pericarditis: Impairs ventricular filling, mimicking restrictive cardiomyopathy.
- Pericardial effusion and cardiac tamponade: Compression of the heart reduces cardiac output.

Noncardiac causes of heart failure

Hypertension
- Long-standing high blood pressure increases afterload, leading to left ventricular hypertrophy (LVH) and eventually diastolic dysfunction (HFpEF).

Infectious and inflammatory causes
- Viral myocarditis: Coxsackievirus, adenovirus, parvovirus B19.
- Bacterial infections: Endocarditis, Lyme disease.
- Autoimmune disorders: Systemic lupus erythematosus (SLE), rheumatoid arthritis, sarcoidosis.

High output states
- Hyperthyroidism → high output failure due to increased metabolism.
- Severe Anemia: Causes high-output heart failure.
- Pregnancy-related (peripartum cardiomyopathy): Dilated cardiomyopathy during or after pregnancy.

Pulmonary causes leading to right heart failure (Cor Pulmonale)
- Chronic obstructive pulmonary disease (COPD)
- Pulmonary hypertension (PAH)
- Obstructive sleep apnea (OSA)

- ***Infective endocarditis:*** Valvular damage, anemia, fever, and myocarditis which may occur in infective endocarditis may precipitate HF.

Classification of Heart Failure

- HF can be classified in many ways based on onset, ejection fraction, ventricle involved, etc.

Based on Ejection Fraction (EF)

- *Heart failure with reduced ejection fraction (HFrEF)* (EF ≤40%): Was earlier known as systolic heart failure. The left ventricle has weak contractility and cannot pump blood effectively. Examples are myocardial infarction, dilated cardiomyopathy.
- *Heart failure with preserved ejection fraction* (HFpEF) (EF ≥50%): Was earlier known as diastolic heart failure. The left ventricle has normal contraction but impaired relaxation, leading to poor ventricular filling. Examples LV hypertrophy due to HTN and HOCM, restrictive cardiomyopathy.
- *High-output heart failure:* Here cardiac output is more than normal with reduced systemic vascular resistance. High-output states by themselves are seldom responsible for HF, but their development in the presence of underlying cardiovascular disease can precipitate HF. Examples of high output states causing heart failure are severe anemia, thyrotoxicosis, AV fistula, Paget's disease, pregnancy, etc.

Based on Clinical Presentation

- *Acute heart failure* (AHF): Sudden onset of heart failure symptoms. Causes are massive myocardial infarction, valve rupture, arrhythmias, or infections.
- *Chronic heart failure* (CHF): Here there is progressive decline in cardiac function over time. Causes include valvular heart disease, dilated cardiomyopathy, and systemic hypertension.

Based on Ventricular Dysfunction

- *Left-sided heart failure (most common type):* In left ventricular failure, there is pulmonary congestion resulting in dyspnea, orthopnea, and paroxysmal nocturnal dyspnea (PND). Important causes are myocardial infarction, mitral and aortic valve disease.
- *Right-sided heart failure:* In right-sided failure, systemic congestion leads to raised jugular venous pulse, congestive hepatomegaly, ascites, and lower limb edema. Often secondary to left-sided HF or pulmonary hypertension (cor pulmonale).
- Failure of both left and right ventricles is called congestive cardiac failure (CCF) and is seen in long-standing valvular heart disease (aortic and mitral valve), myocarditis, cardiomyopathies, and hypertension.

Pathophysiology

- In the normal ventricle, stroke volume increases over a wide range of end-diastolic volumes (the Frank-Starling effect). In the failing heart with depressed contractility, there is relatively little increment in systolic function with further increases in left ventricular volume, and the ventricular function curve is shifted downward and flattened. Systolic dysfunction causes pulmonary congestion (left heart failure) or systemic congestion (right heart failure), or both pulmonary and systemic congestion (CCF), effort intolerance, and organ dysfunction.
- The reduction in cardiac output leads to activation of compensatory mechanisms viz. increased sympathetic activity, stimulation of the renin-angiotensin-aldosterone system (RAAS) and secretion of antidiuretic hormone (ADH). This neurohumoral activation causes tachycardia, peripheral vasoconstriction, sodium and water retention. The result of these compensatory mechanisms is increase in blood pressure (for tissue perfusion) and blood volume (enhancing preload, stroke volume, and cardiac output by the Frank-Starling mechanism). These compensatory mechanisms help to normalize the hemodynamic disturbances to some extent, but increase the myocardial oxygen and energy requirements. In the long run, these compensatory responses perpetuate myocardial damage and worsen heart failure.

  Other compensatory mechanisms are activation of vasodilatory molecules, such as atrial and brain natriuretic peptides (ANP and BNP), prostaglandins (PGE_2 and PGI_2), and nitric oxide (NO), that offset the excessive peripheral vascular vasoconstriction. ANP and BNP cause natriuresis, vasodilation and inhibition of angiotensin II, aldosterone and ADH secretion, thereby reversing some of the harmful effects.
- Persistent compensatory mechanisms lead to pathological cardiac remodeling, worsening heart failure.

Clinical Features

Symptoms

Dyspnea

- *Exertional dyspnea* is seen in early heart failure. As heart failure advances, dyspnea occurs with progressively less strenuous activity and ultimately it is present even at rest.
- PND is discussed in detail later.
- *Orthopnea* is dyspnea in lying down position and is a later manifestation than exertional dyspnea and PND. Orthopnea is due to redistribution of fluid from the abdomen and lower extremities into the chest in lying position, which increases the pulmonary capillary pressure, combined with elevation of the diaphragm.
- *Acute pulmonary edema* results from transudation of fluid into the alveolar spaces because of acute rise in capillary hydrostatic pressures due to sudden decrease in cardiac function. Patient may present with cough or progressive dyspnea. Wheezing is common due to bronchospasm. If acute pulmonary edema is not treated earlier, patient may begin coughing up pink (or blood-tinged), frothy fluid and become cyanotic and acidotic. Some patients may present with Cheyne-Stokes respiration (periodic respiration or cyclic respiration) which is characterized by periods of apnea, hypoventilation and hyperventilation.

Fatigue

- This is due to reduced perfusion of skeletal muscles.

Cerebral symptoms

- Are due to reduced cerebral perfusion and include altered mental status, confusion, lack of concentration, memory impairment, headache, anxiety and insomnia.

Abdominal symptoms

- Like nausea, anorexia, and pain abdomen are due to congested gastric mucosa, liver and portal venous system. Abdominal distension may occur due to ascites in right heart or congestive cardiac failure.

Oliguria, nocturia

- Reduced renal perfusion during day causes sodium and water retention and oliguria. Renal perfusion increases at night due to shift of fluid from the extravascular to the intravascular compartment, resulting in increased excretion of sodium and water and nocturia.

NYHA classification of heart failure (staging of heart failure)

- The New York Heart Association (NYHA) classification system is the simplest and most widely used method to gauge symptom severity. The classification system is a well-established predictor of mortality and can be used at diagnosis and to monitor treatment response.

TABLE 3.22: New York Heart Association (NYHA) Functional Classification

Functional class	Description
Class I	Ordinary physical activity does not cause undue fatigue, dyspnea, palpitations, or angina
Class II	Comfortable at rest. Ordinary physical activity (e.g. carrying heavy packages) may result in fatigue, dyspnea, palpitations, or angina.
Class III	Comfortable at rest. Less than ordinary physical activity (e.g. getting dressed) leads to symptoms.
Class IV	Symptoms of heart failure or angina are present at rest and worsened with any activity.

Physical Examination

Vital signs

- Pulse is fast and of low volume. Pulsus alternans may be seen in LVF.
- BP is low in severe heart failure.
- Respiratory rate may be high due to pulmonary edema. Advanced HF may be associated with periodic breathing or Cheyne-Stokes respirations.

General examination

- In acute heart failure or decompensated chronic heart failure, patient is dyspneic and orthopneic. However, in stable chronic heart failure, patient may be asymptomatic.
- Peripheries may be cold and cyanosed.
- JVP is usually elevated with positive abdomino-jugular reflux.
- Pitting pedal edema may be present. Sacral edema is seen in bed-ridden patients.
- In chronic, severe heart failure, weight loss may occur, leading to a syndrome of cardiac cachexia. Cardiac cachexia is due to elevated levels of cytokines.

CVS

- Cardiac enlargement (apex beat shifted down and out) may be seen. S1 may be diminished in intensity. Third and fourth heart sounds are often audible. Pansystolic murmur may be heard due to incompetence of mitral and tricuspid valve due to dilatation of ventricles.

RS

- Tachypnea may be present due to pulmonary edema. Bilateral fine basal crepitations and rhonchi may be heard due to pulmonary edema. Sometimes signs of pleural effusion may be present.

Abdomen

- Liver may be enlarged and tender due to congestion. Ascites may be present.

NS

- Confusion, memory disturbances may be seen due to reduced brain perfusion.

Investigations

- *Chest X-ray:* The presence of cardiomegaly (a cardiothoracic ratio >0.5 and especially >0.60) is a strong indicator of heart failure. Pulmonary edema may be seen as bilateral batwing hilar haziness, generalized haze (due to interstitial edema), and Kerley's B lines (due to prominent interlobular lymphatics) at the lung base. Bilateral pleural effusion may be seen which is usually more on right side.
- *Electrocardiogram (ECG):* It can show cardiac rhythm, identify ischemia, prior or recent MI, and detect evidence of left ventricular hypertrophy. It also shows conduction defects and electrolyte disturbances.
- *Echocardiography (gold standard test):* Transthoracic echo can confirm the presence of heart failure and also quantify it. It also provides information on left and right ventricular size, regional wall motion abnormality (as an indicator ischemia or infarction), condition of the heart valves, and ventricular hypertrophy. It can also detect left atrial myxoma, and pericardial effusion.
- *Natriuretic peptide measurements:* Elevated serum levels BNP (brain natriuretic peptide) and NT-proBNP (N-terminal pro-BNP) are seen in heart failure.
- *Troponins:* Detect myocardial injury. Elevated in acute decompensated HF.
- *Cardiac catheterization*: In heart failure, there is increased end-diastolic ventricular pressure, reduced cardiac output and reduced ventricular ejection fraction. Coronary angiogram can identify the extent of coronary artery disease.
- *Cardiac MRI:* Identifies fibrosis, cardiomyopathies. Useful when ECHO is inconclusive.

Treatment of Heart Failure

- The ideal approach would be to treat both the underlying and precipitating causes. Correction of underlying cause (e.g. surgical correction of valvular defects) may dramatically improve heart failure. Correction of underlying cause may not always be possible (e.g. old myocardial infarction). Precipitating causes like infections, severe anemia, hyperthyroidism, etc. should be looked for and corrected.

Lifestyle Measures

- ***Rest:*** Rest reduces the demand on the heart. Adequate rest reduces venous pressure and pulmonary congestion. Absolute bed rest is not required even for patients with severe HF.
- ***Diet:*** The diet should provide adequate calories to maintain ideal weight. Obese patients should have a low-calorie diet. Oils and fats should be cut down. The sodium intake should not exceed 6 g of salt per day. Potassium-rich foods are advised for those receiving diuretics.
- Avoid excessive alcohol intake and smoking should be stopped.

Control of Excessive Fluid

- *Low salt diet and fluid restriction:* Can help in decreasing many of the clinical manifestations of heart failure.
- *Diuretics:* These agents reduce ECF volume expansion and reduce edema. Many agents are available and almost all are effective in controlling fluid retention. These agents include frusemide, torsemide, thiazides, spironolactone and amiloride, etc. A combination of potassium losing and potassium sparing diuretics will prevent hypokalemia. Hyponatremia can occur due to diuretics and should be watched for.

Drugs that Improve Survival and Reduce Hospitalization

- Chronic activation of the renin-angiotensin-aldosterone system (RAAS) and of the adrenergic nervous systems in HF causes ventricular remodeling, further deterioration of cardiac function and/or potentially fatal arrhythmias. Drugs that block these two systems are useful in the management of HF and decrease long-term mortality.

- *Angiotensin-converting enzyme (ACE) inhibitors:* ACE inhibitors slow the maladaptive remodeling of ventricles, and reduce the afterload by causing vasodilatation. ACE inhibitors have been shown to prevent or retard the development of HF in patients with left ventricular dysfunction, enhance exercise tolerance, and reduce long-term mortality and rate of readmission to hospitals. ACE inhibitors inhibit local (tissue) renin-angiotensin systems. ACE inhibitor should be given indefinitely to patients with heart failure. However, ACE inhibition should not be used in hypotensive patients. Examples of ACE inhibitors are captopril, enalapril, lisinopril, ramipril, perindopril, etc.
- *Angiotensin receptor blockers (ARB):* These agents have similar effects as ACE inhibitors. They are used when patients cannot tolerate ACE inhibitors due to cough, angioneurotic edema, and leukopenia. Examples of ARBs are losartan, telmisartan, olmesartan, valsartan, etc.
- *Aldosterone antagonist:* The activation of the RAAS in HF increases the levels of angiotensin II and aldosterone. Aldosterone causes Na^+ retention (hence fluid retention), sympathetic activation, myocardial, vascular, and perivascular fibrosis, and vasoconstriction. Spironolactone is an antagonist of aldosterone and when given to heart failure patients on long-term basis reduces mortality and sudden death. Eplerenone is a new, more selective aldosterone inhibitor that can be used instead of spironolactone.
- *Beta-adrenoceptor blockers:* Beta-blockers have been shown to improve the symptoms of HF, and to reduce long-term mortality, sudden death, and hospitalization for HF. They should be given only for patients with moderately severe HF (classes II and III). They should not be given for patients with class IV heart failure, hypotension (systolic pressure <90 mm Hg), severe fluid overload, recent treatment with an intravenous inotropic agent, sinus bradycardia, atrioventricular block, or a bronchospastic condition. Beta-blocker should be started after starting ACE inhibitors and continued indefinitely. Examples are atenolol, metoprolol, bisoprolol, and carvedilol.
- *Vasodilators:* Direct vasodilators are helpful in patients with severe heart failure who have systemic vasoconstriction despite ACE inhibitor therapy. Decrease in periphearal resistance enhances cardiac output by decreasing afterload. Sodium nitroprusside, nitroglycerin, hydralazine and nesiritide are vasodilators, which have to be given by continous IV infusion. Hydralazine and isosorbide dinitrate are useful for chronic oral administration.
- *Angiotensin receptor neprilysin inhibitor (ARNI):* A new therapeutic class of agents acting on the RAAS and the neutral endopeptidase system has been developed. This is called angiotensin receptor neprilysin inhibitor (ARNI)]. This is a combination of valsartan and sacubitril. Sacubitril is a neprilysin inhibitor and valsartan is angiotensin-II receptor inhibitor. By inhibiting neprilysin, sacubitril slows the degradation of ANP, BNP, and other peptides. This results in high circulating levels of ANP and BNP which enhance diuresis, natriuresis, and myocardial relaxation. ANP and BNP also inhibit renin and aldosterone secretion. Because neprilysin breaks down angiotensin II, inhibiting neprilysin will result in accumulation of angiotensin II. For this reason, neprilysin inhibitor sacubitril cannot be used alone; it must always be combined with an ARB to block the effect of the excess angiotensin II. Sacubitril/valsartan combination should be used in patients who are symptomatic even after using an ACEI (or ARB). The ACEI or ARB should be stopped and then Sacubitril/valsartan should be added.
- *Ivabradine:* Ivabradine slows the heart rate through inhibition of the 'If' channel in the sinus node. It reduces heart rate without affecting contractility, blood pressure, or conduction. It should be used only for patients in sinus rhythm. Ivabradine can be used to reduce the risk of hospitalization in symptomatic patients with heart failure with a resting heart rate ≥70 bpm despite using beta-blocker.

Enhancement of Myocardial Contractility

- *Cardiac glycosides (digitalis and digoxin):* Cardiac glycosides enhance myocardial contractility and hence improve symptoms of heart failure. They inhibit Na^+, K^+-ATPase and increase intracellular sodium The latter, in turn, increases intracellular calcium through a Na^+-Ca^{2+} exchange mechanism. The increased calcium augments myocardial contraction. Although, dgoxin reduces symptoms of HF it does not improve long-term survival. Digoxin is not useful in heart failure due to hypertrophic cardiomyopathy, mitral stenosis, chronic constrictive pericarditis, and diastolic HF.
- *Sympathomimetic amines:* These are dopamine and dobutamine which act on beta-adrenergic receptors and improve myocardial contractility. They have to be given by constant intravenous infusion and can be given for several days. They are especially useful in patients with intractable, severe HF, patients with acute myocardial infarction and shock or pulmonary edema or in refractory HF as a "bridge" to cardiac transplantation. Dopamine is useful in heart failure with hypotension since at higher doses it also stimulates alpha-adrenergic receptors and elevates arterial pressure. Dobutamine is useful in the treatment of acute HF without hypotension since it lowers arterial pressure.
- *Phosphodiesterase inhibitors:* Examples are amrinone and milrinone. Both these drugs exert positive inotropic and vasodilator actions by inhibiting phosphodiesterase III, which increases intracytoplasmic cyclic AMP mediating adrenergic stimulation. These agents are administered by continuous intravenous infusion. Indications are same as dopamine and dobutamine.

Antiarrhythmics

Premature ventricular contractions and episodes of asymptomatic ventricular tachycardia are common in advanced HF. Sudden death can occur due to ventricular fibrillation. Amiodarone, a class III antiarrhythmic, is the drug of choice for patients with heart failure.

Anticoagulants and Antiplatelets

- Routine use of anticoagulants (e.g. warfarin) is not recommended in patients with heart failure in sinus rhythm who do not have demonstrated left ventricular thrombus. Anticoagulation is recommended if there is atrial fibrillation or a previous thromboembolic event.
- Antiplatelets such as aspirin should be used only if there is coronary artery disease.

Treatment of Diastolic Heart Failure

- The underlying cause such as ventricular hypertrophy, fibrosis, or ischemia should be treated. Dietary sodium restriction and diuretics are useful to reduce pulmonary and/or systemic venous congestion.

Device Therapy

- *Implantable cardioverter-defibrillator* (ICD): Prevents sudden cardiac death in HFrEF (LVEF ≤35%).
- *Cardiac resynchronization therapy* (CRT): For HF patients with LVEF ≤35% and wide QRS (>150 ms). Intraventricular conduction defects are seen in some patients with heart failure leading to dyssynchrony of cardiac contraction. For example, when there is left bundle branch block (LBBB), right and left ventricles do not contract simultaneously, which impairs cardiac contraction and aggravates HF. "Resynchronization" with a device that has three pacing leads (right atrium, right ventricle, and cardiac vein, which provides left ventricular stimulation) has been shown to improve heart failure symptoms.

Surgical Interventions

- *Heart transplantation:* Considered in refractory end-stage HF.
- *Coronary artery bypass graft (CABG):* For ischemic cardiomyopathy with CAD.
- *Valve repair/replacement: If valvular disease contributes to HFLeft ventricular assist device* (LVAD): Bridge to transplant or destination therapy in end-stage HF.

Q. Describe the genetic basis of some forms of heart failure.

- Heart failure (HF) has a multifactorial etiology, with both genetic and environmental factors playing roles. While common HF forms (e.g. ischemic cardiomyopathy) are largely influenced by lifestyle and comorbidities, several inherited cardiomyopathies have strong underlying genetic basis.

Genetic Cardiomyopathies Leading to Heart Failure

- ***Dilated cardiomyopathy (DCM):*** 30–50% of cases have a genetic basis. Mostly autosomal dominant, but also X-linked, autosomal recessive, and mitochondrial forms exist. Mutations in sarcomere, cytoskeleton, nuclear envelope, and ion channels impair contractility, leading to ventricular dilation, systolic dysfunction, and heart failure.
- ***Hypertrophic cardiomyopathy (HCM):*** ~60–70% of cases are familial. Inheritance is autosomal dominant. Sarcomere protein mutations → Myocyte disarray and fibrosis → Diastolic dysfunction, LV hypertrophy, and risk of sudden cardiac death (SCD).
- ***Arrhythmogenic right ventricular cardiomyopathy (ARVC):*** ~50% familial cases. Autosomal dominant (some autosomal recessive forms exist). There is desmosome protein mutations → Impaired cell adhesion → Myocyte detachment, inflammation, and replacement by fibro-fatty tissue → Arrhythmias and heart failure.
- ***Restrictive cardiomyopathy (RCM):*** Some cases are inherited, mostly autosomal dominant. There is sarcomere or cytoskeletal mutations → Diastolic dysfunction (stiff, noncompliant myocardium) → Pulmonary congestion and HF.
- ***Genetic syndromes with heart failure risk:*** Some genetic disorders include cardiomyopathy as part of a broader syndrome:
    - Fabry disease → LV hypertrophy mimicking HCM.
    - Danon disease → Severe HCM with conduction defects.
    - Mitochondrial disorders → DCM and metabolic HF.
    - Noonan syndrome → HCM.

Indications for Genetic Testing in Heart Failure

- In most patients with heart failure, routine genetic testing is not recommended.
- It is indicated in patients with familial cardiomyopathy cases (DCM, HCM, ARVC, RCM), early onset HF (<50 years of age), and if there is family H/o of sudden cardiac death.

Importance of Genetic Counseling and Genetic Testing in HF

- Identifying at-risk family members for early intervention.
- Guiding implantable cardioverter-defibrillator (ICD) decisions.
- Potential for gene-targeted therapies in the future genetic counseling.
- Determination of the genotype is important, since some forms carry a poorer prognosis.

Q. Brain natriuretic peptide (BNP)/NT-proBNP.

- BNP is a peptide hormone that is released primarily by ventricles in response to increased wall stretch, volume overload, and pressure changes.

- A related biomarker, N-terminal proBNP (NT-proBNP), is an inactive fragment of BNP released in equal amounts but has a longer half-life, making it useful for diagnostic purposes.
- BNP is so called because it was initially identified in the brain. It plays a key role in regulating fluid balance, blood pressure, and cardiac function.
- The level BNP is increased in heart failure, as ventricular cells secrete BNP in response to the high ventricular filling pressures. Ventricles also secrete atrial natriuretic peptide (ANP), but measurement of BNP is more helpful than ANP in the diagnosis of heart failure. Clinical experience with BNP is much greater than ANP.

Physiological Role of BNP

- BNP acts to counteract the effects of heart failure (HF) by:
    - Vasodilation → Reduces preload and afterload
    - Natriuresis and Diuresis → Increases sodium and water excretion
    - Inhibition of RAAS (renin-angiotensin-aldosterone system) → Reduces fluid retention
    - Decreased sympathetic activity → Lowers heart rate and myocardial oxygen demand.
- BNP may also protect against collagen accumulation and the pathologic remodeling that contributes to progressive HF.

Clinical Uses of BNP/NT-proBNP

- To differentiate dyspnea due to heart failure from other causes. Most dyspneic patients with HF have values above 100 pg/ml, while values below 100 pg/ml have a very high negative predictive value for HF as a cause of dyspnea.

BNP (pg/ml)	HF probability
<100	Unlikely
100–400	Possible, needs further evaluation
>400	Likely heart failure

- Monitoring treatment of heart failure: The plasma concentrations of BNP fall after effective treatment of HF and can be used to titrate treatment.
- Prognosis of HF: Higher the BNP, poorer the prognosis.
- Nesiritide is a recombinant BNP used in acute decompensated HF (arrely used).

Other Conditions that Elevate BNP/NT-proBNP

- Acute coronary syndrome (ACS)
- Pulmonary hypertension
- Chronic kidney disease (CKD) (due to decreased clearance)
- Sepsis
- COPD
- Liver cirrhosis.

Q. How do you differentiate between left and right heart failure? (Table 3.23)

TABLE 3.23: Differences between left and right heart failure

	Left heart failure	Right heart failure
Common causes	• Myocardial infarction • Systemic hypertension • Aortic stenosis • Aortic regurgitation	• Pulmonary stenosis • Cor pulmonale due to COPD, ILD, bronchiectasis • Pulmonary hypertension • Pulmonary embolism • Mitral stenosis
Symptoms	• Dyspnea, orthopnea, PND • Nocturia • Palpitations	• Anorexia, nausea, vomiting (due to gastric mucosal congestion) • Right hypochondrial pain (due to liver congestion)
Signs	• Pallor • Sweating • Pulsus alternans • Narrow pulse pressure • Left ventricular S3 and S4 gallop • Bilateral basal lung crepitations	• Peripheral edema • Raised JVP • Ascites, pleural effusion • Right ventricular S3 and S4 gallop

Q. Cardiac remodeling (after MI).

- Cardiac remodeling refers to structural and functional changes in the heart after myocardial infarction.
- It involves changes in ventricular size, shape, and function, which can progress to heart failure (HF) and arrhythmias if unchecked.
- Factors which influence remodeling are loss of viable myocardium (after MI), inflammatory response, increased wall stress in the border zone and remote myocardium, and neurohormonal activation.
- The incidence and extent of adverse ventricular remodeling have significantly declined in the current reperfusion era with primary percutaneous coronary intervention and many effective drugs available to prevent remodeling.

Phases of Post-MI Cardiac Remodeling

Acute Phase (hours to days post-MI)

- Necrosis and inflammation: Death of cardiomyocytes in the infarcted area lead to inflammatory response.
- Early ventricular dilatation due to loss of contractile myocardium leads to increased wall stress. Surviving myocardium compensates by hypertrophy.

Subacute Phase (days to weeks post-MI)

- Scar formation and fibrosis: Necrotic area is reolaced by fibrosis and scar formation. There is thinning and expansion of infarcted area → increases ventricular volume and wall stress.

- Hypertrophy and remodeling of non-infarcted myocardium: Surviving cardiomyocytes undergo hypertrophy to compensate. May develop maladaptive remodeling, worsening heart failure.

Chronic Phase (weeks to months post-MI)

- There is progressive ventricular dilatation ("eccentric hypertrophy") → increased chamber size and spherical shape of LV → reduced contractility → HF → neurohormonal activation (RAAS, SNS, BNP release) → leads to fluid retention, volume overload, and further dilation → worsening of HF → risk of ventricular arrhythmias and sudden cardiac death (SCD).

Factors Influencing Adverse Ventricular Remodeling

- *Infarct size:* This is the single most important factor. Bigger the infarct, greater the extent of remodeling.
- *End-diastolic volume:* An increase in end-diastolic volume occurs early in MI to accommodate a larger preload and compensate for the acute decrease in contractility. However, wall stress increases with the increase in chamber size, which increases the chances of the progression to adverse ventricular remodeling and HF ("dilatation begets more dilatation").
- *Neurohormonal activation:* The acute decrease in ventricular contractility and increase in intracavitary pressure cause activation of the renin-angiotensin-aldosterone and the noradrenergic sympathetic nervous systems which in turn leads to release of neurohormones, such as angiotensin II, aldosterone, and norepinephrine. These hormones produce tachycardia and vasoconstriction which helps in the acute stage to maintain cardiac output and perfusion of vital organs. However, the same neurohormones Increase fibrosis, hypertrophy, and sodium retention.

Clinical Consequences of Cardiac Remodeling

- Heart failure (HFrEF): Progressive systolic dysfunction
- Arrhythmias (VT, VF): Risk of sudden cardiac death (SCD)
- Decreased exercise tolerance: Fatigue, dyspnea
- Mitral regurgitation: Due to LV dilatation and papillary muscle displacement.

Strategies to Prevent or Reverse Remodeling

- Prompt reperfusion to reduce infarct size.
- Reduction of wall stress by using diuretics and peripheral vasodilators (such as ACE inhibitors).
- Inhibition of neurohormonal response by using ACE inhibitors (blocks angiotensin), spironolactone (blocks aldosterone) and beta blockers (blocks sympathetic activity).
- SGLT2 inhibitors (dapagliflozin, empagliflozin): Improve cardiac metabolism, reduce HF progression.

Q. Digoxin.

Q. Manifestations and management of digoxin overdosage.

- Digoxin is a purified glycoside from Digitalis lanata (foxglove plant). It has been used for more than 200 years in the treatment of heart failure.

Actions

- It inhibits Na/K ATPase pump in myocardial cells. Increased intracellular sodium promotes sodium-calcium exchange, leading to a rise in the intracellular calcium concentration. This results in improved myocardial contractility.
- Digoxin also exerts antiadrenergic action in patients with HF by inhibiting sympathetic outflow and augmenting parasympathetic tone thereby causing vasodilatation and reduction of afterload.
- It prolongs the refractory period of AV node by increasing parasymphathetic outflow leading to slowing of ventricular rate.

Pharmacokinetics

- Digoxin has oral bioavailability of about 80%.
- Higher concentration is seen in heart than plasma. It is highly protein bound and hence, it is not effectively removed by hemodialysis in case of toxicity.
- Its half life is 1.6 days and the effect lasts 24–36 hours after the last dose.
- It is mainly excreted by the kidneys and small amount in the stools.

Uses of Digoxin

- Severe heart failure in sinus rhythm: It improves the symptoms of heart failure but does not provide any long-term mortality benefit
- Arrhythmias: Such as atrial fibrillation with fast ventricular rate for ventricular rate control.

Dosage and Route of Administration

- 0.125–0.25 mg daily orally. Maintenance dose should be reduced in renal failure.

Overdosage (Toxicity)

Clinical features

- Symptoms of digoxin toxicity are mostly nonspecific, and include fatigue, blurred vision, disturbed color perception (xanthopsia—yellow vision), anorexia, nausea, vomiting, diarrhea, abdominal pain, headache, dizziness, confusion, delirium, and occasionally hallucinations.
- Cardiovascular effects include bradycardia, atrioventricular block with or without concomitant supraventricular tachyarrhythmia, and ventricular tachyarrhythmias. Hyperkalemia also occurs in acute poisoning.

Treatment

- Digoxin: Specific antibodies are used for hemodyamically significant arrhythmias.

- Other supportive measures include atropine, dopamine, epinephrine, phenytoin, and external cardiac pacing for bradyarhythmias and magnesium, lidocaine, phenytoin, and bretylium for ventricular tachyarhythmias.

Q. Cor pulmonale.

Q. Acute cor pulmonale

Q. Discuss the etiology, pathogenesis, clinical features, investigations, and management of chronic cor pulmonale.

- Cor-pulmonale is defined as an alteration in the structure and function of the right ventricle due to respiratory system disease.
- Pulmonary hypertension is the link between respiratory system disease and cor pulmonale. Respiratory diseases cause pulmonary hypertension, which in turn causes cor pulmonale. In cor pulmonale, there is enlargement of the right ventricle (RV) with or without failure.
- Secondary to abnormalities of the lungs, thorax, pulmonary ventilation, or circulation.
- Excludes RV failure due to left heart disease (e.g. left-sided HF, mitral stenosis) or congenital heart defects.
- Cor pulmonale can be acute or chronic. Acute cor pulmonale develops suddenly and is seen in massive pulmonary embolism and ARDS. Chronic cor pulmonale develops slowly.

Causes of Cor Pulmonale and Mechanism

(Table 3.24)

TABLE 3.24: Causes of cor pulmonale and mechanism

Causes	Mechanism
Acute cor pulmonale	
• Massive pulmonary embolism (PE)	Obstruction to right ventricular outflow → RV strain → RV failure
• Acute respiratory distress syndrome (ARDS)	ARDS → pulmonary vasoconstriction → pulmonary HTN → RV failure
Chronic cor pulmonale (most common)	
• Chronic obstructive pulmonary disease (COPD) – Most common cause	Loss of cross-sectional area of the vascular bed (emphysema) → pulmonary HTN Chronic hypoxia → pulmonary vasoconstriction → pulmonary HTN
• Bronchiectasis	Loss of cross-sectional area of the vascular bed
• Cystic fibrosis	Chronic lung disease → chronic hypoxia → pulmonary vasoconstriction → pulmonary HTN
• Interstitial lung disease (ILD, Pulmonary Fibrosis)	Loss of cross-sectional area of the vascular bed → pulmonary HTN
• Obstructive sleep apnea (OSA)	Chronic hypoxia → pulmonary vasoconstriction → pulmonary HTN
• Pulmonary vasculitis (sarcoidosis, scleroderma)	Puolmonary vascular occlusion → pulmonary HTN
• Chest wall disorders (kyphoscoliosis, obesity hypoventilation syndrome)	Decreased lung expansion → Chronic hypoxia → pulmonary vasoconstriction → pulmonary HTN
• Primary pulmonary hypertension	Increased after-load on right ventricle

Pathogenesis

- All the causes of cor pulmonale affect the right heart by producing pulmonary hypertension. Pulmonary hypertension places extra load on right heart and makes it dilate and fail.
- Hypoxia is a strong vasoconstrictor of the pulmonary artery and its branches. Other factors leading to pulmonary hypertension are reduction of the pulmonary vascular bed by fibrotic and thrombotic obliteration of the capillaries and compression of pulmonary capillaries by high intra-alveolar pressures, when there is air trapping.

Clinical Features

- ***Pulmonary symptoms:*** Patients usually have symptoms related to the underlying pulmonary disorder like cough, exertional dyspnea, wheezing, and easy fatigability. In acute corpulmonale due to pulmonary embolism, there may be signs of DVT.
- ***RV failure symptoms:*** With the onset of RV failure, raised JVP, peripheral edema, ascites, and right upper quadrant pain (due to congested liver) appear.
- Examination may reveal cyanosis, clubbing, signs of right ventricular hypertrophy (RV heave, epigastric pulsations, loud P2) an enlarged, and tender liver and dependent edema.

Investigations

Blood Tests

- ABG may show hypoxia (low PaO_2) and hypercapnia (high $PaCO_2$) due to underlying lung disease.
- Brain natriuretic peptide (BNP)/NT-proBNP are elevated in right heart failure.
- Polycythemia (↑ hemoglobin and hematocrit), seen in chronic hypoxia-induced cor pulmonale (COPD, ILD).
- D-dimer elevated in acute cor pulmonale due to pulmonary embolism (PE).

Chest X-ray

- Chest X-ray may show the underlying lung disease, enlarged RV, and dilated pulmonary artery.

ECG

- May show signs of right ventricular hypertrophy such as right axis deviation, peaked P waves, and deep S waves in lead V1.

Echocardiogram (key diagnostic test)

- Echo shows normal LV size and function but RV and RA dilation. There may be tricuspid regurgitation due to right ventricular dilatation. Doppler echo shows pulmonary HTN.

Right Heart Catheterization (gold standard)

- Can confirm the diagnosis of cor pulmonale by demonstrating increased RV and RA pressures and pulmonary HTN (mean pulmonary artery pressure ≥25 mm Hg at rest).

Tests to Diagnose the Underlying Cause of Cor Pulmonale

- Pulmonary function tests (for COPD, ILD).
- CT-pulmonary angiogram (CTPA) to exclude pulmonary embolism.
- Polysomnography → If obstructive sleep apnea (OSA) suspected.
- Lung biopsy to rule out interstitial lung disease.

Treatment

Treat Underlying Lung Disease

- Chronic obstructive pulmonary disease (COPD) → Bronchodilators, inhaled steroids, oxygen therapy.
- Interstitial lung disease (ILD) → Anti-fibrotic therapy (e.g. pirfenidone, nintedanib).
- Obstructive sleep apnea (OSA) → CPAP or BiPAP therapy.
- Pulmonary embolism (acute cor pulmonale) → Anticoagulation (Heparin, Warfarin, DOACs).
- Obesity hypoventilation syndrome → Weight loss, CPAP therapy.

Reduce Pulmonary Hypertension

- Long-term oxygen therapy in patients with chronic hypoxia (PaO_2 ≤55 mm Hg or O_2 saturation <88%).
- Pulmonary vasodilators: Phosphodiesterase-5 Inhibitors (sildenafil, tadalafil), endothelin receptor antagonists (bosentan, ambrisentan).

Relieve Symptoms of Right Heart Failure

- Diuterics: Furosemide, spironolactone.
- Salt and fluid restriction.

Q. Acute pulmonary edema due to LVF.

- Acute pulmonary edema refers to the rapid build-up of fluid in the alveoli and lung interstitium that has extravasated out of the pulmonary circulation.
- As the fluid accumulates, it impairs gas exchange and decreases lung compliance, producing dyspnea and hypoxia. Pulmonary edema can be broadly divided into two types: cardiogenic and non-cardiogenic pulmonary edema.
- ***Cardiogenic pulmonary edema (synonyms: acute left heart failure, cardiac asthma):*** This form of pulmonary edema occurs when left ventricular failure occurs, so that blood returning to the left atrium exceeds that leaving the left ventricle (LV). As a result, pulmonary venous pressure increases, causing the capillary hydrostatic pressure in the lungs to exceed the oncotic pressure of the blood, leading to filtration of fluid out of the capillaries.

Causes of Cardiogenic Pulmonary Edema

- Acute myocardial infarction or severe ischemia.
- Acute decompensated heart failure (ADHF).
- Acute volume overload of the LV (e.g. acute mitral or aortic regurgitation).
- Mitral stenosis.
- Arrhythmias (atrial fibrillation with rapid ventricular rate, ventricular tachycardia).
- Hypertensive emergency.
- Infective endocarditis.

Clinical Features

- Patients present with severe dyspnea, orthopnea, PND, pink frothy sputum, and excessive sweating.
- Examination shows cyanosis, bilateral basal crepitations, and diffuse rhonchi.
- There may be tachycardia and S3 gallop in LVF.
- In addition, there may be findings of underlying disease.

Investigations

- *BNP/NT-proBNP* → Elevated in LVF.
- *Troponins* → To rule out acute MI casuing pulmonary edema.
- *Chest X-ray* → Increased interstitial markings, and batwing appearance of pulmonary edema. Kerley's B lines may be seen due to thick and tense lymphatics. Cardiomegaly may be present.
- *ECG* may show evidence of ischemia, infarction, and arrhythmias.
- *Echocardiography* (main diagnostic test) shows low ejection fraction and elevated atrial pressures in cardiogenic pulmonary edema. Ejection fraction is normal in diastolic dysfunction.
- *Pulmonary capillary wedge pressure (not routinely done)* → Elevated in cardiogenic pulmonary edema usually above 18 mm Hg. In noncardiogenic pulmonary edema, the wedge pressure may be normal or even low.

Treatment of Cardiogenic Pulmonary Edema

Emergency Treatment of Acute Pulmonary Edema (LMNOPQRS approach)

L = loop diuretics

- Intravenous diuretics (furosemide, 40 mg, or torsemide 20 mg—or higher doses) decrease fluid overload and preload. Benefit is seen even before the onset of diuresis due to venodilation.

M = Morphine

- Morphine is very effective in cardiogenic pulmonary edema. It acts by increasing venous capacitance, lowering left atrial pressure. It also relieves anxiety thus increasing the efficiency of ventilation. The initial dosage is 2–8 mg intravenously which can be repeated after 2–4 hours.

N = Nitrates

- Nitrates cause both arterial and venous dilalatation. Arterial dilalation decreases afterload and venous dilalation decreases pre-load, both of which improve cardiac function and reduce pulmonary edema.

- Sublingual nitroglycerin or isosorbide dinitrate, topical nitroglycerin, or intravenous nitrates will decrease dyspnea rapidly.

O = Oxygen/ventilation

- High-flow O_2, CPAP/BiPAP, or intubation if needed will rapidly improve oxygeneation and reduce respiratory distress. CPAP/BiPAP also help in decreasing pulmonary edema.

P = positioning

- Patient should be put in sitting position with legs hanging down the side of the bed. This position decreases venous return to heart and improves pulmonary edema.

Q = Query (what is the underlying cause?)

- Find the underlying cause and treat that. For example, specific treatment for MI, valvular heart disease, hypertensive emergency, etc.

R = Rise the cardiac output

- Inotropic drugs like dopamine, dobutamine, amrinone and milrinone may improve cardiac output and decrease pulmonary edema. Useful in cases not responding to above measures.

S = use of drugs starting from 'S' for long-term management and prevention

- Sacubitril-valsartan → LV remodeling prevention.
- Sympathetic inhibitors (beta-blockers such as carvedilol, metoprolol) → Improve survival in HFrEF.
- Spironolactone → Reduce fluid retention and fibrosis
- SGLT2 Inhibitors (Dapagliflozin, Empagliflozin) → HF protection
- Salt and fluid restriction to prevent fluid overload.

Q. Noncardiogenic pulmonary edema.

- Noncardiogenic pulmonary edema is fluid accumulation in the lungs due to increased capillary permeability, rather than left ventricular failure or elevated pulmonary capillary wedge pressure (PCWP).

Causes of Noncardiogenic Pulmonary Edema

- ARDS (sepsis, pancreatitis, burns, polytrauma).
- Massive blood transfusion (TRALI - transfusion-related acute lung injury).
- Eclampsia.
- Immersion/submersion.
- Toxin or drug-induced pulmonary edema: Opioid overdose (heroin, morphine), salicylate toxicity, inhaled toxins (chlorine gas, ammonia, smoke inhalation).
- High altitude pulmonary edema (HAPE).
- Neurogenic pulmonary edema (NPE): Head Injury/intracranial hemorrhage.

Treatment

- High-flow oxygen (if mild hypoxia).
- Non-invasive ventilation (BiPAP/CPAP) (for moderate cases).
- Mechanical ventilation with PEEP (for ARDS, severe hypoxia).
- Treat the underlying cause.

Q. Right heart failure (RHF).

Definition

- Right heart failure (RHF) occurs when the right ventricle (RV) fails to pump blood effectively into the pulmonary circulation, leading to systemic venous congestion and reduced cardiac output.

Causes of Right Heart Failure

- It may result from cardiac, pulmonary, and miscellaneous causes.

Cardiac causes

- Left heart failure (most common cause) → Increased LV pressures → ↑ Pulmonary venous congestion → ↑ RV afterload → RHF.
- Right ventricular infarction.
- Tricuspid valve disease (tricuspid regurgitation/stenosis).
- Congenital heart diseases (ASD, VSD, Tetralogy of Fallot, Ebstein's anomaly).

Pulmonary causes (cor pulmonale)

- Chronic obstructive pulmonary disease (COPD)
- Interstitial lung disease (ILD, pulmonary fibrosis)
- Pulmonary embolism (PE)
- Obstructive sleep apnea (OSA)
- Pulmonary hypertension (primary or secondary).

Miscellaneous causes

- Pericardial diseases (constrictive pericarditis, pericardial tamponade)
- Severe anemia or thyrotoxicosis (high-output failure leading to RHF)

Pathophysiology of Right Heart Failure (Fig. 3.15)

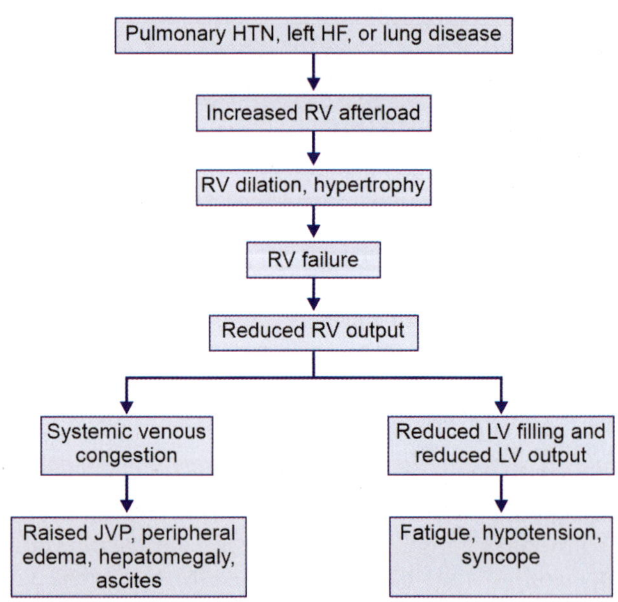

Figure 3.15: Patghophysiology of right heart failure

Clinical Features of Right Heart Failure

Symptoms

- Fatigue and weakness (due to ↓ cardiac output)
- Dyspnea on exertion (if associated with pulmonary HTN)
- Abdominal discomfort (RUQ pain, fullness): Due to hepatic congestion
- Swelling in legs and ankles (pitting edema)

Signs

- Jugular venous distension with prominent "a" Wave
- Congestive hepatomegaly, sometimes pulsatile liver.
- Ascites
- Peripheral edema (bilateral, pitting edema in legs and sacrum)
- Right ventricular heave (palpable at left parasternal border)
- Tricuspid regurgitation murmur (pansystolic at lower left sternal border)
- Key difference from left HF: RHF = Systemic venous congestion (JVD, hepatomegaly, ascites, edema). LHF = Pulmonary congestion (dyspnea, orthopnea, PND)

Investigations

- (BNP/NT-proBNP → Elevated.
- Electrocardiogram (ECG): Evidence of right ventricular hypertrophy (RVH).
- Chest X-ray (CXR): Enlarged right atrium and right ventricle, prominent pulmonary arteries (If pulmonsry HTN present). Clear lung fields (Unlike Left HF).
- Echocardiography (Key diagnostic test): RV Dilation, RV Hypertrophy, tricuspid regurgitation, ↑ pulmonary artery pressure (PAP >25 mm Hg).
- Right heart catheterization (gold standard for pulmonary HTN and RV dysfunction): Mean pulmonary artery pressure (mPAP ≥25 mm Hg) confirms pulmonary HTN.
- Pulmonary function tests (if suspecting COPD, ILD, or OSA).
- CT pulmonary angiography (CTPA), if suspecting pulmonary embolism.

Treatment of Right Heart Failure

- Reduce RV afterload: Treatment of pulmonary HTN (sildenafil, tadalafil, bosentan).
- Improve RV Function (diuretics, inotropes if needed).
- Correct underlying cause (lung disease, left HF, etc.).

Q. What is infective endocarditis? Discuss the etiology, types, pathogenesis, clinical features, and management of infective endocarditis. Add a note on infective endocarditis prophylaxis.

Q. Duke Criteria.

- **Infective endocarditis (IE)** refers to infection of the endocardial surface of the heart.
- It may involve heart valve (native or prosthetic), the lining of a cardiac chamber, a congenital anomaly (e.g. septal defect) or an intracardiac device.
- It is characterized pathologically by the presence of vegetation, which is a mass of platelets, fibrin, microorganisms, and inflammatory cells.
- The same process involving arteriovenous shunts, arterio-arterial shunts (patent ductus arteriosus), or a coarctation of the aorta is called **infective endarteritis**.

Types

Based on Temporal Evolution of Disease

- *Acute IE:* Develops abruptly and progresses rapidly (i.e. over days). It rapidly damages cardiac structures, hematogenously seeds extracardiac sites, and, if untreated, may result in death within weeks.
- *Subacute IE:* Develops insidiously and progresses slowly (i.e. over weeks to months), causes structural cardiac damage only slowly, if at all, and rarely causes metastatic infection.

Based on the Site of Infection

- *Left-sided IE*: Mitral and aortic valves (most common).
- *Right-sided IE*: Tricuspid valve (most common in IVDU).

Based on the Type of Valve Involved

- *Native valve endocarditis (NVE):* Affects natural valves.
- *Prosthetic valve endocarditis (PVE):* Affects mechanical or bioprosthetic valves.

Based on the Mode of Acquisition

- *Community-acquired IE*: No recent hospital exposure.
- *Healthcare-associated IE*: Recent hospitalization, catheter, IV lines.
- *IV drug user (IVDU) IE*: IV drug use, tricuspid valve involvement.

Etiology (Table 3.25)

TABLE 3.25: Etiology of endocarditis
Acute endocarditis
• *Staphylococcus aureus* (most common)
• Group A hemolytic streptococci
• Pneumococci
• Gonococci
Subacute endocarditis
• *Streptococcus viridans*
• *Streptococcus milleri*
• *Streptococcus bovis*
• *Enterococcus fecalis*
• HACEK group
• *Staph. aureus* (rarely)

- The causative organism can be bacteria, rickettsia, chlamydia or fungus.
- However, most cases of infective endocarditis are caused by a small number of bacterial species. These include *Streptococcus viridans*, staphylococci, and HACEK organisms (Haemophilus, Actinobacillus, Cardiobacterium, Eikenella, and Kingella) originating respectively from oral cavity, skin, and upper

respiratory tract. *Streptococcus bovis* originates from GIT, and enterococci from the genitourinary tract.

- Healthcare-associated endocarditis is due to bacteremia arising from IV cannulas and urinary tract infections.
- Candida species is the commonest fungal endocarditis.
- Prosthetic valve endocarditis occurring within 2 months of valve replacement is usually due to intraoperative contamination of the prosthesis or a bacteremic postoperative complication. It can be delayed up to 12 months. Common organisms are coagulase-negative staphylococci, *S. aureus*, facultative gram-negative bacilli, diphtheroids, and fungi. Prosthetic valve endocarditis occurring >12 months after surgery are due to the same organisms causing native valve endocarditis.
- Endocarditis occurring in IV drug abusers is due to *Staph. aureus* strains, and involves tricuspid valve. Polymicrobial endocarditis is common in IV drug addicts.
- About 5–15% of patients with endocarditis have negative blood cultures. Some of these culture negative cases are due to prior antibiotic exposure. Remaining culture negative cases are due to fastidious organisms, such as pyridoxal-requiring streptococci (now designated Abiotrophia species), HACEK organisms, *Bartonella henselae*, or *Bartonella quintana*.

Pathogenesis of IE

- ***Endocardial injury*:** Normal endocardium is resistant to infection and to thrombus formation. Endocardial injury is he starting point in the pathogenesis of IE and occurs due to: turbulent blood flow (congenital heart defects, valvular disease), direct trauma (catheters, prosthetic valves, pacemakers), and inflammation (autoimmune disease, myocarditis).
- ***Formation of nonbacterial thrombotic endocarditis (NBTE):*** Endocardial injury predisposes formation of platelet-fibrin thrombus at the site of injury. This platelet-fibrin thrombus without microorganisms is called nonbacterial thrombotic endocarditis (NBTE) which can subsequently get infected by bacteria during transient bacteremia.
- ***Bacterial entry and adhesion (microbial seeding):*** Transient or persistent bacteremia allows pathogens to adhere to the NBTE. Organisms usually enter the bloodstream from mucosal surfaces, skin, or sites of focal infection. Common sources of bacteremia are dental procedures (viridans streptococci), IV drug use (*Staphylococcus aureus*), GI/GU procedures (Enterococcus). Microorganisms adhere to NBTE but more virulent bacteria (e.g. *S. aureus*) can adhere directly to intact endothelium or exposed subendothelial tissue. If the organisms cannot be removed by defence mechanisms, the organisms proliferate and induce a procoagulant state at the site by eliciting tissue factor from adherent monocytes.
- ***Vegetation formation and growth*:** Once attached, bacteria proliferate within the fibrin-platelet clot, forming vegetations. Vegetations are avascular, limiting immune cell penetration. Vegetations have three layers; an inner layer of RBC, WBC and platelets, a middle layer of bacteria and an outer layer of fibrin. In the absence of host defenses, organisms enmeshed in vegetation proliferate to form dense microcolonies. Organisms deep in vegetations are relatively resistant to killing by antimicrobial agents. Proliferating surface organisms are shed into the bloodstream continuously some of which are cleared by the reticuloendothelial system and others are distributed to all parts of the body **(Fig. 3.17)**.
- ***Systemic dissemination and complications*:** Release of cytokines by inflammatory cells causes constitutional symptoms like fever, malaise. Damage to intracardiac structures leads to valvular incompetence and other manifestations. Embolization of vegetation fragments

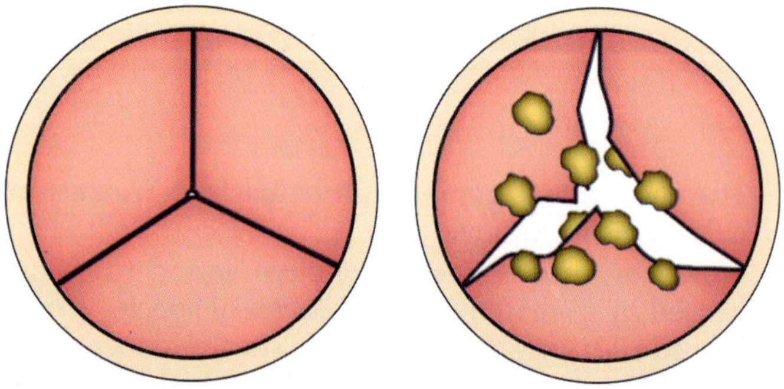

Figure 3.16: Normal valve (left) and valve with IE (right) showing vegetations

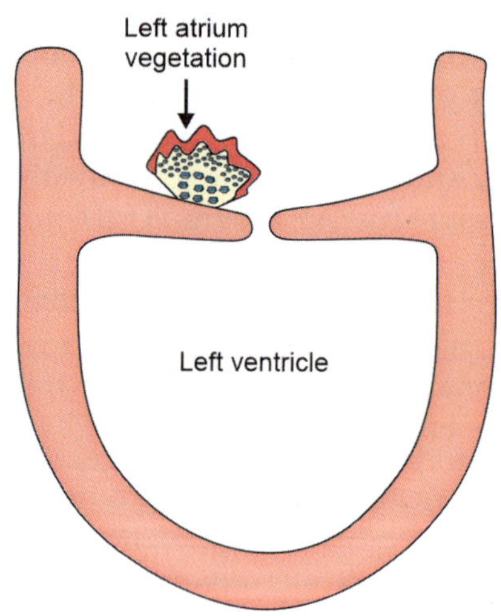

Figure 3.17: Vegetation on mitral valve

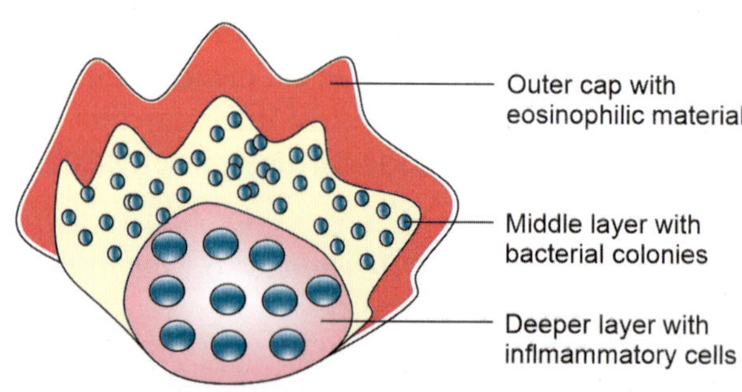

Figure 3.18: Structure of vegetation

leads to infection or infarction of remote tissues. Circulating antigens trigger glomerulonephritis, Osler's nodes, and Roth's spots.

Clinical Manifestations

- The clinical presentation can vary from acute to subacute presentations. Usually, the causative microorganism is responsible for the temporal course of endocarditis.
- IE can present with constitutional symptoms, cardiac manifestations, embolic phenomena, and immunological phenomena.

Constitutional Symptoms

- In patients with acute endocarditis fever is high grade and is usually between 103 and 104°F. In subacute endocarditis, fever is typically low-grade and rarely exceeds 103°F. Fever may be blunted or absent in elderly, debilitated and those with cardiac or renal failure.
- Drenching night sweats, arthralgias, myalgias (especially in the lower part of the back and thighs), and weight loss may accompany fever.

Cardiac Manifestations

- New or changing murmur can occur. Regurgitant murmurs may occur because of damage to valve and its supporting structures. Stenotic murmurs can occur due to large vegetations.
- Valve ring abscess may occur due to local extension of the infection to the valve ring. Valve ring abscesses can cause persistent fever and heart block due to destroyed conduction pathways in the area of the atrioventricular node and bundle of His. Valve ring abscess may burrow into pericardium causing pericarditis or hemopericardium. It can also lead to shunts between cardiac chambers or between the heart and aorta.
- Myocardial infarction may result from coronary artery embolization.
- Diffuse myocarditis can occur and is probably due to immune complex vasculitis.
- Congestive cardiac failure develops in 30–40% of patients due to valvular dysfunction and occasionally due to endocarditis-associated myocarditis or an intracardiac fistula. CHF occurs more frequently with left-sided than right-sided endocarditis and with aortic more than mitral involvement.

Extraoardiao Manifosattions

Embolic and vascular phenomena

- *Embolic events* result in infarction of numerous organs, such as the lung in right-sided endocarditis or the brain, spleen, or kidneys in left-sided endocarditis. Following are the manifestations of embolic events. Most emboli occur before or within the first few days after initiation of antibiotic therapy.
- CNS embolization
  - Ischemic stroke (most common neurological complication).
  - Brain abscess or meningitis (if infected emboli lodge in cerebral vessels).
  - Mycotic aneurysms (infected emboli weaken arterial walls, causing aneurysmal dilation and rupture).
  - Subarachnoid or intracerebral hemorrhage (from ruptured aneurysms)—seizures, stroke, loss of vision.
- Peripheral arterial embolization
  - Limb ischemia/gangrene (due to arterial occlusion).
  - Splenic infarction (left upper quadrant pain, splenomegaly).
  - Renal infarction (flank pain, hematuria, renal dysfunction).
  - Mesenteric infarction (severe abdominal pain, bowel ischemia).
  - Lungs (pulmonary infarction, hemoptyisis, pleurisy and pleural effusion). Occur with right sided IE.
  - Cutaneous embolism—produces **Janeway's lesions**. These are hemorrhagic, nonpainful macules most commonly found on the palms and soles.
  - Nails—splinter hemorrhages. These are nonblanching, linear, brownish-red lesions in the nail beds along the direction of growth of the nail; they may also be seen as a result of local trauma.

Immunologic phenomena

- IE triggers immune system activation, leading to the deposition of immune complexes and inflammation in various tissues. These are more common in subacute bacterial endocarditis due to prolonged infection and immune activation. Immunologic phenomena are different from vascular phenomena (e.g. Janeway lesions and embolic infarcts, which are due to septic emboli rather than immune response). These immunologic phenomena contribute to the clinical features of IE and are considered minor criteria in Duke's diagnostic criteria. Important immunologic manifestations are as follows:
- *Glomerulonephritis:* Hematuria, proteinuria, and renal dysfunction due to immune complex deposition in glomeruli.

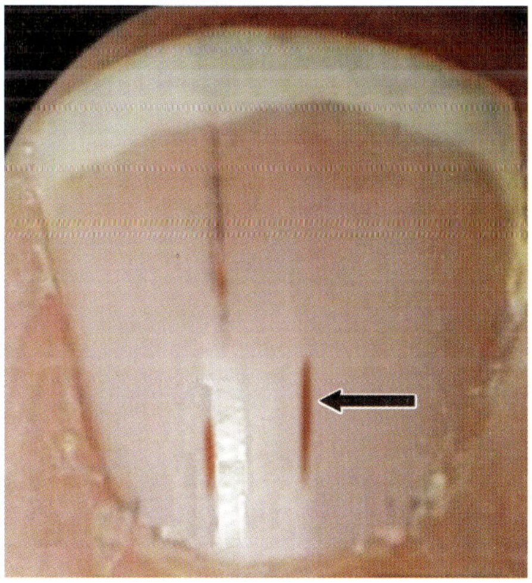

Figure 3.19: Arrow shows splinter hemorrhages

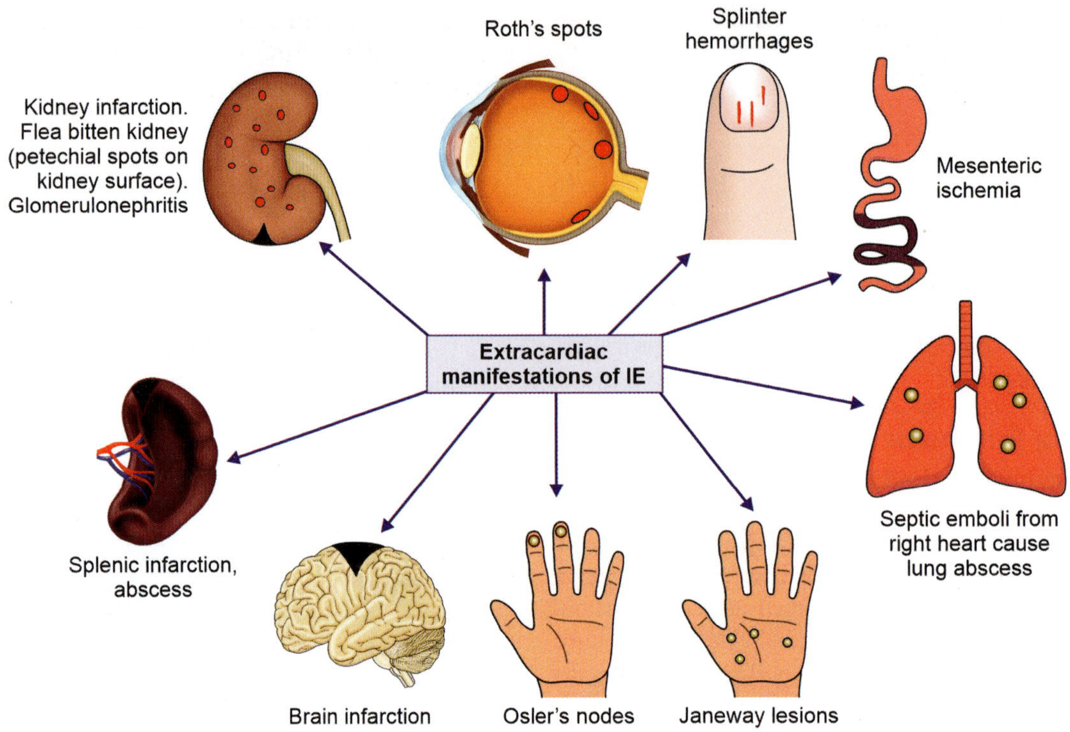

Figure 3.20: Extra-cardiac manifestations of IE

- *Roth's spots:* Circular retinal hemorrhages with white central spot. Result from immune complex-mediated vasculitis and fibrin-platelet deposition in retinal vessels.
- *Osler's nodes*: Painful tender nodules in the pulps of fingers and toes. Caused by immune complex deposition and vasculitis.
- *Immune-complex vasculitis:* Small vessel vasculitis due to circulating immune complexes. Contributes to skin manifestations (palpable purpura) and splinter hemorrhages.
- Hepatosplenomegaly may develop with prolonged illness.

Diagnosis

- The diagnosis of infective endocarditis (IE) relies on a combination of clinical, microbiological, and imaging findings. The modified Duke criteria is the most widely accepted diagnostic tool.

Modified Duke Criteria (Modified again in 2023) (Table 3.26)

- Duke criteria are based on clinical, laboratory, and imaging findings. Now modified Duke Criteria is used to diagnose infective endocarditis.
- Definitive IE
  - 2 major criteria, or
  - 1 major plus 3 minor criteria, or
  - 5 minor criteria
- Possible IE
  - 1 major plus 1 minor criteria or
  - 3 minor criteria

TABLE 3.26: Modified Duke Criteria

<u>Major Criteria</u>

1. Microbiologic criteria (either positive blood cultures or positive laboratory test)

Positive blood cultures (1 of the following):

- Microorganisms that commonly cause IE isolated from 2 or more separate blood culture sets
- Microorganisms that occasionally or rarely cause IE, isolated from 3 or more separate blood culture sets

Positive laboratory test (1 of the following):

- Positive PCR or other nucleic acid-based technique from blood for *Coxiella burnetii*, Bartonella spp, or *Tropheryma whipplei*
- *Coxiella burnetii* IgG antibody titer >1:800 or *Coxiella burnetii* isolated from a single blood culture
- Indirect immunofluorescence assays for detection of IgM and IgG antibodies to *Bartonella henselae* or *Bartonella quintana*, with IgG titer >1:800

2. Imaging criteria (1 of the following):

Echocardiography and/or cardiac CT imaging (any of the following):

- Echocardiography and/or cardiac CT demonstrating vegetation, or valve damage.
- Significant new valvular regurgitation on echocardiography, compared with previous imaging.
- New partial dehiscence of prosthetic valve (compared with previous imaging)

FDG PET/CT imaging

- Abnormal metabolic activity involving a native or prosthetic valve (at least 3 months after implantation) or other intracardiac prosthetic devices.

3. Surgical major criterion

- Evidence of IE observed by direct inspection during cardiac surgery (vegetations, abscesses, valvular destruction).

(Contd.)

TABLE 3.26: Modified Duke Criteria *(Contd.)*

Minor Criteria

1. **Predisposition** (Previous history of IE, valvular stenosis or regurgitation, congenital heart disease, injection drug use, etc.).
2. **Fever** (Temperature ≥38.0°C, 100.4°F).
3. **Vascular phenomena:** Arterial emboli, pulmonary infarcts, mycotic aneurysms, intracranial bleed, conjunctival hemorrhages, Janeway lesions.
4. **Immunologic phenomena:** Positive rheumatoid factor, Osler nodes, Roth spots, or immune complex-mediated glomerulonephritis.
5. **Microbiologic evidence (falling short of major criteria)** Positive blood cultures for a microorganism consistent with IE but not meeting requirements for major criteria. Positive culture or PCR test for an organism consistent with IE from a sterile body site other than cardiac tissue, cardiac prosthesis, or embolus.
6. **Imaging criteria:** Abnormal metabolic activity detected by FDG PET/CT within 3 months of implantation of prosthetic valve, ascending aortic graft (with concomitant evidence of valve involvement), intracardiac device leads or other prosthetic material.
7. **Physical examination criteria (if echocardiography is not available):** New valvular regurgitation identified on auscultation (based on expert opinion); worsening or changing of pre-existing murmur not sufficient.

Mnemonic to remember the major and minor criteria

'**M**y **I**ntelligent **S**ister **P**aints **F**antastic **V**ivid **I**mages **M**aking **I**nspiration **P**ossible'.

- My → **Microbiologic criteria**
- Intelligent → **Imaging criteria**
- Sister → **Surgical major criterion**
- Paints → **Predisposition**
- Fantastic → **Fever**
- Vivid → **Vascular phenomena**
- Images → **Immunologic phenomena**
- Making → **Microbiologic evidence not meeting major criteria**
- Inspiration → **Imaging criteria not meeting major criteria**
- Possible → **Physical examination criteria**

Blood Cultures

- Isolation of the causative microorganism from blood cultures is important not only for diagnosis but also for treatment. At least two sets of blood cultures should be obtained from separate venipuncture sites prior to initiation of antibiotic therapy. Three or more blood culture sets are ideal for distinguishing IE from non-IE bloodstream infections. Patients with IE typically have continuous bacteremia; therefore, blood cultures may be collected at any time and need not necessarily be obtained at the time of fever or chills.
- Obtain follow-up blood cultures 24–72 hours after antimicrobial therapy is begun, and repeat every one to three days until clearance of bacteremia is documented.
- Empirical antimicrobial therapy should be withheld in hemodynamically stable patients with subacute endocarditis, especially those who have received antibiotics within the preceding 2 weeks. This will allow additional blood cultures to be sent without the confounding effect of antibiotic therapy.
- Antibiotics should be started immediately in acute endocarditis and in those with hemodynamic instability after the initial sets of blood culture are obtained.
- Culture negative endocarditis occurs in some cases. This may be due to fastidious organisms and prior antibiotic therapy.

ECG

- Should be done for all to serve as a baseline and to detect any complications like conduction abnormalities, MI, and pericarditis.

Echocardiography

- Echocardiography can identify the presence and size of vegetations, detect intracardiac complications, and assess cardiac function. Echocardiograpy should be done for all patients with a clinical diagnosis of endocarditis.
- Transthoracic echocardiography (TTE), in general, is the first diagnostic test for patients with suspected IE. However, it cannot detect vegetations <2 mm in diameter. It is also not very useful in obese and emphysema patients. TTE is not adequate for evaluating prosthetic valves or detecting intracardiac complications.
- Transesophageal echocardiograpy (TEE, gold standard for IE) is more sensitive than TTE. It can detect small vegetations; detect prosthetic endocarditis and intracardiac complications like myocardial abscess, valve perforation, or intracardiac fistulae.
- Data obtained by TTE and TEE are complementary, so both studies are useful in most patients.

Cardiac CT

- Cardiac CT can be useful in cases where TEE does not provide definitive evidence of infective endocarditis (IE) or its complications. It is also valuable for surgical planning, particularly in patients with extravalvular involvement. While less sensitive than echocardiography for detecting vegetations, Cardiac CT has higher sensitivity for identifying paravalvular abscesses and pseudoaneurysms. Additionally, it may offer superior imaging in cases where TEE is limited by artifacts.
- If clinically indicated, CT imaging of the brain and/or torso can be performed concurrently to assess for systemic embolization.

FDG PET/CT

- 18F-fluorodeoxyglucose positron emission tomography/computed tomography (FDG PET/CT) is an advanced imaging modality which can identify infection especially in challenging cases such as prosthetic valve endocarditis (PVE) and device-related infections as well as extracardiac sites of infection. Helps in detecting the source of infection when blood cultures are negative. More sensitive than

echocardiography for perivalvular complications. Identifies silent embolic events in brain, spleen, kidney, and lungs. Helps assess for vascular complications like mycotic aneurysms.
- It has become one of the major criteria in 2023 updated Duke criteria for diagnosis of IE.

Histopathological Study

- Valve tissue microscopy, culture and PCR (if surgery is done)—improves detection of fastidious organisms.

Molecular Tests

- Confirms IE in culture-negative cases. Polymerase chain reaction (PCR) for bacteria, *Coxiella burnetii* (Q fever IE), Bartonella, *Tropheryma whipplei* (Whipple's disease).

Other Tests

- *Serologic tests* are useful for organisms, which are difficult to culture such as Brucella, Bartonella, Legionella, and *Coxiella burnetii*.
- Complete blood count may show anemia and increased WBC counts.
- *Urine examination* may show microscopic hematuria (due to renal emboli or focal glomerulonephritis) or macroscopic hematuria (due to renal infarction).
- *Urea and creatinine* may be elevated due to glomerulonephritis.
- *Chest X-ray* may show emboli, cardiac enlargement, and other abnormalities.
- *ESR, CRP, circulating immune complex titer, and rheumatoid factor* concentration are commonly increased in endocarditis.
- *Cardiac catheterization* is useful to assess coronary artery patency in older individuals who are to undergo surgery for endocarditis because CABG also can be done in the same sitting.

Treatment

Antimicrobial Therapy

- Effective antimicrobial therapy for endocarditis requires identification of the specific pathogen and assessment of its susceptibility to various antimicrobial agents. Therefore, every effort must be made to isolate the pathogen before initiating antimicrobial therapy, if clinically feasible.
- In patients with acute endocarditis and hemodynamic instability, empirical antibiotic therapy should be started as soon as possible after obtaining blood cultures. Befire giving empiric therapy, at least two (preferably three) sets of blood cultures should be obtained from separate venipunctures and ideally spaced over 30–60 minutes. However, we need not wait for the blood culture reports to start antibiotics in acutely ill patients. Empirical therapy should be targeted at the most likely pathogens in that particular clinical setting.
- In stable patients with suspected IE, empiric therapy is not always necessary and can be deferred until blood culture results are available, because accurate microbiologic diagnosis is a critical first step in planning the treatment strategy.
- It is difficult to eradicate bacteria from the avascular vegetation in infective endocarditis because this site is relatively inaccessible to host defenses. Bactericidal drugs should be used to kill all the bacteria in the vegetations. Antibiotics should be given parenterally in high doses. Prosthetic valve endocarditis requires longer duration of therapy.
- In most patients, effective antibiotic therapy results in subjective improvement and resolution of fever within 5–7 days. Obtain follow-up blood cultures 24–72 hours after antimicrobial therapy is begun, and repeat every one to three days until clearance of bacteremia is documented.
- If fever persists for 7 days in spite of appropriate antibiotic therapy, patients should be evaluated for complications of infective endocarditis such as paravalvular abscess, and extracardiac abscesses (spleen, kidney).
- Vegetations become smaller with effective therapy, but some may remain unchanged. Patients who become afebrile during therapy without any complications can complete remaining therapy as outpatients.
- Serologic abnormalities (e.g. erythrocyte sedimentation rate, rheumatoid factor) resolve slowly and do not reflect response to treatment.

Antibiotic regimens for infective endocarditis

Empirical antibiotic therapy (before culture results)

- Empirical antibiotics are chosen based on whether the patient is having acute or subacute endocarditis, and native valve or prosthetic valve endocarditis.
- In general, empiric therapy should cover staphylococci (methicillin-susceptible and methicillin-resistant), streptococci, enterococci, and gram-negative bacilli.

TABLE 3.27: Initial empirical antibiotic regimens for infective endocarditis

Type of endocarditis	Antibiotic choice
Native valve endocarditis (NVE)	Vancomycin PLUS ceftriaxone (for 4 weeks)
Prosthetic valve endocarditis (PVE)	Vancomycin PLUS cefepime Or Vancomycin PLUS piperacilling-tazobactum (for 6 weeks)

Antibiotic choices based on the organism isolated from blood culture (**Table 3.28**).

Surgery

Indications for surgery

- Patients with direct extension of infection to myocardial structures.
- Prosthetic valve dysfunction.
- Congestive heart failure from valvular damage.
- Badly damaged valve (requires replacement).
- Endocarditis caused by fungi or resistant organisms.

TABLE 3.28: Antibiotic choices based on the organism isolated from blood culture

Organism	Antibiotic	Alternatives
Streptococcus viridans	**Penicillin-G** (18 million units IV in 4–6 divide doses for 4 weeks) OR **Ceftriaxone** (2 g IV OD for 4 weeks)	Use **vancomycin** if patient does not tolerate pencicillin-G or ceftriaxone For viridans streptococci relatively resistant to penicillin, use higher dose of **penicillin G** (24 million units per day) combined with **gentamicin** (3 mg/kg IV OD for the first 2 weeks).
Enterococci	**Penicillin-G** (18 million units IV in 4–6 divide doses for 4 weeks) plus **gentamicin** (1 mg/kg IV 8th hourly) **OR** **Ampicillin** (2 g 4-hourly and gentamicin) plus **Ceftriaxone** (2 g IV 12th hourly) for 4–6 weeks. This is useful for patients with kidney disease as gentamicin which is nephrotoxic is not used.	For patients who cannot tolerate penicillin or ampicillin or enterococci resistant to these agents, use **vancomycin and gentamicin**
Staphylococci	*Methicillin susceptible* Use **nafcillin or oxacillin**, 12 g intravenously daily given continuously or in four to six divided doses, or **cefazolin**, 6 g intravenously daily given continuously or in three divided doses for 6 weeks. *Methicillin resistant (common with prosthetic valve endocarditis)* **Vancomycin** (30 mg/kg/day IV divided in two or three doses for 6 weeks) Plus **Rifampicin** (300 mg IV every 8 hours for 6 weeks) Plus **Gentamicin** (3 mg/kg intravenously every 8 hours for the first 2 weeks)	If patient does not tolerate nafcillin or oxacillin use **vancomycin** or **daptomycin** Rifampicin has excellent biofilm penetration, making it crucial in prosthetic valve endocarditis (PVE) and device-related infections.
HACEK organisms	**Ceftriaxone** (or another third-generation cephalosporin), 2 g intravenously once daily for 4 weeks. Prosthetic valve endocarditis should be treated for 6 weeks.	In penicillin-allergic patients, experience is limited, but fluoroquinolones have in vitro activity and should be considered.

- Patients with recurrent (two or more) embolic events.
- Large vegetations (>10 mm) on echocardiography.
- Emergency surgery is required for new onset acute aortic regurgitation and mitral valve and sinus of Valsalva abscess ruptured into right heart.

Complications of Infective Endocarditis

- *Heart failure:* This is the most frequent major complication of IE.
- *Embolization:* The brain and the spleen are the most common sites of embolization in left-sided IE, whereas septic pulmonary emboli are common in right-sided IE.
- *Mycotic aneurysms:* These occur due to septic embolization to the arterial vasa-vasorum, with subsequent spread of infection and weakening of the vessel wall. They occur most frequently in the intracranial arteries and have a particular predilection for the middle cerebral artery and its branches. Mycotic aneurysms are extremely dangerous, because they can rupture and produce sudden intracranial hemorrhage.
- *Periannular extension of infection:* Leads to abscess formation, perforation, fistula development, and hemodynamic deterioration. Persistent fever and bacteremia despite antibiotic therapy, heart failure, or new conduction block should raise suspicion for this complication.
- *Renal dysfunction:* is a common complication of IE and is often multifactorial due to immune complex deposition, drug-induced nephrotoxicity, and hemodynamic perturbations.

Prognosis

- Poor prognosis is seen in older age, severe comorbid conditions, delayed diagnosis, involvement of prosthetic valves, antibiotic-resistant pathogen, intracardiac complications, and major neurologic complications.

Key points in infective endocarditis treatment
- Early blood cultures before antibiotics.
- IV antibiotics for 4–6 weeks based on the organism.
- Surgical intervention for complications like heart failure, large vegetations, or prosthetic valve IE.
- Neurological monitoring for stroke or embolism.
- Follow-up blood cultures and echocardiography to confirm treatment success.

Q. Infective endocarditis prophylaxis.

- Since bacteremia is the first step in the causation of infective endocarditis, prevention of bacteremia can prevent the occurrence of infective endocarditis.

Bacteremia is prevented by the administration of antibiotics prior to any procedure known to produce bacteremia. However, not all cardiac lesions are prone for infection. Hence, prophylaxis is recommended only in specific lesions.

- The revised guidelines have narrowed the number of procedures for which antibiotic prophylaxis is recommended. Antibiotic prophylaxis is no longer recommended for GI/genitourinary tract procedures (including diagnostic upper GI scopy or colonoscopy) **(Table 3.29)**.

TABLE 3.29: Infective endocarditis prophylaxis

Cardiac conditions associated with highest risk of adverse outcome from IE. Antibiotic prophylaxis required prior to invasive dental or invasive oral procedures
• Prosthetic heart valve or valve repair with prosthetic valve material.
• Durable mechanical circulatory support device (ventricular assist device or artificial heart).
• Previous infective endocarditis.
• Congenital heart disease (CHD)
– Unrepaired cyanotic CHD, including palliative shunts and conduits.
– Completely repaired congenital heart defect with prosthetic material or device, whether placed by surgery or by catheter intervention, during the first 6 months after the procedure
– Repaired CHD with residual defects at the site or adjacent to the site of a prosthetic patch or prosthetic device (which inhibits endothelialization)
• Cardiac transplantation recipients with cardiac valvular disease
Intermediate risk (patients at intermediate risk of adverse outcomes from IE). Antibiotic prophylaxis is not routinely recommended
• Acquired valve disease (due to RHD or other causes)
• Congenital valve disease (bicuspid aortic valve, MVP etc)
• Hypertrophic cardiomyopathy
• Cardiovascular implanted electronic device

Procedures Which Require Infective Endocarditis Prophylaxis

- ***Invasive dental or oral procedures:*** All dental procedures that involve manipulation of gingival tissue or the periapical region of teeth or perforation of the oral mucosa. The following procedures and events do not need antibiotic prophylaxis: Routine anaesthetic injections through noninfected tissue, taking dental radiographs, placement of removable prosthodontic or orthodontic appliances, adjustment of orthodontic appliances, placement of orthodontic brackets, shedding of deciduous teeth, and bleeding from trauma to the lips or oral mucosa.
- ***Respiratory tract:*** Invasive procedures of the respiratory tract that involve incision or biopsy of the respiratory mucosa, such as tonsillectomy or adenoidectomy. Routine prophylaxis for bronchoscopy is not recommended unless the procedure involves biopsy.
- ***Infected skin or musculoskeletal:*** Surgical procedures that involve infected skin, skin structure, or musculoskeletal tissue.

Antibiotic Regimens for IE Prophylaxis (Table 3.30)

TABLE 3.30: Antibiotic regimens for IE prophylaxis (single dose 30–60 min before procedure)

No penicillin allergy
• Amoxicillin 2 g oral OR
• Ampicillin 2 g IM or IV *or* Cefazolin or Ceftriaxone 1 g IM or IV (if unable to take orally)
Alternatives to above if patient is allergic to pencillins
• Azithromycin *or* clarithromycin 500 mg OR (oral or IV)
• Doxycycline 100 mg (oral or IV)

- *Note that clindamycin is no longer recommended forIE prophylaxis because of severe adverse reactions (Cl. difficile infection).*

Q. Janeway leisons.

- ***Janeway lesions*** are due to septic microemboli to skin seen in infective endocarditis.
- They are macular, blanching, nontender (unlike Osler's nodes, which are painful), erythematous lesions seen on the palms and soles. Usually bilateral and multiple. They may persist for days to weeks, but resolve once the infection is controlled.

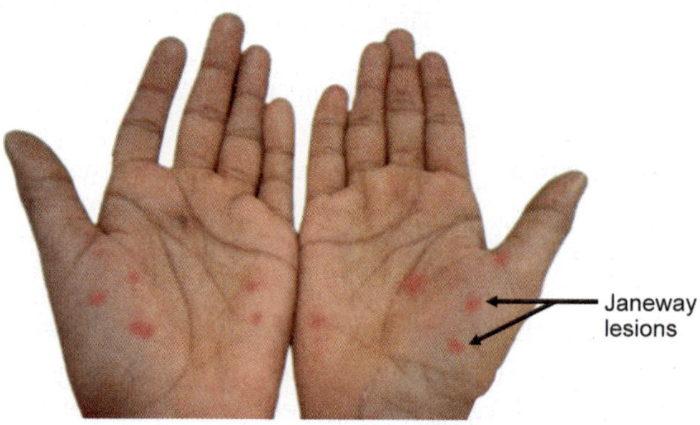

Figure 3.21: Janeway lesions

Q. Osler's nodes.

Osler's nodes are painful, violaceous nodules found in the pulp of fingers and toes and are seen more often in subacute than acute cases of IE. They are due to immune complex deposition in the skin leading to vasculitis in small vessels. This leads to tissue necrosis and painful, raised nodules.

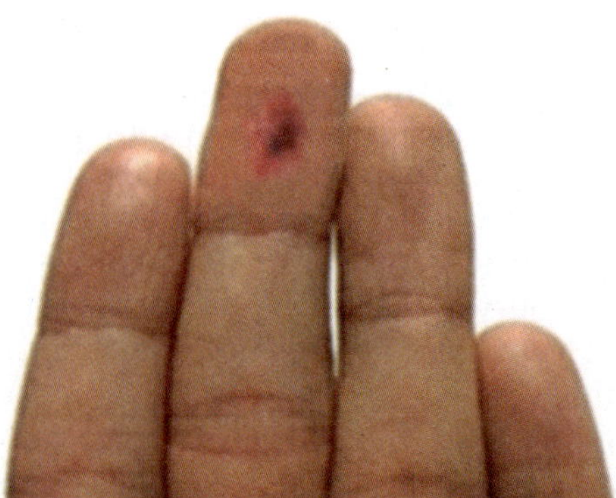

Figure 3.22: Osler's nodes

Q. Roth's spots.

- Roth's spots are round or oval retinal hemorrhages with a pale or white center, seen in the fundus of the eye. They are a sign of immune complex-mediated vasculitis, commonly associated with infective endocarditis (IE) but can also occur in other systemic conditions (leukemia, anemia).
- Pathophysiology: Microemboli to retinal vessels → occlusion of retinal capillaries → local ischemia and hemorrhage. Pale center formation—consists of fibrin, platelet aggregates, or inflammatory infiltrates.

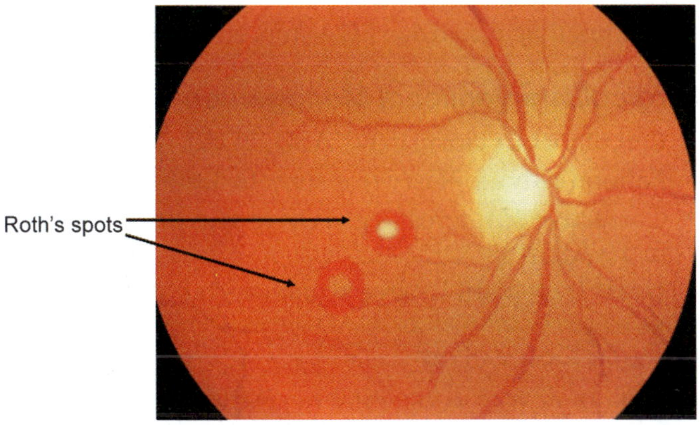

Figure 3.23: Roth's spots

Q. Libman-Sacks endocarditis (verrucous, marantic, or nonbacterial thrombotic endocarditis).

- Libman-Sacks endocarditis (otherwise known as verrucous, marantic, or nonbacterial thrombotic endocarditis) was first described by Libman and Sacks. It is characterized by atypical, sterile, verrucous vegetations.
- Libman-Sacks endocarditis is the most characteristic cardiac manifestation of the autoimmune disease systemic lupus erythematosus. It also occurs in association with antiphospholipid antibody (APLA) syndrome, malignancy and hypercoagulable states.
- The sterile vegetations are common on the aortic and mitral valves and usually affect the edge of the valves. They typically form on both sides of the valve leaflets, unlike bacterial endocarditis, which usually affects only one side. They consist of accumulations of immune complexes, mononuclear cells, hematoxylin bodies, and fibrin and platelet thrombi.
- Healing leads to fibrosis, scarring, and calcification. If the scarring is extensive, it may lead to valve deformity, stenotic or regurgitant lesions.
- Verrucous endocarditis is usually asymptomatic. However, the verrucae can fragment and produce systemic emboli, and infective endocarditis can develop on already damaged valves.
- Treatment involves the management of underlying condition. Anticoagulation may be required if there is atrial fibrillation. Valve surgery may be required for hemodynamically significant valvular dysfunction.

Q. Discuss the etiology, classification, and general clinical features of congenital heart diseases.

- Congenital heart disease (CHD) refers to structural abnormalities of the heart or great vessels present at birth, resulting from improper embryonic development.
- It is the most common congenital anomaly, affecting approximately **1% of live births**.
- Males are affected more commonly except atrial septal defect (ASD) and persistent ductus arteriosus (PDA) which are more common in females.
- Because of improved medical and surgical management, more children with congenital heart disease are surviving into adolescence and adulthood.

Etiology

- Congenital heart diseases are due to abnormal development of a normal structure, or failure of a normal structure to develop fully. Such maldevelopments are due to multifactorial genetic and environmental causes. The recognized risk factors include:
- *Maternal infections,* e.g. rubella infection (persistent ductus arteriosus, pulmonary stenosis).
- *Drugs:* Alcohol abuse (septal defects), phenytoin (associated with pulmonary stenosis) and radiation.
- *Genetic abnormalities,* e.g. familial form of atrial septal defect and congenital heart block.
- *Chromosomal abnormalities,* e.g. septal defects and tetralogy of fallot are associated with Down syndrome (trisomy 21) or coarctation of the aorta in Turner's syndrome (45, XO).

Classification of Congenital Heart Diseases (Table 3.31)

TABLE 3.31: Classification of congenital heart diseases

Cyanotic congenital heart diseases	Acyanotic congenital heart diseases
• Tetralogy of Fallot • Transposition of the great vessels • Tricuspid atresia • Truncus arteriosus • Total anomalous pulmonary venous connection (TAPVC) *Mnemonic to remember above is "five T's"*	• Atrial septal defect (ASD) • Ventricular septal defect (VSD) • Patent ductus arteriosus (PDA) • Coarctation of the aorta • Aortic stenosis • Congenital pulmonary valve regurgitation • Pulmonary stenosis

General Clinical Features of Congenital Heart Diseases

- Congenital heart disease (CHD) should be recognized as early as possible, since early treatment is associated with better outcome. Some general clinical features of congenital heart diseases are as follows:
- In as many as 80% of infants with critical disease, congestive heart failure is the presenting symptom. Difficulty in feeding is common and is often associated with tachypnea, sweating and subcostal retraction. Suspicion of CHD should be raised if feeding takes

more than 30 minutes. A history of feeding difficulty often precedes overt congestive heart failure. On examination, signs of congestive heart failure include an S3 gallop and crepitations in the lungs.

- *Central cyanosis* Occurs in cyanotic congenital heart diseases because of right-to-left shunting of blood or because of mixing of systemic and pulmonary blood flow.
- *Pulmonary hypertension* can happen in left-to-right shunts. Blood from left side of the heart under high pressure enters right side and then into pulmonary artery. This leads to pulmonary hypertension. Pressure in the pulmonary arterial system can exceed that on left side of the heart which can cause reversal of blood flow from right side to left side. This reversal of blood flow is reffered to as *Eisenmenger's syndrome.*
- *Clubbing of the fingers* occurs due to prolonged cyanosis in cyanotic congenital heart diseases.
- *Paradoxical embolism* of thrombus can occur from systemic veins to systemic arterial system when there is a communication between the right and left heart (e.g. VSD). This can lead to an increased risk of cerebrovascular accidents and abscesses.
- *Polycythemia* can develop secondary to chronic hypoxemia, which lead to hyperviscosity and increased risk of thromboembolism and strokes.
- *Growth retardation* is common in children with cyanotic heart disease.
- *Syncope* is common when severe right or left ventricular outflow tract obstruction is present. Exertional syncope, associated with deepening central cyanosis, may occur in Fallot's tetralogy. Exercise increases pulmonary vascular resistance and decreases systemic vascular resistance. Thus, the right to left shunt increases and cerebral oxygenation falls.
- *Squatting* posture is often adopted by children with Fallot's tetralogy. It results in decreased venous return and an increase in the peripheral vascular resistance. This leads to decreased pressure in the right side of heart and increased pressure in left side of the heart which results in reduced right-to-left shunt and improved cerebral oxygenation.
- *Endocarditis* can occur at the sites of shunts and damaged valves.
- *Atrial and ventricular arrhythmias, right heart failure* due to pulmonary HTN, *end-stage heart failure and sudden cardiac death* can occur. This may be the first time that the presence of congenital heart disease is noted.

Diagnosis

- **Echocardiography (TTE/TEE)** → Gold standard for diagnosing CHD.
- **Chest X-ray** → Cardiomegaly, pulmonary congestion, or characteristic findings (e.g. "boot-shaped heart" in TOF).
- **ECG** → Can show chamber enlargement or conduction abnormalities.
- **Cardiac MRI/CT angiography** → For complex CHDs.
- **Pulse oximetry screening** → Detects critical CHDs in newborns.
- **Cardiac catheterization** → Used for both diagnosis and intervention.

Management

Medical Management

- Diuretics (e.g. furosemide) for heart failure.
- ACE inhibitors to reduce afterload.
- Prostaglandin E1 (PGE1) to maintain ductal patency (e.g. in TGA).
- Indomethacin to close PDA in preterm infants.

Surgical/Interventional Management

- Percutaneous closure (for ASD, PDA).
- Balloon valvuloplasty (for stenotic lesions).
- Corrective surgeries (e.g. TOF repair, arterial switch in TGA).
- Heart transplant in severe uncorrectable defects.

Genetic Counseling

- A woman with congenital heart disease needs close follow up during pregnancy. Pregnancy is usually safe except if pulmonary hypertension is present when the prognosis for both mother and fetus is poor.
- Fetal ultrasound screening during pregnancy is necessary to r/o any heart malformations since patients with congenital heart disease are more likely to have a baby with congenital heart disease.

Q. Tetralogy of Fallot (TOF).

- Tetralogy of Fallot is the most common cyanotic congenital heart disease.
- It is characterized by 4 features; **(1) Pulmonary stenosis, (2) VSD, (3) Overriding aorta,** and **(4) Right ventricular hypertrophy.** Pulmonary stenosis can be subvalvular (commonest), valvular or supravalvular.
- Presence of ASD along with TOF is called pentology of Fallot.

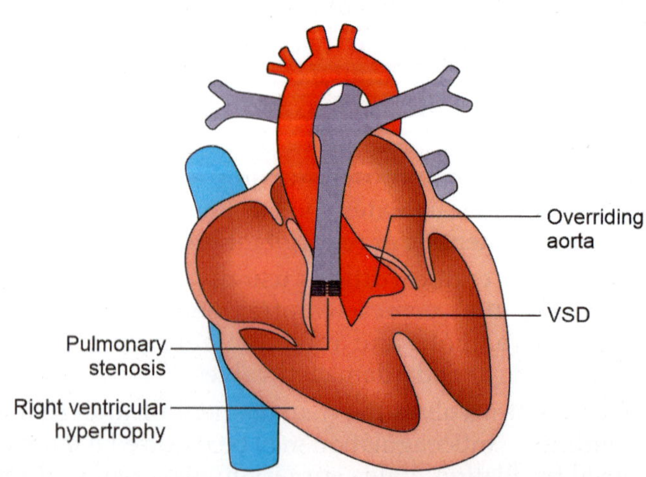

Figure 3.24: Tetralogy of Fallot

Pathophysiology

- Since the right ventricular pressure is more than left ventricle due to pulmonary stenosis, blood is shunted from right to left through the ventricular septal defect, which leads to central cyanosis. Right ventricular hypertrophy (RVH) occurs due to increased pressure load from pulmonary stenosis → leads to a characteristic "boot-shaped heart" on chest X-ray. Squatting episodes increase systemic arterial rsistance and hence reduce the shunt from right to left ventricle. The aorta is displaced to the right and receives blood from both ventricles, contributing to systemic desaturation.

Clinical Features

- Children are usually asymptomatic at birth.
- Children with tetralogy of Fallot may present with dyspnea and fatigue.
- Growth is usually retarded.
- *Cyanotic spells:* Cyanotic spells occur during crying, feeding, exercise and fever. Exercise leads to drop in systemic vascular resistance and increases pulmonary resistance. This leads to shunting of blood from right to left ventricle leading to increased cyanosis and syncope (cyanotic or Fallot's spells). Sudden death can occur during such spells.
- *Squatting episodes* are common because it increases peripheral vascular resistance and decreases right to left shunt.
- Polycythemia and clubbing occur due to chronic hypoxemia which may result in thrombotic strokes.
- A parasternal heave is common due to RVH.
- P2 is faint or inaudible because of pulmonary stenosis. An ejection sound from aortic dilation and a diastolic murmur from consequent aortic regurgitation can be heard. VSD murmur is not heard because it is large.

Investigations

- ***Chest X-ray:*** Shows "boot-shaped heart" heart. This shape results from small concave pulmonary artery and hypertrophied right ventricle coupled with small to normal-sized left ventricle with upturned apex **(Fig. 3.25)**. Pulmonary vascularity is reduced **(Fig. 3.26)**.
- ***ECG:*** Shows right ventricular hypertrophy and right-axis deviation. Right bundle branch block may also be present.
- ***Echocardiogram:*** Can readily identify overriding aorta and VSD. The degree of pulmonary stenosis and VSD are best assessed by Doppler.
- ***Cardiac catheterization:*** Is done for patients in whom operative treatment is contemplated or in whom the integrity of the coronary circulation needs to be verified.

Complications

- Chronic hypoxemia → polycythemia → increased viscosity → increased incidence of intravascular thrombosis and thrombotic stroke.

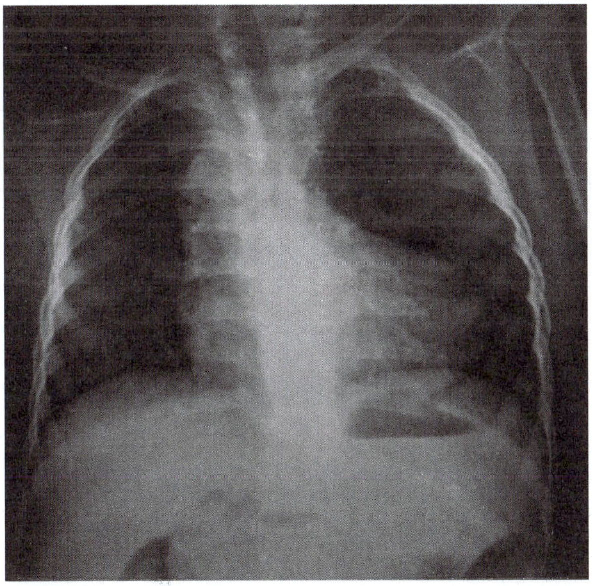

Figure 3.25: X-ray showing boot-shaped heart with upturned apex

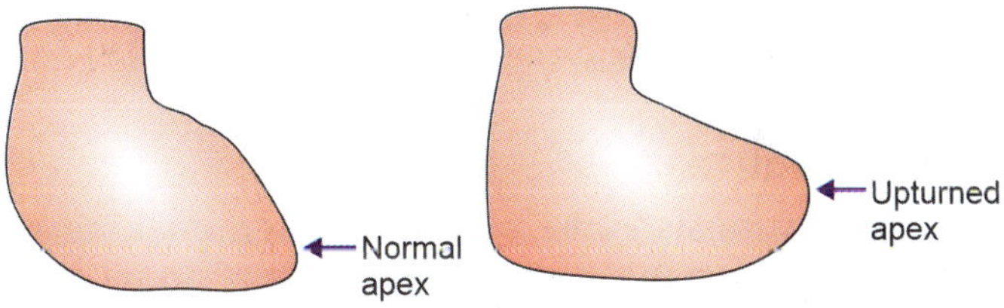

Figure 3.26: Normal and boot-shaped heart

- Brain abscess can occur because organisms entering right ventricle by venous return can enter systemic circulation through VSD and reach brain.
- Infective endocarditis.
- Higher incidence of pulmonary tuberculosis.

Treatment

- Neonates with severe cyanosis may be palliated with an infusion of prostaglandin E1 to open the ductus arteriosus and thereby increase pulmonary blood flow.
- Complete surgical repair consists of patch closure of the VSD and relief of pulmonary stenosis.
- Occasionally a palliative procedure—an anastomosis between subclavian artery and pulmonary artery (Blalock-Taussig shunt)—is performed on very young or premature infants.
- Antibiotic prophylaxis for endocarditis is needed.

Prognosis

- Good prognosis with **early surgical correction** and proper follow-up.

Q. Transposition of the great arteries (TGA).

- Complete TGA is the second most common congenital heart defect.
- Here the aorta arises from the right ventricle and the pulmonary artery arises from the left ventricle. This defect causes deoxygenated blood to enter systemic

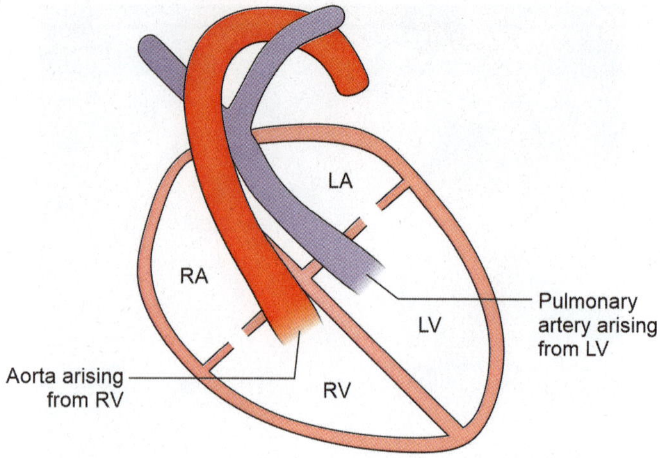

Figure 3.27: Transposition of great arteries (TGA)

circulation, and oxygenated blood to enter pulmonary circulation. Since both systemic and pulmonary circulations are not connected with each other, this condition is incompatible with life unless there is shunt (ASD, VSD, or PDA) which allows mixing of oxygenated and deoxygenated blood **(Fig. 3.27)**.

Clinical Features

- Severe cyanosis is the presenting sign, making its clinical appearance within the first few hours after birth. Neonates who have a communication between right and left heart due to a persistent PDA, ASD or VSD, patent formane ovale, etc. may survive for few weeks and present later.
- Examination shows intense cyanosis and tachypnea. The right ventricular lift is forceful because it is connected to systemic circulation, and the first sound is usually loud at the lower left sternal border. Signs of heart failure may be present.

Investigations

- *Chest X-ray:* Egg-on-a-string" appearance may be seen on chest X-ray (narrow mediastinum due to straightened great arteries). Increased pulmonary vascular markings if VSD or PDA is present.
- *ECG:* may show abnormal right axis deviation and marked right ventricular hypertrophy due to the systemic function of the right ventricle.
- *Echocardiogram:* confirms the presence of TGA.
- *Cardiac catheterization:* Measures oxygen saturation and confirms abnormal circulation patterns.

Treatment

- ***Immediate management (neonatal period):*** Prostaglandin E1 (PGE1) infusion keeps the ductus arteriosus open, allowing oxygenated blood to reach systemic circulation. Balloon atrial septostomy (Rashkind procedure) can be performed in severe cyanosis cases to enlarge the foramen ovale and improve mixing of oxygenated and deoxygenated blood.
- ***Arterial switch operation (Jatene Procedure)—gold standard:*** Transects the aorta and pulmonary artery above their respective valves and switches them to become realigned with their appropriate ventricles. This is the most physiological procedure.
- ***Atrial switch operation (Senning or Mustard procedure).*** Used when arterial switch is not feasible. It involves corrective procedures, which redirect oxygenated blood from the left atrium to the right ventricle so that it may be ejected into the aorta while deoxygenated blood enters the right atrium and heads for the left ventricle and into the pulmonary artery.
- ***Rastelli procedure:*** Performed in patients with TGA with a large VSD and pulmonary stenosis. Reroutes blood at the ventricular level by tunneling the left ventricle to the aorta inside the heart through a VSD. A conduit is placed between the right ventricle and pulmonary artery bypassing pulmonary stenosis.

Q. Ventricular septal defect (VSD).

- VSD is a defect in the inter-ventricular septum.
- VSD is the most common congenital heart disease (1 in 500 live births). It may occur as an isolated anomaly or in association with other anomalies.
- Membranous VSD is the most common type. VSD can close spontaneously or lead to congestive cardiac failure and death in infancy.
- Maladie-de-Roger is a small VSD in muscular portion presenting in older children. It produces a loud pansystolic murmur without any hemodynamic consequences. This defect usually closes spontaneously.

Pathophysiology

- As left ventricular pressure is higher than right ventricular pressure, blood moves from left to right through VSD leading to increased blood flow through pulmonary vasculature. This increased flow leads to pulmonary HTN and increased right ventricular pressure so much that right ventricular pressure may be equal to or more than left ventricular pressure. As a result, the shunt is reduced or reversed (becoming right-to-left) and central cyanosis may develop (Eisenmenger syndrome).

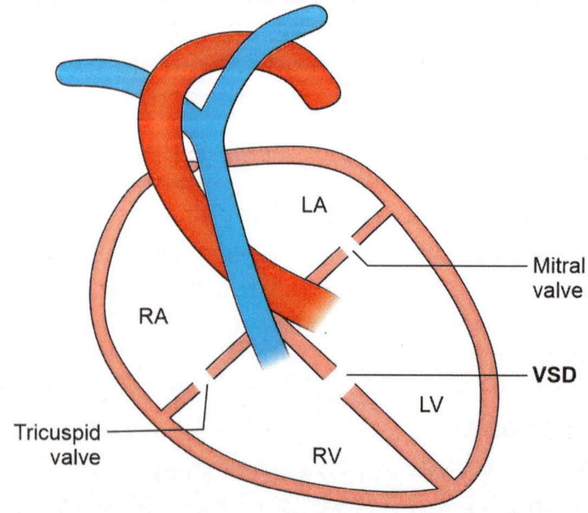

Figure 3.28: Ventricular septal defect (VSD)

Clinical Features

- *Small VSDs* are asymptomatic and 90% of them close spontaneously by 10 years of age.
- *Moderate and large VSD* leads to pulmonary HTN, which causes exertional dyspnea, chest pain, syncope, and hemoptysis.
- When there is reversal of shunt (right-to-left shunt), central cyanosis, clubbing, and polycythemia develop.
- CVS examination reveals cardiac enlargement and hyperdynamic apex. There is often a palpable systolic thrill at the lower left sternal edge. A loud pansystolic murmur is heard in the same area.

Investigations

- *Chest X-ray* may show features of increased pulmonary flow and pulmonary HTN such as prominent pulmonary artery, 'pruned' pulmonary arteries, and right ventricular hypertrophy.
- *ECG* shows features of both left and right ventricular hypertrophy.
- Echocardiography can confirm the presence, size and location of the VSD, and abnormal blood flow.

Treatment

- Surgery is not recommended for patients with small shunts and normal pulmonary arterial pressures.
- Diuretics, digoxin, and ACE inhibitors may be useful to control symptoms of heart failure before cardiac surgery.
- Surgical correction is indicated for moderate to large VSD before the development of severe pulmonary HTN. If severe pulmonary HTN has developed already, it will not reverse or may progress even after surgery.
    - Primary surgical closure (Patch repair): Preferred for large VSDs.
    - Transcatheter device closure (for muscular VSDs if surgery is high risk).

Complications

- Congestive cardiac failure.
- Pulmonary hypertension.
- Eisenmenger syndrome (this is development of severe pulmonary HTN and reversal of left to right shunt causing central cyanosis).
- Infective endocarditis.

Q. Atrial septal defect (ASD).

- ASD is a defect in interatrial septum. It is common in females. This is one congenital heart disease which can present late in 4th or 5th decade of life. Other congenital heart disease which can present very late is bicuspid aortic valve.

Types of ASD

- There are 4 types of ASD, *ostium secundum (most common type), ostium primum, sinus venosus, and coronary sinus defect.*
- Ostium secundum defect is located in the central part of the interatrial septum (fossa ovalis) and is

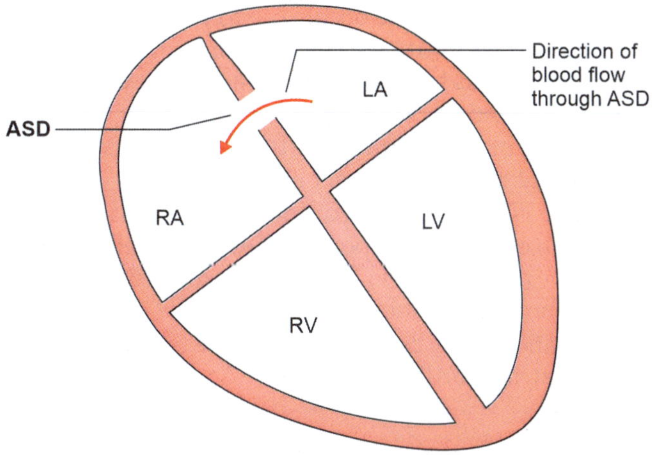

Figure 3.29: Atrial septal defect (ASD)

associated with patent foramen ovale (PFO). This is the most common type of ASD. Patent foramen ovale (PFO) is a normal variant and not a true septal defect. PFO is usually asymptomatic but can be associated with paradoxical emboli and an increased incidence of embolic stroke.
- Ostium primum type septal defect occurs in the lower part of septum, near atrioventricular valves. It is common in patients with Down syndrome.
- Sinus venosus type occurs high in the atrial septum near the entry of superior vena cava.
- Coronary sinus defect (rare): Absent or unroofed coronary sinus, allowing a left-to-right shunt.
- Lutembachers syndrome is a rare combination of ASD with rheumatic mitral stenosis.

Pathophysiology

- ASD allows shunting of blood from high pressure left atrium to low pressure right atrium. Hence, there is increase in right ventricular inflow, right ventricular output, and pulmonary blood flow.
- Increased pulmonary blood flow gives rise to increased pulmonary vascular resistance and pulmonary HTN. This usually happens above the age of 30 years because changes in pulmonary circulation and development of pulmonary HTN happen gradually. Delayed right ventricular systole due to overload leads to wide, fixed split of S2.
- Severe pulmonary HTN may lead to increased right ventricular and right atrial pressure. Consequently, right atrial pressure can be more than left atrium and lead to right to left shunting leading to central cyanosis (Eisenmenger's syndrome). Ultimately, heart failure may develop due to overloading of both ventricles.
- Because of increased blood flow into right side, right atrium and right ventricles dilate and there may be atrial arrhythmias, especially atrial fibrillation.

Clinical Features

Symptoms

- Children with ASD are asymptomatic, but as they reach 3rd decade, they may develop pulmonary HTN as explained above.

- Dyspnea and fatigue occur due to pulmonary HTN.
- Recurrent respiratory infections are common due to increased blood flow through pulmonary vasculature and congestion. Two or more attacks of LRTI per year or 3 or more attacks of LRTI in the past suggest recurrent respiratory tract infections.
- If there is recurrent pneumonia in the past, but now no such episodes, the possibilities are development of CCF or pulmonary HTN both of which decrease the flow through pulmonary circulation.
- Palpitations may be experienced due to atrial arrhythmias (atrial fibrillation).

Signs

- Precordium is hyperdynamic.
- Signs of pulmonary HTN such as left parasternal heave due to RVH, prominent pulmonary artery pulsations may be noted.
- On auscultation, the second heart sound is widely split and fixed (hallmark feature). There is no respiratory variation of gap between A2 and P2. A mid-diastolic rumbling murmur is heard at the fourth intercostal space and along the left sternal border due to increased flow across the tricuspid valve. An ejection systolic murmur may be heard over pulmonary area due to increased blood flow across pulmonary valve.
- Right heart failure may develop and lead to raised JVP and peripheral edema.
- Development of Eisenmenger's syndrome leads to central cyanosis and digital clubbing.

Complications

- Congestive cardiac failure
- Pulmonary hypertension
- Eisenmengers syndrome
- Infective endocarditis
- Atrial fibrillation
- Paradoxical embolism.

Investigations

- ***Chest X-ray*** shows prominent pulmonary artery and pulmonary vascular congestion. It may also show right atrial and right ventricular enlargement.
- ***ECG*** may show right bundle branch block and right axis deviation due to right ventricular hypertrophy and dilatation.
- ***Echocardiogram*** may show right ventricular hypertrophy, dilated pulmonary artery, and abnormal motion of the interventricular septum. It may also show ASD. Abnormal shunt and blood flow can be assessed by color Doppler.
- ***Cardiac catheterization*** can confirm the presence of ASD but usually Echo is enough for confirmation. However, it is especially useful when associated coronary artery disease is present as both coronary arteries and ASD can be assessed in the same sitting. Cardiac catheterization shows increased oxygen content of right atrial blood due to blood flow from left atrium.

Treatment

- Surgical closure should be done between 3–6 years of age or as soon as possible in significant ASD.
- Closure should not be carried out in patients with small defects and trivial left-to-right shunts or in those with severe pulmonary hypertension.
- Angiographic closure is now possible by using a transcatheter device.
- Uncorrected ASD does not usually require antibiotic prophylaxis for endocarditis unless there is another accompanying valvular lesion.

Causes of Recurrent LRTI Other than Congenital Heart Disease

- Bronchial foreign body
- Gastroesophageal reflux
- Asthma
- Immune deficiency
- Swallowing disorder
- Cystic fibrosis
- Rickets (in children).

Q. Patent ductus arteriosus (PDA).

- The ductus arteriosus is a vessel, which connects the pulmonary artery to the descending aorta distal to the subclavian artery.
- In fetal life, the ductus arteriosus is normally open and diverts blood away from the unexpanded and hence high resistance pulmonary circulation into the systemic circulation, where the blood is re-oxygenated as it passes through the placenta.
- The duct normally closes at birth, due to high oxygen in the lungs and the reduced pulmonary vascular resistance. After closure a fibrous band is left behind (ligamentum arteriosum).
- If the duct is defective (e.g. less elastic tissue) it will not close. Prenatal hypoxemia and high-altitude environments may impair closure of ductus.
- PDA is more common in females. It is sometimes associated with maternal rubella. Preterm infants can have PDA which is normal and will close later.

Pathophysiology

- Since pressure in the aorta is more than pulmonary artery, blood flows from aorta to pulmonary artery throughout the cardiac cycle. This leads to increased flow through the pulmonary vasculature leading to pulmonary HTN.
- Left heart also gets overloaded due to increased pulmonary venous return which may result in left heart failure.
- If pulmonary HTN is very severe, it may lead to reversal of flow from pulmonary artery to aorta (Eisenmenger's syndrome).
- One-third of patients with PDA die of heart failure, pulmonary hypertension or endocarditis by the age of 40; two-thirds by the age of 60.

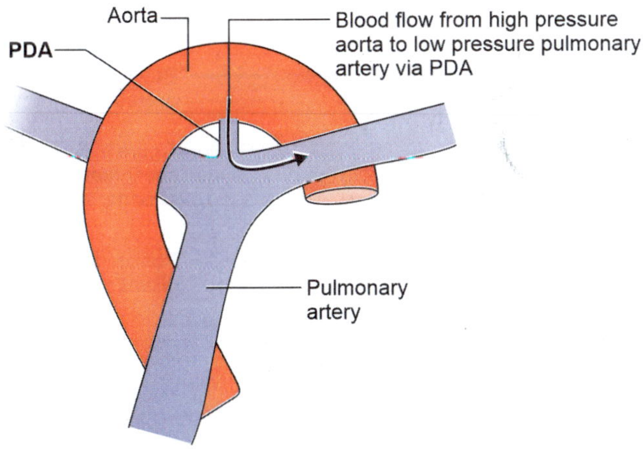

Figure 3.30: Patent ductus arteriosus (PDA)

Clinical Features

- Patients may remain asymptomatic until 20–40 years of age. Symptoms include exertional dyspnea, palpitations (due to atrial fibrillation), and heart failure symptoms. Infective endarteritis risk increases.
- High volume peripheral pulses ('bounding') may be noted due to increased venous return to left heart and hence increased stroke volume. Peripheral signs of wide pulse pressure may be seen just like AR due to increased stroke volume.
- Auscultation reveals a characteristic continuous 'machinery' murmur heard at the first or second left intercostal space. A functional mid-diastolic murmur may be heard at the mitral area due to increased blood flow across mitral valve as the left ventricle receives the blood shunted from aorta into pulmonary circulation via PDA.
- Signs of pulmonary HTN such as loud P2, left parasternal heave and prominent epigatsric pulsations may be present (due to RVH).
- In patients with reversal of shunt (Eisenmenger's syndrome), venous blood from pulmonary artery enters descending aorta (after the origin of left suclavian artery) and leads to differential cyanosis, i.e. a cyanosis in the lower limbs and sparing of upper limbs especially the right arm.

Complications

- Congestive cardiac failure
- Pulmonary hypertension
- Eisenmenger's syndrome
- Infective endocarditis
- Paradoxical embolism
- Aneurysm formation in the ductus and rupture.

Investigations

- *Chest X-ray* may show prominent aorta and pulmonary arterial system. It may also show dilated left atrium and ventricle.
- *ECG* shows left ventricular hypertrophy.
- *Echocardiogram* shows dilated left atrium and left ventricle. Color Doppler can visualize PDA and direction of blood flow.

Treatment

- Premature infants with PDA are treated medically with indomethacin. Indomethacin closes PDA by inhibiting prostaglandin production which maintains patency.
- In other cases, PDA can be closed surgically or via transcatheter methods. Surgery should be done as soon as possible and before the age of 5 years. Closure should not be done if Eisenmenger's syndrome has developed.
- Why we should not close PDA if Eisenmenger's syndrome has developed?
  - In Eisenmenger's syndrome, the right ventricle (RV) is severely hypertrophied and fails due to pulmonary hypertension.
  - PDA allows some deoxygenated blood to bypass the high-resistance pulmonary circulation and reach the systemic circulation.
  - Closing the PDA removes this "relief pathway," worsening right heart failure and causing a sudden cardiovascular collapse.

Q. Coarctation of aorta.

- Coarctation of the aorta refers to narrowing of the aorta. It usually occurs at or just distal to the insertion of ligamentum arteriosum, i.e. distal to the left subclavian artery. Rarely it can occur proximal to the left subclavian artery.
- It is two times more common in men than in women. It is also associated with Turner's syndrome. Other coexisting anomalies are bicuspid aortic valve (most common), VSD and PDA. "Pseudocoarctation" refers to buckling or kinking of the aortic arch without the presence of a significant gradient.

Pathophysiology

- Coarctation causes obstruction of blood flow in the descending thoracic aorta. This leads to the formation of collateral circulation via **internal thoracic, intercostal, and subclavian arteries** to bypass the narrowing.

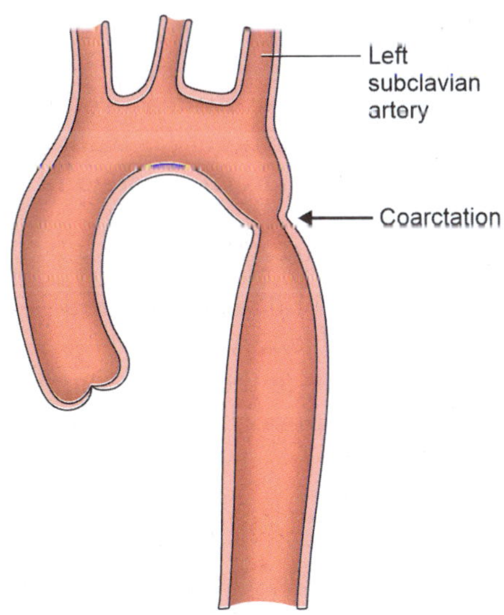

Figure 3.31: Coarctation of aorta

- Increased afterload on the left ventricle (LV) → LV hypertrophy → Risk of heart failure.
- Upper body hypertension (due to increased resistance).
- Lower body hypoperfusion (due to reduced distal blood flow). Decreased renal perfusion activates rennin angiotensin system which leads to the development of hypertension. Lower part of the body may receive less blood supply which leads to growth impairment.

Clinical Features

- Coarctation of the aorta is often asymptomatic for many years. Patients may present with headache, epistaxis (due to hypertension) and claudication, leg fatigue, and cold legs (due to poor blood flow to lower limbs). Older patients may present with angina and symptoms of heart failure.
- There is high pressure in the arms and low pressure in the legs. There are weak pulses in lower limbs and radiofemoral delay. There may be prominent pulsations in the neck.
- Suzman's sign is dilated, tortuous, pulsatile arteries seen around the scapulae and intercostal spaces in the back. It is better seen when the patient bends forward with hands lying down.
- Lower half of the body is less developed than the upper half due to poor circulation. The hips are narrow and the legs are short, in contrast to broad shoulders and long arms. Blood pressure should be measured in both arms and any one leg.
- Signs of LVH may be noted.

Investigations

- Chest X-ray may show figure-3 sign (narrowed segment of aorta with pre- and poststenotic dilation). Dilated intercostal arteries due to collateral flow may erode the undersurfaces of the ribs and cause rib notching (Docks sign).
- ECG shows left ventricular hypertrophy.
- Echocardiography shows the gradient in the descending aorta, LVH and other associated anomalies.
- MRI is the best modality for visualizing the anatomy of the descending aorta.
- Cardiac catheterization can measure pressures and assess collaterals when surgery is planned.
- Aortography can also show the exact site of coarctation.

Complications

- Severe HTN → Cerebral aneurysm and hemorrhage, aortic rupture, heart failure.
- Infective endocarditis at the site of coarctation.
- Aortic aneurysm or dissection of aorta.

Treatment

- Intervention is indicated if the pressure gradient across the coarctation is more than 30 mm Hg.
- Treatment involves surgical excision of the coarctation and end-to-end anastomosis of the aorta.

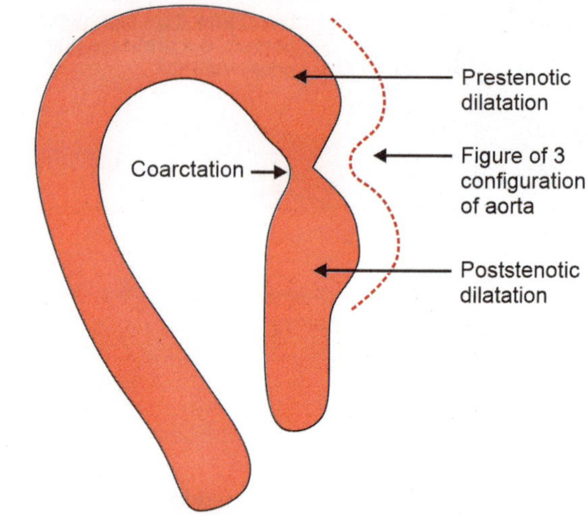

Figure 3.32: Figure 3 sign in configuration of aorta (schematic)

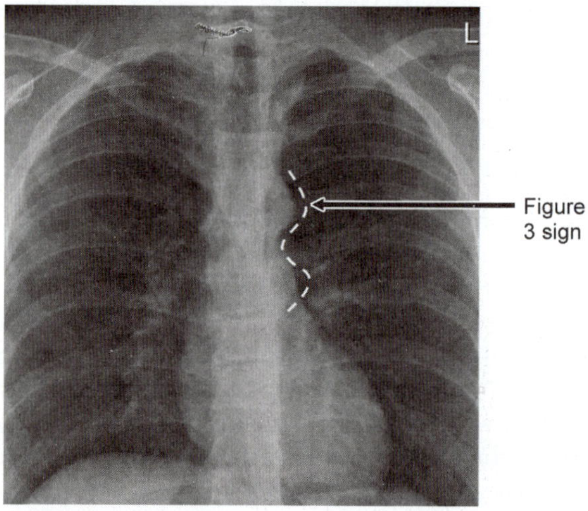

Figure 3.33: Figure 3 sign in coarctation of aorta (X-ray)

- Balloon dilatation is used in some centers either for initial treatment or for recurrence of coarctation. The incidence of incomplete relief and restenosis is decreased by endovascular stent placement.

Q. What is Eisenmenger's syndrome? Discuss the clinical features, investigations and management of Eisenmenger's syndrome.

Definition

- Eisenmenger's syndrome is a severe, irreversible complication of congenital heart defects with a left-to-right shunt, leading to pulmonary hypertension and shunt reversal (right-to-left shunting). This causes cyanosis, clubbing, and secondary complications.
- Congenital heart defects which can cause Eisenmenger's syndrome are ASD, VSD (most common cause), PDA, and atrioventricular septal defect (AVSD).

Pathophysiology

- In congenital heart defects like ventricular septal defect (VSD), atrial septal defect (ASD), or patent ductus arteriosus (PDA), blood flows from the high-pressure left heart to the low-pressure right heart, increasing pulmonary blood flow.

- This chronic increased blood flow through pulmonary circulation leads to remodeling of pulmonary arterioles, causing progressive pulmonary hypertension.
- Due to pulmonary hypertension right heart pressure exceeds that of left heart pressure leading to reversal of blood flow (i.e. from right to left) through the shunt.
- This leads to central cyanosis and hypoxemia.

Clinical Features

- Patients may present with dyspnea on exertion, syncope, chest pain, congestive heart failure, hemoptysis and symptoms related to polycythemia and hyperviscosity.
- On examination, central cyanosis and clubbing are present. Parasternal heave and epigastric pulsations are felt due to right ventricular hypertrophy. Pulmonary artery pulsation is commonly felt. P2 is loud and may be palpable. A tricuspid regurgitation murmur is common, due to right ventricular dilatation. In addition to these, features of underlying congenital heart defect may be noted.

Investigations

- *ECG* shows evidence of right atrial enlargement, right ventricular hypertrophy, and right axis deviation.
- *Chest X-ray* shows dilated pulmonary artery, cardiomegaly, and pulmonary oligemia.
- *Echocardiography* confirms the right-sided pressure overload and pulmonary artery enlargement, as well as the intracardiac defect with right to left shunting.
- *Cardiac catheterization* can directly measure pulmonary artery pressure and also assess the reversibility of the elevated pulmonary vascular resistance after giving vasodilators which is useful to decide whether a patient benefits from surgery.

Treatment

- Eisenmenger's syndrome is the only type of pulmonary artery hypertension, where its development is preventable by early closure of underlying left to right shunt. On the other hand, once it develops, closure of the underlying defect is contraindicated.
- The main interventions are directed toward preventing complications such as influenza vaccine to prevent respiratory infections, iron replacement for iron deficiency; antiarrhythmics for atrial arrhythmias, digoxin and diuretics for right-sided heart failure.
- Pulmonary vasodilators may be tried for pulmonary HTN. Thesea are bosentan, sildenafil, and epoprostenol.
- Phlebotomy can be done for symptomatic polycythemia.
- When patients are severely incapacitated from severe hypoxemia or congestive heart failure, lung transplantation (plus repair of the cardiac defect) or heart-lung transplantation may be considered.

Key Points

- Eisenmenger's syndrome is an irreversible complication of congenital heart defects.
- Pulmonary hypertension leads to shunt reversal (right-to-left shunting), causing cyanosis.
- Closure of the defect is contraindicated once Eisenmenger's syndrome develops.
- Management focuses on symptom relief, pulmonary vasodilators, and preventing complications.

Q. Discuss the etiology (risk factors) of ischemic heart disease (IHD).

OR

Q. Discuss the etiology (risk factors) of atherosclerosis.

- IHD is a life-threatening disease and there are many risk factors for IHD. Some are modifiable and some are non-modifiable.
- Atherosclerosis is responsible for almost all cases of IHD. Most risk factors act by promoting atherosclerosis of the coronary arteries.
- An overview of the established and emerging risk factors for cardiovascular disease is given below.

Risk Factors for IHD

Modifiable Risk Factors (controllable)

- **Dyslipidemia** —Elevated LDL-cholesterol, low HDL-cholesterol, increased total-to-HDL-cholesterol ratio, hypertriglyceridemia are associated with increased risk of IHD.
- **Hypertension**—This is a well-established risk factor for IHD. Both systolic and diastolic blood pressures are important. Isolated systolic hypertension is now established as a risk factor for coronary heart disease and stroke.
- **Diabetes mellitus**—Insulin resistance, hyperinsulinemia, and elevated blood glucose are associated with atherosclerotic cardiovascular disease and IHD.
- **Obesity**—Obesity is associated with a number of risk factors for atherosclerosis, such as hypertension, insulin resistance and glucose intolerance, hypertriglyceridemia, and reduced HDL-cholesterol.
- **Metabolic syndrome**—Patients with the constellation of abdominal obesity, hypertension, diabetes, and dyslipidemia are considered to have the metabolic syndrome (syndrome X). Metabolic syndrome is associated with higher risk of coronary artery disease.
- **Physical inactivity**—This leads to obesity, impaired glucose tolerance and is a risk factor for IHD.
- **Smoking and tobacco use**—Cigarette smoking is an important and reversible risk factor. The incidence of MI increases manifold in people who smoke compared to those who do not.
- **Alcohol onsumption**—Excessive alcohol (>3 drinks/day) increases hypertension, arrhythmias, and heart failure risk.
- **Socioeconomic factors**—low socioeconomic status is associated with higher risk.

- **Chronic kidney disease**—patients with chronic kidney disease have higher risk of IHD.
- **Unhealthy diet**—a diet rich in calories, saturated fat, and transfats is a risk factor for IHD.
- **Psychosocial factors**—Psychological stress can lead to premature atherosclerosis and also aggravate traditional risk factors such as smoking, hypertension, and lipid metabolism. People with depression, anger, stress and other factors have higher chances of developing IHD.
- **C-reactive protein**—a higher level of C-reactive protein (CRP) is associated with higher risk of IHD. CRP is a marker of inflammation which may have a role in promotion of atherosclerosis.
- **Microalbuminuria**—Microalbuminuria reflects vascular damage and is an important risk factor for cardiovascular disease and early cardiovascular mortality.
- **Left ventricular hypertrophy**—Left ventricular hypertrophy (LVH), which is associated with hypertension as well as with age and obesity, is a risk factor for IHD.
- **Hyperhomocysteinemia**—an elevated level of homocysteine is associated with increased risk of IHD.
- **Asymmetrical dimethylarginine (ADMA)**—is an endogenous nitric oxide synthase inhibitor. It is an independent risk factor for endothelial dysfunction and IHD.
- **Lipoprotein(a)—**High Lp(a) levels are a genetic risk factor for premature IHD.
- **Hyperuricemia**—Hyperuricemia is associated with an increased risk of IHD and increased mortality in those with IHD.
- **Infection**—certain infections may play a role in the pathogenesis of atherosclerosis by establishing a low-grade persistent inflammatory process of endohelium. Some organisms suspected are *Chlamydia pneumoniae*, cytomegalovirus, and *Helicobacter pylori*.
- **Collagen vascular disease**—Patients with collagen vascular disease, especially those with rheumatoid arthritis (RA) and systemic lupus erythematosus (SLE), have a significantly increased incidence of cardiovascular disease.
- **Air pollution**—Fine particulate air pollution is associated with increased risk of IHD and cardiopulmonary mortality. This may be due to acute arterial vasoconstriction and myocardial ischemia induced by air pollution.

Nonmodifiable Risk Factors

- **Aging—**As the age advances, atherosclerosis of vessels also increases. Most of the IHD cases occur after 40 years of age. Aging is an independent risk factor for IHD.
- **Sex—**Men have a higher risk compared to premenopausal women due to protective effects of estrogen. After menopause, the risk in women is same as that of men.
- **Family history**—Family history is a significant independent risk factor for IHD, particularly among younger individuals with a family history of premature disease.
- **Ethnicity—**South Asians (Indians, Pakistanis, Bangladeshis) have a higher risk due to genetic factors and high rates of diabetes and dyslipidemia.

Q. Define angina. Describe the etiology, pathogenesis, clinical features, investigations, and management of angina.

Q. Angina equivalents.

Definition

- Angina pectoris may be defined as a discomfort in the chest and/or adjacent area associated with myocardial ischemia but without myocardial necrosis.
- It is a common presenting symptom among patients with coronary artery disease (CAD).

Types

- ***Stable angina*** is usually reproducible and is consistent over time. It is precipitated by effort, and relieved by rest. Stable angina is caused by fixed stenosis in coronary arteries.
- ***Unstable angina*** is diagnosed when a patient has new-onset angina, worsening angina (angina that is more frequent, more prolonged, or precipitated by less effort than before), or angina occurring at rest. This occurs due to plaue rupture leading to platelet aggregation and partial occlusion of coronary artery.
- ***Prinzmetals angina (variant angina)*** is due to coronary vasospasm occurring at rest.
- ***Microvascular angina:*** Dysfunction in small coronary arteries (endothelial dusfunction, microvascular remodeling) impairs blood flow. It is also known as cardiac syndrome X and is more common in women, especially postmenopausal women.

Risk Factors for Angina

- For detailed discussion of risk factors, see above under risk factors for IHD

Nonmodifiable

- Age (>45 in men, >55 in women)
- Family history of IHD
- Male gender (higher risk than premenopausal women).

Modifiable

- Hypertension (increases myocardial workload)
- Dyslipidemia (high LDL, low HDL)
- Diabetes mellitus (accelerates atherosclerosis)
- Smoking (vasoconstriction, thrombosis)
- Obesity and sedentary lifestyle
- Chronic stress and poor sleep.

Etiology

- Angina is due to transient decrease in blood supply to myocardium.

- It may be due to fixed coronary stenosis, clot superimposed on a fixed coronary stenosis, or coronary vasospasm. In the absence of collateral circulation, stenosis of more than 75% of the cross-sectional area (corresponding to >50% lumen diameter by angiography) results in stable angina. Chest pain can occur at rest due to severe stenosis or thrombus formation or due to vasospasm as in Prinzmetal's angina.
- Stenosis is most commonly due to atherosclerosis.
- Angina can also occur when myocardial oxygen demand increases in spite of normal coronary arteries. Examples are patients with aortic stenosis or hypertrophic cardiomyopathy who may experience angina due to markedly increased myocardial oxygen demand because of myocardial hypertrophy. Other factors which increase myocardial oxygen demand are anemia, thyrotoxicosis, aortic regurgitation, exercise, and tachycardia.
- Mental stress, emotions, postprandial state, exposure to cold may reduce coronary flow and lead to angina.
- In syndrome X, patients may experience angina due to failure of coronary vasodilatation with exercise.

Pathophysiology

- Myocardial ischemia is caused by an imbalance between myocardial oxygen supply and oxygen demand. Ischemic myocardium releases active substances, such as adenosine and bradykinin, which stimulate pain receptors and impulses are carried by afferent nerves to upper fifth sympathetic ganglia and upper thoracic spinal cord and from there to thalamus and cortex. When the impulses reach thalamus and cortex, patient perceives the discomfort.
- Myocardial oxygen demand depends mainly on heart rate, wall tension during systole (afterload), the inotropic state of the myocardial cell (contractility), and end-diastolic volume (preload). Whenever there is increased oxygen demand, it is met by coronary vasodilation. Coronary blood flow can increase five to six-fold during exercise from resting values of 0.8 ml/g/min. This increase in flow is due to release of substances like adenosine, and nitric oxide (NO) which are potent vasodilators. Coronary perfusion of the left ventricle occurs mainly in diastole due to decreased wall tension and coronary resistance. Wall tension is highest in the subendocardium and lowest in the subepicardium. Hence, subendocardium is more prone to ischemia than epicardium. However, severe ischemia involves full thickness myocardium from endocardium to the epicardium (transmural ischemia).

Clinical Manifestations

History

- Angina means tightening, not pain. Thus, the discomfort of angina is often described as "pressing," "squeezing," "strangling," "constricting," "bursting," and "burning".
- Angina usually builds up within 30 seconds and disappears in 5–15 minutes. Pain is usually brought on by exertion. The intensity of pain ranges from mild to severe discomfort. The discomfort is most commonly midsternal and radiates to the neck, left shoulder, and left arm. Rarely, it can radiate to the jaw, teeth, right arm, back, and epigastrium.
- The clenching of the fist over the sternum while describing the pain (Levine's sign) is classic.
- Pain may be associated with sweating, palpitations, dizziness and dyspnea.
- There may be history of other comorbid conditions like diabetes and hypertension. Smoking history may be positive.
- *Angina equivalents*: Some patients instead of chest pain or discomfort, experience dyspnea, dizziness, fatigue, or gastrointestinal complaints (epigastric burning, nausea and vomiting). These symptoms are called angina equivalents. When these symptoms occur in response to exercise or other stress, myocardial ischemia should be ruled out.
- *Postprandial angina* develops during or soon after meals because of increased oxygen demand in the splanchnic vascular bed thereby compromising coronary blood flow.

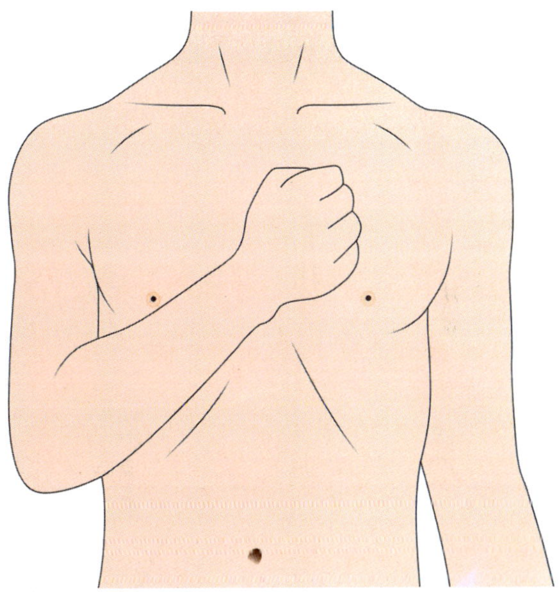

Figure 3.34: Levine's sign

Physical Examination

- *General examination*—may show signs of generalized atherosclerosis like tendon xanthoma, xanthelasmas, thickening of Achilles tendon, locomotor brachialis and corneal arcus. Signs of peripheral vascular disease such as absent peripheral pulses may be noted. Heart rate and BP may be elevated. Excessive sweating may be noted.
- *Systemic examination*—can be completely normal. 3rd and 4th heart sounds, mitral regurgitation murmur (due to ischemic papillary muscle dysfunction) may be heard during ischemia. Paradoxical splitting of S2 (from transient left ventricular dysfunction or left

bundle-branch block) may be noted. Bilateral basal crepitations may be heard during ischemia due to transient left ventricular dysfunction. Pain is promptly relieved by nitroglycerin. Other systems are usually normal.

Investigations

Resting ECG

- This is usually normal between attacks. During an attack, ST depression and T wave inversions in the leads corresponding to ischemic areas may be seen. Changes of old myocardial infarction such as pathological Q waves, and left bundle branch block may be present.

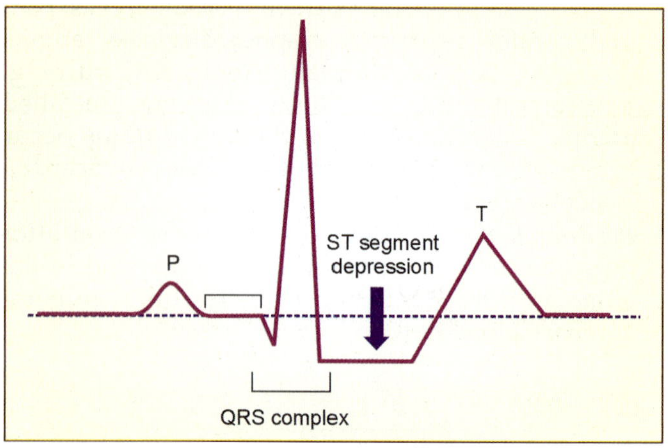

Figure 3.35: ST segment depression

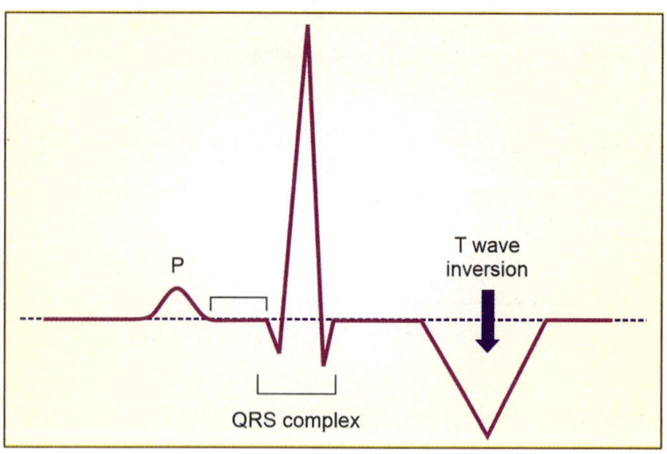

Figure 3.36: T wave inversion

Exercise ECG (stress test)

- Since the resting ECG can be normal in between the attacks, exercise testing can be useful to confirm the diagnosis of angina. Patient is asked to walk on a treadmill and ECG is recorded continuously. Patient may experience chest discomfort during exercise and if ECG shows ST segment depression of >1 mm, it suggests myocardial ischemia. However, a normal test does not exclude coronary artery disease (CAD) (false-negative test) and on the other hand up to 20% of patients with positive exercise tests may not have coronary artery disease (false-positive test).

Echocardiography

- Ischemic or infarcted ventricular wall does not move properly. This is called regional wall motion abnormally (RWMA) and reflect ischemia or previous infarction. Stress echocardiography, can be abnormal if resting echo does not show any abnormalities.

Computed Tomography Angiography (CT-angiogram of coronaries)

- Noninvasive imaging to detect coronary artery disease.
- Helps rule out significant blockages in low-to-intermediate-risk patients.

Myocardial Perfusion Imaging (MPI)/SPECT (Single-photon Emission Computed Tomography)

- Myocardial perfusion scans (using radioactive tracers) at rest and after stress (i.e. exercise or dobutamine), is a sensitive indicator of ischemia and useful in deciding if a stenosis seen at angiography is giving rise to ischemia.

Coronary Angiography (CAG, gold standard test)

- When all the above tests do not provide an answer to chest pain, CAG can be useful. It can delineate the exact coronary anatomy and areas of stenosis. It is always done in patients being considered for revascularization (i.e. coronary artery bypass grafting or coronary angioplasty).
- The indications for coronary angiography are as follows:

- Angina refractory to medical therapy
- Strongly positive exercise test
- Unstable angina
- Angina occurring after myocardial infarction
- Patients under 50 years with angina or myocardial infarction
- Where the diagnosis of angina is uncertain
- Severe left ventricular dysfunction after myocardial infarction
- Non-Q-wave myocardial infarction

Treatment of Angina

- The management of angina aims to relieve symptoms, prevent progression to myocardial infarction, and improve overall quality of life. Treatment includes lifestyle modifications, medications, and invasive procedures when necessary.

Lifestyle Modification

- Quit smoking—reduces cardiovascular risk.
- Healthy diet—low in saturated fats, cholesterol, and salt; rich in fruits, vegetables, and whole grains.
- Regular exercise—at least 30 minutes of moderate-intensity exercise most days (unless contraindicated).
- Weight management—helps reduce strain on the heart.
- Stress reduction—yoga, meditation, or counseling.

Treatment of Comorbid Conditions/Risk Factors

- Treatment of diabetes, hypertension, and hyperlipidemia. Anemia and any thyroid disorder should be corrected.

Medical Treatment

Glyceryl trinitrite (GTN)

- Used sublingually, either as a tablet or as a spray, gives prompt relief (peak action 4–8 minutes and lasts 20–30 minutes). If relief is not obtained within 2 or 3 min after nitroglycerin, a second or third dose may be given at 5-min intervals. It can be given prior to any activity known to induce angina. Transdermal GTN preparations are also available and their action lasts up to 24 hours. All patients with angina require nitrates as regular prophylactic therapy. Oral long-acting preparations of nitrates can be used for daily therapy.

Long-acting nitrates (e.g. isosorbide dinitrate and mononitrate)

- These are helpful for long-term prophylactic therapy. They reduce venous return and hence intracardiac diastolic pressures, reduce afterload and dilate coronary arteries. Tolerance with loss of efficacy develops with 12–24 hours of continuous exposure to long-acting nitrates. To prevent tolerance, patient should be kept free of nitrates for a minimum of 8 hours each day. Nitrates should be used with caution in patients with low BP. Sildenafil can precipitate hypotension if given to patients taking nitrates.

Antiplatelet agents

- Aspirin inhibits cyclooxygenase activity and inhibits platelet aggregation. It reduces the risk of coronary events in patients with coronary artery disease. All patients with angina should be given aspirin (75–325 mg daily) unless contraindicated. Clopidogrel (300 mg loading and 75 mg daily) is another antiplatelet agent which acts by blocking ADP receptor–mediated platelet aggregation. It is as effective as aspirin and especially useful when aspirin is contraindicated due to allergy, dyspepsia and GI bleed. Prasugrel and ticagrelor are other options and are similar to clopidogrel.

Beta-blockers

- Beta-blockers reduce reduce myocardial oxygen demand by decreasing heart rate (negative chronotropic effect) and the force of ventricular contraction (negative inotropic effect). If there is coexistent hypertension, betablockers help in controlling that also. All patients with angina should be given beta-blockers unless there are contraindications (asthma, heartblocks, COPD). Cardioselective beta-blockers like atenolol, metoprolol, carvedilol, nebivolol, and bisoprolol are used commonly.

Angiotensin-converting enzyme (ACE) inhibitors

- Clinical trials have shown that ACE inhibitors reduce major adverse events (death, myocardial infarction, and stroke), angina, and the need for revascularization in patients with CAD.

Statins

- Lipid-lowering drugs such as atorvastatin or rosuvastatin reduce the risk of major cardiovascular events (MI, cardiac arrest, and stroke) in patients with angina.

Calcium-channel blockers

- These drugs block calcium flux into the cell. They relax coronary arteries, cause peripheral vasodilatation and reduce the force of left ventricular contraction, thereby reducing myocardial oxygen demand. The non-dihydropyridine calcium antagonists (e.g. diltiazem and verapamil) also reduce the heart rate and are particularly useful antianginal agents. Long-acting dihydropyridines (e.g. amlodepine, felodepine) are also useful as they have a smooth profile of action with no significant effect on the heart rate. Short-acting dihydropyridines (e.g. nifedipine) can cause reflex tachycardia and worsen angina. Case-control studies have shown that long term nifedipine is associated with adverse outcome and should not be used.

Nicorandil

- This is a potassium-channel activator with a nitrate component. It has both arterial and venous vasodilating properties. It can be used when there are contraindications to other drugs or can be added if angina is not responding to above drugs.

Ranolazine

- This is a cardioselective anti-ischemic agent (piperazine derivative) that partially inhibits fatty acid oxidation. Also inhibits late sodium current into myocardial cells and prolongs QTc interval. Indicated for chronic angina unresponsive to other antianginal treatments. Unlike beta-blockers or calcium channel blockers, it does not reduce blood pressure or heart rate.

Percutaneous Coronary Intervention (angioplasty and stenting)

- Indicated for refractory symptoms despite optimal medical therapy and significant stenosis on coronary angiography.
- Percutaneous transluminal coronary angioplasty (PTCA) is the technique of dilating coronary stenosis by passing and inflating a balloon inside the stenosis. The balloon is threaded into the site of stenosis by a thin catheter inserted through radial or femoral artery. PTCA improves symptoms of angina, but confers no significant prognostic benefit. Complications of PTCA include mortality (1%), acute myocardial infarction (2%), and the need for urgent coronary artery bypass grafting (CABG) (2%). A stent can be placed at the site of stenosis to prevent restenosis. There are many types of stents available in the market. PTCA plus stent implantation is superior to PTCA alone for reducing cardiovascular events and the need for repeat intervention as restenosis is less after stent placement.

Coronary Artery Bypass Grafting (CABG)

- CABG is indicated when patients remain symptomatic despite optimal medical therapy and whose disease is not suitable for PTCA. CABG dramatically improves angina in about 90% of cases. It is also indicated for patients with severe three-vessel disease (significant proximal stenoses in all three main coronary vessels), and in those with left main stem artery disease. CABG provides improved survival in such situations. Usually the left or right internal mammary artery is used in CABG. Long saphenous vein can also be used but is used less commonly now because of higher risk of atheromatous occlusion.

Transmyocardial Laser Revascularization (TMR)

- Patients who remain symptomatic despite optimal medical therapy and are not suitable for PTCA or CABG may benefit from transmyocardial laser revascularization (TMR). Here laser is used to make channels (small holes) in the myocardium to allow direct perfusion of the myocardium from blood within the ventricular cavity. However, studies have not shown much benefit.

Q. Prinzmetal's angina (variant angina).

- Prinzmetal's angina or variant angina is angina pectoris secondary to coronary artery spasm. Many patients with variant angina also have significant fixed obstruction of at least one major coronary artery.

Clinical Features

- Angina mainly occurs during rest, often between midnight and early morning. Not typicaly induced by exertion (unlike stable angina).
- Short duration (~5–15 minutes) but severe.
- May be associated with palpitations, dizziness, or syncope.
- Triggers include cold exposure, emotional stress, smoking, cocaine or amphetamines, hyperventilation, and vasoconstrictive drugs (e.g. triptans).

Diagnosis

- Diagnosis is suspected if ST-segment elevation occurs during the attack (resembles STEMI). Between anginal attacks, the ECG may be normal or show a stable abnormal pattern.
- Ambulatory ECG (Holter monitoring): Detects spontaneous episodes if symptoms occur intermittently.
- Coronary angiography: Confirmation is by provocative testing with ergonovine or acetylcholine, which may precipitate coronary artery spasm during cardiac catheterization. Also confirms absence of significant fixed stenosis.

Treatment

- Calcium channel blockers (diltiazem, verapamil, amlodipine) prevent the attacks. Amiodarone is useful in refractory cases.
- Sublingual nitroglycerin relieves acute attacks.
- Avoid triggers.

Q. What are acute coronary syndromes?

- The term acute coronary syndrome (ACS) is applied to patients in whom there is a suspicion or confirmation of acute myocardial ischemia or infarction. It includes:
    - Unstable angina
    - Non-ST-elevation myocardial infarction (NSTEMI)
    - ST-elevation myocardial infarction (STEMI)

Features of Acute Coronary Syndromes (Table 3.32)

TABLE 3.32: Features of acute coronary syndromes

Feature	Unstable angina (UA)	NSTEMI	STEMI
Cause	Partial occlusion by thrombus	Partial occlusion with myocardial injury	Complete occlusion of a coronary artery
ECG changes	ST depression, T-wave inversion (no ST elevation)	ST depression, T-wave inversion	ST elevation in ≥2 contiguous leads
Cardiac biomarkers (troponin, CK-MB)	Normal	Elevated	Elevated
Myocardial damage	No infarction, just ischemia	Partial-thickness infarction (subendocardial)	Full-thickness infarction (transmural)

Q. Define unstable angina. Describe the etiology, clinical features, investigations, and management of unstable angina.

Definition

- Unstable angina is defined as angina with at least one of three features: (1) it occurs at rest (or with minimal exertion) usually lasting > 10 min, (2) it is severe and of new onset (i.e. within the prior 4–6 weeks), and/or (3) it occurs with a crescendo pattern (i.e. previously diagnosed angina that has become distinctly more frequent, longer in duration, or more severe in nature).
- Note that the widespread use of the high-sensitivity troponin test has changed the diagnosis of unstable angina to NSTEMI in almost all patients formerly diagnosed with unstable angina. Because in all the cases of unstable angina where troponins are negative, high sensitivity troponin will be positive.

Etiology

- Unstable angina is caused by rupture or erosion of the atherosclerotic plaque with formation of partially occlusive thrombus. Progressive atherosclerosis is another cause. Sometimes it is caused by coronary spasm (Prinzmetal's angina) or increase in myocardial oxygen demand superimposed on preexisting CAD.

Clinical Features

- Patients with unstable angina present with substernal chest pain. Characteristics of chest pain are same as those of stable angina but more severe. Pain usually radiates to the neck, left shoulder, and left arm.
- Not relieved by rest or nitroglycerin (unlike stable angina).
- Anginal "equivalents" such as dyspnea and epigastric discomfort may also occur.

- Examination may be normal or may show diaphoresis, pale cool skin, sinus tachycardia, third and/or fourth heart sound, bilateral basal crepitations, and sometimes hypotension.

Investigations

- ECG: Usually shows ST-segment depression, and/or T-wave inversion in the leads corresponding to ischemic area.
- Cardiac biomarkers: CK-MB and troponins are not elevated (unlike NSTEMI). However, high-sensitivity troponin test may be positive in unstable angina.
- Other investigations are same as stable angina.

Treatment

- Patients with unstable angina should be admitted to ICU and placed on bed rest. Oxygen should be started for all patients. Continuous ECG monitoring should be done to detect ST-segment deviation and any arrhythmias. Medical management involves administration of anti-ischemic and antithrombotic treatment. Treatment can be remembered using the mneomonic 'MONA-BASH'.

M → Morphine (For pain relief in severe cases)
O → Oxygen (If SpO_2 <90% or patient is in respiratory distress)
N → Nitroglycerin (For chest pain relief, vasodilation)
A → Antiplatelet agents, Aspirin (162–325 mg, chewable, for antiplatelet effect)
B → Beta-Blockers (Reduces heart rate, myocardial oxygen demand)
A → ACE Inhibitors/ARBs (Reduces cardiac remodeling, blood pressure)
S → Statins (Lowers cholesterol, stabilizes plaques)
H → Heparin (Or other anticoagulants like LMWH/Fondaparinux for clot prevention)

Antiplatelet Agents (aspirin, clopidogrel, Glycoprotein IIB/IIIA inhibitors)

- Platelets play an important role in the formation of thrombus in coronary arteries. When there is rupture of the atheromatous plaque, platelets get exposed to collagen tissue factor, ADP (adenosine diphosphate), thromboxane A2 (TXA2), and thrombin which results platelet activation. Platelet activation leads to the expression of glycoprotein (GP) IIb/IIIa receptors on the platelet surface which leads to platelet aggregation. *Aspirin* prevents platelet aggregation by blocking thromboxane A2 synthesis. All patients with ACS should receive 325 mg loading dose aspirin and then 75–150 mg daily unless contraindicated.
- *Clopidogrel* inhibits ADP-dependent activation of the glycoprotein (GP) IIb/IIIa receptors. A loading dose of 300 mg clopidogrel followed by 75 mg daily along with aspirin is more effective than either drug alone.
- *Ticagrelor* is the first reversible oral antiplatelet agent. It has faster, greater, and more consistent ADP-receptor inhibition than clopidogrel.
- *Abciximab* (a monoclonal antibody), *Eptifibatide, and Tirofiban* are recently developed GP IIb/IIIa receptor antagonists. These are powerful inhibitors of platelet aggregation and can be given intravenously.

Antithrombotic Therapy

- Unfractionated heparin should be started at a dose of 5000 U IV bolus, followed by infusion of 1000 U/h titrated to aPTT 1.5–2.5 times control. Alternatively low molecular weight heparins such as dalteparin or enoxaparin can be used subcutaneously. APTT need not be monitored for low molecular weight heparins.

Other drugs and further treatment for unstable angina is same as stable angina.

Q. Non-ST elevation myocardial infarction (NSTEMI).

- Non-ST-elevation myocardial infarction (NSTEMI) is a type of acute coronary syndrome (ACS) that occurs due to partial occlusion of a coronary artery, leading to myocardial ischemia and infarction without ST-segment elevation on ECG. Unlike unstable angina, NSTEMI results in elevated cardiac biomarkers (Troponins, CK-MB) due to myocardial injury.

Clinical Features

- Are same as that of unstable angina.

Investigations

- Are same as that of unstable angina.

Treatment

- ***Immediate treatment*** same as unstable angina (MONA-BASH). One change in treatment is dual antiplatelet therapy (DAPT) is required for NSTEMI, i.e. aspirin (lifelong) + P2Y12 inhibitor (clopidogrel, ticagrelor, or prasugrel for at least 12 months).
- ***Percutaneous coronary intervention (PCI):*** Preferred for high-risk NSTEMI patients. Involves balloon angioplasty and stent placement.
- ***Coronary artery bypass grafting (CABG):*** Used for severe multivessel disease or left main artery disease.

Complications of NSTEMI

- Arrhythmias (atrial fibrillation, ventricular tachycardia, heart block).
- Heart failure and cardiogenic shock.
- Papillary muscle rupture → Acute mitral regurgitation.
- Ventricular free wall rupture → Cardiac tamponade.
- Dressler's syndrome (Post-MI pericarditis).

Q. Describe the etiopathogenesis, clinical features, diagnosis and management of acute myocardial infarction (STEMI).

- Myocardial infarction (MI) (i.e. heart attack) is the irreversible necrosis of heart muscle secondary to prolonged ischemia. This usually results from an acute reduction in blood supply to myocardium due to plaque rupture and thrombus formation.

- Myocardial injury is reflected by elevated cardiac enzymes CK-MB, troponin I and troponin T. Two patterns of MI can be recognized based on ECG findings.
- *Non–ST segment elevation MI (NSTEMI)*: Here, there will be elevated markers of myocardial injury, such as troponins and CK-MB, but no ST segment elevation in ECG.
- *ST segment elevation MI (STEMI):* When myocardial injury is accompanied by both enzyme and ST segment elevation it is reffered to as *ST segment elevation MI (STEMI).*
- It is important to differentiate between NSTEMI and STEMI because early revascularization therapy improves the outcome in STEMI but not in NSTEMI. NSTEMI has been described above. The following description is about STEMI.

Risk factors for STEMI

- These are same as those described above under atherosclerosis.

Etiology of STEMI

- Atherosclerosis is the disease responsible for most acute coronary syndrome (ACS) cases including myocardial infarction. Approximately 90% of myocardial infarctions result from an acute thrombus that obstructs an atherosclerotic coronary artery.
- Non-atherosclerotic causes of myocardial infarction include: coronary occlusion secondary to vasculitis, hypertrophic obstructive cardiomyopathy, coronary artery emboli, congenital coronary anomalies, coronary trauma, coronary vasospasm (due to cocaine abuse, ephedrine), increased oxygen requirement (as in heavy exertion, fever, or hyperthyroidism); decreased oxygen delivery (severe anemia, carbon monoxide posoning); aortic dissection, with retrograde involvement of the coronary arteries.

Pathogenesis (Figs 3.37 and 3.38)

- Rupture or erosion of an atherosclerotic plaque in the coronary artery induces local thrombus formation which occludes coronary artery leading to myocardial infarction. Initially subendocardium is affected because this is the least supplied area. With continued ischemia the infarct zone extends through to the subepicardial myocardium, producing a transmural Q-wave myocardial infarction. Areas of myocardium which are ischemic but not yet undergone infarction can be salvaged by early reperfusion therapy.
- Microscopy shows coagulative necrosis of myocardial fibers that is ultimately followed by myocardial fibrosis.

Clinical Features

- In up to one-half of cases, a precipitating factor appears to be present before MI, such as vigorous physical exercise, emotional stress, or a medical or surgical illness.

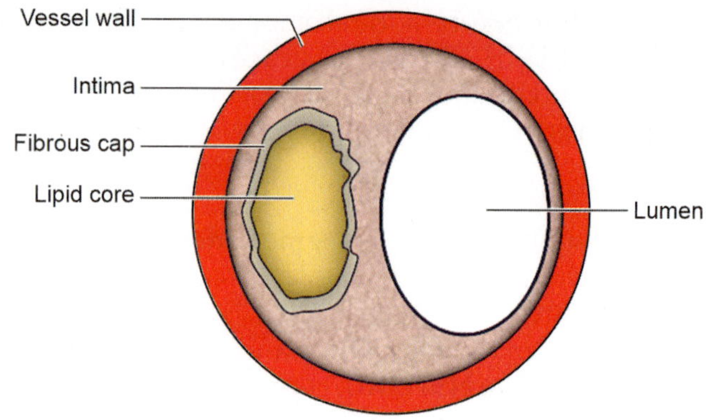

Figure 3.37: Athersclerotic plaque with narrowed lumen of coronary artery

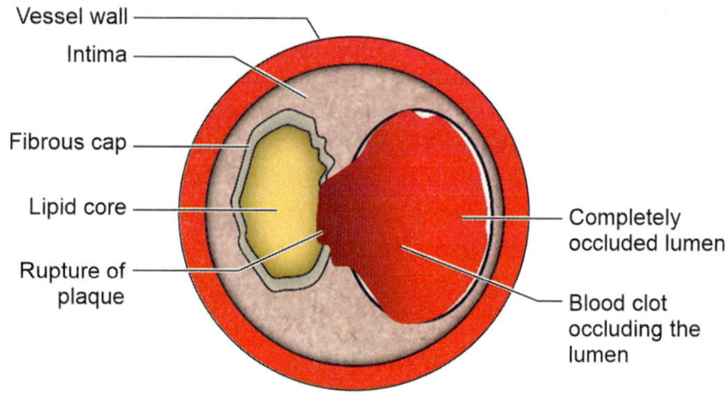

Figure 3.38: Complete occlusion due to rupture of plaque with thrombus formation

- Patients usually present with chest pain, located in the substernal region which frequently radiates to the neck, left shoulder, and left arm. Chest pain of MI is more severe than angina and lasts for more than 30 minutes. Patient may also have dizziness, syncope, dyspnea, and fatigue.
- Anginal "equivalents" such as dyspnea and epigastric discomfort may also occur.
- Elderly, diabetics, and women may present with silent MI (no pain, just weakness or breathlessness).
- Examination may reveal diaphoresis, pale cool skin, tachycardia, a third and/or fourth heart sound, bilateral basal crepitations (due to pulmonary edema), and sometimes hypotension. A transient systolic murmur may be heard over the apex due to ischemic dysfunction of the mitral valve apparatus.

Investigations

Electrocardiogram (ECG)

- Performed within 10 minutes of arrival for suspected MI. Initial ECG may be normal. If normal, it should be repeated every 15 minutes. ECG shows ST elevation in MI. Complete heart block, bundle branch block and arrhythmias may be seen. ECG changes are seen in leads which correspond to the infarcted region of myocardium **(Fig. 3.39)**.

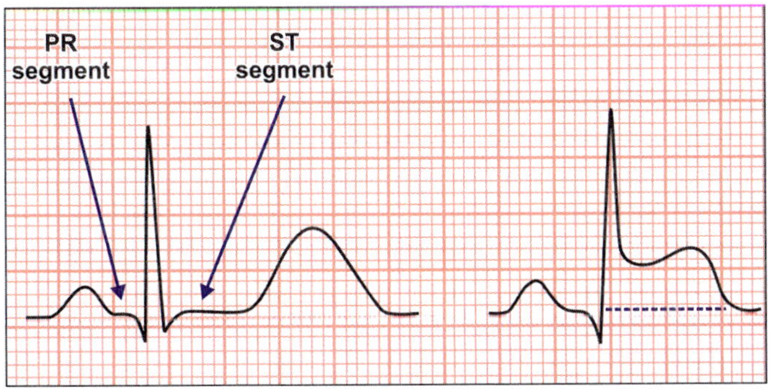

Figure 3.39: Normal ECG (left) and abnormal ECG with ST elevation (right)

- **ECG changes in MI**

ECG changes	STEMI
ST-segment changes	The presence of new ST elevation >2 mm in chest leads and >1 mm in other leads suggests MI
Q waves	May develop later (indicating full thickness infarction)
Reciprocal changes	Present (ST depression in opposite leads)
LBBB (New-onset)	Considered equivalent to STEMI

- **STEMI localization by ECG Leads**

ECG leads showing ST, T changes	Correspond to
• V3, V4, V5, V6	• Anterior wall MI
• V2, V3	• Septal MI
• II, III, aVF	• Inferior wall MI
• I, aVL, V5, V6	• Lateral wall MI

Cardiac Biomarkers

- CK–MB, troponin-I and troponin-T levels are elevated whenever there is myocardial injury (in STEMI and NSTEMI). Troponins rise in 2–4 hours, peak at 1–2 days, and remain elevated for 7–10 days. Troponins are more specific for myocardial injury because elevated CK-MB levels may be found in skeletal muscle damage also. CK-MB helps detect reinfarction because it normalizes faster than troponin and elevation again after normalization indicates reinfarction. New markers are becoming available such as myeloperoxidase and glutathione peroxidase-1.

Echocardiogram

- Hypokinesia or akinesia of ventricular wall may be present due to ischemia or infarction. Echocardiogram can assess left ventricular (LV) function and also identify the presence of right ventricular (RV) infarction, ventricular aneurysm, pericardial effusion, and LV thrombus. VSD and mitral regurgitation may develop in MI, which can be identified by echocardiogram.

Coronary Angiography (CAG)

- It can identify the site of block and allow percutaneous coronary intervention.

Other Investigations

- Full blood count, renal function tests, serum electrolytes, glucose, and lipid profile should be done for all patients.
- Brain natriuretic peptide (BNP/NT-proBNP) is elevated in heart failure post-MI.

Management of Myocardial Infarction

Immediate Measures

- Note that time is muscle and treatment should be initiated as early as possible. More delay means more myocardial damage.
- Again, the mnemonic 'MONA BASH' can be used to remember the treatment of STEMI. It is same as unstable angina and NSTEMI with additional details as follows.

Morphine

- Since there is no proven benefit, morphine is not routinely recommended for all patients with STEMI. It should be used only when chest pain is refractory to nitrates and other medical therapy. The available data suggest that routine use of morphine does not reduce mortality, and morphine may diminish the effect of P2Y12 inhibitors. It is given as 2–5 mg intravenously.

Oxygen

- Give oxygen only if the oxygen saturation is <94%. In patients who have an oxygen saturation ≥94% and no signs of respiratory distress, there is no need to give oxygen. Oxygen is given by nasal prongs or face mask (2–4 liters/min for 6–12 hours after infarction).

Nitrates

- Sublingual glyceryl trinitrate 0.4 mg. Repeat at 5 min intervals up to 3 doses. This relieves chest pain and improves coronary circulation.

Antiplatelet agents

- All patients with STEMI should receive loading doses of two antiplatelet agents (dual antiplatelet therapy). One of the antiplatelet chosen is always aspirin (unless there is aspirin allergy). Aspirin (162–325 mg of uncoated aspirin) should be given as soon as possible to all patients with STEMI, irrespective of further treatment strategy. The first tablet should be chewed or crushed to establish a high blood level quickly. Uncoated aspirin gets absorbed quickly and hence that should be used rather than enteric-coated formulations. After the loading load, aspirin should be continued at a lower dose (75–81 mg) daily, life long.
- Another antiplatelt agent chosen in addition to aspirin is one of the P2Y12 receptor blocker (e.g. prasugrel or ticagrelor or clopidogrel). The choice between different P2Y12 receptor blockers depends on the type of reperfusion therapy chosen next. If fibrinolytic therapy is the reperfusion strategy chosen, then use clopidogrel instead of prasugrel or ticagrelor, because pretreatment with ticagrelor or prasugrel is a relative contraindication to fibrinolytic therapy due to higher

risk of bleeding. However, if percutaneous coronary intervention (PCI) is planned, then prasugrel or ticagrelor are preffered over clopidogrel.

Beta blockers

- Intravenous beta-blocker, e.g. metoprolol, 5 mg every 2–5 min for a total of three doses. Beta-blockers decrease heart rate and sympathetic over activity and hence reduce myocardial oxygen demand. Beta-blockers should be avoided if PR interval is >0.24 s, 2nd or 3rd degree atrioventricular block is present, heart rate is <60 beats/min, systolic blood pressure <90 mm Hg, h/o asthma or COPD is present and severe left ventricular failure is present.

ACE inhibitors/angiotension receptor blockers

- Reduce ventricular remodeling, prevent heart failure, and improve survival. Initiate within 24 hours unless contraindicated (hypotension, renal failure, hyperkalemia).
- *Examples*: Ramipril, enalapril, losartan.

Statins

- In patients with STEMI who are not already taking a statin, a statin is started soon after presentation to the hospital. High-intensity statin therapy (atorvastatin 80 mg daily or rosuvastatin 20 or 40 mg daily) is recommended and is continued lifelong.

Heparin (anticoagulation)

- Intravenous unfractionated heparin is the anticoagulant of choice in STEMI. It should be given to all patients with STEMI whether they undergo reperfusion therapy or not, unless there is a contraindication.
- However, enoxaparin is an alternative in patients who are not undergoing PCI and also in those who are undergoing fibrinolytic therapy.

Reperfusion Therapy

- For patients diagnosed with STEMI, the primary goal of acute management is to rapidly restore blood flow to the acutely occluded coronary artery (i.e. culprit artery) with a reperfusion therapy. Thus, a reperfusion strategy should be chosen within minutes of arrival.
- Coronary reperfusion can be established by two ways; (1) percutaneous coronary intervention (PCI) and (2) fibrinolytic therapy.

Patients with symptom onset less than 12 hours

- First choice is PCI if it can be done within 2 hours of first medical contact (FMC). i.e. time from first medical contact (FMC) to PCI (balloon inflation) should be approximately 2 hours or less.
- If PCI is expected to be delayed by >2 hours, then fibrinolysis should be done first followed 6–24 hours later by angiogram and if required PCI. This is called pharmacoinvasive strategy since it includes both pharmacological intervention (fibrinolysis) as well as invasive intervention (PCI).
- Patients with continued chest pain or failure to resolve ST-segment elevation by about 90 min after fibrinolysis should be referred for rescue PCI.

Patients with symptom onset >12 hours and ≤48 hours

- First choice is PCI as soon as possible.

Patients with symptom onset >48 hours

- Both PCI and fibrinolysis are not effective. However, PCI can stll be considered for ongoing chest pain or heart failure with cardiogenic shock.

Fibrinolysis

Indications

- Fibrinolysis is indicated in people with acute STEMI presenting within 12 hours of onset of symptoms if primary PCI cannot be delivered within 2 hours of onset of symptoms. If PCI can be done within 2 hours, then the preferred therapy is PCI. Fibrinolytic therapy reduces infarct size, limits LV dysfunction, and reduces the incidence of complications such as septal rupture, cardiogenic shock, and malignant ventricular arrhythmias.
- Highest benefit is obtained if fibrinolysis is done within 1–3 hours of the onset of symptoms. Modest benefit is seen if given 3–6 h after the onset of infarction. Benefit may be seen up to 12 hours if chest pain is persisting and ST segment remains elevated without Q waves. Fibrinolytic agents activate plasminogen to plasmin which breaks down the thrombus. Currently available fibrinolytic agents include streptokinase, Alteplase (tPA), reteplase and tenecteplase.
- Most experts prefer **tenecteplase or reteplase** because of ease of administration and less chances of bleeding. **Streptokinase** use is becoming less now a days due to allergic reactions and less efficacy. Streptokinase is not fibrin specific hence has more chances of hemorrhage whereas other agents are fibrin specific and have less chances of hemorrhage.

Drugs and dosage

- **Streptokinase** is given in a dose of 1.5 million Units as intravenous infusion over 1 hour.
- **Alteplase (tPA)** is given as 15 mg bolus i.v. followed by 0.75 mg/kg i.v. over 30 minutes followed by 0.5 mg/kg i.v. over the next 60 minutes.
- **Tenecteplase** is given as single bolus (30–50 mg based on weight) IV over 5–10 seconds.
- **Reteplase** is given as 10 units over 2 minutes then repeat 10-unit bolus at 30 minutes.

Complications of fibrinolysis

- The major risk of thrombolytic therapy is bleeding. Intracerebral hemorrhage is the most serious and frequently fatal complication.
- Note that fibrinolysis is not useful in NSTEMI and may be harmful.

Contraindications to thrombolysis **(Table 3.33)**

TABLE 3.33: Contraindications to thrombolysis

Absolute contraindications
• Hemorrhagic stroke or stroke of unknown origin at any time and ischemic stroke in preceding 6 months
• Intracranial or spinal cord neoplasms
• Active bleeding or bleeding diathesis
• Suspected or known aortic dissection

(Contd.)

TABLE 3.33: Contraindications to thrombolysis *(Contd.)*

Relative contraindications
• Severe uncontrolled hypertension (systolic blood pressure >180 mm Hg)
• Recent major trauma/surgery/head injury (within preceding 3 weeks)
• Active peptic ulcer disease
• Old ischemic stroke
• Oral anticoagulant therapy
• Pregnancy or within 1 week postpartum
• Recent non-compressible vascular punctures
• Recent retinal laser therapy

Percutaneous Coronary Intervention (PCI)

- PCI includes angioplasty and/or stenting. If PCI is done without preceding fibrinolysis, it is referred to as primary PCI. Primary PCI is the preferred reperfusion strategy for ST-elevation myocardial infarction (STEMI) when performed within 2 hours first medical contact (FMC) at an experienced center. Disadvantages of PCI are increased cost, limited availability and requirement of experts.

Coronary Artery Bypass Grafting (CABG)

- CABG is indicated for patients with left main stem or triple vessel disease with impaired left ventricular function.

Post-MI Drug Therapy

- Extensive clinical trials have shown that many drugs taken indefinitely by MI patients reduce the incidence of recurrent MI and cardiovascular death. Therefore, all post-MI patients should be taking the following medications unless there are contraindications.
- *Antiplatelet agents*: Aspirin is recommended indefinitely (mostly lifelong) in all patients who have had an acute MI. Aspirin is given at a dose of 75–150 mg/day. Along with aspirin, a P2Y12 receptor blocker such as clopidogrel is indicated in all patients after acute STEMI for at least 12 months, regardless of the reperfusion strategy. Clopidogrel is given at a dose of 75 mg/day.
- *Beta blocker*: Example metoprolol, carvedilol, atenolol, and bisoprolol. They decrease myocardial oxygen demand and should be given to all patients with MI unless there is a contraindication like asthma or severe LV dysfunction.
- *Oral nitrates*: Example—isosorbide dinitrate or mononitrate. They improve the symptoms of angina and heart failure and should be considered for all patients. However, nitrates should be avoided in patients with a right ventricular MI in whom the reduction in preload can lower the cardiac output.
- *ACE-inhibitors*: Example—enalapril, ramipril, lisinopril, perindopril. They prevent adverse myocardial remodeling after acute MI and reduce heart failure and death. They also reduce atherosclerosis progression and acute MI recurrence. All patients should be given ACE inhibitor lifelong unless there is a contraindication like renal failure and hypotension.
- *Statins*: Example—atorvastatin, rosuvastatin, etc. LDL-cholesterol should be brought down to less than 100 mg/dl. In addition to cholesterol lowering effect, statins also help in plaque stabilization and regression of atherosclerosis. Recent data show statins are effective in secondary prevention regardless of age or baseline lipid levels, even when the LDL is less than 100.
- *Control of comorbid conditions*: like diabetes and hypertension help in reducing recurrent MI. For HTN, ACE inhibitors or β-blockers are the first choice because they also reduce cardiovascular mortality and morbidity as described above. Angiotensin receptor blockers (ARBs) can be considered when ACE inhibitors are not tolerated. ACE inhibitors and ARBs also reduce the long-term complications of diabetes. Diabetes should be strictly controlled by oral drugs or insulin or both.
- *Calcium channel blockers*: They have negative inotropic effect and are not routinely given. They may be given to selected patients without LV dysfunction (ejection fraction greater than 40%) who are intolerant of β-blockers. Preffered agents are diltiazem and verapamil. Short acting nifedipine should be avoided as it causes reflex tachycardia has been shown to increase mortality rate.
- *Smoking cessation*: Continued smoking doubles subsequent mortality risk after acute MI and cessation reduces risk of reinfarction and death.

Complications of Myocardial Infarction

Heart Failure

- Cardiac failure can happen after MI if significant myocardium is damaged.

Myocardial Rupture and Aneurysmal Dilatation

- Infarcted myocardium is weak and cannot tolerate the pressure inside the ventricular chamber. This may lead to rupture of the free wall of the left ventricle or aneurysmal dilatation. Rupture is usually an early, catastrophic and fatal event.
- Ventricular aneurysm impairs cardiac output because of paradoxical motion of its wall. Double, diffuse, or displaced apical impulse is noted on physical examination.

Ventricular Septal Defect (VSD)

- Infarcted septum may perforate and lead to VSD. It is common in elderly and hypertensive patients and after delayed thrombolysis. It requires emergency surgical repair.

Mitral Regurgitation

- Severe mitral regurgitation can occur early in the course of MI. Three mechanisms are responsible for mitral regurgitation in MI, which are as follows.
- Left ventricular dysfunction and dilatation, causing annular dilatation of the valve and subsequent regurgitation.

- Infarction of the inferior wall, producing dysfunction of the papillary muscle.
- Infarction and rupture of the papillary muscles, producing sudden severe mitral regurgitation, pulmonary edema and cardiogenic shock.
- If there is rupture of papillary muscles, emergency surgery should be undertaken.

Cardiac Arrhythmias

- *Ventricular tachycardia and ventricular fibrillation (VT and VF):* Both are common after MI, especially after reperfusion therapy. VF is a common cause of death after MI in first 24 hours. Hemodynamically unstable (hypotension, cyanosis) VT and VF should be treated with DC shock. Hemodynamically stable VT should be treated with intravenous beta-blockers (metoprolol, esmolol), IV lidocaine, or IV amiodarone. Refractory VT and VF may respond to IV magnesium sulphate.
- *Atrial fibrillation:* Is common after MI and can be treated with beta-blockers and digoxin. DC shock may also be given provided there is no clot in the heart. Intravenous diltiazem or verapamil can be used if there is any contraindication to β-blocker use. Amiodarone can be used daily to prevent recurrence.
- *Bradyarrhythmias:* These are common following MI and may be due to sinus node dysfunction and conduction disturbances. AV block may occur during acute MI, especially after inferior wall MI (the right coronary artery usually supplies the SA and AV nodes). Heart block, with hemodynamic compromise (hypotension) requires treatment with atropine or a temporary pacemaker. AV blocks are usually transient and recover later. Permanent pacemaker may be needed if they persist even after 2 weeks.

Acute Pericarditis

- It happens with large, "transmural" infarctions causing pericardial inflammation and presents on days 2–4 after MI. Pericardial effusion may devlop and cause tamponade. Pericarditis developing later (2 to 10 weeks) after acute MI may represent ***Dressler's syndrome***, which is immune-mediated. Treatment includes aspirin or other NSAIDs (indomethacin). Corticosteroids may be required for severe pericarditis.

Post-MI Assessment

- Patients, in whom primary angioplasty has not been performed need to undergo exercise test to identify residual ischemia and to determine the need for coronary angiography. This can be done prior to discharge in patients without angina or 6 weeks later. A positive test requires diagnostic/therapeutic coronary angiography/stenting. Alternatively, nuclear scintigraphy or dobutamine stress echocardiography can be used at 5 days to determine the amount of viable myocardium and the extent of myocardial ischemia.

Q. Biomarkers in acute myocardial infarction.

- Cardiac biomarkers are substances that are released into the blood when the heart is damaged or stressed. Measurements of these biomarkers are used to help diagnose acute coronary syndrome (ACS) and cardiac ischemia.
- This topic is discussed in previous pages.

Q. Pain relief in acute coronary syndrome.

- Prompt treatment of chest pain in MI is an essential part of MI management. Rapid and effective pain relief in acute MI is necessary to prevent detrimental pathophysiologic effects, such as increases in blood pressure, heart rate, and stroke volume. These changes may disrupt the balance between myocardial oxygen supply and demand, and therefore result in the extension of infarction. Persistent, unrelieved pain can also initiate catecholamine release producing an increased workload on an already compromised coronary circulation.
- Morphine: This is the usual drug of choice in MI. However, many studies have shown that there is no mortality benefit. On the other hand it has been shown to be associated with higher risk of death in patients presenting with NSTEMI and perhaps a higher infarct size in patients presenting with STEMI. When using morphine, the goal of therapy should be to use the lowest effective dose with minimal side effects.
- Nitrates: These drugs are especially useful in the setting of persistent ischemia, heart failure or hypertension. Nitroglycerin infusion is commonly used.
- Beta-blockers: These drugs decrease the heart rate and decrease myocardial oxygen demand which is useful in myocardial ischemia and myocardial infarction.

Q. How do you differentiate between stable angina, unstable angina, and myocardial infarction based on clinical features and lab investigations?

See **Table 3.34.**

Q. Cardiac rehabilitation.

- Cardiac rehabilitation (CR) is a structured program designed to improve cardiovascular health in patients recovering from myocardial infarction (MI), heart failure, cardiac surgery, or PCI.
- It includes exercise training, lifestyle modifications, psychosocial support, and medical therapy optimization.

Goals of Cardiac Rehabilitation

- Reduce cardiovascular mortality and morbidity.
- Improve functional capacity and quality of life.
- Prevent recurrent cardiac events (e.g. recurrent MI, stroke).
- Enhance medication adherence and risk factor control.
- Support psychological well-being and stress management.

Indications for Cardiac Rehabilitation

- Acute coronary syndrome (ACS)—STEMI, NSTEMI, unstable angina.
- Post-PCI or CABG.

TABLE 3.34: Differences between stable angina, unstable angina, and MI

Characteristics	*Stable angina*	*Unstable angina*	*Myocardial infarction*
Definition	Angina that is reproducible and consistent over time. It is precipitated by effort, and relieved by rest.	Angina that occurs at rest, severe and new onset angina or previous angina that has clearly worsened.	Myocardial infarction (MI) (i.e. heart attack) is the irreversible necrosis of heart muscle secondary to prolonged ischemia.
Chest pain	Occurs on physical exertion and lasts <10–15 min.	Occurs at rest, lasts >20 minutes.	Chest pain of MI is more severe and lasts for more than 30 minutes.
Response to nitroglycerin	Relieved by nitroglycerin.	Partial or no relief	No relief
Pathology	Fixed stenosis of a coronary artery leading to ischemia. No myocardial necrosis	Ischemia due to dynamic obstruction of coronary artery, resulting from rupture of athersosclerotic plaque with partial thrombus formation.	Plaque rupture with thrombus formation completely occluding a coronary vessel leading to myocardial necrosis
Predictability	Predictable	Not predictable	Not predictable
ECG	Often normal. Tread mill test (TMT) is usually positive.	Usually shows ST segment depression and T wave inversions, but no pathological Q waves	Usually shows ST segment elevation (STEMI). Sometimes no ST elevation (NSTEMI). Pathological Q waves usually seen.
Cardiac markers (CK-MB, troponin I and troponin T)	Normal	Normal or only mildly elevated	Elevated
Echocardiogram	Usually normal	May show regional wall motion abnormalities (RWMA)	Usually show regional wall motion abnormalities (RWMA)
Treatment	Lifestyle changes, aspirin, statins, beta blockers, nitrates	Urgent evaluation, DAPT (dual antiplatelet therapy), anticoagulation, possible PCI.	Primary PCI or thrombolysis

- Chronic stable angina.
- Heart failure (HFrEF, EF ≤40%).
- Post-heart valve surgery or transplant.
- Cardiomyopathy.

Components of Cardiac Rehabilitation

- Exercise training
- Risk factor modification: Smoking cessation, blood pressure control (target <130/80 mm Hg), diabetes management (maintain HbA1c <7%), cholesterol reduction—LDL <55 mg/dl (for high-risk patients), weight management—BMI target <25 kg/m^2.
- Psychosocial support and mental health.
- Nutritional counseling: Mediterranean or DASH diet (high in fruits, vegetables, whole grains, nuts, and lean protein). Limit saturated fats, trans fats, and processed foods. Reduce sodium intake.
- Medication optimization
  - Aspirin lifelong + P2Y12 inhibitors (for 12 months post-MI).
  - Beta-blockers (metoprolol, carvedilol) to reduce cardiac workload.
  - Statins (atorvastatin, rosuvastatin) for lipid control.
  - ACE inhibitors/ARBs (lisinopril, losartan) for LV dysfunction and BP control.

Rehabilitation Team

- Rehabilitation requires help from a team of different professionals and family members. The team may include cardiologist, physician, general practitioner, nurse, physiotherapist, dietitian, psychologist, physiotherapist, occupational therapist, and family members.

Barriers to Cardiac Rehabilitation Participation

- Poor patient adherence
- Lack of endorsement by a doctor
- Multiple morbidities, leading to poor functional capacity
- Poor exercise habits
- Problems with transport
- Poor social support
- Lack of leave from work to attend centre-based sessions.

Q. Killip classification of acute myocardial infarction.

- The Killip classification is used to assess the severity in patients with MI. It has prognostic value.

Class I	No evidence of heart failure
Class II	Findings consistent with mild to moderate heart failure (e.g. S3 gallop, lung rales less than one-half way up the posterior lung fields, or jugular venous distension)
Class III	Overt pulmonary edema
Class IV	Cardiogenic shock

Q. Cardiogenic shock.

- Cardiogenic shock (CS) is a state of severe cardiac pump failure resulting in inadequate tissue perfusion, leading to multi-organ dysfunction and high mortality.

Causes of Cardiogenic Shock

- Acute MI (most common cause)
- Acute mitral regurgitation
- Acute aortic regurgitation
- Acute ventricular septal defect due to rupture of interventricular septum
- End stage cardiomyopathy
- Severe myocarditis
- Left ventricular free wall rupture
- Pericardial tamponade.

Clinical Features

- Sinus tachycardia.
- Severe systemic hypotension (systolic blood pressure below 90 mm Hg). This is due to acute decrease in stroke volume.
- Signs of systemic hypoperfusion (e.g. cool extremities, oliguria, elevated lactate due to tissue hypoxia).
- Dyspnea due to pulmonary congestion.

Differential Diagnosis

- Massive pulmonary embolism (obstructive shock)
- Pericardial tamponade
- Sepsis-induced myocardial dysfunction
- Tension pneumothorax
- Hemorrhagic shock
- Septic shock
- Neurogenic shock.

Investigations

- *ECG:* May show acute MI or other causes of cardiogenic shock.
- *Echocardiography:* It can assess ventricular function, detect tamponade, severe mitral and aortic regurgitation, and ventricular septal rupture.
- *Coronary angiography:* To assess the coronary anatomy should be performed in all patients with cardiogenic shock who are candidates for percutaneous coronary intervention or coronary artery bypass graft surgery.
- *Troponins:* Elevated in AMI
- *BNP/NT-proBNP*: Elevated in heart failure
- *Arterial blood gas (ABG)*: Metabolic acidosis, high lactate.
- *Renal and liver function tests*: Elevated creatinine (AKI), elevated liver enzymes.

Management

General Measures

- Admit in ICU
- Strict bed rest
- High flow oxygen
- Endotracheal intubation and mechanical ventilation if required.

Pharmacologic Agents

- Dopamine or norepinephrine infusion or both can be used to correct hypotension. Amrinone or milrinone infusion can be used if there is myocardial pump failure. Dobutamine should be used cautiously in the presence of hypotension as it has peripheral vasodilating action.

Mechanical Devices

- IABP (intra-aortic balloon pump) can produce rapid, although temporary, stabilization of the patient with cardiogenic shock. It is usually inserted through the femoral artery and placed in the descending thoracic aorta distal to the left subclavian artery. The balloon inflates during diastole and deflates during systole (in a synchronous fashion with the cardiac cycle), resulting in diastolic blood flow augmentation and systolic reduction in afterload. The decline in afterload is due to a brief vacuum effect created by rapid balloon deflation.
- Other circulatory support devices are left ventricular and biventricular assist devices and percutaneous cardiopulmonary bypass support with use of an extracorporeal membrane oxygenator.

Temporary Biventricular Pacing

- May help improve the symptoms and survival of cardiogenic shock.

Treatment of Underlying Cause

- Underlying cause such as acute MI, acute mitral and aortic regurgitations, etc. require specific therapy. Emergency PCI or CABG is required for STEMI. Surgery may be required for ventricular septal rupture and paillary muscle rupture.

Q. Coronary artery bypass grafting (CABG).

- Coronary artery bypass grafting (CABG) involves bypassing native coronary arteries that have high-grade stenosis or occlusion not amenable to angioplasty with stent insertion.
- There are two types of CABG surgical procedures: on-pump and off-pump. In on-pump technique, heart lung machine is used to bypass the heart and is heart is arrested using cardioplegic drugs during surgery. In off-pump technique, there is no use of heart lung machine and surgery is done on beating heart. CABG is usually done through a mid strnotomy incision.
- The conduits used as bypass grafts are routinely the left internal mammary artery (LIMA) and the saphenous vein grafts (SVG). Other conduits that may be grafted include the right internal mammary artery (RIMA), the radial artery, and the gastroepiploic artery **(Fig. 3.40)**.

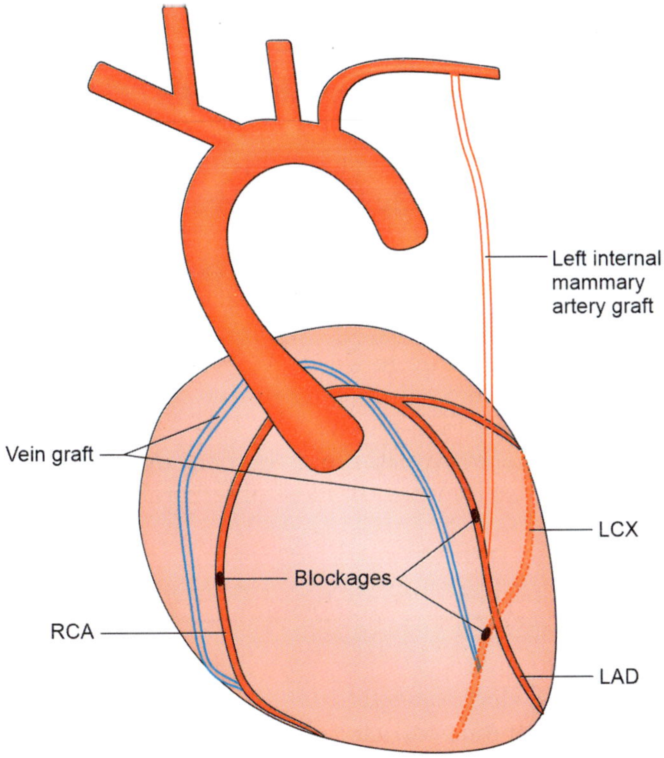

Figure 3.40: Coronary artery bypass grafting (CABG)

Indications for CABG

- Left main coronary artery stenosis >50% (both PCI and CABG have almost similar results).
- Left main equivalent: >70% stenosis of proximal left anterior descending (LAD), and proximal circumflex artery (PCA).
- Triple vessel disease particularly in diabetics.
- One or two vessel disease with extensive myocardium at risk, and not suitable for percutaneous transluminal coronary angioplasty (PTCA).
- Failed PCI or coronary occlusive complications during PCI.
- Surgery for life-threatening complications after acute MI, including VSD, ventricular free-wall rupture or acute MR. CABG can be clubbed along with these corrective surgeries.

Contraindications to CABG

- Severe diffuse CAD (no suitable graft targets).
- Severe comorbidities (e.g. advanced CKD, liver failure, dementia).
- Poor surgical candidates due to frailty or advanced malignancy.
- Lack of viable myocardium in the target area.

Complications of CABG

- Stroke
- Infection
- Graft failure
- Renal failure
- Postoperative atrial fibrillation
- Death.

Q. Sudden cardiac arrest (SCA).

Q. Sudden cardiac death (SCD).

Definition

- Sudden cardiac arrest (SCA) refers to refer to sudden cessation of cardiac activity due to a life-threatening arrhythmia or abrupt loss of myocardial pump function that requires emergency medical intervention for restoration of effective circulation.
- If the patient does not survive an SCA, the death is classified as a sudden cardiac death (SCD).

Etiology

- Most of the time, it is due to cardiac arrhythmias (ventricular tachycardia and ventricular fibrillation) or asystole.
- It is more common in men.
- Preexisting heart disease may or may not to be present, but the time and mode of death are unexpected. Risk factors for SCD are identical to those for coronary artery disease and include old age, male gender, hypertension, tobacco use, hypercholesterolemia, and left ventricular hypertrophy.

Cardiac Diseases Associated with Sudden Cardiac Death

- Ischemic heart disease
- Cardiomyopathies
- Congenital long QT syndrome
- Brugada's syndrome
- Cardiac failure
- Acute myocarditis
- Valvular heart disease (aortic stenosis, mitral valve prolapse).
- Congenital heart disease (tetralogy of Fallot, transposition of great arteries, VSD, PDA).

Noncardiac Causes associated with Sudden Cardiac Death

- Pulmonary embolism—acute RV failure → Cardiac arrest.
- Massive hemorrhage (e.g. ruptured aneurysm, GI bleeding).
- CNS events (stroke, subarachnoid hemorrhage, seizures).
- Electrolyte imbalances—hypokalemia, hyperkalemia, hypocalcemia, hypomagnesemia.
- Drug overdose—cocaine, methamphetamine, opioid toxicity, QT-prolonging drugs.

Clinical Presentation

- Sudden loss of consciousness (syncope)
- No pulse, no breathing
- Gasping or agonal breathing (within first minutes)
- Possible preceding symptoms:
  - Chest pain (if due to MI)
  - Palpitations (suggesting arrhythmia)
  - Dyspnea (if due to heart failure).

Immediate Management of Suspected Cardiac Arrest

- Follow cardiac arrest algorithm: Basic life support (BLS) and advanced cardiac life support (ACLS).

Step	Action
Confirm unresponsiveness	Tap/shout, check pulse and breathing
Call for help (code blue)	Activate EMS, get defibrillator (AED)
Start CPR (CAB sequence)	Compressions (100–120/min, 5–6 cm deep)
Attach defibrillator (AED/ manual)	Check rhythm
Shockable rhythm (VF/VT)?	Deliver shock if yes
Non-shockable rhythm (PEA/ asystole)?	Continue CPR + epinephrine

Investigations

- *ECG:* should be done in all patients. Evidence of MI, prolonged QT interval, short QT interval, epsilon wave, short PR interval, a WPW pattern, or other conditions should be sought.
- *Echocardiogram:* May show evidence of underlying heart disease.
- *Cardiac enzymes (CK-MB, troponins):* Elevations in these enzyme levels may indicate acute coronary syndrome.
- *Electrolytes, calcium, and magnesium:* Severe metabolic acidosis, hypokalemia, hyperkalemia, hypocalcemia, and hypomagnesemia are some of the conditions that can increase the risk for arrhythmia and sudden death.
- *Quantitative drug levels (quinidine, procainamide, tricyclic antidepressants, digoxin):* Drug levels higher than the levels indicated in the therapeutic index may have a proarrhythmic effect. Subtherapeutic levels of these drugs in patients being treated for specific cardiac conditions also can lead to an increased risk for arrhythmia. Most of the antiarrhythmic medications also have a proarrhythmic effect.
- *Toxicology screen:* Drugs such as cocaine can lead to vasospasm-induced ischemia.
- Thyroid function tests: Hyperthyroidism can lead to tachycardia and tachyarrhythmias. Over a period, it also can lead to heart failure. Hypothyroidism can lead to QT prolongation.
- *Brain natriuretic peptide (BNP):* Raised level indicates cardiac failure.

Prevention of Sudden Cardiac Death

- An implantable cardioverter-defibrillator (ICD) prevents sudden death due to ventricular arrhythmias and cardiac arrest in people with high risk.
- Antiarrhythmic drugs such as amiodarone may be used as an alternative to an implantable cardioverter-defibrillator but are less effective.
- Beta blockers, ACE inhibitors and spironolactone have been shown to reduce the risk of sudden cardiac death.

Q. Define cardiac arrest. Discuss the causes and management of cardiac arrest.

Q. Cardiopulmonary resuscitation (CPR).

- Cardiac arrest is is defined as sudden loss of pumping ability of the heart. This leads to abrupt loss of consciousness due to lack of cerebral blood flow. It leads to death in the absence of an active intervention, although spontaneous reversions occur rarely.
- Cardiac arrest occurring in hospital has better chances of suvivval than out of hospital arrest. Similarly cardiac arrest due to VT or VF has better chances of survival than cardiac arrest due to asystole and pulseless electrical activity.
- The onset of irreversible brain damage usually begins within 4 to 6 minutes after loss of cerebral circulation.

Causes of Cardiac Arrest

- VF (ventricular fibrillation)
- VT (ventricular tachycardia)
- Asystole
- Pulseless electrical activity
- Rupture of the ventricle
- Cardiac tamponade
- Massive pulmonary embolism
- Acute disruption of a major blood vessel
- Myocardial infarction
- Electrolyte imbalance (hypkalemia and hyperkalemia)
- Drugs.

Management of Cardiac Arrest (Cardiopulmonary Resuscitation)

- The most important step which increases the survival after cardiac arrest is immediate CPR. The sooner it is initiated, the better is the prognosis.
- The goals of CPR in cardiac arrest are (i) restoring a spontaneous circulation as quickly as possible; and (ii) maintaining continuous artificial circulatory support until return of a spontaneous circulation has been achieved.
- The keys to survival from sudden cardiac arrest are early recognition, early CPR, early defibrillation and early transfer to hospital.
- *CPR consists of 4 main parts:*
  1. Circulation (C)
  2. Airway (A)
  3. Breathing (B)
  4. Defibrillation (D)
- Note that as per new American Heart Association guidelines, the sequence of CPR is CAB and not ABC. The management strategy for cardiac arrest can be divided into five steps:
  1. Initial assessment and activation of emergency medical services
  2. Basic life support (BLS)
  3. Early defibrillation by a first responder (if available)
  4. Advanced life support (ALS)
  5. Post-resuscitation care.

Initial Assessment and Activation of Emergency Medical Services

- Assess the victim for response. Tap the person and shout, "Are you okay?" If no response, call for help. If you are alone activate emergency services and get an automated external defibrillator if available.

BLS

- Check for pulse. This is best done by feeling for carotid pulse at the neck. You should not take more than 10 seconds to assess pulse.
- If there is no carotid pulse, chest compressions should be started at a rate of 100/minute. Chest should be compressed in the middle of chest at the level of nipple line.
- Open the victim's airway and check for breathing. Airway can be opened by head tilt - chin lift manuere.
- If there is no breathing, give 2 breaths (either mouth to mouth or by using a face mask). The breaths should make the chest rise and fall.
- This cycle of 30 compressions and 2 breaths should be continued until the return of spontaneous circulation and breathing or till the patient is declared dead. Breaths can be given by mouth to mouth breathing or by using bag and mask device. Patient can also be intubated using endotracheal tube for more effective ventilations.

Early Defibrillation by a First Responder

- Since the terminal event in most cases of cardiac arrest is ventricular fibrillation, defibrillation as early as possible is very important for successful resuscitation of the victim. For this purpose, automated external defibrillators (AED) can be made use of in a setting outside the hospital. Such AEDs are kept at public places such as airports, railway stations, shopping malls, etc. AED can be used even by lay people.

Advanced Life Support (ALS)

- This involves use of various drugs during CPR such as injection adrenaline (1 mg of 1:10,000 solution) and atropine (1 mg). These drugs are given intravenously. Adrenaline can be repeated many times. Atropine can be given up to three times. Other drugs which are useful in cardiac arrest are calcium gluconate, sodium bicarbonate, magnesium sulphate (2 g IV for torsades-de-pointes), and amiodarone (for ventricular tachycardia). Bag mask ventilation or endotracheal intubation is done for maintaining airway and breathing. Manual defibrillators are used inside the hospital for defibrillation because the rescuer needs to have knowledge of advanced life support and ECG interpretation skills.

Post-resuscitation Care

- After revival, patient should be kept in recovery position and monitored in ICU. The cause of cardiac arrest should be established and treated.

Q. Cardioversion and defibrillation.

- Cardioversion is the delivery of electrical shock that is synchronized to the R wave of QRS complex, while defibrillation is nonsynchronized delivery of shock (delivered randomly during the cardiac cycle). The machine used for cardioversion and defibrillation is called defibrillator.
- During defibrillation and cardioversion, electrical current travels from the negative to the positive electrode by traversing myocardium. It causes all of the heart cells to contract simultaneously. This interrupts and terminates abnormal electrical rhythm. This, in turn, allows the sinus node to resume normal pacemaker activity.
- Old defibrillators delivered energy in a monophasic waveform, meaning that electrons flowed in a single direction. Latest defibrillators deliver a biphasic waveform. Biphasic defibrillators successfully terminate arrhythmias at lower energies than monophasic defibrillators.

Indications

- Atrial fibrillation
- Atrial flutter
- Supraventricular tachycardia
- VT (ventricular tachycardia)
- VF (ventricular fibrillation).

Precautions

- Patient should be anesthetized or sedated before elective cardioversion. This does not apply to emergency situations.
- Patients with chronic atrial fibrillation should be anticoagulated for 6 weeks before elective cardioversion.

Method

- There are two electrodes in the defibrillator. One is applied below the right clavicle. Another is applied on the lower part of left axilla. Required amount of energy is selected. After clearing everybody from the patient, shock is delivered by pressing the shock button.

Complications

- ECG changes (ST segment and T wave changes).
- Precipitation of new arrhythmias.
- Embolization (pulmonary or systemic embolization). This complication is more likely to occur in patients with AF who have not been anticoagulated prior to cardioversion.
- Myocardial dysfunction and necrosis.
- Transient hypotension.
- Pulmonary edema.
- Skin burns.

Q. Define and enumerate the causes of left ventricular hypertrophy (LVH) and LV dilatation.

- LVH is defined as an increase in the mass of the left ventricle, due to increase in wall thickness.
- Left ventricular dilatation refers to increase in cavity size (**Fig. 3.41**).

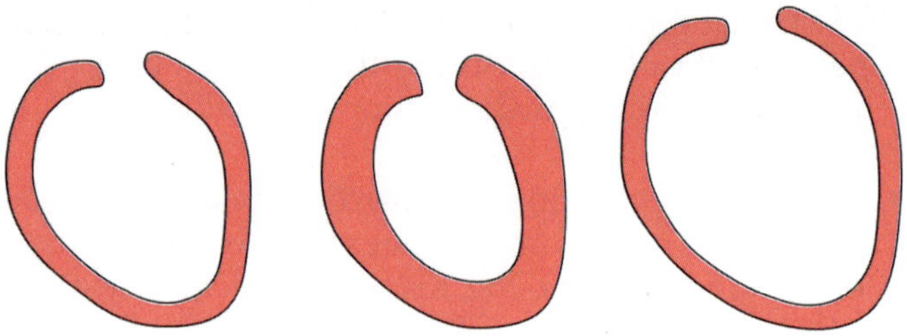

Figure 3.41: LV hypertrophy and LV dilatation

Causes of LVH

- Hypertension
- Aortic stenosis
- Coarctation of aorta
- Hypertrophic obstructive cardiomyopathy.

Causes of Left Ventricular Dilatation

- Aortic regurgitation
- Mitral regurgitation
- VSD
- PDA
- Dilated cardiomyopathy
- Myocardial infarction
- Cardiac failure
- Hyperkinetic circulatory states (anemia, thyrotoxicosis, beriberi, AV fistula).

Q. Discuss the etiology, clinical features, investigations, and management of acute rheumatic fever.

Q. Aschoff nodule.

Q. Erythema Marginatum.

Q. Rheumatic chorea (Sydenham's chorea; St. Vitus Dance).

Q. Jones criteria.

Q. Rheumatic fever prophylaxis.

Definition

- Rheumatic fever is an autoimmune inflammatory process that develops as a sequela of group A Streptococcus (GAS) infection.
- Rheumatic fever involves the heart, joints, central nervous system, skin, and subcutaneous tissues with varying frequency. Involvement of the heart, though rarely fatal during the acute stage, may lead to rheumatic valvular disease, which can lead to cardiac disability or death many years after the initial event.

Etiology

- Rheumatic fever follows pharyngeal infection with group A streptococcus (GAS). It usually occurs 2–3 weeks after the attack of pharyngitis. However, at least one-third of patients deny previous sore throat, and cultures of the pharynx are often negative for group A streptococci at the onset of rheumatic fever. However, antibody response against Streptococcus can be demonstrated in almost all the cases.
- Skin infections are not associated with rheumatic fever but they can cause post-streptococcal glomerulonephritis.

Epidemiology

- Rheumatic fever is a major health problem in the developing countries of Asia, Africa, the Middle East, and Latin America.
- The incidence of rheumatic fever has decreased now because of the availability of antibiotics.
- Outbreaks of rheumatic fever closely follow epidemics of streptococcal pharyngitis or scarlet fever with associated pharyngitis. Patients who have suffered an initial attack tend to experience recurrences of the disease following group A streptococcal infections. Adequate treatment of streptococcal pharyngitis markedly reduces the incidence of rheumatic fever. Recurrence is rare beyond age 34.
- Acute rheumatic fever is most common among children in the 5–15-year age group. There is no clear-cut sex predilection, although there is a female preponderance in rheumatic mitral stenosis and in Sydenham's chorea.

Pathogenesis

- Molecular mimicry is thought to play an important role in tissue injury. There are shared epitopes between cardiac myosin and streptococcal M protein that lead to cross-reactive humoral and T-cell immunity against group A streptococci and the heart. Epitopes of streptococcal M protein also share antigenic determinants with heart valves, sarcolemmal membrane proteins, synovium, and articular cartilage. Circulating antibodies against group A streptococcal cell membranes which cross react with neurons of the caudate and subthalamic nuclei have been found in children with Sydenham's chorea.
- Host factors may also play a role. Associations between disease and human leukocyte antigen (HLA) class II alleles have been identified. Certain B-cell alloantigens are expressed to a greater level in patients with rheumatic fever.
- During active rheumatic carditis, there is T-cell and macrophage infiltration of heart valves, and the production of interleukin-1 and interleukin-2 is increased. All these result in scarring and collagen deposition in the valves and destruction of myocytes. There will be exudative and proliferative inflammatory lesions in the connective tissue of the heart, joints, and subcutaneous tissue. All the three layers of the heart are involved (pancarditis).

Pericardium

- Pericarditis is common and fibrinous pericarditis is occasionally present. Thick exudate gives bread and butter appearance macroscopically. Pericarditis usually heals without any sequelae. Tamponade is rare.

Myocardium

- In the myocardium, there is fragmentation of collagen fibers, lymphocytic infiltration, fibrinoid degeneration and the presence of Aschoff nodules, which are considered pathognomonic of acute rheumatic fever.
- The Aschoff nodule consists of an area of central necrosis surrounded by lymphocytes, plasma cells, and large mononuclear and giant multinucleate cells. Many of these cells have an elongated nucleus with a clear area just within the nuclear membrane ("owl-eyed nucleus").
- Aschoff nodules may also be found in endomyocardial biopsy specimens obtained from patients with acute rheumatic carditis.

Endocardium

- Endocarditis is responsible for chronic rheumatic valvulitis. Small vegetations, 1–2 mm in diameter, are seen on the atrial surface of valve margins and chordae tendineae. There is edema and inflammation of the valve leaflets.
- A thickened and fibrotic patch (MacCallum's patch) may be found in the posterior left atrial wall. It is believed to be due to mitral regurgitant jet impinging on the left atrial wall.
- Healing of the valvulitis leads to fibrosis of the leaflets and fusion of the chordae resulting in valvular stenosis or incompetence.
- The mitral valve is affected most commonly, followed by the aortic valve. Tricuspid and pulmonic valves are rarely affected.

Extracardiac Lesions

- Inflammation can affect the joints (rheumatic arthritis). Skin (subcutaneous nodules), lung (rheumatic pneumonitis) and brain.

Clinical Features

General

- High fever, lassitude, prostration, tachycardia. Fever is usually low grade and rarely lasts for more than 3–4 weeks.

Sore Throat

- Only two-thirds of patients give history of preceding sore throat.

Cardiac

- Carditis occurs in 40–50% of patients with rheumatic fever. Carditis usually occurs within the first 3 weeks of the illness.
- Carditis is the only manifestation of acute rheumatic fever that has the potential to cause long-term disability and death. Cardiac failure can occur due to severe mitral regurgitation or severe myocarditis
- It involves all the three layers of the heart i.e endocardium, myocardium and pericardium.

Endocarditis

- Valvulitis is associated with characteristic murmurs.
- Mitral regurgitation produces a pansystolic murmur best heard at the apex and radiating to the axilla.
- Increased flow across the mitral valve in the presence of valvulitis may produce a middiastolic murmur (Carey Coombs murmur). Carey Coombs murmur can be differentiated from the diastolic murmur of mitral stenosis by the absence of an opening snap, absence of presystolic accentuation, and absence of loud S1.
- Aortic regurgitation produces a high-pitched decrescendo early diastolic murmur.

Myocarditis

- Inappropriate tachycardia.
- S3, S4, or summation gallops may be audible.
- Cardiomegaly.
- Acute congestive heart failure can develop leading to hepatic congestion and right upper-quadrant pain and tenderness. Congestive heart failure is usually caused by left ventricular volume overload associated with severe mitral or aortic regurgitation.

Pericarditis

- Pericardial friction rub.
- Muffled heart sounds due to pericardial effusion. Large effusions leading to tamponade are rare.

Polyarthritis

- Arthritis is the most frequent major manifestation of rheumatic fever (occurs in approximately 75% of patients). Arthralgia is pain in the joints without signs of inflammation.
- It is migratory polyarthritis (joints are involved in quick succession, and each for a brief period of time).
- Usually larger joints such as knees, ankles, elbows, and wrists are involved.
- Small joints and spine are involved rarely.
- Polyarthritis responds dramatically to salicylate therapy.
- Inflammation of any one joint subsides spontaneously within a week and the entire bout of polyathritis rarely lasts more than 4 weeks. Resolution is complete with no residual deformity. However, rarely Jaccoud deformity of the metacarpophalangeal joints can occur after repeated attacks of rheumatic fever. This is a periarticular fibrosis and not a true synovitis.

Subcutaneous Nodules

- It occurs in less than 10% of patients. These are usually associated with carditis and isolated occurrence of nodules is rare.
- They are round, firm, painless, freely movable subcutaneous lesions varying in size from 0.5 to 2 cm.
- Common sites of occurrence are over bony surfaces and over tendons such as elbows, knees, and wrists, the occiput and vertebrae.
- They last for 1–2 weeks and disappear spontaneously.
- Similar nodules also occur in rheumatoid arthritis and SLE.

Erythema Marginatum

- It occurs in less than 10% of patients. This rash is usually found on the trunk and proximal parts of the extremities. Face is spared.
- It appears as erythematous macule or papule with clear center. Lesions may merge and form serpiginous patterns.
- They are not pruritic, nonindurated and blanch on pressure.
- The rash is transient, migrating from place to place without leaving residual scarring. Erythema marginatum has also been reported in sepsis, drug reactions, and glomerulonephritis.

Chorea (Sydenham's chorea; St. Vitus Dance)

- It occurs in 15% of rheumatic fever cases. It can occur in isolation, several months after the attack of rheumatic fever.
- It is most common in the age group 7–14 years and is rare after puberty.
- It is characterized by rapid, purposeless, involuntary movements, most noticable in the extremities and face. The speech is usually slurred and jerky.
- The involuntary movements disappear during sleep and may be suppressed by sedation. Emotional lability is characteristic of Sydenham's chorea and may often precede other neurologic manifestations.
- Most patients recover in 6 months.

Other Clinical Features

- Abdominal pain in rheumatic fever is due to peritoneal inflammation and may be confused with acute appendicitis or sickle cell crisis.
- Epistaxis has been reported in some patients.

Jones Criteria for the Diagnosis of the initial attack of Rheumatic Fever

Major criteria (J♥NES Mnemonic)
• Joint involvement (Migratory polyarthritis)
• ♥ (Heart) Carditis (Pancarditis)
• Nodules (Subcutaneous nodules)
• Erythema marginatum
• Sydenham's chorea (St. Vitus' dance)
Minor criteria
• Fever >38.5°C (101.3°F) in acute phase
• Arthralgia: Joint pain (without swelling), seen when arthritis is absent.
• Elevated inflammatory markers ↑ ESR, ↑ CRP (active inflammation).
• Prolonged PR Interval on ECG
Evidence of preceding streptococcal infection (any one of the following)
• Increased or rising anti-streptolysin O titer or other streptococcal antibodies (anti-DNASE B)
• A positive throat culture for group A B-hemolytic streptococci
• A positive rapid group A streptococcal carbohydrate antigen test in a child whose clinical presentation suggests a high pre-test probability of streptococcal pharyngitis

Diagnosis

Definite ARF

- 2 major OR
- 1 major + 2 minor criteria, plus evidence of preceding GAS infection.

Recurrent ARF

- In patients with prior ARF or RHD: 2 major or 1 major + 2 minor, or 3 minor criteria.

Differential Diagnosis

- Rheumatic fever may be confused with the following:
  - Rheumatoid arthritis
  - Osteomyelitis
  - Infective endocarditis
  - Chronic meningococcemia
  - SLE
  - Lyme disease
  - Sickle cell anemia

Laboratory Findings

General Tests

- Mild to moderate normochromic normocytic anemia
- Polymorphonuclear leukocytosis
- Elevated CRP and ESR are usually present.

Evidence of Preceding Streptococcal Infection

- Throat cultures are usually negative for group A streptococci by the time rheumatic fever appears.
- Rapid antigen detection test (RADT) for GAS: Faster but less sensitive than culture. Used when throat culture is unavailable.
- Streptococcal antibody tests (antistreptolysin O (ASO), anti-DNAse B, antihyaluronidase and antistreptozyme test). ASO titre is elevated in 80% or more of patients with rheumatic fever. ASO titers greater than 200 IU/ml in adults and 333 IU in children are considered elevated. Rising titers are more significant than a single test. Antistreptozyme test (ASTZ) which measures 5 different streptococcal antibodies including ASO and anti-DNAse is a very sensitive test for recent streptococcal infection.
- Recent scarlet fever.

ECG

- Persistent sinus tachycardia that does not resolve during sleep is common in carditis. Prolongation of the PR interval is a consistent finding.
- AV conduction abnormalities, atrial flutter and fibrillation can occur due to carditis.
- Low QRS voltage may be noted if a large pericardial effusion is present.

Echocardiogram

- Gold standard for detecting subclinical carditis.
- Rheumatic mitral valvulitis associated with annular dilation resulting in mitral regurgitation.

- Valvular thickening and the presence of nodular lesions on the body and tips of the mitral leaflet have been described.
- Aortic regurgitation.
- Pericardial effusion (if pericarditis present).
- Left ventricular dysfunction (in severe myocarditis cases).

Endomyocardial Biopsy

- It has limited role in the diagnosis of rheumatic fever. Presence of Aschoff nodules, interstitial mononuclear infiltrates with or without myocyte necrosis is seen in biopsy specimens. Biopsy can be done by percutaneous transvenous route.

Treatment

Management of Acute Episode of Rheumatic Fever

- The patient should be kept at strict bed rest until the fever subsides and ESR, pulse rate, ECG have all returned to baseline.

Antibiotics

- Although evidence of active infection is unusual during the acute phase, it is recommended that patients receive a single dose of benzathine penicillin or a 10-day course of penicillin-V (or erythromycin if penicillin allergic) to curtail exposure to streptococcal antigens. After completion of the course, secondary prophylaxis should be commenced.

Anti-inflammatory drugs

- They provide symptomatic relief of fever, and joint pain. They are not curative and do not prevent the development of rheumatic heart disease. Aspirin is the drug of choice and is very effective for fever and joint inflammation. Aspirin is given for 2–4 weeks, and then tapered off. Other NSAIDs such as naproxen or ibuprofen can be used instead of aspirin.
- Corticosteroids are used in patients with severe carditis manifest by heart failure and in patients who do not tolerate aspirin. Prednisone 40–60 mg per day is given for 2–3 weeks and then gradually tapered over the next 3 weeks. Intravenous dexamethasone can also be used instead of prednisolone.

Management of cardiac failure

- Cardiac failure is managed by diuretics, ACE inhibitors, and betablockers. Digoxin should be used cautiously in the presence of myocarditis due to risk of arrhythmias. Mitral valve repair or replacement may be lifesaving in acute intractable heart failure.

Management of Sydenham's chorea

- *Mild cases*: No treatment needed (self-limiting in 1–6 months).
- *Severe cases*: Valproic acid, or carbamazepine, or haloperidol can be used to control involuntary movements. Steroids are also useful in severe cases.

Prevention of Recurrence (secondary prophylaxis)

- Patients who have already suffered an attack of rheumatic fever are at risk of developing recurrent attacks of rheumatic fever. Recurrent attacks lead to progressive cardiac damage. Hence, rheumatic fever patients should be protected from subsequent streptococcal infections by giving continuous antimicrobial prophylaxis. The risk of recurrence decreases as the age advances.

Drugs used for prophylaxis

Benzathine penicillin G 1.2 million units deep IM (buttocks) every month. However, injections every three weeks may be more effective in preventing recurrences of acute rheumatic fever.

OR

Penicillin V 250 mg twice daily oral (for patients who cannot be given IM injection such as patients on anti-coagulation).

OR

Erythromycin 250 mg twice daily oral for patients who are allergic to penicillin.

The WHO recommendations for the duration of secondary prophylaxis are shown in Table 3.35.

TABLE 3.35: Rheumatic fever prophylaxis

Type	*Duration of prophylaxis after last attack*
Rheumatic fever with carditis and residual heart disease (persistent valvular disease	10 years or until age 40 years (whichever is longer); lifetime prophylaxis may be needed
Rheumatic fever with carditis but no residual heart disease (no valvular disease	10 years or until age 21 years (whichever is longer)
Rheumatic fever without carditis	5 years or until age 21 years (whichever is longer)

Q. Discuss the etiology, clinical features, investigations, complications, and management of mitral stenosis.

- Mitral stenosis (MS) is a narrowing of the mitral valve opening, leading to obstruction of blood flow from the left atrium (LA) to the left ventricle (LV).
- Mitral valve has two leaflets (bicuspid), one anterior and one posterior leaflet.
- In normal adults, the cross-sectional area of the mitral valve orifice is 4–6 cm^2. If the orifice is reduced to less than this, it is called mitral stenosis. Usually, patients will not experience any symptoms until the valve area is reduced to les than 2.5 cm^2. Based on the the mitral valve area (MVA), MS can be
  - **Mild MS:** MVA >1.5 cm^2
  - **Moderate MS:** MVA 1–1.5 cm^2
  - **Severe MS:** MVA <1 cm^2

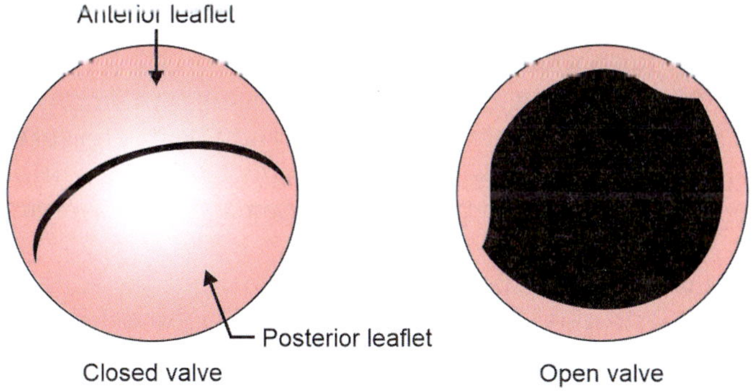

Figure 3.42: Normal mitral valve

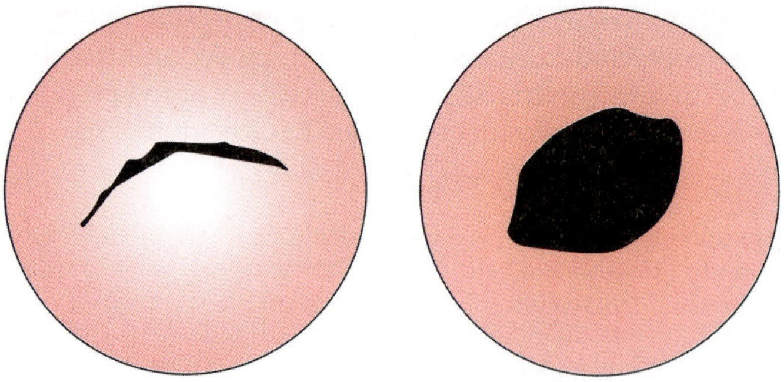

Figure 3.43: Mitral stenosis

Etiology (Table 3.36)

TABLE 3.36: Etiology of mitral stenosis

- Rheumatic heart disease (most common cause).
- Congenital mitral stenosis.
- Carcinoid tumors (*neuroendocrine tumors which secrete various substances which can cause* fibrosis and thickening of the valve leaflets as they pass through the heart).
- Systemic lupus erythematosus (inflammation can affect the heart valves, leading to a condition called Libman-Sacks endocarditis and valve damage).
- Radiation induced fibrosis
- Rare causes
  - Mucopolysaccharidoses (Hurler syndrome; stenosis occurs due to accumulation of glycosaminoglycans in the heart valves).
  - Fabry's disease (genetic disorder characterized by the deficiency of an enzyme alpha-galactosidase A (α-GAL A), which results in the accumulation of certain fatty substances, in multiple organs including heart valves).
  - Whipple's disease (caused by the bacteria *Tropheryma whipplei*. It causes inflammation and fibrosis of heart valve leading to mitral stenosis).

- Rheumatic heart disease is the most common cause of MS, but only 50% patients remember the attack of rheumatic fever. MS is the most common valve lesion due to rheumatic fever. Rheumatic mitral stenosis is more common in women.

Pathophysiology

- When there is mitral stenosis, blood from left atrium cannot flow easily into left ventricle. Hence, blood collects in the left atrium and pressure increases in the left atrium. Because of increased pressure, left atrial hypertrophy and dilatation occur. Left atrial dilatation may lead to atrial fibrillation and left atrial clot formation.
- Due to increased left atrial pressure, pulmonary venous, pulmonary arterial and right heart pressures also increase. Increase in pulmonary vascular pressure leads to pulmonary edema and pulmonary hypertension.
- Pulmonary hypertension leads to right ventricular hypertrophy, dilatation and failure. Right ventricular dilatation results in tricuspid regurgitation.
- An increase in heart rate shortens diastole and hence the time available for ventricular filling. In the presence of MS (in which already there is problem with ventricular filling due to stenosis), any increase in heart rate reduces ventricular filling and raises left atrial pressure.

Clinical Features

History

- Patients are usually asymptomatic until the valve orifice is moderately stenosed. Patient gradually becomes symptomatic as the severity of mitral stenosis increases. The latent period between the initial attack of rheumatic carditis and the development of symptoms due to MS is generally about 20 years. Once the patient becomes seriously symptomatic, death occurs in 2–5 years unless the stenosis is corrected.
- MS usually presents with exertional dyspnea and/or decreased exercise tolerance. Dyspnea results from elevation in left atrial pressure and pulmonary venous hypertension, which leads to reduced compliance of the lungs, a decrease in vital capacity, and increased work of breathing. Dyspnea also may be related to an inability to increase the cardiac output with increased metabolic demands. Dyspnea is exertional initially, but as the severity of MS increases, it may be present at rest also.
- Orthopnea and paroxysmal nocturnal dyspnea can occur because of increased venous return in supine position and consequent congestion of pulmonary vasculature due to left atrial failure (note that in pure MS, left ventricular failure does not occur, but right ventricular failure occurs due to pulmonary HTN).
- Recurrent lower respiratory infections are common. Hemoptysis can occur due to rupture of bronchial veins due to pulmonary hypertension.
- When RV failure occurs, ascites and edema develop.
- Dilated left atrium may lead to atrial fibrillation, giving rise to symptoms such as palpitations. Atrial fibrillation may result in left atrial clot formation and systemic emboli, most commonly to the cerebral vessels resulting in stroke.
- An enlarged LA may impinge on the left recurrent laryngeal nerve, causing hoarseness (Ortner's syndrome).

Physical Examination

- Patients may have a typical look called "mitral facies" or malar flush. This is a bilateral, cyanotic or dusky pink discoloration over the cheeks due to arteriovenous anastomoses and vascular stasis.
- Pulse is low volume and may be irregularly irregular due to atrial fibrillation.
- When right heart failure develops, there may be jugular venous distension, ascites, and pedal edema. Prominent '*a*' wave may be noted in JVP due to pulmonary HTN provided there is no atrial fibrillation. 'a' wave disappears if there is atrial fibrillation.
- Cardiac apex is tapping in nature due to palpable first heart sound.

- Parasternal heave may be present due to right ventricular hypertrophy.
- Loud first heart sound and opening snap may be heard on auscultation. P2 component of S2 may be loud due to pulmonary HTN. A low-pitched mid-diastolic 'rumbling' murmur is heard with the bell of the stethoscope over the apex with the patient lying on the left side. Murmur becomes louder at the end of diastole as a result of atrial contraction (presystolic accentuation). Presystolic accentuation is absent in atrial fibrillation due to loss of atrial contraction.
- An opening snap may precede the mid-diastolic murmur. The gap between S2 and the opening snap provides an estimation of the severity of the mitral stenosis. More severe MS causes higher left atrial pressure. Higher left atrial pressure makes the mitral valve open earlier (i.e. immediately after S2). Hence, mitral valve opening snap becomes closer to S_2. More severe the MS, lesser the gap between S2 and opening snap. Other findings which indicate the severity of MS are presence of pulmonary hypertension (implies severe mitral stenosis), and length of the mid-diastolic murmur which is proportional to the severity of MS. When the valve cusps become immobile, the loud first heart sound softens and the opening snap disappears.
- Pulmonary hypertension can cause pulmonary valvular regurgitation resulting in an early diastolic murmur in the pulmonary area known as Graham Steel murmur.
- Other findings include, tender hepatomegaly, pleural effusions due to right heart failure.

Complications of Mitral Stenosis

- Atrial fibrillation with clot formation and systemic embolization.
- Pulmonary hypertension and right heart failure.
- Recurrent chest infections.
- Hemoptysis.
- Dysphagia due to esophageal compression by the enlarged left atrium.
- Infective endocarditis (rare).
- Death from MS is usually due to progressive right-sided heart failure and/or pulmonary edema in over 60 percent of cases.

Investigations

Chest X-ray

- Chest X-ray shows left atrial enlargement, which produces straightening of the left heart border and a double density at the right heart border due to combined shadows of the right atrium and left atrium. Increased pulmonary vascularity is seen due to pulmonary venous hypertension. Kerley B lines, which represent distended interlobular septa and lymphatics, may be seen due to pulmonary venous engorgement. Calcified mitral valve may be visible in advanced MS.

Electrocardiogram

- ECG usually shows a bifid P wave due to left atrial enlargement and consequent delayed activation. Atrial fibrillation is frequently present. If pulmonary hypertension has developed, there may be features of right ventricular hypertrophy (right axis deviation and tall R waves in lead V1).

Echocardiogram (gold standard test)

- This is the most important tool to diagnose and confirm MS. It can assess the mitral valve apparatus, calculate mitral valve area, left atrial and right ventricular size and function. Estimation of pulmonary artery pressure can be made through measurement of the degree of tricuspid regurgitation. In most cases, echocardiography is enough to judge the severity of mitral stenosis and to make decisions regarding surgery. Transesophageal echocardiography (TEE) is required to detect LA thrombus before intervention.

Cardiac Catheterization

- This is required only if coexisting coronary artery disease is suspected or cardiac surgery is anticipated. If there is coronary artery disease, both CABG and mitral valve replacement can be done in the same sitting.

Treatment

Medical Therapy

- Mild mitral stenosis in sinus rhythm does not require any treatment.
- If the patient develops atrial fibrillation, it should be treated with oral digoxin, a beta-blocker, or a calcium channel blocker (verapamil, diltiazem) to control heart rate.
- Anticoagulation with warfarin should be done (target INR of 2.5–3.5) to prevent clot formation if there is atrial fibrillation.
- Although infective endocarditis in pure mitral stenosis is rare, antibiotic prophylaxis is advised before any invasive procedures.
- Early symptoms of mitral stenosis such as mild dyspnea and orthopnea can usually be treated with diuretics. When symptoms worsen to more than mild or if pulmonary hypertension develops, mechanical correction of the stenosis is necessary.

Percutaneous Balloon Mitral Valvotomy (PBMV)

- A catheter is passed into the right atrium via the femoral vein. The interatrial septum is then punctured and the catheter is advanced into the left atrium and then across the mitral valve. A balloon is then passed over the catheter into the mitral valve and inflated briefly to split the fused valve commissures. This procedure is performed under local anesthesia in the cardiac catheter laboratory. This procedure may result in mitral regurgitation which may require mitral valve replacement.
- Contraindications to the procedure include more than mild mitral regurgitation, calcified mitral valve (valve cannot be opened), and involvement of subvalvular apparatus. The presence of thrombus in the left atrium is also a contraindication to balloon valvotomy because it can be dislodged leading to

systemic emboli. Hence, presence of clot should be ruled out by transesophageal echocardiography prior to this technique. The short- and long-term results of this procedure are similar to surgical valvotomy, with less morbidity and mortality rate. Hence, this has become the procedure of choice for suitable patients.

Surgical Intervention

Surgical Valvotomy

- This procedure is done for patients in whom percutaneous valvotomy is not possible, unsuccessful, or in those with restenosis. Here, the cusps are carefully dissected apart under direct vision. Cardiopulmonary bypass is required for this procedure.

Mitral Valve Replacement

- Replacement of the mitral valve is necessary when:
  - Significant mitral regurgitation is present.
  - Mitral valve is badly damaged and calcified, hence cannot be opened without producing significant regurgitation.
  - There is thrombus in the left atrium.
- Either mechanical prosthetic valves or bioprosthetic valves can be used to replace the mitral valve.
- Mechanical prosthetic valves include caged-ball valve (Starr Edwards prosthesis) and tilting disc valve (Bjork-Shiley valve). Mechanical prosthetic valves require lifelong anticoagulation.
- Bioprosthetic valves include porcine bioprosthetic valve and pericardial xenograft prosthetic valve. Bioprosthetic valves do not last long and hence are not used for patients below 35 years. Bioprosthetic valves do not require anticoagulation and hence are especially useful in pregnancy when oral anticoagulants are contraindicated.

Q. Discuss the etiology, clinical features, investigations and management of mitral regurgitation.

- Mitral regurgitation (MR) is defined as an abnormal reversal of blood flow from the left ventricle (LV) to the left atrium (LA).

Etiology

See **Table 3.37.**

Out of these causes, ruptured chordae tendinae, ischemic papillary muscle dysfunction or rupture, infective endocarditis, cardiac surgery and chest trauma cause acute severe mitral regurgitation

Pathophysiology

- Regurgitation of blood into the left atrium increases the left atrial pressure and leads to left atrial dilatation. In long standing mitral regurgitation, increase in left atrial pressure may not be present due to atrial dilatation which accommodates the regurgitant blood. However, in acute regurgitation there can be significant increase in left atrial pressure leading to pulmonary venous congestion, pulmonary edema and pulmonary HTN.
- Pulmonary HTN leads to right ventricular hypertrophy and right heart failure.
- Regurgitated blood as well as blood coming from pulmonary veins both enter the left ventricle in diastole leading to volume overload. Volume overload of left ventricle leads to left ventricular hypertrophy, dilatation and failure.

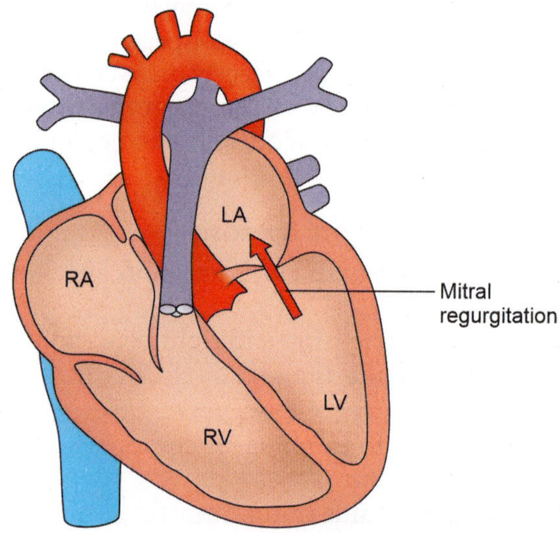

Figure 3.44: Mitral regurgitation

TABLE 3.37: Etiology of mitral regurgitation

- Rheumatic heart disease (most common cause).
- Mitral valve prolapse.
- Ischemic heart disease (due to papillary muscle dysfunction or rupture of chordae tendinae).
- Infective endocarditis-mitral regurgitation may result from destruction of the mitral valve leaflets.
- Myocarditis (due to dilatation of left ventricle).
- Dilated cardiomyopathy (due to dilatation of left ventricle).
- Aortic valve disease (due to dilatation of left ventricle).
- Hypertrophic cardiomyopathy—left ventricular contraction is disorganized and mitral regurgitation often develops.
- Connective tissue disorders—systemic lupus erythematosus (SLE) may cause mitral regurgitation due to Libman-Sacks endocarditis.
- Marfan's syndrome and Ehlers-Danlos syndrome cause mitral regurgitation due to myxomatous degeneration of the valve.
- Trauma (after balloon mitral valvotomy and blunt chest trauma)
- Congenital (endocardial cushion defects, endocardial fibroelastosis)
- Cardiac surgery
- Chest trauma
- Drugs, e.g. fenfluramine.

Clinical Features

History

- Mild mitral regurgitation can remain silent for many years.
- Patients may c/o palpitations due to increased stroke volume or due to development of atrial fibrillation.
- Dyspnea, orthopnoea and PND can occur due to pulmonary venous congestion, pulmonary edema and left ventricular failure.
- Fatigue and lethargy develop due to reduced cardiac output as the blood regurgitates back into left atrium during systole.
- Patients c/o peripheral edema in the late stages of the disease due to right heart failure.
- Clot formation in the dilated left atrium leading to systemic emboli can occur but less common than in mitral stenosis.
- Patients may present with fever due to Infective endocarditis.

Physical Examination

- Bounding pulse (severe MR with high output). Pulse may be irregularly irregular if there is atrial fibrillation.
- Cardiac apex is displaced laterally and outward due to dilated and hypertrophied left ventricle.
- Palpation may reveal a hyperdynamic (due to volume overload), diffuse apex beat (due to dilated LV) and a systolic thrill (due to mitral regurgitation). Parasternal heave may be present due to right ventricular hypertrophy.
- Auscultation reveals soft S1 due to incomplete opposition of the mitral valve, pansystolic murmur (PSM) due to regurgitation of blood throughout the systole. PSM is loudest at the apex and may radiate to other areas and axilla. S-3 may be heard due to rapid filling of the left ventricle in diastole by the large volume of blood coming from left atrium. Sometimes a short mid-diastolic flow murmur may follow the third heart sound due to increased flow across the mitral valve. Loud P2 may be present due to pulmonary HTN. Bilateral basal lung crepitations may be present due to pulmonary venous congestion.
- Signs of right heart failure such as raised JVP, and peripheral edema, congestive hepatomegaly may be present.

Investigations

Chest X-ray

- Chest X-ray may show cardiomegaly due to left atrial and left ventricular enlargement. Prominent pulmonary artery and vasculature may be seen due to pulmonary HTN.

Electrocardiogram

- The ECG usually shows LV hypertrophy and left atrial enlargement. Atrial fibrillation may be present.

Echocardiogram (gold standard test)

- This is the investigation of choice to confirm and assess the extent of mitral regurgitation. It shows the dilated left atrium and left ventricle. Color flow Doppler can determine the severity of regurgitation. Echo can also show the cause of regurgitation (like chordal or papillary muscle rupture) and also the complications of mitral regurgitation (like left atrial clot formation, infective endocarditis and pulmonary HTN). Transesophageal echocardiography can more exactly assess the anatomy and abnormalities of mitral valve which is useful before surgery.

Cardiac Catheterization

- This is helpful to accurately assess the severity of the lesion and to to assess coronary arteries in patients above 40 years of age.

Complications

- Atrial fibrillation with clot formation → Systemic embolism
- Infective endocarditis
- Left ventricular failure
- Pulmonary HTN → Right ventricular failure.

Treatment

Medical Therapy

- Mild mitral regurgitation without any symptoms can be managed conservatively by following the patient with serial echocardiograms.
- Infective endocarditis prophylaxis if indicated.
- ACE inhibitors or ARBs reduce afterload and hence decrease mitral regurgitation.
- Diuretics, beta-blockers and dogoxin are helpful to treat heart failure.
- When atrial fibrillation develops, long-term anticoagulation is required to prevent clot formation.

Surgical Therapy

- Mitral valve repair or replacement is indicated if there is evidence of progressive cardiac enlargement. Most patients with the symptoms of dyspnea, orthopnea, or fatigue should undergo surgery.
- Acute mitral regurgitation, as seen with chordal or papillary muscle rupture or infective endocarditis, requires emergency mitral valve replacement.
- Percutaneous mitral valve repair can be tried in selected patients.

Q. Mitral valve prolapse (MVP).

- Mitral valve prolapse (MVP) is a valvular heart disorder characterized by the bulging of one or both mitral valve leaflets into the left atrium during systole, often leading to mitral regurgitation.
- MVP is also known as systolic click-murmur syndrome, Barlow's syndrome, floppy-valve syndrome, and billowing mitral leaflet syndrome.

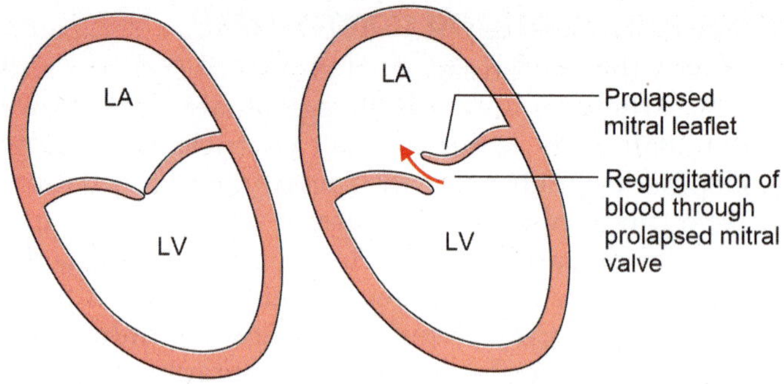

Figure 3.45: Normal mitral valve (left) and prolapsed mitral valve (right)

Etiology

Primary MVP (Idiopathic)
- Myxomatous degeneration of the mitral valve.
- Associated with connective tissue disorders (e.g. Marfan syndrome, Ehlers-Danlos syndrome).
- Genetic predisposition (autosomal dominant inheritance in some cases).

Secondary MVP
- Associated with ischemic heart disease, rheumatic heart disease, or hypertrophic cardiomyopathy.
- Can occur due to papillary muscle dysfunction or ruptured chordae tendineae.

Pathophysiology

- During ventricular systole, a mitral valve leaflet (most commonly the posterior leaflet) prolapses into the left atrium. This may result in abnormal ventricular contraction, papillary muscle strain and some mitral regurgitation. Usually, the syndrome is not hemodynamically serious. Thromboembolism can occur rarely.

Clinical Features

History

- Most patients with MVP are asymptomatic.
- Some patients complain of chest pain, palpitation, light-headedness and syncope.
- Chest pain is the most common symptom and is usually felt in substernal area with stabbing quality. Exact cause of chest pain is not known but may be due to papillary muscle ischemia because of excessive tension on the papillary muscles during systole.
- Palpitation and syncope may be due to autonomic dysfunction which is common in MVP.
- Transient ischemic attacks may occur due to platelet aggregation and emboli formation.
- Sudden cardiac death due to fatal ventricular arrhythmias is a very rare but recognized complication.

Physical Examination

- The most common sign is a mid or late systolic click, which occurs due to sudden prolapse of the valve and the tensing of the chordae tendineae during systole. This click may be followed by a late systolic murmur owing to some regurgitation. With more regurgitation, the murmur becomes pansystolic. Maneuvers that make the left ventricle smaller, such as the Valsalva maneuver, or standing position due to decreased venous return, make the click and murmur more prominent. This happens because of increased prolapse of mitral valve leaflets into the left atrium when the ventricular volume is less. Conversely, squatting and isometric exercise, which increase LV volume, diminish the click and murmur.

Investigations

ECG

- Is usually normal but sometimes nonspecific ST-T changes in leads II, III and aVF may be seen.

Echocardiogram

- This is the investigation of choice to confirm MVP. Two-dimensional echo-cardiography shows posterior movement of one or both mitral valve cusps into the left atrium during systole. Echo can also show if there is any associated mitral regurgitation.

Treatment

- Most patients with MVP have a benign clinical course. No treatment is required for asymptomatic patients
- However, some may progress to have mitral regurgitation and infective endocarditis. Infective endocarditis prophylaxis before invasive procedures is not required inless there is severe MR.
- Palpitations and chest pain can be controlled by beta-blockers like propranolol or metoprolol.
- Antiplatelet agents such as aspirin should be given to patients with transient ischemic attacks.

Q. Classify aortic stenosis (AS). Describe the etiology, clinical features, investigations, and management of valvular aortic stenosis.

Q. Clinical assessment of severity of aortic stenosis.

- Aortic stenosis is narrowing of aortic valve leading to obstruction to blood flow across the aortic valve.
- The normal aortic valve area is 3–4 cm^2. When the area is less than this, it is called aortic stenosis. In severe aortic stenosis, valve area is less than 1 cm^2.
- AS can be valvular, subvalvular or supravalvular.

Etiology (Table 3.38)

TABLE 3.38: Etiology of aortic stenosis
Valvular • Congenital bicuspid valve with superimposed calcification • Age-related degenerative calcific AS (aortic sclerosis) • Rheumatic heart disease
Subvalvular • Membranous diaphragm • Tunnel deformity • Hypertrophic obstructive cardiomyopathy
Supravalvular • Williams syndrome • Familial hypercholesterolemia • Hourglass constriction of aorta • Hypoplasia of aorta

- *Congenital aortic valve stenosis:* Congenitally abnormal (usually bicuspid) aortic valve can undergo progressive narrowing due to turbulent blood flow. Such congenitally abnormal aortic valves are common in men.
- *Rheumatic fever:* Rheumatic endocarditis produces commissural fusion, thickening and calcification of aortic valve leading to narrowing. Rheumatic AS is almost always associated with involvement of the mitral valve and by associated severe AR.
- *Age-related degenerative calcific AS (also known as senile AS or aortic sclerosis):* About 30% of persons >65 years exhibit aortic valve sclerosis. An ejection systolic murmur may be heard but true stenosis is rare. Valve changes are due to inflammatory reaction similar to atherosclerosis.
- *Hypertrophic cardiomyopathy:* This condition is associated with massive hypertrophy of the interventricular septum which blocks the ventricular outflow during systole. It causes subaortic obstruction.

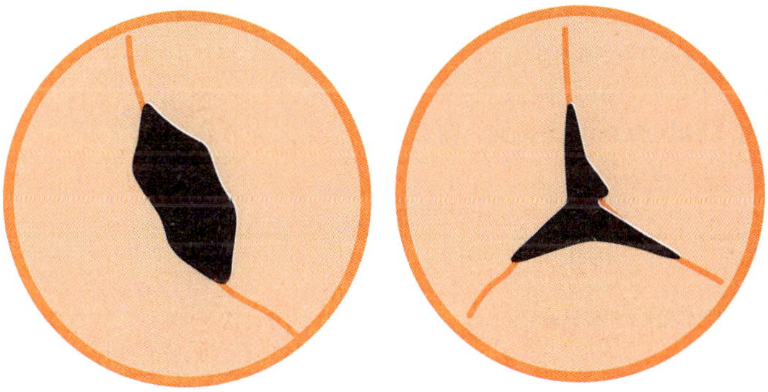

Figure 3.46: Bicuspid (left) and tricuspid aortic valve (right) with stenosis

Pathophysiology

- Obstruction to left ventricular outflow leads to increased left ventricular pressure and compensatory concentric hypertrophy. The hypertrophied LV muscle mass elevates myocardial oxygen requirements. In addition, coronary vessels may be compressed by increased intraventricular pressure leading to decreased blood flow. Both these factors lead to ischemia of myocardium which increases on exertion.
- Since there is obstruction to LV outflow, cardiac output cannot increase on exertion, which leads to exertional syncope, chest pain and dyspnea. Syncope and lightheadedness is due to decreased cerebral perfusion.
- BP may also drop during exertion due to peripheral vasodilation.
- Ultimately, left ventricle may dilate and fail.

Clinical Features

History

- Patient is usually asymptomatic until aortic stenosis is moderately severe (aortic orifice is one-third of its normal size).
- When the AS is moderate to severe, exercise-induced syncope, angina and dyspnea develop. Orthopnea and PND may be present if there is heart failure. When these symptoms develop, prognosis is poor and death usually occurs within 2–3 years unless surgical intervention is done.

Physical Examination

- Pulse is of low volume and slow-rising in nature.
- The apex beat is usually not displaced unless there is LV failure and dilatation. Apex is diffuse and well sustained.
- A systolic thrill may be felt in the aortic area due to turbulent blood flow through narrowed aortic valve.
- Auscultation shows a classic ejection systolic murmur which is usually 'diamond shaped' (crescendo-decrescendo). More severe the AS, the longer the murmur because longer ejection time is needed. The murmur is rough in quality, best heard in the aortic area with patient leaning forward and breath held in expiration. It radiates to carotid arteries especially to the left carotid. The murmur peaks in the mid or late systole because the flow is maximum during the middle of systole. The intensity of the murmur and the severity of AS do not have any correlation because in severe cases, the murmur may be inaudible due to reduced flow. Sometimes the murmur may not be heard in aortic area and heard only over the LV apex, mimicking mitral regurgitation (Gallivardan's phenomenon).
- A systolic ejection click may be heard before the mumur. Presence of an ejection click suggests aortic valve involvement and excludes supravalvular or subvalvular causes of stenosis.
- Aortic component of second heart sound (A2) is delayed, resulting in narrow splitting of second heart sound in mild to moderate AS. Reversed splitting of the second heart sound may be seen in severe AS.
- When the aortic valve becomes immobile due to severe stenosis or calcification, aortic second heart sound becomes soft or inaudible.
- Left ventricular S3 may be heard in left heart failure. An S-4 gallop is common due to stiff left ventricle.

Clinical Assessment of Severity of Aortic Stenosis

Severe aortic stenosis is suggested by one or more of the following findings:

- Low systolic BP
- Heaving apex
- Soft A2 or single second heart sound
- Paradoxical splitting of S2
- Harsh, loud, long ESM with late peaking
- Orthopnea, PND and S3.

Investigations

Chest X-ray

- In the initial stages of AS, chest X-ray shows a normal sized heart. But in later stages, when there is dilatation of heart due to failure, there is cardiomegaly. Ascending aorta shows dilatation because turbulent blood flow above the stenosed aortic valve produces so-called 'post-stenotic dilatation'. Sometimes aortic valve calcification may be visible on X-ray.

ECG

- ECG shows left ventricular hypertrophy. In advanced cases, left ventricular 'strain' pattern due to 'pressure overload' (depressed ST segments and T wave inversion in leads orientated towards the left ventricle (i.e. leads I, AVL, V5 and V6) is seen.

Echocardiogram

- Echo shows LV hypertrophy and thickened, calcified, immobile aortic valve cusps. Transesophageal echo shows the obstructed aortic orifice very well. Echo can also show other valvular abnormalities such as MS and AR, which may accompany AS, and to identify nonvalvular causes of LV outflow obstruction such as obstructive hypertrophic cardiomyopathy.

Cardiac Catheterization

- Catheterization of the left side of the heart and coronary angiography should be done in patients with severe AS who are being considered for surgery. Aortic valve replacement and CABG can be carried out at the same time if there is coronary artery disease.

Natural Course of AS

- AS is a progressive disease, with 0.1 cm^2/year reduction in the valve area. Symptomatic patients usually die within 4 years after the onset of symptoms.
- Death usually occurs due to congestive heart failure or arrhythmias.

Treatment

Medical Treatment

- Patients with severe AS should avoid strenuous physical activity.
- Nitrates can be used for angina.
- Sodium restriction, diuretics and digoxin can be used to treat congestive heart failure.
- HMG-CoA reductase inhibitors (statins) have been shown to slow the progression of leaflet calcification and aortic valve area reduction. Hence, treatment with these agents should be considered for all patients.
- Infective endocarditis prophylaxis.

Balloon Aortic Valvotomy

- This procedure can be used in children and young adults with congenital, noncalcific AS. It is not recommended for adults because of high restenosis rate, except as a "bridge to operation" in patients with severe LV dysfunction who are too ill to tolerate surgery.

Surgical Treatment

- Patients with severe calcific AS (valve area <1.0 cm^2) who are symptomatic, those with LV dysfunction, and those with an expanding poststenotic aortic dilatation require aortic valve replacement. Asymptomatic patients should be followed up regularly for development of symptoms and echocardiography should be done to assess the progression of AS.

Q. Aortic sclerosis (age-related degenerative calcific aortic sclerosis or senile aortic sclerosis).

- Aortic sclerosis refers to aortic valve thickening (sclerosis) without significant obstruction to blood flow. It is considered a precursor to aortic stenosis (AS) but does not always progress to severe obstruction.
- Pathologically it is characterized by fibrosis and thickening of valve leaflets. Calcification can also occur.

Etiology and Risk Factors

Degenerative (most common cause)

- Age-related fibrosis and calcification of the aortic valve.
- Common in elderly individuals (>65 years).

Risk Factors (similar to atherosclerosis)

- Hypertension
- Hyperlipidemia
- Diabetes mellitus
- Smoking
- Chronic kidney disease
- Metabolic syndrome

Clinical Features

- It is usually asymptomatic. Physical examination may show an ejection systolic murmur, best heard over the aortic area. In general, the murmur is brief and not very loud. Carotid pulse and S2 are normal indicating the absence of aortic stenosis.
- Echocardiography shows leaflet thickening, stiffness, and/or increased echogenicity (calcification) of the aortic valve. Leaflet excursion is normal as the commissures are not fused.

Management

- Statins and ACE inhibitors may slow the progression of calcification and prevent future aortic stenosis. There is no need for endocarditis prophylaxis.
- Echocardiographic monitoring every 3–5 years to assess progression.

Q. Discuss the etiology, clinical features, investigations and management of aortic regurgitation (AR).

Q. Peripheral signs of aortic regurgitation (AR).

- Aortic regurgitation (AR), also known as aortic insufficiency, is a condition where the aortic valve fails to close completely during diastole, leading to backflow of blood from the aorta into the left ventricle (LV).
- Aortic regurgitation can be either due to problem in the valve itself or problems in the aortic root. It can be acute or chronic. Rheumatic fever and infective endocarditis are the commonest causes of AR.

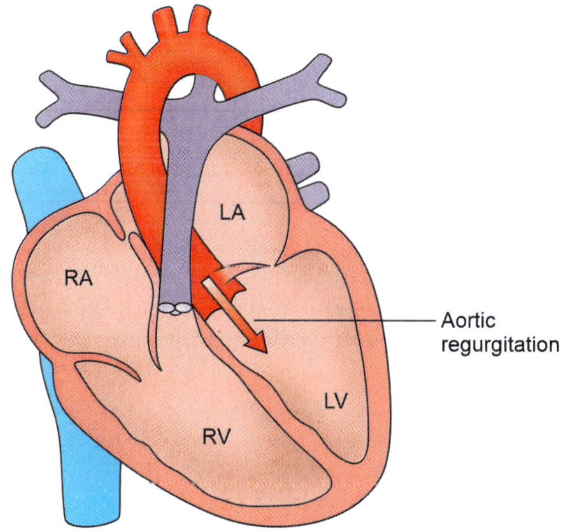

Figure 3.47: Aortic regurgitation

Etiology of AR (Table 3.39)

TABLE 3.39: Etiology of AR

Aortic valve disease
• Bicuspid aortic valve
• Rheumatic heart disease
• Anorexigenic drugs (fenfluramine)
• Severe hypertension
• Osteogenesis imperfecta
• Infective endocarditis
• Failure of prosthetic heart valve
• Trauma
Aortic root disease
• Aneurysm of aorta
• Marfan's syndrome
• Syphilis
• Ankylosing spondylitis
• Psoriatic arthritis
• Takayasu disease
• Aortic dissection
• Ruptured sinus of Valsalva aneurysm
• Idiopathic dilatation of the aorta

- Out of these, acute aortic regurgitation is caused by acute rheumatic fever, infective endocarditis, aortic dissection, ruptured sinus of Valsalva, and failure of prosthetic heart valve.

Pathophysiology

- In AR, some of the blood pumped into the aorta by the left ventricle comes back into the left ventricle through the aortic valve during diastole. This is also joined by the blood coming from left atrium which leads to volume overload of left ventricle (increase in end diastolic volume). There is increase in stroke volume of left ventricle due to this volume overload.
- Increase in stroke volume causes all the peripheral signs of aortic regurgitation. Chronic volume overload causes eccentric hypertrophy and dilatation of left ventricle, which may ultimately fail.
- Increased stroke volume leads to increase in systolic BP and high-volume pulses. Since the blood ejected into the aorta regurgitates back into left ventricle, there is drop in diastolic BP. Rise in systolic BP and fall in diastolic BP leads to increased pulse pressure
- An early diastolic murmur is produced due to blood regurgitating back into left ventricle.
- In advanced cases of AR, there may be increase in left atrial and pulmonary venous pressures leading to right heart failure.
- Myocardial ischemia may occur in patients with AR because myocardial oxygen requirement is elevated by both LV hypertrophy and systolic HTN.
- Acute AR may lead to left ventricular failure because left ventricle is not prepared to handle this sudden volume overload.

Clinical Features

Symptoms

- In early stages, patients may remain asymptomatic.
- Patients may c/o palpitations and head pounding due to increased stroke volume.
- When left ventricular dysfunction appears, symptoms such as exertional dyspnea, orthopnea, PND and fatigue appear. Thickened left ventricular wall also leads to diastolic dysfunction which can also cause above symptoms even if systolic function is normal.
- Anginal chest pain may occur in patients with severe AR due to increased myocardial oxygen demand but less common than in aortic stenosis.

Signs

- Aortic regurgitation produces a myriad of signs due to increased stroke volume and hyperdynamic circulation.
- The pulse is bounding or collapsing. Systolic BP is typically high and diastolic BP low leading to wide pulse pressure. Systolic pressure in the upper limb is at least 40 mm Hg or more than the lower limb (Hill's sign).
- The following peripheral signs may be present in aortic regurgitation.

Peripheral Signs of Aortic Regurgitation (Table 3.40)

TABLE 3.40: Peripheral signs of aortic regurgitation

Sign	Description
Corrigan's neck sign or dancing carotids	Prominent carotid pulsations in the neck
Quincke's sign	Systolic plethora and diastolic blanching in the nail bed when gentle pressure is applied on the nail
De Musset's sign	Head nodding with each heartbeat
Duroziez's sign	Combined systolic and diastolic bruits created by compression of the femoral artery with the stethoscope. It is seen in severe AR

(Contd.)

TABLE 3.40: Peripheral signs of aortic regurgitation *(Contd.)*

Traube's sign (pistol shot femorals)	A sharp bang heard on auscultation over the femoral arteries in time with each heartbeat
Hill's sign	Systolic pressure in the upper limb is at least 40 mm Hg or more than the lower limb
Collapsing pulse (water hammer pulse)	This is characterized by rapid upstroke, rapid down stroke and high volume
Pulsus bisferiens	This is a pulse with double peak. It is seen in severe AR
Mullers sign	Pulsations of the uvula
Lighthouse sign	Alternate flushing and blanching of the forehead
Beckers sign	Visible pulsations of retinal artery and pupil
Rosenbach's sign	Systolic pulsations of the liver
Gerhard's sign	Systolic pulsations of the spleen
Mayne's sign	More than a 15-mm Hg decrease in diastolic blood pressure with arm elevation from the value obtained with the arm in the standard position.

- Note that all the above peripheral signs may be absent in acute aortic regurgitation.
- All these peripheral signs are not specific for AR, since they can be seen in any condition associated with a marked increase in stroke volume and a hyperdynamic circulation. Examples are sympathetic hyperactivity, anemia, fever, pregnancy, thyrotoxicosis, large arteriovenous fistula, patent ductus arteriosus, and severe bradycardia.
- The apex beat is displaced laterally and downwards and is forceful in quality.
- On auscultation, S1 and S2 are usually normal. S2 is followed by an early diastolic high pitch blowing murmur heard best along the left sternal border with the patient sitting and leaning forward.
- The regurgitant jet can impinge on the anterior mitral valve leaflet making it vibrate and cause a mid-diastolic murmur (Austin Flint murmur). Austin Flint murmur can be mistaken for mid-diastolic murmur of mitral stenosis. However, MS murmur is usually accompanied by a thrill, which is, absent in Austin flint murmur.
- Because of increased stroke volume, there can be a functional ejection systolic murmur mimicking aortic stenosis. However, absence of slow rising pulse differentiates functional ejection systolic murmur from true AS.

Clinical Assessment of Severity of AR

- Presence of one or more of the following features suggests that AR is severe:
  - Peripheral signs.
  - Pulsus bisferiens.
  - Hills sign more than 60 mm Hg.
  - Hyperdynamic apex.
  - Early diastolic murmur lasting more than two-third of diastole.
  - Presence of Austin flint murmur.

Investigations

Chest X-ray

- Chest X-ray shows cardiomegaly due to left ventricular enlargement. Post-stenotic dilatation of the aorta may be visible. Aortic valve calcification may be visible in some cases.

ECG

- The ECG features of left ventricular hypertrophy with strain pattern (tall R waves in the left-sided chest leads, deep S waves in the right-sided leads, ST-segment depression and T-wave inversion in leads I, aVL, V_5, and V_6).

Echocardiogram

- Echo can confirm the diagnosis and cause of AR. It can also assess LV function and the status of other valves. The regurgitant jet causing fluttering of anterior mitral leaflet can be detected by color flow Doppler.

Cardiac Catheterization

- It is the most accurate way of confirming and assessing the degree of AR. It can also assess LV function and status of coronary arteries.

Other Tests

- VDRL and TPHA to rule out syphilitic etiology.
- ANA, RA factor, CRP and ESR to rule out connective tissue disease.
- ASO titer and throat swab culture if rheumatic etiology is suspected.

Treatment

Medical

- For asymptomatic patients with normal LV function, afterload reduction is recommended because it delays or reduces the need for aortic valve surgery. Vasodilators like ACE inhibitors, nitrates, hydralazine and nifedifine are helpful to reduce afterload.
- Digoxin, diuretics, ACE inhibitors and salt restriction are useful if there is heart failure.
- The underlying cause of aortic regurgitation (e.g. rheumatic, syphilitic or infective endocarditis) requires specific treatment.
- Infective endocarditis prophylaxis is recommended for AR.

Surgical

- Surgical aortic valve replacement is necessary after the onset of LV dysfunction but before the development of severe symptoms. Valve replacement is needed immediately in acute AR.

- In general, operation should be carried out in patients with left ventricular ejection fraction (LVEF) <55% or a LV end-systolic volume >55 ml/m^2. These parameters have been referred to as the "55/55 rule." However, newer guidelines recommend a more individualized approach based on LV size indexed to body surface area, symptoms, and imaging findings rather than relying solely on the 55/55 rule.
- Surgical treatment is also necessary in patients with acute severe AR.

Q. Hill's sign in aortic regurgitation.

- Hill's Sign is a clinical sign seen in aortic regurgitation (AR). It refers to the exaggerated difference in systolic blood pressure between the lower and upper extremities.
- Normally, the systolic blood pressure in the legs is 10–20 mm Hg higher than in the arms.
- In severe aortic regurgitation, this difference increases to >60 mm Hg, which is known as Hill's sign.

Mechanism

- Elevated blood pressure in the lower limbs arises from the summation of reflected pressure waves. This phenomenon is more pronounced in the legs due to their vessels being more muscular and directly continuous with the aorta, unlike the upper limb vessels which branch off at a 90-degree angle. Consequently, the pressure wave travels rapidly down the lower limb arteries, reflects at their distal ends, and reinforces the incoming wave, leading to the observed higher pressure.

Clinical Relevance

- It can be measured using upper and lower limb blood pressure recordings.
- Hill's sign is considered one of the most sensitive signs of severity of AR.
    - Mild AR: 20–40 mm Hg difference between lower limb and upper limb systolic BP.
    - Moderate AR: 40–60 mm Hg difference.
    - Severe AR: >60 mm Hg difference.

Q. Austin flint murmur.

- This is a mid-diastolic, low-pitched, rumbling murmur heard over the apex in severe aortic regurgitation.
- It is due to the aortic regurgitant jet impinging on anterior mitral leaflet causing it to vibrate.

Characteristics of the Murmur

- Timing: Mid-to-late diastolic
- Location: Best heard at the apex
- Pitch: Low-pitched, rumbling murmur
- Best heard with: Bell of the stethoscope (due to low frequency)
- No opening snap (helps differentiate from mitral stenosis)
- May disappear after vasodilator therapy (amylnitrate inhalation) which reduce AR severity.

Clinical Relevance

- It may be confused with mid-diastolic murmur (MDM) of mitral stenosis. MDM of mitral stenosis is characterized by loud S1, opening snap, and presystolic accentuation. All these features are absent in Austin Flint murmur.

Q. Tricuspid stenosis (TS).

- This is an uncommon valve lesion, seen more often in women than in men.

Etiology

- TS is usually due to rheumatic heart disease and is frequently associated with mitral and/or aortic valve disease. Rarely can it be due to carcinoid syndrome or congenital. Infective endocarditis with large vegetations is another cause especially in IV drug abusers.

Pathophysiology

- Tricuspid valve stenosis results in collection of blood in the right atrium raising its pressure. Rise in right atrial pressure causes systemic venous congestion resulting in hepatomegaly, peripheral edema and ascites.
- Reduced blood flow into right ventricle results in reduced blood flow into left ventricle and hence reduced cardiac output.
- Cardiac output cannot increase on exertion because TS will not allow increased venous return into right and then left ventricle.

Clinical Features

- Patients usually c/o dyspnea and fatigue due to reduced cardiac output.
- Abdominal pain may be there due to congestive hepatomegaly. JVP is raised and shows a prominent 'a' wave. Ascites and peripheral edema may be present.
- A mid-diastolic murmur may be heard at the lower left sternal border, which becomes louder on inspiration. A tricuspid opening snap may occasionally be heard.
- Patients usually develop atrial fibrillation due to right atrial dilatation.

Investigations

- Chest X-ray shows prominent right atrial bulge.
- ECG shows features of right atrial enlargement such as tall, peaked, P waves (>3 mm) in lead II and prominent, upright P waves in lead V_1.
- Echo may show a thickened and immobile tricuspid valve.

Treatment

- Systemic venous congestion can be brought down by diuretics and salt restriction.
- Percutaneous balloon valvotomy (if feasible).
- Surgical repair should be carried out in patients with moderate or severe TS. If repair is not possible tricuspid valve replacement is necessary with preferably a bioprosthetic valve.

Q. Tricuspid regurgitation.

Etiology

- Tricuspid regurgitation (TR) is the backflow of blood from the right ventricle (RV) to the right atrium (RA) during systole due to improper closure of the tricuspid valve.
- Tricuspid regurgitation is usually functional, secondary to dilatation of the tricuspid annulus. Dilatation of the tricuspid annulus occurs whenever there is right ventricular dilatation, e.g. in cor-pulmonale, myocardial infarction and pulmonary hypertension.
- Organic tricuspid regurgitation may occur with rheumatic heart disease, infective endocarditis, carcinoid syndrome, and congenital abnormalities.

Clinical Features

- The symptoms of tricuspid regurgitation are those of right-sided heart failure, including ascites, edema, and right upper quadrant pain due to congested liver. JVP is raised with prominent '*v*' wave.
- Regurgitation into the hepatic veins causes hepatic enlargement and liver pulsation.
- Right ventricular enlargement produces a parasternal heave in the left sternal border.
- A blowing pansystolic murmur is heard at the lower left sternal edge, which increases on inspiration.
- Atrial fibrillation is common due to right atrial enlargement.

Investilgations

- Chest X-ray shows right atrial and ventricular enlargement.
- ECG shows features of right ventricular hypertrophy.
- Echo can confirm the presence and severity of TR and show right atrial and ventricular enlargement.

Treatment

- Functional tricuspid regurgitation usually disappears with treatment of underlying disease.
- Severe organic tricuspid regurgitation may require operative repair or replacement of the tricuspid valve.
- In drug addicts with infective endocarditis of the tricuspid valve, surgical removal of the valve is recommended to eradicate the infection.

Q. Pulmonary stenosis.

Etiology

- Pulmonary stenosis (PS) is the narrowing of the pulmonary valve, leading to obstruction of blood flow from the right ventricle to the pulmonary artery. PS is usually a congenital lesion due to maternal rubella infection during pregnancy. Congenital pulmonary stenosis may be isolated or associated with tetralogy of Fallot.
- Other causes are rheumatic fever and carcinoid syndrome.
- Pulmonary stenosis may be valvular, subvalvular or supravalvular (just like aortic stenosis).

Clinical Features

- PS causes obstruction to right ventricular emptying and results in right ventricular hypertrophy, right heart failure and right atrial enlargement. Patients may have signs and symptoms of right heart failure. JVP is raised with prominent *a* wave.
- PS decreases the blood flow from right side of the heart to left side of the heart and hence causes decreased cardiac output which does not increase on exertion. This causes fatigue and syncope on exertion.
- A midsystolic ejection murmur is heard in the pulmonary area which increases on inspiration. The murmur is often associated with a thrill. There is wide but variable split of S2 (due to delayed pulmonary valve closure).

Investigations

- Chest X-ray shows a prominent pulmonary artery due to post-stenotic dilatation.
- ECG shows features of right atrial and right ventricular hypertrophy.
- Echo can confirm the diagnosis and assess the severity of PS.
- Cardiac catheterization can also assess the level and degree of the stenosis by measuring the systolic pressure gradient across pulmonary valve.

Treatment

- Mild to moderate PS does not require endocarditis prophylaxis.
- Treatment of severe pulmonary stenosis requires balloon valvotomy or surgery.

Q. Pulmonary regurgitation (PR).

- Pulmonary regurgitation (PR) is the backflow of blood from the pulmonary artery into the right ventricle during diastole due to incomplete closure of the pulmonary valve.

Causes of Pulmonary Regurgitation

- Pulmonary valve dysplasia
- Rheumatic heart disease
- Infective endocarditis
- Pulmonary hypertension leading to annular dilatation
- Idiopathic pulmonary artery dilatation
- Marfan's syndrome or other connective tissue disorders
- Carcinoid syndrome affecting the pulmonary valve.

Pathophysiology

- During diastole, the pulmonary valve fails to close completely.
- Blood leaks back into the right ventricle, leading to volume overload.
- Chronic regurgitation causes right ventricular dilatation, hypertrophy, and eventually right heart failure.

Clinical Features

- Fatigue
- Dyspnea on exertion

- Peripheral edema (in severe cases with right heart failure)
- Palpitations
- Graham Steell murmur: A high-pitched, decrescendo diastolic murmur at the left upper sternal border, best heard during inspiration
- Right ventricular heave (suggestive of RV enlargement)
- Signs of right heart failure in advanced cases.

Diagnosis

- Echocardiography (standard test)
- Cardiac MRI (used for detailed assessment of right ventricular function and pulmonary artery dilatation)
- Electrocardiogram (ECG)
- Chest X-ray: May reveal right heart enlargement or pulmonary artery dilation.

Treatment

- Mild PR: No specific treatment; regular monitoring.
- Moderate to severe PR (especially if symptomatic or causing RV dysfunction).
  - Diuretics (for right heart failure symptoms).
  - Pulmonary vasodilators if pulmonary hypertension is present.
  - Pulmonary valve replacement (mechanical or bioprosthetic).

Q. Discuss the causes and differential diagnosis of ejection systolic murmur (ESM).

- An ejection systolic murmur (ESM) is a murmur that occurs during ventricular systole, starting after S1 and ending before S2. It is caused by turbulent blood flow across the semilunar valves (aortic or pulmonary) or through an outflow tract obstruction **(Fig. 3.48)**.
- The ejection of blood begins after closure of the atrioventricular (mitral and tricuspid) valves and is preceded by the time it takes for the ventricular pressures to sufficiently exceed the aortic and pulmonary diastolic pressure and force open the aortic and pulmonary valves. Because of this delay, there is a silent interval between the first heart sound (S1 is produced by closure of the AV valves) and onset of the murmur.

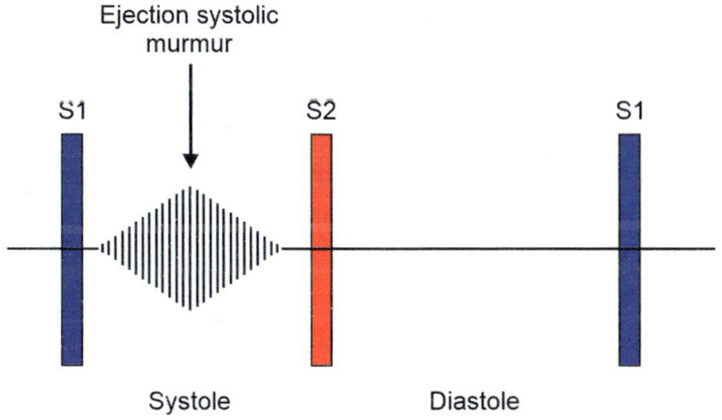

Figure 3.48: Ejection systolic murmur

Characteristics of Ejection Systolic Murmur

- Timing: Begins after S1 and ends before S2 (mid-systolic).
- Crescendo-decrescendo pattern (increases and then decreases in intensity).
- Best heard over the aortic or pulmonary areas.
- Does not obscure S1 or S2.

Causes (Table 3.41)

TABLE 3.41: Causes of ejection systolic murmurs
Valvular diseases • Aortic stenosis • Pulmonary stenosis • Aortic sclerosis • Hypertrophic cardiomyopathy • Tetralogy of Fallot (pulmonary stenosis)
Flow murmurs (functional murmurs) • Hyperdynamic states (thyrotoxicosis, anemia, AV fistula) • Pregnancy • Increased systolic flow across the valve (ASD, aortic regurgitation, mitral regurgitation)
Miscellaneous • Coarctation of aorta • Straight back syndrome • Aneurysm of ascending aorta

Differential Diagnosis

Aortic Valve Sclerosis

- The murmur is brief and not very loud. It is usually best heard over the right second interspace.
- It is not associated with hemodynamic consequences. Carotid pulse and S2 are normal.

Aortic Stenosis

- Murmur is harsh and best heard in the right second intercostal space. It radiates to carotids especially to right carotid.
- Aortic ejection click sound may be heard.
- It produces hemodynamic consequences such as slow rising pulse and low systolic BP.
- LVH is present and apex is heaving type.
- Systolic thrill at right second intercostal space may be present.
- S2 may be normal, narrowly split or paradoxically split with decreased intensity of A2.

Pulmonary Stenosis

- Murmur is harsh and best heard over the left second interspace. It may radiate to the left side of the neck and is frequently accompanied by a palpable thrill.
- Signs of RVH may be present such as left parasternal heave and prominent epigastric pulsations.
- Pulmonary ejection sound may be heard.
- S2 is widely split with a decreased intensity of P2.

Atrial Septal Defect (ASD)

- ESM is produced due to increased flow across pulmonary valve. Murmur is short and soft. It is heard over pulmonary area.

- S2 is widely split and fixed.
- Mid-diastolic rumble over the tricuspid area due to increased flow across tricuspid valve.
- Pulsation in the pulmonary area due to dilated pulmonary artery.
- Hyperdynamic left parasternal impulse due to volume overload of right ventricle.

Coarctation of Aorta

- Murmur can extend beyond the second heart sound, at the left paravertebral inter-scapular area, due to flow across the narrow coarctation area.
- Continuous murmurs may be due to flow through large collateral vessels.
- Cardiac examination is usually normal. S1 and S2 are usually normal.
- Underdeveloped lower segment of the body.
- Differential pressures between the upper and lower limbs (hypertension in the upper limbs).
- Radiofemoral delay.
- Heaving apical impulse.

Hypertrophic Cardiomyopathy (HCM)

- Murmur is best heard at the apex and left lower sternal border.
- Murmur increases with maneuvers which increase the obstruction. These are standing, Valsalva maneuver, and nitroglycerin. Murmur decreases on sitting or squatting, with handgrip, and following passive elevation of the legs.
- Rapidly rising (jerky) carotid pulse.
- Double apical impulse.

Q. Discuss the causes and differential diagnosis of pansystolic murmur (PSM).

- Pansystolic murmur (holosystolic murmur) is heard throughout the systole. PSM occurs when the blood flows from a chamber whose pressure throughout systole is higher than pressure in the chamber receiving the flow.

Causes of Pansystolic Murmur

- Mitral regurgitation.
- Tricuspid regurgitation.
- Ventricular septal defect.

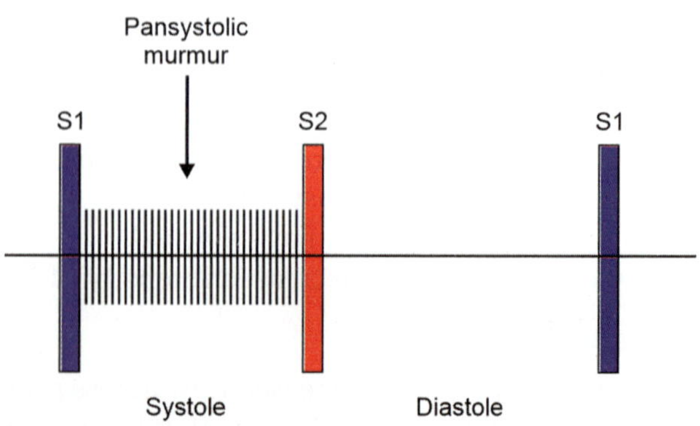

Figure 3.49: Pansystolic murmur

Differential Diagnosis of Pansystolic Murmur

Mitral Regurgitation

Murmur

- Murmur is high pitched, blowing.
- It is best heard at the apex with the diaphragm of the stethoscope with the patient in the left lateral decubitus position.
- It usually radiates to left axilla, and inferior angle of the left scapula.

Associated features

- Apex is shifted out and laterally due to left ventricular enlargement in significant MR. Apex is hyperdynamic in character.
- Systolic thrill at the apex.
- S1 is soft, S2 is widely split but mobile.
- There may be an S3 gallop due to high diastolic flow across the mitral valve.
- Loud P2, parasternal heave and epigastric pulsations due to pulmonary HTN and RVH.
- There may be findings of left heart failure.

Tricuspid Regurgitation

Murmur

- Murmur is best heard with the diaphragm of the stethoscope over the lower left second and third intercostal spaces and along the left sternal border. It may radiate to the epigastrium.
- Intensity of the murmur varies with respiration. It increases during inspiration (Carvallo's sign) due to increase in regurgitant flow following the inspiratory increase in right ventricular volume.

Associated features

- Prominent '*v*' wave and rapid '*y*' descent in the jugular venous pulse.
- Hepatomegaly and systolic hepatic pulsation.
- Right ventricular S3 gallop and a mid-diastolic flow murmur in severe TR.

Ventricular Septal Defect

Murmur

- Murmur is harsh and is best heard along the left sternal border.

Associated features

- High volume collapsing pulse.
- Apex is shifted down and out and is hyperdynamic.
- S2 is normal and pulmonary hypertension is absent.

Q. Discuss the causes and differential diagnosis of early diastolic murmur (EDM).

- An early diastolic murmur (EDM) is a murmur that begins immediately after S2 and gradually decreases in intensity (decrescendo pattern).
- It occurs due to regurgitation of blood from a high-pressure artery (aorta or pulmonary artery) back into the ventricle during diastole.

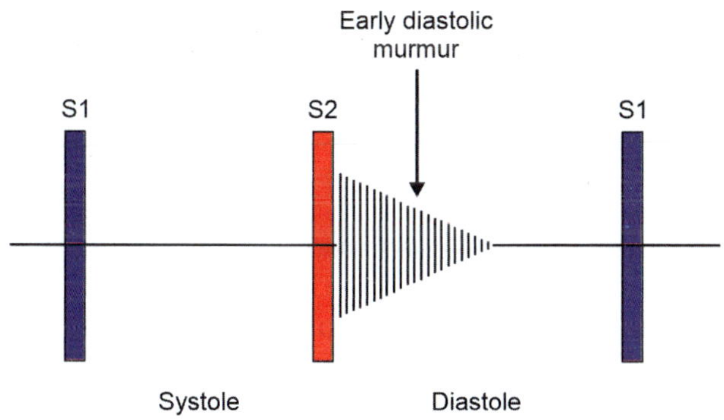

Figure 3.50: Early diastolic murmur

Causes

- Aortic regurgitation.
- Pulmonary regurgitation.

Differential Diagnosis of EDM

Aortic Regurgitation

- Murmur is high-pitched, blowing decrescendo murmur.
- It begins with A2 and usually terminates before S1.
- It is best heard with the diaphragm of the stethoscope over the aortic area or over the left sternal border, with the patient sitting and leaning forward and the breath held in full expiration.
- Murmur radiates towards cardiac apex.
- Apex is hyperdynamic and shifted out and downwards.
- Wide and collapsing pulse.
- Peripheral signs of aortic regurgitation present.

Pulmonary Regurgitation

- The murmur of pulmonary regurgitation due to pulmonary hypertension (Graham-Steell murmur) is high-pitched and "blowing." It is decrescendo type.
- The murmur begins with P2 and is best heard over the left second and third interspaces.
- It may increase in intensity during inspiration.
- P2 is loud.

Q. Discuss the causes and differential diagnosis of mid diastolic murmur (MDM).

- MDM is a low-frequency murmur in mid diastole that results from obstruction to blood flow through stenotic mitral or tricuspid valve or increased blood flow through normal mitral or tricuspid valve **(Fig. 3.51)**.

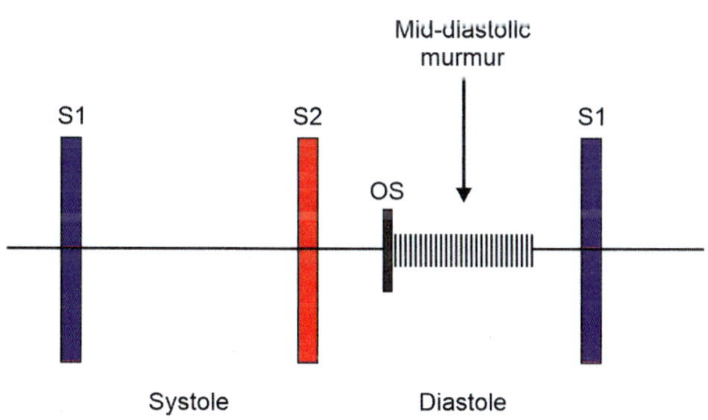

Figure 3.51: Mid-diastolic murmur (MDM) and opening snap (OS)

Causes of Mid-diastolic Murmurs

- Mitral stenosis
- Tricuspid stenosis
- Atrial myxoma
- Austin Flint murmur
- Carey-Coombs murmur
- Increased flow across mitral and tricuspid valves (TR, MR, ASD, VSD, PDA)

Differential Diagnosis

Mitral Stenosis

Murmur

- It is low pitched, rumbling MDM, best heard with the bell of the stethoscope over the apex with the patient in the left lateral decubitus position.
- It starts with an opening snap. Its duration correlates with the severity of mitral stenosis. The longer the duration of the murmur, the more severe is the mitral stenosis.
- Presystolic accentuation (if sinus rhythm is present).

Associated features

- Tapping apex
- Mitral valve opening snap
- Diastolic thrill at the apex
- Loud first heart sound
- Features of pulmonary HTN (parasternal heave, loud P2)
- Presence of atrial fibrillation.

Tricuspid Stenosis

Murmur

- Low-pitched, rumbling, mid-diastolic murmur
- Best heard along the left sternal border
- Intensity of the murmur increases with inspiration (Carvallo's sign).

Associated features

- Peripheral edema and ascites
- Tricuspid opening snap
- Wide splitting of S1 due to delayed closure of the tricuspid valve.
- Presence of atrial fibrillation
- Prominent 'a' wave and slow y descent in the JVP
- Presystolic hepatic pulsation.

Atrial Myxoma

- Atrial myxoma may cause obstruction of the atrio ventricular valves and a mid-diastolic murmur.

Murmur

- Murmur has presystolic accentuation and crescendo character.
- The character and intensity of the murmur may change with position.

Associated features

- A "tumor plop" sound may be present.
- Atrial fibrillation is usually absent.

- No opening snap.
- Systemic features such as fever, fatigue and weight loss may be present.

Austin Flint Murmur

Murmur

- This is an apical diastolic rumbling murmur seen in aortic regurgitation. It is best heard at the apex.

Associated features

- Amyl nitrate inhalation decreases the murmur due to decrease in afterload which decreases aortic regurgitation.
- No opening snap unlike mitral and tricuspid stenosis.
- Peripheral signs of aortic regurgitation present.
- Hyperdynamic apex which is shifted out and downwards.

Carey-Coombs Murmur

Murmur

- This is seen in acute rheumatic fever, due to acute mitral valvulitis.
- Murmur is best heard over the apex.

Associated features

- There may be features of rheumatic fever such as joint pains, erythema marginatum, subcutaneous nodules, etc.

Flow Murmurs

- Mid-diastolic murmurs may occur due to increased flow across the atrioventricular valve even when there is no stenosis. Examples are mitral regurgitation, ASD, VSD, and PDA.

Mitral regurgitation

- Mid-diastolic rumbling murmur is best heard over the apex.
- Hyperdynamic apex, which is shifted down and out.
- Left ventricular S3
- Systolic thrill at the apex
- Soft S1
- Pansystolic murmur best heard over the apex and radiating to axilla.

VSD

- Mid-diastolic rumbling murmur is best heard over the apex.
- Hyperdynamic apex which is shifted down and out.
- Left ventricular S3
- Systolic thrill at the 3rd or 4th left intercostal space.
- Widely split but mobile S2.
- Pansystolic murmur best heard over the 3rd or 4th left intercostal space radiating all over the precordium.

Patent ductus arteriosus (PDA)

- Mid-diastolic rumbling murmur is best heard over the apex.
- Hyperdynamic apex which is shifted down and out.
- Left ventricular S3
- Continuous thrill at the left sternal angle.
- Continuous machinery murmur with late systolic accentuation at the left sternal border.

Tricuspid regurgitation (see differential diagnosis of pansystolic murmurs).

ASD

- Murmur is best heard over the lower left sternal border.
- Visible pulmonary artery pulsations in the left second intercostal space.
- Wide, fixed, splitting of S2.

Q. Define continuous murmur. Enumerate the causes of continuous murmurs.

- **Continuous murmurs** occur throughout the cardiac cycle, spanning **both systole and diastole**, due to a persistent pressure gradient between two chambers or vessels.
- They often indicate abnormal connections between high- and low-pressure systems.

Causes

Patent ductus arteriosus

- Classic "machinery" murmur (Gibson murmur)
- Best heard at left infraclavicular area
- Loudest at S2 and continues into diastole
- Associated with bounding pulses and wide pulse pressure.

Aortopulmonary window

- Abnormal connection between aorta and pulmonary artery.
- Loud continuous murmur at left upper sternal border.
- Often presents with signs of heart failure in infancy.
- Rupture of aneurysm of sinus of Valsalva.

Arteriovenous fistulas

- High-output states due to abnormal artery-vein communication.
- Can be congenital or acquired (e.g. dialysis fistula, trauma, Osler-Weber-Rendu syndrome).
- Murmur over affected site; may have thrill and palpable pulsations.

Pulmonary arteriovenous malformations (AVMs)

- Abnormal shunting between pulmonary artery and vein.
- Continuous murmur over lung fields.
- Associated with hypoxia and clubbing.

Coarctation of aorta

- Continuous murmur over intercostal spaces due to collateral circulation.
- Rib notching seen on chest X-ray.
- Associated with hypertension in upper limbs and weak lower limb pulses.

Mammary souffle

- Soft continuous murmur over breasts.
- Due to increased mammary blood flow in pregnancy.
- Disappears after delivery.

Ruptured sinus of Valsalva aneurysm

- Continuous murmur if rupture creates a shunt between the aorta and right atrium or ventricle.
- Best heard at right sternal border.
- Often presents with acute heart failure symptoms.

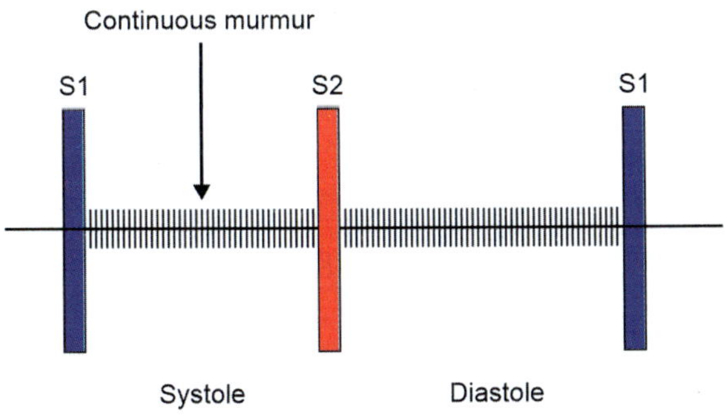

Figure 3.52: Continuous murmur

Q. Define arrhythmia. Classify different types of arrhythmias.

- Arrhythmia refers to any abnormality in the rate, rhythm, or conduction of electrical impulses in the heart.
- Arrhythmias may cause sudden death, syncope, heart failure, dizziness, and palpitations or can be asymptomatic. They can be either transient or sustained.
- Arrhythmia can be classified based on the site of origin (supraventricular or ventricular) and the effect on heart rate (tachyarrhythmias or bradyarrhythmias) **(Table 3.42)**.

TABLE 3.42: Classification of arrhythmias

Based on heart rate
- Bradyarrhythmias: Heart rate <60 per minute
- Tachyarrhythmias: Heart rate >100 per minute

Based on site of origin

Supraventricular arrhythmias (arise above the ventricles)
- Sinus arrhythmias (sinus bradycardia, sinus tachycardia, sick sinus syndrome)
- Atrial arrhythmias (atrial flutter, atrial fibrillation, multifocal atrial tachycardia)
- A-V nodal arrhythmias
  - A-V nodal block: First degree, second degree (Wenckebach), Third degree (complete heart block)
  - Paroxysmal supraventricular tachycardia (PSVT), WPW syndrome

Ventricular
- Ventricular tachycardia
- Ventricular flutter
- Ventricular fibrillation
- Idioventricular rhythms (ventricular escape rhythm)

Q. Sinus arrhythmia.
Q. Sinus bradycardia.
Q. Sick sinus syndrome.

Sinus Arrhythmia

- Fluctuation of autonomic tone due to respiration results in phasic changes of the sinus discharge rate. During inspiration, para-sympathetic tone falls and the heart rate increases, whereas on expiration the heart rate falls. This is known as sinus arrhythmia.
- Sinus arrhythmia is a normal phenomenon and results in a regularly irregular pulse (Note: Irregularly irregular pulse is seen in atrial fibrillation). It is more prominent in children and young adults.
- Loss of sinus arrhythmia is seen in autonomic neuropathies (e.g. due to diabetes) and also in transplanted heart.

Sinus Bradycardia

- A heart rate of less than 60 beats per minute originating in sinus node is called sinus bradycardia. It is usually asymptomatic unless the rate is very slow.

Causes of Sinus Bradycardia (Table 3.43)

TABLE 3.43: Causes of sinus bradycardia

Physiological
- Sleep (due to decreased sympathetic tone)
- Elderly
- Athletes (due to increased vagal tone)

Pathological
- Hypothyroidism
- Cholestatic jaundice
- Raised intracranial pressure
- Myocardial infarction (due to ischemia or infarction of sinus node)
- Hypothermia
- Typhoid fever
- Brucellosis
- Vasovagal syncope
- Severe hypoxia, hypercapnia, acidosis
- Acute hypertension
- Idiopathic
- Drugs (beta blockers)

- Treatment of symptomatic bradycardia includes insertion of temporary pacemaker if there is a reversible cause or permanent pacemaker if the cause is irreversible. Injection of atropine may help temporarily.

Sick Sinus Syndrome

- This refers to episodes of sinus bradycardia, sinoatrial block, or sinus arrest.
- It is caused by idiopathic fibrosis of the sinus node. Other causes are ischemic heart disease, cardiomyopathy, myocarditis and drugs.
- Patient experiences a combination of symptoms (dizziness, confusion, fatigue, and syncope). These symptoms are due to cerebral hypoperfusion and reduced cardiac output.
- Usually, these episodes are intermittent. If the symptoms are recurrent, permanent pace maker insertion is required.

Q. Discuss the etology, clinical features, investigations and management of atrioventricular blocks (heart blocks).

- The specialized cardiac conducting system normally ensures synchronous conduction of each sinus impulse from the atria to the ventricles. Heart block or conduction block may occur at any level in the conducting system. Block in either the AV node or the His bundle results in atrioventricular (AV) block, whereas block lower in the conduction system produces bundle branch block.

Atrioventricular Block

- AV block is defined when some or all impulses are delayed or do not reach the ventricle during normal sinus rhythm or sinus tachycardia.
- Conduction through AV node may be delayed (first degree AV block), intermittent (second-degree AV block) or absent (third-degree AV block).

First-degree AV Block

- This is simple prolongation of the PR interval to more than 0.20 seconds. Here all sinus impulses are conducted to the ventricles but with delay.

Second-degree AV Block (intermittent AV block)

- This occurs when some P waves conduct and others do not. It can be further divided as follows.
- *Mobitz type I block (Wenckebach phenomenon):* Here there is progressive PR interval prolongation until a P wave fails to conduct. Usually it does not progress to complete AV block.
- *Mobitz type II block*: Here the conduction fails suddenly and unexpectedly without a preceding change in PR intervals. It can progress to complete AV block. If the ventricular rate is slow and patient is symptomatic pace maker insertion is necessary.

Third-degree AV Block (complete AV block)

- Here no atrial impulse is conducted to ventricles. Usually there is escape rhythm originating either from bundle of His or ventricles. Atria and ventricles beat independently. Heart rate is usually less than 55 beats/min.
- ECG shows constant P-P and R-R intervals but with complete AV dissociation i, e, atria and ventricles beat independently and there is no relation between P waves and QRS complexes. QRS complexes may be broad if the escape rhythm is originating from ventricles.

Etiology of Atrioventricular Blocks (Table 3.44)

TABLE 3.44: Etiology of atrioventricular blocks

- Fibrosis and sclerosis of the conduction system
- Ischemic heart disease (especially inferior wall MI)
- Drugs (digitalis, calcium channel blockers, beta blockers, amiodarone)
- Increased vagal tone
- Valvular disease
- Congenital heart disease (VSD)
- Cardiomyopathies
- Myocarditis
- Hyperkalemia
- Infiltratve diseases (sarcoidosis, amyloidosis)
- Inflammatory diseases (SLE, scleroderma)

Clinical Features

- First and second degree heart blocks are usually asymptomatic.
- Third degree heart block may present with dizziness, syncope and hemodynamic instability.

Investigations

- Serum electrolytes (sodium, potassium)
- Drug levels (e.g. digoxin)
- ECG
- ECHO
- Electrophysiological testing.

Treatment

- First degree heart block requires no specific treatment other than correcting the underlying cause.
- In symptomatic second and third degree heart blocks, atropine (0.5–2.0 mg intravenously) and isoproterenol (1–4 μg/min intravenously) are useful to temporarily increase the heart rate. Temporary pacemaker insertion may help stabilize the patient if there is a reversible cause such as myocardial ischemia. For long-term treatment permanent pace maker insertion is the treatment of choice.
- Underlying cause should be identified and treated.

Q. Bundle branch blocks.

- The bundle of His divides into right and left bundle branches. The left bundle subdivides into the anterior and posterior divisions. Various conduction disturbances can occur in these bundle branches and are called bundle branch blocks.
- *Right bundle branch block (RBBB)*: Since the right bundle branch supplies right ventricle, its block produces late activation of the right ventricle. This is manifested in ECG as deep S waves in leads I and V6 and tall late R wave in lead V1.
- *Left bundle branch block (LBBB):* This produces delayed activation of left ventricle which is manifested in ECG as deep S wave in lead V1 and a tall late R wave in leads I and V6.

Causes (Table 3.45)

TABLE 3.45: Causes of bundle branch blocks

RBBB

- Congenital heart disease (ASD, Fallot's tetralogy, pulmonary stenosis, VSD)
- Acute myocardial infarction
- Cardiomyopathy
- Conduction system fibrosis
- Cor pulmonale
- Pulmonary embolism

LBBB

- Acute myocardial infarction
- Severe coronary disease (two- to three-vessel disease
- Aortic stenosis
- Hypertension

Clinical Features

- Bundle branch blocks are usually asymptomatic. RBBB produces widely split second heart sound. LBBB may produce reverse splitting of the second sound.

Treatment

- Usually, no treatment is required. LBBB may indicate an underlying coronary artery disease which should be investigated.

Q. Define supraventricular tachycardias. List all supraventricular tachycardias.

- Supraventricular tachycardias (SVTs) are tachyarrhythmias which arise above the ventricle, i.e. from the atrium or the atrioventricular junction.
- Since the conduction is via the His-Purkinje system, QRS shape is normal (narrow QRS complex).
- Following is a list of supraventricular tachycardias.
  - Sinus tachycardia
  - Paroxysmal supraventricular tachycardias (PSVTs) (AV nodal re-entry tachycardia and AV reciprocating tachycardia)
  - Atrial fibrillation
  - Atrial flutter
  - Atrial tachycardia
  - Multifocal atrial tachycardia
  - Accelerated junctional tachycardia

Q. Sinus tachycardia.

- A heart rate of more than 100 beats per minute originating in sinus node is called sinus tachycardia. In the ECG, it is characterized by normal P waves, PR interval and QRS complexes. QRS complexes may be broad if there is intraventricular conduction defect. Sinus tachycardia may be experienced as palpitations.

Causes of Sinus Tachycardia (Table 3.46)

TABLE 3.46: Causes of sinus tachycardia

Physiological (normal response)
• Anxiety, fear
• Exertion
• Fever
• Pregnancy
• Hypoxia
Pathological
• Anemia
• Hypovolemia
• Hypotension
• Heart failure
• Myocardial infarction (MI)
• Pericarditis, myocarditis
• Hyperthyroidism
• Pheochromocytoma
• Sympathomimetic drugs (ephedrine, pseudoephedrine, ß-adrenoceptor agonists)

- Management includes treating the underlying cause or beta blockers.

Q. Pre-excitation syndromes.

Q. Wolff-Parkinson-White (WPW) syndrome.

- Pre-excitation syndromes are due to accessory pathways between the atria and the ventricle that avoid the conduction delay of the AV node. This results in earlier activation (pre-excitation) of the ventricles. Accessory pathways allow the impulses to enter into the ventricles or allow the impulses to travel back to atria thus predisposing to reentrant arrhythmias.

Lown-Ganong-Levine Syndrome

- Due to an accessory pathway (James fiber) that bypasses the AV node but connects the atria to the His bundle, leading to rapid conduction. The QRS complex is normal, since ventricular activation is via the normal conduction pathway (His Purkinje system).

Wolff-Parkinson-White (WPW) Syndrome

- WPW syndrome occurs due to the presence of an accessory pathway (AP), called the Bundle of Kent, which bypasses the AV node, leading to pre-excitation of the ventricles. It is the most common accessory pathway SVT.
- Accessory pathway can be left-sided (Type A WPW) or right-sided (type B WPW). It directly connects the atria to the ventricles, allowing conduction that bypasses the AV node. It conducts impulses faster than the AV node because it lacks the normal conduction delay.
- If the accessory pathway allows bidirectional conduction, a reentrant loop can form between the AV node and the accessory pathway.
- This leads to paroxysmal supraventricular tachycardia (PSVT), specifically AV reentrant tachycardia (AVRT).
- There are types of AVRT; orthodromic AVRT (90%) and antidromic AVRT (10%).
- Orthodromic AVRT: Here, the impulse travels down the AV node → His-Purkinje system → Ventricles → Re-enters via the accessory pathway → Atria. Results in a narrow QRS complex (normal ventricular activation). Appears like supraventricular tachycardia (SVT).
- Antidromic AVRT: Impulse travels down the accessory pathway → Ventricles → Re-enters via AV node → Atria. Produces wide QRS complexes (mimics ventricular tachycardia), because ventricles are not activated through the normal pathway. This type is more dangerous because it can degenerate into ventricular arrhythmias.
- Most patients present during young adulthood or middle age. Typical symptoms are abrupt onset palpitations with abrupt termination with symptoms of hemodynamic compromise (e.g. dyspnea, chest discomfort, light-headedness). Attacks may last only a few seconds or persist for several hours. Heart rate is usually 140–220 beats/minute during palpitations.

Investigations

- ECG
- Electrophysiological studies.

Treatment

- Vagotonic maneuver during SVT.
- Adenosine for emergency management of SVT.
- Verapamil or diltiazem if narrow QRS complex. These drugs increase the refractory period of accessory pathway and reduce conduction rate through it.
- For frequent recurrence, radiofrequency catheter ablation is the procedure of choice.

Q. Paroxysmal supraventricular tachycardia (PSVT).

- Paroxysmal supraventricular tachycardia (PSVT) is a sudden-onset, regular, rapid tachycardia originating above the ventricles (supraventricular).
- PSVT is paroxysmal and recurrent and often seen in young patients with no structural heart disease. Heart rate is usually 150–250 per minute with 1:1 conduction.

Etiology

- PSVT is triggered by a reentry mechanism. This may be induced by premature atrial or ventricular ectopic beats. Other triggers include anxiety, hyperthyroidism and stimulants, including caffeine, drugs, and alcohol.
- It can be idiopathic also or rarely may be associated with congenital heart diseases such as Ebstein's anomaly, atrial septal defect, and Fallot's tetralogy.

Mechanism

- The most common mechanism for paroxysmal supraventricular tachycardia is reentry, which may be initiated or terminated by a fortuitously timed atrial or ventricular ectopic.
- Based on the mechanism there are two types of PSVT; AVNRT and AVRT.
- ***AVNRT (AV nodal reentrant tachycardia):*** This, the most common type, occurs due to dual AV nodal pathways (slow and fast pathways). The impulse loops within the AV node, leading to narrow QRS tachycardia.
- ***AVRT (Atrioventricular reentrant tachycardia):*** This is less common. Here, the reentry is due to due to an accessory pathway between the atria and ventricles, referred to as AV reentrant tachycardia (AVRT). Example is WPW syndrome.

Clinical Features

- It is usually seen in young people. The first presentation is common between ages 12 and 30.
- Attacks may occur spontaneously or may be precipitated by exertion, excess coffee, tea and alcohol.
- Most common symptom of PSVT is rapid regular palpitations, usually with abrupt onset, which can occur spontaneously or precipitated by factors described above. Palpitations are usually terminated by Valsalva maneuvers.
- Other symptoms may include anxiety, dizziness, dyspnea, neck pulsation, chest pain, and weakness.
- Very fast heart rate may compromise cardiac output and cause hypotension and congestive heart failure.
- Polyuria may occur because of release of atrial natriuretic peptide in response to increased atrial pressures during the tachycardia.

ECG

- Rate is usually 150–250 per minute.
- P waves are not visible and are buried within the QRS complex.
- QRS complexes are narrow and occur at regular intervals **(Fig. 3.53)**.

Management

- Patients with hemodynamic instability (e.g. hypotension, pulmonary edema) require emergency cardioversion.
- If the patient is hemodynamically stable, vagal maneuvers, including right carotid massage, Valsalva maneuver, and facial immersion in cold water can be tried. Of these, Valsalva maneuver is the best and often easier for the patient to perform.
- If these maneuvers are not successful, intravenous adenosine (6 mg IV fast bolus) should be tried. If required, a second and third dose of 12 mg can be repeated in 1–2 minutes. Adenosine is very short-acting (half-life <10 s) and causes complete heart block for a fraction of a second and terminates SVT. Side effects of adenosine include bronchospasm, flushing, and chest pain which are transient. It is contraindicated in patients with a history of asthma.

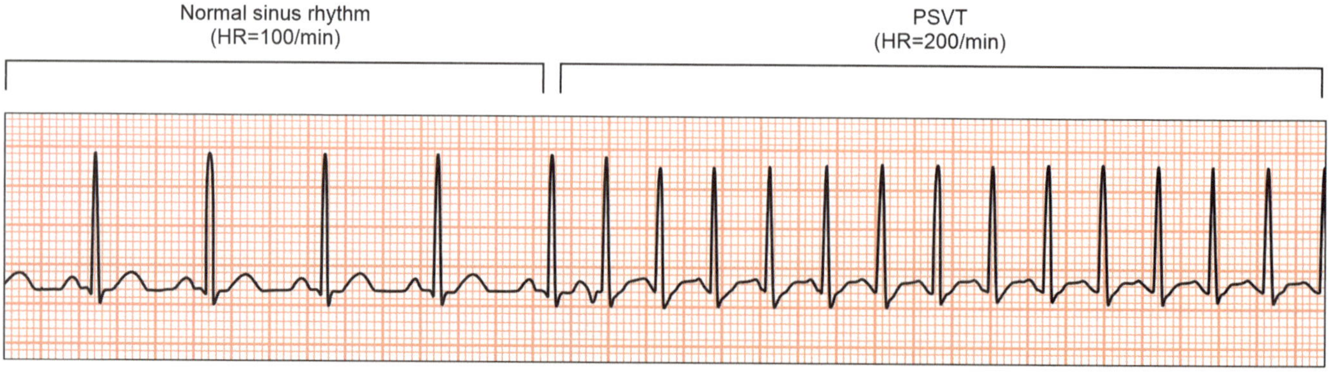

Figure 3.53: Paroxysmal supraventricular tachycardia (PSVT)

- An alternative treatment is verapamil 5–10 mg iv over 5–10 minutes, iv diltiazem, or beta-blockers (esmolol, propranolol, metoprolol).
- Verapamil, diltiazem, beta-blockers or amiodarone can be given to prevent reccurence of SVT.
- Radiofrequency catheter ablation of accessory pathway can cure SVT.

Q. Describe the etiology, clinical features, investigations, and management of atrial fibrillation.

- Atrial fibrillation (AF) is a supraventricular tachyarrhythmia characterized by disorganized atrial electrical activity, leading to loss of coordinated atrial contraction.
- AF is the most common arrhythmia in adults.

Types of AF (Table 3.47)

TABLE 3.47: Types of AF

Type	Features
Paroxysmal AF	Episodes last less than 7 days and terminate spontaneously
Persistent AF	Lasts more than 7 days and may require intervention for termination
Long-standing AF	Lasts more than 1 year and is continuous. Refractory to treatment
Permanent AF	AF persists and is accepted as irreversible. Rate control is the only strategy.

Etiology (Table 3.48)

TABLE 3.48: Etiology of AF

Cardiac causes
• Rheumatic heart disease (especially mitral stenosis or mitral regurgitation) • Coronary artery disease (CAD) • Hypertension • Heart failure • After coronary artery bypass surgery • Cardiomyopathy • Pericardial disease • Pulmonary embolism
Noncardiac causes
• Hyperthyroidism • Alcohol excess ("Holiday heart syndrome") • COPD • Chronic kidney disease • Sepsis/infections • Excessive catecholamine release (stress, stimulants) • Idiopathic (lone atrial fibrillation)

Pathophysiology

- During AF, the atria have disorganized, rapid, irregular electrical activity (300–600 per minute). The ventricular response is also irregular and variable (irregularly irregular).
- There is no coordinated mechanical contraction of atria giving rise to turbulence and stasis of blood in the atria leading to clot formation. With subsequent resumption of atrial contraction, clot can go into left ventricle and then into systemic circulation causing embolism.
- Excessive ventricular rate does not allow proper filling of ventricles, which leads to reduced cardiac output, pulmonary congestion, or angina pectoris.

Clinical Features

Symptoms

- Atrial fibrillation can be asymptomatic and detected incidentally in some patients.
- Patients may complain of anxiety, palpitations, fatigue and dyspnea.
- Chest pain (if CAD is present).
- Patients may also present with stroke due to systemic embolism.

Signs

- Irregularly irregular pulse which is usually 100–150 per minute.
- Varying volume of pulse.
- Apex pulse deficit.
- Loss of 'a' wave in JVP due to absent atrial contraction.
- Variable intensity S1.
- Signs of cardiac failure such as bilateral basal lung crepitations may be there due to fast heart rate.
- There may be features of underlying disease which is responsible for atrial fibrillation.

Complications

- Stroke and thromboembolism—due to atrial blood stasis and clot formation.
- Tachycardia-induced cardiomyopathy—persistent rapid AF can weaken the heart.
- Heart failure—due to tachycardia-induced cardiomyopathy or worsening of pre-existing HF.

Investigations

- ECG shows varying RR intervals. P waves are absent and there may be undulating baseline instead of P waves **(Fig. 3.54)**.
- Echocardioagram can detect underlying condition such as mitral stenosis and atrial dilatation and clot formation.
- Other tests include complete blood count (to identify anemia), thyroid function tests (to identify hyperthyroidism), serum electrolytes (to identify electrolyte imbalance) and chest X-ray (to identify pneumonia, COPD).

Management

- The management of atrial fibrillation (AF) focuses on four key areas:
  - Rate control: Controlling ventricular rate
  - Rhythm control: Restoring sinus rhythm
  - Stroke prevention: Anticoagulation based on risk
  - Management of underlying conditions

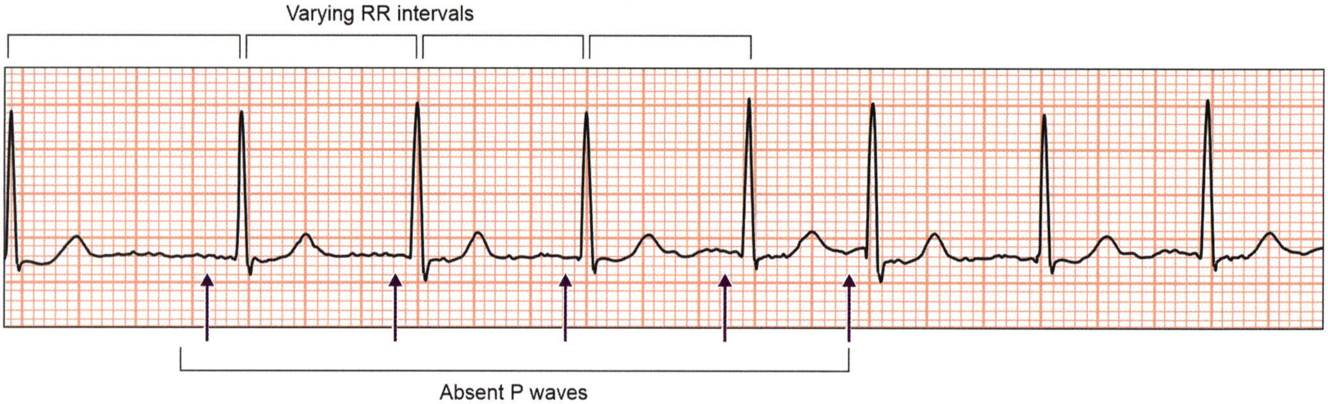

Figure 3.54: ECG showing atrial fibrillation

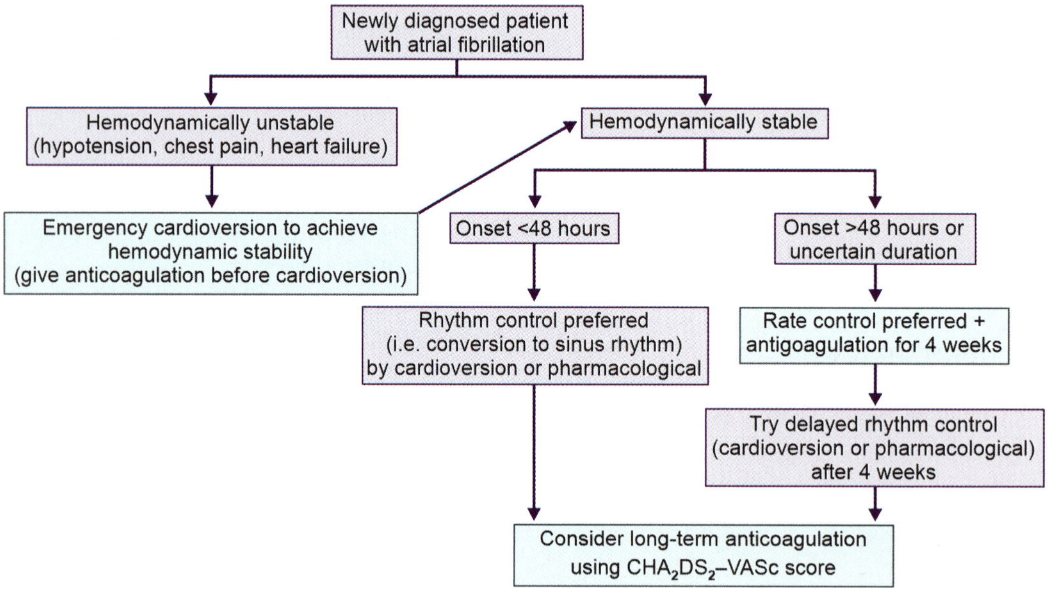

Figure 3.55: Management of atrial fibrillation

- For AF of any duration with hemodynamic instability (as evidenced by hypotension, hypoxia, pulmonary edema, angina), immediate anticoagulation and electrical cardioversion (DC shock with 100–200 joules) is the treatment of choice. If sinus rhythm is not restored, an additional attempt with 360 J is tried. If this also fails, cardioversion may be successful after loading with intravenous ibutilide or intravenous procainamide **(Fig. 3.55)**.
- For hemodynamically stable patients, treatment depends on whether the duration of AF is less than 48 hours or ≥48 hours. If AF duration is less than 48 hours, anticoagulation and cardioversion can be attempted **(Fig. 3.55)**.
- If AF duration is ≥48 hours, cardioversion is risky, because clot formation can occur in the atria, which can be dislodged by cardioversion. For these patients, anticoagulation and rate control (slowing of ventricular rate) should be the initial goal. Ventricular rate control is achieved by intravenous β-blockers (esmolol, metoprolol) and/or calcium-channel blockers (*verapamil* or *diltiazem*). Both prolong the refractory period of the AV node and slow conduction through it. Digoxin is an alternative but is not effective in preventing exercise induced increase in heart rate. After 3 weeks of anticoagulation rhythm control (i.e. conversion to sinus rhythm can be attempted by DC shock or antiarrhythmic drugs (amiodarone, flecainide, or ibutilide). Trans-esophageal echo is the best way to rule out atrial clot for atrial fibrillation of ≥48 hours duration before attempting DC shock.
- If there is a precipitating factor such as alcohol intoxication, fever, thyrotoxicosis, etc. it should be treated.
- Antiarrhythmic drugs are not recommended to maintain sinus rhythm after converting to sinus rhythm, because the risks outweigh the benefits. However, amiodarone can be used in patients with heart failure, moderate-to-severe systolic dysfunction, or hypertension with substantial left ventricular hypertrophy. Most of the recent guidelines favour rate control rather than rhythm control in atrial fibrillation, i.e. no need to convert the AF into sinus rhythm, only the ventricular rate needs to be controlled.
- **Stroke prevention:** Chronic anticoagulation is required for these patients to prevent clot formation.

The need for anticoagulation in patients with nonvalvular AF can be assessed by using CHA_2DS_2-VASc score. Long-term oral anticoagulant therapy is recommended for patients with rheumatic mitral stenosis, mechanical artificial heart valve, and for nonvalvular atrial fibrillation patients with a CHA_2DS_2-VASc score of ≥ 2. Warfarin or other newer oral anticoagulants should be used to maintain INR between 2 and 3.

		Points
C	Congestive heart failure	1
H	Hypertension	1
A	Age (75 or greater)	2
D	Diabetes	1
S	Stroke (prior stroke or TIA)	2
V	Vascular disease (prior heart attack, peripheral artery disease or aortic plaque)	1
A	Age 65–74	1
Sc	Sex category (female)	1

- Patients with poor rate control despite optimal medical therapy should be considered for AV node ablation and pacemaker implantation (*'ablate and pace' strategy*).

Choice of Long-term Therapy

Rhythm control preferred	Rate control preferred
• Younger patients (<65 years) • Symptomatic despite rate control • First episode of AF • Paroxysmal AF • AF secondary to reversible causes (e.g. hyperthyroidism) • Presence of heart failure with reduced EF (HFrEF)	• Older patients (≥65 years) • Minimal symptoms • Long-standing or permanent AF • High risk of stroke • Presence of heart failure with preserved ejection fraction (HFpEF)

Q. Atrial flutter.

- Atrial flutter is an organized atrial rhythm with an atrial rate between 250 and 350 beats per minute.

Etiology

- Causes of atrial flutter are same as atrial fibrillation.

Mechanism

- Atrial flutter is due to impulses traveling through a re-entrant circuit within the right atrium and causing repeated activation of atria. Because of refractoriness of AV node all impulses are not conducted into ventricles. Typically, the ventricular rate is half the atrial rate, i.e. ~150 beats/min because of 2:1 block in the AV node.

Clinical Features

- Patients usually complain of palpitations. Very fast heart rate due to 1:1 AV response may cause angina and hemodynamic instability.

Investigations

- ECG shows regular sawtooth-like atrial flutter waves (F waves) between QRS complexes **(Fig. 3.56)**.
- TSH, Electrolytes: Rule out reversible causes (hyperthyroidism, hypokalemia).
- Holter monitoring: If paroxysmal flutter is suspected.

Management

- Electrical cardioversion is the treatment of choice if the patient is hemodynamically unstable (as evidenced by hypotension, ischemia, or heart failure).
- If atrial flutter duration is more than >48 hours or unknown, patients should be anticoagulated for 4 weeks prior to cardioversion.
- Recurrent attacks may be prevented by antiarrhythmic drugs (amiodarone). In persistent atrial flutter ventricular rate control can be achieved by AV nodal blocking agents (β-blockers and/or calcium channel blockers).
- However, the treatment of choice for patients with recurrent atrial flutter is radiofrequency catheter ablation. Catheter ablation is superior to rate-control and rhythm-control strategies with antiarrhythmic drugs.

Q. Ventricular tachycardia (VT).

- VT is a lifethreatening arrhythmia which originates from the ventricles characterized by a heart rate of ≥100 beats per minute (bpm). Since it does not conduct through the normal conducting system, it is a wide-complex rhythm.

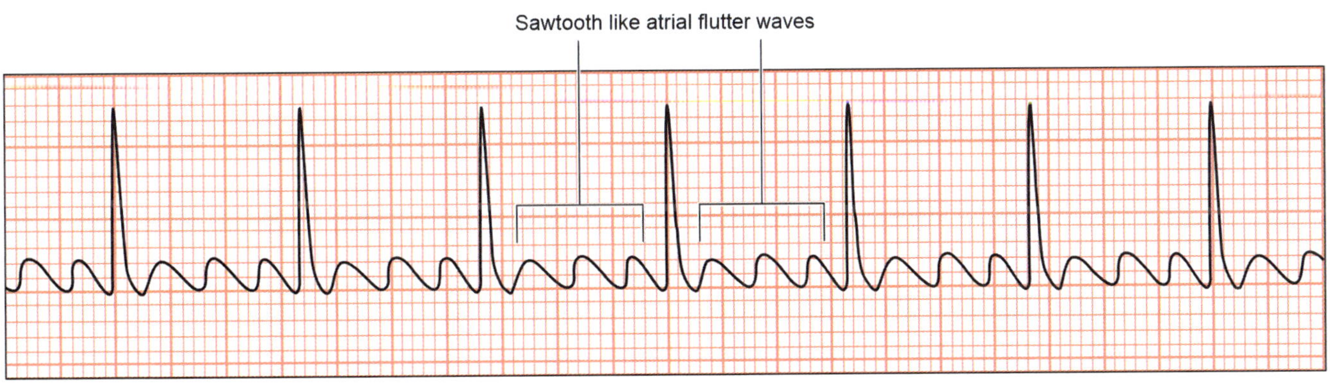

Figure 3.56: ECG showing atrial flutter

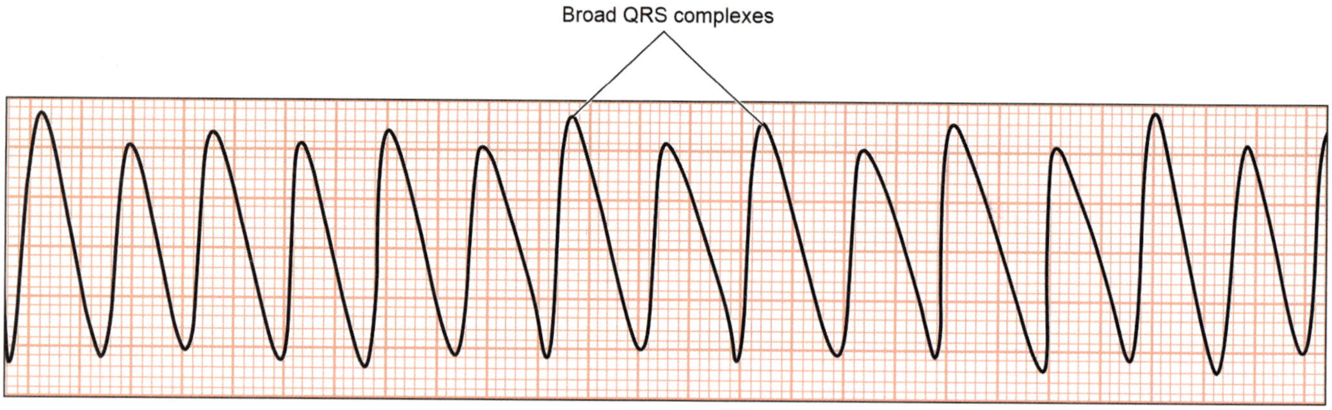

Figure 3.57: ECG showing VT (regular broad complex tachycardia)

- It can be monomorphic (uniform QRS complexes) or polymorphic (QRS morphology varies).
- Sustained VT persists for 30 seconds or more. Sustained polymorphic VT is usually unstable and often degenerates into ventricular fibrillation. Sustained monomorphic VT can also degenerate into ventricular fibrillation but usually stable for long periods.
- Torsades de pointes (TdP) is a polymorphic VT with varying axis. It has a characteristic morphology ("twisting around an axis") and is associated with prolonged QT interval.

Causes (Table 3.49)

TABLE 3.49: Causes of ventricular tachycardia
• Ischemic heart disease
• Dilated cardiomyopathy
• Myocarditis
• Hypertrophic cardiomyopathy
• MVP
• Electrolyte abnormalities (hypokalemia or hypomagnesemia)
• Drugs which prolong QT interval (antiarrhythmics, antipsychotics, macrolides)
• Acid-base disturbance
• Other causes (WPW syndrome, post-cardiac surgery)

Clinical Features

- Palpitations
- Pulse rate is usually between 120 and 220 per min.
- Sustained VT often results in presyncope (dizziness), syncope, hypotension and cardiac arrest.
- Since the atria and ventricles beat independently, there are clinical signs of atrioventricular dissociation (cannon 'a' waves in JVP, and variable intensity of the first heart sound).

Investigations

- *ECG:* It shows a rapid ventricular rhythm with broad QRS complexes. Supraventricular tachycardia with bundle branch block may resemble ventricular tachycardia on the ECG. However, if a broad complex tachycardia is due to SVT with either right or left bundle branch block, then the QRS morphology should resemble a typical RBBB or LBBB pattern. Since most of the cases of broad complex tachycardias are due to ventricular tachycardia, whenever there is a doubt between VT and SVT with aberrant intraventricular conduction, VT should be diagnosed and treated **(Fig. 3.57)**.
- *Serum electrolytes:* Calcium, magnesium, sodium, potassium. Hypokalemia, hypomagnesemia, and hypocalcemia may predispose patients to either monomorphic VT or torsades de pointes.
- *Drug levels,* e.g. digoxin, toxicology screens.
- *Cardiac biomarkers (troponin I or T levels and CK-MB):* To evaluate for myocardial ischemia or infarction.
- *Electrophysiologic study:* It is required in patients at high risk for sudden death as a result of significant underlying structural heart disease.

Treatment

- If the patient is hemodynamically unstable (syncope, hypotension, pulmonary edema, angina), emergency cardioversion is required.
- If hemodynamically stable, intravenous amiodarone or lidocaine can be used to terminate VT. First-line treatment consists of amiodarone (150 mg over 10 minutes, followed by 1mg/min over the next 6 hours, then 0.5 mg/min over 18 hours) or lidocaine (50–100 mg iv over 5 minutes) followed by a lidocaine infusion (2–4 mg iv per minute). Cardioversion is necessary if medical therapy is unsuccessful.
- After resuscitation from VT, the cause of VT should be looked into and treated.
- In the absence of a transient or reversible cause, patients who have had an episode of sustained VT typically require an ICD (implantable cardioverter defibrillator) to prevent further attacks. Most patients with sustained VT and a significant structural heart disorder should also receive a beta-blocker. If an ICD cannot be used, amiodarone can be used to prevent further attacks.
- Magnesium sulfate (if torsades de pointes).

Q. Torsades de pointes (TdP).

- Torsades de pointes refers to ventricular tachycardia (VT) characterized by polymorphic QRS complexes that change in amplitude and cycle length, giving the appearance of oscillations around the baseline **(Fig. 3.58)**.

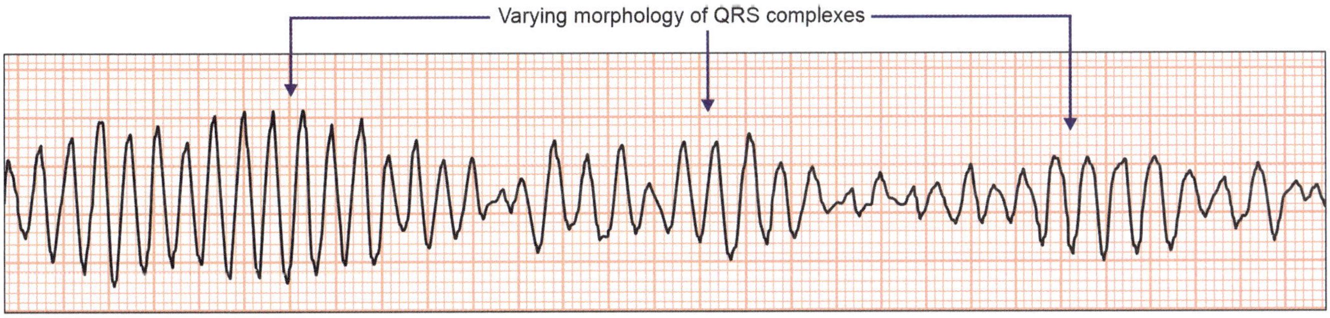

Figure 3.58: Torsades de pointes

Causes

- It arises when ventricular repolarization (QT interval) is prolonged. The causes of torsades de pointes thus include causes of long QT syndrome which are as follows.
- ***Electrolyte disturbances***: Hypokalemia, hypocalcemia and hypomagnesemia.
- ***Drugs:*** Phenothiazines, tricyclic antidepressants, digoxin, quinidine, disopyramide, sotalol, amiodarone, macrolide antibiotics, fluoroquinolones and organophosphates.
- ***Bradycardia and AV block:*** TdP is more likely in patients with sinus bradycardia or heart block, as slow heart rates further prolong the QT interval.
- ***Structural and ischemic heart disease:*** Myocardial infarction, heart failure.
- ***Congenital syndromes:*** Jervell-Lange-Nielsen and Romano-Ward syndrome.
- ***Miscellaneous:*** Bradycardia, acute myocardial infarction, liquid protein diets, dystrophia myotonica, intracranial events.
- Torsades de pointes can be precipitated by increased adrenergic drive (exertion or emotion), sudden arousal (e.g. being woken from sleep by an alarm) or it can occur even when asleep.
- In acquired long QT syndrome, QT prolongation and torsades de pointes are usually provoked by bradycardia.

Investigations

Electrocardiogram (ECG)

- QT interval prolongation in the baseline ECG.
- Polymorphic VT with a sinusoidal "twisting" QRS pattern.
- Changing QRS axis every few beats.
- Pause dependent onset: Typically follows a premature ventricular contraction (PVC).

Other Investigations

- Are same as that of VT.

Clinical Features

- Torsades de pointes causes palpitations and syncope but usually terminates spontaneously.
- It can degenerate to ventricular fibrillation and cause sudden death.

Treatment

Acute Management

- Defibrillation should be done for hemodynamically unstable (hypotension or cardiac arrest) Torsades de Pointes.
- Magnesium sulfate is the drug of choice for Torsades de pointes. Magnesium is given at 1–2 g IV initially over 15 minutes, which can be followed by an infusion. Magnesium sulfate is effective even in patients with normal magnesium levels.
- Any underlying precipitating factor should be addressed, i.e. correcting any electrolyte imbalances, and stopping drugs causing prolonged QT interval.
- Temporary transvenous pacing: based on the fact that the QT interval shortens with a faster heart rate, pacing can be effective in terminating torsade.

Long-term Management

- For congenital prolonged QT interval syndrome, β-adrenergic blocking agents and drugs which shorten QT interval (phenytoin) are useful.
- ICDs with dual-chambered pacing capability have become the treatment of choice for patients with recurrent episodes in spite of using beta blockers.

Q. Ventricular fibrillation (VF).

- Ventricular fibrillation (VF) is a life-threatening arrhythmia characterized by disorganized, rapid, and chaotic electrical activity of the ventricles, leading to loss of coordinated contraction and cardiac output.
- If untreated, VF rapidly leads to sudden cardiac death (SCD).

Causes

Coronary artery disease (most common cause)
• Acute myocardial infarction (STEMI, NSTEMI) → Ischemia leads to re-entry circuits • Previous MI with scar tissue → Causes electrical instability
Structural heart diseases
• Heart failure (dilated cardiomyopathy, HFrEF) • Hypertrophic cardiomyopathy (HCM) • Arrhythmogenic right ventricular cardiomyopathy (ARVC)
Primary electrical disorders (without structural heart disease)
• Long QT syndrome (LQTS) → Torsades de Pointes → VF • Brugada syndrome

(Contd.)

(Contd.)

Metabolic and electrolyte abnormalities
- Severe hypokalemia, hyperkalemia
- Hypocalcemia, hypomagnesemia
- Acidosis (DKA, sepsis, lactic acidosis)
- Drug and toxin-induced VF
- Class I and III antiarrhythmics (flecainide, sotalol, amiodarone overdose)
- QT-prolonging drugs (antipsychotics, antibiotics, antidepressants)
- Cocaine, methamphetamine (sympathomimetic toxins)

Other causes
- Electrocution/Lightning strike
- Commotio cordis (blunt chest trauma at T-wave peak)

Clinical Features

- The patient is pulseless and becomes rapidly unconscious, and respiration ceases (cardiac arrest).
- ECG shows shapeless, rapid oscillations without any organized complexes.

ECG Findings

- Chaotic, irregular, fibrillatory waves
- No P waves, QRS complexes, or T waves
- Amplitude may decrease over time ("coarse" → "fine" VF) **(Fig. 3.59)**.

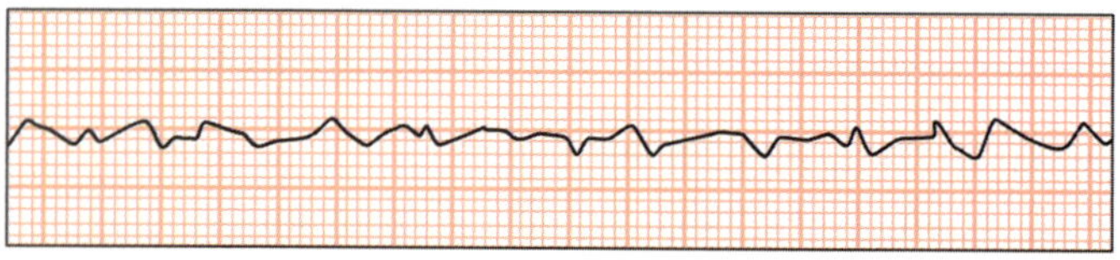

Figure 3.59: Ventricular fibrillation

Treatment

- VF usually ends in death within minutes unless prompt corrective measures are instituted. The rate of survival in out-of-hospital cardiac arrest has increased with expansion of community-based emergency rescue systems, widespread use of automated external defibrillators (AEDs), and increasing numbers of laypersons trained in bystander cardiopulmonary resuscitation (CPR).
- VF rarely reverses spontaneously and requires immediate electrical defibrillation. Basic and advanced cardiac life support is needed.
- If ventricular fibrillation occurs after acute myocardial infarction, it usually does not require any prophylactic therapy to prevent future attacks. However, if the VF has occurred spontaneously without any cause, such patients are at high risk of sudden death and require implantable cardioverter defibrillators (ICDs) to prevent further attacks.

Q. Define ectopic beats (extrasystoles; premature beats). What are the types of ectopic beats?

Q. Supraventricular ectopics (atrial ectopics; atrial premature beats).

Q. Ventricular premature beats (ventricular ectopics, ventricular premature complexes, VPCs).

- A heart beat occurring as a result of an impulse arising in an area other than SA node is called ectopic beat.
- Types—ectopic beats can be classified based on the area from which they arise: atrial, junctional, and ventricular.

Atrial Ectopics

- Atrial ectopic also known as atrial premature beat (APB) or premature atrial contractions (PACs), is a premature activation of the atria arising from a site other than the sinus node.

Etiology

- Idiopathic.
- Mitral valve prolapse (MVP).
- IHD.
- Valvular heart disease (mitral stenosis).
- Hypertrophic cardiomyopathy.
- Smoking, alcohol and excess coffee.

Clinical Features

- Atrial ectopics may be asymptomatic or cause symptoms such as a sensation of "skipping" or palpitations.
- Atrial ectopics are usually benign but rarely may cause atrial fibrillation and ventricular arrhythmias.

ECG

- Atrial ectopic appears as a P wave that occurs relatively early before the next expected sinus P wave, which has a different morphology from the sinus P wave.
- PR interval may be shorter or longer depending on the site of origin of the atrial ectopic.

Treatment

- Treat the underlying cause
- Asymptomatic patients do not require any treatment
- Symptomatic patients with frequent atrial ectopics may benefit from beta-blockers.

Junctional Ectopics

- These arise within the AV junction. They may conduct both anterograde to the ventricles and retrograde to the atrium, or may demonstrate anterograde and/or retrograde conduction block.

Causes

- Idiopathic
- Hypokalemia
- Digitalis toxicity
- Chronic lung disease
- Acute myocardial infarction.

Clinical Features

- They can be asymptomatic or lead to symptoms such as palpitations and missed beats.

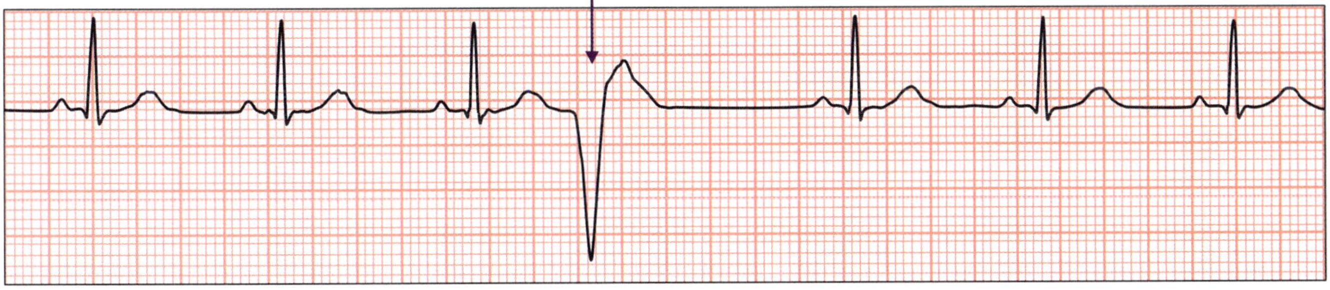

Figure 3.60: Ventricular ectopic

ECG

- Junctional ectopics appear as premature beat with a normal QRS complex.
- PR interval of the junctional ectopic is short. P wave is inverted in ECG leads II, II, aVF due to retrograde activation of atria. Sometimes, P wave may not appear on ECG due to burial of the wave within the QRS complex or lack of retrograde atrial activation.

Treatment

- Treat the underlying cause.
- Asymptomatic patients do not require nay treatment.
- Symptomatic patients may benefit from beta-blockers and calcium channel blockers.

Ventricular Ectopics

- Also known as premature ventricular contractions (PVCS) or ventricular premature complexes (VPC), or ventricular premature beat. These arise from the ventricle and are one of the most common arrhythmias seen.
- Two consecutive PVCs are termed a *couplet*.
- Three or more consecutive PVCs at a rate of 100 beats per minute or more are termed *ventricular tachycardia* (VT).
- Single PVCs may occur sporadically or as bigeminy (every other beat is a PVC), trigeminy (every third beat is a PVC), or higher order periodicities.
- In normal persons, PVCs are not associated with any increase in mortality and morbidity. However, in patients with MI, if frequent (>10 per hour) or complex VPCs (couplets) occur, they are associated with increased mortality.

Etiology

- Idiopathic
- Myocardial infarction
- Drug toxicity (e.g. digitalis intoxication)
- Electrolyte disturbances (e.g. hypokalemia)
- Coronary artery disease
- Heart failure
- Hypertension
- Valvular heart disease.

Clinical Features

- Can be asymptomatic.
- Patient may complain of extra beats, missed beats or heavy beats because it may be the premature beat, the post-ectopic pause or the next forceful sinus beat that is noticed by the patient.
- The pulse is irregular due to premature beats. When a premature beat occurs regularly after every normal beat, 'pulsus bigeminus' occurs.

ECG

- Ventricular ectopics have a broad (> 0.12 s) and bizarre QRS complex, not preceded by P waves because the impulse arises from an abnormal (ectopic) site in the ventricle and travels through abnormal path (does not travel through normal conducting pathway such as Purkinje fibers). It is oriented in opposite direction to other normal QRS complexes **(Fig. 3.60)**.
- Following a premature beat there is usually a complete compensatory pause because the AV node or ventricle is refractory to the next sinus impulse.
- If the VPC comes early ('R on-T' ventricular premature beat occurring simultaneously with the upstroke or peak of the T wave of the previous beat), it may induce ventricular fibrillation in patients with heart disease, particularly in patients following myocardial infarction.

Treatment

- No treatment required for asymptomatic patients.
- Symptomatic patients are treated with beta-blockers or amiodarone.
- Underlying cause should be treated.

Q. Brugada syndrome.

- Brugada syndrome is a genetic disease that predisposes patients to fatal cardiac arrhythmias such as ventricular fibrillation and sudden cardiac death.
- It is an autosomal dominant condition caused by mutations affecting cardiac ion channels, particularly the SCN5A gene, which encodes the cardiac sodium channel.It is common in young males (mean age 30 to 40 years) in South East Asia.

Clinical Presentation

- Often asymptomatic until sudden cardiac arrest. It can present as sudden death or ventricular fibrillation.

- Syncope or near-syncope (due to polymorphic VT/VF).
- Palpitations (due to ectopic beats or non-sustained VT).
- Family history of sudden cardiac death (often in young males <40 years).

ECG Changes

- Classic ECG changes are right bundle branch block with coved ST segment elevation in right precordial leads (V1–V3). These ECG changes may be present spontaneously or provoked by the administration of sodium channel blockers (flecainide or amiodarone). The QT interval is normal.

Treatment

- The only successful treatment is an implantable cardioverter defibrillator (ICD). However, quinidine can be used if ICD insertion is not feasible.

Q. Classify antiarrhythmic drugs with appropriate examples.

- Antiarrhythmic drugs are agents that modify the rhythm and conduction of the heart and are used to treat cardiac arrhythmias.
- However, these drugs can also produce arrhythmias (proarrhythmia) and hence have to be used with caution.
- They are classified based on their mechanism of action as follows.

Classification of Antiarrhythmic Drugs (Table 3.50)

TABLE 3.50: Classification of antiarrhythmic drugs

	Mechanism of action	Examples
Class I	These drugs reduce maximal velocity of depolarization (V_{max}) by blocking Na^+ channels	
IA	↓ V_{max} and prolong action potential duration	Quinidine, procainamide, disopyramide
IB	↓ V_{max} and decrease action potential duration.	Lidocaine, phenytoin, tocainide, mexiletine
IC	↓ V_{max} at normal rates in normal tissue. No change in action potential duration	Flecainide, propafenone, moricizine
Class II	Beta blockers. ↓ SA nodal automaticity, ↑ AV nodal refractoriness, and ↓ AV nodal conduction velocity	Metoprolol, atenolol, bisoprolol, carvedilol and acebutalol
Class III	These drugs prolong action potential duration in tissue with fast-response action potentials	Bretylium, amiodarone, sotalol, ibutilide, dofetilide
Class IV	Calcium (slow) channel blocking agents: ↓ conduction velocity and ↑ refractoriness in tissue with slow-response action potentials	Verapamil, diltiazem

Class I Drugs

- These drugs reduce the excitability of membrane by reducing the rate of entry of sodium into the cell (sodium-channel blockers). They may slow conduction, delay recovery, or reduce the spontaneous discharge rate of myocardial cells.
- Class I agents have been found to increase mortality compared to placebo in postmyocardial infarction patients with ventricular ectopy and in patients treated for atrial fibrillation. In view of this, class I drugs should be avoided in patients with coronary artery disease, left ventricular dysfunction, or other forms of significant structural heart disease.

Class II Drugs

- These are antisympathetic drugs and prevent the effects of catecholamines on the action potential. Most are cardioselective beta-blockers and include metoprolol, atenolol and acebutalol.
- Beta-blockers suppress AV node conduction, and are effective in preventing attacks of junctional tachycardia, and are useful to control ventricular rates in supraventricular tachycardia and atrial fibrillation. They prevent ventricular fibrillation in myocardial infarction and congestive heart failure.

Class III Drugs

- These prolong the action potential and do not affect sodium transport through the membrane. Important drugs in this class are amiodarone and sotalol. Sotalol is also a beta-blocker.
- Amiodarone is the most commonly used drug. It can be used to treat atrial fibrillation, SVT, and ectopic beats. Sotalol may result in acquired long QT syndrome and torsades de pointes. Dofetilide has been used to treat atrial fibrillation and flutter in patients with recent myocardial infarction and poor LV function.

Class IV Drugs

- The nondihydropyridine calcium antagonists decrease conduction velocity and increase refractoriness in tissue with slow-response action potentials and are particularly effective in slowing conduction in nodal tissue.
- These drugs can prevent attacks of junctional tachycardia (AVNRT and AVRT) and may help to control ventricular rates during atrial fibrillation.

Q. Implantable cardioverter-defibrillator (ICD)

- ICD is a lifesaving device that continuously monitors heart rhythm and delivers electrical shocks to terminate life-threatening arrhythmias, such as ventricular tachycardia (VT) and ventricular fibrillation (VF), thereby preventing sudden cardiac death (SCD).
- Life-threatening arrhythmias can cause sudden death in up to 40% of patients within 1 year of diagnosis.
- Modern ICDs are only a little larger than a pacemaker and are implanted in the infraclavicular area. The ICD

recognizes ventricular tachycardia or fibrillation and automatically delivers pacing or a shock to the heart to cause cardioversion to sinus rhythm. The device may have leads to sense and pace both the right atrium and ventricle, and the lithium batteries employed are able to provide energy for over 100 shocks each of around 30 J.

- The use of ICD has reduced the death rate to 2% per year in patients with history of serious ventricular arrhythmias or cardiac failure. Many trials have shown the superiority of ICDs in preventing sudden cardiac death compared to revascularization, antiarrhythmics, beta-blockers, and angiotensin-converting enzyme inhibitors.
- ICD discharges are painful if the patient is conscious. However, ventricular tachycardia may often be terminated by overdrive pacing of the heart, which is painless.
- ICDs are now first-line therapy in the secondary prevention of sudden death. Even selected patients at high risk of sudden death who have never experienced a life-threatening ventricular arrhythmia are also advised to undergo ICD implantation.
- Following are general indications for ICD insertion.

- Spontaneous sustained VT in association with structural heart disease.
- Nonsustained VT in patients with coronary disease, prior myocardial infarction, LV dysfunction, and inducible VT or sustained VT at electrophysiological study
- Dilated and hypertrophic cardiomyopathy
- Long QT syndrome
- Brugada syndrome
- Arrhythmogenic Right Ventricular Cardiomyopathy (ARVC)

Q. Describe the etiology, pathophysiology, clinical features, and management of pulmonary hypertension.

Definition

- Pulmonary hypertension is defined as a mean pulmonary artery pressure of **≥20 mm Hg at rest** (earlier the cutoff was ≥25 mm Hg).

Etiology

- Causes of pulmonary HTN can be grouped into 5 groups as per WHO.

Group 1—Pulmonary arterial hypertension (PAH)
- Idiopathic
- Heritable PAH
- Drug/toxin induced (e.g. anorexigens, methamphetamines)
- Associated with diseases (e.g. connective tissue diseases, HIV, congenital heart disease, portal hypertension, schistosomiasis)

Group 2—PH associated with left heart disease
- Heart failure with preserved/reduced ejection fraction (HFpEF, HFrEF)
- Valvular heart diseases (mitral/aortic stenosis or regurgitation)

(Contd.)

(Contd.)

Group 3—PH associated with lung diseases and/or hypoxia
- COPD
- Interstitial lung diseases (ILDs)
- Other parenchymal lung diseases (bronchiectasis, bilateral fibrocavity)
- Pneumonectomy
- Obstructive sleep apnea (OSA)
- High-altitude exposure

Group 4—PH associated with pulmonary artery obstructions
- Chronic thromboembolic PH
- Other pulmonary artery obstructions (angiosarcoma)

Group 5—PH due to unclear and/or multifactorial mechanisms
- Hematological disorders (hemolytic anemia, myeloproliferative disorders)
- Sarcoidosis
- Metabolic disorders (e.g. glycogen storage diseases)
- Chronic kidney failure with or without hemodialysis

Pathophysiology

- Pulmonary HTN leads to right ventricular hypertrophy and right heart failure. Right ventricular failure leads to peripheral edema. Right ventricular dilatation leads tricuspid annular dilatation leading to functional TR.

Clinical Features

Symptoms

- Patients usually present with exertional dyspnea (commonest symptom), chest pain, syncope and fatigue.
- Exertional dyspnea, fatigue and syncope are due to the inability of the heart to increase cardiac output because of decreased blood flow from right to left side of the heart. Chest pain may be due to right ventricular ischemia.
- Hemoptysis can occur due to rupture of distended pulmonary vessels.
- In addition, there can be symptoms of underlying disease causing pulmonary HTN.

Signs

- JVP is raised with a prominent 'a' wave.
- A right ventricular (parasternal) heave is present, and a loud P2 is heard.
- Other findings include a right ventricular fourth heart sound, and an early diastolic murmur due to pulmonary regurgitation (*Graham Steell murmur*). This murmur is heard over the second and third left intercostal spaces, close to the sternum.
- Tricuspid regurgitation may develop and indicates right ventricular failure. If TR develops, there is a pansystolic murmur and a large jugular '*v*' wave.
- Features of right ventricular failure such as ascites, peripheral edema and hepatomegaly may be present.

Investigations

- ***Chest X-ray:*** It may show right ventricular and right atrial enlargement. Pulmonary arteries are enlarged and taper rapidly. There is peripheral pruning of pulmonary arteries. Peripheral lung fields are oligemic. X-ray may also show the underlying disease causing pulmonary HTN.

- *ECG:* It demonstrates right ventricular hypertrophy (right axis deviation, dominant R wave in lead V1, and inverted T waves in right precordial leads) and right atrial enlargement (tall peaked P waves in lead II).
- *Echocardiography:* It shows right ventricular dilatation and/or hypertrophy, reduction in left ventricular (LV) cavity size, and tricuspid regurgitation. Echocardiogram may also reveal the cause of pulmonary hypertension, such as mitral stenosis or an intracardiac shunt.
- *HRCT (high-resolution CT) scan of lung:* Useful to rule out interstitial and other parenchymal lung disease.
- *Pulmonary function tests:* Are helpful in documenting underlying obstructive airway disease or severe restrictive lung disease.
- *Ventilation/perfusion (V/Q) scan:* Gold standard for detecting chronic thromboembolic pulmonary hypertension.
- *Other investigations:* Hypoxemia and an abnormal diffusing capacity for carbon monoxide are common findings of pulmonary hypertension. ANA to identify connective tissue diseases and HIV testing should be done in unexplained pulmonary HTN. Sleep studies are helpful to rule out obstructive sleep apnea.

Treatment

Treatment of the underlying cause

- Wherever possible, underlying cause should be identified and treated. For example, if pulmonary HTN is due to mitral valve disease, it should be corrected.

General Measures

- Patients should avoid strenuous exercise since it increases pulmonary HTN dramatically. Digoxin and diuretics are useful if there is right heart failure causing peripheral edema and ascites. Oxygen supplementation helps to decrease dyspnea and improves pulmonary hypertension.

Anticoagulant Therapy (e.g. warfarin)

- This is indicated for patients with primary pulmonary hypertension (PPH) because thrombin deposition occurs in the pulmonary circulation and serves as a growth factor to promote the disease process.

Calcium Channel Blockers

- These drugs are useful for patients who have reversible vasoconstriction of pulmonary vasculature (reversibility can be identified by cardiac catheterization and injecting short-acting vasodilators). High doses of calcium channel blockers are required (e.g. nifedipine, 240 mg/day, or amlodipine, 20 mg/day).

Prostaglandins

- Epoprostenol (prostacyclin) and treprostinil (an analogue of epoprostenol) are useful in treating patients who are unresponsive to other therapies. Clinical trials have demonstrated improvement in symptoms, exercise tolerance, and survival with these drugs. Epoprostenol can only be administered intravenously and requires placement of a permanent central venous catheter and infusion through an ambulatory infusion pump system. Treprostinil can be administered subcutaneously through a small infusion pump.

Endothelin Receptor Antagonists

- Endothelin receptor antagonists such as ambrisentan, bosentan, and macitentan bind to endothelin and inhibit vasoconstriction caused by endothelin. These drugs can cause increase in liver enzymes, hence liver function should be monitored monthly throughout the duration of use.

Phosphodiesterase 5 (PDE-5) Inhibitors (tadalafil, sildenafil, vardenafil)

- These drugs have vasodilator action. They dilate pulmonary arteries and lower pulmonary vascular pressure.

Soluble Guanylate Cyclase (sGC) Stimulators

- Riociguat (for PAH and CTEPH).

Atrial Septostomy

- Creates right-to-left shunting to decompress the right heart.

Lung Transplantation

- This is considered in patients who remain symptomatic inspite of all the above treatments. Acceptable results have been achieved with heart-lung, bilateral lung, and single lung transplant.

Q. Describe the etiology, clinical features, diagnosis, complications and management of deep vein thrombosis (venous thrombosis).

Q. Prophylaxis for deep vein thrombosis (DVT).

- Thrombus formation within deep veins, especially of the lower limbs is termed deep venous thrombosis (DVT).
- The presence of thrombus within a superficial vein and the accompanying inflammatory response in the vessel wall is termed *thrombophlebitis*.

Common Sites of DVT

- Deep venous system of lower limbs (most cases of pulmonary embolism are due to this).
- Pelvic veins.

Etiology (risk factors)

- Virchow described three factors (Virchow triad) in the causation of venous thrombosis. These are (**Table 3.51**):
  1. Stasis of blood
  2. Endothelial injury
  3. Hypercoagulable state
- Any one or more of the above factors may be present in DVT.

TABLE 3.51: Risk factors for DVT

Stasis of blood
• Prolonged travel
• Prolonged immobilization (due to surgery, fractures, stroke, illness)
• Congestive heart failure
• Obesity
Endothelial injury
• Presence of a central venous catheter
• Surgery
• Trauma
• Cigarette smoking
Hypercoagulable state
Inherited
• Factor V Leiden mutation
• Prothrombin gene mutation
• Protein S deficiency
• Protein C deficiency
• Antithrombin (AT) deficiency
• Dysfibrinogenemia
Acquired
• Dehydration
• Drugs (Oral contraceptives, steroids, tamoxifen)
• Pregnancy
• Postmenopausal hormone replacement
• Antiphospholipid antibody syndrome
• Cancer
• Chronic obstructive pulmonary disease (because of hypoxia induced polycythemia)
• Hyperhomocysteinemia
• Myeloproliferative disorders (essential thrombocytosis, Polycythemia vera)
• Paroxysmal nocturnal hemoglobinuria
• Inflammatory bowel disease
• Nephrotic syndrome
• Hyperviscosity (Waldenstrom's macroglobulinemia, multiple myeloma, leukocytosis in acute leukemia, sickle cell anemia)

Clinical Features

- DVT may be asymptomatic in 50% of cases.
- Classic symptoms of DVT include swelling, pain, and discoloration in the involved limb. Superficial veins are dilated. Affected limb is usually warm.
- Thrombosed vein may be palpable as a cord.
- There may be pain and tenderness along the course of the affected vein.
- There may be pain in the calf on forceful dorsiflexion of the foot (Homan's sign).
- There may be pain on squeezing the calf muscles (Moses sign).
- In advanced cases, there may be cyanosis and venous gangrene in the affected limb.
- Patient may present with pulmonary embolism symptoms such as sudden dyspnea, pleuritic chest pain, hemoptysis (coughing up blood), tachycardia, hypotension (if massive embolism)

Wells Clinical Prediction Guide for Diagnosis of DVT (Table 3.52)

TABLE 3.52: Wells clinical prediction guide for diagnosis of DVT

Clinical variable	Score
• Active cancer	1
• Paralysis, paresis, or recent cast	1
• Bedridden for >3 days; major surgery <12 weeks	1
• Tenderness along distribution of deep veins	1
• Entire leg swollen	1
• Unilateral calf swelling >3 cm	1
• Pitting edema	1
• Collateral superficial nonvaricose veins	1
• Alternative diagnosis at least as likely as DVT	–2

Low probability = score ≤0, moderate probability = score 1 or 2, high probability = ≥3

Diagnosis of DVT

D-dimer

- D-dimer levels are elevated in DVT (more than 500 ng/ml in most patients with DVT). It is a breakdown product of fibrin and is present whenever clot formation occurs. It is more elevated in pulmonary embolism than DVT because the clot is bigger in pulmonary embolism.
- D-dimer is a useful "rule out" test. A negative D-dimer test almost rules out DVT, but a positive test has to be further investigated by Doppler ultrasonography.
- The D-dimer assay is not specific to DVT. Levels can also increase in patients with myocardial infarction, pneumonia, sepsis, cancer, the postoperative state, and second or third trimester of pregnancy.

Venous Doppler Ultrasonography

- Loss of vein compressibility with gentle manual pressure from the ultrasound transducer suggests thrombosis. Loss of compressibility is due to passive distension by thrombus.
- Thrombus may appear as homogeneous and low echogenicity mass. The vein itself often appears mildly dilated, and collateral channels may be absent.
- Other features of DVT are loss of augmentation of flow on compression and loss of normal respiratory variation. If ultrasound is inconclusive, CT or magnetic resonance imaging of veins may help.

Magnetic Resonance (MR) (Contrast-enhanced)

- When ultrasound is equivocal, MR venography is an excellent imaging modality to diagnose DVT.

Contrast Venography

- This is a **gold standard test**, but **rarely used** now because of availability of Doppler ultrasound and MR venography.

Treatment of DVT

- The objectives of DVT treatment are—prevention of further clot extension, prevention of acute pulmonary embolism, reduction of recurrent thrombosis, reduction of late complications such as postphlebitic syndrome, chronic venous insufficiency, and pulmonary hypertension.

Anticoagulant Therapy

- Anticoagulation is the main treatment for DVT.
- *Oral anticoagulation*—for most patients with DVT, direct oral anticoagulants (DOACs) are the first-choice therapy. These are rivaroxaban, apixaban, dabigatran, edoxaban, betrixaban which can be used instead. Onset of action is within few hours and hence there is no need to use parenteral anticoagulants such as heparin or low molecular weight heparin initially. Warfarin and low molecular weight heparins are alternatives. If warfarin is used, during the initial 5 – 7 day period, heparin or low molecular weight heparin should also be started along with warfarin, because the effect of warfarin comes after few days. After 5–7 days heparin can be discontinued and warfarin continued. Usual starting dose of warfarin is 5–10 mg. it should be adjusted to achieve a target INR of 2.0–3.0. However, due to the availability of DOACs, most clinicians are now using DOACs instead of warfarin, since the onset of action of DOACs is within few hours and there is no need to monitor PT-INR.
- Anticoagulation should be continued for 3–6 months if there is a reversible risk factor. For idiopathic DVT, anticoagulation should be given for 6–12 months. For patients at risk of recurrent DVT (e.g. hypercoagulable disorders), anticoagulation should be given indefinitely.

Inferior Vena Caval (IVC) Filters

- IVC filter is helpful to prevent pulmonary embolism. It is indicated when anticoagulation is contraindicated because of active bleeding and in recurrent venous thrombosis despite intensive anticoagulation.

Elastic Compression Stocking

- Use of an elastic compression stocking for first 2 years prevents postphlebitic syndrome. It should be used as soon as DVT is diagnosed. Stockings need not be worn when patient is in bed.

Leg Elevation

- Elevation of affected leg to 15 degrees reduces pain and edema.

Early Ambulation

- Once anticoagulation has been started and the patient's symptoms (i.e. pain, swelling) are under control, patient is encouraged to ambulate.

Prophylaxis of Deep Vein Thrombosis

- DVT prophylaxis is indicated in patients at high risk of developing DVT. Such patients are as follows **(Table 3.53)**:

TABLE 3.53: Indications for DVT prophylaxis
High-risk surgical patients
• Fracture of pelvis or lower limb bones • Hip and knee joint replacement • Major abdominal and gynecologic surgery • Multiple trauma • Acute spinal cord injury
High-risk medical patients
• Acute coronary syndrome • Cardiac failure • Active cancer • Sepsis • ARDS • Severe infections (pneumonia) • Stroke • Paraplegia • Patients on mechanical ventilator

- Measures useful for DVT prophylaxis are as follows:
  - Limb physiotherapy.
  - Early mobilization.
  - Graduated compression stockings.
  - Intermittent pneumatic compression devices to both legs.
  - Unfractionated heparin, 5000 units subcutaneously 12th hourly or low molecular weight heparin subcutaneously.
  - All the above methods can be combined in high-risk patients.
  - Oral warfarin after initial heparin therapy if the risk factor persists for a long time.

Differential Diagnosis of DVT

- Ruptured Baker's cyst
- Cellulitis
- Postphlebitic syndrome/venous insufficiency
- Calf muscle pull or tear
- Lymphatic filariasis.

Complications

- Pulmonary embolism
- Venous gangrene
- Postphlebitic syndrome (edema, venous claudication, skin pigmentation, dermatitis, and ulceration)
- Chronic venous insufficiency
- Chronic thromboembolic pulmonary hypertension.

Q. What is pulmonary embolism?

Q. Discuss the etiology, pathophysiology, clinical features, diagnosis, and management of acute pulmonary embolism.

Definition

- Pulmonary embolism (PE) refers to obstruction of the pulmonary artery or one or more of its branches by material (e.g. thrombus, tumor, air, or fat) that originated elsewhere in the body.

- This leads to a potential spectrum of consequences, including hypoxia, dyspnea, chest pain, hemodynamic instability, and right heart failure if untreated.

Types

- *Based on temporal pattern:* Acute, subacute, or chronic.
- *Based on anatomic location:* Saddle (at the bifurcation of main pulmonary artery), main, lobar, segmental, or subsegmental.
- *Based on clinical severity*: Massive PE (high-risk PE), Submassive PE (intermediate-risk PE), low-risk PE.

Etiology and Risk Factors

- Etiology of pulmonary thromboembolism is same as that of DVT.
- Thrombus from deep veins of lower limbs is the most common material embolizing to the lungs. Emboli can also occur from tumor, fat (long bone fractures), amniotic fluid, and foreign material during IV drug abuse.
- The following discussion refers to pulmonary embolism due to deep vein thrombosis.

Pathophysiology

- After pulmonary embolism, lung tissue is ventilated but not perfused—producing an intrapulmonary dead space and impaired gas exchange. After few hours, the non-perfused lung no longer produces surfactant leading to alveolar collapse, which exacerbates hypoxemia.
- Pulmonary embolism causes a reduction in the cross-sectional area of the pulmonary arterial bed leading to elevation of pulmonary arterial pressure and dilatation of right ventricle and right atrium.
- A massive pulmonary embolism obstructing the main branches of pulmonary artery may cause sudden hemodynamic collapse and death.
- Embolism into a small peripheral artery may produce pulmonary infarction leading to hemoptysis and pleuritic chest pain. Infarction may not always occur because oxygen continues to be supplied by the bronchial circulation and the airways.

Clinical Features

Massive Pulmonary Embolism

- This leads to sudden hemodynamic collapse due to acute obstruction of the right ventricular outflow.
- Patients present with hypotension and shock
- Central chest pain may be complained of due to cardiac ischemia due to lack of coronary blood flow. This is because of sudden decrease in blood flow from right side of the heart to left side of the heart → sudden fall in cardiac out → decreased coronary flow.
- Syncope and sudden death may occur due to sudden reduction in cardiac output.
- On examination, the patient appears pale, sweaty and tachypnoeic.
- Tachycardia and hypotension are usually present.
- JVP is raised with a prominent *'a'* wave due to right heart failure.
- There is a right ventricular heave, a gallop rhythm and a widely split-second heart sound because P2 is delayed due to right ventricular failure. Tricuspid regurgitation murmur may be present due to right ventricular dilatation.

Small Peripheral Artery Embolism

- This leads to sudden onset of dyspnea, pleuritic chest pain, and hemoptysis. Chest pain and hemoptysis are due to pulmonary *infarction.*
- Other symptoms are palpitations, cough, anxiety, and lightheadedness.
- Many pulmonary emboli occur silently without any symptoms.
- On examination, the patient may be tachypnoeic with a localized pleural rub and often coarse crepitations over the area involved. Pleural effusion can develop on the affected side.

Multiple Recurrent Pulmonary Emboli (chronic pulmonary thromboembolism)

- This leads to insidious onset breathlessness, over weeks to months and pulmonary HTN.
- Patient has symptoms of pulmonary HTN such as exertional dyspnea, weakness, exertional syncope, and occasionally angina.
- On examination, there are signs of pulmonary HTN such as right ventricular heave and loud P2.

Evidence of Deep Vein Thrombosis

- Erythema, warmth, pain, swelling, or tenderness may be present in one or both legs.
- Pain with dorsiflexion of the foot (Homans' sign) may also be present.

Wells Scoring System (Table 3.54)

- This is used to determine the probability of pulmonary embolism (PE).
- Clinical probability of PE: high if score >6; intermediate if 2–6; low if <2.

TABLE 3.54: Wells scoring system for pulmonary embolism

Clinical variable	Score
• Signs and symptoms of DVT	3.0
• Alternative diagnosis less likely than PE	3.0
• Heart rate >100/min	1.5
• Immobilization >3 days; surgery within 4 weeks	1.5
• Prior PE or DVT	1.5
• Hemoptysis	1.0
• Malignancy present	1.0

Differential Diagnosis

- Since the symptoms and signs of pulmonary embolism are non-specific, other diagnoses with similar presentation should be kept in mind. These are,

- Acute coronary syndrome, including unstable angina and acute myocardial infarction
- Pneumonia
- Acute exacerbation of asthma or COPD
- Congestive heart failure
- Pericarditis
- Pneumothorax
- Primary pulmonary hypertension
- Anxiety with hyperventilation.

Diagnosis

D-dimer

- Is elevated (>500 ng/ml) in more than 90% of patients with pulmonary embolism (PE). D-dimer is a product of endogenous fibrin breakdown and indicates presence of clot in the vascular system.
- It is not specific for PE because it is also positive in myocardial infarction, sepsis, or almost any systemic illness. However, it has high sensitivity of 96% and a negative predictive value of 99%.
- If D-dimer is negative, it essentially rules out PE. If it is positive, PE must be confirmed by other tests.

ABG (arterial blood gas) Analysis

- Usually shows hypoxemia and low arterial CO_2 level, i.e. type-1 respiratory failure pattern.

Troponins and BNP

- Elevated in massive PE (indicates right ventricular strain).

ECG

- Sinus tachycardia: New-onset atrial fibrillation or flutter.
- S1-Q3-T3 pattern (S wave in lead I, Q wave in lead III, and an inverted T wave in lead III).
- Right axis deviation and right ventricular strain (T-wave inversion in leads V1 to V4).
- ECG is also useful to rule out other diagnoses such as myocardial infarction.

Chest X-ray

- Common radiographic findings include pleural effusion, atelectasis, pulmonary infiltrates, and mild elevation of hemidiaphragm.
- Classic signs of pulmonary infarction, such as Hampton's hump (wedge shaped opacity above the diaphragm with base towards pleura) or decreased vascularity (Westermark's sign) may be present.
- Dilatation of pulmonary artery and right ventricle.
- Abrupt cutoff of a vessel.
- Chest X-ray is also useful to rule out other diagnoses such as pneumothorax, pneumonia or rib fracture.

Doppler Ultrasound

- This is done to detect thrombosis of pelvic, iliofemoral or calf veins.

Echocardiography

- May reveal abnormalities of right ventricular size or function that may support the diagnosis of pulmonary embolism. It can occasionally show the clot in the proximal pulmonary arteries.

Ventilation-perfusion Scanning (V/Q scan)

- This is a very good test, but nowadays is being replaced by CT-angiogram. V/Q scanning may be used when CT scanning is not available or if the patient has a contraindication to CT scanning or intravenous contrast material.
- Perfusion scan is obtained by 99mTc scintigraphy which demonstrates underperfused areas. Ventilation scan is obtained by inhalation of radioactive xenon gas. If there is a perfusion defect in the normally ventilated area, it is highly suggestive of a pulmonary embolism.
- However, there are some limitations to the test. For example, a similarly matched defect may be seen in emphysematous bulla. Hence, this test should be interpreted in the context of the history, examination and other investigations.

CT Pulmonary Angiography (CTPA) (gold standard test)

- This has remained the accepted "gold standard" technique for the diagnosis of acute pulmonary embolism. It is an extremely sensitive, specific, and safe test. Nowadays it is done only if surgery is considered in acute massive embolism. The test is performed by injecting contrast material through a catheter inserted into the main pulmonary artery. Filling defects or obstructed vessels can be visualized.
- MR imaging gives similar results and is used if CT angiography is contraindicated.

Other Tests

- Troponin levels are usually elevated in pulmonary embolism due to right ventricular damage.
  Algorithm for the diagnosis of pulmonary embolism (Fig. 3.61).

Treatment

General Measures

- High-flow oxygen (60–100%) should be given to all patients. All patients should be admitted to intensive care unit. Intravenous fluids and inotropic agents (dopamine and noradrenaline) should be started if there is hypotension. Intubation and mechanical ventilation should be considered in all patients if there is respiratory compromise.

Anticoagulation (mainstay of treatment)

- Anticoagulants prevent the progression of thrombus and further emboli.
- Either low-molecular-weight heparin (LMWH) (e.g. dalteparin, enoxaparin) or unfractionated heparin

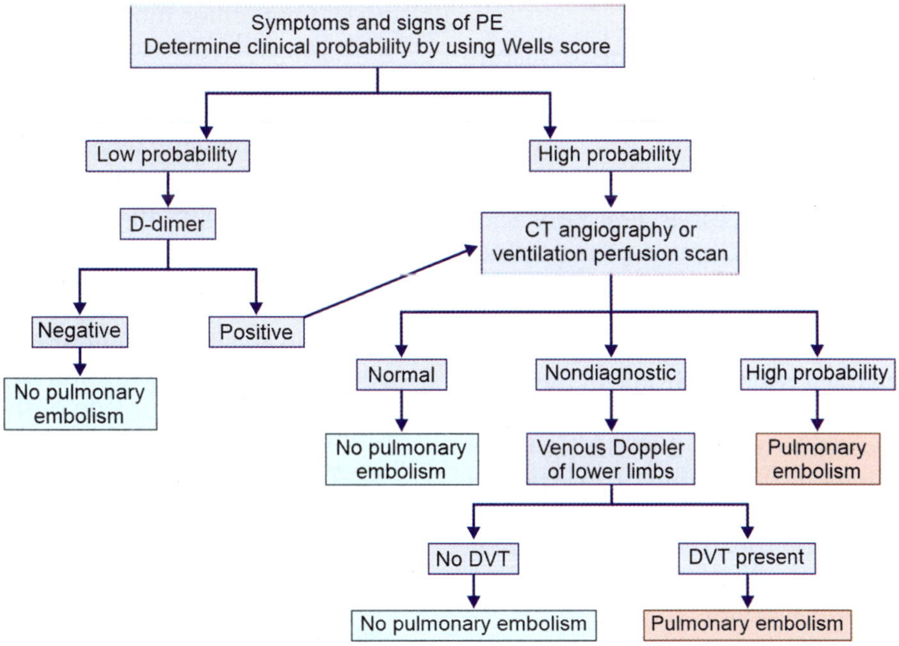

Figure 3.61: Diagnostic algorithm for pulmonary embolism

can be used for this purpose. Unfractionated heparin is given at an initial dose of 5000–10,000 units intravenously, followed by continuous infusion of 1000 units per hour.

- LMWHs have the advantage of less frequent dosing, and aPTT need not be monitored. The chances of heparin induced thrombocytopenia (HIT) is also less with LMWHs.
- Newer oral anticoagulants (direct oral anticoagulants (DOACs) such as apixaban, rivaroxaban, dabigatran can also be started as initial treatment instead of heparin as the action of these DOACs starts immediately.
- Oral anticoagulant (preferably one of the DOACs) has to be continued for 6 weeks to 6 months, depending on the likelihood of recurrence of venous thrombosis or embolism. Lifelong anticoagulation is indicated in recurrent embolism.
- Bleeding due to excess heparin can be corrected by injecting protamine sulphate and due to warfarin by injecting vit-K.

Thrombolytic Therapy

- In addition to anticoagulation, thrombolytic therapy is also indicated in patients with massive pulmonary embolism with hemodynamic compromise such as hypotension. **Alteplase (tPA)** (tissue plasminogen activator can be used for thrombolysis. Catheter-directed thrombolysis can be used in select cases of submassive PE. Thrombolysis has been shown to clear pulmonary emboli more rapidly and to confer a survival benefit in massive PE.

Surgery

- Surgical pulmonary embolectomy may be appropriate in patients who have massive embolism occluding the main or proximal branches uld be considered in all patients if they are not able to mantain and cannot receive thrombolytic therapy or when thrombolysis fails.

Vena Caval Filters (Fig. 3.62)

- Indications for IVC filter placement include contra-indications to anticoagulation and recurrent embolism while on anticoagulant therapy. IVC filters are sometimes placed in the setting of massive PE when it is believed that any further emboli might be lethal, particularly if thrombolytic therapy is contraindicated. Greenfield filter has been most widely used. Filters can be inserted via the jugular or femoral vein.

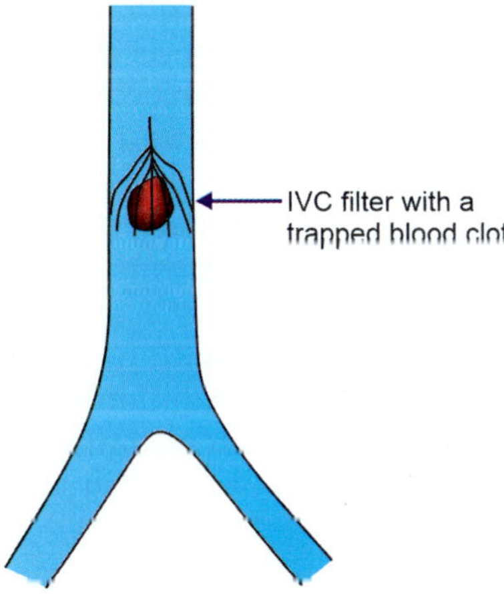

Figure 3.62: IVC filter

Prevention of Pulmonary Embolism

- This is same as prophylaxis for DVT.

Q. Nonthrombotic pulmonary embolism.

- Pulmonary embolism can also result from substances other than thrombus. These include fat, air, amniotic fluid, and foreign bodies.

Fat Embolism

- Fat embolism usually occurs in the setting of fracture of long bones and major surgery. Trauma to other fat-rich tissues such as the liver or subcutaneous tissue can occasionally result in fat embolism.
- The fat particles which enter into vascular system cause obstruction of multiple vessels. Free fatty acids released from neutral fat by lipases cause diffuse vasculitis with capillary leakage from cerebral, pulmonary, and other vascular beds.
- Symptoms develop 24–48 hours after the event which include a characteristic syndrome of dyspnea, petechiae, and mental confusion.
- The diagnosis is made from the clinical and radiographic findings in the setting of risk factors such as surgery or trauma. Fat droplets (by oil red O stain) may be found in bronchoalveolar lavage fluid in fat embolism. However, the diagnosis of fat embolism remains a diagnosis of exclusion.
- Treatment is supportive, including oxygen and mechanical ventilation, and the prognosis is generally good.

Amniotic Fluid Embolism

- Although uncommon, amniotic fluid embolism is one of the causes of maternal death during or after delivery. The delivery may be either spontaneous or by cesarean section and usually without any complication.
- Amniotic fluid may gain access to uterine venous channels during or after delivery. It then travels to pulmonary and general circulations. Amniotic fluid has thromboplastic activity and leads to extensive fibrin deposition in the pulmonary vasculature and other organs. A severe consumptive coagulopathy ensues, with marked hypofibrinogenemia. After the acute event, an enhanced fibrinolytic state often develops. ARDS develops frequently.
- Clinical features are sudden onset dyspnea. There may be hypotension and death can occur. Left ventricular dysfunction may occur, due to the myocardial depressant effect of amniotic fluid.
- Examination of the pulmonary arterial blood may reveal the amorphous fragments of vernix caseosa, squamous cells, or mucin.
- Treatment is supportive, with oxygen, mechanical ventilation, and inotropes. Administration of heparin, antifibrinolytic agents such as α-aminocaproic acid, and cryoprecipitate may be useful in selected patients.

Air Embolism

- Air embolism occurs when large amount of air gains access into the venous system.
- The incidence has increased due to frequent invasive surgical and medical procedures, frequent use of indwelling venous and arterial catheters, and the frequency of thoracic and other forms of trauma.
- Air embolism may be asymptomatic or result in death if severe. If there is patent foramen ovale, air can cross from right to left side and result in systemic embolization. In the absence of a patent foramen ovale, lungs filter most of the air, but large amount of air can still gain access to the systemic circulation.
- Symptoms include dyspnea, wheezing, chest pain, cough, agitation, confusion, tachycardia, hypotension and seizures. A "mill wheel murmur" due to air in the right ventricle may sometimes be heard.
- Arterial blood gas analysis reveals hypoxemia and hypercapnia in severe cases. Chest X-ray may show pulmonary edema or air fluid levels.
- Treatment includes immediate placement of the patient in the Trendelenburg/left lateral decubitus position and administration of 100% oxygen. If air is present in the right side of the heart, it should be aspirated by a central venous catheter. Occasionally, hyperbaric oxygen is indicated. Anticonvulsants are given to control seizures.

Q. Define and classify hypertension. Describe the etiology, pathophysiology, clinical features, diagnosis, and management of essential hypertension.

Q. Joint National Committee VII (JNC-VII) classification of blood pressure.

Q. Secondary hypertension.

- Hypertension is defined as persistently elevated BP more than the defined normal level.
- It is a major risk factor for cardiovascular disease, stroke, kidney failure, and other complications.
- As per the latest guidelines, BP classification is as follows.

Normal blood pressure: Systolic <120 mm Hg and diastolic <80 mm Hg

Elevated blood pressure: Systolic 120–129 mm Hg and diastolic <80 mm Hg

Hypertension (BP ≥130 systolic and ≥ 80 diastolic):

- Stage 1 – Systolic 130–139 mm Hg or diastolic 80–89 mm Hg
- Stage 2 – Systolic at least 140 mm Hg or diastolic at least 90 mm Hg

- Isolated systolic hypertension is defined as a blood pressure ≥130 mm Hg systolic and <80 mm Hg diastolic.
- Isolated diastolic hypertension is defined as a blood pressure <130 mm Hg systolic and ≥80 mm Hg diastolic.
- Hypertension is very common in the developed world and is present in 20–30% of the adult population. Hypertension rates are much higher in black Africans (40–45%of adults). The risk of mortality or morbidity rises progressively with increasing systolic and diastolic pressures.
- BP should be measured at least twice at different times before classifying a patient as hypertensive. Blood pressure should be measured at least twice after 5 minutes of rest with the patient seated, the back supported, and the arm at heart level. The cuff should not be too small for the arm, and tobacco and caffeine should be avoided for at least 30 minutes before measuring BP.

- When assessing the cardiovascular risk, the average blood pressure at separate visits is more accurate than measurements taken at a single visit.

Types of Hypertension

Primary HTN (essential HTN)

Here, a single reversible cause of hypertension cannot be identified. Primary HTN accounts for the majority (95%) of cases of HTN. The term "essential hypertension" was used earlier because it was thought that progressive increase in blood pressure with advancing age was essential to maintain blood flow through atherosclerotic arteries.

Secondary HTN

- Here, a definite reason for hypertension can be found such as renal disease, endocrine problems, etc.

Etiology of Hypertension

Primary HTN (essential HTN, idiopathic HTN)

- There are many risk factors for essential hypertension.

Genetic factors

- Blood pressure tends to run in families and children of hypertensive parents tend to have higher blood pressure than age-matched children of people with normal blood pressure. Concordance of blood pressure is greater within families than in unrelated individuals, greater between monozygotic than between dizygotic twins. However, the exact genetic loci and mutations are unknown.

Age (>55 years)

- Advancing age is a risk factor for HTN, especially above 55 years.

Gender and ethnicity

- Before age 50, the prevalence of hypertension is lower in women than in men, probably due to a protective action of estrogen. After menopause, the prevalence of hypertension increases rapidly in women and exceeds that in men. African Americans have higher prevalence of hypertension than other races.

Obesity

- Fat people are more prone to develop hypertension than thin people. The underlying mechanisms by which obesity leads to hypertension are incompletely understood, but there is mounting evidence for an expanded plasma volume plus sympathetic over activity.

Smoking and alcohol consumption

- Chronic smokers and people who consume large amount of alcohol have higher blood pressure than those who do not smoke and drink. However, small amount of alcohol intake is actually associated with lower blood pressure.

Sodium intake

- High sodium intake is associated with hypertension. Studies of the restriction of salt intake have shown a beneficial effect on blood pressure.

Stress

- Acute stress can temporarily raise blood pressure. However, the relationship between chronic stress and blood pressure remains to be proven.

Humoral mechanisms

- Abnormalities in the autonomic nervous system, and renin-angiotensin system have been also implicated in the pathogenesis of essential HTN. Some hypertensive patients have been defined as having low-renin and others as having high-renin essential hypertension based on plasma rennin activity. However, there is no convincing evidence that the above systems are directly involved in the maintenance of hypertension.

Insulin resistance

- Insulin resistance and/or hyperinsulinemia have been suggested as being responsible for the increased arterial pressure in some patients with hypertension. A syndrome called the 'metabolic syndrome' has been described which consists of hyperinsulinemia, glucose intolerance, reduced levels of HDL cholesterol, hypertriglyceridemia and central obesity in association with hypertension.

Secondary HTN (Table 3.55)

TABLE 3.55: Causes of secondary HTN

Renal causes	Renal artery stenosis, glomerulonephritis, polycystic kidney disease, acute and chronic renal failure
Endocrine causes	Pheochromocytoma, hypothyroidism, hyperthyroidism, Cushing's syndrome, hyperaldosteronism, acromegaly, hyperparathyroidism, congenital adrenal hyperplasia
Drugs	Oral contraceptives, steroids, NSAIDs, sympathomimetics (phenylephrine, phenylpropanolamine)
Miscellaneous	Coarctation of aorta, obstructive sleep apnea, preeclampsia and eclampsia

Pathophysiology

- If hypertension remains uncontrolled for a long time, many changes take place in blood vessels and various organs.
- The resistance vessels (the small arteries and arterioles) show structural changes in the form of increased wall thickness and reduced lumen diameter. The number of these resistance vessels may also decrease. These changes result in an increased peripheral vascular resistance.
- In large arteries, there is thickening of the media, increase in collagen and deposition of calcium. These changes result in loss of arterial compliance, leading to a more pronounced arterial pressure wave. Over a period of time atherosclerotic changes develop in large arteries due to mechanical stress and endothelial injury.
- Left ventricular hypertrophy develops due to increased left ventricular load (increase in afterload). Left

ventricular failure can happen in long standing uncontrolled HTN.

- Thickening and atherosclerotic changes in blood vessels supplying various organs results in damage to those organs. Changes in the renal vasculature lead to a reduced renal perfusion, reduced glomerular filtration rate and, finally, a reduction in sodium and water excretion. Changes in blood vessels of brain may lead to stroke. Changes in blood vessels of heart may lead to myocardial infarction.

Clinical Manifestations

Symptoms

- Hypertension has been termed the "silent killer," because it hardly produces any symptoms. If it is undetected in this long asymptomatic phase, it damages the heart, brain, kidneys, and blood vessels.
- Headache may be a complaint in hypertension, but usually rare and episodes of headaches do not correlate with fluctuations in ambulatory blood pressure.
- Attacks of sweating, headache, and palpitations may point towards the diagnosis of pheochromocytoma.
- Sometimes patients may experience epistaxis when BP is very high.
- Breathlessness may be present due to left ventricular hypertrophy, diastolic dysfunction, or heart failure.
- Angina and leg claudication may be experienced due to atherosclerotic narrowing of coronary and lower limb arteries.
- Malignant hypertension may present with severe headache, vomiting, visual disturbances, seizures, altered sensorium, or symptoms of heart failure.

Signs

- BP is elevated (systolic ≥130/80 mm Hg).
- Signs of an underlying cause should be sought, such as renal artery bruits in renovascular hypertension, or radiofemoral delay in coarctation of the aorta.
- Cardiac examination reveals left ventricular hypertrophy and a loud A2.
- Enlarged, palpable kidneys may be found in polycystic kidney disease.
- A bruit may be heard over the abdomen in lumbar area in renal artery stenosis.
- Nonpitting edema, hoarse voice, and coarse skin may be present in hypothyroidism.
- Cushingoid features (lemon on stick appearance) may be present in Cushing's syndrome.
- Optic fundus should be examined in all patients for hypertensive retinopathy changes. In malignant hypertension, there is papilledema.

Complications of Hypertension

- Hypertension is associated with a number of serious adverse effects.

Cardiovascular Complications

- Coronary artery disease (angina, myocardial infarction)
- Heart failure
- Left ventricular hypertrophy and sudden cardiac death
- Aortic aneurysm
- Aortic dissection
- Premature atherosclerosis of blood vessels.

CNS Complications

- Transient ischemic attacks
- Stroke: Hypertension is the most common and most important risk factor for stroke.
- Intracerebral hemorrhage
- Subarachnoid hemorrhage
- Hypertensive encephalopathy: This is characterized by very high blood pressure, papilledema, blurring of vision, headache, altered sensorium and focal neurological deficits.

Renal Complications

- Proteinuria
- Chronic renal failure: Hypertension is a risk factor for and end-stage renal disease.
- Hypertensive nephrosclerosis.
- Hypertension can accelerate the progression of a variety of underlying renal diseases.

Ophthalmic Complications

- Arteriolosclerosis: Localized or generalized narrowing of vessels.
- Copper wiring and silver wiring of arterioles as a result of arteriolosclerosis.
- Arteriovenous (AV) nicking as a result of arteriolosclerosis.
- Retinal hemorrhages.
- Nerve fiber layer losses.
- Increased vascular tortuosity.
- Remodeling changes due to capillary nonperfusion, such as shunt vessels and microaneurysms.
- Choroidal damage.

Malignant Hypertension

- This is characterized by very high blood pressure with papilledema and end organ damage.

Investigations

Routine Tests

- Urea, creatinine and electrolytes (to assess renal function).
- Urine examination for protein and blood.
- Lipid profile.
- Blood glucose (to rule out diabetes).
- Echocardiography: May show LV hypertrophy.
- ECG usually shows evidence left ventricular hypertrophy.
- Chest X-ray usually shows cardiomegaly and rib notching if there is coarctation of aorta.

Additional Tests (done only if required)

- Renal artery Doppler may be indicated if renovascular hypertension is suspected.

- 24-hour urinary cortisol and VMA is indicated if there is clinical suspicion of Cushing's and pheochromocytoma.
- T3, T4 and TSH, if hypo or hyperthyroidism is suspected.
- Growth hormone levels and skull X-ray if acromegaly is suspected.
- Ultrasound abdomen if polycystic kidney or other renal problems are suspected.
- Ambulatory blood pressure monitoring is used to monitor blood pressure throughout the day. For this, an automatic BP measuring device is worn by the patient throughout the day. It is useful to confirm the diagnosis of hypertension in patients with 'white -coat' hypertension. These devices can also be used to monitor the response of patients to drug treatment and, in particular, can be used to determine the adequacy of 24- hour control with once-daily medication.

Treatment

Nonpharmacologic Treatment

- Weight reduction: BMI should be <25 kg/m^2.
- Diet: low fat, low sodium diet (<6 g sodium chloride per day). Fruit and vegetable consumption should be increased. Potassium rich diet is known to reduce HTN, unless there is chronic kidney disease which is a contraindication for potassium supplementation. Dietary approaches to stop hypertension (DASH) dietary pattern is high in vegetables, fruits, low-fat dairy products, whole grains, poultry, fish, and nuts and low in sweets, sugar-sweetened beverages, and red meats. The DASH dietary pattern is consequently rich in potassium, magnesium, calcium, protein, and fiber but low in saturated fat, total fat, and cholesterol. The DASH diet lowers blood pressure, and combining the DASH dietary pattern with modest sodium restriction produced an additive antihypertensive effect.
- Habits: Alcohol consumption should be cut down and smoking should be stopped.
- Exercise: Regular exercise, preferably aerobic type for at least 30 minutes per day.
- Relaxation techniques, yoga, meditation.

Antihypertensive Agents

- Antihypertensive drugs should be started if blood pressure is persistently above the defined normal ranges. In general, the goal treatment is to bring down the BP to <130 mm Hg systolic and <80 mm Hg diastolic. A goal of <140 mm Hg systolic and <90 mm Hg diastolic is OK for patients who are >75 years of age and patients with labile blood pressure or postural hypotension.
- Initial antihypertensive treatment should include a thiazide diuretic or calcium channel blocker or ACE inhibitor or ARB or beta blocker. There are reports that beta-blockers increase the risk of stroke. Hence, other antihypertensive agents should be preferred over beta-blockers.
- Initially treatment should be initiated with one drug. This drug is increased to maximum tolerated dose gradually till BP is in the desirable range.
- If BP is not controlled within one month with a single drug, addition of a second drug should be considered. Most patients will require a combination of antihypertensive drugs to achieve the recommended targets.
- An easy way to remember the anthypertensive drugs is the mnemonic "ABCD" (A = ACE inhibitor or angiotension receptor blocker, B = beta-blocker, C = calcium channel blocker, D = diuretics).

Angiotemsin-converting Enzyme (ACE) Inhibitors

- Examples are captopril, ramipril, enalapril, perindopril, and lisinopril.
- These drugs block the conversion of angiotensin I to angiotensin II, which is a potent vasoconstrictor. They also block the degradation of bradykinin, a potent vasodilator.

Compelling Indications

- Diabetics with nephropathy: ACE inhibitors slow the progression of diabetic nephropathy and decrease proteinuria.
- Ischemic heart disease: All patients with IHD should be put on ACE inhibitors because these drugs have been shown to reduce long-term mortality and morbidity of IHD.

Contraindications

- Bilateral renal artery stenosis
- Preexisting renal failure.

Side Effects

- Hypotension following the first dose
- Deterioration of renal function in those with severe bilateral renovascular disease
- Dry cough due to their effect on bradykinin
- Angioneurotic edema.

Angiotensin II Receptor Blockers (ARBs)

- Examples: Losartan, candesartan, valsartan, irbesartan, telmisartan and olmesartan.
- These drugs block angiotensin II receptors. Their mechanism of action is same as ACE inhibitors but, since they do not have any effect on bradykinin, they do not cause cough. They can be used instead of ACE inhibitors especially in those who cannot tolerate ACE inhibitors because of persistent cough. Angioneurotic edema and renal dysfunction are also less common with these drugs than ACE inhibitors.
- Compelling indications, contraindications and side effects are same as those of ACE inhibitors.

Beta Blockers

- Examples: Atenolol, metoprolol, bisoprolol, oxprenolol, nebivolol, pindolol, carvedilol, and labetalol.

- These drugs act by inhibiting sympathetic and renin-angiotensin systems. They reduce the force of cardiac contraction, as well as resting and exercise-induced increase in heart rate. Beta-blockers differ among themselves in terms of cardioselectivity, intrinsic sympathomimetic activity and lipid solubility. Some are cardioselective (e.g. metoprolol and bisoprolol), some have intrinsic sympathomimetic activity and cause less bradycardia (e.g. oxprenolol and pindolol). Some are more lipid soluble and produce CNS side effects like depression (propranolol) while some are less lipid soluble (atenolol).

Compelling Indications

- Ischemic heart disease: Beta-blockers have been shown to improve the symptoms of angina and heart failure and reduce long-term mortality and morbidity in these patients. Hence, any patient having IHD and HTN should be put on beta-blockers if BP is uncontrolled even after starting ACE or ARBs.

Contraindications

- Asthma and COPD
- Peripheral vascular disease
- Heart block
- Diabetes (a relative contraindication because beta-blockers can mask hypoglycemia symptoms).

Side Effects

- Bronchospasm, bradycardia, fatigue, bad dreams, depression (propranolol) and hallucinations.

Calcium-channel Blockers

- Examples: nifedipine, amlodepine, s-amlodepine, felodipine, benidipine.
- These agents reduce BP by causing arteriolar dilatation, and some (verapamil, diltiazem) also reduce the force of cardiac contraction.

Side Effects

- Headache, pedal edema, flushing. All these side effects are common with short acting agents such as nifedipine. Verapamil and diltiazem may worsen heart failure.

Diuretics

- Examples: Chlothalidone, hydrochlorthiazide, frusemide.
- Diuretics act by enhancing sodium excretion from the body.

Compelling Indications

- Renal failure with fluid retention.
- Heart failure with fluid retention.

Side Effects

- Increased serum cholesterol, impaired glucose tolerance, hyperuricemia, and hypokalemia. All these are common with higher doses of thiazide diuretics.

Alpha Blockers

- Examples: Prazosin, doxazosin, terazosin, tamsulosin.
- These agents block the action of norepinephrine on alpha receptors resulting in vasodilatation and BP reduction.

Compelling Indications

- Patients having urinary obstructive symptoms due to benign prostate hyperplasia (BPH) along with hypertension will especially benefit from these drugs. They control BP as well as BPH symptoms.

Side Effects

- Postural hypotension.

Direct Vasodilators

- Examples: Hydralazine, and minoxidil.
- These drugs relax vascular smooth muscle and cause vasodilation thus reducing the BP. These drugs are used for patients resistant to other forms of treatment.

Side Effects

- Hydralazine can cause reflex tachycardia, fluid retention and a systemic lupus erythematosus-like syndrome. Minoxidil can cause edema and excessive hair growth.

Centrally Acting Drugs

- Examples: Reserpine, methyldopa and clonidine.
- These drugs stimulate alpha-2 adrenergic receptors in the CNS lowering central sympathetic outflow. They are used as add on therapy in hypertensives not responding to combinations of other drugs. Methyldopa and clonidine are especially useful in pregnant women with preeclampsia.

Side Effects

- These drugs should not be combined with beta-blockers, because both drugs inhibit sympathetic system and can produce bradycardia. They can cause depression. Rebound hypertension is a problem with these agents especially clonidine. α-Methyldopa can cause autoimmune hemolytic anemia, lupus erythematosus and liver damage.

Contraindications

- Depression is a contraindication to centrally acting sympatholytic agents.

Treatment of underlying cause in secondary hypertension

- Surgery for pheochromocytoma, correction of renal artery stenosis, treatment of any endocrine disorder, etc.

Q. Hypertensive emergency (malignant hypertension) and hypertensive urgency.

Hypertensive Emergency

- *Hypertensive emergency* is acute, severe elevation in blood pressure associated with target organ damage.

Patients with hypertensive emergency usually present with a systolic BP of ≥180 mm Hg and/or diastolic BP of ≥120 mm Hg, though there is no specific threshold since individuals who develop an acute rise in blood pressure (even if less than 180/120) can develop target organ damage if the previous pressure was normal.

- Earlier terms such as malignant hypertension and accelerated hypertension are to be avoided. The term "malignant hypertension" was used earlier, because at that time, patients with this condition had a prognosis that was similar to patients with many cancers. However, now, antihypertensive therapies that can quickly and safely lower blood pressure have improved outcomes.

Clinical Features

- Target-organ damage includes hypertensive encephalopathy, preeclampsia and eclampsia, acute left ventricular failure with pulmonary edema, myocardial ischemia, acute aortic dissection, and renal failure. Damage is rapidly progressive and often fatal. The characteristic vascular lesion is fibrinoid necrosis of arterioles and small arteries, which causes the clinical manifestations of end-organ damage.

Investigations

- Investigations to be done include ECG, cardiac biomarkers, urinalysis, serum BUN and creatinine, and CT head for patients with neurologic symptoms or signs.

Treatment

- Hypertensive emergency requires ICU admission and lowering of blood pressure by intravenous medications.
- Sodium nitroprusside infusion is the drug of choice for hypertensive emergencies. Clevidipine is a new, ultra-short-acting (within 1–2 minutes), 3rd-generation calcium channel blocker that reduces peripheral resistance without affecting venous vascular tone and cardiac filling pressures. In recent trials, it has been shown to be more effective with lower mortality than nitroprusside. Starting dose is 1–2 mg/h, doubling the dose every 90 sec until approaching target BP. Hence, if clevidipine is available, it is the drug of choice and is preferred over sodium nitroprusside. Other alternatives are nitroglycerin or labetalol infusion. Blood pressure should be lowered gradually over many hours to a target of 160/100 mm Hg. In the next 48 hours, BP can be lowered to normal value. Oral drugs can be added and parenteral therapy slowly tapered off.

Hypertensive Urgency

- *Hypertensive urgency* is acute, severe elevation in blood pressure to ≥180/120 mm Hg without evidence of target organ damage. Thus, the main difference between hypertensive emergency and urgency is the presence (hypertensive emergency) or absence (hypertensive urgency) of target organ damage.
- Hypertensive urgency is often asymptomatic or may be accompanied by mild headache.
- Hypertensive urgency can be managed by oral drugs. For immediate reduction of BP in hypertensive urgency, labetalol and clonidine are useful.

Q. Define cardiomyopathy. Classify cardiomyopathies.

- Cardiomyopathies are defined as diseases of the myocardium associated with cardiac dysfunction.
- Cardiomyopathies can lead to heart failure, arrhythmias, and sudden cardiac death.

Classification

- The traditional classification of cardiomyopathies into three categories (i.e. hypertrophic, restrictive and dilated cardiomyopathy) has many shortcomings, because, there are multiple overlaps between the etiologies and presentations of the three types. There can be mixed features and same etiology can produce different types of cardiomyopathy. The following classification is the latest one.

Classification of Cardiomyopathies (Table 3.56)

TABLE 3.56: Classification of cardiomyopathies
Primary cardiomyopathies (idiopathic or genetic)
• Dilated cardiomyopathy (DCM)
• Hypertrophic cardiomyopathy (HCM)
• Restrictive cardiomyopathy (RCM)
• Arrhythmogenic right ventricular cardiomyopathy (ARVC)
Secondary cardiomyopathies (due to systemic diseases)
• Ischemic cardiomyopathy (Post-MI heart failure)
• Hypertensive cardiomyopathy (due to long-standing high BP)
• Alcoholic, drug-induced cardiomyopathy (e.g. cocaine, anthracyclines)
• Infiltrative cardiomyopathies (e.g. amyloidosis, sarcoidosis)
• Metabolic cardiomyopathies (e.g. hemochromatosis, thyroid disease)
• Peripartum cardiomyopathy (during or after pregnancy)
• Toxic/drugs (doxorubicin, daunorubicin, cyclophosphamide, radiation, heavy metals; chemical agents)
• Myocarditis (Coxsackie B virus, Chaga's disease)
• Nutritional deficiencies (beriberi; pellagra; scurvy; selenium; carnitine; kwashiorkor)

Q. Hypertrophic cardiomyopathy (hypertrophic obstructive cardiomyopathy (HOCM); idiopathic hypertrophic subaortic stenosis (IHSS)).

- Hypertrophic cardiomyopathy is characterized by asymmetrical ventricular hypertrophy mainly affecting interventricular (asymmetric septal hypertrophy), but in some cases the hypertrophy is localized to mid ventricle or to the apex. The LV is usually more involved than the RV.

Etiology

- It is a familial disease (autosomal dominant with variable penetrance).

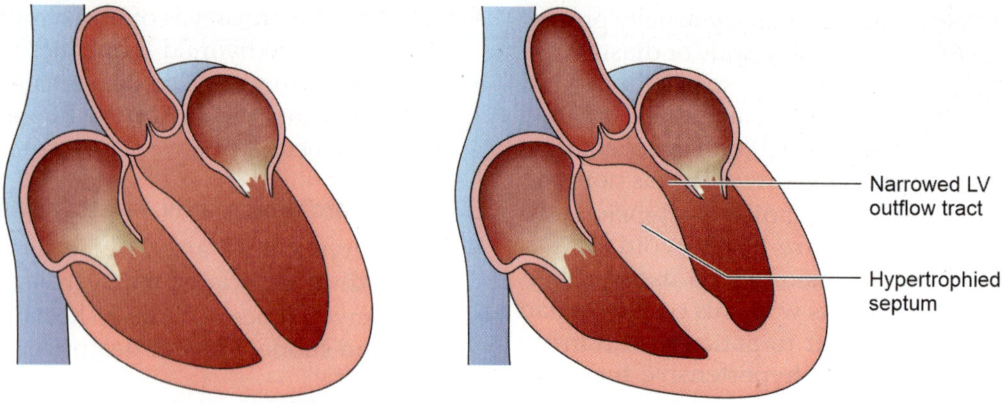

Figure 3.63: Hypertrophic cardiomyopathy (right), left (normal)

Pathophysiology

- Asymmetric LV hypertrophy → Thickened interventricular septum → Left ventricular outflow tract obstruction. There is dynamic obstruction to LV outflow during systole because the outflow tract is narrowed between the bulging septum and the anterior mitral valve leaflet. Smaller enddiastolic volume increases the obstruction (sympathetic stimulation, digoxin, post-extrasystolic beat) and increased end diastolic volume decreases the obstruction.
- Diastolic dysfunction → Impaired relaxation and filling (HFpEF).
- Myocardial ischemia and fibrosis → Risk of ventricular arrhythmias and sudden death.

Clinical Features

Symptoms

- Patients may be asymptomatic
- Family history may be present
- Dyspnea and chest pain
- Syncope occurs usually after exercise, when diastolic filling diminishes and outflow obstruction increases.
- Arrhythmias (atrial fibrillation due to elevated LA pressure, ventricular arrhythmias).
- Most common cause of sudden cardiac death (SCD) in young athletes during exertion.

Signs

- Pulsus bisferiens.
- Prominent *a* wave in JVP due to reduced RV compliance.
- Triple apical impulse (due to the prominent atrial filling wave and early and late systolic impulses).
- Loud S4
- Loud systolic murmur along the left sternal border that increases with upright posture or Valsalva's maneuver and decreases with squatting due to dynamic outflow obstruction.
- Pansystolic murmur may be present due to associated mitral regurgitation.

Investigations

- Chest X-ray is usually normal.
- ECG shows left ventricular hypertrophy and exaggerated septal Q waves.
- Echocardiogram shows asymmetric LVH, a small and hypercontractile LV. Interventricular septum is thickened. Doppler ultrasound reveals dynamic obstruction in the LV outflow tract and usually mitral regurgitation.
- Myocardial perfusion imaging may suggest septal ischemia in the presence of normal coronary arteries.
- Cardiac MRI confirms the hypertrophy.

Natural History

- It is variable.
- Malignant arrhythmias and death can happen in some patients.
- Some patients may progress to dilated cardiomyopathy.

Treatment

- Beta-blockers slow the heart rate and hence increase diastolic filling time. This increases end-diastolic volume which decreases outflow obstruction. Beta-blockers also reduce dyspnea, angina, and arrhythmias.
- Calcium channel blockers (especially verapamil) are also effective in symptomatic patients.
- **Mavacamten** is a is a groundbreaking therapy that directly targets the underlying cause of HCM—sarcomere hypercontractility. It is a first-in-class cardiac myosin inhibitor approved for the treatment of symptomatic obstructive hypertrophic cardiomyopathy (HOCM). It reduces hypercontractility and left ventricular outflow tract obstruction (LVOTO) by modulating myosin-actin interactions.
- Diuretics are generally avoided as they decrease the preload and worsen obstruction. Similarly, vasodilators (ACEi, ARBs, nitrates, digoxin) decrease the afterload, decrease end diastolic LV volume → worsens LV outflow tract obstruction.
- Treatment of arrhythmias (amiodarone, ICD implantation).
- Nonsurgical septal ablation by injection of alcohol into septal branches of the left coronary artery in selected patients.
- Surgical resection of the outflow myocardial septum (myotomy–myomectomy) in patients with severe symptoms.

Q. Dilated Cardiomyopathy (congestive cardiomyopathy).

- Dilated cardiomyopathy (DCM) is characterized by dilation and impaired contraction of one or both ventricles.
- LV dilation and systolic dysfunction are essential for the diagnosis of dilated cardiomyopathy.

Causes of Dilated Cardiomyopathy

It can be familial or acquired. Some important causes of dilated cardiomyopathy are given below:

- Idiopathic (most common cause)
- Genetic (familial DCM)
- Alcoholic
- Myocarditis
- Postpartum
- Nutritional (thiamine and selenium deficiency)
- Drugs (doxorubicin, cyclophosphamide)
- Endocrinopathies (thyrotoxicosis, hypothyroidism)
- Genetic diseases (hemochromatosis, glycogen storage diseases).

Clinical Features

- Clinical features are due to left and right heart failure.
- In most patients, symptoms of heart failure develop gradually.
- Symptoms are dyspnea, fatigue, peripheral edema.
- Sudden death can occur due to arrhythmias.
- Physical examination reveals signs of left heart failure such as basal lung crepitations, cardiomegaly, S3 gallop rhythm and sometimes murmur of functional mitral regurgitation. Signs of right heart failure are elevated JVP, peripheral edema, ascites, and sometimes functional tricuspid regurgitation murmur. In severe cases, Cheyne-Stokes breathing, pulsus alternans, pallor, and cyanosis may be present.

Investigations

- Chest X-ray: It shows cardiomegaly, evidence for left and/or right heart failure, and pleural effusions.
- ECG: Sinus tachycardia, left bundle branch block and ventricular or atrial arrhythmias.
- Echocardiogram: It shows ventricular dilatation, global LV and RV systolic dysfunction. It can also exclude other diagnoses.
- Cardiac MRI: It identifies fibrosis (late gadolinium enhancement), helps differentiate ischemic vs. non-ischemic DCM.
- BNP/NT-proBNP: Elevated in HF.
- Tests to identify underlying cause: Troponins (if myocarditis or MI suspected), thyroid function tests (hyper/hypothyroidism), iron studies (ferritin, TIBC) (hemochromatosis), genetic testing (familial DCM).

Treatment

- Standard therapy for heart failure (ACE inhibitor, beta-blockers, diuretics, and digoxin).
- ARNI = Angiotensin receptor-Neprilysin inhibitor. Sacubitril/Valsartan (ARNI) is a combination drug approved for the treatment of heart failure with reduced ejection fraction (HFrEF). Sacubitril blocks neprilysin, leading to vasodilation, natriuresis and diuresis (via ANP, BNP), reduced cardiac fibrosis and remodeling. RAAS blockade (valsartan component) inhibits angiotensin II AT1 receptors, leading to reduced vasoconstriction, reduced aldosterone → decreased sodium and water retention.
- Sodium restriction and avoidance of excessive physical activity.
- Anticoagulation to prevent thromboembolic episodes.
- Prevention and treatment of arrhythmias (antiarrhythmics, implantable cardioverter-defiberillator (ICD).
- Treatment of underlying cause if any.
- Cardiac transplantation in severe cases not responding to above treatment.

Q. Restrictive cardiomyopathy (obliterative cardiomyopathy)

- Restrictive cardiomyopathy (RCM) is a rare myocardial disorder characterized by diastolic dysfunction due to reduced ventricular compliance (stiff, non-dilated ventricles).
- Hallmark feature is impaired ventricular filling with normal or near-normal systolic function (EF is typically preserved in early stages).

Causes

- Amyloidosis (most common cause)
- Endomyocardial fibrosis
- Hemochromatosis
- Carcinoid syndrome
- Connective tissue diseases (e.g. scleroderma)
- Chemotherapy or radiation
- Hypereosinophilic syndrome
- Post open-heart surgery.

Clinical Features

- It can present at any age and is more common in women than men.
- Symptoms are due to both pulmonary and systemic congestion and include dyspnea, peripheral edema, palpitations, fatigue, weakness, and exercise intolerance.
- Pulse is either normal or of low volume with tachycardia.
- JVP is elevated with prominent y descent. An inspiratory increase in venous pressure may be seen (Kussmaul sign).
- Congestive hepatomegaly, ascites, and peripheral edema may be present.
- The first and second heart sounds are usually normal. A third heart sound (S3 gallop) is frequently present because of the abrupt cessation of the rapid ventricular filling.
- Murmurs of functional mitral and tricuspid regurgitation may be present.

Investigations

- ECG may show non-specific ST-T changes, low voltage QRS complexes and conduction disturbances.
- Echocardiogram shows ventricular hypertrophy. Low voltage complexes in ECG but ventricular hypertrophy in ECHO is highly suggestive of restrictive cardiomyopathy.
- Cardiac MRI can show ventricular wall thickening and a distinctive pattern in amyloidosis.

Treatment

- There is no specific treatment.
- Diuretics to relieve pulmonary and systemic venous congestion.
- Digoxin may precipitate arrhythmias and should be used with caution.
- Beta-blockers and calcium channel blockers help slow heart rates and improve filling.
- Excision of fibrotic endocardium (in endomyocardial fibrosis).
- Underlying cause should be treated.
- Cardiac transplantation should be performed in patients with intractable heart failure.

Q. Define myocarditis. Discuss the etiology, clinical features, investigations, and management of acute myocarditis.

- *Myocarditis* is an inflammation of the myocardium, the middle layer of the heart wall leading to cardiac dysfunction, heart failure and sudden death. It can be acute, subacute, or chronic, and there may be either focal or diffuse involvement of the myocardium.

Etiology (Table 3.57)

TABLE 3.57: Etiology of myocarditis
Infections
• *Viral*: Coxackie, influenza, HIV, dengue, parvovirus B-19, hepatitis-C, corona
• *Bacterial:* Acute rheumatic fever, diptheria, tuberculosis, salmonella, brucellosis
• *Protozoal:* Chagas' disease, leishmaniasis
• *Spirochetal:* Syphilis, leptospirosis, lyme disease
• *Rickettsial:* Scrub typhus, Rocky Mountain spotted fever, Q fever
• *Fungal:* Candidiasis, histoplasmosis, coccidiomycosis
• *Helminthic:* Trichinosis, schistosomiasis
Systemic disorders
• Scleroderma, sarcoidosis, SLE, Wegener's granulomatosis, giant cell myocarditis
Toxins and poisons
• Alcohol, arsenic, aluminum phosphide, insect bites (bee, wasp, spider, scorpion), snake bites
Drugs
• Anthracyclines, cyclophosphamide, antibiotics, diuretics, lithium

Clinical Features

- Myocarditis usually presents as acute congestive heart failure (CCF).
- Signs and symptoms of CCF cuch as dyspnea, orhopnea, raised JVP, peripheral edema, hypotension, S3 and S4 may be present.
- Inappropriate tachycardia.
- There may be preceding febrile illness or respiratory tract infection.
- Heart blocks can occur if the conduction system gets involved.
- If the epicardium is involved, there may be pleuritic chest pain and pericardial effusion.

Investigations

- There may be leukocytosis and raised ESR.
- CK-MB and troponins are elevated.
- Chest X-ray shows cardiomegaly. Pulmonary edema may be present.
- ECG may show nonspecific ST–T changes, conduction blocks, and ventricular ectopics.
- Echocardiography can assess the ventricular function and can exclude other diseases.
- Gallium-67 scintigraphy may reveal increased cardiac uptake in myocarditis. MRI with gadolinium enhancement reveals areas of injury throughout the myocardium.
- Endomyocardial biopsy can confirm the diagnosis, but is rarely done.

Complications

- Arrhythmias
- Heart blocks
- Congestive heart failure
- Chronic myocarditis
- Dilated cardiomyopathy.

Treatment

- Cardiac failure should be treated as per standard guidelines with ACE inhibitors, beta-blockers, digoxin and diuretics.
- Patients with fulminant myocarditis require aggressive short-term support including an intra-aortic balloon pump or an LV assist device.
- Immunosuppressive agents (steroids, azathioprine) may help myocarditis of autoimmune etiology (SLE, sarcoidosis).
- Patients with severe myocarditis, without any improvement with above therapies may be eventual candidates for cardiac transplantation.

Q. What is aortic aneurysm? What are the types of aortic aneurysms?

- Aortic aneurysm is a permanent localized dilatation of the aorta having a diameter of at least 1.5 times the normal diameter of that given aortic segment.

Types

- Based on the morphology, aortic aneurysm can be,
- ***Fusiform***—here the aneurysm is of uniform shape, with symmetrical dilatation that involves the full

circumference of the aortic wall. This is the most common type.

- ***Saccular***—here, the dilatation is more localized and appears as an outpouching of only a portion of the aortic wall.
- ***Pseudoaneurysm*** or ***false aneurysm*** refers to dilatation of only the outer layers of the vessel wall, such as occurs with a contained rupture of the aortic wall. It is not actually an aneurysm.

Q. Discuss the etiology, clinical features, investigations, complications and management of aortic aneurysm.

- Aortic aneurysm can occur in any part of aorta, but commonly involves abdominal aorta. Thoracic aorta is less common than abdominal aorta aneurysm. Abdominal aortic aneurysm is four to five times more common in men than in women.
- The infra-renal aorta is the most common site to get affected because atherosclerosis is common there.
- Thoracic aorta aneurysm can occur in the ascending aorta, arch of aorta, or descending aorta **(Fig. 3.64)**.

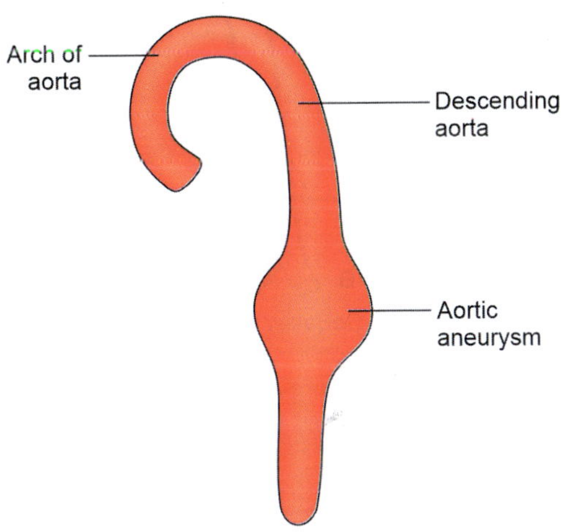

Figure 3.64: Aortic aneurysm

Etiology (Table 3.58)

TABLE 3.58: Etiology of aortic aneurysm

- Atherosclerosis (most common cause)
- Aging
- Smoking
- Bicuspid aortic valve and aortic coarctation
- Inflammatory/infectious disorders (giant cell arteritis, syphilis, mycotic aneurysm)
- Hypertension
- Genetic predisposition
- Marfan syndrome
- Ehlers-Danlos syndrome

Clinical Features

- Most patients are asymptomatic and are discovered incidentally on a routine physical examination or imaging study.
- Systemic thromboembolism due to thrombus formation within the aneurysm.

Abdominal Aorta Aneurysm

- Pain in the hypogastrium or lower back. Pain is steady gnawing type and may last for hours to days.
- Aneurysm expansion or impending rupture may be heralded by new or worsening pain, often of sudden onset.
- Physical examination may reveal a pulsatile mass at or above the umbilicus.
- An arterial bruit may be heard over the abdomen if there is atherosclerotic narrowing.
- When the aneurysm ruptures, patient presents with abdominal pain, hypotension and a pulsatile abdominal mass.

Thoracic Aorta Aneurysm

- Pain in the chest or back.
- Symptoms due to compression or distortion of adjacent structures or vessels by ascending and arch aneurysms. These include:
  - Hoarseness of voice due to compression of left vagus or left recurrent laryngeal nerve
  - Diaphragmatic paralysis due to compression of the phrenic nerve
  - Wheezing, cough, hemoptysis, dyspnea, or pneumonitis due to compression of the tracheobronchial tree
  - Dysphagia due to compression of esophagus
  - Superior vena cava syndrome due to compression of SVC.
- Tracheal tug is descent of trachea with every heartbeat. It is seen in arch of aorta aneurysm due to pulsatile pressure on the left bronchus.
- Ascending aorta aneurysms can present with heart failure due to aortic regurgitation from aortic root dilatation and myocardial infarction due to compression of a coronary artery.

Investigations

- X-ray of chest may show mediastinal widening in thoracic aorta aneurysm. X-ray abdomen may show calcified outline of aortic aneurysm.
- Ultrasound abdomen
- Echocardiogram
- CT or MR angiography
- Conventional angiography.

Complications

- Rupture (most lethal, 90% mortality if untreated).
- Aortic dissection—Intimal tear → False lumen formation.
- Thromboembolism—Can cause distal limb ischemia.

Treatment

- Risk factor reduction (stop smoking, control hypertension).
- Beta-blockers reduce the rate of expansion and chances of rupture by reducing aortic pressure and the abrupt rise in pressure during systole.

- Asymptomatic—size >5.5 cm – surgical repair. Less than this—serial monitoring with ultrasound
- Symptomatic aneurysms—surgical repair irrespective of size.
- Percutaneous placement of an expandable endovascular stent graft inside the aneurysm is another new technique.
- Ruptured aneurysm—emergency surgery.

Q. What is aortic dissection? Discuss the etiology, clinical features, investigations, and management of aortic dissection.

- Aortic dissection is a life-threatening condition where the blood penetrates into the media through a tear in the intima, cleaving it into two layers longitudinally and producing a blood-filled false lumen within the aortic wall.
- This false lumen propagates distally (or sometimes retrograde) to a variable distance along the aorta from the site of intimal tear.

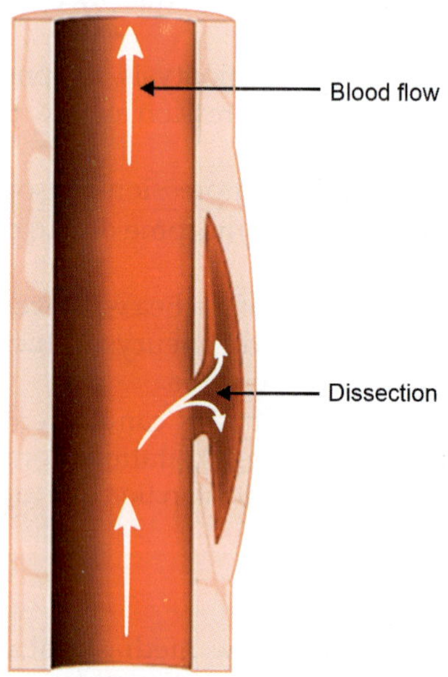

Figure 3.65: Aortic dissection

Etiology

- Systemic hypertension (commonest cause).
- Cystic medial necrosis.
- Preexisting aortic aneurysm.
- Vasculitis (Takayasu arteritis, giant cell arteritis, syphilis).
- Marfans syndrome.
- Ehlers-Danlos syndrome.
- Bicuspid aortic valve.
- Coarctation of aorta.
- Third trimester of pregnancy.
- Trauma.
- High-intensity weight lifting or other strenuous exercise.
- Cardiac catheterization.

Classification

Daily or Stanford Classification

- Type A: Dissection involving the ascending aorta (± descending aorta), regardless of the site of the primary tear.
- Type B: Dissection confined to descending aorta.

DeBakey Classification

- Type 1: Involves both ascending and descending thoracic aorta
- Type 2: Confined to ascending aorta
- Type 3: Confined to descending aorta

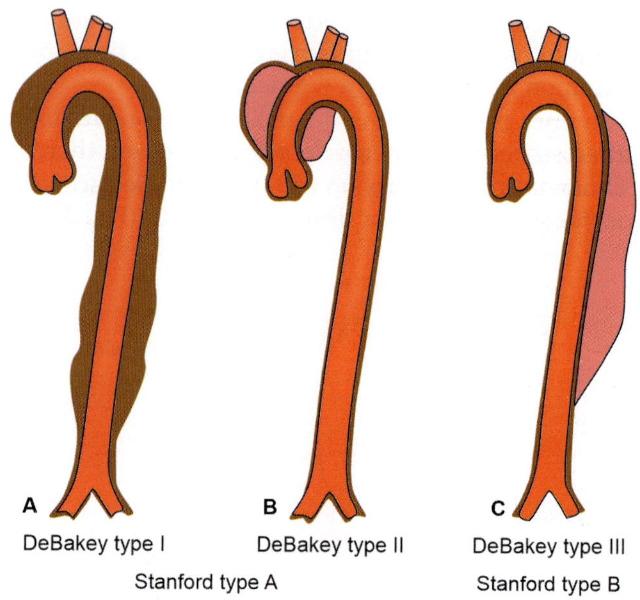

Figure 3.66: Types of aortic dissection

Clinical Features

- Sudden onset severe pain in the chest, in the neck or throat, interscapular, in the lower back, or abdominal depending on the location of the aortic dissection. Pain is described as "tearing," "sharp," or "stabbing."
- There may be asymmetry of pulses.
- Hypertension is present in most patients. Rarely hypotension may be present.
- A dissection involving the ascending aorta can produce the following:
  - Acute aortic regurgitation—due to proximal aortic dissection propagating into a sinus of Valsalva with resultant aortic valve insufficiency, leading to early diastolic murmur, hypotension, or heart failure.
  - Acute myocardial ischemia or MI due to coronary occlusion.
  - Cardiac tamponade and sudden death due to rupture of the aorta into the pericardial space.
  - Neurologic deficits, including stroke or decreased consciousness due to carotid artery occlusion.
  - Horner syndrome due to compression of the superior cervical sympathetic ganglion.
  - Vocal cord paralysis and hoarseness due to compression of the left recurrent laryngeal nerve.

- A dissection that involves the descending aorta can lead to splanchnic ischemia, renal failure, lower limb ischemia, or focal neurologic deficits due to spinal artery involvement and spinal cord ischemia.

Investigations

- *ECG*—shows nonspecific changes. Can rule out myocardial infarction
- *Chest X-ray*—may show widening of the aorta and mediastinum.
- *Echocardiography*—has limited utility for evaluation of the thoracic aortic dissection. Useful for proximal dissections. It is most useful for the assessment of cardiac complications of dissection, including aortic insufficiency, pericardial effusion/tamponade, and heart failure.
- *Aortography*—less commonly used now due to the availability of noninvasive imaging methods. It can identify the site of dissection, the relationship between the dissection and the major branches of the aorta, and the communication site between the true and false lumen.
- *CT angiography with three-dimensional (3D) reconstruction*—is rapidly becoming the diagnostic test of choice to identify aortic dissection.
- *MR angiography*—is as accurate as CT and is useful in patients who have contraindications to the use of intravenous (IV) contrast agents (such as renal failure or allergy).
- *Smooth muscle myosin heavy-chain assay*—increased levels in the first 24 hours are 90% sensitive and 97% specific for aortic dissection. levels are highest in the first 3 hours.

Treatment

- Aortic dissection is a life-threatening emergency.
- Admit the patient in ICU
- Emergency treatment: The goal of initial treatment is to halt any further progression of the aortic dissection and to reduce the risk of rupture. Blood pressure and the force of ventricular contraction should be reduced (systolic blood pressure to 100–120 mm Hg). Intravenous labetalol, which acts as an α-blocker and a β-blocker, is particularly useful in aortic dissection for controlling hypertension and contractile force. Intravenous nitroprusside should be added to if BP is not controlled with labetalol. If β-blockers are contraindicated, calcium channel blockers (diltiazem) may be useful.
- After initial medical therapy, further treatment depends on the type of dissection.
- If the dissection involves the ascending aorta, emergency surgical repair is indicated to minimize the risk of life-threatening complications.
- If the dissection is confined to the descending aorta, medical therapy is as good as surgical therapy. However, if there is complication such as end-organ ischemia, surgery is indicated.
- Surgical therapy involves reconstruction of the aorta. Endovascular stent-grafting has been tried as an alternative to surgery in dissections involving descending aorta.

Q. What is pericarditis? How do you classify pericarditis?

- Pericarditis is inflammation of the pericardium.
- The pericardium is a protective covering for the heart. It has two layers, the outer parietal layer, and inner visceral layer. Between these two layers there is a space called pericardial sac which contains 15–50 mL of pericardial fluid. This fluid is an ultra-filtrate of plasma produced by visceral layer.
- The pericardium lubricates the surface of the heart, prevents deformation and dislocation of the heart and acts as a barrier to the spread of infection. However, the absence of pericardium does not produce any obvious clinical disease.
- Pericarditis can be classified as acute (<6 weeks), sub-acute (6 weeks to 6 months) and chronic (>6 months).

Q. Discuss the etiology, clinical features, investigations, and management of acute pericarditis.

- This refers to acute inflammation (<6 weeks) of the pericardium. Acute pericarditis has many causes and in some cases, the cause is unknown.

Etiology of Pericarditis

- *Idiopathic*
- *Infectious conditions*: viral (coxsackievirus, mumps, varicella, rubella, HIV), bacterial (tuberculosis, staphylococcus, streptococcus, pneumococcus, Legionella, syphilis), fungal (histoplasmosis, coccidioidomycosis, candida), and parasitic.
- *Inflammatory conditions*: rheumatoid arthritis, SLE, scleroderma, and rheumatic fever.
- *Metabolic disorders*: uremia, hypothyroidism, and hypercholesterolemia.
- *Cardiovascular disorders:* acute MI, post-myocardial infarction (Dressler's syndrome), aortic dissection, cardiovascular procedures.
- *Miscellaneous causes:* neoplasms (primary or secondary), drugs (doxorubicin, cyclophosphamide), irradiation, and trauma.

Clinical Features

- Sharp retrosternal and left precordial pain sometimes referred to back and left shoulder. Pain is exacerbated by movement, respiration and lying down. It is typically relieved by sitting forward. The main differential diagnoses are angina and pleurisy.
- The classical clinical sign is a triphasic pericardial friction rub corresponding to atrial systole, ventricular systole, and ventricular diastole. It may also be heard as a biphasic 'to and fro' rub corresponding to systole and diastole. It is high-pitched, scratching, and grating and heard best when firm pressure with the diaphragm of the stethoscope is applied to the chest wall at the left lower sternal border at the end of expiration with the patient leaning forward.
- There is usually fever when infection is present. Features of pericardial effusion may also be present.

Investigations

- Total leukocyte count and ESR may be elevated due to infection.
- ECG shows concave-upwards (saddle shaped) ST elevation in multiple leads, which is characteristic of pericarditis. This has to be differentiated from myocardial infarction where ST elevation is convex upwards. PR segment is depressed. Low voltage QRS complexes and electrical alternans (varying axis) may be seen if there is pericardial Effusion.
- Cardiac enzymes (CK-MB and troponins) are usually normal unless there is associated myocarditis.
- Chest X-ray may show widening of cardiac shadow if there is pericardial effusion.
- Echocardiogram can show pericardial effusion clearly and help detect other cardiac abnormalities.
- Pericardiocentesis: If pericardial effusion is present, it should be removed and analyzed for red blood cells (RBCs), WBCs, total protein level, LDH level, and adenosine deaminase activity. Gram's stain, AFB stain, culture (ordinary and Loewenstein media) and cytology should also be done.
- CT and MRI scan of the heart should be done if the cause is not clear from the above studies.

Management

- If a cause is found, it should be treated (e.g. tuberculosis, uremia).
- Pericardial inflammation can be decreased by NSAIDs (high-dose aspirin or indomethacin or ibuprofen). Steroids (prednisone, 20–60 mg/day) can be used in resistant situations. These anti inflammatory drugs should be given until the patient is afebrile and asymptomatic for 1 week, followed by a gradual taper over the next few weeks.
- Some patients may have recurrent pericarditis. For recurrent pericarditis, treatment with colchicine, or pericardiectomy should be considered.

Q. Constrictive pericarditis.

- Here the pericardium becomes thick, fibrous and calcified, which interferes with relaxation of the heart during diastole leading to many hemodynamic consequences.
- Constrictive pericarditis should be distinguished from restrictive cardiomyopathy because the former is treatable, whereas most cases of the latter are not.

Etiology

- Tuberculosis (most common cause)
- Hemopericardium
- Mediastinal irradiation
- Neoplastic disease
- Bacterial infection
- Rheumatic heart disease
- Rheumatoid arthritis and SLE
- Open-heart surgery.

Clinical Features

- Many clinical features are similar to cardiac tamponade.
- Ascites, dependent edema, hepatomegaly, and raised JVP develop due to reduced ventricular filling and systemic venous congestion.
- Kussmaul's sign and pulsus paradoxus may be positive.
- Pulmonary venous congestion produces dyspnea, cough, and PND.
- Reduced ventricular filling leads to reduced cardiac output, which causes fatigue, hypotension, and reflex tachycardia.
- A 'pericardial knock' may be heard in early diastole at the lower left sternal border due to rapid ventricular filling.
- Atrial fibrillation may develop in some cases due to atrial dilatation.

Investigations

- ***Chest X-ray***—shows a relatively small heart. There may be pericardial calcification.
- ***ECG***—shows low-voltage QRS complexes with generalized T wave flattening or inversion.
- ***Echocardiography***—shows thickened calcified pericardium and small ventricular cavities with normal wall thickness.
- ***CT and MRI***—are useful to assess pericardial anatomy and thickness.

Treatment

- Pericardial resection is the only definitive treatment of constrictive pericarditis. This should be carried out early before severe constriction, myocardial atrophy and liver damage develops.
- In cases of tuberculous constriction, antituberculous therapy should also be given.
- Treatment of any other underlying cause.

Q. Tuberculous pericarditis.

- Tuberculous pericarditis is invariably secondary to tuberculosis elsewhere in the body. It may occur via extension of infection from the lung or tracheobronchial tree, adjacent lymph nodes, spine, or via hematogenous spread.

Clinical Features

- Low grade fever, weight loss, and night sweats.
- Symptoms and signs of pericarditis usually insidious onset.
- There may be signs and symptoms of pulmonary tuberculosis such as cough, hemoptysis, etc.
- In late stages, patients may present with findings of constrictive pericarditis.

Investigations

- *Chest X-ray* shows cardiomegaly and pleural effusions. Pericardial calcification may be seen in late stages. Evidence of concurrent pulmonary tuberculosis may be present.

- *ECG:* Low voltage QRS complexes, inverted T waves and electrical alternans may be present.
  Echocardiogram: Can confirm the presence of pericardial effusion, tamponade and pericardial thickening.
- *Pericardiocentesis:* Fluid is exudative in nature with low sugar and elevated ADA. Fluid should be sent for culure of tubercle bacilli and PCR.
- *Pericardial biopsy:* May show the presence of granulomas and tubercle bacilli.
- *Montoux test:* Most patients will have positive skin test. A negative test suggests low probability of pericardial tuberculosis.

Treatment

- Antituberculous therapy for 6–9 months. 4 drugs should be given for initial 2 months (isoniazid, rifampicin, pyrazinamide, ethambutol) followed by 2 drugs (isoniazid and rifampicin) for 4–7 months.
- Steroids along with antituberculous drugs reduce mortality, the need for subsequent pericardiocentesis and the chances of constrictive pericarditis.
- Therapeutic aspiration may be needed to relieve symptomatic effusion or tamponade.
- If constrictive pericarditis develops, pericardiectomy may be needed.

Q. Pericardial effusion and cardiac tamponade.

- Accumulation of excessive fluid in the pericardial space is called pericardial effusion **(Fig. 3.67)**.
- When large amount of fluid collects in this space, ventricular filling is compromised leading to embarrassment of the circulation. This is known as cardiac tamponade. Tamponade is a medical emergency, which can lead to pulmonary edema, shock, and death.
- The fluid is usually an exudate but blood (hemopericardium), lymph (chylopericardium) and serosanguineous fluid (TB, malignancy) can also accumulate in the space.

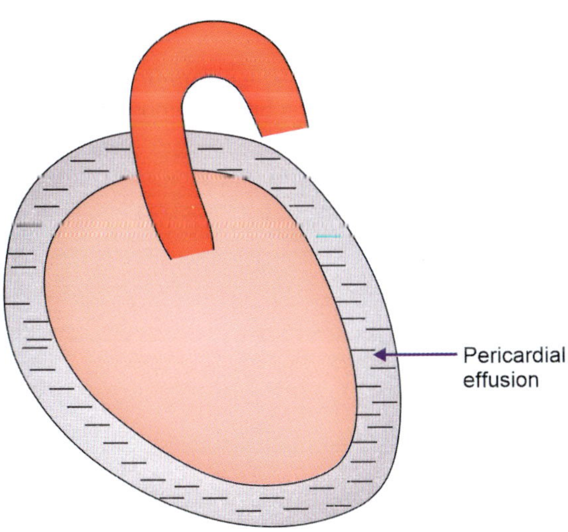

Figure 3.67: Pericardial effusion

Etiology

- Is same as acute pericarditis.

Clinical Features

- Pericardial effusion may present with symptoms similar to acute pericarditis.
- Heart sounds are faint and distant (muffled).
- Apex beat is obscured or palpable medial to the left border of cardiac dullness.
- Pericardial rub may be heard due to pericarditis in the early stages, but this becomes quieter as fluid accumulates and separates the layers of the pericardium.
- The base of the left lung may be compressed by pericardial effusion, producing an area of dullness to percussion below the angle of the left scapula (Ewart's sign).
- If there is cardiac tamponade following additional symptoms and signs may be present:
  - Dyspnea and orhopnea
  - Hypotension
  - Raised JVP with sharp rise and × descent (Friedreich's sign)
  - Kussmaul's sign (rise in JVP during inspiration)
  - Pulsus paradoxus
  - Reduced cardiac output.

Investigations

- ***Echocardiography:*** This is the most useful investigation for demonstrating the effusion and looking for evidence of tamponade.
- ***ECG:*** Shows low-voltage QRS complexes.
- ***Chest X-ray:*** Shows large globular or pear shaped heart with sharp outlines (water bottle appearance).
- ***CT or MRI:*** Is superior to echocardiogram and is especially useful in detecting loculated pericardial effusions and pericardial thickening.
- ***Pericardiocentesis:*** Emergency pericardiocentesis is indicated for cardiac tamponade under echocardiographic guidance. Pericardiocentesis is also indicated when a tuberculous, malignant or purulent effusion is suspected.
- ***Pericardial biopsy:*** May be needed if tuberculosis is suspected and pericardiocentesis is not diagnostic.

Treatment

- Underlying cause should be identified and treated
- Pericardial effusion without tamponade usually resolves spontaneously with the treatment of underlying cause. Pericardiocentesis is indicated to relieve the pressure if there is tamponade. A flexible drainage catheter may be left in the pericardial space for several days to avoid early re-accumulation.
- Recurrent effusions (commonly due to malignancy) may require pericardial fenestration, i.e. creation of a window in the pericardium to allow the slow release of fluid into the surrounding tissues.

Chapter 4

Diseases of Gastrointestinal System

Q. Define the terms nausea, vomiting, retching, regurgitation, rumination and indigestion.

- *Nausea* is the subjective feeling of need to vomit. It may or may not ultimately lead to vomiting.
- It precedes vomiting and may happen alone, with retching or vomiting.
- *Vomiting* (or *emesis*) is the forceful ejection of upper gastrointestinal contents through the mouth resulting from contractions of gut and thoracoabdominal muscles.
- *Retching* or dry heaving, refers to the repetitive, involuntary contractions of the diaphragm and abdominal muscles **without the expulsion of stomach contents.** It often precedes vomiting but does not always lead to it.
- *Eructation (belching)* is the expulsion of swallowed gastric air.
- *Regurgitation* is the sudden, effortless return of small volumes of gastric or esophageal contents into the pharynx. **There is no contraction of thoracoabdominal muscles.** Usually there will be some physical cause for regurgitation such as lax lower esophageal sphincter, or esophageal or gastric motility disorders.
- *Rumination* (merycism) is effortless but purposeful regurgitation of food from the stomach into the mouth, where it is re-chewed and re-swallowed. Often it is a type of eating disorder.
- *Indigestion* is a nonspecific term that encompasses a variety of upper abdominal complaints including nausea, vomiting, heartburn, regurgitation, and dyspepsia (upper abdominal discomfort or pain).

Q. Discuss the causes and mechanism of vomiting. How do you approach and manage a case of vomiting?

- *Vomiting* (or *emesis*) is the forceful ejection of upper gastrointestinal contents through the mouth resulting from contractions of gut and thoracoabdominal wall musculature.
- Vomiting can be projectile or non-projectile. In projectile vomiting, vomiting is not preceded by nausea whereas in nonprojectile vomiting, there is preceding nausea. Projectile vomiting is seen in CNS diseases which increase intracranial pressure such brain tumor, meningitis, and intracranial bleed.

Causes of Vomiting (Table 4.1)

TABLE 4.1: Causes of vomiting

GI diseases
• Acute gastritis
• Peptic ulcer disease
• Mechanical obstruction
▫ Gastric outlet obstruction following peptic ulcer or malignancy
▫ Small intestinal obstruction, e.g. volvulus, adhesions, malignancy
• Motility disorders (gastroparesis due to diabetes, drugs, postvagotomy or idiopathic
• Infections/Inflammation
▫ Food poisoning
▫ Appendicitis
▫ Acute pancreatitis
• Gastrointestinal irritants (alcohol and drugs)
Hepatobiliary causes
• Acute hepatitis (viral, alcoholic, toxic)
• Acute cholecystitis
• Acute cholangitis
• Biliary colic
CNS disorders
• Raised intracranial pressure, e.g. tumors, hydrocephalus, subdural hematoma, subarachnoid hemorrhage, meningitis, encephalitis
• Migraine
CVS
• Acute MI
• CHF
Renal
• Uremia in renal failure
• Ureteric colic
• UTI, pyelonephritis
Endocrinal
• DKA, hypo- or hyperparathyroidism, thyrotoxic crisis, adrenal crisis

(Contd.)

TABLE 4.1: Causes of vomiting *(Contd.)*

Vestibular
• Labyrinthitis, Meniere's disease, motion sickness
Medication/toxin-related
• Chemotherapy, opioids, antibiotics • Alcohol intoxication
Miscellaneous
• Systemic infections (dengue, malaria, typhoid) • Pregnancy • Psychogenic • Radiation therapy • Postoperative

- Most common causes of nausea and vomiting are acute gastroenteritis, systemic febrile illnesses and medications.

Mechanism of Vomiting (Fig. 4.1)

- Vomiting is a reflex mechanism that enables the expulsion of ingested toxins or poisons from the body. It can be triggered by a variety of neuronal or humoral stimuli and involves multiple afferent and efferent pathways. The key components of these pathways include:
- **Area postrema:** Located in the floor of the fourth ventricle, this region houses the "chemoreceptor trigger zone," which is highly sensitive to numerous humoral factors, including neurotransmitters, peptides, drugs, and toxins.
- **Vomiting center:** Found in the medulla, this area comprises the nucleus tractus solitarius and the reticular formation. It integrates signals from humoral factors relayed via the area postrema and visceral afferents transmitted through the vagus nerve. The vomiting center then projects to various motor nuclei to initiate the act of vomiting.
- Vomiting is mediated by five primary neurotransmitter receptors:
  - Muscarinic M1 receptors
  - Dopamine D2 receptors
  - Histamine H1 receptors
  - 5-Hydroxytryptamine (HT) 3 serotonin receptors, and
  - Neurokinin 1 (NK1) substance P receptors.

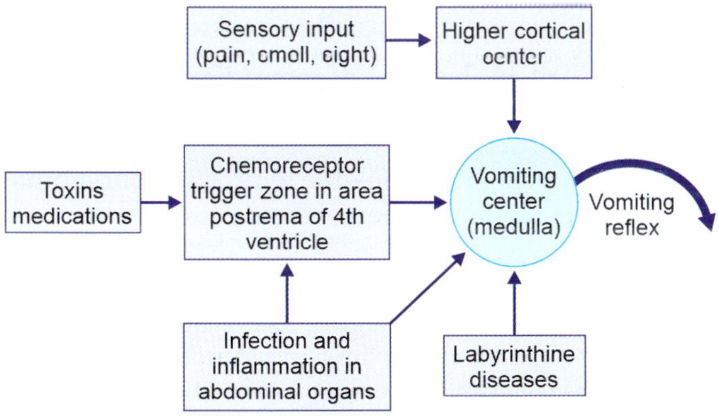

Figure 4.1: Pathophysiology of vomiting

Approach to a Case of Vomiting

History

- *Duration*: Acute vomiting refers to vomiting of few hours or few days. Causes of acute vomiting include obstruction, ischemic, toxic, metabolic, infectious, neurological and postoperative reasons. Chronic vomiting refers to vomiting lasting more than 1 month. Causes of chronic vomiting include partial intestinal obstruction, motility disorder, chronic neurological conditions (such as chronic meningitis, brain tumor), pregnancy or functional reasons.
- *Time of onset*: Early morning vomiting seen in raised intracranial tension, pregnancy, and uremia. Vomiting 1 hour after eating suggests gastric outlet obstruction or gastroparesis. Vomiting few hours after eating suggests gastric or intestinal obstruction.
- *Content of the vomitus:* If bilious then gastric outlet obstruction can be ruled out since bile from duodenum cannot come back to stomach if there is gastric outlet obstruction. Undigested food suggests achalasia or stricture. If hematemesis, suspect upper GI bleed with its causes. If fecal matter is present, suspect distal bowel obstruction.
- *Associated symptoms*: Chronic headache associated with vomiting is seen in intracranial lesion and migraine. Vomiting without preceding nausea (projectile vomiting) is typical of central nervous system pathology. Vertigo suggests a labyrinthine or vestibular problem. Associated diarrhea suggests gastroenteritis. Fever suggests an infection. Severe colicky abdominal pain suggests biliary, ureteric or intestinal obstruction. H/o of missed period in a woman of childbearing age suggests pregnancy.
- *Past medical and surgical history:* The past medical history will reveal the presence of any GI disease or previous surgeries. H/o past abdominal surgery may suggest recurrence of the previous disease or intestinal obstruction due to peritoneal adhesions.

Physical Examination

- Assessment of the patient's hydration status and vital signs. Tachycardia and hypotension may be present if there is hypovolemia. Fever can be present in infections.
- Abdomen should be examined for any abnormality such as distension (seen in intestinal obstruction, peritonitis), tenderness, guarding (seen in abdominal infections), bowel sounds (increased in intestinal obstruction and decreased in peritonitis and paralytic ileus).
- Other systems should be examined for any abnormality.
- Red flags: The following findings are of particular concern and require immediate evaluation and treatment:
  - Signs of hypovolemia (immediate hydration required).
  - Headache, stiff neck, or mental status change (suggest CNS infection).

- Peritoneal signs (suggest peritonitis).
- Distended, tympanitic abdomen (suggest acute abdomen, intestinal obstruction, etc.).

Investigations

- *CBC*: If Hb and hematocrit are high, it indicates dehydration. Leukocytosis is seen in infections.
- *Serum electrolytes*: To rule out hypochloremia, hypokalemia, etc. which can occur due to vomiting.
- *Urea, creatinine*: Renal failure can cause vomiting due to uremia. On the other hand, vomiting itself can cause renal failure if there is dehydration.
- *Urine pregnancy test:* In women of childbearing age to rule out pregnancy.
- *Serum amylase, lipase*: Elevated in pancreatitis which can present with vomiting and abdominal pain.
- *Liver function tests*: To rule out hepatitis. Acute hepatitis can cause nausea and vomiting.
- *Erect abdomen X-ray*: If any intra-abdominal pathology suspected. Dilated bowel loops with multiple air fluid level seen in peritonitis and intestinal obstruction.
- *Ultrasound abdomen*: To rule out any intra-abdominal pathology.
- *Upper GI endoscopy*: If peptic ulcer or gastric outlet obstruction is suspected or if hematemesis is present.
- *CT abdomen*: If the cause of vomiting is not clear from above investigations.
- Other tests as indicated.

Complications of Vomiting

- *Aspiration:* Vomiting in a patient with altered mental status, low or depressed level of consciousness, or persistent vomiting can lead aspiration of vomitus to the lungs and cause asphyxia or aspiration pneumonia.
- *Mallory Weiss syndrome:* Due to severe and repetitive retching and vomiting a partial tear of the mucosa and submucosa in the stomach and gastroesophageal junction can occur and lead to hematemesis.
- *Boerhaave's syndrome:* This is a full thickness tear of all the layers of the esophagus, commonly in the lower part of the esophagus due to repetitive, bouts of retching and vomiting. It is a medical emergency.
- *Hypovolemia:* Recurrent vomiting can cause dehydration and hypovolemia due to loss of water content.
- *Electrolyte imbalance:* Hypokalemia occurs due to hypovolemia which stimulates renin-angiotensin-aldosterone system (RAAS) leading to sodium absorption and potassium excretion in the urine.
- *Hypochloremic metabolic alkalosis:* This occurs due to loss of hydrogen ions and chloride which are present in the gastric juice in the vomitus.

Treatment of Vomiting

- Underlying cause should be treated.
- In severe persistent vomiting, patient should be kept nil by mouth and IV fluids administered.
- Antiemetics can be used for symptomatic control of vomiting, e.g. domperidone 10 mg TID, or metoclopramide 10 mg TID, or ondansetron 4 mg TID. Metoclopramide and ondansetron can be given parenterally and are useful in persistent vomiting.

Q. Causes of loss of appetite (Table 4.2).

TABLE 4.2: Causes of loss of appetite
• **Infections:** HIV, tuberculosis or any other infection
• **Gastrointestinal diseases:** Peptic ulcer, pancreatitis, celiac disease
• **Liver diseases:** Hepatitis, cirrhosis
• **Renal diseases:** Renal failure
• **Endocrine causes:** Hypothyroidism, Addison's disease, hyperparathyroidism
• **Cardiac conditions:** Heart failure
• **Respiratory conditions:** COPD, lung cancer
• **Neurological disorders:** Parkinson's disease, dementia, stroke
• **Malignancies:** Carcinoma stomach, pancreas or any other malignancy, leukemias, lymphomas
• **Psychiatric disorders:** Depression, anorexia nervosa
• **Drugs:** Chemotherapy, certain antibiotics

Q. Define diarrhea, pseudodiarrhea and fecal incontinence.

Q. What are the causes of acute diarrhea? How do you evaluate and manage a case of acute diarrhea.

Diarrhea

- Diarrhea is defined as the passage of loose or watery stools, typically at least three times in a 24-hour period. It results from increased water content in the stool, caused by either reduced water absorption or increased water secretion by the intestines.
- Depending on the duration, diarrhea may be classified as **acute if <2 weeks, persistent if 2–4 weeks, and chronic if >4 weeks** in duration.
- Diarrhea should be differentiated from pseudodiarrhea, and fecal incontinence.

Pseudodiarrhea (false diarrhea)

- This is condition where a patient reports frequent passage of small stool amounts, often mistaken for diarrhea, but without an actual increase in stool volume. Unlike true diarrhea, pseudodiarrhea does not involve excessive fluid loss or increased stool weight.
- Causes: Irritable bowel syndrome (diarrhea-predominant IBS), chronic constipation with overflow (hard stools obstruct the rectum, leading to liquid stool leakage), rectal irritation–due to proctitis (inflammation of the rectum) or hemorrhoids.

Fecal Incontinence

- This is involuntary passage of fecal matter and is seen in neuromuscular disorders and structural anorectal problems. Examples are spinal cord injury leading to loss of sphincter control, physical damage to sphincter due to trauma, surgery or child birth.

Causes of Acute Diarrhea (Table 4.3)

TABLE 4.3: Causes of acute diarrhea

Bacterial
Preformed enterotoxin production
• *Staphylococcus aureus*
• *Bacillus cereus*
• *Clostridium perfringens*
Enterotoxin production
• Enterotoxigenic *E. coli* (ETEC)
• *Vibrio cholerae*
Cytotoxin production
• Enterohemorrhagic *E coli* O157:H5
• *Vibrio parahaemolyticus*
• *Clostridium difficile*
Mucosal invasion
• Shigella
• Salmonella
• *Campylobacter jejuni*
• Enteroinvasive *E. coli* (EIEC)
• *Yersinia enterocolitica*
• Chlamydia
• *Neisseria gonorrhoeae*
• *Listeria monocytogenes*
Viral
• Noroviruses
• Rotavirus
• Cytomegalovirus
Protozoal
• *Giardia lamblia*
• Cryptosporidium
• Cyclospora
• *Entamoeba histolytica*

Pathophysiology of Diarrhea

- Diarrhea is the reversal of the normal net absorptive status of water and electrolyte absorption to secretion. Such a derangement can be the result of either an osmotic force that acts in the lumen to drive water into the gut (osmotic diarrhea) or the result of an active secretory state induced in the enterocytes (secretory diarrhea).
- Example of osmotic diarrhea is lactulose induced diarrhea. In secretory diarrhea, the epithelial cells' ion transport processes are turned into a state of active secretion. Example of secretory diarrhea is bacterial infection of the intestine. Pathogens can induce secretary diarrhea through multiple mechanisms such as production of enterotoxins or cytotoxins, release of cytokines, etc.

Evaluation of a Patient with Acute Diarrhea

History

- Residence: In developing countries, there is higher rates of infectious diarrhea (cholera, rotavirus, amebiasis) due to inadequate sanitation and waterborne pathogens.
- Occupational exposure: Sewage and wastewater workers are at high risk of exposure to waterborne pathogens (e.g. *Vibrio cholerae*, hepatitis A, Shigella). Farmers, veterinarians, livestock handlers are at risk of exposure to zoonotic enteric infections (e.g. Cryptosporidium, Giardia, Salmonella).
- Recent and remote travel (suspect diseases endemic in the area of travel)
- Duration of diarrhea (whether acute or chronic, because the causes are different).
- Frequency and quantity of stools (to assess the severity of diarrhea).
- Appearance of stools: Rice water stool is seen in cholera, pea soup appearance in enteric fever, brown colored in amebiasis, red currant jelly stools in shigella.
- Presence of blood and /or mucus (suggests invasive infection. Fresh blood and mucus is seen in large intestinal diarrhea).
- Any associated vomiting (suggests food poisoning or gastroenteritis).
- H/o pain abdomen (suggests invasive infection).
- Urine output (to assess dehydration).
- H/o fever (suggests infection with invasive organisms).
- Food history can give clue about food poisoning and possible pathogen.
- Recent antibiotic use (may suggest antibiotic induced diarrhea due to clostridium difficile).
- H/o immunocompromised state (suspect diarrhea due to unusual organisms such as Cryptosporidia, *Isospora belli*, etc.).
- H/o animal exposure: Exposure to young dogs or cats is associated with *Campylobacter* organisms. Exposure to turtles is associated with Salmonella organisms.

Examination

- Look for any signs of dehydration. Assess pulse, BP, postural hypotension, skin turgor, dryness of mucus membranes.
- Assess conscious level as patient can be in altered sensorium due to electrolyte imbalance.
- Examine the abdomen for any distension, tenderness and bowel sounds.

Investigations in Acute Diarrhea

- Most cases of acute diarrhea improve spontaneously with supportive treatment and do not require investigations. However, acute diarrhea should be investigated if it is severe with dehydration, associated with bloody stools, fever, lasts more than 2 days without improvement, new community outbreaks, severe abdominal pain and in immunocompromised patients.

Complete Blood Count CBC)

- Hemoconcentration and leukocytosis is commonly seen. High leukocyte count suggests infectious diarrhea.

Urea/Creatinine, Serum Electrolytes

- Urea and creatinine may be elevated due to prerenal azotemia. Electrolyte disturbances such as hyponatremia and hypokalemia occur in severe diarrhea.

Stool Analysis

- Stool should be sent for bacterial and viral cultures, microscopy for ova and parasites, immunoassays for bacterial toxins (*C. difficile*), viral antigens (rotavirus), and protozoal antigens (Giardia, *E. histolytica*). Pathogens can also be identified by detecting their DNA sequences.

Ultrasound Abdomen

- Useful if there is severe abdominal pain or abdominal distension or any mass is felt.

GI Endoscopy

- If stool analysis does not reveal the cause of diarrhea, then flexible sigmoidoscopy with biopsies and upper endoscopy with duodenal aspirates and biopsies may be indicated.
- Colonoscopy may be indicated to identify any growth, or to exclude inflammatory bowel disease.

CT Scan Abdomen

- Is useful in the evaluation of ischemic colitis, diverticulitis, or partial bowel obstruction.

Assessment of Dehydration (Table 4.4)

TABLE 4.4: Assessment of dehydration

Feature	Mild dehydration	Moderate dehydration	Severe dehydration
General appearance	Well	Restless	Lethargic
Oral mucosa	Moist	Dry	Very dry
Skin	Normal	Cool	Cool
Skin turgor	Normal	Reduced	Markedly reduced
Capillary refilling	Normal	Slow	Very slow
Eyes	Normal	Sunken	Markedly sunken
Pulse rate	Normal	Tachycardia	Markedly increased
JVP	Normal	Collapsed	Collapsed
BP	Normal	Postural drop or reduced	Hypotension/ shock
Respiration	Normal	Normal	Increased
Urine output	Normal	Reduced	Markedly reduced
Urine specific gravity	<1.020	>1.020	>1.035
Blood urea	Normal	Normal or high	High

Treatment

Fluid and Electrolyte Replacement

- This is very important in acute diarrhea since dehydration is the major cause of death. If the patient is able to take orally, oral fluid replacement (in the form of ORS or any other fluid) can be given in mild to moderate dehydration. Intravenous rehydration is required if the patient is not able to take orally, in severe dehydration, in infants, and elderly.

Antimotility Agents

- Agents like loperamide, diphenoxylate/atropine combination decrease the frequency and quantity of diarrhea. They can be used in diarrhea without fever and without blood in stools. These agents should be avoided in infective diarrhea (febrile dysentery), which may be exacerbated or prolonged by them.

Antisecretory Agents

- Example is racecadotril.
- Inhibits secretion of water and electrolytes into the intestinal lumen.
- It acts by inhibition of the enzyme neutral endopeptidase (also known as enkephalinase), a cell membrane peptidase enzyme found on the epithelium of the small intestine.
- Dose is 100 mg TID.
- It is useful in acute watery diarrhea.
- It is contraindicated in renal failure, pregnancy and breast feeding.

Antispasmodics

- Such as dicyclomine, mebeverine, hyoscine, etc. can be used in patients with crampy abdominal pain.

Antibiotics

- Moderately to severely ill patients with febrile dysentery may be empirically treated with a quinolone, such as ciprofloxacin (500 mg bid for 3–5 days).
- Empirical treatment with metronidazole can also be given for suspected giardiasis or amebiasis (400 mg TID for 5–7 days).
- Antibiotic therapy may be modified when specific pathogen is identified.
- Antibiotics should also be given to patients who are immunocompromised, have mechanical heart valves or recent vascular grafts, or are elderly even if the organism is not identified.

Q. Traveler's diarrhea

- Traveler's diarrhea refers to diarrhea occurring in persons traveling from resource-rich to resource-poor regions of the world. It is common among travelers to developing countries.
- Food and water contaminated with fecal matter are the main sources of infection. Bacteria such as enterotoxigenic *Escherichia coli*, enteroaggregative *E. coli*, Campylobacter, Salmonella, and Shigella are common causes of traveler's diarrhea.
- Most cases are benign and self-limited, but occasionally can be severe enough to cause dehydration and other complications.

Causes (Table 4.5)

TABLE 4.5: Causes of traveler's diarrhea

Bacteria (80–90% of cases)
• Enterotoxigenic *Escherichia coli* (most common cause)
• *Campylobacter jejuni*
• Salmonella
• Shigella
• *Vibrio parahaemolyticus*
• *Vibrio cholerae*
• *Yersinia enterocolitica*
Viruses
• Rotavirus
• Norovirus
• Adenovirus
Parasites
• *Giardia lamblia*
• *Entamoeba histolytica*

- These organisms are often transmitted by food and water.
- More than 90% cases are due to bacteria; the most common being enterotoxigenic *Escherichia coli* (ETEC).

Risk Factors

- ***Travel to high-risk areas:*** South Asia, Southeast Asia, Africa, Latin America, Middle East.
- ***Poor food and water hygiene:*** Street food, raw or undercooked meats, unpasteurized dairy.
- ***Weakened immunity***: Older adults, young children, immunocompromised individuals.
- ***Low stomach acidity***: Proton pump inhibitor (PPI) or H_2 blocker use increases risk.

Clinical Features

- Most cases occur within first 2 weeks of travel.
- Abdominal cramps followed by sudden onset, watery diarrhea. Diarrhea may last from few hours to few days.
- Malaise, anorexia, nausea, vomiting, and fever.
- Diffuse tenderness over abdomen.
- Additional specific features may be present depending on the organism.

Treatment

- *Fluid replacement:* Most cases are self-limited and resolve on their own within three to five days of treatment with fluid replacement only. Oral fluid replacement is enough in most cases. Broth, fruit juice, or similar fluids may be used. ORS is especially useful in severe diarrhea.
- *Antibiotics:* Shorten the disease duration to about one day. Antibiotics are indicated in patients with severe diarrhea associated with fever, blood, pus, or mucus in the stool. Ciprofloxacin or norfloxacin may be used. Metronidazole/Tinidazole is used for protozoal infections.
- *Antimotility agents:* Antimotility agents such as loperamide (Imodium) or diphenoxylate (Lomotil) can be used to reduce severity of diarrhea. However, caution should be exercised in using these agents in bloody diarrhea.

Prevention

- *Improving food and drink selection:* Avoid raw food items such as chutney, salads, buttermilk, and curds. Use only boiled or bottled water. Avoid fresh fruit juices with ice.
- *Prophylactic antibiotics:* Not routinely necessary. Quinolones or doxycycline 100 mg/day for a few weeks. Bismuth subsalicylate 60 ml four times a day is an alternative. Rifaximin may prove to be the preferred antibiotic because it is not absorbed and is well tolerated.
- *Probiotics:* Such as Lactobacillus and *Saccharomyces boulardii* have been shown to decrease the incidence of diarrhea in travelers.

Q. Enumerate the indications for stool cultures and blood cultures in patients with acute diarrhea.

Indications for stool cultures in acute diarrhea

- Fever
- Blood in stools
- Leukocytes in stool
- Pain resembling that associated with appendicitis (Yersinia)
- Diarrheal illness associated with partially cooked hamburger (cytotoxigenic *E. coli* O157:H7)
- Prolonged diarrhea (more than 4–7 days)
- Immunocompromised host
- For epidemiologic purposes, such as cases involving food handlers.

Indications for blood cultures in acute diarrhea

- Fever
- Pain abdomen
- Patients with sepsis, shock
- Immunocompromised patients

Q. Enumerate the parasites causing diarrhea.

- Amebiasis
- Giardiasis
- Trichuriasis
- Strongyloidiasis
- Balantidiasis
- Microsporidia
- Isospora belli
- *Cryptosporidium parvum*
- *Schistosoma mansoni*
- Capillariasis

Q. Define chronic diarrhea. What are the causes of chronic diarrhea? How do you investigate and manage a case of chronic diarrhea.

- Chronic diarrhea is defined as diarrhea lasting for more than 4 weeks.

Causes of Chronic Diarrhea (Table 4.6)

TABLE 4.6: Causes of chronic diarrhea

Secretory diarrhea • Hormonally mediated: VIPoma, carcinoid, medullary carcinoma of thyroid (calcitonin), Zollinger-Ellison syndrome (gastrin) • Villous adenoma
Inflammatory conditions • Inflammatory bowel disease (ulcerative colitis and Crohn's disease) • Radiation enteritis
Malabsorption syndromes • Celiac sprue, tropical sprue, Whipple's disease, eosinophilic gastroenteritis, small bowel resection (short bowel syndrome), chronic pancreatitis, lactose intolerance
Chronic infections • Giardiasis • Chronic amebiasis • Intestinal tuberculosis • HIV related infections by *Mycobacterium avium* complex, Microsporida, Cryptosporidium, *Isospora belli*
Motility disorders • Blind loop with bacterial overgrowth • Diabetes mellitus • Hyperthyroidism • Irritable bowel syndrome
Malignancy • Lymphoma of intestine, adenocarcinoma colon
Medications • Laxatives, angiotensin receptor blockers

Investigations in Chronic Diarrhea

- In contrast to acute diarrhea, most cases of chronic diarrhea are noninfectious.
- All the tests described for acute diarrhea are required for chronic diarrhea.
- 24-hour stool fat estimation, testing for presence of laxatives, and estimation of stool osmolality (normal osmotic gap in secretory diarrhea, increased in osmotic diarrhea) should be done.
- Intestinal aspirates and quantitative cultures to rule out small bowel bacterial overgrowth.
- If suggested by history or other findings, hormonal excesses should be ruled out by appropriate tests (serum gastrin, VIP, calcitonin, thyroid function tests, etc.).
- Low fecal pH suggests carbohydrate malabsorption; lactose malabsorption can be confirmed by lactose breath testing or by a therapeutic trial with lactose exclusion and observation of the effect of lactose challenge.
- Pancreatic disease should be excluded by secretin-cholecystokinin stimulation test, or by assay of fecal chymotrypsin activity or a bentiromide test.
- Ultrasound abdomen to rule out pancreatitis, malignancy, and pancreatitis.
- Colonoscopy to rule out ileocecal TB, Ca colon, inflammatory bowel disease, etc.
- CT abdomen if malignancy or pancreatitis or abdominal TB is suspected.

Treatment Chronic Diarrhea

- Treatment of chronic diarrhea depends on the specific etiology. For example, elimination of lactose containing foods in lactase deficiency or gluten in celiac sprue, use of steroids or anti-inflammatory agents in inflammatory bowel diseases, etc.

Q. Define constipation. Enumerate the causes of constipation. How do you investigate and treat a case of constipation?

- Constipation may be defined as infrequent stools (less than 3 times in a week), hard stools, excessive straining, or a sense of incomplete evacuation.
- Risk factors for constipation include female sex, older age, inactivity, low caloric intake, low fiber diet, and taking a large number of medications. The incidence of constipation is three times higher in women.

Causes of Constipation in Adults (Table 4.7)

TABLE 4.7: Causes of constipation in adults

Primary functional) constipation	Occurs without a clear medical cause, often due to motility disorders, inadequate fiber or fluid intake, sedentary lifestyle, irregular bowel habits
GI diseases	Intestinal obstruction, colonic neoplasm, colonic stricture, anal fissure, painful hemorrhoids, anal sphincter spasm, pelvic floor dysfunction, descending perineum syndrome, rectal mucosal prolapse, rectocele, Hirschsprung's disease, Chagas' disease, irritable bowel syndrome (constipation predominant), scleroderma with GI involvement
Endocrinopathies	Hypothyroidism, hyperparathyroidism, hypercalcemia, diabetes mellitus
Psychiatric disorders	Depression, eating disorders
Neurologic diseases	Parkinsonism, multiple sclerosis, spinal cord injury, stroke, autonomic neuropathy, myotonic dystrophy
Metabolic	Hypokalemia, hypercalcemia, uremia, porphyria
Drugs	Calcium-channel blockers, antidepressants, opioids, anticholinergics, clonidine, calcium and iron supplements

Approach to a Case of Constipation

History

- Confirm what exactly the patient means and whether there is really constipation. A constipated patient may be otherwise totally asymptomatic or may complain of one or more of the following: straining, lumpy or hard stools, sensation of anorectal obstruction, sensation of incomplete defecation, manual maneuvering required to defecate, abdominal bloating, pain on defecation, and rectal bleeding.
- Ask about the frequency of stools, consistency (lumpy/hard), excessive straining, or prolonged defecation time.

- Presence of blood in the stool and weight loss should be taken seriously as it can indicate carcinoma colon. Similarly presence of vomiting, inability to pass flatus and pain abdomen indicates intestinal obstruction.
- Ask about the symptoms of any underlying disease (see the causes above).
- Ask about food habits, activity, and drug intake.

Examination

- Do a complete physical examination and rectal examination.
- Look for any hernias which can cause constipation or the result of chronic constipation.
- Look for any mass in the abdomen.
- Look for any evidence of endocrine (hypothyroidism) or neurological abnormalities.

Investigations

- Based on the history and examination findings investigations are ordered as follows:

Blood Tests

- Serum calcium, blood sugar, thyroid and parathyroid function tests, etc. if clinically indicated.

Stool Examination

- Look for occult blood (presence of blood may suggest Ca colon).

Sigmoidoscopy, Barium Enema, Colonoscopy

- These are indicated to rule out local anorectal abnormalities. Colonoscopy is especially important in patients above 40 years with h/o of weight loss, rectal bleeding, or anemia to rule out colonic cancer.

Colon Transit Time

- This is measured by performing an abdominal radiograph 120 hours after ingestion of radiopaque markers. Retention of >20% of the marker indicates prolonged transit.

Balloon Expulsion Testing, Anal Manometry, and Defecograph

- These tests can be used to assess pelvic floor dysfunction and anorectal disorders.

Treatment

- *General measures:* Increase fluid intake, high fiber diet and regular physical activity. If these measures fail use the following pharmacological therapies.
- *Bulk laxatives:* These include psyllium (ispaghulla), methylcellulose, and calcium polycarbophil. They exert their laxative effect by absorbing water and increasing fecal mass. They are well tolerated. They may be used alone or in combination with dietary changes. Side effects are impaction above strictures, gas and bloating.
- *Emollients (stool softeners):* Include docusate sodium and liquid paraffin. Docusate sodium acts by lowering the surface tension of stool, thereby allowing water to easily enter the stool. Liquid paraffin works by lubricating the stool. They are generally inferior to bulk laxatives, but more useful in patients with anal fissures and hemorrhoids which cause painful defecation. They are generally well tolerated. Liquid paraffin can cause depletion of fat soluble vitamins if used for long time.
- *Osmotic laxatives:* Include magnesium sulfate, lactulose, polyethylene glycol, sorbitol, and glycerine. These agents are poorly absorbed and act as hyperosmolar solutions which retain water in the intestinal lumen. Magnesium sulfate can cause hypermagnesemia in patients with renal failure. Other agents can cause flatulence and abdominal bloating.
- *Stimulant laxatives:* These include castor oil, bisacodyl and senna. They increase intestinal motility and secretion of water into the bowel. They can cause electrolyte imbalance such as hypokalemia.
- *Prokinetic agents:* Metoclopramide, mosapride, prucalopride. They increase intestinal motility.
- *Enemas:* Enemas act within 5–15 min and are given rectally. These include tap water enema, soap water enema and sodium phosphate enema, etc. Rarely if stools are impacted, digital evacuaton has to be done.
- *New agents:* Newer therapies for constipation include prucalopride, a prokinetic agent that stimulates colonic motility and decreases transit time, and the osmotic agents lubiprostone and linaclotide, which stimulate intestinal fluid secretion by acting on the intestinal mucosa. Lubiprostone and linaclotide are useful in chronic idiopathic constipation and constipation caused by irritable bowel syndrome. Naloxegol and methylnaltrexone are useful in opioid induced constipation.

Q. Enumerate the causes of occult blood in the stool.

- Occult bleeding refers to positive fecal occult blood test without visible fecal blood either to the patient or physician.

Causes (Table 4.8)

TABLE 4.8: Causes of occult blood in the stool
Upper GI lesions
• Esophagitis
• Peptic ulcer disease
• Gastritis/erosions
• Duodenitis/erosions
• Angiodysplasia
• Esophageal or gastric varices
• Gastric cancer
• Gastric or duodenal polyps
Lower GI lesions
• Colon polyps
• Colon cancer
• Angiodysplasia
• Colonic ulcers
• Hemorrhoids
• Anal fissure
Worm infestation
• Hook worm
Drugs
• Aspirin or other NSAIDs

Q. Enumerate the causes of weight loss (Table 4.9).

TABLE 4.9: Causes of weight loss

Involuntary weight loss
• Endocrine disorders (hyperthyroidism, pheochromocytoma, adrenal insufficiency)
• Uncontrolled diabetes mellitus
• Malignancy
• Chronic infections (tuberculosis, HIV, subacute bacterial endocarditis)
• GI disorders (malabsorption syndromes, chronic pancreatitis, IBD, parasitic infestation)
• COPD
• Chronic renal failure
• Psychiatric disorders (depression, mania, anorexia nervosa, schizophrenia)
• Chronic alcoholism
• Drugs (opiates, amphetamines, digoxin, metformin, NSAIDs, anticancer drugs)
Voluntary weight loss
• Treatment of obesity
• Anorexic drugs—amphetamines and derivatives
• Distance runners, models, ballet dancers, gymnasts
• Marked increase in physical activity
• Prolonged fasting

Q. Aphthous ulcers.

- Aphthous ulcers, commonly known as canker sores, are recurrent ulcerations of the oral mucosa without an infectious cause. They are among the most common oral lesions, affecting up to 25% of the general population. These are painful, localized, shallow, round to oval, with a grayish base **(Fig. 4.2)**.
- Aphthous ulcers are common in childhood and adolescence and become less frequent in adulthood. They usually heal within 10–14 days without scarring.

Etiology

- Exact cause of aphthous ulcers is not well known. Alterations in local cell mediated immunity may play a role in the causation.
- Local trauma due to biting, dental procedures, and sharp food may cause aphthous ulcers.
- A genetic basis exists for some recurrent aphthous ulcerations. This is shown by a positive family history in about one third of patients with recurrent aphthous ulcerations.

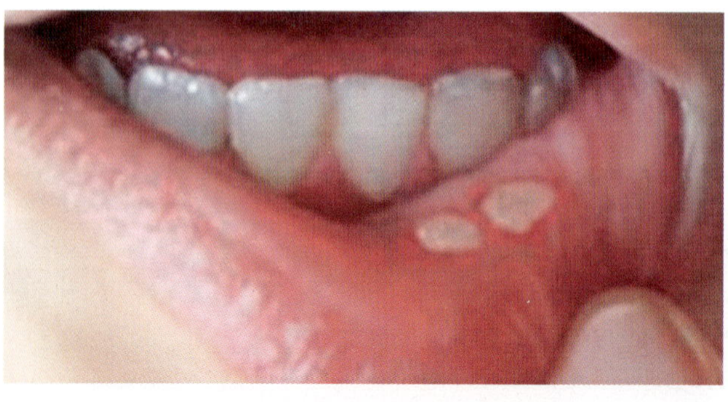

Figure 4.2: Apthous ulcers

- Recurrent aphthous ulcers are seen in stress, infections, food allergy, HIV infection, celiac sprue, gluten sensitive enteropathies, inflammatory bowel diseases, Behcet's disease and vitamin and mineral deficiencies (B vitamins, iron, folic acid, and zinc). Drugs like methotrexate may induce oral ulcers.

Treatment

- *Topical anesthetics:* Lidocaine 2% gel and benzydamine mouthwash (anti-inflammatory) are helpful in reducing pain.
- *Topical corticosteroids:* Local corticosteroid application (triamcinolone gel and hydrocortisone pellets) and other topical analgesics are adequate. These are applied to the ulcer two to four times daily until the ulcer is healed.
- *Antiseptic rinses:* Chlorhexidine gluconate mouth rinses reduce the severity and pain of ulceration but not the frequency. Hydrogen peroxide rinse (diluted 1:1 with water).
- *Systemic therapy (for severe cases):* Oral corticosteroids are indicated for severe disease. Colchicine, dapsone, pentoxifylline, interferon alpha, and levamisole are beneficial in severe recurrent aphthous ulcers. Thalidomide is useful for severe recurrent aphthous ulcers, especially in patients with HIV infection.

Q. What is hiatus hernia? Discuss the causes, clinical features, diagnosis and management of hiatus hernia.

Q. S/N. Sliding hiatus hernia.

Q. S/N. Paraesophageal or rolling hernia.

- Hiatus hernia is herniation of a part of the stomach into the thoracic cavity through the esophageal hiatus of the diaphragm. There are two types: (i) *sliding hiatus hernia* and (ii) *paraesophageal or rolling hernia* **(Fig. 4.3)**.
- **Sliding hiatus hernia:** Here, the gastroesophageal junction and fundus of the stomach slide upward through the hiatus and lie above the diaphragm.
- **Paraesophageal or rolling hernia:** Here, the gastro-esophageal junction remains fixed in its normal location but a small part of the fundus of the stomach rolls up through the hiatus alongside the esophagus.

Etiology

- Incidence increases with increasing age.
- Weakening of the anchors of the gastroesophageal junction to the diaphragm and longitudinal contraction of the esophagus.
- Increased intra-abdominal pressure (ascites, pregnancy, obesity).
- Trauma.
- Post-surgical (e.g. after antireflux procedures, esophagomyotomy, or partial gastrectomy).
- Congenital malformation.
- Connective tissue disorders (Marfan's syndrome, Ehlers-Danlos syndrome).

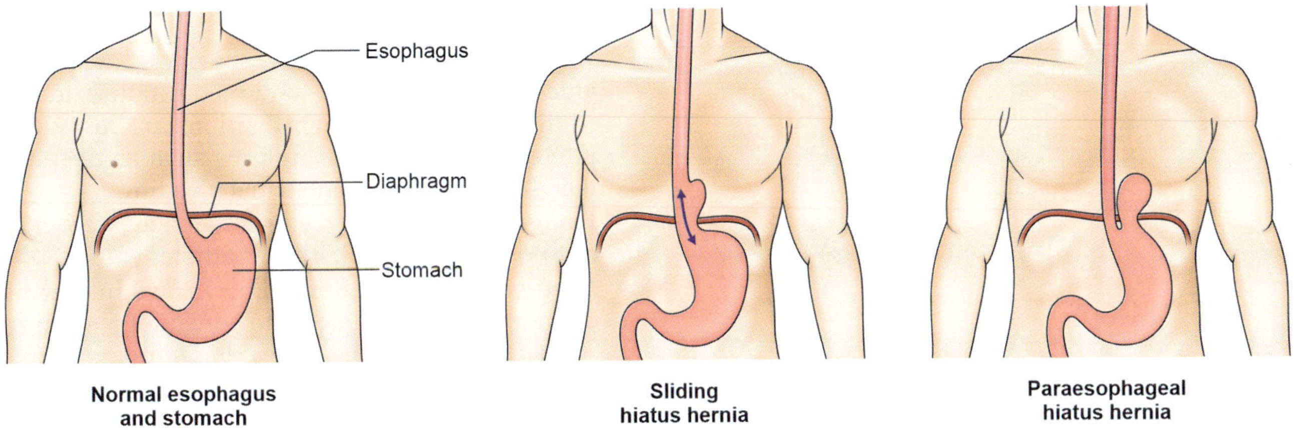

Figure 4.3: Hiatus hernia

Clinical Features

- Asymptomatic in many cases, especially small sliding hernias.
- Heartburn (GERD symptoms)—due to LES dysfunction.
- Regurgitation—especially at night or when lying down.
- Dysphagia (difficulty swallowing).
- Chest pain—can mimic cardiac pain but is relieved by sitting upright.
- Epigastric pain, bloating
- Iron deficiency anemia (chronic occult bleeding from gastric ulceration—Cameron's ulcers).
- Severe cases: Gastric obstruction and gastric strangulation → sudden severe pain, tachycardia (surgical emergency).

Investigations

- Chest X-ray: May show retrocardiac air fluid level or intrathoracic stomach.
- Barium swallow will demonstrate the presence of gastric herniation.
- Endoscopy: Identifies esophagitis, ulcers, or Barrett's esophagus.

Management

- Asymptomatic sliding hiatus hernia does not require any treatment.

Lifestyle Modifications

- Weight loss (reduces intra-abdominal pressure)
- Elevate the head of the bed (prevents nocturnal reflux)
- A avoid spicy foods, caffeine, alcohol, and smoking.
- Smaller, frequent meals (prevent gastric distension).

Medical Management

- Proton pump inhibitors (PPIs): Examples are omeprazole, pantoprazole—First-line therapy.
- Prokinetics (metoclopramide, domperidone)—If there is delayed gastric emptying.
- Antacids for symptomatic relief.

Surgical Treatment

- Symptomatic large hiatus hernia requires surgical treatment. Surgical treatment involves repair of the diaphragmatic defect, and fixing the stomach in the abdominal cavity (fundoplication) combined with an anti-reflux procedure.

Q. What is gastroesophageal reflux disease (GERD)? Describe the etiology, pathophysiology, clinical features, investigations, complications and treatment of reflux esophagitis.

- Gastroesophageal reflux is the movement of gastric contents into the esophagus. It occurs in everyone, multiple times every day.
- It becomes pathological, when the antireflux mechanisms fail sufficiently to allow gastric contents to make prolonged contact with the lower esophageal mucosa causing damage (GERD). Reflux esophagitis is the most common form of GERD, most often recognized by recurrent heartburn.

Etiology of GERD

- Pregnancy, obesity, ascites and weight lifting act by increasing intra-abdominal pressure.
- Fat, chocolate, smoking, coffee, large fatty meals or alcohol ingestion reduce lower esophageal sphincter tone.
- Drugs: Calcium-channel blockers, nitrates reduce sphincter tone.
- Systemic sclerosis reduces sphincter tone and esophageal motility.
- After treatment for achalasia (reflux increases).
- Sliding hiatus hernia predisposes to reflux because the gastroesophageal junction lies above the diaphragm and hence the sphincter effect of diaphragm is lost.

Pathophysiology (Fig. 4.4)

- Esophagus is a 25-cm conduit whose upper third is skeletal muscle and lower two third is smooth muscle. There is a sphincter in the lower esophagus (lower esophageal sphincter) formed by the lower 4 cm of esophageal smooth muscle. It relaxes after swallowing to allow food to enter the stomach and closes after swallowing thereby preventing reflux. Sphincter tone can increase in response to rises in intra-abdominal and intragastric pressures. Reflux is also prevented by

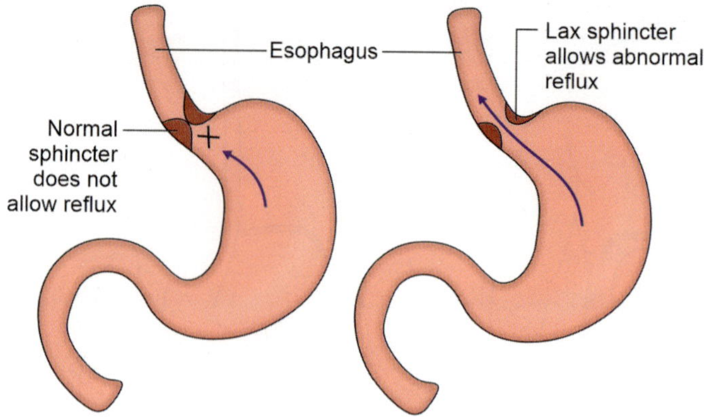

Figure 4.4: Pathology in GERD

contraction of the crural diaphragm which surrounds lower end of esophagus and exerts a 'pinchcock-like' action at the LES.

- When these mechanisms fail, abnormal acid reflux occurs and damages the lower end of esophagus. Damage to esophagus produces mild esophagitis (mild erythema) and erosive esophagitis (mucosal damage, bleeding, superficial linear ulcers, and exudates). Erosive esophagitis may heal by intestinal metaplasia (Barrett's esophagus), which is a risk factor for adenocarcinoma.

Clinical Features

- Regurgitation of sour material into the mouth and heartburn are the main features of GERD. Angina like pain can occur in some patients. Heartburn is due to contact of refluxed material with the sensitized or ulcerated esophageal mucosa. The correlation between heartburn and esophagitis is poor. Patients with severe esophagitis may have mild pain and patients with mild esophagitis may have severe pain. The burning is aggravated by bending, stooping or lying down and on drinking hot liquids or alcohol. It is usually be relieved by antacids.
- Reflux into the pharynx, larynx, and tracheobronchial tree can cause chronic cough, bronchoconstriction, pharyngitis, laryngitis, bronchitis, or pneumonia.
- Dysphagia may develop due to stricture of lower end of esophagus or development of adenocarcinoma in Barrett's esophagus.
- Mucosal erosions may produce bleeding, hematemesis and anemia.

Differentiating GERD from angina (Table 4.10)

TABLE 4.10: Differentiating GERD from angina

GERD	Angina
Burning pain	Gripping or crushing pain
Pain produced by bending, stooping or lying down	Pain produced by exercise
Pain relieved by antacids	Pain relieved by rest and nitrates
Radiates to retrosternal area and not to shoulders and arms	Pain radiates into neck, shoulders and both arms
No dyspnea, sweating and tachycardia	Accompanied by dyspnea, tachycardia and sweating

Investigations

- A history of recurrent heartburn and response to antacids or acid-suppressant medication is adequate to diagnose GERD. Investigations are reserved for patients with alarm symptoms such as dysphagia, weight loss, or gastrointestinal bleeding.
- ***Endoscopy*** is used to confirm damage to esophagus or to rule out other alternate pathology.
- ***Barium swallow*** followed by X-rays in the head-down position can detect movement of barium from stomach to esophagus suggesting reflux.
- ***24-hour esophageal pH monitoring*** is the gold standard test for identifying reflux. This is done by fixing a small pH probe in the esophagus, 5 cm above the LES, and recording all episodes of acid reflux (drop in pH <4) over a 24-hour period. Total number and duration of each reflux event yield a total esophageal acid contact time.
- ***Bernstein test*** can tell whether the symptoms are due to acid reflux. This test is done by perfusing acid (0.1 N Hcl, pH 1.1) or saline (control) through a catheter positioned in mid-esophagus. If symptoms develop during acid, but not saline perfusion, the test is considered positive for GERD.
- ***Resting and stress ECG*** to rule out angina.

Complications of GERD

- Esophagitis
- Peptic stricture
- Barrett esophagus
- Carcinoma of esophagus
- Aspiration pneumonia
- Iron deficiency anemia due to chronic blood loss from esophageal ulcers.

Treatment

General Measures

- Weight reduction if overweight
- Head end elevation of the bed at night
- Reduction in alcohol consumption and cessation of smoking
- Avoid trigger foods (fatty, spicy, caffeine, carbonated drinks)
- Eat smaller meals and avoid eating 2–3 hours before bedtime.

Medical Management

- This is the preferred treatment. The goal of treatment is to relieve symptoms and prevent complications. Most patients obtain symptom relief with the following treatment, but symptoms usually return when treatment is stopped and long-term therapy is then required.
- *Antacids:* antacids neutralize the acid in the stomach and immediately relieve heart burn. Most antacid preparations contain combination of magnesium sulphate and aluminum hydroxide. Magnesium sulfate tends to cause diarrhea while aluminum

hydroxide causes constipation. Combining both of them will have neutral effect on bowel movements. Antacids are available in both liquid and tablet forms. These preparations can be taken as and when required (10 ml 3–6 times daily). Alginate-containing antacids form a gel or 'foam raft' on top of gastric contents and thereby reduce reflux.

- *H_2-receptor antagonists* (e.g. ranitidine, famotidine and nizaladine) are used for acid suppression along with antacids. They should be given for 6–8 weeks.
- *Proton pump inhibitors* (PPIs) (e.g. omeprazole, rabeprazole, lansoprazole, pantoprazole, esomeprazole): they inhibit gastric hydrogen/potassium-ATPase and reduce gastric acid secretion by 90%. These are more effective than H_2 blockers and are preferred over them. 8 weeks of therapy can heal erosive esophagitis in up to 90% of patients. Patients with severe symptoms need prolonged treatment, often for years. Rebound increased acid secretion is a problem with these agents.
- *Prokinetic agents* (metoclopramide, mosapride, cintapride and domperidone): They increase lower esophageal sphincter tone and speed gastric emptying. They are only occasionally helpful. Cisapride increases QT interval and predisposes to cardiac arrhythmias. It has been withdrawn from market. Acotiamide is a novel prokinetic agent which acts by increasing acetylcholine release from enteric neurons through acetylcholinesterase (AChE) inhibition.

Surgery

- Anti-reflux surgery can be considered for patients with severe reflux symptoms confirmed by pH monitoring and with esophagitis on esophagoscopy. But even these patients respond to medical therapy which should be reinforced. Surgery can also be an alternative for patients who require long-term, high-dose PPIs.
- In antireflux surgery, the gastric fundus is wrapped around the esophagus (modified Nissen fundoplication), which increases lower esophageal sphincter pressure and prevents reflux.
- Complications of GERD like stricture require repeated dilatations or surgical resection.

Q. Barrett's esophagus.

- This is metaplasia of esophageal squamous epithelium to columnar epithelium.
- It is a complication of long standing severe reflux esophagitis and is a risk factor for developing esophageal adenocarcinoma. Barrett's epithelium progresses through a dysplastic stage before developing into adenocarcinoma.
- Metaplastic columnar epithelium develops because it is more resistant to acid-pepsin damage than squamous epithelium.
- It is more common in men and older age groups.
- Endoscopically, Barrett's epithelium may be seen as a continuous sheet, a finger like projection into the esophagus or as islands of columnar mucosa.
- An indocarmine spray down the endoscope can detect intestinal metaplasia and possibly dysplasia. Biopsies should be obtained from all four quadrants of the Barrett's segment.

Treatment

- Regular endoscopy can detect dysplasia before development of adenocarcinoma. Hence, endoscopic surveillance every 2–3 years, with four-quadrant biopsies of Barrett's segment is recommended.
- If high-grade dysplasia is found on biopsy, esophagectomy of the involved segment is advised before it turns into adenocarcinoma. Photodynamic laser or thermocoagulative mucosal ablation and endoscopic mucosal resection are being evaluated as alternatives.
- There is no evidence that treatment with PPIs or antireflux surgery leads to Barrett's regression.

Q. Define dysphagia. What are the causes of dysphagia? How do you approach a case a dysphagia?

- Dysphagia means difficulty in swallowing.
- Odynophagia is pain while swallowing.
- It is a symptom, not a disease, and can result from neuromuscular, structural, or functional disorders.

Types of Dysphagia

Oropharyngeal dysphagia (difficulty initiating swallowing)

- Affects the oral cavity, pharynx, and upper esophageal sphincter.
- Patients report choking, coughing, nasal regurgitation, aspiration.

Esophageal dysphagia (food sticking in the esophagus)

- Affects the esophagus and lower esophageal sphincter (LES).
- Patients feel food getting stuck in the chest after swallowing.

Etiology

See **Table 4.11**.

Approach to a Case of Dysphagia

History

- The type of food causing dysphagia gives useful information. Dysphagia only for solids implies mechanical dysphagia with partial obstruction. Dysphagia only for liquids implies neurological cause of dysphagia (classical example is rabies). Dysphagia for both solids and liquids from the onset occurs in severe obstructive lesions.
- H/o difficulty in initiating swallowing suggests oropharyngeal dysphagia. H/o food "sticking" after swallowing indicates esophageal dysphagia.
- The duration and course of dysphagia are also helpful in diagnosis. Transient dysphagia is usually due to an inflammatory process. Sudden onset dysphagia

TABLE 4.11: Etiology of dysphagia

Oropharyngeal dysphagia

Painful diseases of mouth and pharynx
- Stomatitis
- Tonsillitis
- Pharyngitis
- Retropharyngeal abscesses
- Diphtheria

Structural abnormalities
- Head and neck cancer—Tumors in the oropharynx or larynx obstruct the passage.
- Radiation therapy effects—Fibrosis and reduced tissue mobility post-radiation.
- Zenker's diverticulum—Pouch formation in the pharyngeal wall causes food trapping.

Neuromuscular disorders
- Bulbar paralysis
- Pseudobulbar palsy
- Myasthenia gravis
- Multiple sclerosis
- Parkinson disease
- Oculopharyngeal muscular dystrophy
- Rabies

Functional
- Functional dysphagia

Esophageal dysphagia

Mechanical (obstructive) causes
- Congenital stenosis of esophagus
- Tracheoesophageal fistula
- Congenital web
- Strictures
- Carcinoma esophagus
- Diverticulum
- Esophagitis (reflux, Candida)
- Achalasia cardia
- Plummer-Vinson syndrome
- Scleroderma
- Post-surgical or radiation-induced fibrosis
- Extrinsic compression: Thyroid swelling, secondaries in the neck, mediastinal mass, lymphadenopathy, or abscess, aortic aneurysm, left atrial enlargement, osteophytes in cervical spine

Neuromuscular (motility) disorders
- Achalasia cardia
- Scleroderma
- Diffuse esophageal spasm
- Hypertensive lower esophageal sphincter
- Chagas' disease—Infectious cause of achalasia-like esophageal dysfunction due to *Trypanosoma cruzi* infection.
- Nutcracker esophagus (hypertensive peristalsis)—Excessively strong peristaltic contractions, causing pain and dysphagia.
- Parkinson's disease and multiple sclerosis may contribute to esophageal dysmotility (these conditions can cause both oropharyngeal and esophageal dysphagia).

occurs due to obstructive foreign bodies. Progressive dysphagia may be due to carcinoma esophagus or scleroderma or neuromuscular disorders (e.g. Parkinson's, ALS). Intermittent dysphagia is seen in diffuse esophageal spasm.

- Dysphagia with nasal regurgitation is seen in pharyngeal paralysis.
- H/o regurgitation of old food and halitosis suggests Zenker's diverticulum.
- Tracheobronchial aspiration with dysphagia is seen in tracheoesophageal fistula.
- Weight loss and progressive dysphagia in elderly is highly suggestive of carcinoma. When hoarseness precedes dysphagia, the primary lesion is usually in the larynx. When hoarseness appears after dysphagia it suggests involvement of the recurrent laryngeal nerve by extension of esophageal carcinoma. Sometimes hoarseness may be due to laryngitis secondary to gastroesophageal reflux.
- Chest pain with dysphagia occurs in diffuse esophageal spasm and related motor disorders.
- A prolonged history of heartburn preceding dysphagia indicates peptic stricture.
- If odynophagia is present, it suggests inflammatory or infectious conditions such as pharyngitis or esophagitis.

Risk Factors and Past Medical History

- Neurological disorders—stroke, Parkinson's, ALS, multiple sclerosis, myasthenia gravis.
- Autoimmune diseases—scleroderma, polymyositis, Sjögren's syndrome.
- GERD history—risk for esophageal stricture, Barrett's esophagus.
- Head and neck cancer or radiation therapy—structural damage, fibrosis.
- Connective tissue disorders—can affect esophageal motility (e.g. scleroderma).
- Medication history—pill esophagitis (e.g. bisphosphonates, NSAIDs, tetracyclines).
- Anticholinergics, opioids (can impair motility).
- History of surgery—esophageal or cervical spine surgeries may cause structural abnormalities.

Physical Examination

- Weight loss suggests malignancy or malnutrition due to chronic dysphagia.
- Pallor is present in Plummer-Vinson syndrome due to iron deficiency.
- Neck should be examined for thyromegaly, lymphadenopathy or any other abnormality.
- Mouth and pharynx should be examined for any local pathology.
- Skin should be examined for evidence of scleroderma.
- Neurological examination should be done looking for evidence of bulbar or pseudobulbar palsy.
- Abdomen should be examined for any distension, mass.
- Cancer spread to lymph nodes and liver may be evident.
- Respiratory system examination may reveal complications of dysphagia such as aspiration pneumonia.

Investigations

- Hemoglobin and peripheral smear to check for anemia (iron deficiency causes anemia and Plummer-Vinson syndrome).
- Barium swallow: Filling defect may be seen in tumors as filling. Rat tail appearance seen in stricture. Corkscrew appearance is seen in diffuse esophageal spasm. "Bird beak" appearance is seen in achalasia. Pouch-like structure is seen in Zenker's diverticulum.
- Endoscopy and biopsy of any lesions.
- Esophageal manometry: Indicated for motility disorders (achalasia, esophageal spasm, scleroderma). Measures esophageal peristalsis and lower esophageal sphincter (LES) pressure.
- Chest X-ray to rule out mediastinal mass or bronchogenic ca.
- CT scan of neck and chest to rule out any mass lesions.
- MRI brain/spine: If stroke, multiple sclerosis, or brainstem pathology is suspected.

Management of Dysphagia (Table 4.12)

- Management of dysphagia depends on the underlying cause.

TABLE 4.12: Management of dysphagia

Cause	Management
	Oropharyngeal dysphagia
Neurological disorders (stroke, Parkinson's, ALS, MS, myasthenia gravis)	• Swallowing therapy (speech therapy) • Modified diet (thickened liquids, pureed food) • Postural techniques (chin tuck, head turn) • Feeding alternatives (NG tube or PEG if severe) • Disease-specific treatment (e.g. levodopa for Parkinson's, pyridostigmine for myasthenia gravis)
Structural causes (Zenker's diverticulum, tumors, radiation fibrosis)	• Endoscopic or surgical removal (if symptomatic) • Esophageal dilation or stenting (for strictures) • Dietary modifications (if surgery not feasible)
	Esophageal dysphagia
Mechanical obstruction (strictures, rings, webs, cancer)	• Esophageal dilation (for strictures, Schatzki ring) • PPIs (for GERD-induced strictures) • Endoscopic resection or stenting (for esophageal cancer)
Motility disorders (achalasia, diffuse esophageal spasm, scleroderma)	• **Achalasia:** Pneumatic dilation, botulinum toxin, Heller myotomy, calcium-channel blockers • **Diffuse esophageal spasm:** Calcium-channel blockers, nitrates, PPIs (if GERD component) • **Scleroderma:** PPIs for GERD, prokinetics (metoclopramide)
GERD and eosinophilic esophagitis	• **GERD:** PPIs (omeprazole), lifestyle changes, Nissen fundoplication (if refractory) • **Eosinophilic esophagitis:** Elimination diet (allergens), topical corticosteroids (fluticasone, budesonide), PPIs

Q. Plummer-Vinson syndrome (Paterson-Kelly syndrome).

- The combination of esophageal webs, dysphagia, and iron-deficiency anemia is called Plummer-Vinson syndrome.
- It is considered a premalignant condition because it increases the risk of esophageal squamous cell carcinoma.
- It is usually seen in middle-aged women.
- Esophageal webs are thin, diaphragm-like membranes of squamous mucosa. They are usually seen in the upper esophagus and may be multiple.
- Most cases are asymptomatic. Solid food dysphagia may occur. Dysphagia is intermittent and not progressive.
- Investigations include barium esophagogram and endoscopy.
- Treatment involves passage of a large (> 16-mm-diameter) bougie dilator to disrupt the lesion. Repeated dilations are required in many patients. Underlying iron deficiency should be treated.

Q. Define hiccups (singultus). What are the causes of hiccups? Add a note on its treatment.

Definition

- Hiccups, medically known as singultus, are involuntary, repetitive contractions of the diaphragm, followed by a sudden closure of the vocal cords (glottis), producing a characteristic "hic" sound.
- Hiccups have no known physiological function. They are usually benign and self-limiting. However, occasionally they may be a sign of serious underlying illness.

Mechanism

- **Diaphragmatic spasm** → Sudden, involuntary contraction of the diaphragm.
- **Rapid inhalation** → Air rushes into the lungs.
- **Glottic closure** → The vocal cords snap shut, creating the "hic" sound.

Causes

See **Table 4.13**.

Investigations

- Most cases of hiccups are benign and require no investigations.
- Persistent hiccups (lasting >48 hours) require detailed neurologic examination, serum creatinine, liver function tests, and a chest X-ray.
- If the cause is still not clear, CT of the head, chest, and abdomen, echocardiography, bronchoscopy, and upper GI scopy may help. Chest fluoroscopy helps in studying diaphragmatic movement and diagnosing unilateral hiccups.

Treatment

- Idiopathic hiccups can often be terminated by simple measures such as stimulation of nasopharynx,

TABLE 4.13: Causes of hiccups

CNS diseases
Neoplasms, infections, cerebrovascular accident, trauma.
Toxic and metabolic problems
Alcohol intoxication, uremia, diabetic ketoacidosis, hyponatremia
Irritation of the vagus or phrenic nerve
• Sudden temperature changes (hot then cold liquids, hot then cold shower) • Foreign body in ear • RS: Pneumonia, empyema • CVS: Myocardial infarction, pericarditis, aneurysm, reflux esophagitis • Abdomen: Subphrenic abscess, hepatitis, pancreatitis, cholecystitis, gastric or pancreatic malignancy, sudden gastric distension (carbonated beverages, air swallowing, overeating).
Surgical
General anesthesia, postoperative
Psychogenic
Excitement, stress, laughing
Idiopathic

pressure on eyeballs, breath holding, Valsalva's maneuver, sneezing, or rebreathing into a bag, stimulation of the vagus by carotid massage.

- If there is gastric distention, it should be relieved by belching or insertion of a nasogastric tube.
- Drugs: Many drugs can help to control hiccups.
  - Chlorpromazine, 25–50 mg orally or intramuscularly
  - Baclofen 10 mg TID
  - Other useful drugs are metoclopramide, domperidone, phenytoin, diazepam, and gabapentin.

Q. Define dyspepsia. What are the causes of dyspepsia? How do you investigate and manage a case of dyspepsia?

- Dyspepsia is pain or discomfort in the upper abdomen especially in the epigastrium. Patient may describe it as abdominal fullness, early satiety, burning, bloating, belching, nausea, retching, or vomiting.
- Dyspepsia may be functional dyspepsia (without any identifiable cause) or organic dyspepsia (with an identifiable cause).
- Functional dyspepsia accounts for the majority of cases.

Causes of Dyspepsia

- ***Food related***: Overeating, eating high-fat foods, drinking too much alcohol or coffee.
- ***GI tract problems***: Gastritis, peptic ulcer, GERD, gastric cancer, gastroparesis (in diabetes mellitus), infections (*Helicobacter pylori*, Giardia, Strongyloides).
- ***Pancreatic diseases***: Pancreatitis. pancreatic carcinoma
- ***Biliary tract disease***: Cholelithiasis.
- ***Other conditions***: Diabetes, renal insufficiency, myocardial ischemia, hiatus hernia and pregnancy.
- ***Drugs***: NSAIDs. metformin, corticosteroids, erythromycin.
- ***Functional dyspepsia (also known as non-ulcer dyspepsia)***: No identifiable cause.

Differential Diagnosis

Peptic Ulcer Disease

- Discomfort occurs predominantly in the epigastrium, but can also occur in the right or left upper quadrants.
- Pain is usually burning type or hunger-like in quality. It can be vague or cramping.
- Gastric ulcer pain is aggravated by food while duodenal ulcer symptoms occur two to five hours after meals or on an empty stomach. Symptoms also occur at night, between 11 PM and 2 AM, when the circadian stimulation of acid secretion is maximal.
- Antacids, H_2 blockers and proton pump inhibitors relieve the pain.

Gastroesophageal Reflux Disease

- Most common symptoms of GERD are heartburn and regurgitation.
- Symptoms are aggravated by stooping or lying flat and relieved by antacids.

Gastric Malignancy

- Usually occurs in patients over 50 years of age.
- Other features include progressive dysphagia, weight loss, hematemesis, anemia, persistent vomiting and abdominal mass.

Biliary Tract Disease

- Dull aching pain in the epigastrium or right upper quadrant. Pain may radiate to the back or scapula.

Pancreatitis

- Pain is mainly in the epigastric region, severe and dull aching. It often radiates to back and associated with nausea and vomiting, It increases on lying down and decreases by bending forward.

Irritable Bowel Syndrome

- Chronic abdominal pain and altered bowel habits is characteristic of IBS.

Drug-induced Dyspepsia

- Dyspeptic symptoms appear after the intake of offending drugs.

Investigations

- If the patient is less than 50 years, he is likely to be having functional dyspepsia hence empiric therapy with H_2 blockers (ranitidine, famotidine) or proton pump inhibitors (omeprazole, pantoprazole) may be tried.
- However, if the history or examination is pointing towards any specific cause listed above, investigations should be done to rule out the same.

- Ultrasound abdomen and CT abdomen is helpful to rule out pancreatic or biliary tract disease.
- Esophageal pH monitoring may help if gastroesophageal reflux is suspected.
- Noninvasive tests for *H. pylori* (IgG serology, fecal antigen test, or urea breath test) help in ruling out *H. pylori* infection.
- Upper GI scopy should be done in patients above 50 years with persistent dyspepsia and in all patients with "alarm" features such as weight loss, dysphagia, recurrent vomiting, evidence of bleeding, or anemia to rule out carcinoma stomach.

Treatment

- If any underlying cause is found, it should be treated.
- For functional dyspepsia, 2–4 weeks of therapy with H_2 blockers (ranitidine, famotidine) or proton pump inhibitors (omeprazole, pantoprazole) may be tried.

Q. Discuss the etiology, clinical features, investigations and management of functional dyspepsia (nonulcer dyspepsia; idiopathic dyspepsia).

- Nonulcer dyspepsia is defined as chronic dyspepsia (pain or upper abdominal discomfort) in the absence of organic disease.
- It is a diagnosis of exclusion after ruling out ulcers, GERD, and other gastrointestinal diseases.

Etiology

- Exact etiology is unknown. However, following factors have been implicated.
  - Abnormal gastric motor function (delayed gastric emptying, reduced gastric compliance).
  - Visceral hypersensitivity.
  - *Helicobacter pylori* infection.
  - Psychosocial factors (anxiety, somatization, neuroticism, and depression).
  - Dietary and lifestyle factors: Excessive caffeine, alcohol, spicy foods, eating large or fatty meals, smoking

Clinical Features

- Patients are usually young (<40 years) and women are affected twice as commonly as men.
- Patients c/o postprandial fullness, early satiation, and epigastric pain. Any one or more of these symptoms may be present.
- Morning symptoms are characteristic and pain or nausea may occur on waking.
- Symptoms of irritable bowel syndrome such as pellet-like stools and feeling of incomplete evacuation after defecation may be present.
- Examination is usually normal except for epigastric tenderness. There is no weight loss. Patients often appear anxious.
- A drug history (NSAIDs) should be taken and depressive illness should be ruled out.

Rome IV Criteria for Functional Dyspepsia

- Functional dyspepsia is defined by the presence of one or more of the following symptoms in the absence of structural disease using imaging or endoscopy.

Symptoms must be present for at least 3 months, with onset ≥6 months prior, and include one or more of the following:

Postprandial distress syndrome (PDS) (meal-related symptoms)
- Early satiety (feeling full quickly)
- Postprandial bloating or discomfort

Epigastric pain syndrome (EPS) (meal-independent symptoms)
- Burning or gnawing epigastric pain
- No improvement with bowel movements

No structural disease found on endoscopy

Investigations

- All organic causes should be ruled out by appropriate tests.
- Alarming features which merit thorough investigations include dysphagia, anemia, weight loss, anorexia, hematemesis or melena.
- In women, pregnancy should be ruled out by urine pregnancy test and ultrasound.
- Upper GI scopy to rule out peptic ulcer, malignancy and hiatus hernia.
- Ultrasound abdomen if required to rule out gallstone disease and other mass lesions.
- Tests to rule out *H. pylori* infection.

Management

- Explain the nature of illness and reassure.
- Address any underlying psychological stress.
- Avoid cigarette smoking and alcohol abuse. Reduce intake of fatty foods.
- The first-line treatment is with a proton pump inhibitor or H_2 receptor antagonist for at least four weeks. Then, if symptoms persist, treatment with tricyclic antidepressants, or prokinetic agents are tried. Prokinetic agents include itopride, metoclopramide (10 mg 8-hourly), mosapride and domperidone (10 mg 8-hourly). Acotiamide is a new upper gastrointestinal motility modulator useful in functional dyspepsia.
- *H. pylori* should be eradicated if the tests are positive.

Q. Describe briefly esophageal motility disorders.

Q. Achalasia

Esophageal motility disorders include:
- Achalasia
- Diffuse esophageal spasm
- Nutcracker esophagus
- Hypertensive lower esophageal sphincter
- Scleroderma (systemic sclerosis)

Achalasia (Esophageal Aperistalsis; Megaesophagus)

- Achalasia (a Greek term which means "does not relax") is neurogenic esophageal motility disorder characterized by impaired esophageal peristalsis and a lack of lower esophageal sphincter (LES) relaxation during swallowing.

Etiology

- There is loss of inhibitory neurons in the distal esophagus leading to impaired relaxation of smooth muscle.
- Primary idiopathic achalasia accounts for most of the patients.
- Secondary achalasia occurs due to malignant infiltration of the esophagus, lymphoma, Chagas' disease, eosinophilic gastroenteritis, and neurodegenerative disorders.

Clinical Features

- Achalasia occurs at any age but usually begins between ages 20 and 60.
- Dysphagia, chest pain, and regurgitation are the main symptoms. Dysphagia is insidious onset and gradually progressive over months to years. Dysphagia occurs with both liquids and solids. Aspiration may occur due to regurgitation of retained food and saliva in the esophagus. Weight loss is also common.

Investigations

- *Esophageal manometry* is the preferred investigation of choice. It shows elevated resting esophageal pressure and failure of LES to relax on swallowing. Cholecystokinin (CCK), which causes relaxation of LES in normal people, causes contraction of the LES in achalasia. This happens because of loss of inhibitory neurons.
- *Barium swallow* shows proximal esophageal dilation and beak-like narrowing of terminal esophagus **(Fig. 4.5)**.
- *Chest X-ray* may show absence of the gastric air bubble. An air-fluid level in the mediastinum in the upright position represents retained food in the esophagus.

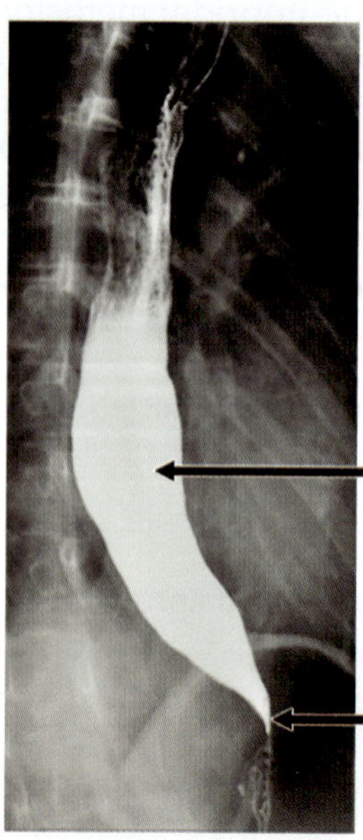

Figure 4.5: Beak-like appearance of achalasia on barium swallow

- *Fluoroscopy* shows loss of peristalsis in the lower two-thirds of the esophagus.
- *Endoscopy* is helpful to exclude other causes of dysphagia, particularly gastric carcinoma.

Treatment

- Balloon dilatation and laparoscopic Heller's myotomy of the LES.
- Endoscopic myotomy is also an effective procedure.
- Nitrates and calcium channel blockers provide short-term benefit. Nitroglycerin, 0.3–0.6 mg, or isosorbide dinitrate, 2.5–5 mg sublingually or 10–20 mg orally is used before meals. The calcium channel blocker nifedipine, 10–20 mg orally or sublingually before meals, is also effective.
- Endoscopic injection of botulinum toxin into LES can provide temporary relief. Botulinum toxin relaxes LES by blocking cholinergic excitatory nerves in the sphincter.

Diffuse Esophageal Spasm

- Diffuse esophageal spasm (DES) is a rare esophageal motility disorder characterized by uncoordinated, simultaneous contractions of the esophageal muscles. These abnormal contractions disrupt the normal peristalsis (the wave-like motion that moves food down the esophagus), leading to symptoms and functional problems.
- The exact cause is unclear but may involve dysfunction in the enteric nervous system.
- Normal peristalsis is disrupted; instead, multiple simultaneous contractions occur, mostly in the distal (lower) esophagus.

Clinical Features

- Diffuse esophageal spasm presents with chest pain and dysphagia. Chest pain is retrosternal and may radiate to both arms, and the sides of the jaw mimicking the pain of myocardial ischemia. However presence of dysphagia should help distinguish the pain from myocardial ischemia.

Investigations

- Esophageal manometry (gold standard test) shows increased luminal pressure.
- Barium swallow shows "corkscrew" or "rosary bead" appearance of the esophagus due to uncoordinated simultaneous contractions of the esophagus **(Fig. 4.6)**.
- Endoscopy: Often normal; used to rule out structural lesions.

Treatment

- Smooth muscle relaxants such as sublingual nitroglycerin (0.3–0.6 mg) or longer-acting agents such as isosorbide dinitrate (10–30 mg orally before meals) and nifedipine (10–20 mg orally before meals) are helpful.

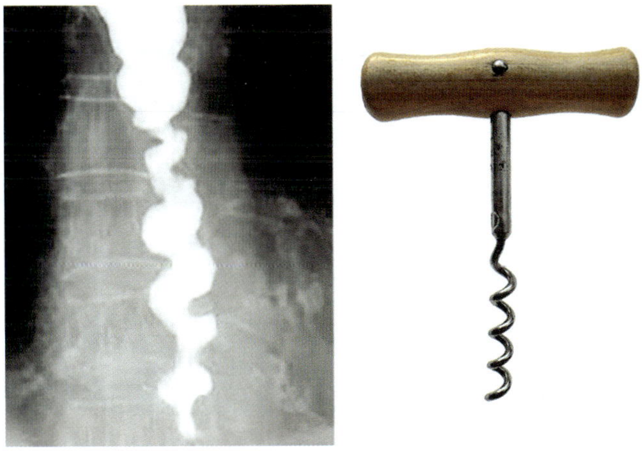

Figure 4.6: Corkscrew appearance of esophagus on barium swallow in diffuse esophageal spasm

- Botulinum toxin injection (temporary relief).
- Surgical/Interventional: Esophageal myotomy (rare, for refractory cases). Peroral endoscopic myotomy (POEM) is an emerging procedure.

Nutcracker Esophagus

- Here, there are coordinated peristalsis, but contractions are of very high amplitude and prolonged duration (hypertensive peristaltic contractions).
- Hypertensive peristaltic contractions may be due to cholinergic or myogenic hyperactivity.
- Patients present with chest pain, dysphagia, or both. Chest pain usually occurs at rest but may be brought on by swallowing. Dysphagia for solids and liquids may occur.
- Barium swallow shows pattern resembling nutcracker instrument used to crush nuts.
- Other investigations and treatment is same as diffuse esophageal spasm.

Hypertensive Lower Esophageal Sphincter

- This refers to spastic contraction of LES and failure to relax. This leads to dysphagia. Investigations and treatment are same as diffuse esophageal spasm.

Scleroderma

- Esophageal involvement is present in up to 90% of patients with scleroderma. Scleroderma primarily involves the smooth muscle layer of the gut wall, resulting in atrophy and sclerosis of the distal two-thirds of the esophagus. This produces aperistalsis or low amplitude contractions, and low or absent lower esophageal sphincter pressure.
- The proximal esophagus (striated muscle) is spared and exhibits normal motility.
- Patients commonly present with dysphagia.

Treatment

- Prokinetic drugs such as metoclopramide and mosapride increase esophageal sphincter pressure, improve peristalsis, and enhance gastric emptying.
- Erythromycin is also beneficial in scleroderma. It acts as a motilin agonist which increases gastric contractions and lowers esophageal sphincter pressure.

Q. Discuss the etiology, clinical features, investigations and management of peptic ulcer disease.

- Peptic ulcer is a break in the gastric or duodenal mucosa that penetrates through the muscularis mucosae.
- Peptic ulcer arises when there is decrease in mucosal defensive factors or increase in ulcerogenic factors such as acid and pepsin.
- Peptic ulcers occur more commonly in duodenum than stomach but can also occur in the jejunum after anastomosis to stomach and ileum adjacent to Meckel's diverticulum.
- They are more common in men than women.
- Duodenal ulcers occur commonly between 30 and 55 years of age, whereas gastric ulcers occur commonly between 55 and 70 years of age.

Etiology (Table 4.14)

TABLE 4.14: Etiology of peptic ulcer
• *H. pylori* infection (produces mucosal damage)
• NSAIDs and aspirin
• Gastrinoma (Zollinger-Ellison syndrome)
• Malignancy (gastric, lymphoma)
• Vascular insufficiency including crack cocaine use (produces mucosal ischemia and damage)
• Radiation therapy (mucosal damage)
• Carcinoid syndrome
• Crohn's disease
• Stress (acute illness, burns, head injury)
• Smoking and alcohol intake
• Idiopathic

Pathophysiology

- Most cases of peptic ulcer are due to *Helicobacter pylori* infection and use of nonsteroidal anti-inflammatory drugs (NSAIDs).
- Most duodenal ulcer patients have increased acid secretion whereas acid secretion is normal or even decreased in patients with gastric ulcer. Hence, increased acid may play an important role in the causation of duodenal ulcer and impaired mucosal defense may play an important role in the causation of gastric ulcer.
- NSAIDs inhibit the synthesis of protective prostaglandins which play an important role in the mucosal defense, and lead to ulcer formation.
- *H. pylori* infection causes chronic inflammation of gastric mucosa which overwhelms the gastric mucosal defense mechanisms and leads to gastric ulcer formation.

Clinical Features

- Epigastric pain (dyspepsia) is the most common symptom of peptic ulcer. However, some patients may have silent ulcers which come to attention due to bleeding or perforation. Pain is well localized, felt in the epigastrium and not severe. It is usually burning type but can also be gnawing, dull, aching, or "hunger-like."
- Pain occurs in episodes (periodicity), lasting 1–3 weeks every time, 3–4 times a year. In between, patient can be free of pain.
- The typical pain pattern in duodenal ulcer occurs 2–3 hours after a meal and is frequently relieved by antacids or food whereas gastric ulcer pain is worsened by intake of food. Pain that awakes the patient from sleep (between midnight and 3 AM) is the most discriminating symptom, and is seen in two-thirds of duodenal ulcer patients and one-third of gastric ulcer patients.
- Nausea and weight loss are common in gastric ulcer whereas weight gain may be present in duodenal ulcer patients because pain relief from food in duodenal ulcer makes them eat more frequently.
- Epigastric pain which becomes constant, and radiates to the back may indicate ulcer penetration into pancreas.
- Sudden onset of severe, generalized abdominal pain may indicate ulcer perforation with consequent peritonitis.
- Pain worsening with meals, nausea, and vomiting of undigested food suggest gastric outlet obstruction.
- Tarry stools or coffee ground vomitus indicate bleeding from ulcer.
- Physical examination is often normal in uncomplicated peptic ulcer except mild epigastric tenderness. Sometimes pallor may be present due to chronic blood loss from ulcer. In peptic ulcer perforation board like rigidity of abdominal wall is found.

Differences between Gastric and Duodenal Ulcer (Table 4.15)

TABLE 4.15: Differences between gastric and duodenal ulcer

Factors	Gastric ulcer	Duodenal ulcer
Age	Older patients (55–70 years)	Younger patients 30–55 years
Sex	Equal in both sexes	More in males
Acid secretion	Normal or decreased	Increased
Course of the illness	Less remittent	More remittent
Episodes of pain	Immediately after food	Occur 1–3 hours after a meal
Antacids	Inconsistent relief of pain	Prompt relief of pain
Food	Provokes the pain	Relieves the pain
Night pains	Rare	Common
Effect on weight	Weight loss	Weight gain

Investigations

Blood Tests

- Anemia may be present due to acute or chronic blood loss from the ulcer. Increased WBC count and increased amylase and lipase suggests ulcer penetration into the pancreas. Serum gastrin levels may be high in patients with Zollinger-Ellison syndrome.

Upper GI Endoscopy

- This is the procedure of choice for the diagnosis of duodenal and gastric ulcers. Biopsy can also be taken during endoscopy. Duodenal ulcers are virtually never malignant and do not require biopsy.

Barium Swallow

- Can be used for screening patients with uncomplicated dyspepsia. However, it is less commonly used now because of wide availability of endoscopy.

Tests for H. pylori

- Mucosal biopsies can be obtained during endoscopy for rapid urease test and for histologic examination. Noninvasive tests for *H. pylori* include stool antigen test and urea breath test.

Complications of Peptic Ulcer

- Hemorrhage
- Perforation
- Penetration into adjacent structures
- Gastric outlet obstruction due to scarring
- Gastric ulcers may turn into malignancy.

Differential Diagnosis

- Peptic ulcer disease must be distinguished from other causes of epigastric distress (dyspepsia).

Treatment

- The goal of treatment is to provide relief of symptoms (pain or dyspepsia), promote ulcer healing, and ultimately prevent ulcer recurrence and complications.

General Measures

- Avoid smoking and spicy food
- Cut down or quit alcohol intake
- Avoid aspirin and NSAIDs.

Acid Neutralizing/Inhibitory Drugs

Proton pump (H^+, K^+-ATPase) inhibitors

- Proton pump inhibitors (PPIs) are the most potent acid inhibitory agents available and are the drug of choice to treat peptic ulcer. They covalently bind and irreversibly inhibit H^+ K^+-ATPase which is the final pathway in acid secretion. These are given for 4 to 6 weeks.
- Examples are omeprazole, esomeprazole, lansoprazole, rabeprazole, and pantoprazole.

H_2 receptor blockers

- These agents decrease acid secretion. Examples are ranitidine, famotidine, and nizatidine. All are equally

effective. They are less commonly used now because of availability of PPIs.
- These agents are given for 4–6 weeks.

Antacids

- They relieve the pain by neutralizing the acid. They are mainly used for symptomatic relief of epigastric pain.
- Commonly used antacids are mixtures of aluminum hydroxide and magnesium hydroxide. Aluminum hydroxide can produce constipation and phosphate depletion; magnesium hydroxide may cause loose stools. Combining both will neutralize the side effects of each other.
- Dose is 15–30 ml 4–6 times per day.
- Calcium carbonate and sodium bicarbonate are other potent antacids.

Mucosal Protective Agents

Sucralfate

- Sucralfate is a complex sucrose salt which becomes a viscous paste within the stomach and duodenum in acidic pH. Thus it forms a coating on ulcers and helps in healing. It does not act in alkaline pH. Hence, giving it along with other acid suppressing agents may render it ineffective.

Bismuth-containing preparations

- These agents coat the ulcer, prevent further pepsin/acid induced damage and stimulate prostaglandins, bicarbonate, and mucus secretion.
- Colloidal bismuth subcitrate (CBS) and bismuth subsalicylate (BSS) are the most widely used preparations. These compounds are commonly used as one of the agents in an anti *H. pylori* regimen.

Prostaglandin analogs

- These agents enhance mucosal defense and repair. They also enhance mucous bicarbonate secretion and stimulate mucosal blood flow. Example is prostaglandin E1 derivative misoprostal.
- Misoprostol is contraindicated in pregnant women because it can cause uterine bleeding and contractions.

H. pylori Eradication

- *H. pylori* should be eradicated in patients with documented peptic ulcer disease. *H. pylori* eradication prevents the recurrence of peptic ulcer and also helps in remission of gastric MALT lymphoma. The agents used with the greatest frequency include amoxicillin, metronidazole, tetracycline, clarithromycin, and bismuth compounds. Combination therapy should be used to eradicate *H. pylori*. Treatment should be given for 10–14 days.

Surgical Treatment

- Less commonly used now because of the availability of effective medical therapy.
- Partial gastrectomy with Bilroth I anastomosis for gastric ulcer.
- Options for duodenal ulcer are truncal vagotomy plus pyloroplasty, selective vagotomy plus pyloroplasty, and highly selective vagotomy.
- Emergency surgery is indicated in penetrating or perforating peptic ulcers.

Q. Stress ulcers.

- They are superficial, multiple erosions (*vs* single, deeper peptic ulcers), usually found in the stomach or proximal duodenum, triggered by physiological stress, not emotional stress. They are usually shallow but deeper lesions can cause massive hemorrhage and/or perforation.
- Examples are Curling's ulcer in duodenum due to severe burns and Cushing's ulcer in stomach, esophagus, or duodenum in CNS injury.
- Stress ulcers are the most common cause of gastrointestinal (GI) bleeding in intensive care unit (ICU) patients.

Risk Factors for Development of Stress Ulcers (Table 4.16)

TABLE 4.16: Risk factors for development of stress ulcers
• Shock
• Sepsis
• Liver failure
• Renal failure
• Multiple trauma
• Head or spinal trauma (Cushing's ulcer)
• Burns (Curling's ulcer)
• Organ transplant recipients
• Prior history of peptic ulcer disease or upper GI bleeding
• Mechanical ventilation

Pathogenesis

- Erosions begin to develop within hours of major trauma or serious illness. They are thought to result from derangements in the balance between gastric acid production and mucosal protective mechanisms. Hypersecretion of acid due to excessive gastrin stimulation of parietal cells is seen in patients with head trauma.
- In critically ill patients, increased concentrations of refluxed bile salts or the presence of uremic toxins can denude the glycoprotein mucous barrier and lead to ulcer formation.
- Ischemia in shock, sepsis, and trauma can lead to impaired perfusion of the gut and lead to ulcer formation.

Clinical Features

- The most common presentation of stress ulcers is the onset of acute upper GI bleed like hematemesis or melena in a patient with an acute critical illness.
- Hypotension may occur due to severe bleeding and there may be drop in hemoglobin concentration requiring blood transfusions.

Evaluation

- Gastric lavage can identify the presence of blood in the upper GI tract.
- Endoscopy will show multiple shallow erosions in the stomach/duodenum.

Treatment

- H_2 blockers (ranitidine, famotidine, nizatidine). Less commonly used nowadays.
- Proton pump inhibitors (omeprazole, pantoprazole, esomeprazole). Most commonly used treatment.
- Sucralfate.
- Prostaglandin analogs (misoprostol).
- Bleeding ulcers require endoscopic therapies (epinephrine injection, electro-cauterization, or clipping of the bleeding vessels).

Prevention of Stress Ulcers

- Antacids.
- H_2 blockers (ranitidine, famotidine, nizatidine).
- Sucralfate.
- Proton pump inhibitors (omeprazole, pantoprazole, esomeprazole).
- Prostaglandin analogs (misoprostol).
- Early enteral nutrition.

Q. Role of *Helicobacter pylori* in peptic ulcer.

Q. Tests to detect *Helicobacter pylori*.

Q. *Helicobacter pylori* eradication regimens.

- *H. pylori* **(Fig. 4.7)** is a spiral-shaped, flagellated, gram-negative, urease-producing bacterium. It lives in the mucus layer of stomach. Some bacterial cells are found adherent to the mucosal cells.
- It has several acid resistance mechanisms of which the most important is production of urease enzyme which hydrolyses urea to produce buffering ammonia.

Epidemiology

- *Helicobacter pylori* is the most common chronic bacterial infection in humans.
- Prevalence of *H. pylori* is more in developing countries and low socioeconomic groups. Prevalence is high in the older population-presumably acquired in their childhood when hygiene was less good than today.
- Humans are the only important reservoir of *H. pylori*. Colonization is common in childhood institutions suggesting direct person-to-person spread.
- It spreads by fecal-oral or oral-oral route.

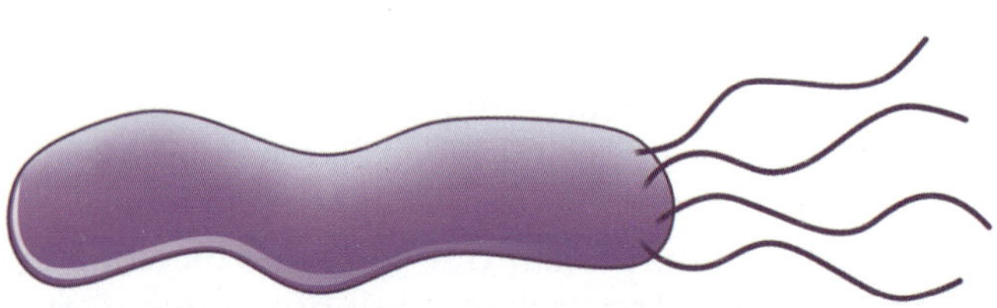

Figure 4.7: *H. pylori*

Pathogenesis

- *H. pylori* does not invade the mucosa. Instead, it damages the mucosa by disrupting the mucous layer, liberating enzymes and toxins, and adhering to the gastric epithelium. Urease is an important enzyme secreted by it. Urease converts urea into ammonia, thus alkalinizing the surrounding acidic medium so that *H. pylori* can survive, but simultaneously produces ammonia-induced mucosal damage.
- *H. pylori* produces toxins, Vac A (vacuolating toxin) and Cag A (cytotoxic associated protein) as well as urease and adherence factors. *H. pylori* infection produces superficial gastritis characterized by inflammatory cell infiltration of the mucosa. These inflammatory cells release cytokines which damage the mucosa.
- Effects of *H. pylori* infection depend on the location within the stomach. The antral-predominant infection results in increased gastrin production, probably via local impairment of somatostatin release. Increased gastrin stimulates increased acid production leading to duodenal ulcer formation. Body predominant infection leads to diffuse gastritis, gastric atrophy and decreased acid production. Patients with body-predominant infection are predisposed to gastric ulcer and gastric adenocarcinoma. Some patients have mixed infection of both antrum and body with varying clinical effects. The mucosa appears red endoscopically, and histologically there is epithelial cell damage.
- *H. pylori* colonization increases the lifetime risk of peptic ulcer disease, gastric cancer, and B cell non-Hodgkin's gastric lymphoma. Smoking increases ulcer and cancer risk in *H. pylori*–positive individuals.

Diseases caused by *H. pylori*

- Gastroesophageal reflux disease and dyspepsia.
- Gastritis.
- Peptic ulcer disease.
- Gastric adenocarcinoma.
- MALT (mucosal-associated lymphoid tissue) lymphoma.

Tests to Detect *H. pylori* Infection

Noninvasive Tests

- *Urea breath test (UBT):* This is a quick and simple test which can be used as a screening test. The urea is labeled with isotope 13C (Carbon-13). The patient drinks a solution of this labeled urea and then blows into a tube. If *H. pylori* urease is present, the urea is hydrolyzed and labeled carbon dioxide is detected in breath samples. The test is very sensitive (97%) and specific (96%). The breath test is also used to demonstrate eradication of the organism following treatment.
- *H. pylori fecal antigen test: H. pylori* antigen can be detected in the stool by immunoassay. This is less accurate than urea breath test but useful in children. Can be used to detect posttreatment eradication.

- *Serological tests:* Detect IgG antibodies by enzyme-linked immunosorbent assay (ELISA) or immunoblot. These tests may be positive even after eradication therapy and therefore are not useful for confirming eradication or the presence of a current infection. These are especially useful for epidemiological studies.

Invasive Tests

- These tests require endoscopy.
- *Biopsy urease test.* Gastric biopsies are added to a urea solution containing phenol red. If *H. pylori* are present, the urease enzyme splits the urea to release ammonia which raises the pH of the solution and causes a rapid color change.
- *Culture.* Biopsy specimens can be cultured and antibiotic sensitivity ascertained.
- *Histology.* Biopsy specimens can be stained (Giemsa) and looked for the presence of *H. pylori*.

Treatment

- There are many triple drug regimens for eradication of *H. pylori* infection. These are as follows.
- Omeprazole, amoxicillin, and clarithromycin (OAC)
- Bismuth subsalicylate, metronidazole, and tetracycline (BMT)
- Lansoprazole, amoxicillin, and clarithromycin (LAC)
- These triple drug combinations come as kits and are given for 10–14 days.

Q. Describe and enumerate the indications, pharmacology and side effects of pharmacotherapy of acid peptic disease including *Helicobacter pylori*.

Indications for Pharmacotherapy in Acid Peptic Disease (APD)

Pharmacologic treatment in acid peptic diseases is indicated for:

- Peptic ulcer disease (PUD): Gastric and duodenal ulcers due to any reason.
- *Helicobacter pylori* infection: Confirmed infection with associated ulcer disease or dyspepsia.
- Gastroesophageal reflux disease (GERD): Symptomatic reflux or erosive esophagitis.
- Zollinger-Ellison syndrome: Gastrin-producing tumor causing hyperacidity.
- NSAID prophylaxis: In patients at risk for NSAID-induced ulcers.
- Stress ulcer prophylaxis: Critically ill patients (e.g. ICU, mechanical ventilation).

Major Drug Classes Used in APD and *H. pylori* Infection

Proton Pump Inhibitors (PPIs)

- *Examples*: Omeprazole, esomeprazole, pantoprazole, lansoprazole.
- *Pharmacology*: Irreversibly inhibit H^+/K^+-ATPase in gastric parietal cells. Profound and long-lasting reduction in gastric acid secretion.
- *Side effects*:
  - Headache, nausea, diarrhea
  - Long-term: B_{12} deficiency, hypomagnesemia, increased fracture risk, increased risk of infections (e.g. *C. difficile*, pneumonia).

H_2-receptor Antagonists (H2RAs)

- *Examples*: Ranitidine (withdrawn in many places), famotidine, nizatidine
- *Pharmacology*: Competitively inhibit histamine at H_2 receptors in parietal cells. Reduce basal and stimulated acid secretion
- *Side effects*:
  - Headache, dizziness, diarrhea, fatigue.

Antacids

- *Examples*: Magnesium hydroxide, aluminum hydroxide, calcium carbonate
- *Pharmacology*: Neutralize existing stomach acid. Provide symptomatic relief of dyspepsia
- *Side effects*:
  - Magnesium: Diarrhea
  - Aluminum: Constipation
  - Calcium carbonate: Rebound hyperacidity, kidney stones

Mucosal Protective Agents

Sucralfate

- Forms protective barrier at ulcer site
- Requires acidic pH to activate
- *Side effects*: Constipation, drug binding interactions (space dosing)

Bismuth Subsalicylate

- Antibacterial against *H. pylori*, protective coating
- *Side effects*: Black stools/tongue, salicylate toxicity with overuse.

Misoprostol

- Prostaglandin E1 analog—enhances mucus, bicarbonate secretion, inhibits acid
- Used for NSAID ulcer prevention
- *Side effects*: Diarrhea, abdominal cramps, contraindicated in pregnancy (uterine contractions)

H. pylori Eradication Regimens

Triple therapy (14 days)

1. PPI (e.g. omeprazole)
2. Clarithromycin
3. Amoxicillin or Metronidazole (if penicillin allergy)

Quadruple therapy (14 days) (indications: Clarithromycin resistance or prior treatment failure)

1. PPI
2. Bismuth subsalicylate
3. Tetracycline
4. Metronidazole

Summary of Treatment of Acid Peptic Disease

See **Table 4.17**.

TABLE 4.17: Treatment of acid peptic disease

Drug class	Examples	Mechanism	Key side effects
PPIs	Omeprazole, pantoprazole	Inhibit proton pump (H^+/K^+-ATPase)	B_{12} deficiency, hypomagnesemia, fractures
H_2RAs	Famotidine	Block histamine H_2 receptor	Confusion (elderly), gynecomastia (cimetidine)
Antacids	Mg/Al hydroxide, Ca carbonate	Neutralize gastric acid	Diarrhea (Mg), constipation (Al), kidney stones (Ca)
Mucosal protectants	Sucralfate, bismuth, misoprostol	Barrier formation, mucus/bicarb enhancement	Constipation, black stools, diarrhea (Misoprostol)
Antibiotics (*H. pylori*)	Clarithromycin, amoxicillin	Antibacterial (protein or cell wall)	GI upset, rash, QT prolongation, *C. difficile* risk

Q. Define hematemesis. What are the causes of hematemesis? How do you investigate and manage a case of hematemesis?

Q. Causes of upper gastrointestinal (GI) bleeding.

Q. Causes of lower GI bleeding.

Q. Describe the approach to a case of acute GI bleeding. How do you differentiate between upper and lower GI bleeding based on clinical features?

- *Hematemesis* is vomiting of blood which may be obviously red or have an appearance similar to "coffee-grounds". Usually the source of bleeding in hematemesis is GI tract above the ligament of Treitz. Ligament of Treitz **(Fig. 4.8)** corresponds to the junction of duodenum and jejunum.
- Lower GI bleeding is described as bleeding that occurs below the level of ligament of trietz.
- Hematochezia refers to presence of fresh blood in stool.
- Melena refers to passage of black, tarry, and foul smelling stool.

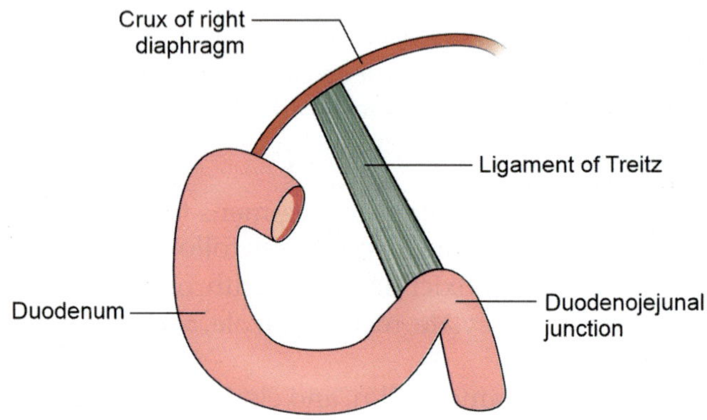

Figure 4.8: Ligament of Treitz

Etiology of GI Bleed

See **Table 4.18**.

TABLE 4.18: Etiology of GI bleeding

Etiology of upper GI bleeding (hematemesis)
• Peptic ulcers (responsible for the majority of cases)
• Esophageal varices due to portal HTN
• Portal hypertensive gastropathy
• Mallory-Weiss tears
• Vascular anomalies (hereditary hemorrhagic telangiectasia)
• Ca esophagus
• Ca stomach
• Erosive gastritis (due to NSAIDs, alcohol, or severe medical or surgical illness)
• Erosive esophagitis (due to GERD)
• Aortoenteric fistulas
• Post-surgical (anastomosis)
• Systemic causes; hemophilia, thrombocytopenia
Etiology of lower GI bleeding
• Dysentery (bacillary, amebic)
• Lower GI malignancy (Ca colon, Ca rectum)
• Inflammatory bowel disease (Crohn's disease, ulcerative colitis)
• Hemorrhoids
• Diverticulitis
• Necrotizing enterocolitis
• Mesenteric vascular disease
• Angiodysplasia
• Radiation-induced telangiectasia
• Radiation enteritis
• Polyp
• Post-biopsy or polypectomy

Clinical Presentation

History

- Vomiting of red blood or coffee ground vomitus **(Fig. 4.9)**. Red blood indicates fresh bleeding and coffee ground indicates bleeding sometime back. Other causes of red colored vomitus are food coloring, colored gelatin or drinks, red candy, beets, and tomato skins.
- Patient may give h/o of melena. Melena refers to black, tarry, foul smelling stool. It indicates bleeding in upper GI tract. Other causes of black colored stool are bismuth or iron preparations, spinach, blueberries, black grapes, and licorice.
- Guaiac test can be performed if there is doubt whether red color is due to blood or some other substance. It will be positive in the presence of blood.
- H/o syncopal attack (due to hypotension) may be present if there is massive bleeding.

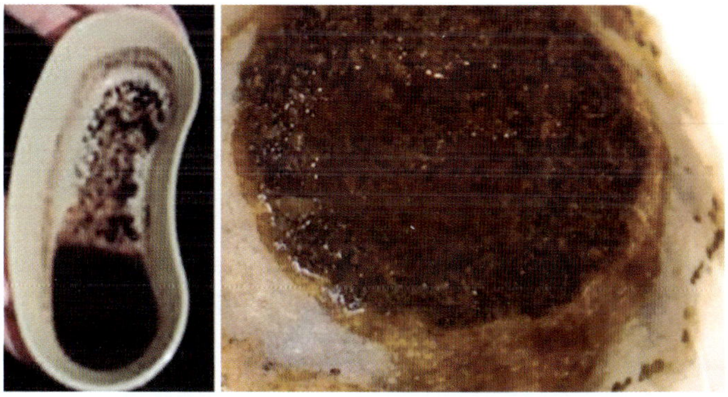

Figure 4.9: Coffee ground appearance of hematemesis.

- NSAID use or previous h/o peptic ulcer or dyspepsia suggests peptic ulcer.
- H/o heavy alcohol ingestion or retching before hematemesis suggests a Mallory-Weiss tear.
- H/o chronic liver disease with portal hypertension suggests esophageal varices as the cause of hematemesis.
- H/o dysphagia and weight loss prior to hematemesis suggests esophageal or gastric malignancy.
- H/o constipation or pain while passing stool suggests hemorrhoids or anal fissure as the cause of blood in stool.

Examination Findings

- Heart rate and blood pressure can give an idea of amount of bleed. Significant bleeding leads to tachycardia and postural hypotension. A systolic blood pressure less than 100 mm Hg suggests severe bleeding. Pallor may be present.
- Patient may present in a state of shock with hypotension, cold peripheries, excessive sweating, in severe bleeding.
- Signs of liver disease such as jaundice, and ascites may be present.

Differences between Upper and Lower GI Bleeding

See **Table 4.19**.

Investigations

Complete Blood Count with Differential Count

- Hb, PCV are important to know the amount of bleed. Hemoglobin does not fall immediately after bleeding because hemodilution takes some time (up to 72 hours). MCV (mean corpuscular volume) may be low due to development of iron deficiency anemia due to recurrent blood loss.

Coagulation Profile

- Bleeding time, clotting time, and prothrombin time. Sometimes a bleeding diathesis may be the cause of hematemesis or it may exacerbate bleeding due to other causes.

Blood Grouping and Cross Matching

- This is required because patient may require blood transfusion in case of massive hematemesis.

Liver Function Tests and Renal Function Tests

- To rule out liver disease and renal failure. Renal failure (prerenal azotemia) can occur in case of massive hematemesis and hypotension. Preexisting renal failure can cause uremic gastropathy and cause hematemesis.

Endoscopy

- Upper GI endoscopy is the investigation of choice in hematemesis. It is diagnostic as well as therapeutic.
- Colonoscopy is useful to identify the causes of lower GI bleed.
- Endoscopy can identify the source of bleeding, determine the risk of re-bleeding and render endoscopic therapy.

Ultrasound Abdomen

- To identify liver disease such as cirrhosis and any GI malignancy.

Angiography

- If bleeding persists and endoscopy fails to identify a bleeding site.

TABLE 4.19: Differences between upper and lower GI bleeding

	Upper GI bleeding	Lower GI bleeding
Site of bleed	Above ligament of Treitz	Below ligament of Treitz
Common causes	Peptic ulcer, esophageal varices, erosive gastritis, carcinoma stomach, Mallory-Weiss tear	Diverticulosis, hemorrhoids, carcinoma colon, inflammatory bowel disease
Presentation	Vomiting of blood (fresh blood or coffee ground) Melena	Fresh blood in stool
Bowel sounds	Increased	Normal
Nasogastric aspiration	Shows blood	Clear
Investigation of choice	Upper GI endoscopy	Lower GI endoscopy
BUN/creatinine ratio	Increased (because of absorption of blood which is rich in proteins)	Normal
Proton pump inhibitors	Useful in treatment	No benefit

Management of Hematemesis

Initial Stabilization

- Take care of ABCs first.
- A = Airway: Assess consciousness and airway protection.
- Intubate if: Altered mental status, massive bleeding, or aspiration risk.
- B = Breathing: Administer high-flow oxygen if hypoxic. Monitor SpO_2 and respiratory effort.
- C = Circulation: In patients with significant bleeding, two intravenous lines should be inserted. Blood should be sent for grouping and cross-matching for 2–4 units or more of packed red blood cells. Aggressive fluid replacement with normal saline or Ringer lactate should be started till blood is available. In mild to moderate bleeding fluid replacement is enough and blood transfusion is not required.
- A nasogastric tube (Ryle's tube) should be placed in all patients with hematemesis. The aspiration of red blood or "coffee grounds" confirms an upper gastrointestinal source of bleeding. Periodic aspiration of the nasogastric tube can identify ongoing bleeding or rebleeding.
- In actively bleeding patients, platelets are transfused if the platelet count is below 50,000/µl. Uremic patients (who have platelet dysfunction) with active bleeding are given three doses of desmopressin (DDAVP), 0.3 µg/kg intravenously, at 12-hour intervals. Fresh frozen plasma is given if prothrombin time is prolonged and INR (international normalized ratio) is >1.5.

Pharmacological Measures to Control Bleeding

Intravenous proton pump inhibitors (PPIs)

- Intravenous proton pump inhibitors (omeprazole, lansoprazole, or pantoprazole) reduce bleeding in patients with peptic ulcer. They can be used in bleeding due to other causes. PPIs also reduce the recurrence of bleeding after endoscopic therapy. Example, pantoprazole is given as 80 mg IV bolus, then 8 mg/hr infusion for minimum 46 hours.

Octreotide or vasopressin infusion

- Continuous intravenous infusion of octreotide (50 µg IV bolus, followed by 50 µg/hour for 2–3 days) reduces splanchnic blood flow and bleeding pending endoscopy. Octreotide is especially useful for variceal bleed, but can also be used for upper GI bleeding of any cause. Vasopressin can also be used but not as effective as octreotide.

Endoscopic Therapy

- Urgent endoscopy is done in patients with active bleeding not responding to conservative measures. Otherwise it can be done once the patient is hemodynamically stable, usually within 24 hours after admission.
- Hemostasis can be achieved in actively bleeding lesions with endoscopic therapies such as cautery, injection, or ligation. Actively bleeding varices can be treated with sclerosant injection or rubber band ligation of the bleeding varix. Actively bleeding ulcers, angiomas, or Mallory-Weiss tears can be controlled with either injection of epinephrine, cauterization, or application of an endoclip.
- Colonoscopy should be done in lower GI bleed and appropriate endoscopic therapy should be done to stop bleding (application of clips, epinephrine injection, or laser photocoagulation).

Intra-arterial Embolization or Vasopressin

- Angiographic treatment is used rarely in patients with persistent bleeding even after endoscopic therapy.

Transvenous Intrahepatic Portosystemic Shunts (TIPS)

- Placing a stent from the hepatic vein to the portal vein through the liver reduces portal venous pressure and helps in control of acute variceal bleeding. It is used when endoscopic modalities have failed.

Surgery

Surgery is indicated in:

- Severe, life-threatening hemorrhage from peptic ulcer not responsive to other measures.
- Coexisting reason for surgery (e.g. perforation, obstruction, malignancy)
- Aortoenteric fistula.

Q. Enumerate the indications for endoscopic interventions and surgery in patient with GI Bleeding.

Endoscopy is the first-line diagnostic and therapeutic tool in GI bleeding, especially for upper GI bleeding (UGIB).

Indications for Endoscopy in UGI Bleed

- All patients with suspected UGIB (e.g. hematemesis, melena).
- Active bleeding seen on presentation (hematemesis, melena, hematochezia).
- Hemodynamic instability or recent signs of bleeding (after initial stabilization).
- Suspected variceal bleeding (in patients with liver disease/portal hypertension).
- Confirmed peptic ulcer with high-risk of bleeding.
- Diagnosis and therapy of lesions: Ulcers, varices, Mallory-Weiss tears, Dieulafoy lesions, neoplasms, angiodysplasia.
- Recurrent bleeding after initial stabilization.

Indications for Surgical Intervention in GI Bleeding

- Surgery is reserved for life-threatening or refractory bleeding not controlled by endoscopy or interventional radiology.

- Massive GI bleeding with hemodynamic instability unresponsive to resuscitation.
- Failure of endoscopic therapy to control bleeding
- Recurrent bleeding after two endoscopic attempts

- Bleeding from a source inaccessible to endoscopy
- Complicated peptic ulcer disease (e.g. bleeding + perforation or obstruction)
- Bleeding neoplasms requiring resection
- Persistent transfusion requirement (e.g. >4–6 units of blood within 24 hours)
- Unavailability of endoscopy/interventional radiology in an emergency setting

Q. Indications for colonoscopy in GI bleed

- Unclear source of bleeding after normal upper GI scopy.
- Passage of fresh blood per rectum (hematochezia), if brisk UGI bleed is ruled out. In brisk UGI bleeding, blood can rapidly transit to the colon, making colonoscopy appear falsely positive.
- Occult bleeding or iron deficiency anemia with negative upper GI scopy.
- Mixed presentation (UGI bleeding cannot be excluded entirely).

Q. Determine appropriate level of specialist consultation as per clinical, hemodynamic status of the patient with GI bleed

- GI bleeding can range from mild to life-threatening, and appropriate consultation needs to be decided based on the severity.

Stable Patient with Mild-to-moderate GI Bleeding

Clinical Features

- Stable vitals (HR <100, SBP >100 mm Hg).
- No ongoing active bleeding.
- Mild anemia, no signs of shock.
- Coffee-ground vomiting or melena without hemodynamic compromise.

Action

- Gastroenterologist (within 24 hours) for diagnostic/therapeutic endoscopy.
- Outpatient or inpatient nonurgent endoscopy if fully stable and low-risk.

Hemodynamically Unstable or Ongoing Active Bleeding

Clinical Features

- Tachycardia, hypotension, syncope.
- Ongoing hematemesis, melena, or hematochezia.
- Requires resuscitation or transfusion.

Action

- Urgent gastroenterology consultation for emergency endoscopy (within 6–12 hours).

Massive or Refractory Bleeding (uncontrolled or recurrent)

Clinical Features

- Persistent hemodynamic instability despite fluids/blood.
- Recurrent bleeding after endoscopy.
- High transfusion requirement (e.g. >4–6 units/24 hours).

Action

- Gastroenterologist (STAT).
- Interventional radiologist for angiographic embolization (if endoscopy fails).
- Surgeon (emergency) for potential operative intervention.
- Critical care/intensivist for ICU admission.

Multidisciplinary Consultations (as needed)

Specialist	Indication
Gastroenterologist	All confirmed or suspected GI bleeds
Surgeon	Failed endoscopic therapy, perforation, or massive bleed
Interventional radiologist	Failed endoscopy, inaccessible lesions
Hepatologist	Variceal bleeding, liver disease
ICU/intensivist	Unstable or critically ill patient
Hematologist	Coagulopathy, bleeding diathesis

Q. Generate a differential diagnosis of GI bleed based on the presenting symptoms and clinical features.

Suspect UGI bleed if patient presents with any of the following:

- Hematemesis (vomiting blood).
- Melena (black, tarry stools).
- Epigastric pain, history of NSAID use, alcohol or liver disease.
- Note that hematochezia can also occur if there is massive UGI bleed.

Differential Diagnosis of UGI Bleed Based on Clinical Features (Table 4.20)

TABLE 4.20: Differential diagnosis of UGI bleed based on clinical features

Clinical features	Possible diagnosis
Epigastric pain, NSAID use, *H. pylori*, melena or hematemesis	Peptic ulcer disease
History of liver disease, portal hypertension, severe hematemesis	Esophageal varices
NSAIDs, alcohol, stress; less severe bleeding	Gastritis/gastroduodenitis
Repeated retching or vomiting, followed by sudden hematemesis	Mallory-Weiss tear
GERD history, odynophagia, less severe bleeding	Esophagitis
Older age, dysphagia, weight loss, anorexia, chronic bleeding	Esophageal or gastric cancer
Sudden massive bleeding, normal mucosa on scope	Dieulafoy's lesion
Intermittent bleeding, often in elderly	Angiodysplasia
Post-aortic surgery, herald bleed followed by massive hemorrhage	Aortoenteric fistula

Differential Diagnosis of Lower GI Bleed Based on Clinical Features (Table 4.21)

TABLE 4.21: Differential diagnosis of lower GI bleed based on clinical features

Clinical features	Possible diagnosis
Painless, bright red bleeding	Hemorrhoids, diverticulosis (especially in elderly), angiodysplasia
Painful bleeding, tenesmus	Fissures, inflammatory bowel disease, ischemic colitis
Diarrhea with blood and mucus, fever	Infectious colitis (dysentery)
Chronic diarrhea with blood and mucus, no fever	IBD
Elderly patient, weight loss, altered bowel habits	Colorectal cancer, malignancy
Elderly patient, sudden onset pain abdomen with blood in stool	Ischemic colitis
Young patient with abdominal pain	IBD, infectious colitis
Chronic bleeding/anemia	Polyps, hemorrhoids
Bleeding + NSAID use	NSAID-induced colitis, diverticular bleed
Post-polypectomy or post-scope	Iatrogenic bleeding

Q. Pharmacotherapy of vasopressors in upper GI bleeding.

- Vasopressors are primarily used in esophageal/gastric variceal bleeding due to portal hypertension (e.g. in cirrhosis).
- These agents reduce portal venous pressure, thereby decreasing bleeding.

Indications for Vasopressors in UGI Bleeding

- Suspected or confirmed variceal bleeding
- Hemodynamic instability or shock in UGIB
- As a bridge to endoscopy
- Patients with known liver cirrhosis and bleeding
- To prevent early rebleeding after endoscopic treatment.

Vasopressor Agents: Pharmacology and Side Effects

Terlipressin

- **Mechanism:** Synthetic analog of vasopressin; causes **splanchnic vasoconstriction**, reducing portal pressure.
- **Dose:** 2 mg IV every 4–6 hours initially, then 1 mg every 4–6 hours (up to 48–72 hours)
- **Advantages:** Effective for **variceal bleeding and hepatorenal syndrome**
- **Side effects:** Abdominal cramps, hypertension, bradycardia, ischemia (cardiac, mesenteric, limb), hyponatremia.

Octreotide

- Preferred due to fewer side effects than vasopressin.
- **Mechanism:** Somatostatin analog; reduces splanchnic blood flow and portal pressure.
- **Dose:** 50 μg IV bolus, followed by continuous infusion of 50 μg/hour for 3–5 days.
- **Side effects:** Hyperglycemia or hypoglycemia, bradycardia, abdominal discomfort, gallstones (with prolonged use).
- Octreotide has been discussed in detail as a separate question (*see* next section).

Somatostatin

- Less commonly used due to short half-life and cost.
- **Mechanism:** Natural hormone; inhibits release of vasodilators like glucagon → reduces portal blood flow.
- **Dose:** 250 μg IV bolus, then infusion at 250–500 μg/hour.
- **Side effects:** Nausea, abdominal pain, hyperglycemia, bradycardia, rare ischemia.

Vasopressin (rarely used now)

- **Mechanism:** Potent vasoconstrictor that reduces splanchnic and portal blood flow.
- **Dose:** 0.2–0.4 units/min (requires central monitoring).
- Often combined with nitroglycerin to counteract ischemia.
- **Side effects:** Severe hypertension, cardiac ischemia, arrhythmias, bowel or limb ischemia.

Q. Octreotide.

- Octreotide is a long-acting analogue of somatostatin. Its pharmacological actions are similar to somatostatin which is a natural hormone.

Pharmacokinetics

- Octreotide acts on somatostatin receptors. It is administered through a subcutaneous or intravenous route. It is absorbed quickly and completely after subcutaneous and intravenous injection.

Pharmacological Actions

- Inhibits secretion of many hormones, such as gastrin, cholecystokinin, glucagon, growth hormone, insulin, secretin, pancreatic polypeptide, TSH, and vasoactive intestinal peptide.
- Reduces intestinal and pancreatic secretion.
- Reduces gastrointestinal motility and inhibits contraction of the gallbladder.
- Causes vasoconstriction.
- Reduces portal vein pressure by decreasing splanchnic blood flow via splanchnic vasoconstriction.

Uses of Octreotide

- Treatment of growth hormone producing tumors (acromegaly and gigantism), when surgery is contraindicated.

- Treatment of diarrhea and flushing episodes associated with carcinoid syndrome.
- Treatment of diarrhea in people with vasoactive intestinal peptide secreting tumors (VIPoma).
- Treatment of mild cases of glucagonoma when surgery is not an option.
- Bleeding esophageal varices (given as intravenous infusion, acts by reducing portal venous pressure).
- Radiolabeled octreotide is used in nuclear medicine imaging to noninvasively image neuroendocrine and other tumors expressing somatostatin receptors.
- Radiolabeled octreotide can also be used in the treatment of unresectable neuroendocrine tumors expressing somatostatin receptors.
- Hypoglycemia: Octreotide is also used in the treatment of refractory hypoglycemia in neonates and sulphonylurea-induced hypoglycemia in adults.

Adverse Effects

- Gastrointestinal side effects are common and include diarrhea, nausea, abdominal discomfort, gallbladder abnormalities, such as cholelithiasis and microlithiasis.
- Bradycardia, conduction abnormalities, and arrhythmias.
- Hypoglycemia and hyperglycemia occur due to alteration in glucose metabolism.
- Hypothyroidism
- Skin itching
- Pain at the injection site
- Headache and dizziness
- Rare side effects include acute anaphylactic reactions, pancreatitis and hepatitis.

Q. Discuss the etiology, classification, clinical features, investigations and management of malabsorption syndrome.

Q. What are the disorders causing malabsorption? How do you approach a case of suspected malabsorption?

- Malabsorption refers to impaired absorption of nutrients.
- Malabsorption occurs mainly due to diseases of small intestine since this is the major site of absorption of nutrients.
- Fat is the most difficult to absorb and hence most malabsorption syndromes have steatorrhea (excess fat in feces). A stool test for fat is the best screening test for malabsorption.
- There are three stages of nutrient absorption: Luminal, mucosal, and postabsorptive.
  - The luminal phase involves mechanical mixing and digestive enzymes.
  - The mucosal phase requires a properly functioning mucosal membrane for absorption.
  - The postabsorptive phase becomes facilitated by an intact blood supply and lymphatic system.
- Malabsorption can occur due to problems in any of these three phases.

Causes of Malabsorption (Table 4.22)

TABLE 4.22: Causes of malabsorption
Disorders of luminal phase
• *Enzyme deficiency*: Chronic pancreatitis, cystic fibrosis.
• *Enzyme inactivation*: Zollinger-Ellison syndrome.
• *Diminished bile salt synthesis*: Parenchymal liver diseases.
• *Impaired bile secretion*: Bile duct obstruction, chronic cholestasis
• *Increased bile salt loss*: Ileal disease or resection
• *Reduced luminal availability of specific nutrients:* Intrinsic factor deficiency in Pernicious anemia causing B_{12} deficiency
• *Bacterial consumption of nutrients*: Bacterial overgrowth causing vitamin B_{12} deficiency
Disorders of mucosal phase
• *Defects in brush border hydrolysis*: Sucrase-isomaltase deficiency, Lactase deficiency
• *Defects in mucosal absorption (villous atrophy):* Celiac sprue, tropical sprue, lymphoma, Whipple's disease, radiation enteritis, AIDS, giardiasis, Crohn's disease
Disorders of postabsorptive, processing phase
• *Defects in enterocyte processing:* Abetalipoproteinemia
• *Defects in lymphatic transport:* Intestinal lymphangiectasia, intestinal tuberculosis
Systemic diseases causing malabsorption
• Thyrotoxicosis (rapid transit through gut)
• Hypothyroidism (impaired intestinal motility, bacterial overgrowth)
• Diabetes mellitus (impaired intestinal motility, bacterial overgrowth)
• Scleroderma (impaired intestinal motility, bacterial overgrowth)
Drugs causing malabsorption
• Antibiotics (Vitamin B_{12} and vitamin K deficiency)
• Methotrexate (Folic acid antagonist, causes inhibition of crypt cell division).
• Cholestyramine (binds bile salts)
• Laxatives (rapid transit through gut. Liquid paraffin causes fat soluble vitamin deficiency).
Surgical causes
• Resection of terminal ileum → B_{12} and bile salt malabsorption
• Short bowel syndrome after surgical resection and re-anastomosis
• Gastric bypass

Clinical Features

Diarrhea

- Diarrhea is the most common complaint. It is due to the osmotic load received by the intestine because of unabsorbed carbohydrates and solutes.
- Bacterial action producing hydroxy fatty acids from undigested fat also can increase fluid secretion from the intestine, further worsening the diarrhea.

Steatorrhea

- Steatorrhea is due to fat malabsorption.
- The hallmark of steatorrhea is the passage of pale, bulky, and foul-smelling stools, which float on top of the toilet water and are difficult to flush. Also, patients find floating oil droplets in the toilet following defecation.

Weight Loss and Fatigue

- Weight loss is due to protein energy malnutrition from malabsorption. Fatigue is due to weight loss plus coexisting anemia.

Flatulence and Abdominal Distention

- Bacterial fermentation of unabsorbed food substances releases gases, such as hydrogen and methane, causing flatulence.
- Flatulence often causes uncomfortable abdominal distention and cramps.

Edema

- Protein malabsorption causes hypoalbuminemia which causes peripheral edema.
- With severe protein depletion, ascites may develop.

Anemia

- Anemia develops due to iron deficiency (microcytic anemia), folic acid or vitamin B_{12} deficiency (macrocytic anemia). Iron deficiency is common in celiac disease. Vitamin B_{12} deficiency is common in Crohn's disease with ileal involvement or ileocecal TB.

Bleeding Disorders

- Bleeding tendency is due to vitamin K malabsorption and decreased production of vitamin K dependent clotting factors. Ecchymosis is usually seen but patient can also have melena and hematuria.

Bone Pain and Pathologic Fractures

- This is due to vitamin D deficiency causing osteopenia or osteomalacia.
- Malabsorption of calcium can lead to secondary hyperparathyroidism.

Neurologic Manifestations

- Electrolyte disturbances, such as hypocalcemia and hypomagnesemia, can lead to tetany, manifesting as the Trousseau sign and the Chvostek sign.
- Vitamin malabsorption can cause generalized motor weakness (pantothenic acid, vitamin D) or peripheral neuropathy (thiamine, vitamin B_{12}), a sense of loss for vibration and position (vitamin B_{12}), night blindness (vitamin A), and seizures (biotin).

Investigations

Imaging Studies

- *Endoscopy:* Upper GI scopy is helpful to visualize stomach, duodenum and upper jejunum. A cobblestone appearance of the duodenal mucosa is seen in Crohn's disease. Reduced duodenal folds and scalloping of the mucosa may be seen in celiac disease. Small bowel biopsy can also be taken during endoscopy.
- *CT and ultrasound abdomen:* May be helpful in the diagnosis of chronic pancreatitis and other abnormalities in the abdomen.

TABLE 4.23: Summary of features of specific nutrient malabsorption
Carbohydrates: Watery diarrhea, flatulence, acidic stool pH, milk intolerance.
Protein: Edema, muscle atrophy, amenorrhea.
Fat: Pale, bulky, foul smelling stool which floats on water and difficult to flush. Diarrhea without flatulence. Weight loss.
Vitamins *Vitamin A*: Follicular hyperkeratosis, night blindness *Vitamin B_{12}*: Anemia, neuropathy, subacute combined degeneration of the spinal cord. *Vitamin B_1, B_2*: Cheilosis, painless glossitis, acrodermatitis, angular stomatitis *Folic acid:* Megaloblastic anemia. *Vitamin D:* Tetany, pathologic fractures due to osteomalacia, muscular irritability. *Vitamin K:* Bleeding tendency
Minerals and electrolytes *Iron:* Anemia, glossitis, pica *Calcium:* Tetany, pathologic fractures due to osteomalacia, muscular irritability. *Zinc:* Anorexia, weakness, tingling, impaired taste.

- *Barium studies:* An upper gastrointestinal series with small bowel follow-through or enteroclysis (a double contrast study performed by passing a tube into the proximal small bowel and injecting barium and methylcellulose) can provide information about the gross morphology of the small intestine. For example, small bowel diverticula and mucosal abnormalities can be identified.
- *Wireless capsule endoscopy:* Wireless capsule endoscopy allows for visualization of the entire small bowel. Because of the risk of retention, it should be avoided in patients with suspected small bowel strictures.

Tests for Fat Absorption

- Fecal fat estimation: Increase in stool fat excretion is known as steatorrhea. A 72-hour fecal fat estimation can detect steatorrhea. More than 6 g/day of fat in stool is pathologic.
- Sudan III stain: Sudan stain on a spot stool sample can detect more than 90% of patients with steatorrhea.
- Measurement of fat soluble vitamin levels in the blood (A,D,E, K); prothrombin time.
- Near infrared reflectance analysis (NIRA): This may become the procedure of choice in future. NIRA can simultaneously measure fecal fat, nitrogen, and carbohydrates in a single sample.
- 14C-triolein breath test: The test involves measurement of breath CO_2 after ingestion of the radiolabeled triglyceride triolein, and provides a measure of fat absorption.

Tests for Carbohydrate Absorption

- *Oral glucose tolerance test:* There will be failure of blood glucose levels to rise after glucose loading.
- *D-xylose test:* Patient ingests 25 g of D-xylose, and urine is tested for the presence of D-xylose. Excretion

of lesser amounts of D-xylose suggests abnormal absorption (as in celiac sprue).

- *Lactose tolerance test:* After ingestion of 50 g lactose, blood glucose levels are monitored. Insufficient increase in blood glucose plus the development of symptoms is diagnostic of lactose intolerance. Another test is measurement of breath hydrogen after lactose ingestion. An increase in breath hydrogen is diagnostic.
- *Breath tests:* Breath tests using hydrogen, $14CO_2$, or $13CO_2$ can be used to diagnose specific forms of carbohydrate malabsorption (e.g. lactose, fructose, sucrose isomaltase and others). All of these breath tests rely on bacterial fermentation of nonabsorbed carbohydrate and therefore concurrent antibiotic administration often alters the results.

Tests for Protein Absorption

- Serum albumin will be low.
- Intravenous radioactive chromium is used to label circulating albumin. In case of protein losing enteropathy radioactivity appears in stools.
- Measurement of nitrogen in the stool will be more than 2.5 g.
- Excretion of alpha-1 antitrypsin in the stool (normally it is absent in the stool).

Tests for Absorption of Other Substances

- Complete blood count (anemia), serum iron, ferritin, folate, vitamin B_{12} level, Schilling test (for vitamin B_{12} malabsorption), serum calcium, sodium, potassium, β-carotene, and prothrombin time should be obtained in all patients with suspected malabsorption.

Tests for Bacterial Overgrowth

- The gold standard for diagnosis of bacterial overgrowth is the direct quantitative measurement of bacterial counts from aspirated intestinal fluid. However this is invasive and hence the following tests are used more commonly.
- ***Hydrogen breath test.*** This is used to detect bacterial overgrowth in the intestine. Oral lactulose or glucose is metabolized by bacteria with the production of hydrogen. An early rise in the breath hydrogen indicates bacterial overgrowth in the small intestine.
- ***14C-glycocholic acid breath test.*** It is rarely done now and has been replaced by the hydrogen breath test. Patient is given radiolabeled bile acid (14C-glycocholic acid) orally. Bacteria in the intestine deconjugate the bile acid, releasing [14C]-glycine, which is metabolized and appears in the breath as $14CO_2$.

Serologic Tests

- IgA endomysial antibody and IgA anti-tTG antibody both are found in celiac disease. IgG or IgA antigliadin antibodies are also present in celiac sprue.

Intestinal Mucosal Biopsy and Histopathology

- Villous atrophy is seen in celiac disease, and tropical sprue.

Treatment

- Treat the underlying cause.
- Avoid milk and milk products in lactose intolerance.
- Gluten-free diet in celiac disease.
- Pancreatic enzyme supplements in pancreatic insufficiency.
- Reduction of long chain fatty acids and low fat diet in fat malabsorption.
- Antibiotics are the therapy for bacterial overgrowth.
- Corticosteroids, anti-inflammatory agents such as mesalamine, are used to treat inflammatory bowel disease such as Crohn's disease.
- Replacement of specific nutrients which are deficient such as folic acid, iron and vitamin B_{12}, vitamin D, etc.
- Caloric and protein replacement.

Q. Schilling test.

- This test is performed to determine the cause for vitamin B_{12} malabsorption. Vitamin B_{12} is absorbed in the terminal ileum.
- Causes of vitamin B_{12} malabsorption are intrinsic factor defficiency, atrophic gastritis, small intestinal bacterial overgrowth, exocrine pancreatic insufficiency, and ileal disease.
- Schilling test is performed by administering 1 mcg of radiolabeled vitamin B_{12} orally, followed by an intramuscular injection of 1000 microgram of vitamin B_{12} one hour later to saturate vitamin B_{12} binding sites so that absorbed radiolabeled B_{12} is excreted in the urine.
- A 24-hour urine is then collected for determination of the percent excretion of the oral dose. Normally at least 10% of the radiolabeled vitamin B_{12} is excreted in the urine. In patients with pernicious anemia or impaired absorption, less than 10% of the radiolabeled vitamin B_{12} is excreted.
- Next, the above step is repeated after the addition of intrinsic factor. If this second urine collection is normal, it proves intrinsic factor deficiency or pernicious anemia.
- If urinary excretion of vitamin B_{12} is still less than 10% after adding intrinsic factor, then the test is repeated after a course of antibiotics. Small intestinal bacterial overgrowth is suggested if an abnormal test is normalized after a course of antibiotics. If the absorption is abnormal even after addition of intrinsic factor and exclusion of bacterial overgrowth, it suggests terminal ileal disease. The Schilling test can also be abnormal in pancreatic insufficiency and celiac disease. Normalization after pancreatic enzyme substitution or a gluten-free diet is useful for diagnosis of these causes of malabsorption.
- The Schilling test can also be used to determine the functional integrity of the ileal mucosa after treatment of ileal Crohn's disease.
- Many labs have stopped doing the Schilling test, due to lack of production of radiolabeled-B_{12} test substances. Also, the treatment remains same (i.e. injection of vitamin B_{12}), even if the exact cause were

identified. Moreover, upper GI scopy can detect many causes of vitamin B_{12} deficiency. Hence, Schilling test it is not being performed now.

Q. Celiac sprue (celiac disease, gluten-sensitive enteropathy).

- Celiac sprue is an inflammatory condition of the small intestine precipitated by the ingestion of wheat, rye, and barley in individuals with genetic predispositions.
- It occurs throughout the world but common in Northern Europe. There is increased incidence of celiac disease within families but the exact mode of inheritance is unknown.

Etiology

- Inflammatory damage to the intestinal mucosa is due to gluten protein of wheat. Gluten is also present in barley, rye and oats. The toxic component in gluten is gliadin.
- It is strongly associated with HLA-DQ2 and HLA-DQ8. However environmental factors also play an important role.

Pathogenesis

- Gluten is found in wheat, barley, and rye.
- The toxic component is gliadin (a protein fragment in gluten).
- Gliadin is partially digested in the intestinal lumen. Gliadin is rich in glutamine. Some of the glutamines in gliadin are deamidated by the enzyme tissue transglutaminase (tTG), generating negatively charged glutamic acid residues.
- These altered gliadin peptides are recognized by local intestinal T cells as foreign, thereby stimulating an immune response. B-cells are also activated and produce various antibodies such as antigliadin, anti-endomysial, and antitissue transglutaminase (tTG) antibodies.
- This immune response causes damage to intestinal mucosa resulting in mal-digestion and malabsorption of nutrients.
- Summary of pathogenesis: Gluten → Gliadin → Deamidation by tTG → Presented by HLA-DQ2/8 → CD4+ T-cell activation → Cytokine release → Villous atrophy + crypt hyperplasia → Malabsorption.

Pathology

- The mucosa of the jejunum is predominantly affected, and the damage decreases towards the ileum.
- There is absence of villi, making the mucosal surface flat **(Fig. 4.10)**. Histological examination shows crypt hyperplasia with chronic inflammatory cells in the lamina propria and subtotal villous atrophy. In the lamina propria there is an increase in lymphocytes and plasma cells.

Clinical Features

- Celiac disease can present at any age but usually in infancy after weaning on to gluten-containing foods. It has a female preponderance.

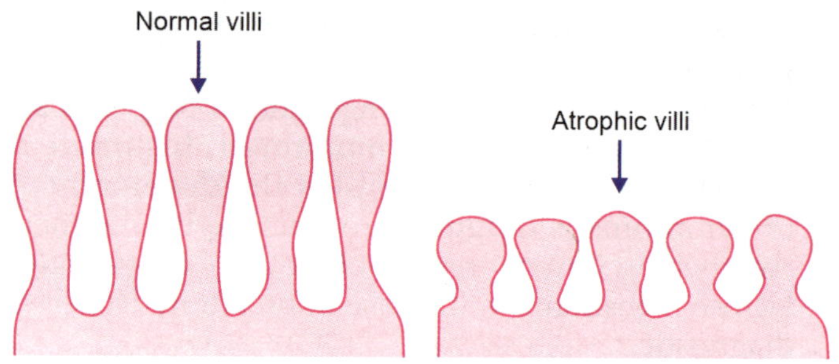

Figure 4.10: Normal and abnormal villi

- Many patients present with anemia or osteoporosis without gastrointestinal symptoms. These individuals usually have proximal intestinal disease that impairs iron, folate, and calcium absorption.
- Patients with significant mucosal involvement present with diarrhea, abdominal distension and bloating after eating, weight loss or growth retardation, and features of vitamin and mineral deficiencies. Absorption of all nutrients, electrolytes, fat-soluble vitamins, calcium, magnesium, iron, folate, and zinc, is affected. Diarrhea is due to decreased surface area for water and electrolyte absorption and the osmotic effect of unabsorbed luminal nutrients.
- There is an increased incidence of other autoimmune diseases, like thyroid disease, type-1 diabetes, primary biliary cirrhosis and Sjogren's syndrome.
- Extraintestinal manifestations of celiac disease include rash (dermatitis herpetiformis), neurologic disorders (myopathy, epilepsy), psychiatric disorders (depression, paranoia), and reproductive disorders (infertility, spontaneous abortion).

Investigations

- *Duodenal/jejunal biopsy* shows characteristic changes of celiac sprue.
- *Serologic markers:* Useful in supporting the diagnosis. An IgA antitissue transglutaminase antibody (IgA TTG), detected by ELISA is the best first test for suspected celiac sprue. Antigliadin IgA and IgG antibodies are sensitive but not specific. Antiendomysial IgA antibodies are highly sensitive and specific for celiac disease.
- *Tests for malabsorption of proteins, carbohydrate, fat and vitamins:* All patients with celiac disease should be screened for vitamin and mineral deficiencies and have bone densitometry.

Treatment

- Treatment consists of a lifelong gluten-free diet. Wheat, rye, and barley should be excluded from the diet.
- A lactose-free diet is also recommended until symptoms improve because of secondary lactase deficiency.
- Any deficient vitamins and minerals should be replaced. Women of childbearing age should be given folic acid supplements.
- 90% of patients on gluten-free diet experience symptomatic improvement within 2 weeks. A small

percentage of patients do not improve on a strict gluten-free diet (refractory sprue). Such patients may have atrophic mucosa. Lymphoma should be ruled out in refractory sprue. Steroids may be of help in refractory sprue if there is persistent inflammation.

Complications

- Intestinal lymphoma.
- Ulcerative jejunitis.

Q. Dermatitis herpetiformis.

- Dermatitis herpetiformis is a chronic, intensely itchy skin condition associated with celiac disease, caused by IgA deposition in the skin.
- Triggered by gluten sensitivity, just like in celiac disease. It is characterized by an itchy papular vesicular eruption on the skin. These blisters rupture due to scratching, dry up, and leave an area of pigmentation and scarring.
- IgA antibodies against tissue transglutaminase (tTG) cross-react with epidermal transglutaminase (eTG). This leads to granular IgA deposition in the skin which results in neutrophilic infiltration and blister formation.
- The presence of dermatitis herpetiformis is pathognomonic of gluten sensitivity → always screen for celiac disease.
- The diagnosis can be confirmed by the demonstration of granular IgA deposition in the skin in an area not affected by blistering.
- Treatment includes dapsone in addition to gluten free diet.

Q. Tropical sprue.

- Tropical sprue is a chronic diarrheal disease, possibly of infectious origin, that involves the small intestine and is characterized by malabsorption of nutrients, especially folic acid and vitamin B_{12}.
- It was called tropical sprue because it is common in residents or visitors of a tropical area. Tropical sprue is endemic in most of Asia, some Caribbean islands, Puerto Rico and parts of South America. In India, it is mainly seen in south India. Epidemics of tropical sprue occur, lasting up to 2 years in these areas.

Etiology

- Exact cause is unknown, but is likely to be due to an infectious agent because it responds to antibiotics.
- Often follows an episode of acute gastroenteritis.
- Some of the implicated bacteria include *E. coli*, Klebsiella and Enterobacter.

Pathophysiology

- Affects the entire small intestine, particularly the distal portion.
- Chronic infection leads to:
  - Inflammation of small intestinal mucosa
  - Partial villous atrophy
  - Defective absorption of nutrients including fats, B_{12}, and folate

Clinical Features

- Patients present with diarrhea, anorexia, abdominal distension and weight loss which can be acute or insidious in onset.
- Steatorrhea is common. Nutritional deficiencies, especially of folate and vitamin B_{12} develop after several months to years. Patient may also have glossitis, stomatitis, and peripheral edema.

Investigations

- *Endoscopy and mucosal biopsy:* Endoscopy shows flattening of duodenal folds and "scalloping." The jejunal mucosal biopsy show partial villous atrophy which is usually less severe than celiac disease. Changes are seen in whole of small intestine.
- Other causes of diarrhea must be excluded particularly Giardia and celiac disease, which can mimick tropical sprue.

Treatment

- Broad-spectrum antibiotics and folic acid can cure the condition, especially if the patient leaves the tropical area and does not return. Antibiotic treatment involves tetracycline 1 g daily for up to 6 months. Doxycycline can be used instead of tetracycline.

Q. Whipple's disease.

- Whipple's disease is a chronic multisystem disease caused by the gram-positive bacteria *Tropheryma whipplei*. *Tropheryma whipplei* has high infectivity but low virulence.
- Although the first descriptions of the disorder described a malabsorption syndrome with small intestinal involvement, the disease also affects the joints, CNS, and CVS.

Pathophysiology

- *T. whipplei* infects macrophages in the intestinal lamina propria and lymph nodes.
- Leads to obstruction of lymphatic flow, villous blunting, and impaired absorption.
- Disseminates systemically → affects joints, brain, heart, eyes.

Clinical Features

- The disease is common in middle-aged men and affects multiple systems. Onset is insidious and features include diarrhea, steatorrhea, abdominal pain, weight loss, migratory large-joint arthropathy, fever, dementia and ophthalmologic symptoms. It is a major cause of culture negative endocarditis.

Investigations

- Biopsies from the small intestine and other involved organs show presence of PAS-positive (periodic acid-Schiff) macrophages containing the characteristic small bacilli.
- PCR testing: Detects *T. whipplei* DNA in tissue or CSF (especially helpful in CNS involvement).

Treatment

- Ceftriaxone or penicillin initially followed by trimethoprim/sulfamethoxazole for minimum 1 year. Combination of doxycycline and hydroxychloroquine can be used in patients with sulpha allergy.

Q. Protein-losing enteropathy.

- Protein-losing enteropathy is not a specific disease but refers to many disorders characterized by excess protein loss into the gastrointestinal tract.

Causes of Protein-losing Enteropathy (Table 4.24)

TABLE 4.24: Causes of protein-losing enteropathy
Gastrointestinal mucosal diseases causing protein loss into GIT
• Ulcerative colitis
• Gastrointestinal carcinomas
• Peptic ulcer
• Amyloidosis
• Celiac sprue
• Whipple's disease
• Ménétrier's disease (hypertrophic gastropathy)
Lymphatic dysfunction
• Intestinal tuberculosis
• Obstruction (enlarged mesenteric nodes or lymphoma)
• Lymphangiectasia
Cardiac disorders
• Heart failure
• Chronic pericarditis

Clinical Features

- There is peripheral edema, low serum albumin and globulin levels in the absence of renal and hepatic disease.
- Both albumin and globulin are low in protein losing enteropathy. If only albumin is low with normal globulin, search for renal and/or hepatic disease.
- Patients with increased protein loss into the gastrointestinal tract from lymphatic obstruction often have steatorrhea and diarrhea.

Diagnosis

- Loss of protein into the gastrointestinal tract can be demonstrated by giving radiolabeled proteins and its quantification in stool during a 24 or 48 hours period.

Treatment

- Underlying disease should be treated. For example, gluten-free diet in celiac sprue or mesalamine for ulcerative colitis.

Q. Discuss the etiology, pathophysiology, clinical features, investigations, and management of lactose intolerance.

- The term lactose intolerance refers to the development of GI symptoms such as abdominal pain, bloating, flatulence, diarrhea, and vomiting after the ingestion of lactose. It is due to lactase deficiency which hydrolyses lactose into glucose and galactose.
- Intolerance to lactose-containing foods (e.g. dairy products) is a common problem worldwide.

Etiology of Lactose Intolerance

Primary lactase deficiency

- Racial or ethnic
- Developmental
- Congenital lactase deficiency

Secondary lactase deficiency

- Bacterial overgrowth
- Infectious enteritis
- Giardiasis
- Mucosal injury
- Celiac disease
- Tropical sprue
- Inflammatory bowel disease (especially Crohn's disease)
- Drug-or radiation-induced enteritis

Pathophysiology

- Lactose is hydrolyzed by intestinal lactase to glucose and galactose in the intestine which are then absorbed. If there is lactase deficiency, lactose cannot be hydrolyzed and absorbed. The unabsorbed lactose creates an osmotic load in the intestine, which draws fluid into the intestine. Excess fluid in the intestine causes dilatation of intestine and diarrhea. In the colon, free lactose is fermented by colonic bacteria to yield short-chain fatty acids and hydrogen gas. The combined increase in fecal water, intestinal transit, and generated hydrogen gas accounts for abdominal pain, bloating, flatulence, and diarrhea.

Clinical Features

- Among adults, the age of presentation is 20–40 years.
- Abdominal pain: may be crampy in nature and is often localized to the periumbilical area or lower quadrant.
- Bloating
- Flatulence
- Diarrhea: Stools are usually bulky, frothy, and watery.
- Vomiting
- Borborygmi may be audible on physical examination and to the patient.

Investigations

Lactose Tolerance Test

- 50 g of lactose is given orally and blood glucose levels are measured at 0, 1 and 2 hours. An increase in blood glucose by less than 20 mg/dl plus the development of symptoms is diagnostic.
- This test is cumbersome and time consuming, and has largely been replaced by the lactose hydrogen breath test.

Lactose Hydrogen Breath Test

- This is the most common test done. Oral lactose is given in the fasting state, at a dose of 2 g/kg (maximum dose,

25 g). Unabsorbed lactose is fermented by intestinal bacteria leading to release of hydrogen gas that is absorbed into the blood and excreted by lungs. Breath hydrogen is sampled at baseline and at 30-minute intervals after the ingestion of lactose for three hours.

- Baseline and post-lactose values are compared. A breath hydrogen value of more than 20 ppm is diagnostic of lactose malabsorption.

Genetic Test for Primary Lactose Malabsorption

- Missing gene coding for lactase may be identified.

Intestinal Biopsy and Measurement of Lactase Enzyme Levels

- This is the "gold standard" test for lactose malabsorption. However, it is not routinely required.

Treatment

Dietary Lactose Restriction

- Initially complete restriction of lactose-containing foods should be tried till the symptoms improve. Improvement of symptoms confirms the diagnosis also.
- Small quantities of lactose may subsequently be reintroduced into the diet, with careful monitoring of symptoms. Many patients will tolerate graded increase in lactose containing foods.

Enzyme Replacement

- Commercially available "lactase" preparations are actually bacterial or yeast beta-galactosidases. They can be taken with food and reduce symptoms in many lactose intolerant subjects.

Probiotics

- Lactase-containing probiotics may be beneficial. However, studies have shown mixed results.

Calcium Supplementation

- Avoidance of milk and other dairy products can lead to reduced calcium intake, which may increase the risk for osteoporosis and fracture. Hence, calcium supplementation should be given to all patients. A dose of 1200–1500 mg/day is necessary for adolescents and young adults.
- In addition, the vitamin D status should also be monitored. If necessary, vitamin D supplementation should also be given.

Q. Abdominal tuberculosis.

- Abdominal tuberculosis (TB) is a form of extrapulmonary tuberculosis that affects the gastrointestinal tract, peritoneum, mesenteric lymph nodes, and/or solid abdominal organs like the liver, spleen, or pancreas. One or more of these structures may be affected.
- The **most common site of intestinal involvement is the ileocecal region**. The affinity of *M. tuberculosis* for this site may be due to relative stasis of intestinal contents here, and abundant lymphoid tissue.
- Tuberculosis is being seen more frequently in patients with HIV infection.

Etiology

- *Mycobacterium tuberculosis*.

Routes of Spread

- Intestinal tuberculosis occurs due to swallowing of infected sputum, or hematogenous spread from active pulmonary or miliary TB, or ingestion of contaminated milk or food, or spread from adjacent organs.

Pathology

Intestinal Tuberculosis

- The macroscopic appearance of the intestinal TB can be categorized into 3 types.

Ulcerative (60%)

- This is characterized by multiple superficial ulcers.
- Ulcers are perpendicular to the long axis of intestine. Healing may result in scarring and stricture formation.
- This pattern has been associated with a virulent clinical course.

Hypertrophic (10%)

- This is characterized by scarring, fibrosis, and hypertrophic mass (pseudotumor).

Ulcerohypertrophic (30%)

- This is characterized by an inflammatory mass centering around the ileocecal valve with thickened and ulcerated intestinal walls.
- It is common in ileocecal TB compared to other segments of intestine.

Peritoneal Tuberculosis

- Peritoneum is studded with tubercles.
- Wet type presents with ascites which develops due to "exudation" of proteinaceous fluid from the tubercles. Most patients have this type.
- Dry type is characterized by fibro adhesive form of the disease.
- Patients may have combination of both of the above.

Lymphadenitis (mesenteric or retroperitoneal nodes)

- May present as abdominal mass or vague discomfort.
- Common in children and young adults.

Solid Organ TB

- Involvement of liver, spleen, or pancreas is rare and often part of miliary TB.
- Presents with fever, hepatosplenomegaly, or organ dysfunction.

Clinical Features

- Constitutional symptoms like anorexia, fatigue, fever, night sweats, and weight loss.

- Nonspecific chronic abdominal pain, diarrhea, constipation, or blood in the stool.
- A doughy mass may be palpable in right lower quadrant of abdomen.
- Abdominal distension due to ascites.
- Patients may also present acutely with small intestinal obstruction and colonic perforation.

Complications of Abdominal Tuberculosis

- Intestinal perforation
- Abscess formation
- Fistula formation (between intestinal loops and into the exterior through skin)
- Malabsorption
- Massive bleeding
- Intestinal obstruction.

Differential Diagnosis

- TB must be differentiated from other diseases affecting ileocecal region such as Crohn's disease, *Yersinia enterocolitica*, *Y. pseudotuberculosis* infection and cecal carcinoma.
- Peritoneal TB presenting with ascites must be differentiated from malignant ascites, pancreatic ascites, cirrhosis, etc.

Diagnosis

- *Routine laboratory tests* reveal mild anemia, increased ESR and hypoalbuminemia.
- *LFTs* may be altered in hepatic TB or due to systemic illness.
- *HIV* test important due to high TB-HIV co-infection.
- *Chest X-ray* may show evidence of active or old tuberculosis.
- *Plain X-ray* abdomen may show calcified lymph nodes and dilated bowel loops.
- *Tuberculin skin* test is positive in most patients.
- *Ascitic fluid analysis*
  - High leukocyte count of 150–4000/mm^3, with predominant lymphocytes.
  - Fluid is exudative (protein content is >3.0 mg/dl, low SAAG <1.1).
  - AFB stain and culture may be positive but have low yield rate.
  - Polymerase chain reaction (PCR) assay can rapidly detect mycobacteria.
  - Adenosine deaminase (ADA) levels in ascitic fluid has high sensitivity and specificity for detecting tuberculosis (>33 U/L is suggestive of TB).
  - Cartridge based nucleic acid amplification test (CB-NAAT/GeneXpert) of ascitic fluid.
- *Barium meal* and small bowel follow-through may show mucosal ulcerations, strictures (string sign), and hypersegmented bowel loops.
- *Barium enema* may show deformed cecum, a gaping and incompetent ileocecal valve with narrowing of terminal ileum (inverted umbrella sign).
- *Ultrasound abdomen* may show ascites, thickened ileocecal region, ileocecal mass and lymphadenopathy.
- *CT scan*: Better detail than ultrasound. May show concentric mural thickening of the ileocecal region, with or without proximal intestinal dilatation. Adjacent mesenteric lymphadenopathy may be seen on CT.
- *Colonoscopy* shows ulcers, strictures, nodules, pseudopolyps, fibrous bands, fistulas, and deformed ileocecal valves. Biopsy can be obtained from lesions.
- *Laparoscopy:* Laparoscopy examination is an effective method of diagnosing peritoneal tuberculosis because it can directly visualize tubercles and biopsy of the peritoneum can be taken. Biopsy specimens may be tested for AFB by staining, culture and PCR.

Treatment

- Treatment is similar to that for pulmonary TB. Conventional antitubercular therapy for at least 6 months including initial 2 months of HRZE (e.g. isoniazid, rifampicin, pyrazinamide, and ethambutol) followed by 4 month HR is recommended in all patients.
- Surgery is required for complications such as intestinal perforation, abscess or fistula, massive bleeding, and intestinal obstruction.

Q. What are inflammatory bowel diseases (IBD)? Discuss the etiology of IBD.

- Inflammatory bowel disease (IBD) is an immune mediated chronic intestinal inflammation. There are two major types of IBD–ulcerative colitis (UC) and Crohn's disease.
- Ulcerative colitis (UC) affects only the colon and Crohn's disease (CD) can affect any part of the GI tract. There is overlap between these two conditions in their clinical, histological and radiological features and sometimes differentiation between the two is not possible. It is possible that these conditions represent two aspects of the same disease.

Epidemiology

- IBD occurs worldwide but more common in the West. Both Crohn's disease (CD) and ulcerative colitis (UC) have an incidence of approximately 5–10 per 100 000 annually. Whites are affected more commonly than non-white races. Jews are more affected than non-Jews, and the Ashkenazi Jews have a higher risk than the Sephardic Jews.

Etiology (common for both Crohn's disease and ulcerative colitis)

- The exact etiology of IBD is unknown. But the pathogenesis involves three factors: genetic susceptibility, environmental factors and host immune response. Many risk factors have been identified which are as follows.
- *Familial and genetic factors:* IBD is more common amongst relatives of patients than in the general population. There is increased concordance for IBD in monozygotic twins than dizygotic twins.

- *Environmental factors:* Good domestic hygiene has been shown to be a risk factor for CD but not for UC. It is suggested that in a clean environment, intestinal immune system is not exposed to many pathogens and hence, may not be able to handle an infection. Hence, even minor infections trigger prominent inflammation.
- *Psychosocial factors:* Major life events such as illness or death in the family, divorce or separation, interpersonal conflict, or other major loss are associated with an increase in IBD symptoms.
- *Nutritional factors:* High sugar and fat intake is suspected to be associated with IBD, but more studies are needed to confirm it.
- *Smoking:* Patients with CD are more likely to be smokers, and smoking has been shown to exacerbate CD. In contrast, there is an increased risk of UC in nonsmokers and nicotine has been shown to be an effective treatment of UC.
- *Appendicectomy:* Appendicectomy is protective for the development of UC, particularly if performed before the age of 20. In contrast, appendicectomy may increase the risk of development of CD.
- *Intestinal microflora:* IBD is characterized by an overaggressive immune response to luminal bacterial antigens and other products, occurring against a background of genetic susceptibility. There is an alteration in the bacterial flora, with an increase in anaerobic bacteria in CD and an increase in aerobic bacteria in UC.
- *Immunological factors:* Many immunological abnormalities have been described in IBD patients. Many patients lack the ability to appropriately down regulate antigen-specific or antigen nonspecific inflammatory responses to endogenous luminal antigens. There is upregulation of macrophages and T-helper lymphocytes in IBD which release pro-inflammatory cytokines. There is also activation of other cells (eosinophils, mast cells, neutrophils and fibroblasts) which leads to excess production of chemokines (lymphokines, arachidonic acid metabolites, neuropeptides and free oxygen radicals), all of which can lead to tissue damage.

Q. Describe the etiology, pathology, clinical features, investigations and treatment of Crohn's disease.

- Crohn's disease is an idiopathic, chronic inflammatory disease of the gastrointestinal (GI) tract that can affect any part of the tract from the mouth to the anus. It is characterized by exacerbations and remissions.

Epidemiology

- Crohn's disease is slightly commoner in females (M: F = 1:1.2).
- Its incidence has a bimodal distribution with the onset occurring most frequently between ages 15–30 years and 40–60 years old.
- It is more common in western population and in urban areas than rural areas.

Etiology

- Refer previous question on IBD.

Pathology

Macroscopic Changes

- Crohn's disease can affect any part of the gastrointestinal tract from the mouth to the anus but commonly affects the terminal ileum and ascending colon (ileocolonic disease).
- The disease is characterized by skip lesions (normal areas in between affected areas) **(Fig. 4.11)**.
- The involved small bowel is usually thickened and narrowed. There are deep ulcers and fissures in the mucosa of the intestine, producing a cobblestone appearance.
- Fistulae and abscesses may be seen in the colon.

Microscopic Changes

- In Crohn's disease the inflammation extends through all layers (transmural) of the bowel.
- There is an increase in chronic inflammatory cells and lymphoid hyperplasia.
- Noncaseating granulomas may be seen.

Clinical Features

- It is a chronic disease with remissions and exacerbations.
- The disease may present insidiously or acutely.
- The major symptoms are diarrhea, abdominal pain, and weight loss.
- Constitutional symptoms of malaise, lethargy, anorexia, nausea, vomiting and low-grade fever may be present.
- The abdominal pain can be colicky, or felt as discomfort.
- Diarrhea may be associated with blood, making it difficult to differentiate from ulcerative colitis. Steatorrhea may be present due to small intestinal involvement.
- It can present as an emergency with acute right iliac fossa pain mimicking appendicitis.
- It can be complicated by anal and perianal disease and can be the presenting feature, often preceding colonic and small intestinal symptoms by many years.

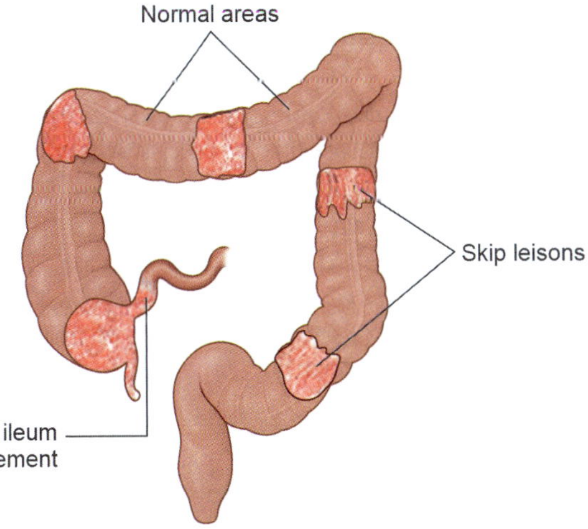

Figure 4.11: Skip lesions in Crohn's disease

- Enteric fistulae, e.g. from intestine to bladder or vagina occur in some cases.
- Examination may show weight loss and general ill-health. Right iliac fossa tenderness and mass are occasionally found. The mass is due either to inflamed loops of bowel that are matted together or to an abscess. Anal fissures or perianal abscesses may be present. Extraintestinal features such as arthritis may be present.

Investigations

- *Blood tests:* Anemia is common due to blood loss. ESR, CRP, and WBC counts are raised indicating inflammation. Hypoalbuminemia is present in severe disease due to protein loss from intestine. Presence of anti-saccharomyces cerevisiae antibodies (ASCA) with absence of anti neutrophil cytoplasmic antibodies (pANCA) is seen in Crohn's disease and can distinguish Crohn's from ulcerative colitis.
- *Stool examination:* This should be done to exclude infective causes of diarrhea.
- *Fecal calprotectin*: this is high in IBD. Calprotectin is a protein released by neutrophils. When there is inflammation in the intestine due to IBD neutrophils infiltrate intestine and release calprotectin, resulting in an increased level in the stool. This test can help distinguish between IBD and IBS (irritable bowel syndrome).
- *Barium meal follow-through:* Examination may show an asymmetrical alteration in the mucosal pattern with deep ulceration, and areas of narrowing or stricturing (string sign). Changes are commonly seen in terminal ileum. Skip lesions with normal bowel in-between.
- *Ultrasound, CT or MRI abdomen:* These are used to define the thickness of the bowel wall and mesentery as well as intra-abdominal and para-intestinal abscesses and also used to rule out alternate pathology in acute presentations.
- *Radionuclide scans:* With radiolabeled leukocytes are used to identify small intestinal and colonic disease and to localize extraintestinal abscesses.
- *Colonoscopy:* Superficial or deep ulceration with **cobblestone appearance** and deep fissures. Skip lesions. Rectal sparing.
- *Video capsule endoscopy:* Can visualize the small bowel when regular endoscopy or colonoscopy cannot reach these areas.
- *Colonic biopsy:* Can be used to confirm the diagnosis of IBD and exclude other diagnoses. The biopsy characteristically reveals crypt abscesses, branching of crypts, atrophy of glands, and loss of mucin in goblet cells in ulcerative colitis.

Treatment

- Treatment is aimed at reducing the intestinal inflammation by using various anti-inflammatory agents. goal of therapy is to induce and then maintain a remission.

General Measures

- Cigarette smoking should be stopped.
- Diarrhea can be controlled with loperamide or codeine phosphate. Diarrhea in long standing inactive disease may be due to bile acid malabsorption and responds to cholestyramine.
- Anemia may be due to B_{12}/folic acid or iron deficiency, which should be replaced.

5-ASA (amino salicylic acid) Agents

- The mainstay of therapy for IBD is 5-ASA agents. These agents are effective at inducing remission in both UC and CD and in maintaining remission in UC. It is unclear whether they can maintain remission in CD also. Example is sulfasalazine.
- Sulfasalazine is not broken down in small intestine and the intact molecule reaches colon where it is broken down by colonic bacteria into sulfa and 5-ASA moieties. 5-ASA acts as local anti-inflammatory agent in the colon.
- There are many side effects of sulfasalazine including folate malabsorption. These side effects are due to sulfa moiety. Patients on sulfasalazine should be given folic acid supplements.
- Newer sulfa-free agents such as mesalamine, olsalazine and balsalazide have less of side effects.
- Topical mesalamine enemas are effective in mild-to-moderate distal CD. Mesalamine suppositories are effective in treating proctitis.

Glucocorticoids

- These are effective in patients with moderate to severe UC and CD. Prednisone 40–60 mg/d is given if there is poor response to 5-ASA therapy.
- Glucocorticoids play no role in maintenance therapy of either UC or CD. Once clinical remission has been induced, they should be tapered slowly.

Immunosuppressive Agents

- *Azathioprine, 6-mercaptopurine,* methotrexate and cyclosporine are mainly employed as steroid sparing agents in the management of glucocorticoid-dependent IBD. Tacrolimus and mycophenolate mofetil are newer immunosuppressive agents.

Biologics

- Infliximab is a monoclonal antibody against TNF that is extremely effective in CD. Two other anti-TNF agents, adalimumab and golimumab may be less immunogenic than infliximab and have shown efficacy in the treatment of Crohn's disease.

Nutritional Therapies

- Patients with active CD respond to bowel rest, along with total enteral or total parenteral nutrition (TPN). Bowel rest and TPN are as effective as glucocorticoids at inducing remission of active CD but are not effective as maintenance therapy. However, UC does not respond to dietary measures.

Surgical Management

- In Crohn's disease surgery is indicated in stricture and obstruction unresponsive to medical therapy, massive hemorrhage and refractory fistula. Unlike UC, surgery is not curative in Crohn's—disease often recurs.

Complications

- Intestinal obstruction
- Fistulas
- Abscesses
- Malabsorption
- Colorectal cancer

Q. Describe the etiology, pathology, clinical features, investigations and treatment of ulcerative colitis.

- Ulcerative colitis is an idiopathic inflammatory condition of the colon which results in diffuse friability and superficial erosions on the colonic wall.
- It is the most common form of inflammatory bowel disease worldwide. There is an increased prevalence of ulcerative colitis in nonsmokers or those who recently quit smoking.

Etiology

- Refer previous question on IBD.

Pathology

Macroscopic Changes (Fig. 4.12)

- UC usually involves only colon and spares small intestine except in a few patients where terminal ileum can also be involved (backwash ileitis).
- Mucosa is erythematous and has a fine granular surface that looks like sandpaper. Mucosal involvement is continuous without skip lesions.
- Rectum is also involved in 95% of cases.

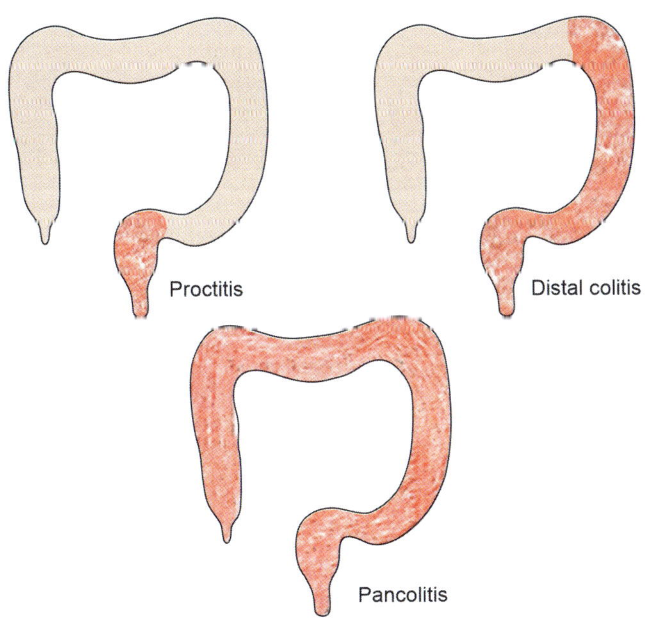

Figure 4.12: Ulcerative colitis

- Inflammatory swollen mucosa gives the appearance of pseudopolyps.
- In severe inflammation, toxic dilatation can occur.
- On healing, the mucosa can return to normal, although there is usually some residual glandular distortion.

Microscopic Changes

- Mucosa shows a chronic inflammatory cell infiltrate in the lamina propria. Crypt abscesses and goblet cell depletion are also seen.
- Inflammation is restricted to the mucosa and submucosa of the colon.

Clinical Features

- The disease can be mild, moderate or severe, and in most patients runs a course of remissions and exacerbations.
- The major symptom in ulcerative colitis is diarrhea with blood and mucus, sometimes accompanied by lower abdominal discomfort. Diarrhea is often nocturnal and/or postprandial.
- General features include malaise, lethargy and anorexia.
- Aphthous ulceration in the mouth is seen.
- When there is proctitis (rectal inflammation) blood mixed with the stool, urgency and tenesmus are seen.
- Extraintestinal manifestations can be seen in some patients and include episcleritis, scleritis, uveitis, peripheral arthropathies, sacroiliitis, ankylosing spondylitis, primary sclerosing cholangitis, erythema nodosum, and pyoderma gangrenosum.

Investigations

Blood Tests

- Anemia is common due to blood loss. ESR, CRP and white cell counts are raised indicating inflammation. Hypoalbuminemia is present in severe disease due to protein loss from intestine. pANCA may be positive in ulcerative colitis.

Stool Examination

- This should be done to exclude infective causes of colitis.

Plain X-ray Abdomen

- To exclude toxic dilatation of colon.

Flexible Sigmoidoscopy and Colonoscopy

- Sigmoidoscopy is enough initially since total colonoscopy may precipitate toxic megacolon or perforation in severe disease. Colonoscopy can be done in mild cases.
- Mucosa is erythematous. In addition, petechiae, exudates, touch friability, and frank hemorrhage may be present.
- Severe cases may have ulcers, profuse bleeding, and copious exudates. Colonic involvement is continuous in ulcerative colitis (skip lesions in Crohn's disease).
- Pseudopolyps may be present.

Barium Enema

- Rarely used in the diagnosis of ulcerative colitis. It may be normal in mild forms of disease.
- It shows ulcers, shortening of the colon, loss of haustrae, narrowing of the lumen, and pseudopolyps. It should be avoided in severely ill patients as it may precipitate ileus with toxic megacolon.

Colonic Biopsy

- Can be used to confirm the diagnosis. It reveals crypt abscesses and chronic changes including branching of crypts, atrophy of glands, and loss of mucin in goblet cells.

Treatment

- Treatment is same as that of Crohn's disease.
- Surgery (total proctocolectomy with ileostomy) is indicated in severe ulcerative colitis associated with toxic megacolon, colonic perforation and massive colonic hemorrhage.

Q. Comparison of ulcerative colitis and Crohn's disease (Table 4.25).

Q. Toxic megacolon.

- Toxic megacolon is total or segmental nonobstructive colonic dilatation (usually ≥6 cm) associated with systemic toxicity. It is a potentially lethal complication of inflammatory bowel disease (IBD) or infectious colitis.
- Colonic dilatation without systemic toxicity is not considered toxic megacolon. (e.g. Hirshsprung's disease, chronic constipation, intestinal pseudo-obstruction, diffuse gastrointestinal dysmotility).

Etiology

TABLE 4.26: Causes of toxic megacolon

Inflammatory bowel disease
• Ulcerative colitis
• Crohn's disease
Infectious
• *Clostridium difficile* pseudomembranous colitis
• Salmonella-typhoid and non-typhoid
• Shigella
• Campylobacter
• Yersinia
• *Entameba histolytica*
• CMV colitis (common in HIV patients)
Ischemia
• Ischemic colitis

Pathogenesis

- Mucosal inflammation leads to the release of inflammatory mediators and bacterial products, increased inducible nitric oxide synthase, which in turn increases nitric oxide. Nitric acid relaxes smooth muscle in colon leading to dilatation.
- Extension of the mucosal inflammation to the smooth muscle layer paralyzes the colonic smooth muscle, leading to dilatation.
- Precipitating factors of toxic megacolon include hypokalemia, antimotility agents, opiates, anticholinergics, antidepressants, barium enema, and colonoscopy. Discontinuing or rapid tapering of corticosteroids, sulfasalazine, or 5-ASA compounds in IBD may contribute to the development of megacolon.

TABLE 4.25: Comparison of ulcerative colitis and Crohn's Disease

	Ulcerative colitis	Crohn's disease
Male: female ratio	Equal	Slightly more common in males
Smoking	May prevent disease	May cause disease
Oral contraceptives	No increased risk	Increased risk
Appendectomy	Protective	Not protective
Gross blood and mucus in stool	Frequent	Occasional
Systemic symptoms	Occasional	Frequent
Pain abdomen	Occasional	Frequent
Abdominal mass	Rare	Yes
Perineal disease	Rare	Frequent
Small intestinal involvement	No (only backwash ileitis)	Yes
Stricture of intestine	Occasional	Frequent
Intestinal obstruction	Rare	Frequent
Response to antibiotics	No	Yes
Recurrence after surgery	No	Yes
pANCA-positive	Frequently	Rarely
Presence of anti-*Saccharomyces cerevisiae* antibodies	No	Yes
Rectal sparing	Rarely	Frequently
Skip leisons	No	Yes
Cobblestone appearance	No	Yes

Pathology

- Marked dilatation of the colon, thinning of the bowel wall, and deep ulcers **(Fig. 4.13)**.
- Acute inflammation in all layers of the colon.

Clinical Features

- Toxic megacolon affects all ages and both sexes.
- Signs and symptoms of acute colitis may precede the onset of acute dilatation.
- Patients usually present with abdominal pain and distention, nausea, vomiting, diarrhea (may or may not be bloody), and altered sensorium.
- Physical examination reveals a toxic appearing patient with altered sensorium, tachycardia, fever, postural hypotension, lower abdominal distension and tenderness.
- Peritonitis symptoms indicate bowel perforation.
- Large doses of steroids and analgesics may mask the signs or symptoms of toxic megacolon.

Investigations

- Anemia related to blood loss
- Leukocytosis
- Electrolyte disturbances
- Hypoalbuminemia
- ESR and CRP are usually increased.
- Plain X-ray abdomen: Transverse or right colon is commonly affected. Multiple air-fluid levels in the colon are seen. Normal colonic haustral pattern is either absent or severely disturbed.
- Stool specimens should be sent for culture, microscopic analysis, and C. difficile toxin.
- Ultrasonography and computed tomography (CT).
- Limited endoscopy without bowel preparation is useful to diagnose the cause. Only minimal air should be introduced into the colon to avoid worsening ileus or distention and perforation. Full colonoscopy is risky in toxic megacolon. It can lead to perforation.

Treatment

- Initial therapy is medical. However, a surgical consultation should be obtained upon admission, and the patient should be evaluated daily by both the medical and surgical team.

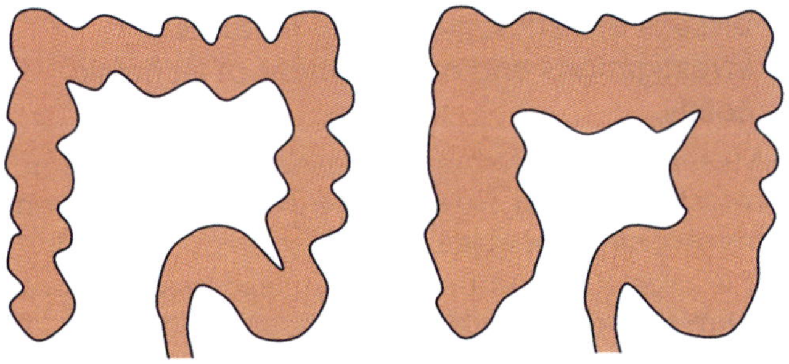

Figure 4.13: Normal (left) and toxic megacolon (right)

Medical Therapy

- Patients with IBD should be kept nil per oral and a nasogastric tube is inserted to decompress the gastrointestinal tract. Enteral feeding is begun as soon as the patient shows signs of improvement.
- Anemia, dehydration, and electrolyte imbalances should be treated aggressively.
- All antimotility agents, opiates, and anticholinergics should be discontinued as they aggravate ileus.
- Intravenous H_2 blockers or proton pump inhibitors should be given to prevent gastric stress ulcers.
- Broad spectrum antibiotics are given to reduce septic complications and to prevent possible peritonitis in case of perforation (third-generation cephalosporin plus metronidazole).
- Intravenous corticosteroids (hydrocortisone 100 mg or equivalent every 6–8 hours or by continuous infusion) should be given to all patients for the treatment of underlying ulcerative colitis or Crohn's disease. Steroids do not increase the risk of perforation. Steroids are not used in toxic megacolon due to C. *difficile* colitis or infective colitis.
- If toxic megacolon is due to severe C. *difficile* colitis (antibiotic induced), the first step is to stop the offending antibiotic, followed by oral vancomycin via a nasogastric tube. Intravenous vancomycin has no effect on C. *difficile* colitis since the antibiotic is not excreted into the colon. If there is response to vancomycin, intravenous metronidazole may be added at a dose of 500 mg every eight hours.

Surgical Therapy

- Perforation, massive hemorrhage, increasing transfusion requirements, worsening signs of toxicity, and progression of colonic dilatation are absolute indications for surgery.
- Subtotal colectomy with end-ileostomy is the procedure of choice for urgent or emergent surgery.

Q. Discuss the etiology, clinical features, investigations, and management of pseudomembranous colitis.

Etiology

- Pseudomembranous colitis is severe inflammation of the inner lining of the colon. It is most often caused by overgrowth of clostridioides (formerly *Clostridium*) *difficile* after prolonged broad spectrum antibiotic therapy.
- Commonly implicated antibiotics are,
  - Ampicillin
  - Clindamycin
  - Tetracycline
  - Third-generation cephalosporins
  - Fluoroquinolones

Pathogenesis

- *C. difficile* is an anaerobic bacterium which colonizes the colon of 3% of healthy adults. It is acquired by fecal-oral transmission. It is readily transmitted from patient to patient by hospital personnel.

- Antibiotics disrupt the normal bowel flora and allow *C. difficile* to flourish.
- After multiplication, it produces two toxins; toxin A and toxin B. Both toxins possess cytotoxic activity and can damage the colon. Both toxins adhere to receptors on the human colonocyte brush border, and cause necrosis and shedding of these cells into the lumen. Both the toxins cause an acute inflammatory diarrhea with massive infiltration of the intestinal mucosa with neutrophils and monocytes.
- Shedding of colonic epithelial cells produces shallow ulcers. Serum proteins, mucus, and inflammatory cells flow outward from the ulcer, creating a pseudomembrane.

Pathology

- Rectum and colon show a yellow or off-white membrane adherent to the eroded mucosa (pseudomembrane). Pseudomembranes are patchily distributed.
- There is edema and hyperemia of the full thickness of the bowel wall.

Clinical Features

- Symptoms usually begin during or shortly after antibiotic therapy but may be delayed for up to 2 months.
- Most patients report mild-to-moderate greenish, foul-smelling watery diarrhea with lower abdominal cramps. With more serious illness, there is abdominal pain and profuse watery diarrhea with up to 30 stools per day. The stools may have mucus but seldom gross blood.
- Physical examination is normal or reveals left lower quadrant tenderness. There may be fever up to 40°C.
- Rarely fulminant colitis with serious complications, such as perforation, prolonged ileus, toxic megacolon, and death can occur.

Investigations

Stool Studies

- Demonstration of *C. difficile* toxins in the stool by cytotoxicity assay (toxin B) or rapid enzyme immunoassays (EIA) for toxins A and B.
- Culture for C difficile is sensitive, but slower (2–3 days), more costly, and less specific than toxin assays, and not used in most clinical settings.
- Fecal leukocytes are present in only 50% of patients with colitis.

Flexible Sigmoidoscopy

- Reveals typical pseudomembranes **(Fig. 4.14)**.

Plain X-ray Abdomen

- To look for evidence of toxic dilation or megacolon but are of no value in mild disease.

Abdominal CT Scan

- Useful in detecting colonic edema, and evaluation of possible complications.

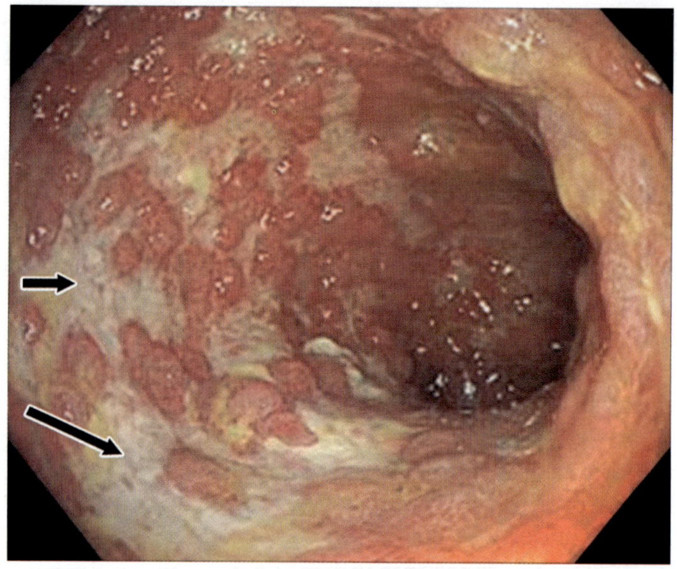

Figure 4.14: Pseudomembranes in colon (arrows)

Treatment

- Offending antibiotic should be discontinued. This alone may lead to resolution of symptoms in mild cases.
- If diarrhea is severe, the drug of choice is oral vancomycin, 125 mg orally four times daily due to faster symptom resolution and fewer treatment failures than metronidazole. Vancomycin is not absorbed and acts directly at the infection site. Intravenous vancomycin should be not be used as it is not effective. Oral or intravenous metronidazole 500 mg three times daily is an alternative. In fulminant cases, both vancomycin and metronidazole can be combined.
- Fidaxomicin is a new macrolide approved for the treatment of *C. difficile*-associated diarrhea. This agent has a narrower antimicrobial spectrum and alters the gut microflora less than do metronidazole and vancomycin.
- Probiotics such as *Saccharomyces boulardii*, and Lactobacillus may help in controlling the disease and also prevent relapses.
- Frequent recurrences despite therapy with oral vancomycin, can be treated with fecal microbiota transplantation.
- Total colectomy may be required in patients with toxic megacolon, perforation, sepsis, or hemorrhage.

Q. Discuss the etiology, clinical features, investigations and management of mesenteric ischemia.

OR

Q. Discuss the etiology, clinical features, investigations and management of ischemic colitis.

- Mesenteric ischemia is caused by a reduction in intestinal blood flow. It can be acute or chronic, involve small or large bowel.
- It is a serious condition and can lead to sepsis, bowel infarction, and death.
- Ischemic colitis is the most frequent form of mesenteric ischemia, affecting mostly the elderly.

Etiology of Mesenteric Ischemia

- Embolic occlusion (emboli arise from heart or aorta)
- Thrombotic occlusion (due to atherosclerosis)
- Hypotension (myocardial infarction, heart failure, arrhythmias or sudden blood loss)
- Vasculitis
- Venous occlusion
- Strangulated hernia
- Colon volvulus.

Clinical Features

Small Bowel Ischemia

- It is due to occlusion of superior mesenteric artery.
- Pathological changes may range from mild ischemia to transmural hemorrhagic necrosis and gangrene.
- Sudden onset abdominal pain with minimal physical signs.
- Abdomen may be distended with diminished bowel sounds.
- Signs of peritonitis may be present.
- Patients may have evidence of cardiac disease and arrhythmia responsible for emboli.

Large Bowel Ischemia (ischemic colitis)

- The splenic flexure and descending colon are prone for ischemic injury since they have little collateral circulation. Ischemic injury can range from transient colitis to gangrene and fulminant pancolitis.
- Patient is usually elderly.
- Sudden onset of cramping, left-sided lower abdominal pain, and rectal bleeding.
- Symptoms usually resolve over 24–48 hours and healing occurs within 2 weeks.
- Some have a residual fibrous stricture or segmental colitis.
- A minority develop gangrene and peritonitis.

Chronic Mesenteric Ischemia

- Postprandial abdominal pain (intestinal angina).
- Food fear → weight loss.
- Seen in patients with atherosclerosis.

Investigations

- Leukocytosis, metabolic acidosis, and high amylase levels.
- Plain X-ray abdomen may show 'thumb-printing' due to mucosal edema.
- Ultrasound abdomen.
- CT abdomen.
- CT angiography shows occluded or narrowed mesenteric artery.
- Investigations for underlying prothrombotic disorders.
- Colonoscopy and barium enema in ischemic colitis.

Treatment

- Patient is kept nil by mouth (NBM)
- IV fluids and electrolytes
- Intravenous antibiotic therapy (ciprofloxacin and metrinidazole)
- Embolectomy and vascular reconstruction if possible.
- Thrombolysis may sometimes be effective in patients at high surgical risk.
- Anticoagulation in mesenteric vein thrombosis
- Laparotomy and resection of the involved segment with end to end anastomosis is required in patients with bowel gangrene and signs of peritonitis.
- Small bowel transplantation can be considered in selected patients.
- Chronic mesenteric ischemia: Elective revascularization (angioplasty/stenting or bypass).

Q. Discuss the etiology, clinical features, investigations and management of irritable bowel syndrome (IBS).

- Irritable bowel syndrome (IBS) is a functional gastrointestinal disorder characterized by chronic abdominal pain and altered bowel habits in the absence of any organic cause.
- Organic causes should be ruled out before making a diagnosis of IBS.

Etiology

- Hereditary and environmental factors.
- Abnormal gastrointestinal motility in the form of exaggerated gastrocolic reflex, altered gastric emptying, increased small bowel contractions and increased small intestinal transit.
- Visceral hypersensitivity.
- Neurotransmitters such as serotonin may be an important factor. It stimulates intestinal secretion and peristalsis in addition to visceral pain receptors via 5-HT3 and 5-HT4 pathways.
- Microscopic inflammation: Detailed immunohistologic investigation has revealed mucosal immune system activation in a subset of patients with irritable bowel syndrome (mostly those with the diarrhea predominant type).
- Role of infection (post-infectious IBS): Gastroenteritis is a common trigger for IBS. The IBS symptoms can be triggered by an enteric infection and can persist for weeks, months and years.
- Psychologic disturbances: many patients with IBS have increased anxiety, depression, phobias, and somatization.
- Certain foods may precipitate an attack, e.g. excess coffee.

Clinical Features

- IBS is common in young people. It is 3 times more common in women.

Rome IV Criteria for the Diagnosis of IBS

- Recurrent abdominal pain on average at least 1 day per week during the previous 3 months associated with two or more of the following:
  - Related to defecation (may be increased or unchanged by defecation)
  - Associated with a change in stool frequency
  - Associated with a change in stool form or appearance

- Four subtypes of IBS have been recognized:
  1. Diarrhea predominant (IBS-D)
  2. Constipation predominant (IBS-C)
  3. Mixed (alternating diarrhea and constipation) (IBS-M)
  4. Unclassified (IBS-U)
- The usefulness of this classification is debatable because the symptoms can change from one type to another in a given patient.
- Abdominal pain in IBS is highly variable in intensity and location. It is frequently episodic and crampy, but may be dull aching also. Pain may be mild or it may interfere with daily activities. Abdominal pain is mainly present during daytime hence sleep disturbance is rare. Pain is often exacerbated by eating or emotional stress and relieved by passage of flatus or stools.
- Alteration in bowel habits usually begins in adult life. The most common pattern is constipation alternating with diarrhea, usually with one of these symptoms predominating. Diarrhea in IBS usually consists of small volumes of loose stools. Nocturnal diarrhea does not occur in IBS. Bleeding, malabsorption and weight loss does not occur in IBS.
- Patients with IBS also complain of increased belching or flatulence. Many patients also complain of dyspepsia, heartburn, nausea, and vomiting.
- Physical examination is usually normal, but palpation of the abdomen may reveal tenderness, particularly in the left lower quadrant.

Red Flag Signs (require further investigation to rule out serious underlying problems other than IBS)

- Age >50 years with new onset symptoms
- Weight loss
- GI bleeding or occult blood
- Nocturnal symptoms
- Anemia
- Family history of IBD or colorectal cancer.

Differential Diagnoses

- Anxiety disorders
- Bacterial overgrowth syndrome
- Malabsorption syndromes (such as celiac sprue)
- Gastroenteritis
- Giardiasis
- Hypercalcemia
- Hyperthyroidism
- Inflammatory bowel disease
- Colon cancer.

Investigations

- Since IBS is a diagnosis of exclusion, following investigations should be done routinely to exclude other diseases with similar presentation.
- Complete blood count
- Stool examination—to look for ova, cysts and occult blood
- Stool calprotectin (to rule out IBD)
- Celiac serology (for IBS-D)
- Colonoscopy—in those older than 50 years to rule out carcinoma colon.
- Hydrogen breath test—if the main symptoms are diarrhea and increased gas to rule out malabsorption.
- Upper GI scopy—if the patient has prominent dyspepsia.
- Ultrasound abdomen.

Treatment

Patient Counseling and Dietary Alterations

- Patients should be reassured and functional nature of the disorder explained. Foods which aggravate symptoms (such as coffee, disaccharides, legumes, and cabbage) should be avoided. Such diet is called low FODMAP diet. (FODMAP stands for fermentable oligo-, di-, mono-saccharides and polyols)

Stool-bulking Agents

- High-fiber diets and bulking agents, such as bran or hydrophilic colloid, are helpful in treating IBS. Dietary fiber has multiple effects on colonic physiology. Because of their hydrophilic properties, stool-bulking agents bind water and thus prevent both excessive hydration and dehydration of stool. Hence these agents can reduce both diarrhea and constipation in IBS patients.

Antispasmodics

- Anticholinergic drugs (e.g. hyoscyamine) may provide temporary relief for symptoms such as painful cramps related to intestinal spasm.

Antidiarrheal Agents

- Peripherally acting opiate-based agents are the initial therapy of choice for diarrhea-predominant IBS.
- Diphenoxylate (Lomotil), 2.5–5 mg every 4–6 hours, can be prescribed. Codeine is also helpful. These agents should be used only temporarily and should be replaced gradually with high-fiber diet.

Antidepressant Drugs

- Tricyclic antidepressants (amitryptyline, imipramine, desipramine) slow jejunal migrating motor complex transit propagation and delays orocecal and whole-gut transit. They improve diarrhea, pain, and depression.
- The selective serotonin reuptake inhibitor (SSRI) paroxetine accelerates orocecal transit, and may be useful in constipation-predominant patients.
- The SSRI citalopram blunts perception of rectal distention and reduces abdominal pain.

5-HT3-receptor Antagonists

- A 5HT3 receptor antagonists such as alosetron, cilansetron, and ramosetron are useful in diarrhea predominant IBS. They reduce abdominal discomfort and improve stool frequency, consistency, and urgency. However a major side effect ischemic colitis has been observed with alosetron and this drug is not commonly used now. Cilansetron was not marketed. Ramosetron is now widely available and commonly used. Ischemic colitis has not been observed with ramosetron.

5HT4 Receptor Agonist

- Tegaserod is a 5HT4 receptor agonist which has been approved for use in constipation predominant IBS.

Lubiprostone

- This agent activates chloride channels in the small intestine. As a result, chloride ions are secreted and sodium and water passively diffuse into the lumen to maintain isotonicity. It is useful in constipation predominant IBS.

Q. Enumerate the causes of acute abdomen. What are the clinical features of acute abdomen? How do you investigate and manage a case of acute abdomen?

- Acute abdomen refers to sudden, severe abdominal pain of less than 24 hours duration that may require urgent medical or surgical intervention. It can arise from a wide range of abdominal or systemic conditions.

Causes of Acute Abdomen (Table 4.27)

TABLE 4.27: Causes of acute abdomen
Surgical causes
Inflammatory
• Appendicitis
• Cholecystitis
• Pancreatitis
• Diverticulitis
Obstructive
• Small or large bowel obstruction
• Volvulus
• Hernia (incarcerated/strangulated)
• Intussusception
Perforation
• Peptic ulcer perforation
• Diverticular perforation
• Typhoid/perforated appendix
Vascular
• Mesenteric ischemia/infarction
• Ruptured abdominal aortic aneurysm (AAA)
Traumatic
• Blunt or penetrating abdominal trauma
• Organ rupture (spleen, liver)
Gynecological/Urological
• Ectopic pregnancy
• Ovarian torsion or rupture
• Testicular torsion
• Ureteric colic
Medical causes
• Acute pyelonephritis
• Diabetic ketoacidosis
• Acute intermittent porphyria
• Lead poisoning
• Hemophilia and other bleeding disorders
• Henoch-Schonlein purpura
• Sickle cell crisis
• Polycythemia vera
• Embolic phenomenon

Clinical Features of Acute Abdomen

History

- Complaints: Acute abdomen usually presents with pain abdomen. Find out the exact location and nature of pain. Pain may be localized (appendicitis, pancreatitis) or diffuse (intestinal obstruction, peritonitis). In general, the pain of an acute abdomen can either be constant (due to inflammation) or colicky because of a blocked hollow organ.
- A sudden onset of pain suggests a perforation (e.g. of a duodenal ulcer), a rupture (e.g. of an aneurysm or ectopic pregnancy), torsion (e.g. of an ovarian cyst), or acute pancreatitis.
- Vomiting is usually present in any acute abdomen but, if persistent, suggests intestinal obstruction. The character of the vomitus should be asked-does it contain blood, bile or small bowel contents.
- Absolute constipation and abdominal distension may be present in intestinal obstruction.
- Past history: enquire about any previous operations, gynecological problems and any concurrent medical condition.

General Examination

- The general condition of the patient should be assessed.
- Most acute abdomen patients look acutely ill.
- Fever suggests an acute infectious process.
- Note pulse rate, respiratory rate, blood pressure and state of hydration. Large volumes of fluid may be lost from the vascular compartment into the peritoneal cavity or into the lumen of the bowel, giving rise to hypovolemia, i.e. a pale cold skin, a weak rapid pulse and hypotension.

Abdomen

- *Inspection:* Note the presence of scars, distension or mass.
- *Palpation:* Tenderness, rebound tenderness, presence or absence of guarding should be noted. Guarding indicates peritonitis. Guarding can be localized or generalized.
- *Bowel sounds:* Increased bowel sounds indicate intestinal obstruction. Absent bowel sounds suggest peritonitis.
- *Special signs:* Rovsing's (appendicitis), Murphy's (cholecystitis), Cullen's/Grey-Turner's (pancreatitis).
- Other systems should be examined to rule out any concurrent disease.

Investigations

- ***Blood count:*** White cell count is raised in inflammatory conditions.
- ***Serum amylase and lipase:*** High levels (more than five times normal) indicate acute pancreatitis.
- ***Urine pregnancy test:*** Should be done in women of child bearing age to rule out ectopic pregnancy and its rupture.

- ***X-ray erect abdomen:*** air under the diaphragm may be seen in abdominal viscus perforation. Multiple air fluid levels are seen in peritonitis and intestinal obstruction.
- ***Ultrasound:*** This is useful in the diagnosis of acute cholangitis, cholecystitis and aortic aneurysm, acute pancreatitis and acute appendicitis. It can detect renal and ureteric stones and ruptured ectopic gestation.
- ***CT scan:*** It is more accurate than ultrasound in most acute emergencies.
- ***Laparoscopy:*** This has gained increasing importance as a diagnostic tool prior to proceeding with surgery. In addition, therapeutic maneuvers, such as appendicectomy, can be performed.

Treatment of Acute Abdomen

- Acute abdomen is a medical emergency.
- Initial treatment involves keeping the patient nil per oral and continuous nasogastric aspiration of stomach contents through a Ryle's tube.
- Hydration should be maintained by intravenous fluids.
- Empirical antibiotis (cephalosporins plus metroinidazole or tinidazole intravenously) should be started pending the identification of cause.
- Once the cause is identified, treatment should be directed towards that.
- Most cases of acute abdomen require surgery for the underlying cause (e.g. acute appendicitis, perforation of peptic ulcer, etc.).

Q. Describe the etiology, clinical features and management of acute peritonitis.

- Peritonitis is an inflammation of the peritoneum.
- It may be acute or chronic, localized or diffuse, primary or secondary.
- Acute peritonitis is most often infectious and is usually related to a perforated viscus.

Etiology (Table 4.28)

TABLE 4.28: Causes of acute peritonitis
Primary peritonitis (spontaneous, infection without perforation)
• SBP—spontaneous bacterial peritonitis in cirrhosis with ascites
Secondary peritonitis (due to perforation or leakage from abdominal organs)
• Penetrating trauma
• Perforated appendicitis
• Perforated peptic ulcer
• Perforated diverticulitis
• Perforated typhoid enteritis
• Strangulated bowel
• Pancreatic necrosis
• Ruptured ectopic pregnancy
• Endoscopic perforation
• Bowel infarction.
Iatrogenic
• Peritoneal dialysis
• After ascitic fluid tapping
• Postoperative

Localized Peritonitis

- This is seen with acute inflammatory conditions of the gastrointestinal tract (e.g. acute appendicitis, acute cholecystitis). There is local pain and tenderness. The treatment is for the underlying disease.

Generalized Peritonitis

- This is a surgical emergency and is usually due to perforation of a hollow viscus (e.g. perforated appendix, perforated peptic ulcer).
- In case of perforated peptic ulcer, acid contents leak into peritoneal cavity and cause chemical peritonitis which gets infected later with bacteria.
- *E. coli* and Bacteroides are the most common organisms responsible for peritonitis since these are present in the intestine.
- The peritoneal cavity becomes acutely inflamed, with production of an inflammatory exudate that spreads throughout the peritoneum, leading to intestinal dilatation and paralytic ileus.

Clinical Features

- The cardinal manifestations of peritonitis are acute abdominal pain and tenderness, usually with fever.
- The location of the pain depends on the underlying cause and whether the inflammation is localized or generalized. In case of localized peritonitis physical findings are limited to the area of inflammation. Generalized peritonitis is associated with diffuse abdominal tenderness and rebound tenderness.
- Rigidity of the abdominal wall is common in both localized and generalized peritonitis.
- Bowel sounds are usually absent due to paralytic ileus.
- Tachycardia, hypotension, and signs of dehydration are common.

Investigations

- Leukocytosis and acidosis.
- Elevated serum amylase and lipase levels may detect pancreatitis.
- Plain abdominal X-ray: Shows dilated and edematous bowel loops with air fluid levels. Gas under the diaphragm may be seen in perforated viscus.
- CT and/or ultrasonography can identify the cause of acute abdomen and the presence of free fluid or an abscess.
- If ascites is present, fluid should be aspirated and sent for cell count cell type, protein, lactate dehydrogenase levels, Gram's stain and culture (>250 neutrophils/µl is usual in peritonitis).

Treatment

- Patient should be hydrated well with IV fluids.
- Continuous nasogastric aspiration should be done in view of paralytic ileus.
- Empirical antibiotics (cephalosporins plus metronidazole or tinidazole intravenously) should be started.

- Treatment of peritonitis is always surgical. Usually, laparotomy is required.
- Surgery has a twofold objective; peritoneal lavage of the abdominal cavity and specific treatment of the underlying condition.

Q. Discuss the causes, clinical features, investigations and management of intestinal obstruction.

- Intestinal obstruction is a blockage of the normal flow of intestinal contents.
- It may be due to mechanical or nonmechanical (e.g. paralytic ileus) causes.

Causes of Obstruction (Table 4.29)

TABLE 4.29: Causes of intestinal obstruction

Mechanical obstruction
• Adhesive bands
• Obstructed hernia
• Diverticulitis
• Intestinal neoplasms
• Regional enteritis
• Gallstone obstruction
• Intussusception
• Volvulus
• Ca colon
Nonmechanical (pseudo-obstruction)
• *Adynamic ileus*-peritonitis, retroperitoneal, lower-lobe pneumonia, electrolyte disturbances (hypokalemia)
• *Spastic ileus, or dynamic ileus*-results from prolonged contraction of the intestine. Seen in heavy metal poisoning, uremia, porphyria, and extensive intestinal ulcerations.

Pathophysiology

- Distention of the intestine is caused by the accumulation of gas and fluid proximal to and within the obstructed segment.
- Most of the air consists of swallowed air. Fluid accumulation is due to ingested fluid, swallowed saliva, gastric juice, and biliary and pancreatic secretions. Fluid from the body may also move into the lumen causing further accumulation of fluid. This may lead to sequestration of large volumes of fluid in the lumen leading to dehydration, hypotension, shock and renal failure.
- Blood supply to the obstructed segment of intestine may get compromised (e.g. in obstructive hernia) and lead to gangrene of intestine and blood loss into the lumen.
- Bacteria may get into the peritoneum through the gangrenous segment leading to peritonitis.
- Massive abdominal distension may compromise breathing and cause inferior vena cava compression.

Clinical Features

- Patient presents with colicky abdominal pain, vomiting and constipation.
- Examination of the abdomen reveals distension with increased bowel sounds.
- Pulse is rapid and there may be dehydration and signs of shock.
- Tenderness of abdomen suggests strangulation or peritonitis, and urgent surgery is necessary.
- Examination of the hernial orifices and rectum must be performed.

Investigations

- Plain X-ray of the abdomen (erect view) shows distended bowel loops with multiple air fluid levels **(Fig. 4.15)**.
- Ultrasound abdomen and CT can identify the cause of obstruction.

Management

- Initial management is by resuscitation with intravenous fluids (mainly isotonic saline with potassium) and continuous nasogastric aspiration through a Ryle's tube. Many cases will settle on conservative management.
- Exploratory laparotomy may be required in serious cases not responding to conservative therapy. If the bowel is gangrenous, that segment has to be resected and end to end anastomosis done.

Q. Ileus (paralytic ileus, functional ileus)

- Ileus, also known as paralytic ileus or functional ileus occurs when there is temporary cessation of peristalsis without any mechanical blockage, leading to accumulation of gas and fluids within the bowel.
- Clinical presentation of ileus is similar to mechanical bowel obstruction.

Causes of Ileus

- Postoperative (especially abdominal surgery, most common cause).
- Intra-abdominal infection/inflammation (sepsis/peritonitis).
- Retroperitoneal or intra-abdominal hematomas (e.g. from ruptured abdominal aortic aneurysm, blunt abdominal trauma).

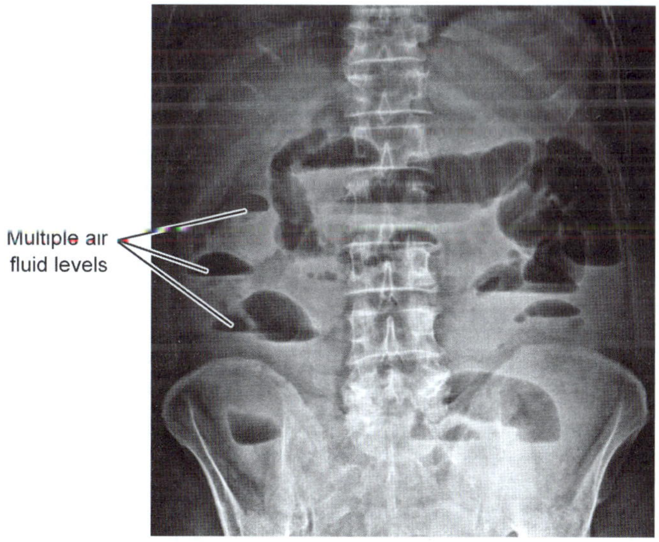

Figure 4.15: Multiple air fluid levels in intestinal obstruction

- Metabolic disturbances (e.g. hypokalemia).
- Drugs (e.g. opioids, anticholinergics).
- Spinal cord injury.

Clinical Features

- Abdominal distension which is of slow onset as compared to the sudden onset seen with mechanical intestinal obstruction.
- Pain abdomen which is usually diffuse without peritoneal signs. Pain is usually less severe and less colicky than mechanical obstruction.
- Nausea and vomiting.
- Decreased or inability to pass flatus.
- Examination shows distended and tympanic abdomen with mild diffuse tenderness. Bowel sounds are usually sparse or absent as opposed to a mechanical obstruction where there is increased bowel sounds in the early phase.

Investigations

- Plain X-ray abdomen usually shows multiple air fluid levels.
- CT abdomen
- RFT and LFT
- Serum amylase and lipase to rule out pancreatitis.
- Serum electrolytes to rule out hypokalemia.
- Complete blood count—anemia is seen in intra-abdominal bleeding, raised WBC count is seen in intra-abdominal infection, abscess, or intestinal ischemia.

Treatment

- Bowel rest is given by keeping the patient nil by mouth and giving intravenous (IV) fluids. Total parenteral nutrition (TPN) is recommended if the patient is unable to tolerate adequate oral intake after 7 days.
- Nasogastric aspiration of stomach contents is done if required.
- Chewing gum has been shown to be a cheap, well-tolerated way to potentially help with ileus as it stimulates the cephalocaudal reflex, which promotes peristalsis and inhibits inflammation.
- Treatment of the underlying condition is very important. Treating the infection, electrolyte abnormalities, decreasing opiate use, can all potentially decrease the durability of an ileus.
- Incidence of ileus can be decreased by using regional anesthesia rather than general anesthesia, using laparoscopic surgery wherever possible, and decreasing the use of opiate analgesics.

Q. Probiotics.

- Probiotics are microorganisms that have beneficial properties for the host. Examples are Lactobacillus, Bifidobacterium, *Clostridium butyricum*, *Streptococcus salivarius*, and *Saccharmomyces boulardii*.

Mechanisms of Benefit

- Suppression of growth or invasion by pathogenic bacteria
- Improvement of intestinal barrier function
- Modulation of the immune system
- Produce antimicrobial substances.

Potential Uses

- Ulcerative colitis
- Crohn's disease
- Antibiotic associated diarrhea
- Infectious diarrhea
- Irritable bowel syndrome
- Lactose intolerance
- Hepatic encephalopathy
- Allergy

Q. Prebiotics.

- Prebiotics are nondigestible food ingredients that selectively stimulate the growth or activity of beneficial gut bacteria, especially probiotics, thereby promoting host health.
- Commonly known prebiotics are: Oligofructose, inulin (present in chicory root, onions, and garlic), galacto-oligosaccharides, lactulose, breast milk oligosaccharides.

Sources of Prebiotics

- Chicory root is the richest natural source. Other dietary sources are beans, raw oats, unrefined wheat, unrefined barley, onion, garlic and raw banana.

Mechanism of Action

- Enhance growth of Bifidobacteria and Lactobacilli.
- Reduce exogenous and endogenous intestinal infection.
- Improved bowel habit.
- Suppress IBD inflammation.
- Immunomodulation (anti-inflammatory).
- Controlled serum lipids and cholesterol.

Q. Carcinoid syndrome.

- Carcinoid syndrome is a collection of symptoms caused by hormone-secreting neuroendocrine tumors (NETs).
- Carcinoid syndrome results from vasoactive substances (including serotonin, bradykinin, histamine, prostaglandins, polypeptide hormones) secreted by carcinoid tumor (neuroendocrine tumor). Serotonin acts on smooth muscle to cause diarrhea, colic, and malabsorption. Histamine and bradykinin cause flushing through their vasodilator effects.
- Carcinoid tumors are neoplastic proliferation of enterochromaffin cells.
- Carcinoid tumors can be found in GIT, bronchi, thyroid, ovary and testes.
- In GIT, the most common site is ileum and appendix.
- These tumors are less aggressive than carcinomas and their growth is usually slow. They can spread locally and also metastasize to other organs especially liver.

- Carcinoid syndrome refers to the systemic symptoms produced by secretory products of carcinoid tumors. The secretory products produced by the primary tumor are metabolized in the liver and hence, do not reach the systemic circulation. However, when there are liver metastases, secretory products from these metastases reach systemic circulation and produce symptoms. **Therefore carcinoid syndrome is seen only when there are liver metastases**.
- These tumors follow the so-called rule of one third, which is as follows:
  - One third of these tumors are multiple.
  - One third of those in the gastrointestinal (GI) tract are located in the small bowel.
  - One third of patients have a second malignancy.
  - One third of these tumors metastasize.

Clinical Features

- Carcinoids occur most frequently in patients aged 50–70 years.
- **Classic triad:** Flushing, diarrhea, and cardiac involvement.
- Episodic cutaneous flushing is the clinical hallmark of the carcinoid syndrome, and occurs in most of patients. It occurs in the face, neck, upper chest and lasts from 0.5 to 30 minutes. There may be associated lacrimation, periorbital edema, tachycardia and hypotension.
- Venous telangiectasias are purplish vascular lesions seen on the face, and occur due to prolonged vasodilatation.
- Secretory diarrhea occurs in most patients. Stools are watery and non-bloody, and may be accompanied by abdominal cramping.
- Wheezing and dyspnea due to bronchospasm often during flushing episodes.
- Cardiac valvular lesions: Occur due to fibrosis from serotonin. Right sided valves (tricuspid regurgitation and pulmonary stenosis) are most often affected, because inactivation of humoral substances by the lung protects the left heart.
- Diversion of tryptophan for synthesis of serotonin can result in the development of pellagra. Normally niacin is produced from tryptophan.
- Hepatomegaly due to hepatic metastases, intestinal obstruction and bleeding from intestinal tumors.
- Other features include increased incidence of peptic ulcer, muscle wasting due to poor protein synthesis and ureteral obstruction due to retroperitoneal fibrosis.

Investigations

- Increased urinary excretion of 5-hydroxyindoleacetic acid (5-HIAA) in 24-hour collection (more than 9 mg). 5-HIAA is the end product of serotonin metabolism.
- Plasma Chromogranin A: Elevated. Marker for neuroendocrine tumors.
- Serotonin level in blood and platelets is high.
- Chest X-ray, CT scan, barium and endoscopic studies are used to localize the tumor.
- Somatostatin receptor imaging with positron emission tomography (PET)/CT is a very useful investigation to localize carcinoid tumors since somatostatin receptors are present on the cell surface of neuroendocrine cells. For this purpose, scan various somatostatin analogues can be labeled with radioisotopes and injected intravenously and then scan is done.
- Echocardiography: To detect valvular lesions.
- Laparotomy and biopsy of the lesion can be attempted in selected cases.

Treatment

Medical Management

- Somatostatin analogs (e.g. octreotide, lanreotide)–first-line
- Interferon-alpha–as adjuvant.
- Antidiarrheals: Loperamide and serotonin-receptor antagonists (cyproheptadine, ondansetron) to control diarrhea.
- Telotristat: Inhibits serotonin synthesis (in refractory diarrhea).
- Bronchodilators for wheeze.
- Avoidance of conditions and diets precipitating flushing and diarrhea.
- Supplementation of food with niacin to prevent pellagra.

Surgical/Interventional

- The treatment of a carcinoid tumor without liver metastases is surgical resection.
- The treatment of carcinoid tumor with liver metastases (carcinoid syndrome) is palliative. However, primary tumor and hepatic metastases can be excised as it decreases the tumor burden and improves the symptoms.
- Hepatic artery embolization, radiofrequency ablation can decrease the size of hepatic metastases.

Q. Zollinger-Ellison Syndrome (Gastrinoma).

- Zollinger-Ellison syndrome is caused by gastrin-secreting gut neuroendocrine tumors (gastrinomas), which result in hypergastrinemia and increased acid secretion.
- Gastrinomas are usually located in the pancreas or the duodenal wall.
- Most gastrinomas are solitary or multifocal nodules that are potentially resectable. Over two-thirds of gastrinomas are malignant, and one-third would have already metastasized to the liver at initial presentation. Multifocal gastrinomas are associated with MEN 1 syndrome.

Clinical Features

- Abdominal pain occurs due to peptic ulcers. Over 90% of patients with Zollinger-Ellison syndrome develop peptic ulcers. Ulcer is usually single and found in the duodenum, but there can be multiple ulcers. These ulcers may be refractory to standard treatment, big (>2 cm), and may recur.

- Symptoms of gastroesophageal reflux.
- Diarrhea and weight loss occur in one-third of patients due to direct intestinal mucosal injury and pancreatic enzyme inactivation by acid, leading to maldigestion, and malabsorption.

Investigations

- Upper GI endoscopy: To look for duodenal ulcerations and hypertrophy of gastric folds.
- Increased fasting serum gastrin concentration (>150 pg/ml): H_2-blocker should be withheld for 24 hours and proton pump inhibitors for 6 days before measuring gastrin levels.
- Measurement of gastric pH: Most patients have very low pH due to high acid output. A gastric pH of >3.0 excludes gastrinoma.
- Secretin stimulation test: Useful to distinguish Zollinger-Ellison syndrome from other causes of hypergastrinemia. Intravenous secretin produces a rise in serum gastrin within minutes in patients with gastrinoma.
- High serum calcium level suggests hyperparathyroidism and MEN 1 syndrome.
- Serum parathyroid hormone (PTH), prolactin, luteinizing hormone (LH), follicle-stimulating hormone (FSH), and growth hormone (GH) level should be obtained to exclude MEN 1.
- Imaging studies are used to locate the site of primary tumor and to identify metastases. Gastrinomas express somatostatin receptors that bind radiolabeled octreotide. Somatostatin receptor imaging with single photon emission computed tomography (SPECT) can identify the site of gastrinomas. Endoscopic ultrasonography (EUS) may be useful to detect small gastrinomas in the duodenal wall, pancreas, or peripancreatic lymph nodes. CT and MRI scans may be helpful to identify liver metastases and primary lesions, but less sensitive than SPECT.

Treatment

- Localized disease is treated with surgical resection.
- In patients with liver metastases, initial therapy should be directed at controlling hypersecretion. Oral proton pump inhibitors (omeprazole, esomeprazole, rabeprazole, pantoprazole, or lansoprazole) are used to decrease the acid secretion. Surgical resection or cryoablation can be tried for single metastases. Other options for liver metastases include somatostatin analogues, interferon alpha, cytotoxic chemotherapy, and hepatic arterial chemoembolization.

Q. Gardner's syndrome (familial adenomatous polyposis).

- This is an uncommon autosomal dominant disorder characterized by multiple adenomatous polyps throughout the colon. Hundreds to thousands of adenomatous colonic polyps will develop by age 15. Most will develop colorectal cancer by the age of 50 years.
- It results from germline mutation of the APC gene on the long arm of chromosome 5 followed by acquired mutation of the remaining allele.
- Many extraintestinal features are also seen in FAP which include; subcutaneous epidermoid cysts, osteomas, dental abnormalities, retinal abnormalities, desmoid tumors, and lipomas.

Investigations

- Colonoscopy and genetic testing: All first-degree relatives of the affected patients should also undergo testing. In families with known FAP, at-risk family members should undergo direct mutation testing at 13–14 years of age.

Treatment

- Affected individuals should undergo colectomy (total proctocolectomy with ileal pouch-anal anastomosis). This will prevent the transformation of polyps into adenocarcinoma.
- Sulindac is a NSAID that has been shown to reduce the number and size of adenomas if given for a long time.
- The selective COX-2 inhibitor celecoxib has also been shown to reduce the adenoma burden.

Q. Peutz-Jeghers syndrome.

- This is characterized by multiple hamartomatous polyps in the small intestine and colon, as well as melanin pigmentation of the lips, mouth and digits **(Fig. 4.16)**.
- The disorder is caused by a mutation on chromosome 19p.
- Most cases are asymptomatic. However, chronic bleeding, anemia or intussusception may be seen. Malignant potential of polyps is low though there is a small risk of adenocarcinoma.
- Management involves surveillance of polyps with colonoscopy and biopsy every 1–3 years.

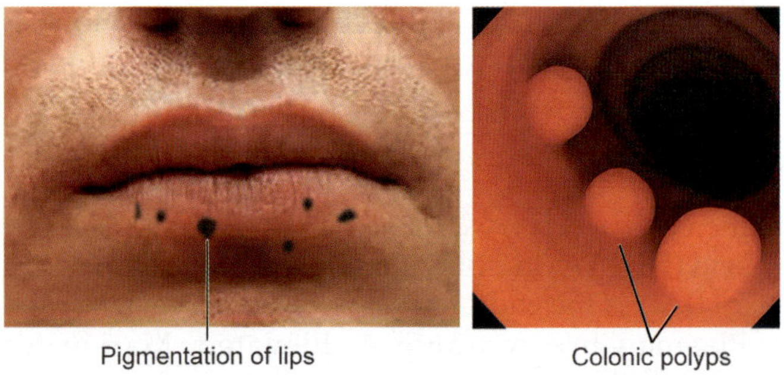

Figure 4.16: Peutz-Jegher syndrome

Q. Discuss the etiology, clinical features, investigations and management of acute pancreatitis. What are the complications of acute pancreatitis?

- Acute pancreatitis is an inflammatory condition of the pancreas characterized by abdominal pain and elevated levels of pancreatic enzymes in the blood.

Etiology (Table 4.30)

TABLE 4.30: Causes of acute pancreatitis

Common causes
• Gallstones
• Alcohol
• Post-ERCP
• Idiopathic
Rare causes
• Post-surgical (abdominal, cardiopulmonary bypass)
• Trauma (blunt or penetrating abdominal injury)
• Drugs (azathioprine, thiazides, sulfasalazine, valproate)
• Metabolic (hypercalcemia, hypertriglyceridemia)
• Pancreas divisum
• Vascular (Ischemia, atheroembolism, vasculitis)
• Infections (mumps, Coxsackie virus, HIV, Leptospira, Ascaris)
• Cystic fibrosis
• Toxins (methanol, scorpion venom, organophosphates)
• Renal failure
• Severe hypothermia

Pathophysiology

- Damage to pancreas by any of the above causes leads to premature activation of zymogen granules, releasing proteases which digest the pancreas and surrounding tissue.
- Pancreas becomes swollen. In severe cases there may be necrosis and hemorrhage.
- Pancreas has a poorly developed capsule, and adjacent structures, including the common bile duct, duodenum, splenic vein and transverse colon, are commonly involved.
- Both the endocrine and exocrine function of the pancreas is altered during an attack of acute pancreatitis which will return to normal if the attack is mild. However, permanent exocrine and endocrine insufficiency may develop in severe pancreatitis (necrotizing pancreatitis).

Clinical Features

Symptoms

- Abdominal pain: Severe, constant upper abdominal pain which radiates to the back. Pain is sudden in onset and gradually increases in severity. Pain decreases if patient sits up and leans forward and increases on lying down. Pain increases on lying down because the weight of stomach falls on the inflamed pancrease.
- Nausea and vomiting.
- Anorexia.

Signs

- Fever (low-grade).
- Tachycardia.
- Tachypnea (due to pleural effusion, inflammation of lungs, or atelectasis).
- Jaundice due to compression of common bile duct.
- Epigastric tenderness.
- Guarding and rebound tenderness in severe cases.
- Bluish discoloration of the flanks (Grey-Turner's sign) or the periumbilical region (Cullen's sign) are features of severe pancreatitis with hemorrhage **(Fig. 4.17)**.
- Absent bowel sounds due to paralytic ileus.
- Hypotension and shock in severe cases.
- Erythematous skin nodules due to focal subcutaneous fat necrosis.
- Ischemic injury to retina seen on fundus examination (Purtscher retinopathy).

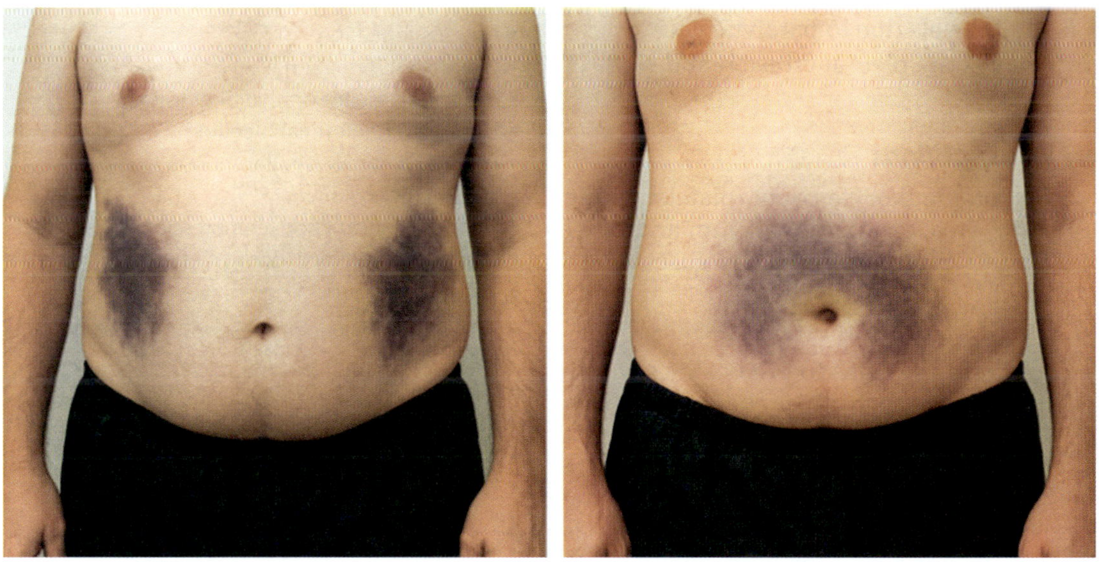

Figure 4.17: Grey-Turner's (left) and Cullen's sign (right)

Investigations

Serum Amylase

- This is elevated in acute pancreatitis for 3–5 days. It is rapidly cleared by kidneys. Hence, levels may be normal if measured after 3–5 days. In this situation the diagnosis can be made by elevated urinary amylase:creatinine ratio. A persistently elevated serum amylase-concentration suggests pseudocyst formation. High amylase levels are also found in pancreatic ascites and pleural effusion. Serum amylase concentration has no prognostic value.
- Elevated amylase is not specific to pancreatitis. High serum amylase levels can also occur in mesenteric ischemia, perforated peptic ulcer, ruptured ovarian cyst, renal failure, DKA, and parotitis.

Serum Lipase

- This is more specific than that of amylase in diagnosing pancreatitis.
- Lipase takes longer time to clear from the blood. Hence, it is helpful to make a diagnosis of pancreatitis even if the patient presents late.

Ultrasound Abdomen

- Shows swollen pancreas. It is also useful to pick up gallstones, biliary obstruction or pseudocyst formation.

CT Scan Abdomen

- This is the most important imaging test for the diagnosis of acute pancreatitis and its local complications. Patients who do not improve with initial conservative therapy or who are suspected of having complications should undergo CT scan of the abdomen.
- MRI is an alternative to CT especially if contrast cannot be used due to renal failure.

Plain X-ray Abdomen and Chest

- To exclude other causes of acute abdominal pain (e.g. gas under diaphragm in perforation).
- Calcification in pancreas in chronic pancreatitis.
- Multiple air fluid levels due to paralytic ileus.
- Chest X-ray may show pleural effusion and signs of ARDS.

Other Blood Investigations

- Blood glucose, total leukocyte count, platelet count, ESR, CRP, blood urea, creatinine, calcium and other electrolytes, triglycerides, arterial blood gases.

Assessment of Severity of Acute Pancreatitis

- There are two scoring systems to predict the severity and mortality in acute pancreatitis. These are Ranson criteria and Bedside Index Severity in Acute Pancreatitis (BISAP) score. BISAP score is easy to calculate and immediate assessment can be done about the severity of pancreatitis. In addition, BISAP score has good predictive performance for both severe acute pancreatitis and mortality.

BISAP Score

- Each of the following parameter carries 1 point.
  - BUN >25 mg/dl (8.9 mmol/l)
  - Abnormal mental status with a Glasgow coma score <15
  - Evidence of SIRS (systemic inflammatory response syndrome
  - Patient age >60 years old (1 point)
  - Imaging study reveals pleural effusion
- 0–2 points: Lower mortality (<2%)
- 3–5 points: Higher mortality (>15%).

Ranson Criteria to Predict Severity of Acute Pancreatitis (Table 4.31)

TABLE 4.31: ***Ranson criteria***

On admission • Age >55 • White blood cell count >16,000/mm^3 • Blood glucose >200 mg/dl • Lactate dehydrogenase >350 U/L • Aspartate aminotransferase (AST) >250 U/L
First 48 hours • Hematocrit fall by >10% • Blood urea increase by 5 mg/dl despite fluids • Serum calcium <8 mg/dl • pO_2 <60 mm Hg • Base deficit >4 MEq/L • Fluid sequestration >6 liters

- Each of the above parameter counts for 1 point toward the score. A Ranson score of 0–2 has a minimal mortality. A Ranson score of 3–5 has a 10–20% mortality rate, and the patient should be admitted to the intensive care unit (ICU). A Ranson score higher than 5 after 48 hours has a mortality of more than 50% and is associated with more systemic complications.

Complications of Acute Pancreatitis (Table 4.32)

TABLE 4.32: Complications of acute pancreatitis

Local • Pancreatic necrosis • Abscess formation • Pseudocyst formation • Pancreatic ascites or pleural effusion • Upper gastrointestinal bleeding • Splenic or portal vein thrombosis • Erosion into colon • Duodenal obstruction (compression by pancreatic mass) • Obstructive jaundice (due to compression of common bile duct)
Systemic • Systemic inflammatory response syndrome (SIRS) and multi-organ failure • DIC • Renal failure • Acute respiratory distress syndrome (ARDS) • Hyperglycemia • Fat necrosis • Hypocalcemia (due to sequestration of calcium in fat necrosis) • Hypoalbuminemia (due to increased capillary permeability)

Differential Diagnosis

- Perforated peptic ulcer
- Perforation of any other hollow viscus
- Acute cholecystitis
- Acute intestinal obstruction
- Leaking aortic aneurysm
- Renal colic
- Acute mesenteric ischemia or thrombosis.

Management

- Nothing by mouth.
- Intravenous fluids to maintain intravascular volume. This is the most important step and Ringer lactate is the preferred fluid.
- Nasogastric aspiration: Not routinely necessary. Required if the patient has persistent abdominal pain in spite of analgesics, paralytic ileus, protracted vomiting or intestinal obstruction.
- Analgesics for abdominal pain. Adequate pain control requires opiates such as meperidine or tramadol.
- Admit severe cases in intensive care unit. Monitor pulse, BP, abdominal girth, urine output, blood glucose and calcium levels.
- Prophylactic systemic antibiotics (imipenem or meropenem or ceftazidime) should be given in severe cases to prevent pancreatic infection.
- Proton-pump inhibitors are used to decrease the acid output.
- The role of somatostatin or octreotide infusion is controversial.
- ERCP with endoscopic sphincterotomy and stone extraction is indicated if pancreatitis results from gallstone particularly if jaundice (serum total bilirubin >5 mg/dl) or cholangitis is present.
- Surgery is indicated for complications such as infected pancreatic necrosis, pancreatic abscess, intestinal obstruction, perforation, etc.

Q. Chronic pancreatitis

- Chronic pancreatitis is persistent inflammation of the pancreas that results in permanent structural damage with fibrosis and ductal strictures, followed by a decline in exocrine and endocrine function (pancreatic insufficiency).

Causes of Chronic Pancreatitis (Table 4.33)

TABLE 4.33: Causes of chronic pancreatitis
• Chronic alcoholism
• Smoking
• Tropical pancreatitis (India)
• Stenosis of the ampulla of Vater
• Pancreas divisum
• Cystic fibrosis
• Familial
• Autoimmune diseases (Sjögren's syndrome, primary biliary cirrhosis)
• Idiopathic

Clinical Features

- Middle-aged alcoholic men are predominantly affected.
- Pain in the upper abdomen is the most common symptom. It may be constant or intermittent. It may radiate to back. Pain may be relieved by leaning forward and worsened by food intake.
- Features of malabsorption: Diarrhea, steatorrhea, and weight loss.
- Diabetes develops in advanced cases.
- Physical examination reveals a thin, malnourished patient with epigastric tenderness. Skin pigmentation over the abdomen and back is common due to chronic use of a hot water bottle to relieve the abdominal pain.

Investigations

- Serum amylase and lipase usually normal.
- Ultrasound abdomen.
- CT (may show atrophy, calcification, ductal stricture or dilatation).
- Abdominal X-ray (may show calcification).
- ERCP accurately demonstrates the anatomy of pancreatic ducts. Magnetic resonance cholangiopancreatography (MRCP) is a noninvasive alternative to ERCP.
- Endoscopic ultrasound.
- Tests of pancreatic function: Secretin/cholecystokinin (CCK) stimulation test, 24-hour fecal fat estimation, oral glucose tolerance test.

Complications of Chronic Pancreatitis

- Pseudocyst
- Pancreatic ascites
- Obstructive jaundice due to stricture of the common bile duct as it passes through the diseased pancreas.
- Duodenal stenosis
- Portal or splenic vein thrombosis
- Peptic ulcer.

Management

- Stop alcohol intake.
- Pain relief: NSAIDs, opiates, celiac ganglion blockade.
- Oral pancreatic enzyme supplements to improve the digestion and absorption of food.
- Patients with severe chronic pain resistant to conservative measures are considered for surgical or endoscopic pancreatic therapy.
- Endoscopic therapy involves dilatation or stenting of pancreatic duct strictures and removal of calculi (mechanical or shock-wave lithotripsy).
- Surgical interventions are partial pancreatic resection preserving the duodenum, total pancreatectomy and pancreatico-jejunostomy.

Q. Discuss the causes and differential diagnosis of acute upper abdominal pain.

Causes of Acute Upper Abdominal Pain

See **Table 4.34.**

TABLE 4.34: Causes of acute upper abdominal pain

- Peptic ulcer perforation
- Acute cholecystitis
- Biliary colic
- Acute pancreatitis
- Lower lobe pneumonia
- Myocardial infarction
- Aortic dissection or rupture
- Splenic abscess and infarct

Peptic Ulcer Perforation

- Previous history of recurrent epigastric pain with relation to food and periodicity.
- After perforation, pain becomes severe and penetrating type. Initially it is felt in the epigastrium, but later spreads to whole abdomen due to generalized peritonitis.
- Tachycardia and hypotension are usually present.
- Abdominal examination shows board like rigidity, guarding and absent bowel sounds due to peritonitis. Liver dullness may be absent or reduced due to gas collection below the diaphragm.
- Plain X-ray abdomen in the erect posture may show gas under the diaphragm and multiple air fluid levels.

Acute Cholecystitis

- Pain is mainly in the right hypochondrium. Pain is constant and may also be felt in the right shoulder tip.
- Associated fever, jaundice, nausea and vomiting.
- Tenderness in the right hypochondrium and rigidity. Murphy's sign present (sudden inspiratory arrest due to pain while palpating right hypochondrium).
- Gallbladder may be palpable.
- Blood tests show leukocytosis, raised bilirubin, and liver enzymes.
- Plain X-ray abdomen may show gallstones.
- Ultrasound abdomen may show gallstones, gall-bladder wall thickening and pericholic fluid collection.
- Cholescintigraphy shows cystic duct obstruction.

Biliary Colic

- Biliary colic is usually due to gallbladder contracting and pressing a stone against the gallbladder outlet or cystic duct opening, leading to increased gallbladder pressure and pain.
- Biliary colic is a misnomer, since the pain is not typically colicky.
- Pain is deep and gnawing type and is occasionally sharp and severe.
- Pain is localized in the right upper quadrant or epigastrium.
- As the gallbladder relaxes, stones often fall back from the cystic duct. As a result, the attack reaches a crescendo over many hours and resolves completely.
- Pain may recur multiple times.

Acute Pancreatitis

- History of precipitating factors like alcohol binge, and gall stones.
- Pain is steady and usually felt in the mid-epigastrium, radiates to back between scapulae. Its onset is rapid, but not as abrupt as that with a perforated viscus.
- Pain of pancreatitis lasts for many days. Pain is accompanied by nausea and vomiting.
- Pain decreases on sitting and leaning forward.
- Cullen's sign and Grey-Turner's sign rarely.
- Amylase and lipase are elevated.
- Ultrasound abdomen and CT scan shows swollen pancreas.

Lower Lobe Pneumonia

- Lower lobe pneumonia causes referred pain to upper abdomen probably due to diaphragmatic irritation.
- Pleuritic chest pain may be present in the lower chest.
- Fever, dyspnea and cough with expectoration are usually present.
- Chest examination reveals crepitations and bronchial breath sounds over the affected area.
- Chest X-ray shows pneumonic patch.
- Abdominal pain is occasionally the sole presenting complaint in a patient with lower lobe pneumonia.

Myocardial Infarction

- Risk factors such as old age, hypertension, diabetes, and smoking may be present.
- Pain is felt more in the left side of chest and retrosternal area. It may radiate to left shoulder and left arm.
- There may be associated symptoms such as dyspnea, sweating.
- Examination may show bilateral basal crepitations over the lungs, third and fourth heart sound.
- ECG shows evidence of MI such as ST segment elevation and pathological Q waves.
- CK-MB and troponins are elevated.
- Echocardiogram shows akinesia or hypokinesia of the involved myocardium.

Aortic Dissection

- Sudden, severe, tearing pain radiating to the back.
- Predisposing factors may be present such as; hypertension, previous aortic aneurysm, Marfan's syndrome, etc.
- Asymmetric pulses may be present.
- Chest X-ray shows mediastinal and/or aortic widening.
- CT, MRI or aortogram can confirm the diagnosis.

Splenic Abscess and Infarct

- Splenic abscesses are associated with fever and tenderness in the left upper quadrant.
- Similar findings may be present in splenic infarction.
- Risk factors for splenic infarction such as atrial fibrillation, hypercoagulable state, sickle cell anemia, etc. may be present.
- Leukocytosis, high ESR in case of abscess.
- Ultrasound abdomen can confirm the presence of splenic abscess.

Q. Discuss the causes and differential diagnosis of acute lower abdominal pain.

Causes of Acute Lower Abdominal Pain

- Appendicitis
- Acute diverticulitis
- Ureteric colic
- Torsion of ovarian cyst
- Rupture of ectopic pregnancy.

Appendicitis

- Common in young individuals.
- Pain is initially periumbilical. Later it shifts to right lower quadrant due to development of local peritonitis.
- Associated nausea and vomiting present.
- Tenderness and rebound tenderness positive in right iliac fossa.
- Ultrasound abdomen reveals swollen appendix or appendicular mass.

Acute Diverticulitis

- Usually occurs in older individuals.
- Pain is often present for several days prior to presentation.
- Pain occurs in the right or left lower quadrant.
- Abdominal tenderness.
- CT scan and contrast enema are helpful in diagnosis.

Ureteric Colic

- Past history of kidney stones may be present.
- Pain is severe and radiates from loin to groin. Pain comes on and off and paroxysms of severe pain last 20–60 minutes. Pain may radiate to the ipsilateral testicle, tip of the penis, or labia.
- Hematuria may be present.
- Nausea, vomiting, dysuria, and urgency may be present.
- Ultrasound abdomen and CT scan can confirm the diagnosis.

Ovarian Cyst

- Sudden onset lower abdominal pain often associated with waves of nausea and vomiting. However, this can occur in other conditions also and hence, nonspecific.
- Previous history of ovarian cyst/mass.
- History of recent vigorous activity.
- Ultrasound and CT-abdomen can confirm the diagnosis.

Rupture of Ectopic Pregnancy

- Women in reproductive age group.
- H/o amenorrhea present.
- Sudden onset lower abdominal pain with vaginal hemorrhage.
- Signs of hypovolemic shock may be present such as hypotension, tachycardia, and pallor.
- Pregnancy test positive. Hemoglobin low.
- Ultrasound abdomen confirms the diagnosis.

Q. Discuss the causes and differential diagnosis of diffuse abdominal pain.

Causes

- Mesenteric infarction
- Ruptured abdominal aortic aneurysm
- Diffuse peritonitis.
- Intestinal obstruction

Mesenteric Infarction

- Acute and severe onset of diffuse and persistent abdominal pain.
- Pain is out of proportion to physical findings.
- Patients have evidence of cardiovascular, ischemic, or atherosclerotic disease.
- Stool occult blood may be positive.
- Angiography or MRI angiography of the celiac artery or mesenteric arteries can confirm the diagnosis.

Ruptured Aneurysm

- Patients present with abdominal or back pain.
- Physical examination shows pallor, hypotension and a pulsatile abdominal mass.
- Ultrasound abdomen, CT or MRI can confirm the diagnosis.

Peritonitis

- Pain is diffuse and constant. It is aggravated by movement, coughing and deep breathing. Hence, patients with peritonitis lie down still, in supine position with the knees flexed.
- Patient appears sick.
- Fever, tachycardia and hypotension.
- Abdominal tenderness, rebound tenderness and guarding present.
- Bowel sounds are absent.
- Plain X-ray abdomen shows multiple air fluid levels and gas under diaphragm in case of visceral perforation causing peritonitis.

Intestinal Obstruction

- Pain is colicky and intermittent. Paroxysms of pain occur every 4 or 5 minutes.
- Associated vomiting, constipation and abdominal distention.
- Hypotension, oliguria, and dry mucous membranes indicate dehydration.
- Tenderness may be present.
- Tympanic note on percussion due to air filled bowel loops.
- Bowel sounds increase initially but later decrease.
- Plain X-ray abdomen shows multiple air fluid levels.
- Ultrasound abdomen, and CT abdomen can confirm the diagnosis and reveal the cause of obstruction.

Chapter 5

Diseases of Nervous System

Q. Enumerate the common symptoms/manifestations of nervous system disease.

The main symptoms of nervous system disease with which patient presents are as follows:

Changes in Higher Mental Functions

- Unconsciousness or alteration of consciousness, delirium
- Loss of memory
- Illusion, delusion or hallucination
- Behavioral abnormality
- Speech problems

Symptoms/Signs of Cranial Nerve Dysfunction

(Table 5.1)

TABLE 5.1: Symptoms/signs of cranial nerve dysfunction

Cranial nerves	Patient complaints in case of cranial nerve dysfunction
Olfactory nerve	Any loss or alteration in sensation of smell
Optic nerve	Blurring of vision or blindness
3rd, 4th, 6th nerves (occulomotor, trochlear, and abduscent nerve)	Diplopia (double vision), squint
Trigeminal nerve	Difficulty in chewing food, loss of sensation over face
Facial nerve	Deviation of angle of the mouth: facial asymmetry: epiphora
Vestibulocochlear nerve	Vertigo, deafness, tinnitus
Glossopharyngeal nerve	Difficulty swallowing; impairment of taste over the posterior one-third of the tongue and palate; impaired sensation over the posterior one-third of the tongue, palate, and pharynx
Vagus nerve	Nasal intonation or regurgitation: • Hoarseness of voice • Dysphagia
Accessory nerve	Difficulty in turning the head and shrugging shoulders
Hypoglossal nerve	Wasting of tongue, dysarthria

Motor system problems

- Weakness in any part of the body
- Wasting/thinning of limbs
- Stiffness of limbs
- Muscle twitching in one or more parts of the body (fasciculations)
- Abnormal (involuntary) movements
- Pain in the muscles

Sensory system problems

- Numbness
- Pins and needles
- Tingling
- Crawling
- Prickling
- Burning
- Tightness
- Itching

Signs/symptoms of increased intracranial tension

- Headache
- Vomiting (projectile)
- Convulsions
- Blurred vision
- Behavioral changes
- Altered sensorium

Cerebellar system problems

- A wide-based, unsteady, lurching walk, often accompanied by a tremor in the trunk of the body.
- Slow, unsteady and jerky movement of the arms or legs.
- Slowed and slurred speech.
- Rapid, small movements of the eyes (called nystagmus)
- Tremor of hands while reaching for objects.

Autonomic nervous system (includes bladder and bowel function)

- Inability to sweat properly, leading to heat intolerance
- Loss of bladder control, leading to infection or incontinence.
- Dizziness, light-headedness or fainting on standing up because of postural hypotension.

- Diarrhea, constipation or incontinence due to dysfunction of autonomic nerves supplying digestive tract
- Difficulty in eating or swallowing
- Sexual dysfunction (impotence)

Miscellaneous

- Fever (CNS infections such as meningitis, encephalitis, brain abscess)
- Neck stiffness (meningitis, subarachnoid hemorrhage, cervical spondylosis)
- Involuntary movements (seizure, chorea, athetosis, ballismus)
- Headache (migraine, meningitis, brain tumor, subarachnoid hemorrhage).

Q. Enumerate the neuroimaging techniques.

- Nowadays many neuroimaging techniques are available which can help pinpoint the location and pathology of nervous system diseases. These include:

- Computed tomography (CT)
- Magnetic resonance imaging (MRI)
- Perfusion CT (pCT)
- Perfusion MRI (pMRI)
- CT angiography (CTA)
- MR angiography (MRA)
- Functional MRI (fMRI)
- MR spectroscopy (MRS)
- MR neurography
- Positron emission tomography (PET)

Q. Computed tomography (CT scan)

- CT is a cross-sectional image created by a computer using the data obtained by passing X-ray beams through a section of the body.
- An X-ray tube rotates axially around the patient, and a diametrically opposed array of detectors detect the radiation traversing the body. This data is converted to cross-sectional images with the help of powerful processors.
- Denser structures (like bone) absorb more X-rays and appear white; less dense areas (like CSF or air) appear darker.
- A modern CT scanner is capable of obtaining sections as thin as 0.5–1 mm. Complete study of the brain can be obtained in 20–60 seconds.
- CT is safe, fast, and reliable. Radiation exposure is between 3 and 5 cGy per study.
- In the helical CT the table with the patient moves continuously through the rotating X-ray beam, generating a "helix" of information that can be reformatted into various slice thicknesses.
- Multiple detectors can be positioned to detect the radiation which results in multiple slices per revolution of the X-ray beam around the patient. These "multidetector" scanners have greatly reduced the time per examination of the patient.
- CT scan can be taken after giving intravenous contrast (contrast-enhanced CT). This is helpful to identify vascular structures and to detect defects in the blood-brain barrier (BBB), which are associated with disorders such as tumors, infarcts, and infections. There are both ionic and nonionic contrast agents. Ionic contrast agents can cause renal failure and allergic reactions which is not seen with nonionic contrasts.

Advantages

- Fast (scans completed in minutes)
- Widely available in most hospitals
- Excellent for acute hemorrhage and bone imaging
- Compatible with implanted devices (e.g. pacemakers).

Disadvantages

- Radiation exposure, especially in repeat scans.
- Lower soft tissue contrast compared to MRI.
- May miss small or early ischemic strokes.
- Contrast risks (e.g. nephrotoxicity or allergic reactions) if iodinated contrast is used.

Indications for CT scan

- Trauma to the head and spine
- Stroke
- Intracranial space occupying lesions
- Suspected subarachnoid hemorrhage
- Conductive hearing loss
- Suspected infections
- Evaluation of a suspected pathology in any part of the body.

Q. Magnetic resonance imaging (MRI)

- Magnetic resonance imaging (MRI) is a powerful, non-invasive imaging technique that uses strong magnetic fields and radiofrequency waves to create images of the body parts.

How MRI works

- The body is placed in a strong magnetic field, which aligns hydrogen protons (mainly from water molecules).
- Radiofrequency pulses temporarily disturb this alignment.
- As the protons realign, they emit signals that are detected and used to create high-resolution images.
- No ionizing radiation is used (unlike CT scans).
- MR images can be generated in sagittal, coronal, axial, or oblique planes without changing the patient's position. Three-dimensional imaging is also possible with MRI.
- The heavy-metal element gadolinium is used as intravenous MR contrast agent. Allergic reactions are rare with this agent and renal failure does not occur.

Advantages of MRI over CT scan

- No radiation exposure
- Better delineation of soft tissue details
- MRI is the gold standard for imaging the brain and spinal cord, offering exceptional soft tissue contrast and the ability to detect subtle abnormalities.
- Clearly differentiates white and gray matter.

- Very useful in the evaluation of posterior fossa lesions where CT is not very accurate due to dense bony structures.
- Particularly useful to recognize demyelinating plaques as in multiple sclerosis.

Disadvantages of MRI

- Expensive
- Time-consuming (30–60 minutes per scan)
- MRI scanning can cause claustrophobia (fear of closed spaces) in some patients because the patient is moved into a long, narrow gap within the magnet. This can be reduced by mild sedation.
- Unlike CT, movement of the patient during an MR sequence distorts the images. Hence, uncooperative patients should either be sedated for the MR study or go for CT scan.
- Contraindicated in people with certain implants (e.g. older pacemakers, cochlear implants).

Contraindications to MRI

The metallic parts of many medical devices and implants can get dislodged due to powerful magnetic field of the MRI. Hence, MRI is contraindicated in the following situations:

- Cardiac pacemaker or permanent pacemaker leads
- Internal defibrillatory device
- Cochlear prostheses
- Metallic bone implants
- Electronic infusion devices
- Intracranial aneurysm clips (metallic)
- Ocular implants (some) or ocular metallic foreign body
- Swan-Ganz catheter
- Magnetic dental implants.

Q. Magnetic Resonance Angiography (MRA).

- MRA uses the same basic technology as MRI but is tailored to highlight flowing blood.
- Through the selection of different imaging parameters, differing blood velocities can be highlighted and selective venous and arterial MRA images can be obtained.
- MRA can also be obtained during infusion of a contrast material called contrast-enhanced MRA which has become the standard for extracranial vascular MRA. Gadolinium is used as contrast.
- MRA is not as good as conventional angiography for the detection of small-vessel detail, such as is required in the workup of vasculitis. MRA is also less sensitive in the presence of slowly flowing blood and thus may not differentiate complete from near-complete occlusions.
- However, despite of these limitations, MRA has become very important in evaluation of the extra-cranial carotid and vertebral circulation as well as of larger-caliber intracranial arteries and dural sinuses. It is also useful in the noninvasive detection of intracranial aneurysms and vascular malformations.

Q. Positron Emission Tomography (PET).

- Positron emission tomography (PET) allows the imaging of structures by virtue of their ability to concentrate molecules labeled with a positron-emitting isotope.
- PET scan is obtained by the detection of positrons emitted during the decay of a radionuclide that has been injected into a patient. The most frequently used moiety is fluoro-deoxy-glucose (FDG), which is an analog of glucose.
- Metabolically active cells, such as malignant cells, utilize and import more glucose than other tissues and thus take up FDG more avidly. Multiple images of glucose uptake activity are formed after 45–60 min. Images reveal differences in regional glucose activity among normal and pathologic brain structures.
- A lower activity of FDG in the parietal lobes is seen in Alzheimer's disease.
- Higher activity may be seen in malignant lesions and areas of seizure focus.

Q. Describe the technique, indications and contraindications of lumbar puncture.

Q. Composition of normal CSF.

- Lumbar puncture (LP) is the technique of obtaining CSF from the lumbar area for analysis. LP is useful in the diagnosis of a variety of infectious and noninfectious neurologic conditions.

Technique

- LP can be performed with the patient in the lateral recumbent position or sitting upright **(Fig. 5.1)**.
- The safe site of puncture is L3/4 or L4/5 interspace since this is well below the termination of the spinal cord which ends at L1–L2 in adults. These spaces can be identified by drawing a line joining the highest points of the iliac crests. This line corresponds to L3/4 space.

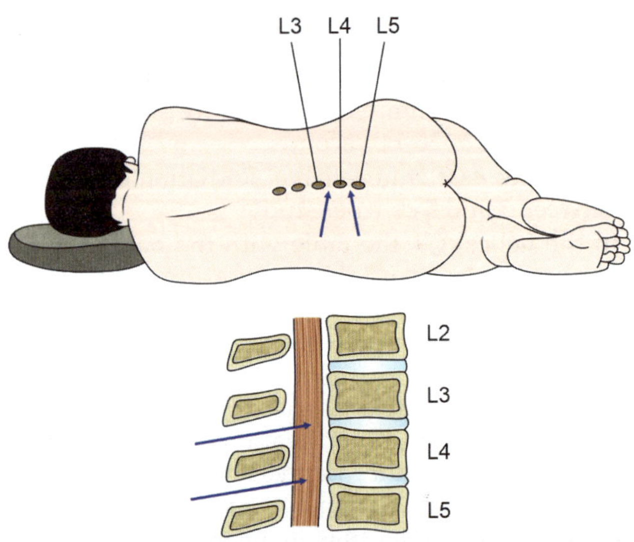

Figure 5.1: Position of patient and site for lumbar puncture

- Correct patient positioning is important for the success of LP. The patient is instructed to remain in the fetal position with the neck, back, and limbs held in flexion. The overlying skin should be cleaned with alcohol and a disinfectant such as povidone-iodine. A sterile drape with an opening over the lumbar spine is then placed on the patient.
- Local anesthesia (lignocaine) is infiltrated into the lumbar intervertebral space and a 20 or 22 gauge spinal needle containing a stylet is inserted into the lumbar intervertebral space.
- The spinal needle should be advanced slowly in the direction of umbilicus. The bevel of the needle should face upwards to allow the needle to spread rather than cut the dural sac (the fibers of which run parallel to the spinal axis).
- As soon as the subarachnoid space is entered, there is loss of resistance to the insertion of needle. The stylet should be withdrawn to check for the CSF flow. If no CSF flow is detected the needle should be manipulated back and forth and rechecked for CSF flow.
- Once CSF begins to flow through the needle, the patient should be instructed to slowly straighten the legs to allow free flow of CSF within the subarachnoid space. A manometer should then be placed over the hub of the needle and the opening pressure should be measured. Fluid is then serially collected in sterile plastic tubes or bottles. A total of 8–15 ml of CSF is typically removed during routine LP.

Indications for lumbar puncture

- Diagnosis of meningitis
- Diagnosis of subarachnoid hemorrhage (RBCs are found in CSF).
- CNS malignancies (malignant cells may be found in CSF).
- Demyelinating conditions such as multiple sclerosis and Guillain-Barré syndrome (albumin-cytologic dissociation is seen where there is increase in CSF albumin without increase in cells).
- For spinal anesthesia
- Administration of intrathecal antibiotics and chemotherapeutic agents
- As therapeutic in NPH (normal pressure hydrocephalus).
- Injection of contrast media for myelography or for cisternography.

Complications

LP is a relatively safe procedure, but following complications can occur rarely:

- Post-LP headache
- Infection (meningitis)
- Bleeding
- Cerebral herniation
- Radicular pain or numbness
- Late onset of epidermoid tumors of the thecal sac.

Contraindications

- Bleeding diathesis (thrombocytopenia, coagulation defects)
- Infected skin over lumbar area
- Raised intracranial pressure.

Composition of normal CSF

Appearance	Clear, colorless
Pressure	60–150 mm of CSF
Proteins	20–40 mg/dl
Sugar	40–70 mg/dl
Chlorides	720–750 mg/dl
Cells (per mm^3)	0–5 (all lymphocytes)
Culture	Sterile

Q. Electroencephalography (EEG)

- EEG is a noninvasive method used to record electrical activity of the brain by electrodes placed on the scalp. The recorded activity represents the postsynaptic potentials of pyramidal cells of cerebral cortex.
- Normal EEG varies according to the patient's age and level of arousal.
- The electrical activity from any electrode pair can be described in terms of amplitude and frequency.

Normal EEG

- Amplitude ranges from 5 to 200 μV. Frequency of EEG activity ranges from 0 Hz to approximately 20 Hz. The frequencies are described by Greek letters: alpha, beta, theta, delta, and gamma **(Table 5.2)**.

TABLE 5.2: Normal EEG waves

Wave type	Frequency	Associated state
Delta	0.5–4 Hz	Deep sleep
Theta	4–8 Hz	Light sleep, drowsiness
Alpha	8–13 Hz	Relaxed wakefulness (eyes closed). They disappear with eyes open. Alpha activity disappears normally with attention (e.g. mental arithmetic, stress, opening eyes)
Beta	13–30 Hz	Active thinking, focus
Gamma	>30 Hz	Higher mental activity, consciousness

Clinical uses

- ***Epilepsy diagnosis***: Detects abnormal, synchronous neural activity (spikes, sharp waves).
- ***Sleep disorders***: Evaluates sleep stages and abnormalities.
- ***Brain death***: Assesses absence of cerebral activity.
- ***Encephalopathies***: Helps identify diffuse brain dysfunction.
- Evoked potentials can be utilized to test the integrity of a pathway in the CNS.

Abnormal EEG

- In routine EEG studies, some "activations" are used to bring out inapparent abnormalities. These activations include, hyperventilation for 3 min, photic stimulation, and sleep deprivation on the night prior to the recording. These provocations are especially useful to activate epileptic activity.

- Increased generalized slow wave (theta and delta) activity is seen in metabolic encephalopathies.
- Focal slow wave activity is seen in focal brain lesions (e.g. tumor, infarct).
- Spike and sharp waves may be seen in epilepsy.
- Evoked potentials can be utilized to test the integrity of a pathway in the CNS. For example in multiple sclerosis where there is demyelination of central neurons, conduction is slow and evoked potentials are delayed.

Q. Nerve conduction velocity (NCV) studies.

- NCV studies are used to evaluate the function and integrity of peripheral nerves.
- Conduction studies can assess the number of functioning axons by measuring the amplitude of action potential since each axon makes a contribution to the magnitude of the electrical field. The state of myelin sheath of axons can be assessed by the conduction velocity of action potential since the conduction velocity depends on intact myelin sheath.
- Basic principle: An electrical stimulus is applied to a nerve. The response is recorded at a different site along the nerve or at the muscle it innervates. The speed (velocity) at which the electrical impulse travels is calculated in meters per second (m/s).
- In patients with axonal degenerative neuropathies, such as diabetic neuropathy, the primary abnormality in NCV study is reduced sensory action potential amplitudes. Slowing of conduction is the primary feature in demyelinating neuropathies such as Guillain-Barre Syndrome and compression and entrapment neuropathies (e.g. carpal tunnel syndrome).

Q. Define weakness. How do you approach a case of weakness? How do you differentiate upper from lower motor neuron weakness?

- Weakness is reduction in normal power of one or more muscles.
- Paralysis and the suffix "plegia" indicate weakness that is complete or nearly complete. "paresis" refers to weakness that is mild or moderate.
- Weakness can be due to lesions anywhere in the motor cortex, corticospinal tracts, anterior horn cells, spinal nerve roots, peripheral nerves, neuromuscular junction, and muscles.
- Weakness should not be confused with fatigue (sense of tiredness without loss of muscle power) or apraxia (inability to perform learned movements despite intact strength).

Approach to a Case of Motor Weakness

Is it really weakness or something else?

- Many patients with a variety of systemic disorders may misinterpret difficulties performing certain tasks or fatigue as weakness. Fatigue is tiredness. Examples are cardiopulmonary disease, joint disease, anemia, and cachexia from malignancy. Objective muscle power is normal in such cases, but muscle power is less in weakness.
- Asking about the impact of weakness on routine activities can help determine whether there is true muscle weakness versus decreased effort due to other limitations. Patients with true weakness will typically complain about trouble performing specific tasks. In many cases, the motor examination is required to help determine if there is true muscle weakness versus decreased effort from pain, fatigue, or other limitations.

Is it UMN or LMN type weakness (Table 5.3)

- Motor weakness may be due to a lesion anywhere along the motor pathway starting from motor cortex

TABLE 5.3: Differences between upper and lower motor neuron weakness

Feature	Upper motor neuron lesion	Lower motor neuron lesion
Muscle atrophy	No	Yes
Fasciculations	No	Yes
Muscle tone	Increased	Decreased
Distribution of weakness	Weakness is predominantly distal than proximal. Weakness affects extensors of upper limb and flexors of lower limb predominantly.	Can be generalized (e.g. GB syndrome), predominantly proximal (e.g. myopathies), predominantly distal or focal (in neuropathies). No preferential involvement of corticospinal innervated muscles
Tendon reflexes	Exaggerated	Diminished
Babinski's sign	Extensor	Flexor
Abdominal reflex	Absent depending on the involved spinal level	Present
Clonus	Present	Absent
Sensory loss	Loss of cortical sensations	Peripheral sensations
Site of lesion	Corticospinal or corticobulbar tract	Anterior horn cells, nerve roots, peripheral nerves, neuromuscular junction, muscles

in the brain till the muscles. Upper motor neuron ends in the cranial nerve nuclei in the brainstem and anterior horn cells in the spinal cord. So any lesion above the cranial nerve nuclei or above anterior horn cells is called UMN type lesion and produces UMN type of weakness.

- If you can recognize whether the weakness is UMN or LMN type, then you have solved the first step of localizing the lesion. If UMN type weakness is there, then the lesion is above the cranial nerve nuclei (in case of muscle weakness supplied by cranial nerves) or above the anterior horn cell (in case of muscles supplied by corticospinal tract). Lesions at or below cranial nerve nuclei and anterior horn cells is called LMN type weakness.

Further Localization by Analyzing the Pattern of Weakness Along with Accompanying Features

- Further localization relies on careful clinical assessment to recognize the pattern of weakness, associated signs and symptoms. All these clinical data along with appropriate brain or spinal imaging will help to localize the lesion and possible pathology and etiology. Sudden onset weakness is usually due to stroke which requires urgent evaluation and treatment. However, focal limb weakness can be caused by many non-stroke pathologies and these also should be considered in the differential diagnosis of weakness.
- Following is the description of motor weakness at different levels along the motor pathway starting from motor cortex till the muscles **(Table 5.4)**.

Onset and Course of Weakness

- Sudden onset weakness suggests stroke (ischemic or hemorrhagic) or trauma.
- Maximal weakness at onset followed by rapid recovery suggests embolic stroke. Other features which suggest cardioembolic stroke are H/o valvular heart disease, atrial fibrillation, infective endocarditis, and recent MI.
- Weakness which is worsening or involving more areas (evolving stroke) suggests thrombotic stroke. Evolution of weakness is due to progression of thrombus in the involved vessel.
- If repeated activity tends to worsen the weakness (for example, if there are things that patients can't do at the end of the repeated activity that they could at the beginning), it suggests a diagnosis of myasthenia gravis.
- Sudden onset weakness with complete recovery, with normal imaging, think of transient ischemic attack (TIA).
- If weakness is recurrent with recovery in between, possibility of multiple sclerosis, periodic paralysis, or myasthenia gravis (fluctuating) should be considered.
- If the weakness is insidious onset, starting in lower limbs and gradually ascending upwards to involve upper limbs, it suggests Guillain-Barré syndrome.
- If the weakness is insidious onset and very slowly progressive (over weeks to months), it suggests degenerative disorders (motor neuron disease), slowly progressive peripheral neuropathy, or malignancy.
- If there is sudden onset weakness with pain in a single limb, consider vascular and orthopedic causes such as ischemia of limb, fracture or compartment syndrome.
- Features of raised intracranial pressure (ICP) such as headache, altered sensorium, vomiting, papilledema suggest hemorrhagic stroke. Signs of raised intracranial pressure (ICP) can also occur in massive brain infarct after 1 or 2 days. But in case of brain hemorrhage, signs of raised intracranial pressure (ICP) appear immediately. Other causes of headache and vomiting associated with weakness are meningoencephalitis, space-occupying lesion, and hemiplegic migraine. Meningoencephalitis is usually associated with fever and neck meningeal signs. Stiffness. Space-occupying lesion usually present with insidious onset headache and weakness (however, sudden onset headache and vomiting can occur due to hemorrhage into the tumor which is sudden onset). Patients with migraine usually give H/o recurrent headache.

Family History

- Family history is important in detecting hereditary neuropathies (e.g. Charcot-Marie-tooth-disease) and myopathies (e.g. muscular dystrophies). Some of the familial periodic paralysis problems may be hereditary.

Examination of Patient

- Examination is focused on confirming the pattern of weakness and determining the type of weakness.
- Exaggerated deep tendon reflexes, increased muscle tone (spasticity), and extensor plantar response suggest upper motor neuron (e.g. corticospinal tract) lesion in the brain or spinal cord.
- Absent or decreased deep tendon reflexes, decreased muscle tone, muscle atrophy, and muscle fasciculations suggest lower motor neuron lesion.
- If patients have hyporeflexia and predominantly distal muscle weakness, particularly with distal sensory deficits or paresthesias, suspect polyneuropathy.

Investigations

- Lesions can be vascular events (infarction/hemorrhage), inflammatory/immunologic, infectious, neoplastic, toxic, or metabolic in origin.
- Various investigations may help in identifying the exact nature of lesion. These include CT and/or MRI imaging, NCV studies, etc.
- Serum electrolytes to rule out hypokalemia or hyperkalemia which occurs in periodic paralysis.
- Elevation of muscle enzymes (creatine kinase) occurs in muscle diseases.
- Muscle biopsy may be necessary to determine the precise form of myopathy.
- Nerve conduction studies are important for peripheral neuropathies.

TABLE 5.4: Localization of site of lesion by analyzing the pattern of weakness

Distribution of weakness	Location of lesion	Possible accompanying signs
One side of the body (hemiplegia or hemiparesis). Upper limb and facial weakness > lower limb weakness	Lateral surface of the cortex (parietal cortex) supplied by middle cerebral artery	Exaggerated deep tendon reflexes (DTRs). Cortical sensory loss on the side of weakness. Aphasia (if dominant hemisphere is involved), apraxia, visual field deficit, gaze palsy.
One side of the body (hemiplegia or hemiparesis), but lower limb more weak than upper limb and face.	Medial surface of brain supplied by anterior cerebral artery	Cortical sensory loss in affected leg, frontal lobe signs, sometimes incontinence. DTR increased.
Dense hemiplegia. This means weakness equally affects face, arm, and leg.	Internal capsule	Usually no sensory loss. DTR increased.
Ipsilateral cranial nerve and contralateral body weakness	Brainstem lesion	Accompanying signs and symptoms depend on the level of brainstem lesion. For example diplopia occurs in mid brain and pontine lesions due to involvement of 3rd, 4th, or 6th nerves.
Weakness of both upper and lower limbs (quadriparesis)	Spinal cord lesion above C5 (complete transverse lesion).	Bowel, bladder, or sexual dysfunction common. All modalities of sensation lost below the level of lesion.
Weakness of both lower limbs (paraparesis), UMN type	Thoracic cord lesion (transverse lesion)	Bowel, bladder, or sexual dysfunction common. There is a sensory level below which all modalities of sensation are lost. Lower limb DTR exaggerated
Weakness of both legs, LMN type, asymmetric.	Cauda equina	Occasional bowel, bladder, or sexual dysfunction; radicular pain in multiple nerve root distribution may be present. DTR depressed or absent.
Weakness of one half of the body, UMN type, without any cranial nerve involvement including face. **Contralateral loss of pain, touch, and temperature (due to spinothalamic tract involvement)**	Hemi-cord syndrome (Brown-Séquard syndrome)	Ipsilateral loss of vibration and joint position sense ((due to posterior column involvement).
Patchy weakness, LMN type, asymmetrical	Anterior horn cell involvement (example-poliomyelitis)	Presence of muscle atrophy and fasciculations. DTR depressed or absent.
Weakness of muscles supplied by a nerve root	Single nerve root lesion	Radicular pain common along the involved root. Reflex served by that nerve root may be absent. Dermatomal sensory loss may be present.
Asymmetric weakness of groups of muscles, LMN type	Plexopathy (brachial plexopathy, lumbar plexopathy)	Pain is common, especially with brachial plexopathy, DTRs in the involved limb may be depressed or absent.
Weakness of muscles in the distribution of a single peripheral nerve.	Mononeuropathy	LMN type weakness, muscle atrophy may be present. Sensory impairment in the distribution of involved nerve may be present.
Bilateral distal weakness with little or no proximal weakness, LMN type.	Polyneuropathy (e.g. diabetic peripheral neuropathy)	Distal DTRs depressed or absent. There may be distal sensory impairment (glove and stocking type)
Bilateral weakness of proximal muscles more than distal muscles, with the upper limbs more affected than the lower limbs. **Fluctuating muscle weakness that varies in severity, worsens with physical activity, and improves with rest.**	Myasthenia gravis (neuromuscular junction)	The pupils, deep tendon reflexes, and sensory examinations are normal. There may be extraocular muscle weakness causing diplopia, ptosis, or both. Bulbar muscle weakness may produce difficulty chewing or frequent choking, dysphagia, hoarseness, and dysarthria.
Bilateral weakness, proximal muscles more than distal muscles	Muscle diseases Pain and tenderness of muscles indicate myositis	Sensory examination—normal DTRs—normal Pseudohypertrophy may be present in muscular dystrophies.
Asymmetric weakness which has features of both UMN (DTR exaggerated) and LMN involvement (muscle atrophy, fasciculations)	Motor neuron disease	No sensory involvement. Motor neuron disease purely affects motor system.

Q. Describe the pathway of upper motor neuron.

Q. Pyramidal tract (corticospinal tract).

- Upper motor neuron pathway consists of corticospinal and corticobulbar tracts.
- Upper motor neurons have their cell bodies in layer V of the primary motor cortex (the precentral gyrus, or Brodmann's area 4) and in the supplemental motor cortex (area 6).
- Axons of these neurons descend through the subcortical white matter and the posterior limb of the internal capsule.
- In the brainstem they pass through cerebral peduncle of the midbrain, the basis pontis, and the medullary pyramids.
- At the cervicomedullary junction, most pyramidal axons cross to opposite side and form lateral corticospinal tract. 10–30% remain ipsilateral in the anterior spinal cord to form anterior corticospinal tract.
- Finally, the axons end on anterior horn cells of spinal cord through monosynaptic connections **(Fig. 5.2)**.
- Corticobulbar neurons are similar to corticospinal neurons but innervate brainstem motor nuclei.

Q. Plantar reflex (Babinski sign).

- Plantar reflex is a nociceptive superficial reflex subserved by S1 segment.
- It was first described by Babinski.

Method of Elicitation

- Ask the patient lie supine with the hips and knees extended and heels resting on the bed. If the patient is seated, the knee should be extended, with the foot held either in the examiner's hand or resting on examiner's knee. But supine position is the best.
- Lateral part of sole is stroked with a with a blunt and narrow tip object (e.g. a key, or handle of a reflex hammer), starting near the heel and proceeding to the base of the little toe and then turn medially towards the base of other toes **(Fig. 5.3)**.

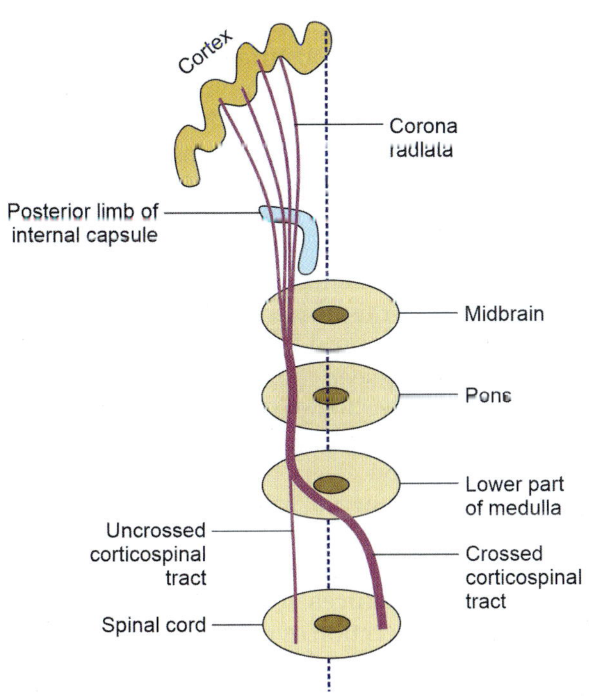

Figure 5.2: Corticospinal tract

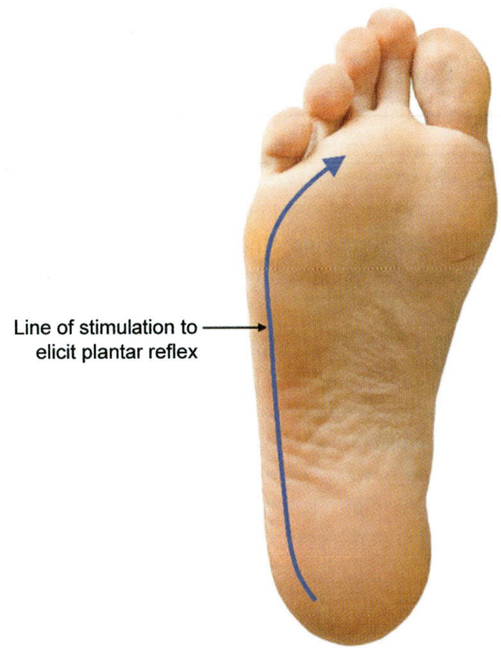

Figure 5.3: Plantar reflex

Normal Response

- Flexion of the big toe and adduction of other toes. This is called flexor plantar response.

Abnormal Response

- Extension of the big toe, with or without fanning out of other toes. It is called extensor plantar response or Babinski sign.

Causes of Extensor Plantar Response

- It is a sign of upper motor neuron lesion. It is found in lesions of corticospinal tract above S1. It is also found in metabolic encephalopathies and after an attack of epilepsy.
- Physiological: in infants, children below 2 years, and during deep sleep.

Equivocal Response

- This is neither flexor nor extensor and is difficult to interpret.

Q. Define coma. Describe the mechanism and causes of coma. How do you investigate and manage a case of coma.

- Coma is a clinical state in which patient is unresponsive to external stimulation and is unarouseable ("unarousable unresponsiveness").

Mechanisms of Coma

- Consciousness is maintained by an interaction of reticular activating system of brainstem and cerebral cortex. Hence, altered consciousness including coma can be produced by any pathology in the brainstem, reticular formation, and cerebral cortex.

Causes of Coma (Table 5.5)

TABLE 5. 5: Causes of coma
Structural causes
• **Trauma:** Extradural/subdural hematoma, contusion
• **Stroke:** Large MCA infarcts, brainstem stroke, hemorrhage
• **Tumors:** Mass effect or herniation
• **Hydrocephalus**, herniation syndromes
• **Brain abscess, encephalitis (e.g. HSV)**
Metabolic causes
• **Hypoglycemia, hyperglycemia**
• **Hypoxia, CO poisoning**
• **Uremia, hepatic encephalopathy**
• **Electrolyte disturbances:** Na^+, Ca^{2+}, Mg^{2+}
• **Drug overdose:** Benzodiazepines, opioids, alcohol
• **Infections:** Meningitis, sepsis
• **Endocrine:** Myxedema coma, Addisonian crisis

Examination of a Patient with Coma

Immediate Assessment

- Take care of ABCs first (airway, breathing circulation). If ABCs are not alright take immediate measures to correct them.
- Record depth of coma by using Glasgow Coma Scale.
- Blood glucose (fingerstick).
- Get a quick short history from those who brought the patient. Ask about previous health of the patient, whether there was a history of diabetes, a head injury, a convulsion, alcohol or drug use, or a prior episode of coma or attempted suicide, and the circumstances in which the person was found. H/o of vomiting and headache, followed by loss of consciousness suggests intracranial hemorrhage. Many patients with diabetes, epilepsy or hypoadrenalism carry identification which may give clue about the cause of coma.
- Next go for full general and neurological examination.

Vital Signs

- Alterations in vital signs (temperature, heart rate, respiratory rate, and blood pressure) can provide important clues to the diagnosis.
- Fever indicates a systemic infection (e.g. pneumonia) or bacterial meningitis or viral encephalitis. An excessively high body temperature with dry skin should arouse suspicion of heat stroke or intoxication by a drug with anticholinergic activity. Hypothermia is seen in patients with alcohol or barbiturate intoxication, drowning, exposure to cold, peripheral circulatory failure, and myxedema.
- Bradycardia may suggest ingestion of medications such as tricyclic antidepressants or anticonvulsants, or raised intracranial pressure.
- Marked hypertension is observed in patients with cerebral hemorrhage and in hypertensive encephalopathy. Hypotension suggests alcohol or barbiturate intoxication, internal hemorrhage, myocardial infarction, dissecting aortic aneurysm, septicemia, or Addison disease.
- Cheyne-Stokes (periodic) respiration is alternating hyperpnea and apnea seen in bilateral cerebral dysfunction, or brainstem problem. It also occurs in metabolic comas and respiratory failure. Kussmaul (acidotic) respiration is deep, sighing hyperventilation seen in diabetic ketoacidosis and uremia.

General Examination

- Many general examination findings may provide clues to the cause of coma.
- Marked pallor suggests internal hemorrhage.
- Cyanosis: Coma may be due to respiratory failure or cardiac failure.
- Cherry-red skin color is seen in carbon monoxide poisoning.
- Jaundice: Coma may be due to liver failure, sepsis.
- Petechiae and purpura: Coma may be due to intracranial bleed due to some bleeding problem.
- Hyperpigmentation: Coma may be due to Addison's disease.
- Injection marks: Coma may be due to drug abuse.
- Coarse and dry skin: Coma may be due to hypothyroidism.
- Excessive sweating suggests hypoglycemia or shock, and excessively dry skin, diabetic ketoacidosis or uremia.
- A macular-hemorrhagic rash indicates the possibility of meningococcal infection, staphylococcal endocarditis, typhus, or Rocky Mountain spotted fever.
- Odor of breath: Look for smell of ketones, alcohol, or ammonia. Arsenic poisoning produces the odor of garlic. OP compound poisoning produces kerosene smell.
- Multiple bruises (particularly a bruise or boggy area in the scalp), bleeding, CSF leakage from an ear or the nose, or periorbital hemorrhage suggests the possibility of head trauma.

Neurological Examination in Coma

- Only a limited examination can be done in comatose patients.
- Note the predominant postures of the limbs and body; the presence or absence of spontaneous movements on one side; the position of the head and eyes.
- ***Head, neck and spine:*** Note trauma, skull burr-holes and bruits, neck stiffness.
- ***Pupils:*** Check size and reaction to light. Unilateral dilated pupil indicates compression of the third nerve due to temporal lobe uncus herniation (coning). This happens in raised intracranial pressure on one side (e.g. an extradural hematoma). Bilateral fixed, dilated pupils are seen in brainstem death, and deep coma of any cause. Bilateral pinpoint pupils are seen in pontine lesions (e.g. a pontine hemorrhage) and opioid intoxication.
- ***Fundi:*** Presence of papilledema suggests raised intracranial tension. Look for retinal hemorrhage.
- ***Ocular movements:*** Vestibulo-ocular reflexes. Passive head turning produces conjugate ocular deviation away from the direction of rotation (doll's eye reflex). This reflex is absent in deep coma and brainstem lesions. In ***caloric stimulation test,*** ocular deviation toward the irrigated ear is seen when ice-cold water

is irrigated into the external auditory meatus. This is also absent in brainstem death.

- ***Abnormalities of conjugate gaze: Lateral deviation*** occurs towards a destructive frontal lesion. Rarely, an irritative lesion in one frontal lobe can make the eyes deviate to opposite side. In a pontine lesion, conjugate lateral deviation occurs away from the lesion. ***Skew deviation*** (one eye deviated up and the other down) indicates a brainstem or cerebellar lesion.
- Decorticate rigidity and decerebrate rigidity (posturing) describe stereotyped arm and leg movements occurring spontaneously or elicited by sensory stimulation. Flexion of the elbows and wrists and supination of the arm (decortication) suggests bilateral damage rostral to the midbrain. Extension of the elbows and wrists with pronation (decerebration) indicates damage to motor tracts in the midbrain or caudal diencephalon.
- ***Other findings:*** Look for any asymmetry in tone, reflexes and plantar responses.

Cardiac Examination

- Cardiac diseases such as atrial fibrillation, infective endocarditis, MI, etc. can produce embolic stroke and cause coma.

Abdominal Examination

- Look for abnormal bowel sounds, organomegaly, masses, and ascites. Bowel sounds are absent in an acute abdominal condition, as well as with anticholinergic poisoning. Increased bowel sounds occur in organophosporus compound poisoning. Hepatomegaly is seen in hepatoma or metastatic disease which indirectly suggests brain metastases as the cause of coma. Look for evidence of cirrhosis such as ascites and splenomegaly which suggests hepatic encephalopathy as the cause of coma.

Respiratory System Examination

- Look for evidence of COPD, pneumonia or any other lung disease which can produce respiratory failure and coma.

Investigations

- Tests should be chosen according to the clues available from history and examination.
- CBC with ESR/CRP: Infection, inflammation
- Routine biochemistry (urea, creatinine, electrolytes, glucose, calcium, magnesium, liver function tests)
- Metabolic and endocrine studies (TSH, serum cortisol)
- Blood cultures, malaria test to rule out cerebral malaria and sepsis.
- Drugs screen (e.g. diazepam, narcotics, etc.)
- Urine examination for ketone bodies
- Arterial blood gas analysis (hypoxia and hypercarbia can cause coma).
- ***Imaging:*** CT or MRI brain should be done to rule out any intracranial pathology.
- ***CSF examination:*** This is helpful to rule out meningitis and subarachnoid hemorrhage.
- ***Electroencephalography:*** EEG is of some value in the diagnosis of metabolic coma, encephalitis and ongoing nonconvulsive seizures.

Management

- The management focuses on immediate stabilization, identifying and treating the underlying cause, and preventing complications.

Immediate Stabilization

- Take care of ABCs (airway, breathing, and circulation).
- *Airway*: Ensure patent airway. Intubate if GCS ≤8 to protect airway.
- *Breathing*: Give oxygen, assist ventilation if needed (bag-valve mask or ventilator).
- *Circulation*: IV fluids for hypotension. Monitor BP, HR. Treat shock.

Identifying and Treating the Underlying Cause

- The underlying cause of coma should be treated. For example, correction of blood glucose in hypoglycemia.
- Give empiric lifesaving treatments if cause is uncertain:
  - Thiamine 100 mg IV (before glucose to prevent Wernicke's encephalopathy)
  - Dextrose 50% IV (if hypoglycemia suspected or unknown glucose)
  - Naloxone 0.4–2 mg IV (if opioid overdose suspected)
  - Flumazenil (for benzodiazepine overdose—use with caution)

General Measures

- Ryle's tube and a urinary catheter should be passed.
- Skin care—frequent turning of patient to avoid pressure sores. Patient should be kept preferably in water bed to prevent pressure sores.
- Oral hygiene—mouth washes, frequent suction
- Eye care—taping of lids, prevention of corneal damage by applying lubricating eye drops and eye ointment.
- Nutrition and hydration—food and water may be given through Ryle's tube. IV fluids may also be used if required.

Q. Glasgow Coma Scale (GCS).

- The Glasgow Coma Scale (GCS) is a way to grade coma severity. It was introduced to assess the conscious level of patients with acute brain injury from head trauma, intracranial hemorrhage and many other causes. The GCS reflects the initial severity of brain dysfunction, while serial assessments demonstrate the evolution of the injury.
- Three parameters are used for this purpose; eye response (E), verbal response (V), and motor response (M). It is easy to use and has good interobserver reliability.
- The GCS is scored between 3 and 15, 3 being the worst, and 15 the best. A score of 13 or higher correlates with mild brain injury; a score of 9–12 correlates with moderate injury; and a score of 8 or less represent severe brain injury (**Table 5.6**).

- The GCS is useful for prognosis, but does not aid in the diagnosis of coma.

TABLE 5.6: Glasgow Coma Scale

Eye opening	
• Spontaneous	4
• To sound	3
• To pain/pressure	2
• No eye opening	1
Verbal response	
• Oriented	5
• Confused	4
• Inappropriate words	3
• Incomprehensible sounds	2
• No verbal response	1
Motor response	
• Obeys commands	6
• Localizing response to pain	5
• Withdrawal response to pain	4
• Flexion to pain	3
• Extension to pain	2
• No motor response	1

[Remember EVM; 4, 5, 6]

Q. Locked-in syndrome.

- Locked-in syndrome (LIS) is a rare but dramatic neurological condition where the patient is conscious and aware, but completely paralyzed except for vertical eye movements and blinking. It is often mistaken for coma or vegetative state—making recognition absolutely vital.
- Clinical tip: If a "comatose" patient blinks on command, always consider locked-in syndrome.
- Pathology in locked-in syndrome: This occurs when a lesion damages the bilateral ventral pons. Examples of such lesions are pontine hemorrhage, pontine abscess, brainstem tumors, and central pontine myelinolysis. Locked-in syndrome most often is observed as a consequence of pontine infarction due to basilar artery thrombosis.
- EEG is normal as the brain is normal. Majority of people die but some may live for many years.
- Management involves supportive measures (ventilator support, nasogastric tube feeding, bladder care, prevention of bedsore) and treatment of underlying cause.
- Even if the patient survives, long-term disability is severe.

Q. Brain death.

- Brain death is the irreversible loss of all brain activity, including the brainstem.
- It is clinically and legally equivalent to death even if the heart beat is present with life support.

Establishing the diagnosis

To declare brain death, all of the following must be met:

1. Coma (unresponsiveness)
    - No eye opening, no response to verbal or painful stimuli
2. Absence of brainstem reflexes
    - Pupils: Fixed and dilated, no light reaction
    - Corneal reflex: Absent
    - Oculocephalic reflex (doll's eye): Absent
    - Oculovestibular reflex (cold caloric test): Absent
    - Gag and cough reflex: Absent
    - No facial movement to pain
3. Apnea (no spontaneous breathing)
    - Confirmed by apnea test (*see* below)

- The apnea test: Preoxygenate with 100% O_2 for 10 min. Disconnect the ventilator from the endotracheal tube. If there is no respiratory movement even after a minimum of 8–10 minutes of ventilator disconnection, it indicates brain death.
- Spinal reflex movements may be present even in brain death and do not exclude the diagnosis.
- Before declaring brain death, there should be normal body temperature, systolic BP >100 mm Hg and no significant electrolyte imbalance. Ongoing seizure activity should be ruled out. Also ensure that no recent neuromuscular blocking agents or CNS depressants have been administered.
- An isoelectric EEG is helpful in confirming the diagnosis but not necessary.
- Brain death should be differentiated from locked-in syndrome (consciousness and eye movements preserved), and vegetative state (eye opening and respiration often preserved).

Prognosis

- Patients with brain death are unlikely to survive for more than a week.

Legal and ethical aspects

- Brain death = legal death.
- Requires documentation by qualified physicians, usually two separate exams.
- At this time, depending on family and patient preference, cardiopulmonary support can be withdrawn, or arrangements for organ harvest may be made.

Q. Persistent vegetative state (unresponsive wakefulness syndrome).

- **Vegetative state** is a clinical condition in which a patient has wakefulness without awareness. They appear awake (eyes open, sleep-wake cycles present) but lack any conscious interaction with the environment. They may show reflex movements but there is no response to commands.
- It occurs due to extensive cortical gray or subcortical white matter lesions with relative preservation of brainstem.
- There are no purposeful or voluntary behavioural responses to visual, auditory, tactile, or noxious stimuli.

- No evidence of language comprehension or expression.
- Brainstem maintains basic autonomic functions (heartbeat, breathing, eye opening).
- There is bowel and bladder incontinence.
- If this state persists for:
  - >1 month, it is called persistent vegetative state.
  - >3 months (non-traumatic) or >12 months (traumatic), it is called permanent vegetative state.
- Vegetative state has no specific treatment. Treatment is mainly supportive.
- Prognosis is poor.

Q. Differences between coma, LIS, vegetative state, and brain death (Table 5.7).

Q. Ptosis (blepharoptosis).

- Ptosis refers to drooping of the upper eyelid (**Figs 5.4 and 5.5**).

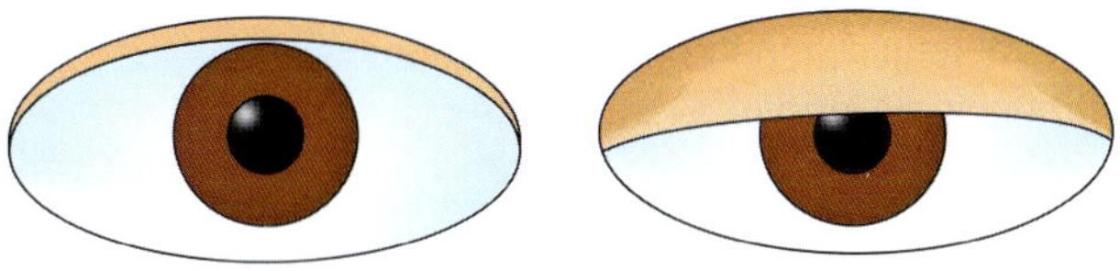

Figure 5.4: Right eye normal, left eye partial ptosis

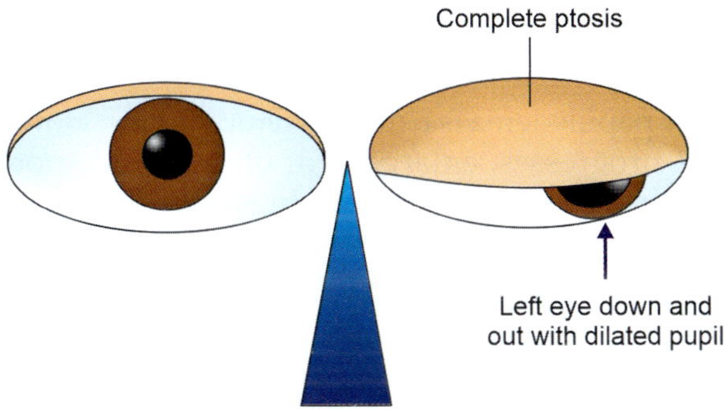

Figure 5.5: Left eye 3rd nerve palsy

- It can be unilateral or bilateral, congenital or acquired, and may indicate neurological, muscular, or mechanical causes.
- Often ptosis is the result of dysfunction of upper eyelid elevator muscles. These elevator muscles are the levator palpebrae superioris and the Mueller muscle. The levator palpebrae superioris is a striated muscle innervated by the oculomotor nerve. The Mueller muscle is a smooth muscle, innervated by sympathetic system.
- Ptosis can be disabling, if it obstructs vision.

Causes of ptosis (**Table 5.8**)

TABLE 5.8: Causes of ptosis

Causes	Features
Congenital ptosis	Usually unilateral Due to dystrophic levator palpebrae muscle Many patients also have amblyopia, strabismus
3rd nerve palsy	Usually unilateral Affected eye position is "down and out" Diplopia present Pupil is dilated on the affected side
Horner's syndrome	Usually unilateral Pupil is constricted on the affected side Anhidrosis on the affected side of face
Myasthenia gravis	Usually bilateral Pupils are normal size Degree of ptosis variable, improves with rest Associated diplopia often present
Muscle disease (e.g. oculopharyngeal dystrophy)	Usually bilateral Pupils are normal size
Mechanical ptosis	Usually unilateral Occurs due to excess weight on the upper lid Examples are eyelid tumors and chalazion

TABLE 5.7: Differences between coma, LIS, vegetative state, and brain death

Feature	Coma	Locked-in syndrome (LIS)	Vegetative state	Brain death
Consciousness	Absent	Preserved	Absent	Absent
Awareness	Absent	Fully aware	Absent	Absent
Sleep-wake cycles	Absent	Present (normal)	Present (eye opening/closing)	Absent
Eye opening	Absent	Spontaneous + on command	Spontaneous (reflexive)	Absent
Eye movements	Absent	Vertical only (voluntary)	Non-purposeful eye movements	Absent
Communication	Absent	Via blinking or eye movement	None	Absent
Motor activity	Absent	Absent except vertical eye movements	Reflexive or posturing only	Absent
Breathing (spontaneous)	Usually absent	Often absent (needs support)	Present	Absent
Brainstem reflexes	Usually present	Present (except voluntary)	Present	Absent
EEG	Slowed or variable	Normal	Slow, nonspecific	Isoelectric (flatline)
Prognosis	Variable (can improve or worsen)	May communicate with support	Poor if persistent >3–12 months	Irreversible (legally dead)

Approach to a Case of Ptosis

History

- Onset (sudden vs gradual): sudden onset → stroke (3rd nerve palsy, Horner's syndrome). Gradual onset → Aponeurotic or congenital ptosis.
- Duration: Congenital ptosis often present since birth.
- Progressive worsening → Myasthenia gravis (MG), muscular dystrophy.
- Variable and worsens with fatigue → Indicates MG.
- Associated diplopia → Suggests extraocular muscle involvement (e.g. 3rd nerve palsy, MG).
- Trauma or surgery history → Suggests traumatic or iatrogenic ptosis.
- Family history → Could point toward hereditary myopathies or congenital ptosis.

Examination

- Fatigue test (sustained upgaze) → Suggests MG if ptosis worsens.
- Ice pack test → Ptosis improves in MG after 2 min.
- Dilated and fixed pupil suggests 3rd nerve palsy.
- Constricted pupil (miosis) suggests Horner's syndrome.
- Extraocular movements (EOM) affected in 3rd nerve palsy, orbital disease, or MG.
- Motor weakness, reflexes and tone: Helps if systemic neuromuscular disease is suspected.

Investigations

- Tensilon test (edrophonium) and serum AChR antibodies: If MG is suspected.
- CT/MRI brain/orbit: If 3rd nerve palsy or mass is suspected.
- Chest X-ray: If Horner's syndrome due to pancoast tumor is suspected.

Treatment

- Treat the underlying cause.
- Patients with obstructed vision can be considered for surgical correction.

Q. Papilledema.

- Papilledema refers to swelling of optic disc.
- In papilledema, there is axonal swelling within the optic nerve, blockage of axonal transport with capillary and venous congestion.
- Pseudopapilledema: Congenital anomalies of the disc, including drusen and myelinated nerve fibers, may cause the appearance of disc swelling or pseudopapilledema.

Causes of Papilledema

Raised intracranial pressure
- Space-occupying lesions (brain tumor, abscess, hematoma)
- Subarachnoid hemorrhage
- Idiopathic intracranial hypertension,
- Meningitis, encephalitis

Optic nerve disease
- Optic neuritis (e.g. multiple sclerosis)
- Optic neuropathy (hereditary, ischemic and toxic)

Venous occlusion
- Cavernous sinus thrombosis
- Central retinal vein thrombosis/occlusion
- Orbital mass lesions

Other causes
- Hypercapnia
- Optic nerve glioma
- Malignant hypertension
- Vasculitis (e.g. SLE)

Clinical Features

- Early papilledema is usually asymptomatic. However, as it progresses, enlargement of the blind spot and blurring of vision develop. In severe papilledema, arterial blood flow falls and infarction of the optic nerve occurs leading to severe and permanent visual loss.
- Diffuse headache and vomiting may be present if the cause of papilledema is due to raised intracranial pressure. The earliest ophthalmoscopic signs of disc swelling are pinkness of the disc followed by blurring of the nasal margin. Later there is loss of normal venous pulsation, and obliteration of physiological cup. Small hemorrhages may be present around the disc **(Fig. 5.6)**.

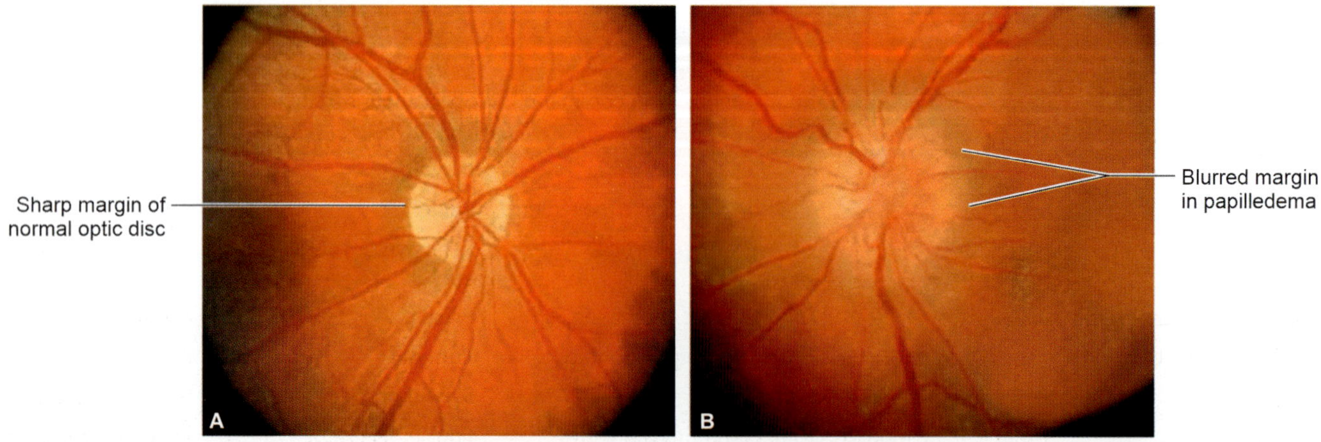

Figure 5.6: Normal (A) and papilledema (B)

Investigations

- Neuroimaging (e.g. CT scan, MRI) of the brain should be done to rule out any mass lesion.
- Magnetic resonance (MR) venography to detect venous sinus thrombosis.
- Lumbar puncture (after ruling out mass lesion) and CSF analysis to identify any infectious or neoplastic disease.
- If there is doubt about disc edema, fluorescein angiography can be used to confirm it. Fluorescein is injected intravenously and if there is edema, it leaks in the retina.

Treatment

- Treat the underlying cause.
- Diuretics: The carbonic anhydrase inhibitor, acetazolamide (Diamox), is useful in selected cases, especially idiopathic intracranial hypertension.
- Lumboperitoneal shunt or ventriculoperitoneal shunt can be used to bypass CSF.

Q. Optic neuritis.

Q. Retrobulbar neuritis.

Optic neuritis is inflammation of the optic nerve.

Types of Optic Neuritis

- *Papillitis*—involvement of optic disc.
- *Retrobulbar neuritis*—refers to optic nerve inflammation behind the eyeball. There is no abnormality seen at the disc but there is severe visual impairment.

Causes

- ***Demyelinating diseases***: The most common cause of optic neuritis is demyelination (e.g. multiple sclerosis).
- ***Infections***: Measles, mumps, influenza, varicella-zoster virus, sinusitis, meningitis, TB, syphilis, HIV.
- ***Autoimmune disorders***: Particularly systemic lupus erythematosus.
- ***Chemicals and drugs***: Lead, methanol, quinine, arsenic, antibiotics.

Clinical Features

- A history of preceding viral illness may be present. Patients are usually young adults and present with impairment of vision in one eye or less commonly, both eyes.
- Dyschromatopsia (change in color perception may be present).
- Presence of retro-orbital or ocular pain, usually exacerbated by eye movement.
- Pupillary light reaction is decreased in the affected eye and various types of visual field defects are present.
- Fundus examination shows swollen optic disc, blurred margins, hyperemia, possible flame hemorrhages.

Investigations

- MRI brain with orbits is very useful in assessing inflammatory changes in the optic nerves and to rule out structural lesions.
- Visual evoked potentials are abnormal in optic neuritis. They may be abnormal even when MRI of the optic nerve is normal.
- Blood tests: ESR/CRP, ANA, NMO-IgG (neuromyelitis optica-IgG), syphilis, etc.
- Lumbar puncture: If systemic/infectious cause suspected.

Treatment

- IV steroids (methylprednisolone 1 g/day × 3–5 days) followed by tapering oral steroids.
- Plasma exchange has been used in patients with no significant improvement with steroids.
- Treat underlying infection if identified.

Q. Optic atrophy.

- Optic atrophy is the degeneration of optic nerve which occurs as an endpoint of many diseases that causes axon degeneration in the retinogeniculate pathway.
- It is not a diagnosis itself but a clinical sign indicating past or ongoing optic nerve damage.
- ***Primary optic atrophy:*** Here the optic nerve fibers degenerate in an orderly manner and are replaced by glial cells without alteration of optic nerve head.
- ***Secondary optic atrophy***:

Causes of Optic Atrophy

- ***Primary optic atrophy:*** It happens due to direct optic nerve damage from many causes. Examples are: Infarction of the nerve from thromboembolism, iinflammation (multiple sclerosis, syphilis), optic nerve compression, trauma, toxic (quinine and methyl alcohol), vitamin B_{12} deficiency.
- ***Secondary optic atrophy***: Refers to optic atrophy secondary to papilledema due to any cause. Examples are raised intracranial pressure due to various reasons, Cavernous sinus thrombosis.

Clinical Features

- The main symptom is vision loss (varies from mild to complete blindness).
- Color vision is markedly reduced.
- Fundoscopy shows characteristic pale optic disc. If the disc is pale and sharp, think primary atrophy. If the disc is pale and blurred, think secondary atrophy (post-papilledema).

Investigations

- Visual field testing
- Color vision testing
- MRI brain and orbits: Rule out compressive or demyelinating causes.
- Blood tests: B_{12}, folate, ESR, CRP, syphilis serology, etc.
- Genetic testing: If hereditary cause suspected.

Treatment

- No treatment can reverse optic atrophy. The goal is to identify and treat the underlying cause early to prevent further damage.

Q. Describe the visual pathway. Describe briefly the field defects produced at various levels with appropriate diagrams.

Visual Pathway

- Whenever we see an object, its image falls on the retina. The image is converted to nerve action potentials by retinal rod, cone and ganglion cells.
- The axons of ganglion cells of retina form optic nerve. From each eye, one optic nerve starts. Both optic nerves cross in the optic chiasma.
- At the chiasma fibers from the nasal portion of retina cross, whereas fibers from temporal side of retina do not cross.
- Crossed nasal fibers join uncrossed temporal fibers and form optic tract. Optic tract reaches lateral geniculate body and synapses there. Some optic tract fibers reaching the lateral geniculate bodies pass to the brainstem to control refraction (lens) and pupillary aperture.
- From the lateral geniculate body, fibers pass in the optic radiation to reach the occipital cortex.
- In the optic radiation fibers from upper part of retina (representing lower visual field) lie above (parietal lobes) and those from lower part of retina (representing upper visual field) lie below in the temporal lobes.

Visual Field Defects due to Lesions at Various Levels of Visual Pathway (Fig. 5.7)

A. Unilateral Anopia

- Complete loss of vision in one eye
- Seen in unilateral optic nerve lesion (trauma, ischemia, aneurysm, tumor, optic neuritis) or ocular pathology (corneal opacification, cataract, vitreal hemorrhage, retinal detachment, retinal artery occlusion, glaucoma).

B. Binasal Hemianopia

- Loss of vision in the nasal (inner) half of both sides of vision. This is a rarely encountered visual field defect.
- Seen in bilateral lesion involving each side of optic chiasma. Examples of such lesions are bilateral internal carotid artery aneurysms, hydrocephalus, intracranial mass lesions, and elevated intracranial pressure, neurosyphilis, ischemic optic neuropathy, optic nerve drusen, and glaucoma.

C. Bitemporal Hemianopia

- Loss of lateral vision in both eyes
- Seen in optic chiasmal compression. Causes are pituitary mass lesion, craniopharyngioma, and pituitary apoplexy. These leisons compress optic chiasma.

D. Homonymous Hemianopia

- Loss of left or right field in both eyes
- The "homonymous" aspect means that the visual field loss occurs on the same side of each eye. Seen with contralateral optic tract lesion. Causes are stroke (infarction or hemorrhage), brain tumors, trauma, and surgical interventions. Uncommon causes are multiple sclerosis and infections (encephalitis, abscess).

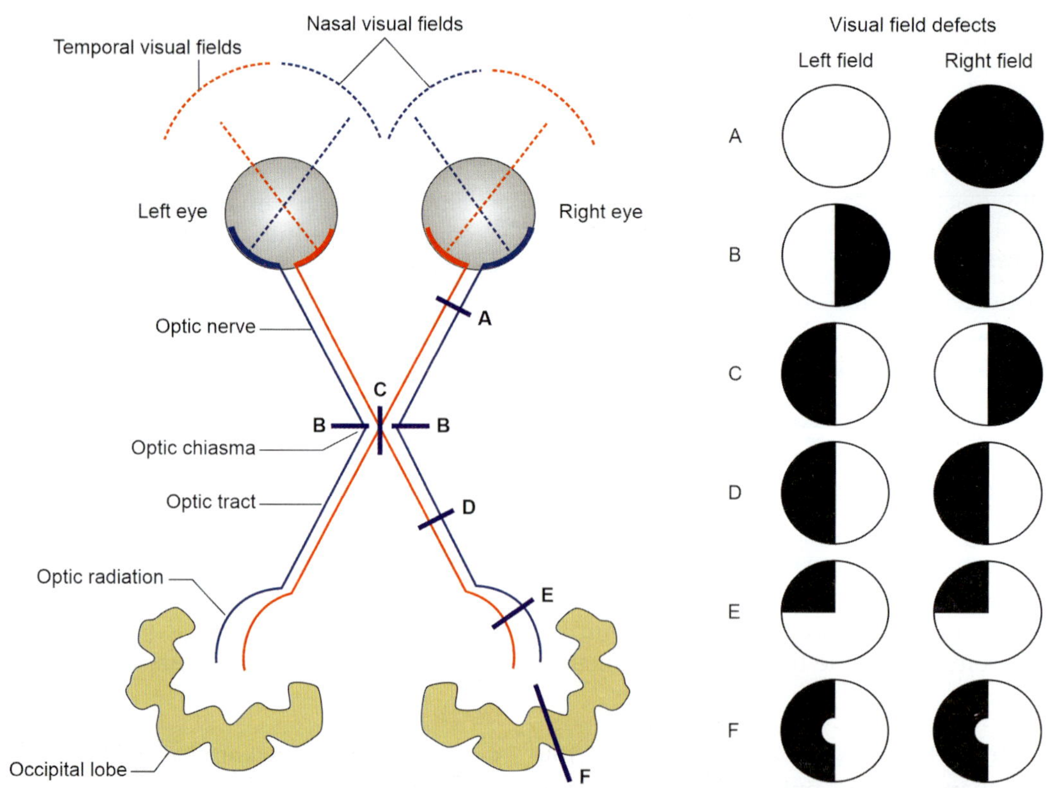

Figure 5.7: Optic pathway and visual field defects

E. Homonymous Quadrantanopia

- Loss of vision in one quarter of the visual field in both eyes, resulting in a similar region of blindness in each eye. It can be right or left, superior or inferior.
- Seen in contralateral optic radiation lesion. Causes are lesions (especially infarcts) that selectively damage the inferior or superior parts of optic radiation or occipital cortex. Examples of lesions are stroke, tumors, and traumatic brain injury.
- ***Homonymous superior quadrantanopia***—loss of the left or right upper quarters of vision in both eyes. Occurs due to lesions involving contralateral superior aspects of optic radiation or occipital cortex.
- ***Homonymous inferior quadrantanopia***—loss of the left or right inferior quarters of vision in both eyes. Occurs due to lesions involving contralateral inferior aspects of optic radiation or occipital cortex.

F. Homonymous Hemianopia with Macular Sparing

- Loss of vision in one half of the visual field in both eyes, with preservation of central vision (the macula) in both eyes. Occurs due to contralateral occipital lobe lesion. Examples of lesions are stroke, tumors, and traumatic brain injury.

Q. Causes of pinpoint pupils.

- Pinpoint pupils (miosis) are small pupils that typically measure less than 2 mm in diameter and do not respond well to changes in light.
- Causes of pinpoint pupils are as follows:

- Pontine hemorrhage
- Opiate poisoning
- Organophosphate poisoning
- Drugs (pilocarpine drops, timolol drops)

Q. Argyll Robertson pupil (ARP).

- ARP refers to pupils which constrict on a near object (they "accommodate"), but do not constrict when exposed to bright light (light reflex absent). (remember the mnemonic ARP = Accommodation reflex present) **(Fig. 5.8)**.
- This finding is highly specific for late-stage syphilis.
- The location of the lesion is believed to be in the dorsal midbrain that interrupts the pupillary light reflex pathway but spares the more ventral accommodation reflex pathway. A partial lesion in the third nerve or the ciliary ganglion has also been considered as a cause.

Causes

- Late-stage syphilis (neurosyphilis)
- Pinealomas
- Multiple sclerosis
- Diabetes mellitus

- Argyll Robertson pupil should not be confused with Adie's pupil, which may yield a similar result. Adie's pupil is caused by ciliary ganglion destruction, and the reaction to light is absent or greatly diminished.

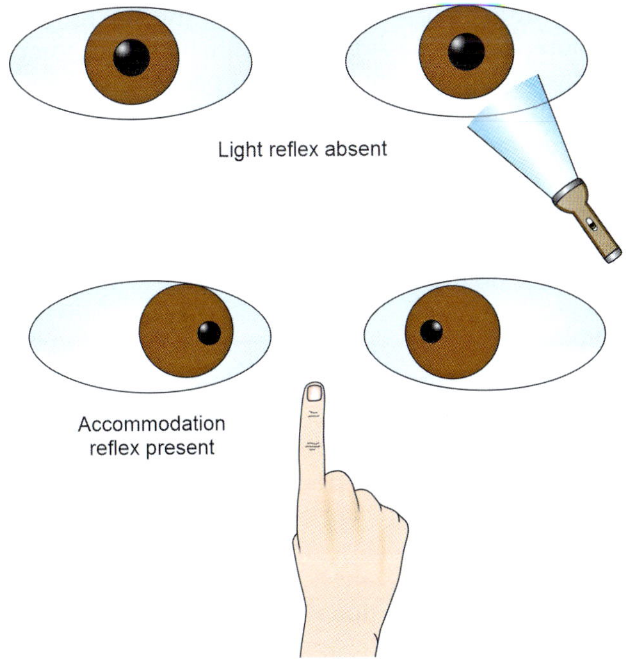

Figure 5.8: Argyl-Robertson pupil

However, Adie's pupil does react slowly with prolonged maximal stimulation. Furthermore, once the Adie's pupil reacts to accommodation, the pupil tends to remain tonically constricted and dilates very slowly.

Q. Horner syndrome.

- Horner syndrome results from an interruption of the sympathetic nerve supply to the eye and is characterized by the classic triad of miosis (i.e. constricted pupil), ptosis, and facial anhidrosis (loss of sweating).
- This sympathetic pathway originates in the hypothalamus, runs through the brainstem and spinal cord, sympathetic trunk, brachial plexus, and carotid plexus.

Causes

- *Central*: Stroke, trauma, demyelination, tumor (brainstem or spinal cord).
- *Peripheral*: Pancoast tumor, cervical adenopathy, neck and skull injuries, aortic or carotid dissection, thoracic aortic aneurysm.

Clinical Features

- Classic signs of a Horner syndrome are ptosis, miosis, and anhidrosis on the affected side.
- Ptosis is due to paralysis of the Müller's muscle, supplied by sympathetic pathway. Miosis is due to loss of sympathetic dilator action on pupil. Anhidrosis happens because sweat glands are supplied by sympathetic system.
- Loss of ciliospinal reflex on the affected side.
- Enophthalmos.

Diagnosis

- ***Confirmation of Horner's syndrome:*** Cocaine drops cause pupillary dilatation in normal eyes whereas it has no effect in eyes with impaired sympathetic

innervation. Cocaine acts by blocking the reuptake of norepinephrine at the sympathetic nerve synapse and causes pupillary dilation in patients with intact sympathetic supply.
- Imaging studies (CT or MRI) may be required to locate the site and nature of lesion.

Treatment

- Depends on the underlying cause.

Q. Diplopia.

- Diplopia is seeing two objects when there is actually one object.
- Diplopia may be monocular or binocular.
- Monocular diplopia is double vision in one eye that persists when the other eye is closed. It is often related to problems within the eye itself, not neurologic or extraocular muscle causes.
- Binocular diplopia is double vision when both eyes are open. Double vison disappears when any one eye is closed. It results from misalignment of the eyes—both eyes are open but looking at different targets, so the brain perceives two images.

Causes of Diplopia

Monocular Diplopia

- Astigmatism (irregular curvature of cornea causes light rays to focus unevenly).
- Keratoconus, corneal distortion or scarring (diplopia due to same reason as above).
- Multiple openings in the iris (causes multiple images on the retina).
- Cataract (light scatter from lens opacity leads to ghosting or double image).
- Subluxation of the lens
- Vitreous abnormalities.

Binocular Diplopia

- Cranial nerve palsies (3rd, 4th, or 6th)
- Extraocular muscle disorders
- Myasthenia gravis
- Orbital infiltration (e.g. thyroid infiltrative ophthalmopathy, orbital pseudotumor).

Evaluation of a Case of Diplopia

History and Examination

- Ask whether diplopia is monocular or binocular. Does covering any one of the eyes make the diplopia disappear? This test helps to rule out monocular diplopia, which persists in the affected eye when the other eye is covered.
- Ask whether the images are separated vertically, horizontally, or both **(Figs 5.9 and 5.10)**. Horizontal diplopia suggests 6th nerve palsy. Vertical diplopia suggests 4th nerve palsy. Intermittent diplopia suggests a waxing and waning neurologic disorder, such as myasthenia gravis.
- Take a detailed neurologic history.

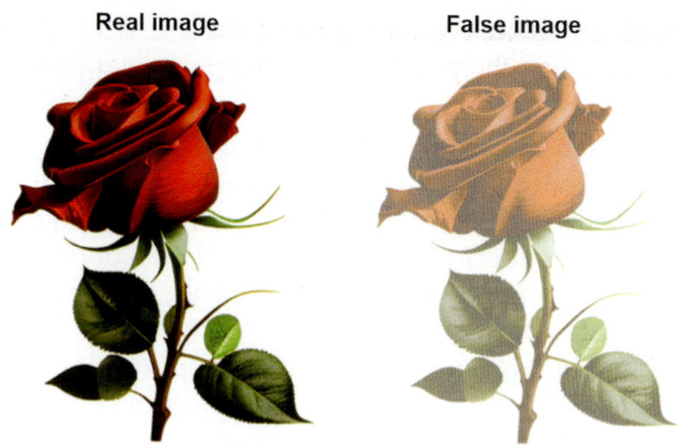

Figure 5.9: Horizontal diplopia

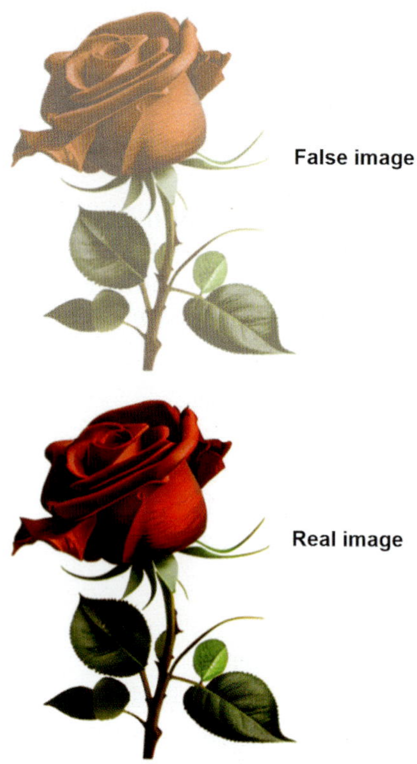

Figure 5.10: Vertical diplopia

- Look for the presence of any squint and check the eyeball movements in all directions. If an eyeball is unable to move in a particular direction it suggests 3rd, 4th or 6th nerve palsy as the cause of diplopia.
- Look for presence of ptosis. Complete ptosis occurs in 3rd nerve palsy along with pupillary dilatation. Partial bilateral ptosis with diplopia is seen with myasthenia gravis.

Investigations

- CT or MRI of the brain and orbit to rule out any intracranial or orbital pathology.
- Tensilon test if myasthenia gravis is suspected.

Treatment

- Treatment of the underlying cause.
- Patching one eye prevents double vision and allows the patient to continue functioning while awaiting resolution or intervention.

- Stick-on occlusive lenses can be applied to glasses to minimize the cosmetic handicap of a patched eye, while blurring one eye to minimize double vision.
- Strabismus surgery is occasionally necessary. Recession/resection of extra ocular muscle, transposition of extraocular muscle, weakening or shortening surgery are helpful in reducing double vision.
- Injection of botulinum toxin into the medial rectus muscle to reduce contracture due to a weak lateral rectus muscle.

Q. Apraxia.

- Apraxia is inability to perform a learned motor act in the absence of pyramidal, extrapyramidal, cerebellar, or sensory dysfunction.
- Apraxia results from damage to parietal lobes or their connections, where memories of learned movement patterns are stored. Less commonly it is due to frontal lobe lesions.
- Apraxia can be elicited by asking the person to perform a motor act which he knew earlier, for example, lighting a cigarette, brushing teeth, etc.

Causes of Apraxia

- *Stroke*: Especially in left parietal lobe or frontal lobe.
- *Neurodegenerative diseases*: Alzheimer's, corticobasal degeneration.
- *Trauma*: Affecting motor planning centers.
- *Tumors/lesions*: In left hemisphere or corpus callosum.
- *Normal pressure hydrocephalus* (*NPH*): Gait apraxia is a classic feature.

Types

- ***Ideomotor apraxia:*** This is the most common type of apraxia. Here the person is unable to carry out a motor command, e.g. lighting a cigarette and brushing teeth. It is seen in left parietal lobe lesions.
- ***Ideational apraxia:*** Here the patient cannot plan or execute the required movements in the correct sequence although individual movements may be performed correctly. For example, they may put their shoes on before their socks.
- ***Constructional apraxia:*** Here the person is unable to copy simple shapes or build simple blocks.
- ***Dressing apraxia:*** Difficulty putting clothes on properly. Puts shirt on backward or pants over head.
- ***Gait apraxia:*** Difficulty initiating or coordinating walking. Often seen in frontal lobe lesions or NPH.

Treatment

- Treatment includes speech therapy, occupational therapy, and physical therapy.
- Underlying cause has to be treated.

Q. Aphasia.

Q. Sensory aphasia.

Q. Motor aphasia.

Aphasia

- Aphasia is the acquired inability to produce and/or understand written and spoken language.
- It must be distinguished from congenital or developmental language disorders like dyslexias.
- This usually manifests as a difficulty speaking or understanding spoken language, but reading and writing are also usually impacted.
- Most individuals are left-hemisphere dominant for language function. Cerebral dominance is influenced by handedness; of the 90–95% of people who are right handed, more than 95% have left-sided language dominance. Even a majority of left handed individuals have left sided language dominance.
- Important types of aphasia are as follows.

Types of Aphasias

Sensory Aphasia (Wernicke's Aphasia)

- Here the person is not able to comprehend verbal or written language. But able to speak fluently though not meaningfully. Hence, also called "empty speech". Patient chooses inappropriate words during speech (paraphasia).
- Reading is also affected because patient cannot comprehend the written language.
- Sensory aphasia is produced by damage to posterior part of the superior temporal gyrus in dominant hemisphere (Wernicke's area or area 22). Damage may be due to infarction, hemorrhage, tumors, trauma and infections.

Motor Aphasia (Broca's Aphasia)

- Here the comprehension of spoken speech is relatively preserved but the speech is non-fluent. Speech consists of few, poorly articulated words described as telegraphic speech. But the speech is meaningful and allows the patient to communicate with others in spite of deficient word output.
- Naming and writing are also affected.
- Motor aphasia is caused by damage to dominant posterior inferior frontal lobe (Broca's area or area 44). Damage may be due to infarction, hemorrhage, tumors, trauma and infections.

Global Aphasia

- Global aphasia is the most severe form of aphasia, characterized by complete impairment of language — including speaking, understanding, reading, and writing. It is a combination of both sensory and motor aphasia.
- It results from large lesions affecting both Broca's and Wernicke's areas (e.g. massive left MCA ischemic stroke, hemorrhage, severe head trauma, etc.).
- Patients may only produce stereotyped utterances (e.g. "da-da" or expletives).

- Often appear mute or nearly mute with poor or no comprehension.
- May show preserved emotional expressions or automatic phrases.

Anomic Aphasia

- While anomia is a common feature in most aphasia syndromes, it can also manifest as an isolated deficit. Anomic aphasia refers to the condition where patients struggle to name or write the word for a specific item. Despite this difficulty, they can often explain the meaning of the word and recall related words. Their spontaneous speech is characterized by pauses, circumlocution (substituting related words or phrases), and occasional paraphasic errors, but remains fluent with intact repetition and sentence comprehension.
- Circumlocution involves using alternative language or descriptions to compensate for difficulty recalling specific words. For example, if someone cannot recall the word "piano," they might say, "It's a large musical instrument with keys that you play with your fingers."
- Paraphasia involves producing incorrect or unintended words during speech, either phonemically or semantically. For example, if someone intends to say "cat," but instead says "dog," it would be considered a semantic paraphasia (inappropriate word substitution). If they say "tat" instead of "cat," it would be a phonemic paraphasia (sounds similar but incorrect).
- Various associated lesions in different anatomical sites have been identified, including the basal temporal lobe, the anterior inferior temporal lobe, the temporo-parieto-occipital junction, and the inferior parietal lobe.

Summary Table of Aphasias

See **Table 5.9**.

Diagnosis

- Exclude other communication problems such as severe dysarthria, impaired hearing, impaired vision (e.g. when assessing reading), or motor writing ability.
- Detailed neurological examination: Bedside speech assessment includes the following:
- **Spontaneous speech:** Speech is assessed for fluency (ease and rapidity of producing words), number of words spoken, ability to initiate speech, presence of spontaneous paraphasic errors (e.g. "fork" for "spoon"), word-finding pauses, hesitations, and prosody (the emotional intonation of speech).
- **Naming:** the patient is asked to name simple objects such as a key, pencil, coin, watch, parts of the body (nose, ear, chin, fingernail, knuckle), or to name colors.
- **Repetition:** Patients are asked to repeat grammatically complex phrases (e.g. "no ifs, ands, or buts"). Patients with impaired repetition may omit words, change the word order, or commit paraphasic errors.
- **Comprehension:** Patients are asked to point to objects named by the clinician, carry out one-step and multistep commands, and answer simple and complex yes-or-no questions.
- **Reading and writing:** Patients are asked to write spontaneously or to dictation and to read aloud in the language they already know.
- Brain imaging (CT or MRI) to identify the brain pathology.

Treatment

- Treatment of cause
- Speech therapy
- Augmentative communication devices (e.g. a book or communication board that contains pictures or symbols of a patient's daily needs, computer-based devices).

Q. Define headache. Enumerate the causes of headache.

- Headache is defined as "pain located in the head or upper neck, above the orbitomeatal line (imaginary line running from the outer corner of the eye to the center of the external ear canal)" **(Fig. 5.11)**. Pain must be localized above the orbitomeatal line, distinguishing headache from neck or facial pain.
- Headache is a very common complaint reported by patients. Most people experience headache at least once during life.

TABLE 5.9: Summary table of aphasias

Aphasia type	Lesion site	Fluency	Comprehension	Repetition	Naming	Reading	Writing
Broca's (expressive)	Inferior frontal gyrus	Non-fluent	Preserved	Impaired	Impaired	Intact	Impaired
Wernicke's (receptive)	Superior temporal gyrus	Fluent	Impaired	Impaired	Impaired	Impaired	Impaired
Global	Large perisylvian lesion	Non-fluent	Impaired	Impaired	Impaired	Impaired	Impaired
Anomic	Diffuse or temporal lesions	Fluent	Preserved	Intact	Impaired	May or may not be impaired	May or may not be impaired

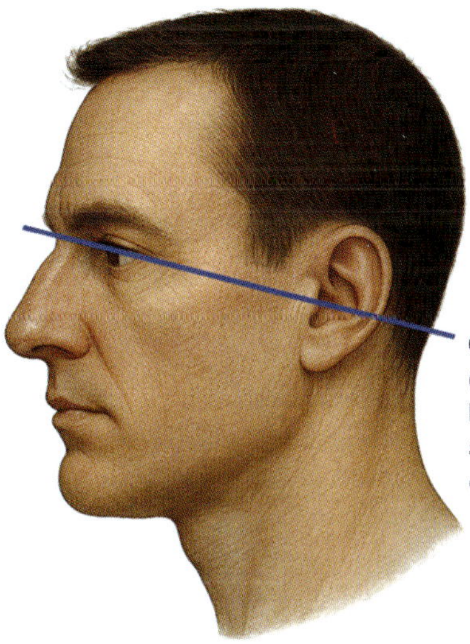

Figure 5.11: Headache area (above orbitomeatal line)

- Most causes of headache are benign, but rarely headache can be due to potentially life-threatening central nervous system (CNS) diseases such as brain tumor, intracranial hemorrhage, etc.

Classification and Causes of Headache

- Headaches are divided into three major categories:

Primary Headache Disorders

Primary headache disorders are defined as headache syndromes that occur independently, meaning they are not caused by any underlying structural, metabolic, or other identifiable medical condition. In these disorders, the headache itself is the primary clinical problem. There is no secondary cause (like trauma, infection, or tumor) responsible for the pain. These include:

- Migraine
- Tension headache
- Cluster headache

Secondary Headache Disorders

Secondary headache disorders are headaches that occur as a result of an underlying condition or external factor, rather than being the primary issue themselves. In other words, the headache is a symptom of another medical problem. These include:

- Head or neck trauma (e.g. post-concussive headache).
- Stroke (intracranial bleed, infarction)
- Intracranial space-occupying lesion (brain abscess, tumor, hematoma, AV malformation)
- Cortical vein thrombosis
- Severe hypertension
- Infection (meningitis, sinusitis)
- Temporal arteritis
- Metabolic disturbances (hypoxia, hypercarbia, hypoglycemia)
- Glaucoma
- Idiopathic intracranial hypertension (pseudotumor cerebri).

Painful Cranial Neuropathies, Other Facial Pain, and Other Headaches

These are headache disorders that involve pain in the cranial nerves or facial structures. These include:

- Trigeminal neuralgia
- Glossopharyngeal neuralgia
- Occipital neuralgia
- Other cranial neuralgias
- Facial pain not associated with headache
- Central causes of facial pain

Q. Describe the classification, pathophysiology, clinical features and treatment of migraine headache.

- Migraine is recurrent headache associated with visual and gastrointestinal disturbance. Though migraine is a benign headache, attacks of headache are usually severe.
- Migraine can be classified into three types:
  - Migraine with aura (old term: classic migraine)
  - Migraine without aura (old term: common migraine)
  - Migraine variants (retinal migraine, ophthalmoplegic migraine, familial hemiplegic migraine, basilar migraine).

Epidemiology

- The prevalence of migraine is high. It is three times more common in women than men. It tends to run in families, and more common in young females. Migraine without aura (common migraine) is the most common type (80% of all migraine cases).

Pathophysiology

- The exact cause of migraine is unknown. However, various theories have been put forward and various brain abnormalities have been found in patients with migraine.
- Migraine has a strong genetic component. Approximately 70% of migraine patients have a first-degree relative with a history of migraine. The risk of migraine is increased 4-fold in relatives of people who have migraine with aura.
- Migraine was previously thought to be a vascular phenomenon that resulted from intracranial vasoconstriction followed by rebound vasodilation. Currently, however, the neurovascular theory considers migraine as primarily a neurogenic process with secondary changes in cerebral perfusion associated with a sterile neurogenic inflammation.
- A phenomenon called cortical spreading depression (CSD) (a wave of neuronal and glial depolarization that slowly spreads across the cerebral cortex) has been found in patients with aura. This cellular depolarization causes aura phase which in turn activates trigeminal fibers, causing the headache phase. Activation of the trigeminovascular system by CSD stimulates nociceptive neurons on dural blood vessels to release plasma proteins and pain-generating substances such as calcitonin gene-related

peptide (CGRP), substance P, vasoactive intestinal peptide, and neurokinin A. The resultant state of sterile inflammation is accompanied by further vasodilation, producing pain. The serotonin receptor (5-hydroxytryptamine [5-HT]) is believed to be the most important receptor in the headache pathway and is found in trigeminal sensory neurons.

- Migraineurs have been found to have neuronal hyperexcitability in the cerebral cortex, especially in the occipital cortex.

Clinical Features

- Three phases of migraine can be recognized:
  - Premonitory symptoms
  - Aura
  - Headache
- ***Premonitory symptoms:*** Precede an attack of migraine. These include fatigue, concentration difficulty, sensitivity to light or sound, nausea, blurred vision, yawning, etc.
- ***Aura:*** Migraine aura is a transient neurologic symptom due to transient focal neurological dysfunction. Auras typically occur before the onset of migraine headache, and the headache usually begins simultaneously with or just after the end of the aura phase. Most auras last for less than one hour. Auras can be visual disturbances (blurring of vision, fortification spectra, light flashes), sensory symptoms, motor weakness and speech disturbances.
- ***Headache:*** it is usually unilateral although it can affect both sides. The pain is usually described as pulsating or throbbing in nature, often severe in intensity. Pain can be debilitating, often making it difficult to perform routine tasks.
- ***Associated symptoms:***
  - Nausea and vomiting: Many individuals experience nausea, and some may vomit during a migraine attack.
  - Photophobia (sensitivity to light) and phonophobia (sensitivity to sound): These are common during a migraine attack, often requiring individuals to seek dark and quiet environments.

IHS (international headache society) criteria to diagnose migraine **(Tables 5.10 and 5.11)**

TABLE 5.10: IHS diagnostic criteria for migraine without aura

A. At least 5 attacks fulfilling criteria B to D
B. Headache attacks lasting 4–72 hours (untreated or unsuccessfully treated)
C. Headache has at least two of the following characteristics:
   1. Unilateral location
   2. Pulsating quality
   3. Moderate or severe pain intensity
   4. Aggravation by or causing avoidance of routine physical activity (e.g. walking or climbing stairs)
D. During headache at least one of the following:
   1. Nausea and/or Vomiting
   2. Photophobia and Phonophobia
E. Not attributed to another disorder

TABLE 5.11: IHS diagnostic criteria for migraine with aura

A. At least 2 attacks fulfilling following criteria (B to C).
B. One or more of the following fully reversible aura symptoms:
   - Visual
   - Sensory
   - Speech and/or language
   - Motor
   - Brainstem
   - Retinal
C. At least 3 of the following 6 characteristics:
   1. At least one aura symptom spreads gradually over ≥5 minutes
   2. Two or more aura symptoms occur in succession
   3. Each individual aura symptom lasts 5–60 minutes
   4. At least one aura symptom is unilateral
   5. At least one aura symptom is positive
   6. Headache appears within 60 minutes of aura symptoms

Migraine Precipitants

Triggers that initiate or start a migraine attack. Knowing the precipitant factors (triggers) helps with prevention or trigger avoidance. Various precipitants of migraine have been identified, which are as follows:

- Hormonal changes, such as those accompanying menstruation (common), pregnancy, and ovulation
- Stress
- Excessive or insufficient sleep
- Excessive exercise
- Eyestrain or other visual triggers
- Medications (e.g. vasodilators, oral contraceptives)
- Exposure to bright or fluorescent lighting
- Loud noises
- Strong odors (e.g. perfumes, colognes, petroleum distillates)
- Weather changes
- Motion sickness
- Certain food items (ice cream, chocolate, cheese)
- Hunger
- Red wine.

Aggravating Factors for Migraine

These are factors that worsen an ongoing migraine attack. Knowing them helps with management during an attack. These include:

- Physical activity
- Exposure to noise or light
- Coughing or straining
- Head movement
- Strong odors.

Investigations

- Migraine is a clinical diagnosis. Hence, investigations are ordered only if an organic pathology is suspected or to rule out any comorbid illness.
- ***Routine blood tests:*** Severe anemia can sometimes cause headache. High ESR is seen in giant cell arteritis (temporal arteritis) which can mimic migraine.

- ***Neuroimaging (CT or MRI of head)***: This is not routinely necessary. It is indicated in following situations: first or worst severe headache, change in the pattern of previous migraine, abnormal neurologic examination, onset of migraine after age 50 years, in immunocompromised patient, headache with fever, and migraine with epilepsy.
- ***Lumbar Puncture:*** is indicated in following situations: First or worst headache of a patient's life (suggests subarachnoid hemorrhage), progressive headache, unresponsive, chronic, intractable headache.
- ***Calcitonin gene-related peptide (CGRP):*** Serum level of CGRP is elevated in most migraine patients. It is a neurotransmitter that causes vasodilation and can aid in the diagnosis of chronic migraine by serving as a biomarker for permanent trigeminovascular activation.

Management

Treatment of an Acute Attack (abortive therapy)

- ***First line:*** Paracetamol or any other simple analgesics should be given, with an antiemetic such as domperidone if necessary. Analgesics are more effective if started in the beginning of headache.
- ***Triptans (5-HT agonists)*** can also abort an attack. These include sumatriptan, zolmitriptan, naratriptan and rizatriptan. Contraindicated in cardiovascular disease, uncontrolled hypertension, and hemiplegic or basilar migraine.
- ***Ditans:*** This is new class of drugs which are serotonin 5-HT1F receptor agonists. The advantage of ditans over triptans is that they do not cause vasoconstriction, hence safe in patients with cardiovascular disease and uncontrolled hypertension. *Examples*: Lasmiditan.
- ***CGRP antagonists (gepants):*** These are also a new class of drugs. Examples are ubrogepant and rimegepant. Useful in patients who cannot tolerate triptans or have cardiovascular contraindications.
- ***Ergot alkaloids:*** Less commonly used today due to side effects such as prominent vasoconstriction. *Examples*: Ergotamine, dihydroergotamine.
- During an attack rest in a dark and quiet room.
- For more details of abortive therapy *see* below.

Prophylaxis

- Migraine prophylaxis involves using medications regularly to reduce the frequency, severity, and duration of migraine attacks and improve the patient's quality of life. It is not used for aborting acute attacks, but for long-term management.

Indications for prophylaxis

- ≥4 migraine days/month
- ≥2 attacks/month that are disabling
- Poor response or contraindication to acute medications
- Patient preference or overuse of acute meds
- Hemiplegic, basilar-type, or prolonged aura migraines

Medications for prophylaxis

- Avoid precipitating factors.
- Beta-blockers such as atenolol, metoprolol, and propranolol. Propranolol 40–120 mg in divided doses. Useful in patients with coexisting hypertension or anxiety, because these drugs can treat both migraine and hypertension simultaneously.
- Antidepressants: Amitriptyline, clomipramine, mirtazapine, venlafaxine. Good for comorbid anxiety/depression.
- Calcium-channel blockers: Verapamil, nifedipine. Useful for patients with comorbid hypertension.
- Antiepileptics: Sodium valproate, topiramate. Especially useful for patients with comorbid epilepsy.
- Calcitonin gene-related peptide (CGRP) inhibitors: Erenumab, fremanezumab, galcanezumab, eptinezumab.

Duration of prophylaxis

- Typically continued for 6–12 months, then reassess. Gradually taper, if migraines are well controlled.

For more details on prophylactic therapy, see subsequent pages

Q. Describe the indications, pharmacology, dose, side effects of abortive therapy in migraine.

Indications for Abortive (acute) therapy in Migraine

- Relieve an ongoing migraine attack.
- Stop progression from mild to severe attack. Abortive medications are most effective when taken early in the attack.

Main Classes of Abortive Drugs

NSAIDs

- *Pharmacology*: Inhibit cyclo-oxygenase → ↓ prostaglandins → ↓ inflammation and pain.
- *Examples/doses*:
  - Paracetamol, 650 mg 3–4 times daily.
  - Aceclofenac 100 mg PO
  - Ibuprofen, 400–600 mg PO
  - Naproxen, 500–550 mg PO
  - Diclofenac, 50–100 mg PO or suppository
  - For moderate to severe headache, some of the above drugs can be given IM (paracetamol, diclofenac).
- *Side effects*: Gastric irritation, dyspepsia, GI bleeding, renal impairment.

Triptans

- *Pharmacology*: Selective 5-HT1B/1D agonists. Reduce pain by causing vasoconstriction of cranial vessels, and inhibition of trigeminal nerve activation.
- *Examples/doses*:
  - Sumatriptan 50–100 mg PO or 6 mg SC or intranasal spray.
  - Rizatriptan 10 mg PO
  - Zolmitriptan 2.5–5 mg PO

- Eletriptan 40 mg PO
- Naratriptan 2.5 mg PO
- *Side effects*: Chest tightness, flushing, dizziness, drowsiness. Contraindicated in ischemic heart disease, stroke, uncontrolled hypertension.

Triptans with NSAIDs

- The best-studied combination is sumatriptan-naproxen. This combination is more effective than either drug used alone.
- Other combinations include rizatriptan plus acetaminophen and frovatriptan plus dexketoprofen.

Ergot Derivatives

- *Pharmacology*: Non-selective 5-HT1 agonists and vasoconstrictors.
- *Examples/doses*:
  - Ergotamine tartrate 1–2 mg sublingual.
  - Dihydroergotamine (DHE) 1 mg IM/SC/IV or nasal spray.
- *Side effects*: Nausea, vomiting, vasospasm. Contraindicated in pregnancy, IHD, peripheral vascular disease, and uncontrolled hypertension.

Antiemetics

- *Pharmacology*: Dopamine receptor antagonists. These drugs can be used along with other agents or as monotherapy for acute migraine headache.
- *Examples/doses*:
  - Domperidone 10 mg PO
  - Metoclopramide 10 mg IV
  - Prochlorperazine 10 mg IV or IM
- *Side effects*: Drowsiness, extrapyramidal symptoms, QT prolongation.

CGRP Antagonists

- *Pharmacology*: They modulate calcitonin gene-related peptide (CGRP) activity which reduces trigeminovascular pain transmission in migraine.
- *Examples/doses*:
  - Ubrogepant, 50 or 100 mg oral. The dose may be repeated in two hours with a maximum daily dose of 200 mg.
  - Rimegepant, 75 mg PO.
  - Zavegepant, 10 mg intranasally as a single spray.
- *Side effects*: Nausea, somnolence, dry mouth. worsening hypertension and Raynaud's phenomenon.

Ditans (Lasmiditan)

- *Pharmacology*: Lasmiditan is a selective serotonin 1F receptor agonist that lacks vasoconstrictor activity and therefore can be used for patients with relative contraindications to triptans due to cardiovascular risk factors.
- *Dose*: 50 or 100 mg PO.
- *Side effects*: Dizziness, paresthesia, somnolence, fatigue, and nausea. Patients should avoid driving after taking this drug.

Q. Describe the indications, pharmacology, dose, side effects of prophylactic therapy in migraine.

Indications for Prophylaxis

- ≥4 migraine days/month
- ≥2 attacks/month that are disabling
- Poor response or contraindication to acute medications
- Patient preference or overuse of acute meds
- Hemiplegic, basilar-type, or prolonged aura migraines.

Pharmacology of Common Prophylactic Agents

Beta-blockers

- *Pharmacology*: Block β-adrenergic receptors, modulating vascular tone and reducing cortical excitability.
- *Examples/dose*
  - Propranolol: 40–160 mg/day (divided doses)
  - Metoprolol: 50–200 mg/day
- *Side effects*: Fatigue, hypotension, bradycardia, depression, cold extremities, contraindicated in asthma.

Antiepileptics

- *Pharmacology*: Enhance GABAergic inhibition and inhibit excitatory neurotransmission.
- *Examples/dose*
  - Topiramate: Start at 25 mg/day, titrate to 50–100 mg/day.
  - Valproate: 500–1000 mg/day.
- *Side effects*
  - Topiramate: Weight loss (topiramate), paresthesia, cognitive issues, kidney stones.
  - Valproate: Teratogenicity, weight gain, hepatotoxicity.

Tricyclic Antidepressants

- *Pharmacology*: Inhibits reuptake of serotonin and norepinephrine.
- *Examples/dose*
  - Amitriptyline: 10–25 mg at bedtime, titrate up to 75–150 mg/day.
- *Side effects*: Sedation, dry mouth, constipation, weight gain, orthostatic hypotension.

Calcium Channel Blockers

- *Pharmacology*: Inhibits calcium influx, stabilizes vascular tone.
- *Examples/dose*:
  - Flunarizine: 5–10 mg daily at night.
  - Verapamil: 120–240 mg daily oral in divided doses.
- *Side effects*: Weight gain, depression, fatigue, constipation, bradycardia.

CGRP (Calcitonin Gene-related Peptide) Antagonists

Pharmacology: Inhibit CGRP receptor or ligand, involved in migraine pathogenesis.

Monoclonal antibodies against CGRP

- *Examples/dose*:
  - Erenumab: 70–140 mg subcutaneously once monthly
  - Fremanezumab: 225 mg monthly or 675 mg every 3 months
- *Side effects*: Injection site reactions, constipation, hypertension (erenumab).

CGRP receptor antagonist

- *Rimegepant*: 75 mg every other day
- *Side effects*: Nausea, somnolence, dry mouth. worsening hypertension and Raynaud's phenomenon.

Q. Differences between migraine with aura (classical) and migraine without aura (nonclassical migraine) (Table 5.12).

TABLE 5.12: Differences between migraine with aura and migraine without aura

Feature	Migraine with aura (classical migraine)	Migraine without aura (nonclassical or common migraine)
Aura	Present (visual, sensory, speech, etc.)	Absent
Headache onset	During or after aura	Begins without warning
Visual symptoms	Common (flashing lights, zig zag lines, scotoma)	Rare
Sensory/speech disturbance	May be present	Usually absent
Prevalence	~25–30% of migraine cases	~70–75% of migraine cases
Risk of stroke	Slightly higher	Lower

Q. Cluster headache.

- The definition of cluster headaches is a unilateral headache with at least one autonomic symptom ipsilateral to the headache.
- Cluster headache (CH) is characterized by repetitive headaches that occur for weeks to months at a time (i.e. occurring in clusters), followed by periods of remission.

Etiology

- The exact cause of CH is unknown. The disorder is sporadic but rarely can be inherited.
- Several factors can provoke CH attacks. Subcutaneous injection of histamine provokes attacks in many patients. Stress, allergens, seasonal changes, or nitroglycerin and alcohol may trigger attacks. Many patients with CH are heavy smokers and alcoholics.

Pathophysiology

- The exact pathophysiology of CH is incompletely understood. There is involvement of the trigeminovascular system and the parasympathetic nerve fibers. Vasodilatation may be responsible for the pain and autonomic features of cluster headaches.
- Some studies have shown a defect in the central pathway of pain control and autonomic nervous system dysregulation leading to dysfunction in supraspinal control of pain and cognitive processing.
- Activation of hypothalamus has been noted during the attack of headache.

Clinical Features

- It usually affects males between 30 and 40.
- Headache is strictly unilateral, usually deep, excruciating, felt around one eye and may last for several hours. Headaches occur every day usually at the same time. They most often occur at night usually one to two hours after going to bed. Most attacks are episodic, with daily attacks for weeks to months (cluster), followed by a remission for months to years.
- CH is associated with ipsilateral autonomic symptoms such as lacrimation and redness of the eye, stuffy nose, rhinorrhea, sweating, pallor, and Horner's syndrome **(Fig. 5.12)**.
- Nausea and vomiting can also occur.
- Diagnostic criteria for cluster headache **(Table 5.13)**.

TABLE 5.13: Diagnostic criteria for cluster headache

A. At least five attacks fulfilling criteria B–D

B. Severe or very severe unilateral orbital, supraorbital, and/or temporal pain lasting 15–180 minutes (when untreated)

C. The headache is accompanied by at least one of the following ipsilateral symptoms:
- Conjunctival injection and/or lacrimation
- Nasal congestion and/or rhinorrhea
- Eyelid edema
- Forehead and facial sweating
- Miosis and/or ptosis
- A sense of restlessness or agitation

D. Attack frequency: From one every other day to 8 per day

E. Not better accounted for by another diagnosis

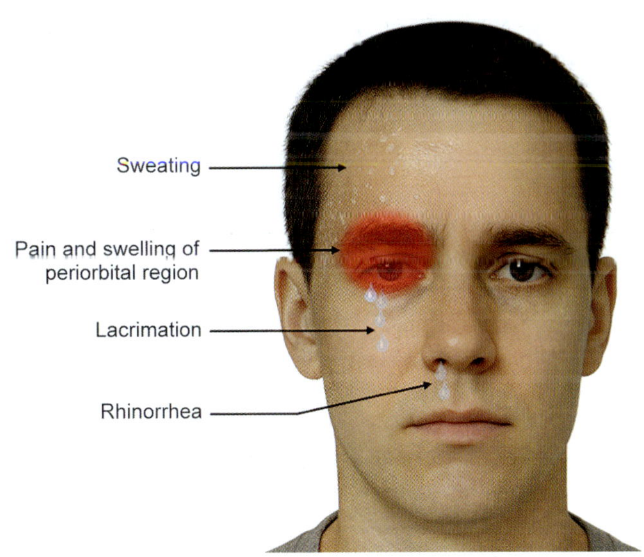

Figure 5.12: Clinical features of cluster headache

Treatment

Acute Attack

- Oxygen inhalation (100% oxygen via a face mask) is the most effective therapy. It is effective in less than 10 minutes.
- Triptans (e.g. sumatriptan, 6 mg subcutaneously) can also be used to abort an attack.
- Dihydroergotamine can be an effective abortive agent.

Prevention of Attacks

- The best treatment is to prevent cluster attacks until the bout is over by using prophylactic medications.
- Prophylactic drugs are verapamil, prednisolone, lithium, methysergide, ergotamine, and sodium valproate. Verapamil is the most widely prescribed prophylactic drug. A 10-day course of prednisone, beginning at 60 mg daily for 7 days followed by a rapid taper, may prevent headache.
- Ergotamine can also prevent the attacks if given 1–2 hours before an expected attack. Various invasive nerve blocks and ablative neurosurgical procedures (e.g. percutaneous radiofrequency ablation, trigeminal gangliorhizolysis, and rhizotomy) can be considered in refractory CH.

Q. Enumerate the indications for emergency care admission and describe Immediate supportive care in patients with headache.

Indications for Emergency Care Admission in Patients with Headache

A patient with headache should be admitted to the emergency department (ED) for urgent evaluation and management if any of the following red flag features are present:

- **Sudden onset ("Thunderclap headache"):** Severe headache reaching peak intensity within seconds to minutes → Suspect subarachnoid hemorrhage (SAH).
- **Altered mental status or loss of consciousness:** Suggests raised ICP, encephalitis, or intracranial bleeding.
- **Meningeal signs:** Fever, neck stiffness, photophobia → Meningitis or encephalitis.
- **Focal neurological deficits:** Weakness, aphasia, vision changes → Stroke, mass lesion, or CNS infection.
- **Seizures:** First-time seizure or new-onset seizure with headache.
- **Papilledema:** Sign of raised intracranial pressure.
- **New headache in immunocompromised patients:** Risk of opportunistic infections or malignancy (e.g. cryptococcal meningitis, CNS lymphoma).
- **Headache with systemic signs:** Fever, weight loss, myalgia → Suggests giant cell arteritis, infection, or malignancy.
- **New or different headache in pregnancy/postpartum:** Risk of preeclampsia/eclampsia, cortical venous sinus thrombosis.
- **Headache after trauma:** Rule out intracranial hemorrhage.

Immediate Supportive Care in Patients with Headache

Once admitted for evaluation of headache, immediate supportive care involves the following:

Airway, Breathing, Circulation (ABC)

- Ensure patient is stable.
- Provide oxygen if hypoxic.
- IV access for fluids and medications.

Pain Control

- Paracetamol or NSAIDs (if no contraindications)
- Antiemetics if nausea/vomiting is present.

Neurological Monitoring

- Regular checks of **Glasgow Coma Scale (GCS)**
- Look for evolving signs of raised ICP or seizures.

Seizure Precautions

- If history of seizure or at risk (e.g. encephalitis, SAH), consider prophylactic **antiepileptics.**
- Keep suction, oxygen, and benzodiazepines ready.

Manage Raised Intracranial Pressure (if suspected)

- Head elevation (30 degrees)
- Avoid hypotension or hypoxia
- Consider mannitol or hypertonic saline if signs of herniation.

Treat Underlying Cause Promptly

- **Antibiotics/antivirals** if meningitis suspected.
- **Antihypertensives** in hypertensive emergency.
- **Steroids** for giant cell arteritis.
- **Neurosurgical consult** if mass lesion or hydrocephalus suspected.

Q. Enumerate the causes of facial pain.

Causes of Facial Pain

- Trigeminal neuralgia
- Postherpetic neuralgia
- Glossopharyngeal neuralgia
- Occipital neuralgia
- Superior laryngeal neuralgia
- Carotodynia
- Carotid artery dissection
- Posttraumatic facial pain
- Sinusitis
- Dental pain
- Persistent idiopathic (atypical) facial pain
- Thalamic pain
- Cancer

Q. Discuss the etiology, clinical features and management of trigeminal neuralgia (tic douloureux).

- Trigeminal neuralgia (TN) is a chronic pain condition affecting the trigeminal nerve.

- It is characterized by recurrent episodes of sudden, severe, usually unilateral, brief, stabbing or electric shock like pain in the distribution of one or more branches of the trigeminal nerve.

Epidemiology

- The annual incidence of TN is 4–5 per lakh population.
- It is one of the most common causes of facial pain in the elderly. Most cases begin after age 50.
- It is slightly more common in women.

Etiopathogenesis

- Most cases of trigeminal neuralgia are caused by compression of the trigeminal nerve root.
- Compression by an aberrant loop of an artery (often by a loop of the superior cerebellar artery) accounts for 80–90% of cases. Other causes of nerve compression include acoustic neuroma, meningioma, epidermoid cyst, saccular aneurysm or arteriovenous malformation.
- Compression leads to demyelination of the nerve in the area around the compression. Demyelination results in ectopic impulse generation and crossing of impulses between fibers. Touch sensation impulses may cross into fibers carrying pain sensation and lead to pain.
- Demyelination may also be caused by multiple sclerosis and lead to trigeminal neuralgia.

Clinical Features

- The pain of trigeminal neuralgia occurs in paroxysms and is maximal at the onset.
- The pain is described as "electric shock-like" or "stabbing" and is unilateral in most cases.
- Pain occurs along the distribution of one or more sensory divisions of the trigeminal nerve, most often the maxillary (**Fig. 5.13**).
- It usually lasts from one to several seconds, and does not awaken the patient at night. Episodes may last weeks or months.

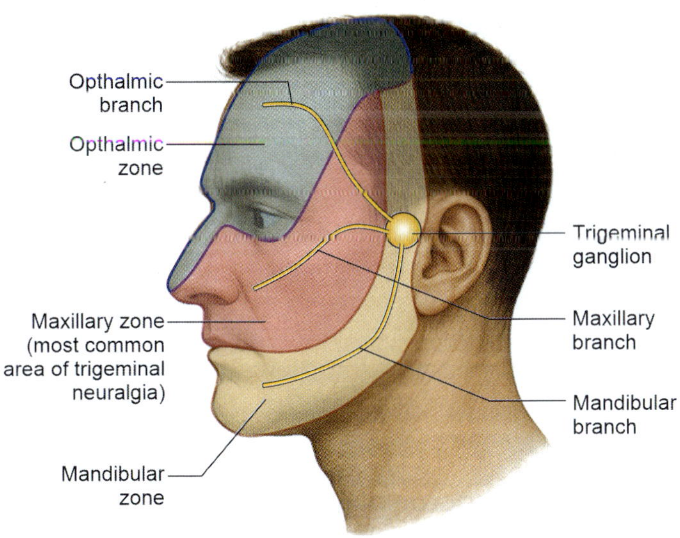

Figure 5.13: Areas of pain in trigeminal neuralgia

- Facial muscle spasms can be seen with severe pain. This finding gave rise to the older term for this disorder, "tic douloureux."
- Trigger zones in the distribution of the affected nerve may be present; lightly touching these areas often triggers an attack. Other triggers include chewing, talking, brushing teeth, cold air, smiling, and shaving.

Investigations

- ***Magnetic resonance imaging/magnetic resonance angiography (MRI/MRA)*** can identify demyelinating lesions, a mass lesion in the cerebellopontine angle, or an ectatic blood vessel which may be responsible for trigeminal neuralgia.
- These investigations are especially indicated for patients with sensory loss and young patients (under the age of 40).

Treatment

- ***Medical therapy:*** Pharmacologic therapy is the initial treatment for most patients with trigeminal neuralgia that is not caused by a structural lesion. Carbamazepine is the drug of choice. Other effective drugs are sodium valproate, phenytoin, baclofen, or clonazepam. Newer antiepileptic drugs such as gabapentin, lamotrigine, and topiramate are also effective. Patients who fail to respond to medication should be considered for microvascular decompression surgery.
- ***Surgical therapy:*** Surgery is reserved for patients who are refractory to medical therapy. A variety of surgical procedures may relieve symptoms in patients refractory to drug therapy. These include, microvascular decompression (involves the removal or separation of vascular structures, often an ectatic superior cerebellar artery, from the trigeminal nerve). Immediate postoperative relief is found in most patients. Percutaneous radiofrequency rhizotomy creates a lesion in the gasserian ganglion of the trigeminal nerve by application of heat. The lesion is thought to selectively destroy pain impulses carried by unmyelinated or thinly myelinated fibers. Other options are gamma knife radiosurgery, glycerol injection or balloon compression.

Q. Glossopharyngeal neuralgia.

- Glossopharyngeal neuralgia is defined as paroxysmal pain in areas innervated by cranial nerves IX and X.

Etiology

- The usual cause of glossopharyngeal neuralgia appears to be microvascular compression, although abscess and tumor are sometimes associated.

Clinical Features

- The pain is paroxysmal, unilateral, sudden in onset, has a jabbing or briefly persistent quality.
- The pain is felt in or around the ear, tongue, jaw, or larynx and it can be triggered by chewing,

swallowing, coughing, speaking, yawning, certain tastes, or touching the neck or external auditory canal.
- Many attacks may occur in a day and may awaken sufferers from sleep. Severe attacks have rarely been associated with bradycardia/asystole resulting in syncope presumably because of intense glossopharyngeal outflow and vagal efferent discharge.

Investigations

- MRI/MRA to rule out a mass lesion or vascular pathology.

Treatment

- Medical treatment is similar to that for trigeminal neuralgia and includes carbamazepine, gabapentin, or baclofen.
- Cases refractory to adequate medical treatment often respond to microvascular decompression.

Q. Postherpetic neuralgia (PHN).

- Postherpetic neuralgia (PHN) refers to pain persisting beyond 3 months after an attack of herpes zoster.

Clinical Features

- The probability of developing postherpetic neuralgia (PHN) increases with advanced age.
- The pain is described as "burning" or brief, recurrent, electric shock like sensation. Most patients have allodynia, defined as pain evoked by nonpainful stimuli such as light touch.
- Patients often have areas of decreased sensation within the affected dermatomes.

Treatment

- There are many ways of treating postherpetic neuralgia: antidepressants (amitryptaline, nortryptaline), analgesics (aspirin, ibuprofen), capsaicin, topical anesthetics, anticonvulsants (carbamazepine, gabapentin), intrathecal corticosteroids, NMDA receptor antagonists (ketamine and dextromethorphan), cryotherapy, and surgery (anterolateral cordotomy, and electrocoagulation of the dorsal root).

Q. Idiopathic intracranial hypertension (pseudotumor cerebri).

- Idiopathic intracranial hypertension (IIH) (pseudotumor cerebri) is a disorder of unknown etiology characterized by elevated intracranial pressure, headache and papilledema.

Etiology

- There is no hydrocephalus or an identifiable cause for increased CSF pressure. Raised intracranial pressure probably results from obstruction of cerebral venous outflow probably because of smaller venous sinuses.
- Strong association with obesity.
- In children, this disorder sometimes develops after corticosteroids are stopped or after growth hormone is used. IIH may also develop after tetracyclines or large amounts of vitamin A are taken.

Clinical Features

- Most cases occur in young women who are obese. Patients with higher body mass indexes (BMIs) and recent weight gain are at increased risk.
- Patients with IIH usually present with symptoms related to increased intracranial pressure and papilledema.
- *Symptoms of increased intracranial pressure:* Diffuse headache worsened by coughing and straining, and worse in the morning. Diplopia can occur due to increased intracranial pressure causing abducent nerve palsy. Tinnitus (pulsatile) can be there and is often described as hearing one's heartbeat in the ear.
- *Symptoms due to papilledema:* Transient visual disturbances, enlarged blind spots and loss of peripheral visual fields. Optic atrophy can lead to permanent loss of vision.

Diagnosis

- The diagnosis is made by lumbar puncture (CSF pressure higher than 250 mm H_2O).
- Normal CSF composition.
- Normal MRI brain with magnetic resonance venography to exclude other pathologies.
- No localizing neurological signs (except abducens nerve palsy).

Treatment

- Weight reduction can help to some extent.
- Intracranial pressure should be reduced to prevent visual loss. Drugs to reduce intracranial pressure include acetazolamide and furosemide.
- Repeated lumbar punctures may be useful, if drug treatment is ineffective.
- If all these measures fail, surgical options include optic nerve sheath fenestration and ventricular-peritoneal shunting of CSF.
- Spontaneous recovery may sometimes occur.

Q. Describe the course of facial nerve. Enumerate the causes and clinical features of facial nerve palsy at various levels.

Facial nerve is a mixed nerve, but predominantly motor. It contains:

- Motor fibers: Innervates muscles of facial expression, the stapedius muscle in the ear, and the posterior belly of the digastric and stylohyoid muscles.
- Parasympathetic fibers to the lacrimal, submandibular, and sublingual salivary glands.
- Afferent fibers for taste from the anterior two thirds of the tongue via the chorda tympani.
- Somatic afferents from the external auditory canal and pinna.

Pathway of Facial Nerve

Origin and Intracranial Course

- Facial nerve originates from multiple brainstem nuclei that are functionally specialized. It begins as two roots; a large motor root arises from the motor nucleus in the pons, and a small sensory root (sensory root is sometimes known as nervus intermedius) arises from the pontomedullary junction.

- After arising, axons of the facial nerve travel dorsomedially and encircle the abducens nucleus and exit from the anterior aspect of pons **(Fig. 5.14)**.
- The motor root and the nervus intermedius then pass through the posterior cranial fossa along with 8th cranial nerve at the cerebellopontine angle, and finally all the three enter into the internal acoustic meatus in the temporal bone. The two roots of facial nerve remain separate till they reach the internal acoustic meatus, but fuse inside the internal acoustic meatus to form facial nerve proper.

Intratemporal Course

- *Facial canal*: Within the temporal bone, the facial nerve travels through the facial canal (also known as the Fallopian canal). Facial canal is a 'Z' shaped structure and is the longest bony canal for any nerve. Within the facial canal, three important events occur:
- Firstly the two roots fuse to form the facial nerve.
- Next, the nerve forms the geniculate ganglion.
- Lastly, the nerve gives rise to:
  - Greater petrosal nerve—parasympathetic fibers to mucous glands and lacrimal gland.
  - Nerve to stapedius—motor fibers to stapedius muscle of the middle ear.
  - Chorda tympani—special sensory fibers to the anterior 2/3rd tongue and parasympathetic fibers to the submandibular and sublingual glands.

Extracranial Course

- Facial nerve exits the skull via the stylomastoid foramen, Just after exit, it gives out posterior auricular, digastric, and stylohyoid branches.
- The nerve then turns forward and enters the parotid gland and gives out following branches which innervate the muscles of facial expression, stylohyoid, and posterior belly of the digastric.
  - Temporal
  - Zygomatic
  - Buccal
  - Mandibular
  - Cervical
- The nervus intermedius (NI) is the sensory and autonomic component of the facial nerve. It runs in between 7th and 8th nerve (hence called nervus intermedius) across the CP angle and enters into internal auditory meatus and then it enters the facial canal. Nervus intermedius joins facial nerve at the geniculate ganglion. Nervus intermedius carries general sensation from external auditory canal and tympanic membrane, and special sensation of taste from the anterior two-thirds of the tongue. Nervus intermedius also carries parasympathetic fibers from the superior salivatory and lacrimal nuclei, to submandibular, sublingual, submaxillary glands, and the lacrimal glands.

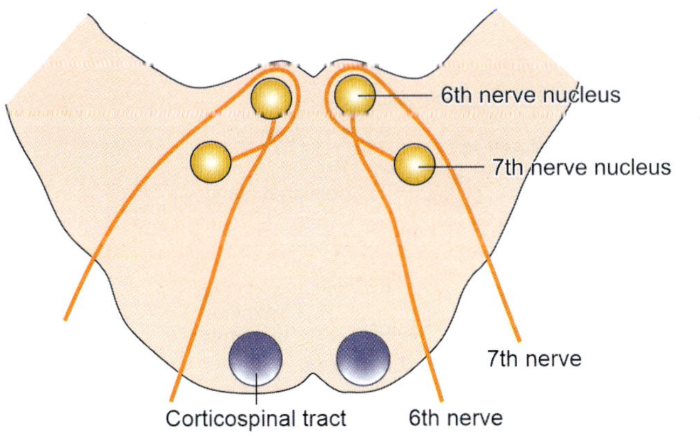

Figure 5.14: Cross section of pons showing origin of facial nerve

Causes and Clinical Features of Facial Nerve Lesions at Various Levels (Table 5.14)

- LMN facial palsy implies a lesion involving the facial nerve at the nucleus in the pons or along the course of the facial nerve ipsilateral to the side of facial weakness. Facial muscle weakness is same with lesions anywhere along the course of the nerve. Localization depends on the associated findings, such as hyperacusis, decreased tearing, impaired taste, and involvement of neural structures in addition to facial weakness. The dictum in neurology "TELL ME WHO YOUR FRIENDS ARE, I WILL TELL YOU WHO YOU ARE" applies very well in localizing the level of facial nerve palsy by looking for the associated signs of facial nerve palsy.
- It is easy to understand and localize the site of LMN lesion if you start from peripheral branches of nerve facial nerve and move upwards till the facial nucleus in the pons.

Clinical Features of LMN Facial Palsy

- Unilateral LMN lesion causes weakness of both upper and lower face on the same side of lesion.
- Drooping of angle of mouth, dribbling of saliva from the angle of mouth, deviation of mouth to normal side.
- There is weakness of frowning (frontalis) and of eye closure since upper facial muscles are weak.
- Corneal exposure and ulceration may occur due to inability of the eyes to close during sleep.
- The platysma muscle is also weak.

Clinical Features of UMN Facial Palsy

- In UMN lesions only the lower part of face is affected and upper part is spared because of bilateral hemispheric representation. Hence, raising eyebrows, wrinkling of forehead, eye closure and blinking are all preserved.
- Clinical features in the lower part of the face are same as those described in LMN facial palsy.

Bilateral UMN Type Facial Palsy

- Cerebrovascular accidents disrupting bilateral corticonuclear fibers.

TABLE 5.14: Causes and clinical features of facial nerve lesions at various levels

Level of lesion	Clinical features	Causes
Facial nerve or its branches after emergence from stylomastoid foramen *(Site A in Fig. 5.15)*	Only ipsilateral facial muscle weakness is seen without any accompanying findings, involvement may be partial because of selective involvement of certain branches of the parotid plexus.	Parotid tumor or abscess, trauma
At or just above the stylomastoid foramen *(Site B in Fig. 5.15)*	It causes weakness of all facial muscles supplied by facial nerve.	Bell's palsy, geniculate herpes (Ramsay-Hunt syndrome), Guillain-Barré syndrome, petrous bone fracture, neoplasm, diabetes mellitus, sarcoidosis, Lyme disease, HIV infection
Above the origin of chorda tympani, but below the origin of nerve to stapedius *(Site C in Fig. 5.15)*	Weakness of facial muscles plus reduced salivation and reduction of taste sensations in the anterior two-third of the tongue. There is no hyperacusis as the lesion is below the origin of nerve to stapedius thus sparing it.	Same as above
Above the origin of nerve to stapedius but below the level of geniculate ganglion *(Site D in Fig. 5.15)*:	All the signs and symptoms of lesion B plus hyperacusis (i.e. increased susceptibility to hearing).	Same as above
Site D at the level of geniculate ganglion: *(Site E in Fig. 5.15)*	All the signs and symptoms of lesion C plus reduction of lacrimation due to additional involvement of greater superficial petrosal nerve which supplies lacrimal gland.	Same as above
Cerebellopontine angle or cisternal course, just peripheral to the pons or between the pons and the facial canal *(Site F in Fig. 5.15)*	Tinnitus, deafness and vertigo (7th nerve involvement), facial pain or sensory dysfunction (5th nerve involvement), loss of taste on the anterior two-thirds of the tongue, decreased salivary and lacrimal secretion (nervus intermedius involvement), hyperacusis (lesion proximal to stapedius branch), ipsilateral ataxia and nystagmus (involvement of the cerebellum or cerebellar connections)	Neoplasm (especially acoustic neuroma), cholesteatoma, head trauma, meningeal inflammation or infiltration
Pons (facial nucleus and fascicle)	Although involvement of only facial nerve nucleus can occur rarely in pontine leisons, usually other structures in the pons also often get involved which provide clue to the pontine level of facial nerve palsy. Associated features to look for are horizontal gaze palsy from ipsilateral 6th nerve nuclear involvement, and contralateral hemiparesis from corticospinal tract involvement. Other possible associations are contralateral ataxia, ipsilateral Horner syndrome, and ipsilateral loss of taste (involvement of nucleus tractus solitaries) and facial sensation (involvement of 5th nerve nucleus).	Infarction, hemorrhage, neoplasm, syringobulbia, abscess, central pontine myelinolysis, tuberculoma, granuloma, trauma, multiple sclerosis; other demyelinating disorders.

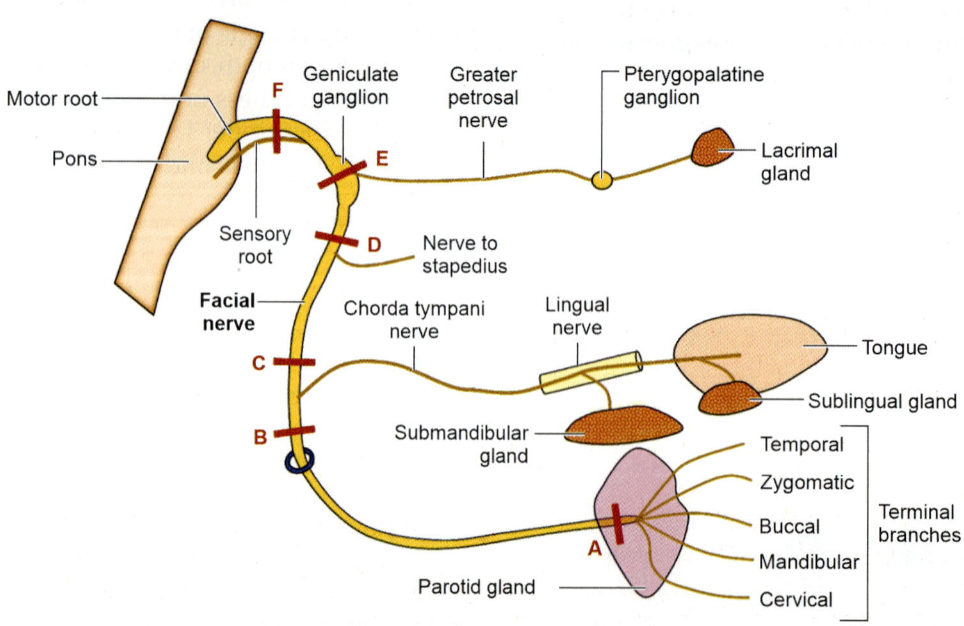

Figure 5.15: Facial nerve course and lesions at various levels (red lines)

- Pseudobulbar palsy
- Brainstem encephalitis
- Demyelinating lesions
- Motor neuron disease.

Bilateral LMN Type Facial Palsy

- ***Muscle diseases:*** Facioscapulohumeral dystrophy, myotonic dystrophy, congential myopathies.
- ***Neuromuscular junction involvement***: Myasthenia gravis, botulism, OP compound poisoning.
- ***Peripheral nerves:*** Guillain-Barré syndrome (Miller fisher variant), Lyme's disease, sarcoidosis, HIV, mumps, amyloidosis, SJS (Sjögren syndrome), acute porphyria, bilateral Bell's palsy (rare).

How to Differentiate Bilateral LMN from Bilateral UMN Facial Palsy

See **Table 5.15.**

TABLE 5.15

	Bilateral LMN facial palsy	Bilateral UMN facial palsy
Upper half of the face	Involved	Involved
Facial reflexes (corneal reflex)	Absent	Present
Emotional facial movements	Absent	Present
Pseudobulbar affect	Absent	May be present
Jaw jerk	Present or absent	Brisk
Other deep tendon reflexes	Absent	Exagereated due to bilateral cortcospinal tract involvement

Features of Chronic LMN Facial Palsy

- *Crocodile tears*: During regrowth of damaged facial nerve fibers, some fibers originally connected with salivary glands, may erroneously connect with lacrimal gland. In such instances patients will shed tears while eating. This is known as crocodile tear syndrome, or Bogorad's syndrome or gustatolacrimal reflex.
- *Retraction of mouth on closure of eyes*: Other example of synkinesis is when the nerves controlling the eye muscles misdirect and regrow connections with the muscles of the mouth. Abnormal movement or different facial muscle group occurs afterwards, since movement of one muscle can now affect the other one. For example, the corner of the mouth can involuntarily lift when the affected individual closes the eye.
- *Jaw winking*: Involuntary closure of eye on lateral movement of the jaw.

Q. Discuss the etiology, clinical features, investigations and management of Bell's palsy.

- Bell's palsy is an acute, idiopathic, LMN type facial palsy. It is the most common cause of unilateral facial paralysis.

Etiology

- Exact cause is unknown.
- It is thought to be due to a viral (often herpes simplex virus-1) infection that causes swelling of the nerve within the facial canal leading to compression of the nerve. Compression of the nerve often occurs at the geniculate ganglion.

Clinical Features

- Patient notices sudden unilateral facial weakness.
- Weakness is LMN type (*see* above for clinical features of LMN facial palsy). Bell's phenomenon is uprolling of eye balls when patient tries to close the eyes.
- Loss of taste (anterior 2/3rd of tongue—via chorda tympani).
- Hyperacusis (paralysis of stapedius).
- Decreased lacrimation.
- Eye irritation or dryness (due to reduced blinking/ closure).
- Weakness progresses over hours or several days. Spontaneous recovery usually starts in the second week. Complete recovery may take 12 months.
- Some patients may be left with residual weakness.

Investigations

- Nerve conduction studies and electromyography (EMG) can be used to assess the severity of lesion and chances of recovery.
- Imaging studies: imaging is indicated if the physical signs are atypical, there is slow progression beyond three weeks, or if there is no improvement at six months. High resolution CT scanning and MRI can be used to rule out other causes of facial palsy such as tumors or vascular events. Pathological geniculate ganglion enhancement is seen in Bell's palsy.

Treatment

- Steroids (prednisolone 60 mg daily tapered over 10 days) is the drug of choice. Antivirals such as acyclovir along with steroids dos not provide any additional benefit compared to steroids alone but can be considered in severe cases.
- Eyes should be protected by applying artificial tears or tarsorrhaphy (suturing the upper to lower eyelid).
- Facial nerve stimulation is useful within two weeks if surgical decompression is planned. Severe degeneration of the facial nerve is irreversible after two to three weeks.
- Surgical decompression of the facial nerve is not a currently recommended treatment. Decompression may be of benefit in patients with profound nerve dysfunction.

Q. Ramsay-Hunt syndrome (Herpes zoster oticus).

- Ramsay-Hunt syndrome (RHS) is a viral neuropathy caused by the reactivation of the varicella-zoster virus (the same virus that causes chickenpox and shingles) in the geniculate ganglion of the facial nerve.

- Ramsay-Hunt syndrome (RHS) was described by Ramsay-Hunt in 1907. Herpes zoster oticus or Cephalicus are the alternate names of this syndrome. RHS is a viral polyneuropathy, occurs after reactivation of varicella zoster virus (VZV) hiding inside dorsal roots and cranial nerve ganglions. Aging, malignancy, chemo radiotherapy exposure, immune deficiency may trigger reactivation of this virus.

Clinical Features

- Clinical features include a triad of ipsilateral LMN type facial palsy, ear pain, and vesicles in the auditory canal and auricle **(Fig. 5.16)**.
- Taste perception in anterior 2/3rd of tongue and lacrimation are affected in some patients.
- Hearing loss, tinnitus, and/or vertigo can be seen with the involvement of the vestibulocochlear nerve.
- Sometimes other cranial nerves (V, IX, X) may be involved in severe cases.

Investigations

- Usually not necessary for the diagnosis.
- Microscopic evaluation with the Tzanck smear can be performed on the fluid obtained from the vesicles. The smear will show multinucleated giant cells using a Giemsa stain.
- PCR or direct fluorescent antibody testing of vesicular fluid can confirm VZV.
- MRI may be useful in showing inflammation near the geniculate ganglion.

Treatment

- High dose steroids together with antiviral drugs (acyclovir, famciclovir, or valacyclovir) are used to treat RHS. The aim is to decrease the degeneration of the nerve.
- Intractable RHS cases resistant to medical therapy usually require surgical decompression of facial nerve.

Q. Define vertigo. Enumerate the causes of vertigo. Discuss the approach to a case of vertigo.

- Vertigo is a false sensation of movement of the self or the sorroundings, usually a spinning or rotating sensation. Almost everyone has experienced vertigo as the transient spinning dizziness immediately after turning around rapidly several times. Vertigo is a symptom, not a diagnosis.
- Dizziness is an imprecise term patients often use to describe various related sensations, including faintness (a feeling of impending syncope), lightheadedness, feeling of imbalance or unsteadiness and a spinning sensation. So dizziness always does not mean vertigo.

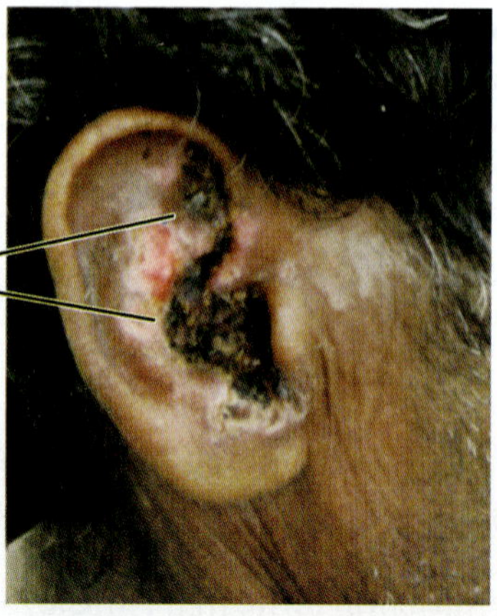

Figure 5.16: Ramsay-Hunt syndrome

Pathophysiology

- The vestibular system is the main neurologic system involved in balance. This system includes: the vestibular apparatus of the inner ear, the 8th (vestibulocochlear) cranial nerve, and the vestibular nuclei in the brain stem and cerebellum.
- Disorders of the inner ear and 8th cranial nerve are considered peripheral disorders. Those of the vestibular nuclei and their pathways in the brain stem and cerebellum are considered central disorders. Any asymmetrical neural activity anywhere in the vestibular system produces vertigo.

Causes of Vertigo

Peripheral causes

- Benign paroxysmal positional vertigo (BPPV)
- Vestibular neuritis
- Acute labyrinthitis
- Meniere's disease
- Herpes-zoster oticus (Ramsay-Hunt syndrome)
- Perilymphatic fistula
- Otitis media
- Otosclerosis
- Acoustic neuroma
- Aminoglycoside toxicity

Central causes

- Migrainous vertigo
- Brainstem ischemia
- Cerebellar infarction and hemorrhage
- Cerebellopontine angle tumors
- Chiari malformation
- Multiple sclerosis

Others

- Drugs (Aminoglycosides, anticonvulsants, alcohol).

Approach to a Case of Vertigo

Clinical History and Findings

- Peripheral vertigo should be distinguished from central vertigo, because central vertigo is of more serious nature.
- Ask the patient to describe what exactly he feels. This will help in differentiating true vertigo from other causes of dizziness such as lightheadedness.
- Nausea, vomiting and imbalance usually accompany vertigo.
- H/o recurrent episodes in the past suggest BPPV.

- Ask about triggers and relievers, i.e. whether triggered by head/body position change which suggests peripheral vertigo.
- Tinnitus and hearing loss suggest middle ear pathology and vertigo of peripheral origin.
- Presence of nystagmus should be noted. In peripheral lesions, nystagmus is usually horizontal with a rotatory component. In central vertigo, nystagmus can be horizontal or vertical and may be associated with other signs of brain stem or cerebellar dysfunction.
- H/o of loss of consciousness, focal neurological findings and cerebellar signs suggests a central cause of vertigo.

Differentiating Peripheral and Central Vertigo

(Table 5.16)

TABLE 5.16: Differences between peripheral and central vertigo

Feature	Peripheral vertigo	Central vertigo
Nystagmus	Unidirectional, horizontal	Multidirectional or vertical
Imbalance	Mild to moderate; able to walk	Severe; unable to stand still or walk
Nausea, vomiting	May be severe	Varies
Hearing loss, tinnitus	Common	Rare
Neurologic deficits	Rare	Common
Latency following provocative maneuver	Longer (up to 20 seconds)	Shorter (up to 5 seconds)
Head impulse test	Abnormal	Abnormal

Investigations

- Audiologic tests, caloric stimulation, electronystagmography, CT scan or MRI, and brain stem auditory evoked potential studies are indicated in patients with persistent vertigo or when CNS disease is suspected.
- These studies will help distinguish between central and peripheral lesions and to identify causes requiring specific therapy.

Treatment

Symptomatic Treatment

- These medications can be used to suppress the vertigo whatever may be the cause. These drugs act by suppressing the vestibular system. Examples are scopolamine, cinnarazine, betahistine, meclizine, dimenhydrinate, diphenhydramine, prochlorperazine, promethazine, metoclopramide, and domperidone.

Disease-specific Treatment

- If any underlying disease is found, treatment should be directed towards that.

Q. Nystagmus.

- Nystagmus is involuntary rhythmic oscillation of the eyes. Due to the involuntary movement of the eye, it is often called "dancing eyes".

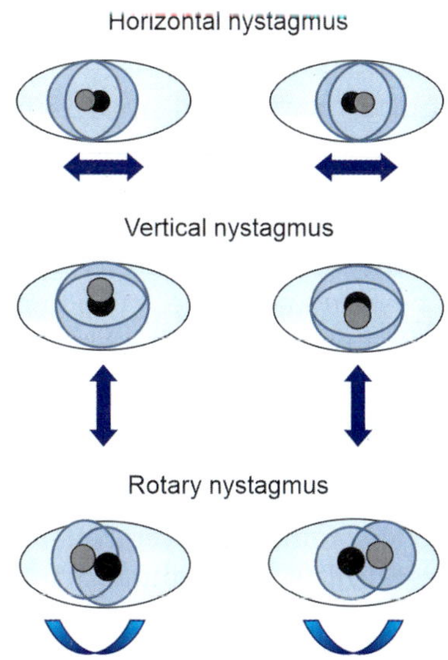

Figure 5.17: Types of nystagmus

- Nystagmus can be horizontal, vertical, torsional or a combination of these **(Fig. 5.17)**. Nystagmus may be unilateral or bilateral, conjugate or disconjugate (dissociated), congenital or acquired.

Pathophysiology

- Eyes move reflexively to adjust for slight movement of head, which stabilizes the image that we are looking at and allows us to see a sharper image. Nervous system maintains position of the eyes by three mechanisms: eye fixation, the vestibulo-ocular reflex, and the neural integrator. Any abnormality in these three mechanisms stimulating the eye movements in the absence of head movement causes nystagmus.

Types of Nystagmus

Physiological Nystagmus (Normal Reflex)

- Occurs in response to certain stimuli (e.g. optokinetic nystagmus, caloric testing).
- Helps maintain visual stability during head movement.

Pathological Nystagmus

- **Congenital (infantile) nystagmus**: Appears within the first few months of life, often horizontal, may be associated with visual deficits.
  - **Causes:** Albinism, bilateral congenital cataract, optic nerve hypoplasia, Noonan syndrome.
- **Acquired nystagmus**: Develops later in life, typically due to neurological or vestibular disorders.
  - **Causes:** Benign paroxysmal positional vertigo (BPPV), brain tumors in the posterior fossa, lateral medullary syndrome, Méniere's disease, Wernicke–Korsakoff syndrome, cerebellar ataxia, alcohol intoxication, phenytoin overdose.

Clinical Features

- The primary symptom of nystagmus is involuntary eye movement. Usually the movement is side-to-side (horizontal nystagmus), but it can also be up and down (vertical nystagmus) or circular (torsional or rotary nystagmus).

- The oscillations may be of approximately equal amplitude and velocity (pendular nystagmus) or, more commonly, with a slow initiating phase and a fast corrective phase (jerk nystagmus).
- Vertigo usually accompanies nystagmus due to peripheral vestibular disease. In such cases, nystagmus is usually horizontal with a fast and slow phase (jerk nystagmus).
- Nystagmus due to central causes (lesions in the brainstem or cerebellum) is often more irregular or vertical. Downbeat nystagmus (fast phase downward) is often linked to brainstem or cerebellar abnormalities. Upbeat nystagmus (fast phase upward) is also associated with central nervous system lesions.
- Oscillopsia (a to-and-fro illusion of environmental motion) and blurred vision occur due to oscillation of retinal image.
- There may be abnormal head position because the patient tends to keep their head in a position which causes least oscillopsia or blurred vision.

Investigations

- Brain imaging (CT or MRI) to rule out any brain pathology.
- Electronystagmographs record eye muscle contractions to evaluate the direction and velocity of nystagmus. It may be used to evaluate low-amplitude nystagmus.

Treatment

- Treatment of underlying cause.
- ***Medications***: Baclofen and gabapentin may reduce nystagmus.
- ***Botulinum injections***: This has been used to weaken the extraocular muscles and diminish the amplitude of nystagmus.
- ***Prism lenses and optical solutions***: These can be used to keep the eyes in a position of gaze in which nystagmus is minimal.
- ***Surgery***: Attachment of the muscles is shifted to maintain a gaze position where nystagmus is minimal or absent.

Q. Discus the causes, clinical features and management of raised ICP (intracranial pressure).

- The CSF pressure, measured at lumbar puncture (LP), is normally 60–200 mm of H_2O (or 5–15 mm Hg). A pressure of more than 200 mm of H_2O is called raised ICP.

Mechanisms of Raised ICP

- The volume of brain parenchyma is relatively constant in adults. The volumes of CSF and blood in the intracranial space are variable. Any abnormal increases in the volume of any of these components may lead to elevation in ICP.
- CSF is produced by the choroid plexus at a rate of 20 ml/h (500 ml/day). CSF is reabsorbed via the arachnoid granulations into the venous system. Increased production or decreased absorption of CSF can lead to raised ICP.
- Cerebral blood flow increases with hypercapnia and hypoxia and may lead to raised ICP.

Causes of Raised ICP

- Intracranial hemorrhage
- Central nervous system infections
- Space-occupying lesions (neoplasm, abscess, hematoma)
- Vasculitis
- Ischemic infarcts with cerebral edema
- Obstruction of venous outflow (e.g. venous sinus thrombosis, jugular vein compression, neck surgery)
- Increased CSF production (e.g. choroid plexus papilloma)
- Decreased CSF absorption (e.g. arachnoid granulation adhesions after bacterial meningitis)
- Obstructive hydrocephalus
- Idiopathic (pseudotumor cerebri).

Clinical Features

- Symptoms of elevated ICP include headache, depressed consciousness and vomiting.
- Signs include 6th nerve palsies, papilledema, and a triad of bradycardia, respiratory depression, and hypertension (Cushing's triad, sometimes called Cushing's reflex or Cushing's response). Cushing's triad may be due to brainstem compression. The presence of this response is an ominous finding that requires urgent intervention.
- Signs and symptoms of underlying disease.

Management

- ***Head end elevation***: It increases venous return from head and lowers ICP.
- ***Hyperventilation***: Use of mechanical ventilation to lower $PaCO_2$ to 26–30 mm Hg has been shown to rapidly reduce ICP through vasoconstriction and a decrease in the volume of intracranial blood.
- ***Hypertonic saline bolus:*** Hypertonic saline given as intravenous bolus doses can acutely lower ICP. Many studies have demonstrated that it is better than mannitol. Although, many centers are preferring this over mannitol, further studies are needed on long-term clinical outcomes.
- ***Intravenous mannitol***: This is an osmotic diuretic. It reduces brain volume by drawing free water out of the tissue into the circulation which is excreted by the kidneys, thus dehydrating brain parenchyma. Dose is 1–1.5 g/kg of 20% mannitol every 6–8 hours.
- ***Corticosteroids:*** Dexamethasone 4 mg 6th hourly is used in raised ICP due to meningitis and brain tumors.
- ***Glycerol:*** 30 ml orally every 6th–8th hourly. Acts osmotically by drawing water from the brain into intrvascular compartment. Use of glycerol has decreased because glycerol has been shown to have a significant rebound effect and to be less effective in ICP control.

- ***Barbiturates:*** It reduces brain metabolism and cerebral blood flow, thus lowering ICP and exerting a neuroprotective effect. Pentobarbital is generally used, with a loading dose of 5–20 mg/kg as a bolus, followed by 1–4 mg/kg per hour.
- ***Therapeutic hypothermia*:** Hypothermia decreases cerebral metabolism and may reduce cerebral blood flow and ICP.
- ***Removal of CSF*:** Removal of CSF reduces ICP which can be done by ventriculostomy.
- ***Decompressive craniectomy*:** Removal of the rigid confines of the bony skull allows the intracranial contents to expand and reduces ICP.
- ***Specific treatment*:** The best treatment of elevated ICP is to correct the underlying cause. Examples are removal of meningioma or intracranial hematoma.

Q. Classify and enumerate the causes of meningitis.

- Meningitis is an inflammatory disease of the arachnoid mater and the cerebrospinal fluid.

Causes of Meningitis (Table 5.17)

TABLE 5.17: Causes of meningitis
Bacteria
• *Neisseria meningitidis*
• *Streptococcus pneumoniae*
• *H. influenza*
• *Mycobacterium tuberculosis*
• *Staphylococcus aureus*
• Group B Streptococcus
• *Listeria monocytogenes*
• *Treponema pallidum*
Viruses
• Enteroviruses
• ECHO
• Coxsackie
• Mumps
• Herpes simplex
• HIV
• Epstein-Barr virus
Fungi
• *Cryptococcus neoformans*
• Candida
• *Coccidioides immitis*
• *Histoplasma capsulatum*
Spirochetal
• Leptospirosis
• Lyme disease
• Syphilis
Rickettsial
• Typhus fever
Protozoal
• Naegleria
Miscellaneous
• Sarcoidosis
• Leukemic meningitis
• Chemical meningitis
• Drug induced—NSAIDs, rofecoxib, intravenous immunoglobulin.

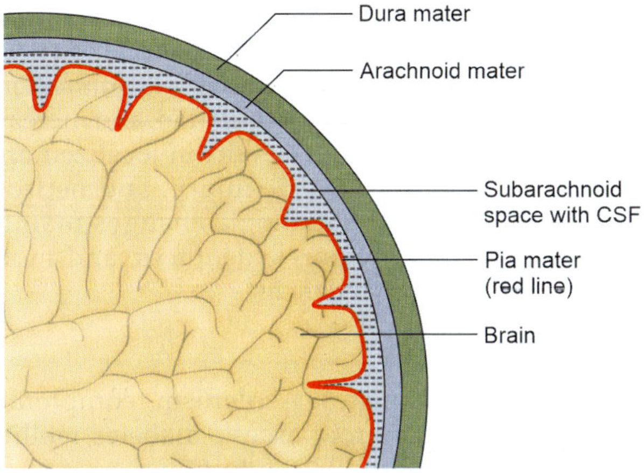

Figure 5.18: Meningeal layers covering the brain

Q. Describe the etiology, clinical features, investigations and management of acute pyogenic meningitis (acute bacterial meningitis).

Q. Causes of neck stiffness.

Q. Kernig's sign; Brudginski's sign.

Q. Prevention of meningitis.

Etiology

Common organisms
- *Neisseria meningitidis*
- *Streptococcus pneumoniae*
- *H. influenza*

Uncommon organisms
- *Staphylococcus aureus*
- Group B *Streptococcus*
- *Listeria monocytogenes*
- Klebsiella
- Proteus
- Pseudomonas
- Salmonella
- *Neisseria gonorrhea*

Pathogenesis

- The organism responsible for meningitis can reach the CSF via three routes: (i) colonization of the nasopharynx with subsequent bloodstream invasion and subsequent central nervous system (CNS) invasion; (ii) invasion of the CNS following bacteremia due to a localized source, such as pneumonia, infective endocarditis or a urinary tract infection; (iii) direct entry of organisms into the CNS from a contiguous infection (e.g. sinuses, mastoid), trauma, or neurosurgery.
- There are many steps involved before frank meningitis develops such as colonization of the host mucosal epithelium by pathogens, invasion into bloodstream, crossing of the blood-brain barrier, and multiplication within the CSF.
- Much of the damage from meningitis results from cytokines (interleukin-1, interleukin-6, and tumor necrosis factor-alpha) released within the CSF due to inflammatory response. Once inflammation is

initiated, a series of injuries occur to the endothelium of the blood-brain barrier (e.g. separation of intercellular tight junctions) that result in vasogenic brain edema, loss of cerebrovascular autoregulation, and increased intracranial pressure. This results in localized areas of brain ischemia, cytotoxic injury, and neuronal apoptosis. All these pathologic changes manifest clinically as coma, seizures, deafness, and motor, sensory, and cognitive deficits.

Predisposing Factors

- Immunodeficient states: Asplenism, complement deficiency, corticosteroid excess, diabetes mellitus, chronic alcoholism and HIV infection.
- Acute otitis media.
- Recent exposure to someone with meningitis.
- Recent travel, particularly to areas with endemic meningococcal disease.
- Injection drug use.
- Recent head trauma with CSF otorrhea or rhinorrhea.

Clinical Features

- Patients with bacterial meningitis usually appear ill. The classic triad of acute bacterial meningitis consists of fever, neck stiffness, and altered mental status.
- Patients are usually febrile but some may have hypothermia.
- Headache is also common and is diffuse and severe.
- ***Neck stiffness:*** Spasm of neck muscles on attempted flexion.
- ***Brudzinski's neck sign:*** Passive neck flexion, while the patient is in supine position, produces involuntary flexion of hips and knees.
- ***Brudzinski's leg sign***: Passive flexion of one leg produces automatic flexion of the other leg.
- ***Kernig's sign:*** Extension of knee from flexed thigh position causes passive resistance. This is due to the spasm of hamstring muscles due to the inflamed sciatic nerve as it passes through the spinal theca.
- Other manifestations include photophobia, vomiting, seizures, focal neurologic deficits (including cranial nerve palsies), and papilledema.
- Certain bacteria, particularly *N. meningitidis*, can cause characteristic skin manifestations, such as petechiae and palpable purpura.
- Arthritis occurs in some patients with bacterial meningitis.

Investigations

- ***Blood counts***: White blood cell count is often elevated with a let shift. However there may be leukopenia in severe infection. Platelet count may be reduced if disseminated intravascular coagulation (DIC) is present or in the face of meningococcal bacteremia.
- ***Blood cultures:*** Blood cultures may be able to identify the causative organism in 50–75% of patients with bacterial meningitis.
- ***Serum procalcitonin*** levels can be used as a guide to distinguish between bacterial and aseptic meningitis in children. Elevated serum procalcitonin levels predict bacterial meningitis.
- ***Lumbar puncture and CSF analysis (gold standard test):*** This is the test of choice to diagnose meningitis. Every patient with suspected meningitis should have LP done unless the procedure is contraindicated. CSF should be sent for protein, sugar, cell count, cell type, Gram's stain, India ink stain, culture sensitivity, AFB stain and culture and PCR studies. Opening pressure should be noted at the time of LP.

CSF Findings in Meningitis of Different Etiology

(Table 5.18)

- ***CT scan head***: A contrast CT shows meningeal enhancement in meningitis. It is also helpful to rule out other pathologies such as subarachnoid hemorrhage, cerebral abscess, mass lesion, middle ear and sinus disease. It should be done before LP in patients with raised ICP or mass lesion to prevent the risk of herniation. CT scan before an LP is indicated in patients with one or more of the following risk factors for a mass lesion.

Indications for CT Scan before LP in Meningitis

- Immunocompromised state (e.g. HIV infection, immunosuppressive therapy)
- History of CNS disease (mass lesion, stroke, or focal infection)
- New onset seizure (within one week of presentation)
- Papilledema
- Abnormal level of consciousness
- Focal neurologic deficit.

Treatment

- Bacterial meningitis is a medical emergency and treatment should be initiated immediately as soon as it is suspected. The mortality rate of untreated disease approaches 100%.

TABLE 5.18: CSF findings in meningitis of different etiology

	Normal	Viral	Bacterial (pyogenic)	Tuberculosis
Appearance	Crystal-clear	Clear/turbid	Turbid/purulent	Turbid/viscous
Pressure	60–200 mm of CSF	Normal	Increased	Increased
WBC count	<5/mm^3, all lymphocytes	10–300/mm^3 Lymphocyte predominant	100–5000; >80% neutrophils	100–500/mm^3, most are lymphocytes
Protein	less than 50 mg/dl	Increased	Increased	Increased >100
Glucose	40–60% of blood glucose	Normal	Low	low

- There are two general principles of antibiotic therapy: use of bactericidal drugs effective against the infecting organism; and the use of drugs that enter the CSF.

Empirical Antibiotic Therapy

- Pending identification of the causative organism, empirical antibiotic therapy should be started.
- Third-generation cephalosporins, such as cefotaxime or ceftriaxone, plus vancomycin are the drugs of choice for this purpose because they have good CSF penetration and also good activity against pathogens. Ampicillin should be added for those above 60 years to cover the possibility of Listeria meningitis.
- Vancomycin is added initially to cover for the possibility of cephalsporin resistant *Streptococcus pneumoniae*. It can be withdrawn later if the organism isolated from CSF is sensitive to ceftriaxone.

Age range	Empirical antibiotics
Adults up to age 60	Ceftriaxone (or cefotaxime) plus vancomycin Dosage: ceftriaxone 2 g IV 12th hourly for 10–14 days. Vancomycin 1 g IV 12th hourly
Above 60 years	Ceftriaxone (or cefotaxime) plus vancomycin, plus ampicillin

Role of Steroids in Meningitis

- Trials have shown that dexamethasone given shortly before or at the same time as the first dose of antibiotics significantly improves outcomes in patients with meningitis.
- Dexamethasone reduces CSF synthesis of cytokines (such as tumor necrosis factor-alpha and interleukin-1), CSF inflammation, and cerebral edema which are responsible for much of the damage and sequelae.

Complications of Meningitis

Neurological

- Cerebrovascular abnormalities (thrombosis, vasculitis, hemorrhage, and aneurysm formation)
- Cerebral edema and raised ICP
- Obstructive hydrocephalus
- Seizures
- Intellectual impairment
- Deafness and cranial nerve palsies
- Subdural abscess.

Systemic

- Septic shock
- ARDS
- DIC.

Prevention of Meningitis

- Some forms of meningitis can be prevented by vaccination and chemoprophylaxis.

Vaccines

- Vaccines are available for *S. pneumoniae*, *N. meningitidis*, and *H. influenzae*.
- Pneumococcal vaccine: Pneumococcal vaccine is administered to chronically ill and older adults (over age 65). Pneumococcal vaccine is administered intramuscularly as a 0.5 ml dose. Effect lasts up to 5–10 years.
- Meningococcal vaccine: A quadrivalent meningococcal polysaccharide conjugate vaccine (serogroups A, C, Y and W-135) is available in many countries. It is given to children and adults as a single intramuscular (IM) 0.5 ml dose. Effect lasts up to 1 year.
- *H. influenzae* vaccine: This vaccine is now routinely administered to children. It is available in combination with hepatitis-B vaccine. For adults, it is indicated only for those with prior splenectomy.

Chemoprophylaxis

- Chemoprophylaxis can prevent the spread of meningococcal and Haemophilus meningitis.
- ***Neisseria meningitides:*** Rifampicin (600 mg PO every 12 hours for a total of four doses in adults), or ciprofloxacin (500 mg PO once), or ceftriaxone (250 mg IM once). Chemoprophylaxis is necessary only in close contacts of an isolated case of invasive meningococcal infection. Close contacts include household members and other intimate contacts, children in school environments, coworkers in the same office, young adults in dormitories, and recruits in training centers.
- ***H. influenza:*** Unvaccinated, young children (less than four years of age) should receive brief course of rifampicin (20 mg/kg with a maximum of 600 mg/day PO for four days) if they are exposed to a case of meningitis.

Q. Aseptic meningitis.

- Aseptic meningitis refers to patients who have clinical and laboratory evidence for meningeal inflammation with negative routine bacterial cultures.

Causes of Aseptic Meningitis

- **Infections:** Viruses (most common cause), fungi, spirochetes, TB.
- **Non-infectious causes:** Drugs (NSAIDs, IV immunoglobulins, carbamazepine, ciprofloxacin, isoniazid), malignancy, SLE, sarcoidosis and Behcet's disease.

Clinical Features

- These are similar to bacterial meningitis (e.g. fever, headache, altered mental status, stiff neck, photophobia).

Investigations

- CSF show increased pressure and lymphocytic pleocytosis. CSF protein and sugar are usually normal.

Treatment

- Involves correction of the underlying cause. However, in contrast to bacterial meningitis, majority of patients with aseptic meningitis have a self-limited course that will resolve without specific therapy.

Q. Describe the etiology, clinical features, investigations and management of tuberculous meningitis (TBM).

- Tuberculous meningitis (TBM) is the most severe type of extrapulmonary tuberculosis, but it is the least common type. It can occur as the sole manifestation of TB or concurrent with pulmonary or other extrapulmonary sites of infection.

Etiology

- *Mycobacterium tuberculosis.*

Pathophysiology

- TBM develops in 2 steps. In the first step ***Mycobacterium tuberculosis*** bacilli enter the host by droplet inhalation, and are phagocytosed by alveolar macrophages. Subsequently bacilli spread to regional lymph nodes to produce the primary complex. During this stage, bacteremia occurs and the tubercle bacilli seed many organs. In persons who develop TBM, bacilli seed the meninges or brain parenchyma, resulting in the formation of subpial or subependymal foci of caseous lesions. These are termed Rich foci, after the original pathologic studies of Rich.
- The second step in the development of TBM is an increase in size of a Rich focus until it ruptures into the subarachnoid space. Tubercles (Rich focus) rupturing into the subarachnoid space cause meningitis. Those deeper in the brain or spinal cord parenchyma cause tuberculomas or abscesses. A severe inflammatory response is elicited by mycobacterial components. A thick exudate, phlebitis, arteritis, thrombosis, infarction and obstruction of CSF flow are common findings. Basal meningitis accounts for the frequent dysfunction of cranial nerves (CNs) III, VI, and VII, eventually leading to obstructive hydrocephalus from obstruction of basilar cisterns. Complications include raised intracranial pressure, cerebral edema, syndrome of inappropriate antidiuretic hormone secretion (SIADH), hydrocephalus, brain infarcts, hemi- or quadriplegia, convulsions, deafness, blindness, mental retardation and other neurological sequelae.

Clinical Features

- TBM presents as a subacute febrile illness associated with headache and neck stiffness. Neck stiffness may be absent in the early stages.
- Features of CNS dysfunction such as personality change, vomiting, lethargy, confusion, and cranial nerve palsies may be present.
- Sudden onset of focal neurologic deficits, including monoplegia, hemiplegia, aphasia, and tetraparesis can occur.
- Involuntary movements may be seen in some patients. Tremor is the most common movement disorder seen. Other abnormal movements such as myoclonus, choreoathetosis, and hemiballismus can also be seen.
- Fundoscopic examination often shows choroidal tubercles.
- If untreated, death occurs within five to eight weeks of the onset of illness.

Diagnosis

- ***CSF examination:*** CSF shows elevated protein and decreased glucose concentration with predominant lymphocytosis. The demonstration of acid-fast bacilli (AFB) in the CSF remains the most rapid and effective means of reaching an early diagnosis. PCR for AFB should be sent in all suspected cases of TB meningitis.
- ***Brain imaging:*** CT scan head may show meningeal enhancements especially basal meninges. Obstructive hydrocephalus may be present. MRI has more sensitivity in detecting the distribution of meningeal inflammatory exudates.
- ***Montoux test:*** is usually positive.
- ***Chest X-ray:*** May show evidence of pulmonary tuberculosis.
- ***Cartridge Based Nucleic Acid Amplification Test (CB-NAAT/GeneXpert):*** This test has high sensitivity and specificity. It can also detect drug resistance.
- ***Other tests:*** HIV test to rule out immunocompromised state, blood sugar, electrolytes, LFT, RFT, and CBP with ESR.

Treatment

- Antituberculous therapy should be started if there is strong clinical suspicion of TB meningitis even if it cannot be confirmed by investigations.
- Treatment involves initial two month period of intensive therapy with 4 drugs (isoniazid, rifampicin, pyrazinamide and ethambutol). This is followed by a continuation phase lasting 7–10 months with 2 drugs (isoniazid, rifampicin). Streptomycin can be used instead of ethambutol but is available only as injection.
- Steroids should be given to all patients with TB meningitis. Dexamethasone is given at a dose of 12 mg/day in divided doses or prednisolone at a dose of 60 mg/day. Steroids should be given in full dose for 3 weeks, and then tapered off gradually over the following 3 weeks.
- Surgery: Patients with hydrocephalus may require surgical decompression to reduce raised intracranial pressure.

Q. Describe the pharmacology, dose, adverse reactions and regimens of drugs used in the treatment of bacterial, tubercular and viral meningitis.

Bacterial Meningitis

Pharmacology and Regimens

See **Table 5.19.**

TABLE 5.19: Drugs used in bacterial meningitis

Drug	Mechanism	Dose (Adult)	Adverse reactions
Ceftriaxone/Cefotaxime	Inhibit cell wall synthesis	Ceftriaxone: 2 g IV q12h Cefotaxime: 2 g IV q4–6h	Hypersensitivity, diarrhea, biliary sludge
Vancomycin	Inhibits cell wall synthesis (Gram + coverage)	15–20 mg/kg IV q8–12h	Nephrotoxicity, "red man" syndrome
Ampicillin	Inhibits cell wall synthesis. Covers Listeria	2 g IV q4h	Hypersensitivity, rash, diarrhea
Dexamethasone	Reduces inflammation and neurological sequelae	10 mg IV q6h × 4 days (adults)	Hyperglycemia, GI bleeding, immunosuppression

Empirical Regimens for Different Age Groups

- <1 month: Ampicillin + Cefotaxime or Gentamicin
- 1 month–50 years: Ceftriaxone + Vancomycin ± Dexamethasone
- >50 years/immunocompromised: Ceftriaxone + Vancomycin + Ampicillin
- Duration of treatment varies from 1 to 3 weeks.

Tubercular Meningitis (TBM)

Pharmacology and Regimen

See **Table 5.20**.

Standard Regimen (WHO Guidelines)

- 2 months intensive phase: HRZE (Isoniazid, rifampicin, pyrazinamide, ethambutol)
- 10 months continuation phase: HR (Isoniazid + Rifampicin)
- Adjunct: Steroids for 6–8 weeks

Viral Meningitis

- Most cases are self-limited and caused by enteroviruses, but treatment is indicated for HSV, VZV, CMV and in immunocompromised patients.

Pharmacology and Regimen

See **Table 5.21**.

Q. Describe the functional and the vascular anatomy of the brain.

Functional Anatomy of the Brain

- The brain is divided into major regions, each with specific functions **(Table 5.22)**.

Cerebrum

- Largest part of the brain
- Divided into two hemispheres and four lobes per hemisphere **(Fig. 5.19)**:

TABLE 5.20: Drugs used in tubercular meningitis

Drug	Mechanism	Dose (Adult)	Adverse reactions
Isoniazid (INH)	Inhibits mycolic acid synthesis	5 mg/kg/day (max 300 mg)	Hepatotoxicity, peripheral neuropathy (prevent with pyridoxine)
Rifampicin	Inhibits DNA-dependent RNA polymerase	10 mg/kg/day (max 600 mg)	Hepatotoxicity, orange discoloration of fluids
Pyrazinamide	Disrupts mycobacterial cell membrane metabolism	20–25 mg/kg/day	Hepatotoxicity, hyperuricemia, GI upset
Ethambutol	Inhibits arabinosyl transferase (cell wall)	15–25 mg/kg/day	Optic neuritis (visual disturbances)
Corticosteroids	Reduce CNS inflammation and edema	Dexamethasone 8–24 mg/day, in divided doses or Prednisolone 1 mg/kg body weight	Hyperglycemia, GI bleeding, immunosuppression

TABLE 5.21: Drugs used in viral meningitis

Drug	Mechanism	Dose (Adult)	Adverse Reactions
Acyclovir	Inhibits viral DNA polymerase (HSV, VZV)	10 mg/kg IV q8h (adjust for renal function)	Nephrotoxicity (crystalluria), CNS toxicity
Ganciclovir	Inhibits viral DNA synthesis (CMV)	5 mg/kg IV q12h	Bone marrow suppression, nephrotoxicity
Foscarnet	DNA polymerase inhibitor (for resistant HSV/CMV)	60 mg/kg IV q8h	Nephrotoxicity, electrolyte imbalances

TABLE 5.22: Normal and abnormal functions of the brain lobes

Lobe	Normal function	Abnormal function due to lesions
Frontal lobe	**Dominant side (usually the left side)** • Voluntary motor control (primary motor cortex) • Executive functions (planning, decision-making, problem-solving) • Speech production (Broca's area – usually in the left hemisphere) • Emotional regulation • Personality • Social behavior • Verbal working memory (remembering numbers, words, instructions)	• Contralateral motor weakness or paralysis • Disinhibition • Obsessive-compulsive behavior • Lack of initiative • Impaired memory • Incontinence • Primitive reflexes (grasp reflex, snout reflex) • Anosmia
	Nondominant side • No role in speech production (but may help with emotional tone of speech) • More involved in social judgment, recognizing humor, and emotional insight • Emotional expression, affect regulation, empathy • Helps in understanding and expressing emotional tone of speech	• Disinhibition, emotional blunting, lack of insight • Antisocial behavior
Parietal lobe	**Dominant side** • Mathematical ability and calculation • Speech, language • Planned movement • Cortical sensations	• Dyscalculia • Dysphasia • Dyslexia • Apraxia • Contralateral homonymous hemianopia • Contralateral loss of cortical sensations
	Non-dominant side • Spatial awareness and orientation (helps you understand your body's position in space) • Visual attention • Directing attention to both sides of the visual field (the right parietal lobe attends to both left and right hemispace, while the left parietal lobe mainly attends to the right side) • Coordinates movements in relation to the environment • Constructional skills: Drawing, building, or assembling objects (like copying a figure or arranging blocks). • Awareness of body and surroundings: • Integrates sensory input to maintain awareness of one's own body in relation to the world (body schema). • Emotional and prosodic processing: Interpretation of the emotional tone in speech (prosody). Understanding nonverbal cues and spatial aspects of communication	• Contralateral hemispatial neglect • Spatial disorientation: Getting lost even in familiar surroundings • Constructional apraxia • Contralateral homonymous hemianopia • Anosognosia: Lack of awareness or denial of one's deficits or illness (e.g. a person may deny paralysis of their left side) • Contralateral loss of cortical sensations
Temporal lobe	**Dominant side** • Language comprehension (Wernicke's area) • Verbal memory (e.g. word lists, facts) • Auditory Processing: Processing of spoken words and language sounds. • Olfaction	• Wernicke's aphasia (fluent but meaningless speech) • Impaired verbal memory • Language comprehension deficits
	Nondominant side • Music, tone sequences • Nonverbal memory (faces, music, etc.)	• Loss of musical skills • Complex hallucinations • Homonymous hemianopia • Inability to recognize familiar faces (prosapognosia) • Difficulty understanding emotional cues
Occipital lobe	**Dominant side** • Analysis of vision • Reading, letter recognition, written word processing	• Contralateral homonymous hemianopia with macular sparing • Alexia (inability to read) • Visual agnosia • Visual hallucinations (lights, zig zags)
	Non-dominant side • Holistic, gestalt processing (e.g. shapes, faces) • Spatial and contextual visual tasks • More dominant for facial recognition and scenic memory	• Contralateral homonymous hemianopia with macular sparing • Prosopagnosia • Visual-spatial disorientation

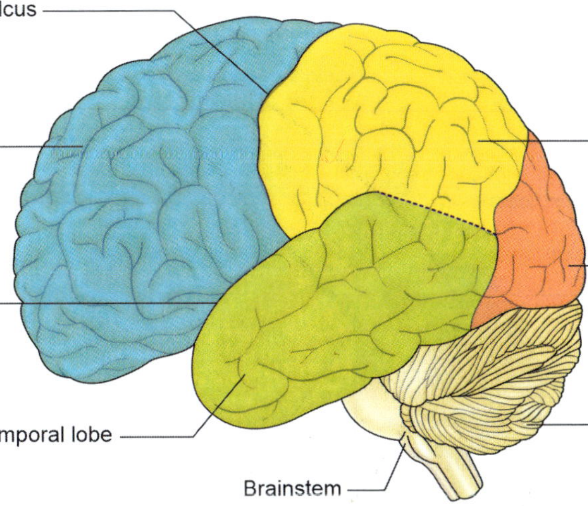

Figure 5.19: Lobes of brain

Diencephalon

- *Thalamus*: Relay center for sensory signals.
- *Hypothalamus*: Homeostasis, hormone regulation, autonomic control.

Cerebellum

Coordinates balance, posture, and fine motor control.

Brainstem

- Includes midbrain, pons, and medulla oblongata.
- Controls vital functions: Breathing, heart rate, consciousness.
- Contains cranial nerve nuclei.

Limbic System

- Includes hippocampus, amygdala, cingulate gyrus.
- Involved in emotion, memory, and motivation.

Vascular Anatomy of the Brain

Arterial supply

- The brain is supplied by two main arterial systems that form the circle of Willis:

Anterior Circulation (from internal carotid arteries)

- Anterior cerebral artery (ACA):
  - Supplies medial frontal and parietal lobes
  - Infarct → leg weakness, personality changes
- Middle cerebral artery (MCA):
  - Supplies lateral cerebral cortex
  - Infarct → face/arm weakness, aphasia (dominant hemisphere), neglect (non-dominant)
- Anterior communicating artery:
  - Connects both ACAs

Posterior Circulation (from vertebral arteries → basilar artery)

- Posterior cerebral artery (PCA):
  - Supplies occipital lobe, inferior temporal lobe
  - Infarct → visual field defects, memory loss
- Basilar artery:
  - Brainstem and cerebellum
  - Branches: Pontine arteries, AICA, SCA
- Vertebral arteries:
  - Give rise to PICA (posterior inferior cerebellar artery)
  - Infarct → Wallenberg syndrome (lateral medullary syndrome)
- Posterior communicating artery:
  - Connects ICA to PCA, part of circle of Willis

Venous Drainage

- Via dural venous sinuses → Internal jugular vein
- Major sinuses: Superior sagittal sinus, straight sinus, transverse sinus, sigmoid sinus

Clinical Correlation (Table 5.23)

TABLE 5.23: Anterior and posterior circulation stroke and clinical features

Anterior circulation stroke	Posterior circulation stroke
• MCA (dominant): Aphasia, contralateral face/arm weakness or hemiplegia. • ACA: Leg weakness, behavioral changes	• Posterior inferior cerebellar artery (PICA): Lateral medullary syndrome (Wallenberg syndrome) • Superior cerebellar artery (SCA): Ataxia, vertigo, dysmetria, tremor • Basilar artery: Locked in syndrome. • Posterior cerebral artery: Contralateral homonymous hemianopia, thalamic syndrome. • Vertebral arteries: Medial or lateral medullary syndromes.

Q. Draw a diagram of internal capsule and the location of fibers running through it (Fig. 5.20).

Q. Draw a diagram of circle of Willis and label the various arterial branches (Fig. 5.21).

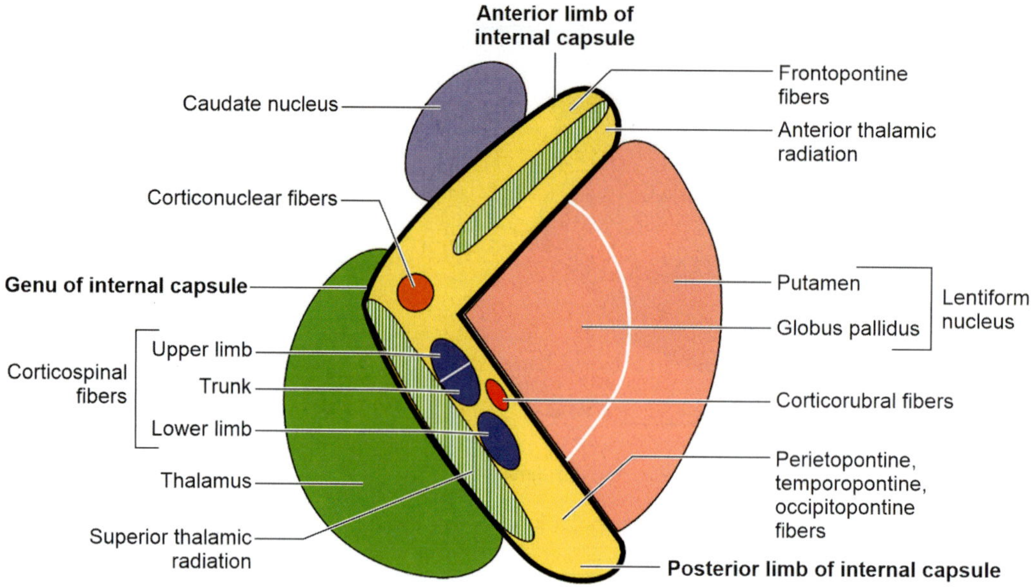

Figure 5.20: Anatomy of internal capsule

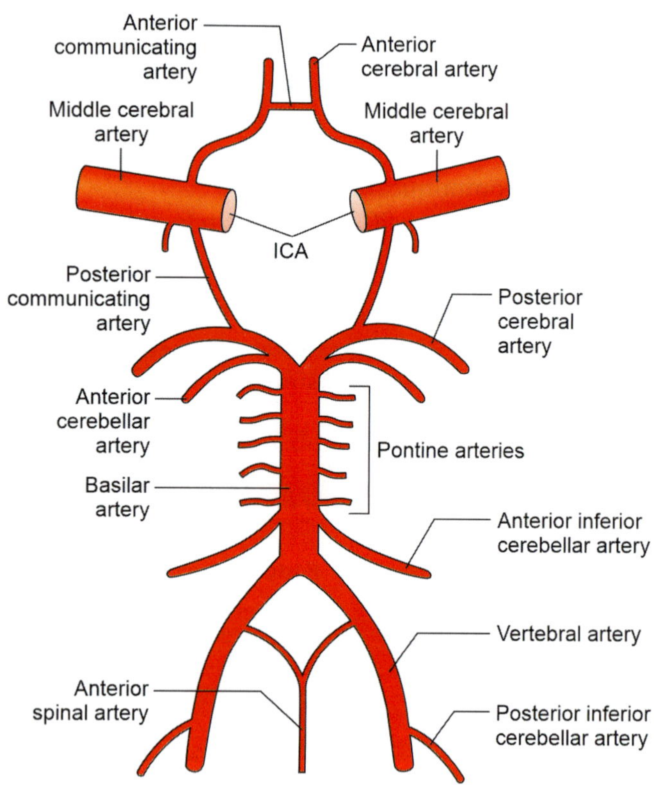

Figure 5.21: Circle of Willis

- Circle of Willis is formed by the anastomosis between two internal carotid arteries and two vertebral arteries. This extensive anastomosis helps in maintaining the blood supply to brain even when a major feeding vessel gets blocked.
- Aneurysms can occur in the circle of Willis especially at the branching points. Most of the aneurysms occur in the anterior circulation of circle of Willis.

Q. Define stroke.

Q. What are the types of stroke (cerebrovascular accident)?

Definition

- Stroke or cerebrovascular accident (CVA) is defined as sudden onset of a neurologic deficit from a vascular mechanism.
- Stroke is the leading cause of neurologic disability in adults. It is more common in males and mainly affects elderly people. Blacks have almost twice the risk of stroke compared to whites.

Types

Ischemic (nonhemorrhagic)

- 85% of strokes are ischemic. Caused by interruption of cerebral blood flow due to thrombosis or embolism. Further classified as follows:
  - Thrombotic stroke—*in situ* occlusion of cerebral artery due to atherosclerosis and thrombus formation.
  - Embolic stroke—emboli from heart or extracranial arteries.
  - Lacunar stroke—occlusion of small penetrating arteries, often due to hypertension.
  - Watershed infarcts—occur in border zones between major cerebral arteries.

Hemorrhagic

- 15% of strokes are hemorrhagic strokes, further classified as follows:
  - Subarachnoid hemorrhage—bleeding into subarachnoid space, often from ruptured aneurysms.
  - Intracerebral hemorrhage—bleeding directly into brain parenchyma.

Etiology

- Refers to the direct cause or origin of a disease or condition.

Ischemic stroke

- Atherosclerosis and thrombus formation
- Cardioembolism (e.g. atrial fibrillation, myocardial infarction)
- Small vessel disease (lipohyalinosis, microatheroma)
- Hypercoagulable states (e.g. antiphospholipid syndrome)
- Arterial dissection
- Vasculitis

Hemorrhagic stroke

- Chronic hypertension
- Cerebral amyloid angiopathy (especially in elderly)
- Aneurysms (e.g. berry aneurysms in circle of Willis)
- Arteriovenous malformations (AVMs)
- Trauma
- Coagulopathies (e.g. anticoagulation therapy, liver disease)
- Illicit drug use (e.g. cocaine, amphetamines)

Q. Describe the initial supportive management of a patient presenting with a cerebrovascular accident (CVA).

- The initial supportive management of a patient presenting with a cerebrovascular accident (CVA)—whether ischemic or hemorrhagic—focuses on stabilization, preventing further injury, and assessing for definitive treatment **(Fig. 5.22)**.

Immediate Assessment (ABCDE Approach)

A: Airway

- Ensure the airway is patent.
- If GCS <8 or the patient is unable to protect their airway (e.g. reduced consciousness, vomiting), consider endotracheal intubation.

B: Breathing

- Assess respiratory rate, oxygen saturation.
- Provide supplemental oxygen to maintain $SpO_2 > 94\%$ if hypoxic.
- Monitor for signs of aspiration pneumonia.

C: Circulation

- Monitor blood pressure, heart rate, ECG.
- Maintain permissive hypertension in ischemic stroke (unless BP > 220/120 mm Hg or contraindications like thrombolysis).
- Treat hypotension aggressively to ensure adequate cerebral perfusion.
- Establish IV access, send routine bloods (FBC, U&E, glucose, coagulation profile).

D: Disability (Neurological Status)

- Identify neurological impairment or deterioration. Assess the following:
- AVPU scale: Alert, responds to voice, pain, or unresponsive.
- GCS (Glasgow Coma Scale).
- Pupils: size, reactivity.
- Blood glucose—check for hypoglycemia (can mimic stroke).
- Treat hypoglycemia immediately with IV glucose.

E: Exposure (to trauma, drugs, toxins, infections)

- Examine the whole body for signs of illness, injury, rash, bleeding, etc.
- Look for rashes, wounds, trauma, limb perfusion, pressure sores.
- Check temperature.
- Treat visible problems.
- Use warming blankets if hypothermic.
- Consider causes like infection, drugs, seizures, head injury.

Rapid Neurological Assessment

- Determine time of onset of symptoms.
- Use a scale like the NIH stroke scale (NIHSS) to quantify stroke severity.
- Perform urgent non-contrast CT brain to differentiate ischemic vs hemorrhagic stroke.
- Time is brain. Once stabilized, rapidly determine eligibility for reperfusion therapy (thrombolysis or thrombectomy).

Blood Glucose

- Hypoglycemia can mimic stroke.
- Check blood glucose immediately.
- If low (<60 mg/dl), administer IV glucose.
- Additional key investigations
  - ECG—to rule out atrial fibrillation or myocardial infarction.
  - Chest X-ray—especially if there are breathing issues.
  - Blood investigations—including lipids, HbA1c, and infection screen.

Other Supportive Measures

- Keep head of bed at 30° to reduce intracranial pressure and improve venous drainage.
- Monitor for and manage fever—antipyretics if >37.5°C.
- Maintain normovolemia—IV fluids if necessary, but avoid overload.
- Insert urinary catheter if retention or incontinence occurs.
- Consider DVT prophylaxis (e.g. compression stockings if not hemorrhagic stroke).

Consult Stroke/Neuroteam Early

- Early involvement is critical for decisions regarding thrombolysis, thrombectomy, or neurosurgical intervention.

Q. Discuss the etiology, risk factors, clinical features, investigations and management of ischemic stroke.

Etiology

- Ischemic stroke is due to sudden occlusion of an intracranial vessel, with reduction in blood flow to the brain area supplied by that vessel. Occlusion happens either due to *in situ* thrombosis or embolus from a distant site.

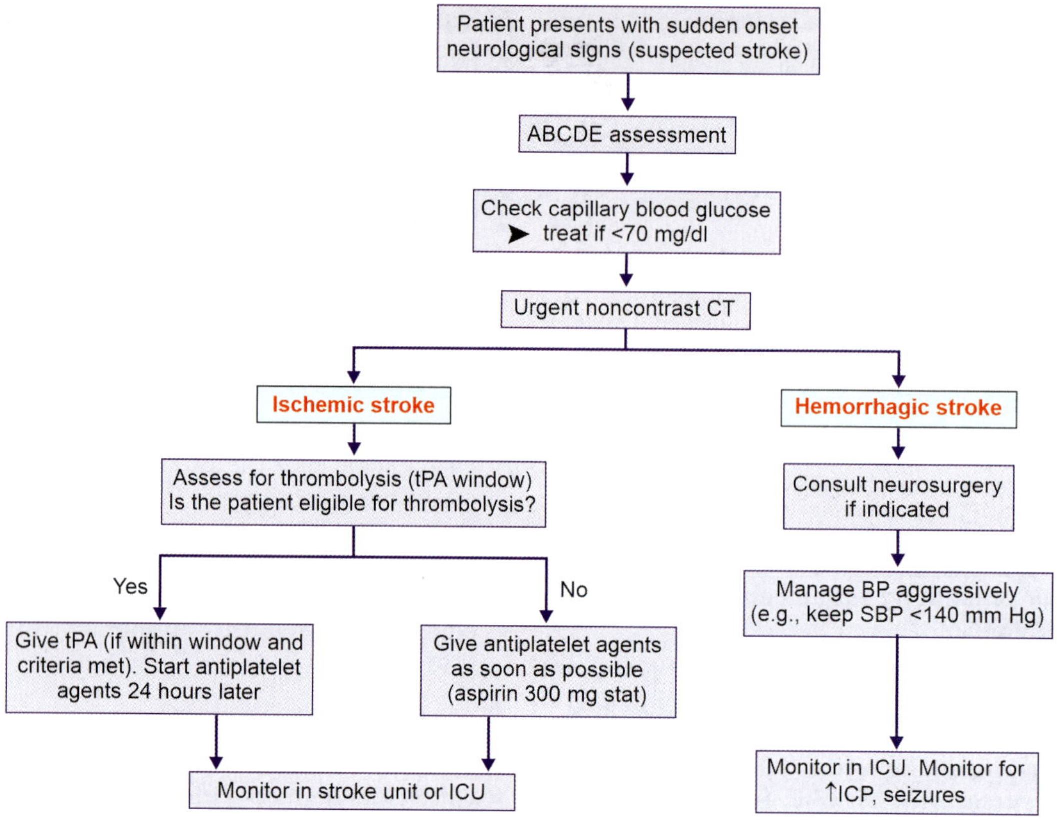

Figure 5.22: Initial stroke management

- *In situ* thrombosis can happen in a previously diseased vessel such as atherosclerotic vessels. Rupture of an atherosclerotic plaque or acute dissection of a large vessel (e.g. internal carotid artery, middle cerebral artery) can also lead to acute thrombosis.
- Emboli can come from distant sites and occlude cerebral vessels. Sources of emboli include heart and other arteries (e.g. the internal carotid and aortic arch).

Causes of Ischemic Stroke (Table 5.24)

- The causes listed under "cardioembolic and uncommon causes" produce stroke in young (<50 years) also.

Pathophysiology of Ischemic Stroke (Fig. 5.23)

- Acute occlusion of an intracranial vessel causes reduction in blood flow to the brain region it supplies. Reduction of blood supply produces ischemia or

TABLE 5.24: Causes of ischemic stroke

Common causes	Uncommon causes
Thrombosis • Small vessel thrombosis (lacunar stroke) • Large vessel thrombosis • Dehydration ***Embolic occlusion*** • Artery-to-artery – Carotid disease – Aortic disease • Cardioembolic – Atrial fibrillation – Mural thrombus – Myocardial infarction – Dilated cardiomyopathy – Valvular lesions (mitral stenosis, mechanical valve) – Infective endocarditis – Paradoxical embolus (ASD, patent foramen ovale)	• Hypercoagulable disorders – Protein C deficiency – Protein S deficiency – Antithrombin III deficiency – Antiphospholipid syndrome – Factor V Leiden mutation – Malignancy – Sickle cell anemia – Polycythemia vera – Essential thrombocytosis – Homocysteinemia – Nephrotic syndrome • Venous sinous thrombosis • Fibromuscular dysplasia • Vasculitis (PAN, Wegener's, Takayasu's, giant cell arteritis, syphilis, tuberculosis) • Atrial myxoma • Drugs: cocaine, amphetamine • Moyamoya disease

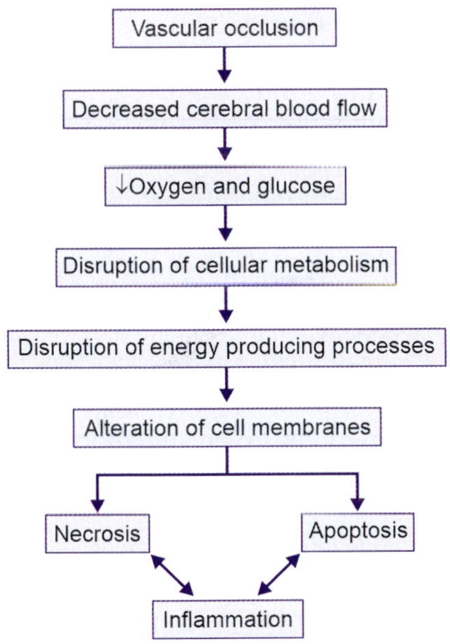

Figure 5.23: Pathogenesis of ischemic stroke

infarction depending on the severity of reduction of blood flow.

- If blood flow is restored before significant amount of cell death, patient may experience only transient symptoms, i.e. a TIA (transient ischemic attack).
- The infarcted area is surrounded by ischemic area the function of which is reversible if blood flow is restored within a reasonable time. This area is called ***ischemic penumbra***. The ischemic penumbra will eventually infarct if blood flow is not restored. Saving the ischemic penumbra is the goal of revascularization therapies.
- Cerebral infarction occurs via two pathways: (1) cellular necrosis and (2) apoptosis in which cells become programmed to die.
- Cellular necrosis happens due to severe reduction in blood supply which results in failure of mitochondria to produce ATP. Loss of ATP production leads to stoppage of membrane ion pumps allowing calcium to accumulate inside cells and glutamate release from synaptic terminals. Excess glutamate also leads to intracellular calcium accumulation. Excess calcium inside neurons produces free radicals by membrane degradation and mitochondrial dysfunction. Free radicals ultimately lead to death of neuronal cells.
- In apoptosis, cells die days to weeks later. It is seen in ischemic penumbra.

Clinical Features of Ischemic Stroke

- Initial symptoms occur suddenly. Generally, they include numbness, weakness, or paralysis of the contralateral limbs and the face, inability to speak (aphasia); confusion; visual disturbances in one or both eyes; dizziness or loss of balance and coordination; and headache.
- Systemic or autonomic disturbances (e.g. hypertension, fever) occasionally occur.
- H/o sudden, severe headache, vomiting, impaired consciousness or coma suggests intracranial bleed.
- Neurologic deficits depend on the vessel blocked and the area of brain involved (**Table 5.25**).

TABLE 5.25: Clinical features of ischemic stroke

	Occluded blood vessel	Clinical manifestations
Anterior Circulation	**Internal carotid artery**	Ipsilateral blindness (variable) and features of MCA territory stroke on the opposite side.
	Middle cerebral artery (MCA)	Contralateral hemiparesis (worse in the arm and face than in the leg), dysarthria, hemianesthesia, contralateral homonymous hemianopia, aphasia (if the dominant hemisphere is affected) or apraxia and sensory neglect (if the nondominant hemisphere is affected)
	Anterior cerebral artery (ACA)	Contralateral hemiparesis (worse in the leg than arm), urinary incontinence, apathy, confusion, poor judgment, mutism, grasp reflex, gait apraxia
Posterior Circulation	**Posterior cerebral artery (PCA)**	Contralateral homonymous hemianopia, unilateral cortical blindness, memory impairment, unilateral 3rd cranial nerve palsy, hemiballismus.
	Vertebrobasilar system	Unilateral or bilateral cranial nerve deficits (producing nystagmus, vertigo, dysphagia, dysarthria, diplopia, blindness), truncal or limb ataxia, spastic paresis, crossed sensory and motor deficits, impaired consciousness, coma, death (if basilar artery occlusion is complete), tachycardia, labile BP.

Investigations

CT Scan Head

- Plain CT head is the imaging modality of choice in acute stroke because it can be done fast and is widely available. An infarct appears as hypointense area. However, infarct may not be visible for 24–48 hours in CT scan. Brainstem lesions may not be visible properly on CT scan.
- CT scan can also exclude hemorrhage, and other pathologies like neoplasms, abscesses, and conditions that mimic stroke.
- Contrast-CT is more useful in subacute infarcts and can also visualize venous structures.

MRI Brain

- MRI is less sensitive in excluding hemorrhage than CT. It is also more expensive and time consuming, not widely available, and limited by claustrophobia. Because of all these reasons, MRI is not preferred in the acute evaluation of stroke.
- However, MRI is more sensitive than CT in picking up infarction in all areas of the brain, including cortex and brainstem (**Fig. 5.24**).

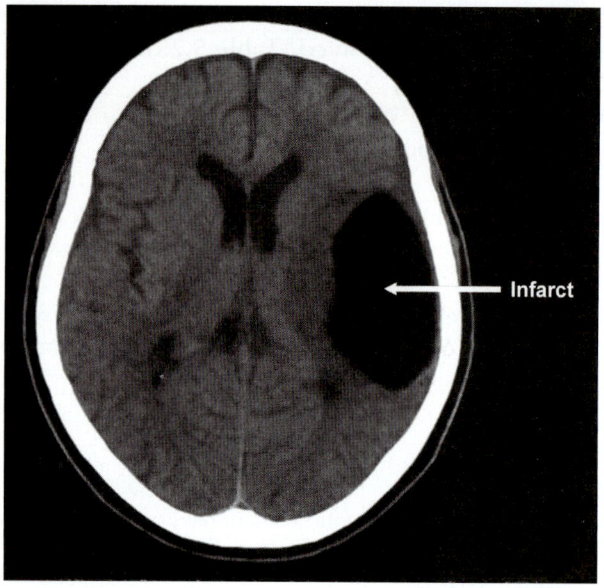

Figure 5.24: CT scan showing hypointense infarction

- It is more sensitive in picking up early brain infarction than CT scan.

CT-angiogram and MR-angiogram

- Can be done to identify the exact location of vessel block.

Carotid and Vertebral Artery Doppler

- Useful to identify diseases of the carotid and vertebral arteries.

ECG and Echocardiogram

- To rule out any heart problem.

Blood Tests

- Blood sugar, urea, creatinine, electrolytes, hemoglobin, cell count, coagulation parameters, lipid profile, toxicology screen (if toxin or overdose suspected).

Treatment

Initial Management

- Assess ABCs (airway, breathing, circulation).
- Secure airway.
- Monitor oxygenation.
- Provide ventilatory support if required.

Antithrombotic Treatment

- Antiplatelet agent, aspirin should be given as soon as the diagnosis of ischemic stroke is confirmed. A loading dose of aspirin 325 mg should be given followed by 75–150 mg daily life long. Aspirin prevents the extension of clot and also reduces the chances of recurrent stroke (secondary prevention). However, withhold these agents before and for 24 hours after thrombolytic therapy.
- If patients have had a TIA or minor stroke, clopidogrel plus aspirin (dual antiplatelet therapy) given within 24 hours of symptom onset and continued for 21 days appears more effective than aspirin alone for reducing risk of subsequent major stroke in the first 90 days and does not increase risk of hemorrhage. However, prolonged (e.g. >3 months) use of clopidogrel plus aspirin is avoided because it has no advantage over aspirin alone in long-term secondary stroke prevention and results in more bleeding complications.

Anticoagulation

- They are not useful in atherothrombotic cerebral ischemia. However, they are indicated in cardioembolic stroke (e.g. in atrial fibrillation) and stroke caused by cerebral venous thrombosis. Heparin or low-molecular-weight heparin can be given subcutaneously and later changed to oral anticoagulant therapy with warfarin.

Intravenous Thrombolysis

- Recombinant tPA (tissue plasminogen activator) has been shown to improve the outcome if given within 3 hours after the onset of stroke. There is a slightly increased risk of intracranial bleed especially if given after 3 hours. tPA is contraindicated in the presence of high BP (>185/110), recent major surgery, prior stroke or head injury within 3 months and gastrointestinal bleeding in preceding 3 weeks.

Mechanical Thrombectomy

- These techniques include intra-arterial thrombolysis and endovascular thrombectomy. They can be used in ischemic stroke due to large-vessel occlusions such as middle cerebral artery (MCA), internal carotid artery, and the basilar artery. Mechanical thrombectomy is recommended within the time frame of 6–16 hours after the stroke onset.

Statins

- High-intensity statins (atorvastatin 80 mg daily or rosuvastatin 20 mg daily) are recommended for patients who have clinical atherosclerotic cardiovascular disease. In addition, patients may be continued on statins if they were on them prior to the ischemic stroke. Statins should be continued lifelong for to prevent stroke recurrence.

Supportive Measures

- Prevent infections (pneumonia, urinary tract, and skin) and deep venous thrombosis (DVT).
- Fever is detrimental and should be treated with antipyretics and surface cooling.
- Blood glucose should be monitored and kept at <110 mg/dl.
- Patients may develop cerebral edema which causes obtundation or brain herniation. Edema peaks on the second or third day. It is likely to develop in large infarcts. It should be reduced by IV mannitol and head end elevation.

Réhabilitation

- Rehabilitation services improve neurologic outcomes. Proper rehabilitation of the stroke patient includes early physical, occupational, and speech therapy.

The goal of rehabilitation is to return the patient to home and to maximize recovery by providing a safe, progressive regimen suited to the individual patient.

Q. Describe thrombolytic therapy in ischemic stroke.

Q. Enumerate the indications and contraindications to thrombolytic therapy in a stroke patient.

- Thrombolytic therapy is the administration of clot-dissolving drugs (fibrinolytics) to re-establish blood flow in an occluded cerebral artery during an acute ischemic stroke.
- The goal is to minimize infarct size, preserve brain tissue, and improve functional outcomes.

Common Agent Used

- **Alteplase (rtPA—recombinant tissue plasminogen activator)**.

Time Window

- **Within 4.5 hours** of symptom onset. Best outcomes if given **as early as possible** (within 90 minutes).
- Some patients may qualify for **extended mechanical thrombectomy** up to 24 hours (not IV thrombolysis).

Mechanism of Action

- Alteplase converts **plasminogen to plasmin**, which breaks down **fibrin** in thrombi.
- This **dissolves the clot** obstructing cerebral blood flow.

Indications for IV Thrombolysis (tPA)

- Clinical diagnosis of acute ischemic stroke.
- Age ≥18 years.
- Time since symptom onset ≤4.5 hours.
- Noncontrast CT brain shows no hemorrhage.
- Measurable neurologic deficit (e.g. NIHSS >4).
- Informed consent obtained (where possible).

Contraindications to Thrombolysis

Absolute Contraindications

- Intracranial hemorrhage on imaging
- History of intracranial hemorrhage
- Known cerebral aneurysm, AV malformation, tumor
- Recent major head trauma or stroke (within 3 months)
- Active internal bleeding
- Platelet count <100,000/mm^3
- Coagulopathy: INR >1.7 or aPTT prolonged
- Use of anticoagulants (e.g. warfarin with INR >1.7, DOACs within 48 hours)
- Uncontrolled hypertension: BP >185/110 mm Hg (despite treatment)

Relative Contraindications (Use Clinical Judgment)

- Minor or rapidly improving stroke symptoms
- Recent major surgery or trauma (within last 14 days)
- Recent GI or urinary tract bleeding (within last 21 days)
- Recent myocardial infarction
- Pregnancy
- Age >80 (still often treated depending on local protocol).

Q. Describe the role of antiplatelet agents in stroke patients.

Q. Enumerate the indications and contraindications of antiplatelet agents in ischemic stroke (non-hemorrhagic stroke).

Role of Antiplatelet Agents in Stroke Patients

- Antiplatelet agents help prevent platelet aggregation, thereby reducing the risk of recurrent thrombotic events (e.g. strokes, TIAs) by maintaining cerebral arterial patency.

Common Antiplatelet Agents Used in Ischemic Stroke and Dosage (Table 5.26)

TABLE 5.26: Antiplatelet agents used in ischemic stroke and dosage

Agent	Dose (Acute)	Dose (Maintenance)	Comments
Aspirin	300 mg stat	75–150 mg daily	Start ASAP if no tPA; delay 24 h post-tPA
Clopidogrel	300 mg loading	75 mg daily	Useful if aspirin-intolerant
Aspirin + Clopidogrel (dual antiplatelet therapy)	300 mg + 300 mg loading	Continue 75 mg + 75 mg fo 21–90 days in selected patients	Effective in minor stroke or TIA to prevent subsequent major stroke

Indications for Antiplatelet Therapy in Stroke (Table 5.27)

TABLE 5.27: Indications for antiplatelet therapy in stroke

Indication	Details
Acute ischemic stroke (not thrombolysed)	Start aspirin 300 mg within 24 hours of stroke onset after CT confirms no bleed
Acute ischemic stroke (thrombolysed)	Start aspirin 24 hours after thrombolysis, once repeat CT excludes hemorrhage
Transient ischemic attack (TIA)	Start aspirin or clopidogrel immediately
Secondary prevention of ischemic stroke	Long-term antiplatelet therapy (aspirin or clopidogrel)
Short-term dual therapy (DAPT)	Aspirin + clopidogrel for 21–90 days in minor stroke or high-risk TIA to prevent subsequent major stroke

Contraindications to Antiplatelet Agents (Table 5.28)

TABLE 5.28: Contraindications for antiplatelet therapy in stroke

Category	Contraindication
Bleeding risk	Active bleeding (e.g. peptic ulcer, GI bleed, hemorrhagic stroke)
Allergy	Hypersensitivity to aspirin or clopidogrel
Platelet disorder	Thrombocytopenia or bleeding diatheses
Concurrent anticoagulation	Use with warfarin or DOACs may increase bleeding risk (assess carefully)
Severe liver disease	Increased bleeding tendency
Post-thrombolysis, for 24 hours	Avoid antiplatelets before 24h post-tPA till CT rules out hemorrhage due to thrombolysis

Special Considerations

- Avoid aspirin in patients with asthma or aspirin-sensitive bronchospasm.
- Clopidogrel may be preferred in patients with GI intolerance to aspirin.
- For patients with atrial fibrillation, anticoagulation is preferred over antiplatelets.

Q. Lacunar infarcts (lacunar stroke).

- Lacunar infarcts are small (<15 mm in diameter) subcortical infarcts caused by occlusion of small penetrating branches that supply deep subcortical structures.
- These branches arise at acute angles from the large arteries of the circle of Willis, stem of the middle cerebral artery (MCA), or the basilar artery.
- They are a type of ischemic stroke, typically affecting the basal ganglia, thalamus, internal capsule, corona radiata, and pons.

Etiology

- Lipohyalinosis
- Microatheroma
- Small emboli.

Risk Factors

- Aging
- Hypertension
- Diabetes mellitus
- Smoking
- Hyperhomocysteinemia
- Genetic factors.

Clinical Features

There are 5 important lacunar stroke syndromes:

1. Pure motor hemiparesis
2. Pure sensory stroke
3. Sensorimotor stroke
4. Ataxic hemiparesis
5. Dysarthria-clumsy hand syndrome.

Pure Motor Hemiparesis

- This is the most frequent lacunar stroke syndrome. It is characterized by hemiparesis without any cortical signs (aphasia, agnosia, apraxia, etc.) or sensory deficit. Sometimes weakness may affect only the arm or leg.
- The site of lesion is posterior limb of internal capsule (carries corticospinal and corticobulbar tracts) or basis pontis.

Pure Sensory Stroke

- Pure sensory stroke is defined as numbness of one side of the body in the absence of motor deficit or cortical signs.
- The site of lesion is thalamus (VPL nucleus).

Sensorimotor Stroke

- This is characterized by both weakness and numbness on one side of the body (contralateral to the lesion) in the absence of cortical signs.
- The site of lesion is posterolateral thalamus and posterior limb of the internal capsule.

Ataxic Hemiparesis

- These patients present with unilateral limb ataxia and weakness. Patients may also exhibit other ipsilateral cerebellar signs such as dysarthria, dysmetria, and nystagmus.
- The site of lesion is posterior limb of internal capsule, or basis pontis.

Dysarthria-clumsy Hand Syndrome

- This is the least common of all lacunar syndromes.
- This is characterized by facial weakness, dysarthria, dysphagia, and weakness and clumsiness of one hand. There are no sensory deficits or cortical signs. All these features are caused by damage to the corticobulbar fibers—the neural pathways that connect the cerebral cortex to the cranial nerve nuclei in the brainstem (e.g. cranial nerves V, VII, IX, X, XII).
- The site of lesion is basis pontis or the genu of internal capsule.

Investigations

- CT scan—less sensitive in picking up lacunar infarcts.
- MRI scan—more sensitive than CT scan.
- CT-angiography or MR-angiography—to rule out major artery block.

Treatment

- Thrombolytic therapy—intravenous recombinant tissue-type plasminogen activator or rt-PA if the patient presents within 3 hours.
- Dual antiplatelet therapy (aspirin plus clopidogrel) for 3 weeks followed by single antiplatelet (aspirin, 75–300 mg daily) lifelong to prevent stroke recurrence.
- Treatment of underlying risk factors such as hypertension, diabetes, hyperlipidemia, etc.

Q. Discuss the etiology, clinical features, investigations and management of hemorrhagic stroke (intracerebral hemorrhage).

- Intracerebral hemorrhage refers to bleeding within the brain parenchyma. This is the most common type of intracranial hemorrhage. Symptoms are due to mass effect of bleeding and associated edema.

Epidemiology

- Intracerebral hemorrhage is common in old age. However, it can also occur in young people due to rupture of arteriovenous malformation. It is more common in men. Incidence is high in Asians and African Americans.

Etiology

- Head injury
- AV malformation or aneurysm rupture
- Cavernous angioma
- Capillary telangiectasias
- Hypertension (usually causes hemorrhage into the putamen)
- Large infarct (bleeding can occur into the infarct).
- Cortical venous sinus thrombosis (can cause hemorrhagic infarct).
- Cerebral amyloid angiopathy (occurs in elderly)
- Drugs: Cocaine, amphetamine, phenylpropranolamine. These drugs can cause sudden increase in BP and lead to hemorrhage.
- Anticoagulant or thrombolytic therapy (warfarin, DOACs, tPA).
- Coagulopathy (e.g. thrombocytopenia, hemophilia)
- Brain tumor (hemorrhage can occur into a tumor)
- Vasculitis (polyarteritis nodosa or SLE)
- Moyamoya disease (it is an occlusive arterial disease which can occasionally cause intracerebral hemorrhage).

Clinical Features

- Patients present with sudden onset of headache, focal neurologic deficits, and impaired consciousness. Headache, vomiting, and impaired consciousness occur due to increased intracranial pressure. Some patients may present in coma.
- Intracerebral hemorrhages especially hypertensive hemorrhages occur when the patient is active.
- Seizures occur in some patients and are more common in lobar hemorrhages involving cerebral cortex (due to irritation of the cortex).
- Patients may complain of a stiff neck and have meningismus on physical examination, if there is extension to ventricles and subarachnoid space.
- Neurologic symptoms and signs vary depending upon the location of the hemorrhage and usually increase gradually over minutes or a few hours.
- Putaminal hemorrhage causes hemiplegia, hemisensory loss, homonymous hemianopia, gaze palsy, stupor, and coma.
- Cerebellar hemorrhage causes an inability to walk due to imbalance, vomiting, headache (which is usually occipital), neck stiffness, gaze palsy, and facial weakness. There is no hemiparesis. Patient may slip into coma due to brainstem compression.
- Thalamic hemorrhage produces hemiparesis, hemisensory loss, and occasionally transient homonymous hemianopsia.
- Lobar hemorrhage produces unilateral hemiparesis and hemisensory deficits. Speech impairment can occur if dominant hemisphere is involved. Occipital hemorrhages present with contralateral homonymous hemianopia.
- Pontine hemorrhage produces deep coma due to disruption of the reticular activating system. There is total paralysis. Pupils are pinpoint and react to a strong light source.

Differential Diagnosis

- Ischemic stroke
- Seizure
- Migraine
- Subarachnoid hemorrhage
- Metabolic encephalopathy.

Investigations

CT Scan Head

- Plain CT head is the investigation of choice to diagnose intracerebral hemorrhage **(Fig. 5.25)**. CT can provide information about the size and location of the hematoma, extension into the ventricular system, the presence of surrounding edema, and shifts in brain contents (herniation). Hyperacute blood will appear hyperdense (white appearance). Over weeks, it will appear isodense and later becomes hypodense.

MRI Head

- MRI and CT are equivalent for the detection of acute intracranial hemorrhage (ICH), but MRI is more accurate for the detection of chronic ICH.

CT Angiography/MR Angiography

- To assess for vascular malformations or aneurysms.

Other Tests

- Routine tests such as blood sugar, urea, creatinine, electrolytes, lipid profile and complete hemogram should be obtained.
- Coagulation profile (PT/INR, aPTT).

Management

- Initial measures: ABCDE approach (*see* previous pages).
- Admit the patient in ICU for continuous neurological and hemodynamic monitoring.
- All anticoagulant and antiplatelet drugs should be discontinued for at least one to two weeks after the onset of hemorrhage and any anticoagulant effect

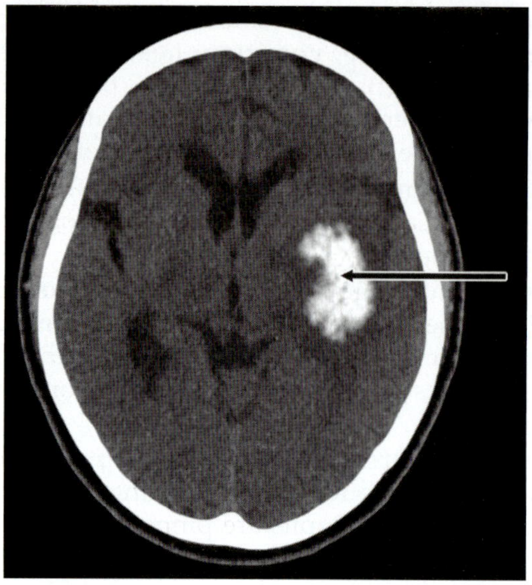

Figure 5.25: Intracerebral bleed (arrow)

should be reversed immediately with appropriate agents.

- ***Blood pressure control:*** BP is often elevated in patients with ICH and in hypertensive hemorrhage. BP should be controlled with intravenous nitroprusside, nicardipine, or labetalol. The goal is to maintain the systolic pressure between 140 and 160 mm Hg. BP less than this may compromise cerebral perfusion.
- ***Surgery:*** Surgical evacuation is indicated for all cerebellar hemorrhages greater than 3 cm in diameter since there is a high risk of brainstem compression and obstructive hydrocephalus. Surgical evacuation is also indicated in lobar hematoma if there is gradual deterioration of neurological deficits.
- ***Managing raised ICP***
  - Hyperventilation
  - Mannitol
  - Inj frusemide 20 mg IV Q 6th hourly
  - Elevation of head of bed.
- ***Prevention of seizures:*** Inj phenytoin 15 mg/kg body weight loading dose given as IV infusion over 30 min, then 100 mg every 8th hourly. Levetiracetam 500 mg 12th hourly is another option.
- ***Hemostatic therapy:*** If the patient presents within 3 hours of onset, treatment with activated recombinant factor VIIa (rFVIIa) may stop the ongoing hemorrhage and hematoma enlargement. Factor VIIa promotes hemostasis at sites of vascular injury.
- ***General measures:*** DVT prophylaxis, nutrition (RT feeds, IV fluids).

Q. Discuss the etiology, clinical features, investigations and management of subarachnoid hemorrhage.

- Subarachnoid hemorrhage (SAH) is bleeding into the subarachnoid space.
- It is classified as:
  - Traumatic SAH (most common)
  - Nontraumatic or spontaneous SAH (usually due to ruptured aneurysms)

Etiology

- Trauma (most common overall cause)
- Rupture of berry aneurysms (most common nontraumatic cause)
- Arteriovenous malformations
- Mycotic aneurysms
- Vasculitis
- Intracranial arterial dissections
- Amyloid angiopathy
- Bleeding diatheses
- Illicit drug use (cocaine and amphetamines)
- Unknown cause

Risk Factors

- Cigarette smoking
- Hypertension
- Alcohol
- Family history
- Phenylpropanolamine (used in cold remedies, increases the risk of hemorrhagic stroke)
- Estrogen deficiency (this may be the cause of increased risk of SAH in postmenopausal women)
- Anticoagulant use.

Clinical Features

- Symptoms of SAH begin abruptly.
- Main symptom is sudden onset, severe headache (thunderclap headache) classically described as the "worst headache of my life." Headache is usually diffuse. Some patients have warning headaches preceding major hemorrhage for many days.
- Headache may be associated with brief loss of consciousness, seizure, photophobia, nausea, and vomiting.
- Examination reveals variable level of consciousness, neck stiffness and Kernig's sign. Subhyaloid hemorrhage is seen on fundoscopy occasionally.
- Blood in the subarachnoid space causes a chemical meningitis which increases intracranial pressure lasting few days to few weeks. Secondary vasospasm may cause focal brain ischemia and stroke.

Investigations

CT Scan Head

- Plain CT head is the cornerstone of SAH diagnosis. Clot is demonstrated in the subarachnoid space in most cases if the scan is done within 24 hours of the bleed. There may be intracerebral and intraventricular extension of blood in some cases. The sensitivity of CT for detecting SAH is highest in the first 12 hours after SAH (nearly 100%) and then decreases over time. Minor bleed may not be picked up on CT scan.

Lumbar Puncture

- Lumbar puncture should be done in all cases if there is a strong suspicion of SAH despite a normal CT scan. The classic findings are an elevated opening pressure and a uniformly blood stained CSF.

- Blood can be present in CSF due to traumatic tap and it should be differentiated from SAH. Clearing of blood (a declining RBC count with successive collection tubes) suggests traumatic tap. If the last tube is normal, it reliably excludes SAH.
- Xanthochromia (pink or yellow tint) represents hemoglobin degradation products. Xanthochromia in CSF is highly suggestive of SAH because blood has to be present in CSF for few hours for it to occur. Hence xanthochromia cannot occur due to traumatic LP.

CT or MR Angiography

- This is a noinvasive way of imaging crebrovascular anatomy. Hence, it has replaced conventional angiogram as the initial diagnostic test of choice.
- Digital subtraction angiography (DSA): Gold standard for detecting aneurysms/AVMs, especially for planning treatment.

Blood Tests

- CBC, coagulation profile
- Renal and liver function tests
- Electrolytes (monitor for hyponatremia from SIADH or cerebral salt-wasting)

Treatment

Immediate Measures

- ABCDE approach (Airway, Breathing, Circulation, Deficits, Exposure; *see* previous pages).

General Measures

- Admit the patient in intensive care unit.
- Bed rest, stool softeners, adequate analgesia to diminish hemodynamic fluctuations.
- Deep venous thrombosis (DVT) prophylaxis with pneumatic compression stockings.
- Discontinue all anticoagulants and antiplatelet agents if the patient is taking any. Anticoagulant effect should be reversed immediately with vitamin K and fresh frozen plasma.

Reduction of Intracranial Pressure (ICP)

- Head end elevation.
- Mannitol 20%, 100 ml IV every 6th–8th hourly.
- Loop diuretics (e.g. furosemide) also can decrease ICP.
- Use of intravenous steroids (e.g. dexamethasone) for decreasing ICP is controversial.

Reduction of Blood Pressure

- If BP is high, it should be lowered by using labetalol infusion. Vasodilators such as nitroprusside or nitroglycerin should be avoided because they increase cerebral blood volume and therefore increase intracranial pressure.

Prevention of Vasospasm

- Nimodipine (oral calcium channel blocker) 60 mg every four hours by mouth or nasogastric tube.

Seizure Prophylaxis

- Antiepileptic drugs (phenytoin or sodium valproate or levetiracetam) should be given to prevent seizures. Long-term seizure prophylaxis is not required.

Treatment of Aneurysms and AV Malformations

- Placement of a clip across the neck of the aneurysm remains the treatment of choice for most aneurysms. Endovascular techniques with coil placement are becoming popular for obliteration of aneurysms and AV malformations.

Complications

- Rebleeding is the most dreaded complication of SAH. It usually occurs within the first 24 hours.
- Vasospasm (presence of blood in the subarachnoid space causes smooth muscle contraction and vasospasm. Vasospasm can lead to brain ischemia and infarction).
- Hydrocephalus can occur due to obstruction of free CSF flow by the presence of blood in the subarachnoid space.

Q. Enumerate the indications for surgery in a hemorrhagic stroke.

Indications for Surgery in Hemorrhagic Stroke

Cerebellar hemorrhage

- Hematoma >3 cm in diameter associated with the following:
  - Neurological deterioration
  - Brainstem compression
  - Hydrocephalus from ventricular obstruction
- Urgent surgical evacuation is recommended (often lifesaving)

Lobar hemorrhage

- Superficial (lobar) hematomas >30 ml with:
  - Clinical deterioration
  - Midline shift or mass effect
  - Accessible location (non-eloquent cortex)

Intraventricular hemorrhage (IVH) with hydrocephalus

- Indication for external ventricular drain (EVD)
- To relieve obstructive hydrocephalus and control intracranial pressure

Elevated intracranial pressure (ICP)

- Refractory to medical management (mannitol, hypertonic saline).
- Surgical decompression (e.g. decompressive craniectomy) may be considered.

Underlying structural lesions

- Hemorrhage associated with arteriovenous malformation (AVM), cavernous malformation, and tumors.
- Surgical resection may be planned electively after stabilization.

Note:
- Deep hemorrhages (e.g. basal ganglia, thalamus, brainstem) are usually not surgically accessible and are managed conservatively.
- Decisions should be individualized based on neurological status, location, size of bleed, comorbidities, and patient/family wishes.

Q. Enumerate and describe the indications and modalities of multidisciplinary rehabilitation of patients with a CVA.

- Multidisciplinary rehabilitation is essential in stroke management and significantly improves functional recovery, psychosocial adjustment, and quality of life. Early, individualized, and goal-directed therapy is the cornerstone of optimal outcomes in CVA patients.
- Early initiation (within 24–48 hours if stable) is associated with better outcomes.
- Can be provided in:
  - Inpatient rehabilitation units.
  - Outpatient rehabilitation centers.
  - Home-based care (for selected patients).

Indications for Multidisciplinary Rehabilitation in Patients with CVA

- All stroke survivors benefit from rehabilitation. However, rehabilitation is specifically indicated in patients who:
  - Have survived the acute phase of stroke.
  - Exhibit residual neurological deficits (e.g. hemiparesis, aphasia, dysphagia).
  - Are medically stable and can participate in a structured rehabilitation program.
  - Demonstrate potential for functional recovery (e.g. conscious, able to follow commands).
  - Have no absolute contraindications (e.g. severe comorbidities, ongoing medical instability).

Goals of Rehabilitation

- Restore function and independence.
- Prevent complications (e.g. contractures, pressure ulcers).
- Improve quality of life.
- Support psychological and social reintegration.

Modalities of Multidisciplinary Rehabilitation

- Rehabilitation requires a team approach, involving several disciplines.

Neurologist/Physician

- Oversees medical stabilization.
- Monitors for complications (e.g. seizures, infections).
- Adjusts medications and preventive strategies (e.g. anticoagulants, antihypertensives).

Physiotherapy

- *Motor retraining*: Strengthening, balance, and coordination exercises.
- *Gait training*: Use of assistive devices (walker, cane).
- *Spasticity management*: Stretching, splinting, sometimes botulinum toxin.

Occupational Therapy

- Focuses on activities of daily living (ADLs): Bathing, dressing, eating.
- Promotes upper limb function recovery.
- Home/workplace modification for accessibility.
- Training in use of adaptive devices.

Speech and Language Therapy

- For patients with:
  - Dysphasia (aphasia): Language re-education
  - Dysarthria: Articulation training
  - Dysphagia: Safe swallowing techniques to prevent aspiration.

Neuropsychology/Psychiatry

- Cognitive rehabilitation (e.g. attention, memory training)
- Management of post-stroke depression, anxiety, or emotional lability
- Counseling for patient and family.

Dietician/Nutritionist

- Nutritional assessment and management
- Enteral feeding if dysphagia present
- Stroke-specific diet planning (e.g. low salt, diabetic diet).

Social Worker

- Assists with discharge planning, home support, financial aid
- Coordinates community-based services and vocational training
- Supports reintegration into society and employment if feasible.

Q. Causes of hemiplegia in an elderly male.

- Hemiplegia is paralysis of one side of the body.

Causes of Hemiplegia (Table 5.29)

TABLE 5.29: Causes of hemiplegia
Acute onset • Stroke (ischemic, hemorrhagic) • Trauma
Subacute onset • Cerebral metastases • Subdural hematoma • Granulomas (tubercular, fungal) • Brain abscess • Cortical vein thrombosis
Chronic • Slowly growing neoplasms

Q. What is stroke in young? Enumerate the causes of stroke in young.

- Stroke in young refers to stroke occurring in individuals of less than 50 years.
- Unlike in older adults, where stroke is commonly due to atherosclerosis and hypertension, young stroke patients often have diverse and less traditional risk

TABLE 5.30: Causes of stroke in young

Hematological diseases	
• Protein C deficiency • Protein S deficiency • Antithrombin III deficiency • Antiphospholipid antibody syndrome (APLA) • Factor V Leiden mutation • Sickle cell anemia • β-thalassemia • Polycythemia vera • Essential thrmbocytosis • Dysproteinemias	All these conditions cause hypercoagulable state and ischemic stroke
• Hemophilia • Thrombocytopenia	These conditions cause hemorrhagic stroke
Connective tissue diseases	
• Systemic vasculitis (PAN, Wegner's, Takayasu's, giant cell arteritis) • Systemic lupus erythematosus • Inflammatory bowel disease	
Infections	
• Syphilis • Meningitis • Tuberculosis • HIV	
Drug abuse	
• Cocaine, amphetamine	
Cardiac disorders (cardioembolic)	
• Atrial fibrillation • Atrial myxoma • Intracardiac tumor • Infective endocarditis • Libman-Sacks endocarditis • Myocardial infarction (mural thrombus) • Dilated cardiomyopathy • Paradoxical embolism (Atrial septal defect, patent foramen ovale) • Valvular heart diseases (MS, MR, AS, AR)	
CNS lesions	
• AV malformations • Aneurysms • Neoplasms	
Genetic and metabolic disorders	
• Cerebral autosomal dominant arteriopathy with subcortical infarcts and leukoencephalopathy (CADASIL) • Mitochondrial encephalopathy, lactic acidosis, and stroke-like episodes (MELAS) • Homocystinuria • Fabry disease	

factors (**Table 5.30**). The underlying cause of stroke in young should be identified and treated. Treatment is same as those in elderly.

Q. Transient ischemic attack (TIA)

Classic Time-based Definition

- TIA was originally defined as sudden onset of a focal neurologic symptom and/or sign lasting less than 24 hours. However, this classic definition of TIA is no longer adequate, because many TIAs satisfying this definition have been shown to have infarction on MRI.

Tissue-based Definition

- In the tissue-based definition, which is now the most widely accepted, TIA is a transient episode of neurologic dysfunction caused by focal brain or retinal ischemia, without evidence of acute infarction.
- TIAs increase the risk of subsequent stroke. TIA can be considered as a serious warning for an impending ischemic stroke; the risk is highest in the first 48 hours following a TIA.

Causes of TIA

Risk factors for TIA are the same as those for ischemic stroke. Modifiable risk factors include the following:

- Hypertension
- Cigarette smoking
- Dyslipidemia
- Diabetes
- Obesity
- Lack of physical activity
- High-risk diet (e.g. high in saturated fats, trans fats, and calories)
- Heart disorders (particularly disorders that predispose to emboli, such as acute MI, infective endocarditis, and atrial fibrillation)
- Drugs (e.g. cocaine, amphetamines)
- Hypercoagulable states
- Vasculitis
- Alcoholism

Unmodifiable Risk Factors

- Prior stroke
- Old age
- Family history of stroke
- Male sex.

Clinical Features

- Neurologic deficits are similar to those of stroke. Symptoms and signs depend on the blood vessel and the brain area that is involved.
- Features of anterior circulation TIA (carotid system) include amaurosis fugax (transient monocular blindness due to ophthalmic artery involvement), aphasia, hemiparesis, hemisensory loss, and hemianopic visual loss.
- Features of posterior circulation TIA (vertebrobasilar system) include diplopia, vertigo, vomiting, dysarthria, ataxia, transient global amnesia, and loss of consciousness.

Differential Diagnosis

- TIAs must be distinguished from other causes which cause transient neurological dysfunction such as following.
  - Stroke (both ischemic and hemorrhagic).
  - Post ictal (Todd) paralysis following an attack of epilepsy.
  - Hypoglycemia.
  - Migraine aura.

Investigations

- MRI or CT head to rule out any intracranial pathology.
- Carotid and vertebral artery Doppler to rule out stenosis.
- MR angiography
- ECG and echocardiogram to rule out cardiac problems.
- 24 hour ECG monitoring (Holter monitoring) to rule out transient arrhythmias.
- Other routine tests (blood sugar, lipid profile, CBC, ESR, electrolytes, urea, creatinine).

Treatment

- The main aim of treatment of TIA is to decrease the risk of subsequent stroke or TIA. Early treatment after a TIA can significantly reduce the risk of stroke.

Antiplatelet Agents

- Give a loading dose of aspirin (300 mg) immediately, followed by aspirin (75 mg daily) lifelong. This will reduce the risk of subsequent stroke. Dual antiplatelet therapy with both aspirin and clopidogrel for the first 4 weeks followed by single antiplatelet therapy (aspirin) lifelong is more effective in preventing subsequent stroke).

Statins

- Statins (such as atorvastatin and rosuvastatin) along with antiplatelet agents reduce the risk of subsequent stroke.

Anticoagulants

- Heparin and warfarin should be given in embolic TIA such as atrial fibrillation.

Surgical Approaches

- ***Internal carotid endarterectomy*** is recommended if internal carotid artery stenosis greater than 70%.
- Percutaneous transluminal angioplasty (stenting) is an alternative procedure.

Treatment of Risk Factors

- Diabetes, hypertension, dyslipidemia, etc. should be treated. Smoking should be stopped.

Q. Clinical differentiation between hemorrhagic, thrombotic and embolic stroke.

See **Table 5.31.**

Q. Amaurosis fugax.

- Amaurosis fugax (from the Greek *amaurosis*, meaning dark, and the Latin *fugax*, meaning fleeting) refers to a transient loss of vision in one or both eyes.
- It is often described as a "curtain coming down over the eye" and then lifting.
- It is considered a form of transient ischemic attack (TIA) involving the retinal circulation.
- Patients with amaurosis fugax are at risk of stroke, myocardial infarction and vision loss. Hence the underlying cause should be identified and treated.

Etiology

- Retinal artery emboli (atherosclerotic plaques from carotid artery (most common)
- Cardiac emboli
- Critical carotid artery stenosis causing low perfusion
- Systemic hypotension
- Retinal vasospasm (e.g. in migraine).
- Giant cell arteritis (especially in elderly)

TABLE 5.31: Differentiation between hemorrhagic, thrombotic and embolic stroke

Feature	Hemorrhagic	Thrombotic	Embolic
• Time of onset	During activity	In sleep	Any time
• Progression	Over minutes and hours	Over hours	Within seconds
• Headache	Present	Usually absent	Usually absent
• Vomiting	Present	Absent	Absent
• Seizures	Usually present	Unusual	Unusual
• Early resolution	Unusual	Variable	Possible
• Presence of known bleeding disorder or on anticoagulation	May be present	Absent	Absent
• Signs of Meningeal irritation	May be present	Absent	Absent
• Severe hypertension	Usually present	May or may not be present	May or may not be present
• Carotid bruit	Does not support the diagnosis	Supports the diagnosis	Supports the diagnosis
• Cardiac disease (valvular heart disease, atrial fibrillation, etc.)	Does not support the diagnosis	Does not support the diagnosis	Highly supportive

- Elevated plasma viscosity, for example with leukemia, multiple myeloma.
- Atherosclerotic cerebrovascular disease.

Clinical Features

- Sudden monocular painless vision loss
- Described as "black curtain" or "shade" descending over vision.
- Lasts seconds to minutes, then fully resolves.
- No residual visual deficit after the episode.

Investigations

- Tests to rule out vascular risk factors such as diabetes, hypertension, dyslipidemia.
- Ophthalmologic evaluation.
- ESR and C-reactive protein to exclude giant cell arteritis (GCA).
- Carotid Doppler.
- MR angiogram to r/o carotid artery dissection.
- ECG and echocardiogram to rule out cardiac disease.
- EEG if seizures are suspected.
- Hypercoagulable testing in patients prior thrombosis, miscarriage, or family history.
- Complete blood count to screen for polycythemia vera and essential thrombocythemia.
- CT or MRI brain to rule out other causes of vision loss.

Management

- Treat as TIA—urgent evaluation is necessary.
- Antiplatelet therapy (e.g. aspirin).
- Statins.
- Carotid endarterectomy/stenting—if high-grade stenosis present.
- Anticoagulation if cardioembolic cause.
- Treatment of underlying vascular risk factors, such as hypertension, diabetes, and dyslipidemia.

Q. Wallenberg's syndrome (lateral medullary syndrome).

- Wallenberg's syndrome (lateral medullary syndrome) is due to lateral medullary infarction (or rarely due to hemorrhage). It can happen due to occlusion of posterior inferior cerebellar artery (PICA) or its parent vessel, the vertebral artery. Most of the cases occur due to PICA occlusion **(Fig. 5.26)**.

Signs and Symptoms

- *Ipsilateral ataxia of limbs, falling to side of lesion*: Due to involvement of inferior cerebellar peduncle, cerebellar hemisphere, cerebellar fibers, spinocerebellar tract.
- *Nystagmus, diplopia, oscillopsia, vertigo, nausea, vomiting*: Due to involvement of vestibular nucleus.
- *Ipsilateral Horner's syndrome (miosis, ptosis, decreased sweating):* Due to involvement of descending sympathetic tract.
- *Dysphagia, hoarseness, paralysis of palate, paralysis of vocal cord, diminished gag reflex:* Due to involvement of nucleus ambiguus, ninth and tenth cranial nerves.
- *Hiccoughs:* Exact cause unknown, but probably due to the involvement of nucleus ambiguus or adjacent areas regulating respiration.
- *Contralateral body loss of pain/temperature/crude touch:* Due to involvement of spinothalamic tract. Note that there is usually preserved light-touch, vibration, and proprioception on the body, because these sensations are carried by dorsal columns and then through medial lemnisci which lie in medial part of medulla.
- *Ipsilateral facial loss of pain/temperature/crude touch:* Due to involvement of the spinal nucleus of 5th nerve and the descending spinal tract of 5th nerve. Note that light-touch, vibration, and proprioception are preserved on the affected side of face because these

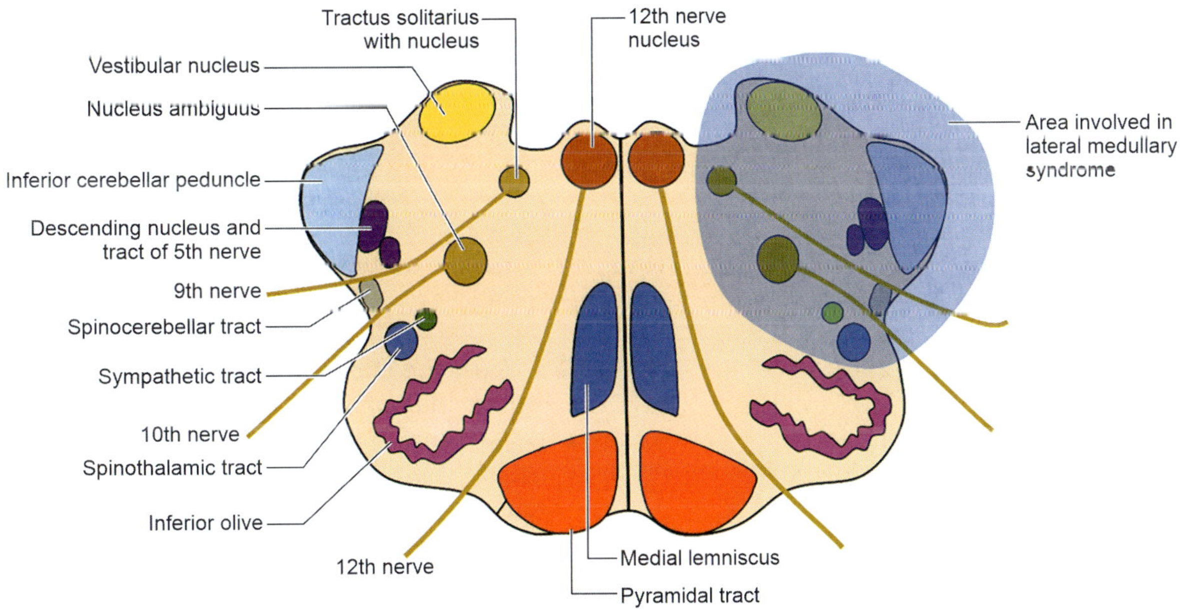

Figure 5.26: Lateral medullary syndrome

sensations are carried by dorsal columns and then through medial lemnisci which lie in medial part of medulla.

- *Occasionally ipsilateral loss of taste in the posterior tongue:* Due to involvement of nucleus and tractus solitaries.

Investigations

- *CT or MRI of the brain:* CT scan can be done within a short time and useful in emergencies. However, significant artifacts can occur due to the bony structures surrounding the brainstem and cerebellum. Brainstem lesions are better identified by MRI scan due to the absence of these artifacts.
- **Other routine tests:** Complete blood count, blood sugar, renal and liver function tests, lipid profile and serum electrolytes.

Treatment

- Admit the patient to ICU.
- Since the patients have dysphagia and are at high risk of aspiration, pass a Ryle's tube and perform endotracheal intubation. Patient should be fed through Ryle's tube to avoid aspiration until there is improvement of lower cranial nerve function.
- Antiplatelets and statins: since infarction is the most common cause of lateral medullary syndrome, antiplatelets such as aspirin plus statins such as atorvastatin should be given lifelong.
- Swallow/voice therapy critical; many recover swallowing within weeks.

Q. How do you decide the side, site and most probable nature of the lesion in a given patient with neurological symptoms/signs.

Upper *vs* Lower Motor Neuron (UMN *vs* LMN) Lesion

- *See* previous pages for details.

Side of Lesion and Symptom Presentation

Lesion location	Clinical side of weakness
Above brainstem (cortex/internal capsule)	Contralateral to lesion
Brainstem (UMN fibers decussate here)	Often contralateral body, ipsilateral cranial nerves
Spinal cord	Ipsilateral to lesion if tract damage is unilateral
Peripheral nerve/root	Ipsilateral to lesion

Site of Lesion and Clinical Features

Site of lesion	Key features
Cerebral cortex	Contralateral weakness, aphasia, seizures, cortical sensory loss, hemineglect
Internal capsule	Dense hemiplegia, contralateral face, arm, leg weakness, no cortical signs
Brainstem	"Crossed" findings (e.g. ipsilateral CN palsy + contralateral hemiparesis)
Cerebellum	Ataxia, dysmetria, intention tremor
Spinal cord	Definite sensory level, bowel bladder involvement, LMN signs at level, UMN signs below
Nerve root	Radicular pain (dermatomal distribution), LMN type motor weakness in muscles supplied by the particular root, loss of reflex served by the root, sensory loss
Peripheral nerve	LMN type weakness of muscles supplied by the peripheral nerve, loss of reflexes supplied by the particular nerve, loss of sensation in the distribution of nerve.
Neuromuscular junction	Fatigable weakness (e.g. myasthenia gravis). Weakness more with exertion and improves after resting, no sensory symptoms
Muscle	Proximal weakness, preserved reflexes, no sensory loss

Nature of Lesion Based on Onset of Symptoms

Onset of symptom	Likely nature of lesion
Sudden (seconds to minutes)	Vascular (stroke, TIA)
Acute (hours to days)	Infectious, inflammatory, or toxic
Subacute (days to weeks)	Neoplastic, immune-mediated
Chronic (weeks to months)	Degenerative, compressive, metabolic
Relapsing-remitting	Multiple sclerosis, autoimmune

Likely Nature of Lesion/Pathology Based on Associated Clinical Features

Associated feature	Possible cause
Fever + meningism	Meningitis, encephalitis, brain abscess
Seizure + focal deficits	Cortical lesion (tumor, stroke, abscess)
Vision loss + weakness	MS (optic neuritis + motor tract involvement)
Back pain + leg weakness	Spinal cord compression, disc prolapse
Sudden headache + focal signs	Hemorrhagic stroke, SAH
Asymmetrical weakness + fasciculations	Motor neuron disease (e.g. ALS)

Q. Discuss the etiology, clinical features, investigations and management of acute viral encephalitis.

- Encephalitis means inflammation of brain parenchyma, usually due to viral infection. Encephalitis can also be caused by bacteria, fungi, protozoa and helminthes.
- If both brain and spinal cord are involved, it is referred to as encephalomyelitis.
- Brain inflammation can be associated with meningitis and is known as meningoencephalitis.

Etiology of Viral Encephalitis

- Herpes simplex
- ECHO viruses
- Coxsackie
- Mumps
- Epstein-Barr virus
- Cytomegalovirus
- Influenza virus
- Japanese encephalitis virus
- West Nile virus
- Rabies
- HIV

- Common viruses causing encephalitis are herpes simplex, ECHO, coxsackie, mumps and Epstein -Barr viruses. Herpes simplex encephalitis is the most common etiology.
- Most of the time viral etiology cannot be confirmed and diagnosis is based on clinical features.
- Viral encephalitis can occur in epidemic and endemic forms in many places. Examples are Japanese encephalitis in South East Asia, California encephalitis in USA, West Nile encephalitis in Egypt and Sudan, etc.
- Rabies is a variety of sporadic viral encephalitis.

Clinical Features

- Symptoms include fever, headache, and altered mental status, often accompanied by seizures and focal neurologic deficits.
- Symptoms and signs of meningeal irritation (photophobia and neck stiffness) are usually absent in encephalitis but may be present in meningoencephalitis.
- Status epilepticus, particularly convulsive status epilepticus, or coma suggests severe brain inflammation and a poor prognosis.
- Specific clinical findings may sometimes suggest the causative virus: Parotitis suggests the mumps; flaccid paralysis suggests West Nile virus infection; findings of hydrophobia, aerophobia, and hyperactivity suggest rabies virus; grouped vesicles in a dermatomal pattern suggest varicella-zoster virus.

Differential Diagnosis

Encephalitis should be differentiated from other causes of altered sensorium which are as follows:

- Meningitis with cerebral edema
- Cerebral venous thrombosis
- Cerebral abscess
- Acute disseminated encephalomyelitis (ADEM)
- Cerebral malaria
- Delirium
- Septicemia.

Investigations

- CT and MRI scan may show areas of cerebral edema, often in the temporal lobes.
- EEG often shows characteristic slow waves.
- CSF shows a raised cell count with predominant lymphocytes. CSF sugar is normal and protein is mildly elevated. PCR for herpes simplex and other viral serology (blood + CSF) is helpful to identify the virus.

Treatment

- If herpes simplex encephalitis is suspected, it should be treated immediately with intravenous acyclovir (10 mg/kg IV Q 8 h) for 14–21 days. Ganciclovir is useful in CMV encephalitis. There is no specific treatment for other viral encephalitis. Oseltamivir in influenza-associated encephalitis.
- Supportive treatment involves anticonvulsants, antiedema measures, bedsore prevention, attention to nutrition through Ryle's tube, IV hydration and Foleys catheterization, etc.
- Prophylactic immunization against Japanese encephalitis is advised for travellers to endemic areas in Asia.

Q. Discuss the etiology, clinical features, investigations and management of brain abscess.

- Brain abscess is a focal collection of pus within the brain parenchyma. It behaves as a space-occupying lesion.

Etiology

Bacteria (most common cause)

- Streptococcus
- *Bacteroides species*
- Staphylococci (after trauma or neurosurgery)
- Listeria

Fungi

- Actinomyces
- Nocardia
- Candida
- Aspergillus
- *Coccidioides immitis*

In HIV infected patients

- Toxoplasmosis
- *Cryptococcus neoformans*

Pathogenesis

- Bacteria can invade the brain either by direct spread, trauma, neurosurgery or hematogenous spread.
- ***Direct spread:*** Organisms come from a contiguous site such as otitis media, mastoiditis, sinusitis and dental infections.
- ***Trauma:*** Bullet wounds to the brain can carry bacteria into the brain. Skull fractures can also expose the brain tissue to infections.
- ***Neurosurgery:*** Brain abscess can also complicate neurosurgical procedures.
- ***Hematogenous spread:*** Bacteria can reach brain through blood from other sources of infection such as lung abscess, empyema, skin infections, pelvic infection, intra-abdominal infection and bacterial endocarditis. Brain abscesses associated with bacteremia usually result in multiple abscesses.

Clinical Features

- Fever and headache are the most complaints. Since abscess is a space occupying lesion, it causes symptoms of raised intracranial pressure such as headache, vomiting, and altered sensorium. Headache is localized to the side of the abscess and severe. Focal signs (e.g. hemiparesis, aphasia, hemianopia) and seizures occur depending on the location of the abscess.
- Third and sixth cranial nerve deficits may develop due to raised intracranial pressure.
- Papilledema is a late manifestation of cerebral edema and usually takes several days to develop.

Differential Diagnosis

- Epidural and subdural empyema
- Septic dural sinus thrombosis
- Mycotic cerebral aneurysms
- Focal necrotizing encephalitis
- Neoplasms
- Pyogenic meningitis.

Investigations

- CT head with contrast or MRI scan shows the ring enhancing abscess.
- Lumbar puncture is better avoided as there is risk of herniation due to raised ICP.
- Aspiration with stereotactic guidance allows the infective organism to be identified.
- Serology: anti-Toxoplasma IgG antibody in blood and anticysticercal antibodies on CSF specimens, can aid in the diagnosis of *Toxoplasma gondii* or neurocysticercosis.

Management

- Treatment of brain abscess usually requires a combination of antibiotics and surgical drainage.
- Streptococcal and anaerobic infections are treated with intravenous cephalosporins plus metronidazole.
- Staphylococcal infections should be treated with flucloxacillin or vancomycin. Other bacteria are treated appropriately.
- Duration of antibiotic therapy is usually 6 – 8 weeks.
- Glucocorticoids (dexamethasone) should be used when there is significant brain edema causing mass effect and altered mental status.
- Antiepileptics may be required to prevent seizures.
- Surgical decompression may be necessary if parenteral antibiotics are unsuccessful.

Q. Neurocysticercosis (NCC).

Etiology

- *Causal agent*: *Taenia solium* pork tapeworm, larval (cysticercus) stage.
- Humans acquire NCC by ingesting eggs (fecal–oral) shed by a human tapeworm carrier—not by eating pork. Man is the definitive host and pig is the intermediate host.
- When man ingests eggs, they develop into larval cysts called oncospheres, which invade the intestine and are carried by the blood to various organs including brain. In the brain, they remain as cysts for many years which is called neurocysticercosis.

Clinical Features

- Common presentation is seizures. Other symptoms include headache, vomiting, focal neurological signs, and raised intracranial pressure.
- Symptoms are due to mass effect, an inflammatory response, or obstruction of the foramina and ventricular system of the brain.

Investigations

- CT scan or MRI scan—can identify cysts. MRI is more sensitive than CT scan.
- Serological studies—detection of antigen or antibodies to cysticerci can support the diagnosis of neurocysticercosis.

Treatment

- ***Neurocysticercosis*** should be treated with albendazole or praziquantel. Dose of albendazole is 15 mg/kg per day (usually 800 mg/day) in two divided doses for 14 days. Combined albendazole plus praziquantel is given if there are multiple (>2) viable cysts. Corticosteroids are usually recommended (30–40 mg prednisolone or 12–16 mg dexamethasone daily in divided doses) for patients during antihelminthic therapy. Anticonvulsants are indicated to prevent seizures.
- Contraindications to antihelminthics—uncontrolled ICP, massive cyst burden, or only calcifications.
- Neurosurgery to removal of cysts—is indicated in case of cysts producing mass effect and cysts present in 4th ventricle producing hydrocephalus.

Q. Define and differentiate between seizures, convulsions and epilepsy.

Seizure

- A ***seizure*** is a transient, sudden, abnormal, synchronous electrical discharge in a group of cerebral neurons.
- May produce motor, sensory, autonomic or psychic manifestations or no outward signs at all; duration seconds to minutes; self-limited.
- Can occur once (e.g. febrile seizure, metabolic insult) without implying a chronic disorder.

Convulsion

- The clinical phenomenon of involuntary, forceful muscle contractions ± loss of consciousness resulting from a seizure involving motor cortex and brainstem pathways.
- Manifests as tonic (stiffening), clonic (jerking) or tonic-clonic movements of limbs/face.
- Some seizures do not have convulsive movements (e.g. absence seizures, focal aware with aura).

Epilepsy

- A chronic disorder characterized by an enduring predisposition to generate epileptic seizures with any of the following features.
  - ≥ 2 unprovoked (or reflex) seizures >24 hours apart, or
  - One unprovoked seizure and a ≥60 % risk of recurrence over next 10 years (based on EEG, imaging, or etiology), or
  - Diagnosis of an epilepsy syndrome (e.g. juvenile myoclonic epilepsy, childhood absence epilepsy) known to carry high recurrence risk.
- Represents the disease state; implies need for long-term management and risk counseling. Requires a persistent tendency to seizures, not a single acute symptomatic event. May include both convulsive and nonconvulsive seizure types.
- Unprovoked seizure means seizure which is not due to any reversible transient cause such as hypoglycemia and electrolyte imbalance.
- Note that in a known epileptic even though the seizures are unprovoked, seizures can also be provoked by transient causes such as hypoglycemia and electrolyte disturbances.

Q. Enumerate the etiological classification of epilepsy (Table 5.32).

Etiological ("STIGMAU") Classification — ILAE 2022 (International League against Epilepsy)

- Note that more than one category may apply in a given patient.

TABLE 5.32: Etiological classification of epilepsy

Category	Causes
Structural	Cortical dysplasia, stroke, tumor, trauma, mesial temporal sclerosis, tuberous sclerosis, etc.
Genetic	Singlegene (SCN1A, KCNQ2), chromosomal (Down), channelopathies; includes "genetic generalized epilepsies."
Infectious	Neurocysticercosis, HIV, HSV encephalitis, cerebral malaria, TB, postmeningitis, etc.
Metabolic	Inborn errors (GLUT1 deficiency, ureacycle defects), systemic derangements (hypoglycemia, hyponatremia).
Immune	Autoimmune encephalitis (antiNMDAR, LGI1), Rasmussen encephalitis.
Unknown	Cause not yet determined.

Q. Clinical classification of epilepsy (ILAE 2025 classification).

- ILAE (international league against epilepsy) has given the latest classification of epilepsy which is as follows **(Table 5.33)**.

TABLE 5.33: Clinical classification of epilepsy

FOCAL
- Focal preserved consciousness seizure (FPC)
- Focal impaired consciousness seizure (FIC)
- Focal unknown state of consciousness seizure (FUSC)
- Focal-to-bilateral tonic-clonic seizure (FBTC)

GENERALIZED
- Absence seizures
- Generalized tonic-clonic seizure (GTC)
  - Generalized tonic-clonic seizure
  - Myoclonic tonic-clonic seizure
  - Absence-to-tonic-clonic seizure
- Generalized motor seizures—other than tonic-clonic
  - Generalized myoclonic seizure (GM)
  - Generalized clonic seizure (GC)
  - Generalized negative myoclonic seizure (GNM)
  - Generalized epileptic spasm (GES)
  - Generalized tonic seizure (GT)
  - Generalized atonic seizure (GA)
  - Generalized myoclonic-atonic seizure (GMA)

UNKNOWN WHETHER FOCAL OR GENERALIZED
- Unknown whether focal or generalized - Preserved Consciousness seizure (UPC)
- Unknown whether focal or generalized - Impaired Consciousness seizure (UIC)
- Unknown whether focal or generalized – Unknown state of Consciousness seizure (UUSC)
- Unknown whether focal or generalized - tonic-clonic seizure (UTC)

UNCLASSIFIED

Q. Discuss the etiology, clinical features, investigations and management of generalized tonic clonic seizures (GTCS).

- A generalized tonic-clonic seizure is a convulsive seizure that begins simultaneously in both cerebral hemispheres and is characterized by an initial tonic phase followed by a clonic phase of rhythmic, synchronous jerks, typically culminating in post-ictal unresponsiveness.
- It was earlier known as grand mal epilepsy.

Etiology

- The *etiology* of epilepsy is usually multifactorial. Both hereditary and environmental factors play a role.
- Following are the common causes of seizures some of which lead to epilepsy.

- Idiopathic (commonest cause of epilepsy)
- Birth trauma
- Developmental abnormalities (e.g. microcephaly, porencephaly, hydrocephalus)
- Metabolic abnormalities (e.g. hypocalcemia, hypoglycemia, hypomagnesemia, hyponatremia, uremia, hepatic encephalopathy, phenylketonuria)
- Infections (meningitis, encephalitis, tuberculosis, congenital syphilis, brain abscess, parasitic infestations)

- Acute brain injury (head injury, acute ischemic or hemorrhagic stroke, subdural hematoma, cerebral venous thrombosis, posterior reversible encephalopathy syndrome, eclampsia, hypoxic-ischemic injury)
- Substance or medication withdrawal (alcohol, benzodiazepines)
- Drug intoxication, poisoning, and overdose (cocaine, amphetamine)
- Space-occupying lesion in brain (neoplasm, abscess)
- Degenerative (Alzheimer's disease)

Pathophysiology of a Seizure

- Ion-channel mutations, cortical malformations, injury, infection, metabolic or immune factors lower the threshold for excitation of neurons. Intrinsic (sleep-wake transitions, hormonal shifts) or extrinsic (fever, flashing lights, missed medication) perturbations tip the balance toward hyperexcitability in a susceptible neural circuit.
- Seizures develop when the balance between excitatory and inhibitory mechanisms is disturbed at the cellular or the synaptic level. Glutamate is the most common excitatory neurotransmitter and gamma-aminobutyric acid (GABA) is the most common inhibitory neurotransmitter involved. Failure of inhibitory processes is increasingly thought to be the major mechanism leading to status epilepticus.
- Spread of electrical activity between neurons is normally restricted. During a seizure, large groups of neurons are activated repetitively, unrestrictedly and hypersynchronously. Inhibitory synaptic activity between neurons fails. This produces high-voltage spike-and wave EEG activity, the electrophysiological hallmark of epilepsy.
- A focal (partial) seizure is epileptic activity confined to one area of cortex. Focal seizure can spread and involve all parts of the brain. This is called focal seizure with secondary generalization. Seizure can be generalized from the onset. This is called generalized onset seizure.
- Significant physiologic changes occur if seizures are prolonged especially in generalized tonic clonic seizures. These are tachycardia, hypertension, cardiac arrhythmias, hyperglycemia which result from catecholamine surge. Blood pressure may decrease as the seizure activity continues. Body temperature may increase as a result of the vigorous muscle activity and increased sympathetic drive. Marked acidosis usually occurs and has both respiratory and metabolic component. It should not be treated, as acidosis is known to have an anticonvulsant effect and resolves with termination of the seizure. Hypoxia occurs due to breathing getting affected by convulsions and also due to aspiration.
- Neuronal death occurs with prolonged seizures due to abnormal neuronal discharges. Neuronal death probably occurs due to the inability to handle large increases in intracellular calcium brought about by prolonged exposure to excitatory neurotransmitters.

Clinical Features of GTCS

- These begin with sudden loss of consciousness.
- All muscles of the arms and legs as well as the chest and back become stiff which is called tonic phase. The patient may begin to appear cyanotic during this tonic phase. A loud cry may occur in the tonic phase as air is forcibly expelled across constricted vocal cords. Incontinence of urine and feces may occur.
- After approximately one minute, there is synchronous clonic muscle jerking.
- Following the seizure the patient may be unconscious, confused, complain of a headache, bodyache or feeling weak, and changes in the mood may be noticed for 24 hours. Injuries include tongue bite, head wounds, dislocation of shoulders, and compression fractures of vertebrae.
- Serum levels of prolactin and creatine phosphokinase are elevated following a seizure.
- The interictal EEG may show generalized spikes, which may or may not be followed by waves, sharp waves and slow waves.

Differential Diagnosis

- Syncope (e.g. cardiac arrhythmia, vasovagal syncope, dysautonomia)
- Metabolic conditions (e.g. hypoglycemia, hyponatremia)
- Migraine (e.g. migrainous aura, migraine equivalent)
- Transient ischemic attacks
- Sleep disorders (e.g. cataplexy, narcolepsy, night terror)
- Movement disorders (e.g. paroxysmal dyskinesia, chorea)
- Psychiatric conditions (e.g. conversion, panic attacks, breath-holding spells, malingering)

Investigations

Neuroimaging

- CT or MRI scan should be done to exclude a structural brain lesion which could be the cause of seizures.
- MRI is better than CT to identify lesions such as cortical dysplasia, infarcts, or tumors. However in an emergency situation CT scan is suitable to exclude a mass lesion, hemorrhage, or large stroke because it can be done faster and also more widely available.
- PET scan (positron emission tomogram) can show the seizure focus as hypermetabolizing area.

Electroencephalography (EEG)

- EEG is an essential study in the evaluation of epileptic seizures. It can help confirm the diagnosis and also differentiate between generalized and partial seizures. However, a normal EEG does not rule out epilepsy. Video-EEG monitoring is very helpful for confirming or classifying the type of seizure or for diagnosing pseudo-seizures. Video-EEG records EEG activity and clinical behavior simultaneously, usually for 2–7 days. However, it is expensive and time consuming, hence monitoring all patients is impractical. Only those who do not respond to treatment or in whom pseudoseizures are suspected should undergo video-EEG.

- Use of provocation techniques such as sleep deprivation, hyperventilation and intermittent photic stimulation, increase the sensitivity of EEG.

Prolactin Levels

- Serum prolactin concentration may rise and remain elevated for upto 6 hours after an epileptic attack.

Lumbar Puncture

- This is helpful to exclude CNS infections such as meningitis if there are clinical features suggestive of meningitis along with seizures.
- It should be done only after a space-occupying brain lesion has been excluded by neuroimaging.

Treatment

During an Attack

- Put the patient in a safe place away from fire and sharp objects.
- Put the patient in lateral position and insert a padded mouth gag.
- Inj lorazpam 4 mg slow IV OR inj diazepam 10 mg slow IV.

Treatment of Underlying Condition

- For example, correcting hypocalcemia or hypoglycemia; removal of a structural lesion such as brain tumor, vascular malformation, or brain abscess.
- If the underlying cause can be corrected fully and there is no risk of further seizure, antiepileptic treatment is not needed. However after the removal of a brain lesion, a scar may form and act as a seizure focus. Hence such lesions require antiepileptic therapy.

Antiepileptic Drug Therapy

- Antiepileptics are indicated for all people when seizures meet the criteria for epilepsy diagnosis (*see* the definition of epilepsy in previous sections).
- Choice of antiepileptic drugs for GTCS are **valproate, topiramate, lamotrigine, and zonisamide**.
- Antiepileptics should be introduced slowly to minimize side effects, and gradually increased to achieve the therapeutic levels. If seizures continue to occur even after the maximum dose of first drug, a second antiepileptic drug should be added to the first drug. If seizures are controlled with the second drug, first drug can be gradually withdrawn.
- An attempt can be made to discontinue antiepileptic drugs if the patient is seizure free for at least 2 years with a normal EEG. Drugs should be withdrawn gradually over 2–3 months.

General Measures

- Avoid precipitating factors such as sleep deprivation, physical stress, blinking lights, loud noise, and alcohol intake.
- Advice the patient to avoid swimming, going to heights, fire and moving machinery.
- Avoid an occupation which puts the patient or public at risk such as driving a public transport vehicle.

Surgical Treatment for Epilepsy

- Surgery is an option for patients with refractory epilepsy not responding to medical therapy.
- Surgical procedures include temporal lobectomy or amygdalohippocampectomy in patients with temporal lobe epilepsy, removal of an identified lesion (lesionectomy) in focal seizures.
- Hemispherectomy or multilobar resection is useful for some patients with severe seizures due to hemispheric abnormalities, and corpus callosotomy has been shown to be effective for tonic or atonic seizures.

Vagus Nerve Stimulation (VNS)

- VNS is a new treatment option for patients with medically refractory epilepsy who are not candidates for resective brain surgery.
- It involves repetitive electrical stimulation of left vagus nerve by a subcutaneous generator placed in the infraclavicular region.
- The exact mechanism of action of VNS is unknown, although it is supposed to increase seizure threshold.

Q. Discuss acute management of a seizure episode.

- Any convulsive activity ≥5 min requires emergency therapy (definition of impending status epilepticus).

Immediate Supportive Care — "ABC + S"

- **Airway:** Turn patient lateral (recovery position), clear secretions, do not insert objects into mouth. Prevent aspiration; tongue biting is usually minor.
- **Breathing:** Administer high-flow O_2 by mask; monitor SpO_2. Hypoxia worsens neuronal injury and prolongs seizures.
- **Circulation:** Check pulse, BP, cardiac monitor; establish IV/IO line. Rapid drug delivery and detect arrhythmias.
- **Safety:** Cushion head, remove nearby hazards, loosen clothing. Limit injury during convulsions.

Abortive Pharmacologic Therapy

- First choice is benzodiazepine (IV lorazepam 0.1 mg/kg, maximum 4 mg).
- If no IV access → IM midazolam 10 mg.
- Pre-hospital caregiver route → Buccal midazolam or rectal diazepam.
- Repeat once after 5 min if seizure persists.

Post-ictal Assessment

- Once the seizure has stopped:
  - Take a detailed history: Witness account, prodrome, duration, focal signs.
  - Rule out mimics: Syncope, psychogenic seizures, TIA, migraine.

Investigations

- *Blood tests*: CBC, glucose, electrolytes, calcium, magnesium, renal/liver function tests. This is to rule out metabolic causes.
- Toxicology screen: Especially in young adults to rule out drug/toxin induced seizures (amphetamine, cocaine).
- EEG (not urgent, ideally within 24–48 hours): Helps classify seizure type.
- Neuroimaging: To detect structural lesions (tumor, infarct, etc.). Non-contrast CT (to urgently rule out major pathologies in the brain), or MRI (more sensitive than CT, done if the patient is stable).

Prevention of Further Seizures

- Most first seizures DO NOT require immediate antiepileptic therapy, unless risk of recurrence is high.
- Start AEDs (antiepileptic drus) if the seizure is unprovoked with high recurrence risk as evidenced by following features:
  - Abnormal EEG
  - Structural brain lesion on imaging
  - Neurological deficit
  - Strong family history of epilepsy
  - Patient has had ≥2 seizures
  - Status epilepticus or prolonged recovery
  - Safety-critical profession (e.g. pilot, driver)
- Do not start AEDs if:
  - Provoked seizure (e.g. alcohol withdrawal, metabolic disturbance like hypoglycemia, hypocalcemia, etc.).
  - Normal neuro exam, EEG, imaging.
  - Full recovery, low risk of recurrence.
- If AED is required, any one of the following drugs can be used.
- **Levetiracetam:** 1 g IV stat followed by 500 mg IV 12th hourly. Levetiracetam is preferred because it does not cause hypotension.
- **Valproate:** Initial dose of oral valproate is 10–15 mg/kg per day. The dose may be increased at one-week intervals by 5–10 mg/kg per day as needed.
- **Phenytoin or fosphenytoin**: The prodrug fosphenytoin has largely replaced phenytoin for IV use. Loading Dose of phenytoin is (for acute management, e.g. status epilepticus) 15–20 mg/kg IV infusion. Maintenance dose is 300–400 mg/day PO or IV in three divided doses. Administer slowly (max rate = 50 mg/min to avoid hypotension and cardiac arrhythmias). Dose of fosphenytoin is same as that of phenytoin.
- **Phenobarbitone:** Loading dose is 15–20 mg/kg IV. Administer slowly (maximum infusion rate 50–75 mg/min to avoid respiratory depression and hypotension). Maintenance dose is 1–3 mg/kg/day IV or PO in 1–2 divided doses. Often used after failure of benzodiazepines and phenytoin/fosphenytoin because of side effects.

Patient Education and Support

- Counseling on driving restrictions (often 6–12 months seizure-free required).
- Avoid high-risk activities (e.g. swimming alone, climbing heights, working with heavy machinary).
- Seizure first aid instructions for family/friends.
- Address underlying cause if identified (e.g. stop alcohol, manage hypoglycemia).

Follow-up

- Neurology referral for further evaluation
- Repeat EEG or imaging if new symptoms occur.

Q. Discuss the general management (long-term management) of epilepsy including different types of antiepileptic drugs, their side effects and drug to drug interactions.

General Approach

- Diagnosis confirmation
  - Detailed history, eyewitness accounts, EEG, and neuroimaging (MRI preferred).
- Classification of seizures
  - Focal seizures (start in one brain area)
  - Generalized seizures (involve both hemispheres)
- Treatment goals
  - Achieve seizure freedom with minimal side effects.
  - Improve quality of life.
- Nonpharmacological management
  - Lifestyle modifications: Regular sleep, stress management, avoiding seizure triggers (like flashing lights, alcohol).
  - Surgery: For drug-resistant epilepsy (e.g. temporal lobectomy).
  - Devices: Vagus nerve stimulator (VNS), responsive neurostimulation (RNS).
  - Diet: Ketogenic diet (especially in refractory childhood epilepsies).

Pharmacological Management

Important antiepileptic drugs (Table 5.34).

First-line AEDs based on seizure type (Table 5.35).

Important drug interactions

- Enzyme inducers (increase metabolism of other drugs → decreased drug levels): Carbamazepine, phenytoin, phenobarbital.
- Enzyme Inhibitors (decrease metabolism → increased drug levels): Valproic acid.
- Some AEDs (e.g. carbamazepine, phenytoin, topiramate at high doses) can reduce effectiveness of hormonal contraceptives. Alternative contraception methods should be considered.
- Teratogenicity: Valproate carries a high risk of neural tube defects and should be avoided in women of childbearing age unless absolutely necessary. Lamotrigine is considered relatively safer.

TABLE 5.34: Important antiepileptic drugs

Drug	Main uses	Key side effects	Notable interactions
Valproic acid	Generalized seizures, absence, myoclonic	Weight gain, tremor, hair loss, hepatotoxicity, teratogenicity	Increases levels of lamotrigine (risk of rash)
Carbamazepine	Focal seizures, trigeminal neuralgia	Diplopia, ataxia, hyponatremia, leukopenia	Autoinducer (induces its own metabolism); reduces efficacy of oral contraceptives
Lamotrigine	Focal and generalized seizures, bipolar disorder	Rash (risk of Stevens-Johnson Syndrome), dizziness	Levels increased by valproate
Levetiracetam	Broad-spectrum use. Works for almost all types of seizures except absence seizures	Behavioral changes (irritability, depression)	Minimal drug interactions
Ethosuximide	Absence seizures	GI upset, fatigue, hiccups	Few interactions
Phenytoin	Focal and generalized seizures (less favored now)	Gingival hyperplasia, hirsutism, neuropathy, ataxia	Strong CYP450 inducer
Topiramate	Focal and generalized seizures, migraine prevention	Cognitive slowing, weight loss, kidney stones	Reduces efficacy of oral contraceptives

TABLE 5.35: First-line AEDs based on seizure type

Seizure type	Preferred drugs
Generalized tonic-clonic	Phenytoin, lamotrigine, levetiracetam, valproate, topiramate, and zonisamide
Focal seizures or secondarily generalized seizures	Lamotrigine, levetiracetam, oxcarbazepine, carbamazepine or lacosamide
Absence seizures	Ethosuximide, valproate, lamotrigine
Myoclonic seizures	Valproate, levetiracetam, zonisamide, clonazepam
Tonic/Atonic seizures	Valproate, lamotrigine, clobazam, zonisamide, levetiracetam

Monitoring Therapy

- Therapeutic drug levels (e.g. for phenytoin, valproate) in certain cases.
- Liver function tests (especially with valproate, carbamazepine).
- Complete blood counts (for drugs like carbamazepine).
- Renal function (for levetiracetam).

When to Consider Withdrawing AEDs

- After 2–5 years of seizure freedom.
- Factors favoring successful withdrawal: Normal EEG, single seizure type, normal neurological examination.
- Slow tapering is essential to avoid withdrawal seizures.

Q. Clinical features of different seizure types.

Focal Preserved Consciousness Seizure (formerly called simple focal)

- Involve a part of the brain and consciousness is not lost.
- It can be motor, sensory, and psychic or associated with autonomic symptoms.
- Focal motor seizure may consist of jerking of one hand or twitching of one half of the face.
- Focal nonmotor seizure may consist of subjective paraesthesiae involving a hand or a leg.
- They have an abrupt onset and usually last for a few seconds. EEG may show focal spikes. If the seizure focus is deep seated EEG may be normal.

Focal Impaired Consciousness Seizure (formerly complex focal seizures)

- These also involve a part of the brain but consciousness is impaired or lost. Most of these seizures arise in the temporal lobe.
- A motionless stare with altered consciousness followed by automatisms is the usual pattern. Automatisms are repetitive, purposeless, complex movements such as picking at clothes, smacking lips or swallowing. EEG usually shows abnormal spikes in the area where the seizures originate.
- Psychic symptoms related to memory known as ***deja vu and jamais vu*** may be seen in complex focal seizures. Deja vu is a feeling of familiarity in an unfamiliar situation, and jamais vu is a feeling of strangeness in a familiar situation.
- ***Todd's paralysis*** refers to reversible neurological deficit, which lasts less than 48 hours, following a focal seizure.

Focal to Bilateral Tonic Clonic Seizure (formerly called focal onset with secondary generalization)

- Here the seizures start in a focal area of the brain and then spread to involve the whole brain to become generalized seizure.
- ***"Jacksonian march"*** refers to orderly progression of focal seizure due to the spread of seizure in the cerebral

cortex (for example, from thumb to fingers to face to leg).

- Patient is conscious initially but later loses consciousness when the seizure becomes generalized.

Generalized Clonic Seizures

- Clonic seizures consist of rhythmic jerking motor movements.

Generalized Tonic Seizures

- These are associated with intense stiffening of the body. There is no convulsive jerking. They occur most often during sleep, usually in children. The cause is usually the Lennox-Gastaut syndrome. Tonic (sustained) contraction of axial muscles may begin abruptly or gradually, then spread to the proximal muscles of the limbs. Tonic seizures usually last 10–15 sec.

Generalized Atonic Seizures (drop attacks)

- Sudden loss of muscle tone typically lasting less than 15 seconds, with falling and brief loss of consciousness.

Generalized Myoclonic Seizures

- Generalized myoclonic seizures are a type of seizure characterized by sudden, brief (1–2 seconds), shock-like muscle jerks. These jerks usually affect both sides of the body and are caused by abnormal electrical activity in both cerebral hemispheres simultaneously. If the seizures evolve into rhythmic jerking movements, they are classified as clonic seizure. Myoclonus is not always pathological. Physiological myoclonus is seen when a person is falling asleep and during early sleep phases. Non-epileptic myoclonus is also seen in hypoxia, drug toxicity and metabolic disturbances. In myoclonic seizure, EEG shows fast polyspike-and–slow wave complexes.

Absence Seizures

- Absence seizures involve brief, sudden lapses of consciousness. There is no aura or postictal confusion. Absence seizures are more common in children and there is significant inherited predisposition for absence seizures.
- The person abruptly stops what they're doing, often staring blankly. Each episode lasts 5–15 seconds. There will be sudden stop in motion without falling as if frozen. There may be automatic movements such lip smacking, eyelid flutters, chewing motions, finger rubbing, etc. Afterward, there's no memory of the incident. Some people have dozens of episodes daily, which interfere with school or daily activities. A decline in a child's learning ability may be the first sign of this disorder. Teachers may comment about a child's inability to pay attention.
- The classic ictal EEG shows 3-Hz generalized spike-and–slow wave complexes.

Q. Status epilepticus.

- Current definition of status epilepticus is as follows:
    - ≥5 minutes of continuous seizures, or
    - ≥2 discrete seizures between which there is incomplete recovery of consciousness.
- For nonconvulsive and focal status epilepticus the time duration is 10 minutes.
- Status epilepticus is an emergency and must be treated immediately.

Causes of Status Epilepticus

- Anticonvulsant withdrawal or noncompliance
- Metabolic disturbances (hypoglycemia, hyponatremia, hypocalcemia, hypomagnesemia)
- Drug intoxication or withdrawal
- CNS infection (encephalitis, abscess)
- CNS lesions (tumors, AV malformations)
- Cerebral hypoxia
- Refractory epilepsy
- Head trauma.

Pathophysiology

- Seizures are sustained by excess excitation and reduced inhibition of neurons. Glutamate is the most common excitatory neurotransmitter and gamma-aminobutyric acid (GABA) is the most common inhibitory neurotransmitter involved. Failure of inhibitory processes is increasingly thought to be the major mechanism leading to status epilepticus.
- Significant physiologic changes occur in status epilepticus especially in generalized tonic clonic seizures. These are tachycardia, hypertension, cardiac arrhythmias, hyperglycemia which result from catecholamine surge. Blood pressure may decrease as the seizure activity continues. Body temperature may increase as a result of the vigorous muscle activity and increased sympathetic drive. Marked acidosis usually occurs and has both respiratory and metabolic component. It should not be treated as acidosis is known to have an anticonvulsant effect and resolves with termination of the seizure. Hypoxia occurs due to breathing getting affected by convulsions and also due to aspiration.
- Neuronal death occurs with prolonged seizures due to abnormal neuronal discharges. Neuronal death probably occurs due to the inability to handle large increases in intracellular calcium brought about by prolonged exposure to excitatory neurotransmitters.

Investigations

- Serum electrolytes, calcium, magnesium
- Blood sugar level
- Complete blood count
- Liver and renal function tests
- Toxicology screen
- Anticonvulsant level
- Arterial blood gas
- Other tests as indicated: Chest X-ray, CT scan or MRI of brain, lumbar puncture, blood cultures
- EEG also should be obtained. Nonconvulsive status epilepticus (NCSE) needs EEG for diagnosis.

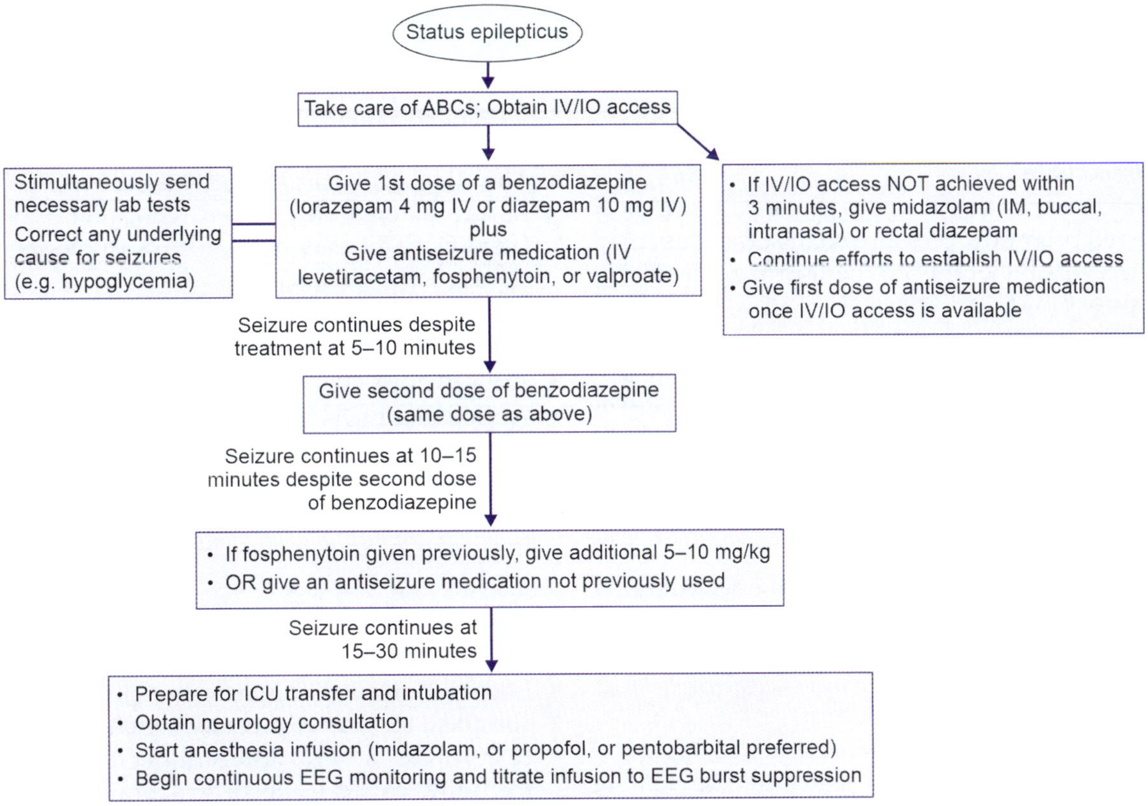

Figure 5.27: Management of status epilepticus

Treatment

- Take care of ABCs (airway, breathing and circulation). Admit the patient in ICU. Intubate the patient. Insert urinary catheter (**Fig. 5.27**).
- Do a brief medical and neurologic examination, establish IV line and send samples for investigations.
- Antiseizure drugs: Intravenous benzodiazepines are the drugs of choice to terminate a seizure attack (examples; lorazepam or diazepam). Further seizures should be prevented by loading the patient with levetiracetam, fosphenytoin or valproate. *See* the following algorithm.
- Always look for and treat underlying causes (stroke, infection, toxins, etc.).
- Earlier treatment = better outcomes.
- Longer seizure = higher brain injury risk.

Complications

- Rhabdomyolysis
- Lactic acidosis
- Aspiration pneumonia
- Neurogenic pulmonary edema
- Respiratory failure
- Cardiac injury (due to massive release of catecholamines)
- Neuronal death (due to repetitive firing).

Q. Extradural hematoma (epidural hematoma).

- Extradural hematoma is accumulation of blood between the skull and the dura mater (extra- or epidural) (**Fig. 5.28**).

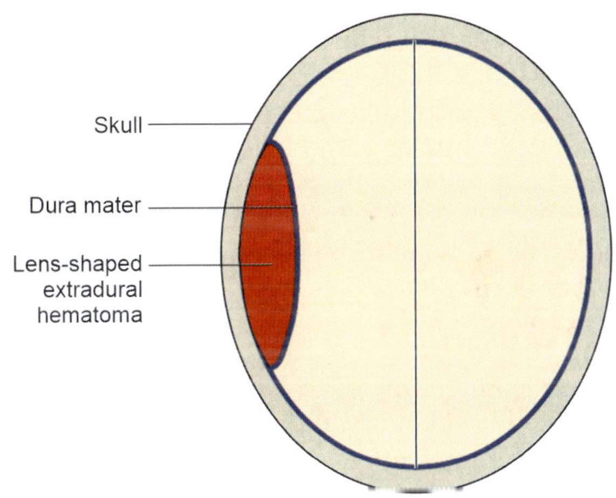

Figure 5.28: Extradural hematoma

- It usually occurs after head injury due to rupture of the middle meningeal artery, its branches or the accompanying veins.

Clinical Features

- Patient may present with classic "lucid interval":
  - Initial loss of consciousness after trauma
  - Followed by a lucid (alert) period
  - Then deterioration (progressive drowsiness, coma).
- "Lucid interval" may last for minutes to hours before coma occurs.
- Other features are severe headache, vomiting, seizures, ipsilateral pupil dilation (due to compression of the oculomotor nerve), and hemiparesis (contralateral body weakness).

- The enlarging hematoma compresses and shifts the underlying brain. The rising intracranial pressure may result in trans tentorial herniation of the medial temporal lobe (uncal herniation) with consequent pressure on the brainstem, the third nerve and the posterior cerebral artery.
- Pressure on brainstem leads to unconsciousness. If not relieved promptly, pressure on the brainstem may lead to irreversible brainstem hemorrhage, resulting in respiratory and cardiac arrest.

Diagnosis

- Immediate CT scan should be done if extradural hematoma is suspected. Extradural hematoma is seen as a biconvex high-attenuating lesion between the skull and the brain, with shift of the midline to opposite side.

Treatment

- Very small hematomas without mass effect may be managed conservatively without surgery.
- Large hematomas with mass effect and midline shift need neurosurgical intervention—craniotomy to evacuate the hematoma.
- Anticonvulsants if seizures occur.

Q. Subdural hematoma (SDH).

- This is accumulation of blood beneath the dura (between the dura mater and the arachnoid mater). It usually results from tearing of bridging veins crossing this space **(Fig. 5.29)**.
- It occurs due to trauma (most common cause). Rarely due to anticoagulants and bleeding disorders.
- It can be acute (manifests within 3 days of injury), subacute (3 days to 3 weeks), and chronic (>3 weeks). The earlier a hematoma becomes symptomatic the more serious it is.

Clinical Features

- Clinical features are due to expanding hematoma and associated brain injury and edema.
- Acute SDH presents with decreased consciousness, headache, confusion, focal neurological deficits (e.g. weakness, speech difficulties), and seizures.

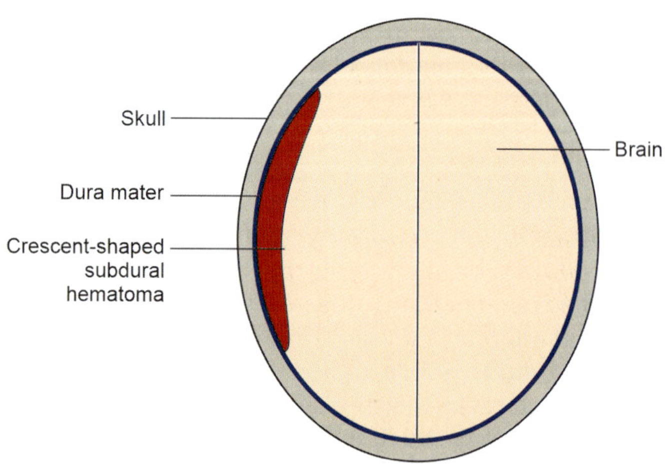

Figure 5.29: Subdural hematoma

- Chronic SDH (especially in elderly) may present with insidious onset personality change, memory issues, and mild weakness. It may mimic dementia or stroke.

Diagnosis

- The diagnosis can be confirmed by CT scan. SDH is seen as crescent-shaped (concave) hyperdensity. Chronic SDH may appear dark (hypodense) rather than white on CT scan.

Treatment

- Antiepileptics.
- Antiedema measures (mannitol, diuretics, head end elevation).
- Surgical evacuation is indicated if the hematoma is big (25–30 ml), causing mass effect and the patient fails to improve on conservative management.

Q. Describe the functional neuroanatomy of the locomotor system of the brain.

- Locomotion (walking, running, posture control) is a complex, coordinated motor function.
- It involves several interconnected brain regions, including cortical, subcortical, brainstem, and spinal cord structures.
- Control is both voluntary (planning, initiating movement) and automatic (rhythm, balance).
- Key components are as follows:

Motor Cortex

- ***Primary motor cortex (precentral gyrus):*** Executes voluntary movements. Neurons (especially upper motor neurons) send signals via the corticospinal tract to the spinal cord.
- ***Premotor cortex and supplementary motor area (SMA):*** Plan and organize movements. SMA is important for initiating locomotion and bilateral coordination (e.g. using both legs together).

Basal Ganglia

- ***Structures:*** Caudate nucleus, putamen, globus pallidus, subthalamic nucleus, substantia nigra.
- ***Functions:*** Regulate movement initiation, speed, and smoothness. Suppress involuntary movements.
- Disorders here (like Parkinson's disease) cause gait freezing, shuffling steps, and postural instability.

Cerebellum

- ***Functions:*** Coordinates timing, precision, and balance. Adjusts locomotor patterns based on sensory feedback (proprioception, vision, vestibular input).
- Damage causes ataxia (unsteady gait), dysmetria, and poor balance.

Brainstem

- ***Mesencephalic locomotor region (MLR):*** Important in gait initiation and modulation. Stimulates reticulospinal tracts, activating central pattern generators (CPGs) in the spinal cord.

- ***Reticular formation:*** Integrates locomotor commands and postural control.
- ***Vestibular nuclei:*** Maintain equilibrium and orientation during movement.

Spinal Cord

- Contains ***central pattern generators (CPGs):*** Neural circuits capable of generating rhythmic, patterned movements (like walking) without needing continuous cortical input. Brain commands start/stop/adjust these rhythms.

Sensory Feedback Systems

- Proprioceptive input (from muscles, tendons, joints) informs the brain about body position and motion.
- Visual and vestibular systems contribute to balance and trajectory control.
- Feedback continuously modifies locomotion to adapt to terrain and avoid obstacles.

Q. What are the movement disorders? Enumerate movement disorders.

Q. Classify involuntary movements.

Q. Mention the CNS disorders characterized by involuntary movements.

- Movement disorders are neurologic syndromes characterized by either an excess of movement or a paucity of voluntary and automatic movements, unrelated to weakness or spasticity.

Classification

- Movement disorders are commonly classified as those with decreased or slow movement (hypokinetic disorders) and increased movement (hyperkinetic disorders).

Hypokinetic disorder

- Parkinson disease

Hyperkinetic disorders

- Tremor
- Myoclonus
- Dystonia
- Chorea
- Hemiballismus (rapid chorea)
- Athetosis (slow chorea)
- Tics
- Fasciculations

Q. Classify Parkinsonism.

- Parkinsonism is a clinical syndrome presenting with any combination of bradykinesia, rest tremor, rigidity, and postural instability. Most common cause of parkinsonism is Parkinson disease which is idiopathic.

Classification of Parkinsonism (Table 5.36)

TABLE 5.36: Classification of parkinsonism
Primary (idiopathic) parkinsonism
• Parkinson's disease
Secondary (acquired) parkinsonism
• Drug or toxin induced
• Vascular (multi-infarct)
• Posttrauma (punch drunk syndrome)
• Postencephalitis
• Normal pressure hydrocephalus (NPH)
Parkinsonism plus syndromes (multisystem degenerations)
• Progressive supranuclear palsy (PSP)
• Multiple system atrophy
• Dementia with Lewy bodies
• Corticobasal syndromes
Heredodegenerative parkinsonism
• Spinocerebellar ataxia
• Wilson disease
• Juvenile onset Huntington's disease

Q. Describe the etiology, clinical features, diagnosis and management of Parkinson's disease (idiopathic parkinsonism; paralysis agitans).

- Parkinson's disease is an idiopathic, slowly progressive, degenerative disorder characterized by resting tremor, stiffness (rigidity), slow and decreased movement (bradykinesia).
- James Parkinson, a physician based in London, first described this condition. He called it as ***the shaking palsy.***

Epidemiology

- Parkinson's disease (PD) is seen worldwide with a prevalence of 150/100 000.
- Its peak age of onset is in the 60s. Rarely, PD begins during childhood or adolescence (juvenile parkinsonism). Onset between ages 21 and 40 years is sometimes called early-onset PD. Genetic causes are more likely in juvenile and early-onset PD.
- It affects both sexes.
- It is less prevalent in tobacco smokers than nonsmokers. Coffee drinking is protective against the disease.

Etiology

- The exact etiology of Parkinson's diseases is unknown. Some factors possibly involved are:
- ***MPTP:*** Minute doses of methylphenyltetrahydropyridine (MPTP) a toxic product of heroin can cause severe parkinsonism. MPTP- like herbicides have been implicated in the causation of PD.
- ***Genetic factors:*** There is clustering of early-onset Parkinson's disease in some families. Mutations in the parkin gene on chromosome 6 have been found in families with autosomal recessive cases of PD and some young apparently sporadic cases.

Pathology

- The main pathology in Parkinson's disease is depletion of the dopaminergic neurons of the substantia nigra and degeneration of the nigrostriatal tract.
- The degenerating neurons contain Lewy bodies (alpha-synuclein) and neurofibrillary tangles. Lewy bodies are round, eosinophilic, intracytoplasmic inclusions. Lewy body is a highly sensitive marker for PD.
- All these changes result in reduction of striatal dopamine, which is the main biochemical abnormality in PD. Normally an equilibrium exists between acetylcholine and dopamine. With dopamine deficiency, there is acetylcholine hyperactivity which can account for some clinical features such as tremors and rigidity.
- Other neurotransmitters such as norepinephrine, serotonin, somatostatin, substance P, and the enkephalins are also decreased in Parkinson's disease. Depression may be related to reduction of noradrenaline and serotonin in the brain.

Clinical Features

- The symptoms start insidiously and tend to be unilateral or asymmetrical at the onset. The rate of progression is very variable, with a benign form running over several decades. Usually the course is over 10–15 years, with death resulting from bronchopneumonia.
- The initial manifestations may be tremor, slowness, stiffness or clumsiness of an arm or, less commonly, of a leg.
- The classical triad of tremor, rigidity and akinesia develop slowly, over months or several years. Limbs and joints feel stiff due to rigidity.
- Fine movements become difficult due to tremors. Writing becomes small (micrographia) due to hypokinesia and spidery due to tremors.

Tremor

- The tremor has a frequency of 4–6 Hz, is present mainly at rest (resting tremor) and is suppressed on voluntary movement. Distal muscles are affected more than the proximal, and the rhythmic tremor at the wrists and fingers resembles "pill-rolling" movement. It disappears during sleep and is aggravated by emotional excitement. This tremor may also be seen in the legs or lower jaw.

Rigidity

- Rigidity is present over the entire range of movement (lead-pipe rigidity) and is present equally in both agonist and antagonistic muscles groups. It is seen mainly in the limbs but can also be present in the neck and axial muscles. When rigidity is associated with tremor, smooth lead pipe rigidity is broken up into a jerky resistance to passive movement - known as cogwheel rigidity.

Akinesia

- There is lack (akinesia) or paucity (bradykinesia) of movement. There is difficulty initiating movement. Motor acts like dressing, feeding and walking show a marked slowing. Rapid fine finger movements, such as piano-playing, become indistinct, slow and tremulous. Facial immobility gives a mask-like appearance. Blinking rate is reduced, producing a stare.

Posture and Gait

- The head and body becomes stooped forwards, often with pronounced kyphosis. The arms become flexed at the elbow and wrists. Flexion also occurs in the joints of the legs. The posture is sometimes called 'simian' to describe the apelike forward flexion, immobility and lack of associated hand movements. The gait may be slow or hurried with diminished arm swing.
- Patients may walk rapidly with short steps (festinating gait) as though they are chasing their center of gravity.
- Sometimes, patient may not be able to initiate walking as if their feet are glued to the floor (called freezing phenomenon).
- Balance deteriorates, and falls are common in later stages of PD.

Speech

- Speech is initially a monotonous and later becomes slurred as a result of akinesia, tremor and rigidity.

Cognitive, Autonomic and Sensory Disturbances

- Patients with PD often become passive and disinterested in daily activities. Slowness of thought process and inattentiveness are often seen. Anxiety and depression is more common. Cognitive disturbances suggestive of frontal lobe dysfunction are common. Dementia may develop in the late stages.
- Autonomic dysfunction such as constipation, increased frequency of micturition, nocturia, and orthostatic hypotension may occur. Skin is greasy and sweating excessive. Subjective sensory dysfunction such as muscle pains, abdominal discomfort, dysaesthesia in feet may be present.

Diagnosis

- Diagnosis is made by clinical features. There is no lab test to confirm the diagnosis. Neuroimaging should be done (CT or MRI) if any other disease is suspected. PD must be differentiated from other diseases shown below which cause slowness and decreased cognitive functions.

Differential Diagnoses

- Alzheimer's disease
- Multi-infarct dementia
- Sequelae of repeated head injury (e.g. in boxers)
- Hypoxic brain damage
- Hypothyroidism
- Depression
- Normal pressure hydrocephalus.

Treatment

- Treatment of Parkinson's disease can be divided into non-pharmacologic, pharmacologic, and surgical therapy.

Non-pharmacologic Treatment

- Education of both patient and his family about the disease.
- Emotional and psychological support to the patient.
- Regular physical exercise, physiotherapy and speech therapy may keep the patient more active.
- Good nutritious diet, rich in fiber.

Pharmacologic Treatment

- All pharmacologic therapies for Parkinson's disease (PD) are symptomatic. Treatment should generally begin when motor symptoms are affecting function and quality of life.

Levodopa/carbidopa combinations (preferred choice)

- For most patients with early PD seeking control of motor symptoms, levodopa is the initial choice therapy. Levodopa converts to dopamine in the brain. Levodopa should be administered at the minimum effective dose to control symptoms. Carbidopa is combined with levodopa because carbidopa blocks the peripheral decarboxylation of levodopa into dopamine and thus reduces the symptoms of nausea and orthostatic hypotension. Also, more levodopa becomes available to cross the blood brain barrier and act in the brain as dopamine cannot cross the blood brain barrier. The usual starting dose of levodopa is carbidopa-levodopa combination (25 mg/100 mg), half tablet two to three times daily with meals. This dose should be adjusted further if required until patient feels adequate symptom relief. Treatment should be started with low dose and gradually increased.

Alternatives to levodopa-based therapy

- The following drugs can be used as monotherapy in selected patients or they can be added along with levodopa to augment the effect of levodopa and to reduce the side effects due to levodopa.
  - Dopamine agonists
  - MAO-B Inhibitors (monoamine oxidase type B inhibitors)
  - Catechol O-methyltransferase (COMT) inhibitors
  - Amantadine
  - Anticholinergics

Dopamine agonists

- Dopamine agonist monotherapy is an alternative to levodopa therapy in select patients. These drugs act directly on postsynaptic dopamine receptors (primarily D_2 type). Compared to levodopa, they are longer acting and thus provide a more uniform action. They can be combined with carbidopa/levodopa and also with anticholinergics and amantadine.
- Examples of dopamine agonists include **pramipexole, ropinirole, pergolide, and bromocriptine. Rotigotine** is a newer agent available as a transdermal skin patch. Dopamine agonists can be considered in the following clinical scenarios:
- Mild symptoms with preference for once-daily medication: In patients of any age who prefer once-daily dosing and only require modest symptomatic relief, monoamine oxidase B (MAO-B) inhibitors offer a reasonable alternative to levodopa.
- Younger patients at high risk of dyskinesia: For patients younger than 50 years who are at increased risk of developing dyskinesias—such as those with younger onset age, lower body weight, or female sex—initial monotherapy with a dopamine agonist may be preferred.
- Patients with tremor-predominant Parkinson's disease: Some patients present with an isolated, symptomatic tremor without significant bradykinesia or gait disturbance. Although levodopa remains the first-line therapy, higher doses may be needed for high-amplitude tremor. In cases of milder tremor, amantadine monotherapy can also be considered.
- Avoid dopamine agonists in patients whose occupations involve driving or using heavy machinery, given the risk of sleep attacks. Also avoid them in older adults due to increased risk of adverse effects, especially cognitive impairment.

MAO-B inhibitors (monoamine oxidase type B inhibitors)

- Examples: Selegiline, rasagiline, safinamide.
- These drugs block the enzyme MAO-B, which is responsible for breaking down dopamine in the brain. By inhibiting this enzyme, these drugs increase dopamine levels in the brain, helping to improve motor symptoms.
- They can be used in early Parkinson's disease as monotherapy in patients with mild symptoms to delay the need for levodopa. In later stages, they can be used as add on therapy to levodopa to reduce "off" time (periods when medication is not working well).
- Selegiline can cause insomnia. Rasagiline is well-tolerated in early and late disease. Advantages of rasagiline over selegiline are once a day dosing and no chance of hypertensive crisis when patients consume tyramine which can happen with selegiline. Safinamide is newer and may be particularly helpful when motor fluctuations are problematic.
- Side effects: Nausea, dizziness, insomnia (especially with selegiline), hallucinations (rare, mainly in elderly).
- Drug interactions: Risk of serotonin syndrome if combined with certain antidepressants (SSRIs, SNRIs, tricyclic antidepressants).

Catechol O-methyltransferase (COMT) inhibitors

- Examples: Entacapone, tolcapone, opicapone.
- These drugs inhibit catechol-O-methyltransferase enzyme, which breaks down levodopa in the periphery. They decrease the wearing-off symptoms of levodopa. Always used with levodopa to prolong its effect and reduce "wearing-off."
- Side effects: Tolcapone can cause hepatotoxicity (needs liver monitoring). Entacapone is safer. Can cause diarrhea and orange-colored urine.

Amantadine

- It is an antiviral drug useful in Parkinson disease.
- Amantadine has both anticholinergic and dopaminomimetic properties and can reduce drug-induced dyskinesias. It is a weak NMDA receptor antagonist; increases dopamine release.
- Used for mild symptoms; also used later for levodopa-induced dyskinesias.
- Side effects: Livedo reticularis (mottled skin), edema, hallucinations.

Anticholinergics

- Examples: Trihexyphenidyl, benztropine.
- Block acetylcholine to correct dopamine-acetylcholine imbalance.
- These drugs can be used along with levodopa. Anticholinergics are useful for controlling rest tremor and dystonia. Best for tremor-predominant Parkinson's (especially younger patients).
- Side effects: Anticholinergic drugs are less well tolerated in older patients because of the risk of cognitive impairment, constipation, and prostatism. Other side effects are dry mouth, blurred vision, and urinary retention.

Neuroprotective therapy

- Many agents can slow down the decline of dopaminergic neurons. These agents include selegeline, coenzyme Q_{10}, vit-E, and L-carnitine. Some trials have shown that these drugs delay the progression of parkinsonism.

Surgical Therapy

- Several surgical procedures have been studied in advanced Parkinson's disease (PD), including deep brain stimulation (DBS), thalamotomy, and pallidotomy.
- Deep brain stimulation (DBS) causes an effect similar to surgery due to high frequency stimulation of subthalamus and pallidum without producing a lesion.

Summary table of doses, side effects, and drug interactions for key Parkinson's drugs

See **Table 5.37**.

Q. Write briefly about dystonia.

- Dystonia is a movement disorder characterized by sustained or intermittent muscle contractions that cause twisting movements and abnormal postures.

TABLE 5.37: Drugs used to treat Parkinson's disease

Class	Drug	Typical Dose	Side effects	Drug interactions
Levodopa/ carbidopa	Levodopa/ carbidopa	25 mg/100 mg, half tablet two to three times daily with meals	Dyskinesias: chorea, dystonia Wearing-off phenomenon "On-off" phenomenon Confusion, hallucinations, vivid dreams, psychosis Orthostatic hypotension	Risk of hypertensive crisis due to excess catecholamines if used along with non-selective MAO inhibitors (e.g. phenelzine, tranylcypromine)
MAO-B inhibitors	Selegiline	5 mg twice daily (oral) or 1.25–2.5 mg once daily	Nausea, dizziness, insomnia (especially with selegiline), hallucinations (rare, mainly in elderly)	Risk of serotonin syndrome if combined with certain antidepressants (SSRIs, SNRIs, tricyclic antidepressants).
	Rasagiline	1 mg once daily		
	Safinamide	Start 50 mg once daily → increase to 100 mg once daily		
COMT inhibitors	Entacapone	200 mg with each dose of levodopa (max ~1600 mg/day)	Tolcapone can cause hepatotoxicity (needs liver monitoring). Entacapone is safer. Can cause diarrhea and orange-colored urine.	Risk of hypertensive crisis if used along with MAO inhibitors. Reduced breakdown of drugs metabolized by COMT (e.g. methyldopa, dobutamine, isoproterenol) → increased effects
	Tolcapone	100–200 mg three times daily		
	Opicapone	50 mg once daily		
Amantadine	Amantadine	100 mg 1–2 times daily (max 400 mg/day if needed)	Livedo reticularis (mottled skin), edema, hallucinations.	Additive anticholinergic effects with other anticholinergic drugs (Trihexyphenidyl, Benztropine, antihistamines)
Anticholinergics	Trihexyphenidyl	Start 1 mg daily → titrate up to 6–10 mg/day in divided doses	Cognitive impairment, constipation, dry mouth, blurred vision, and urinary retention. Can also help with drug-induced extrapyramidal symptoms.	Additive anticholinergic effects with other anticholinergics. Opposing effects with cholinesterase inhibitors (e.g. donepezil, rivastigmine — used for Alzheimer's). Enhanced sedation, confusion if used with other CNS depressants
	Benztropine	0.5–2 mg once or twice daily		

- It can affect a single part of the body (focal dystonia), two or more adjacent parts (segmental dystonia), or the entire body (generalized dystonia).

Etiology of Dystonia

Primary (idiopathic) dystonia
- Genetic

Secondary (acquired) dystonia
- Brain injury (trauma, hypoxia, electrical injury, perinatal brain injury)
- Stroke (ischemic, hemorrhagic)
- Infection (viral encephalitis, HIV, subacute sclerosing panencephalitis)
- Brain tumor
- Wilson disease
- Cerebral palsy
- Brain hypoxia
- Drugs: Antipsychotics, metoclopramide, prochlorperazine
- Functional movement disorder

Types (by location)

- Cervical dystonia (torticollis): Neck muscles contract involuntarily.
- Blepharospasm: Forceful eye closure.
- Writer's cramp: Task-specific dystonia affecting the hand.
- Oromandibular dystonia: Affects jaw, lips, and tongue muscles.
- Generalized dystonia: Affects the trunk and at least two other body regions.

Clinical Features

- Twisting, repetitive movements or abnormal postures.
- Symptoms can worsen with voluntary action and stress, and may temporarily ease with sensory tricks (e.g. touching the chin in cervical dystonia).

Diagnosis

- Mainly by history and physical examination.
- MRI or other tests to rule out secondary causes.
- Genetic testing if hereditary dystonia is suspected.

Treatment

- Treatment depends on the cause.
- Anticholinergics such as trihexyphenidyl are effective for primary dystonia. Other effective drugs include baclofen, benzodiazepines (clonazepam), carbamazepine, valproate, primidone, and lithium.
- Botulinum toxin injections are helpful if drug therapy fails, especially for focal dystonia.
- Neurosurgical treatment, such as stereotactic thalamotomy, or deep brain stimulation (DBS) can help in severe refractory cases.

Q. Chorea.

- Chorea is characterized by rapid, involuntary, irregular, unpredictable, purposeless, random movements that can affect various parts of the body.
- Chorea is often due to dysfunction of the basal ganglia, particularly the striatum (caudate nucleus and putamen), leading to disinhibition of motor pathways.

Causes of Chorea

Hereditary

- Benign hereditary chorea
- Lesch-Nyhan syndrome
- Huntington's disease

Acquired

- Physiologic chorea (seen in infants)
- Cerebral palsy
- Sydenham chorea (chorea minor, rheumatic chorea, St. Vitus' dance): Often associated with rheumatic fever, typically occurring in children and adolescents.
- After cardiac surgery.
- Metabolic disorders: Conditions such as hyperthyroidism, Wilson's disease, systemic lupus erythematosus. Lesch-Nyhan syndrome, Niemann-Pick disease, and gangliosidosis. Chorea is nearly universal in the neuroacanthocytosis syndromes.
- Kernicterus
- Pregnancy: Chorea gravidarum, a rare condition, can occur during pregnancy
- Systemic lupus erythematosus
- Stroke (basal ganglia)
- Drugs: Antipsychotics, antiemetics (metoclopramide), phenytoin, levodopa.

Clinical Features

- Movements are non-rhythmic, rapid, and jerky.
- Movements are often described as dance-like, as the term "chorea" comes from the Greek word *choreia*, meaning "dance." Choreography (dance sequence in movies) also comes from the word "chorea".
- It is not suppressible and involves distal muscles and face commonly.
- Chorea worsens with voluntary movement (e.g. trying to grab an object) and disappears during sleep.
- Chorea and athetosis can occur together (called choreoathetosis).

Investigations

- Diagnosis is mainly by clinical features.
- MRI brain may show atrophy (e.g. caudate nucleus in Huntington's).
- Blood tests to check for metabolic, autoimmune, or infectious causes.
- Genetic testing for Huntington's disease if suspected.

Treatment

- Underlying cause must be treated. Phenothiazines (e.g. haloperidol) and tetrabenazine provide some symptomatic relief.

Q. Sydenham chorea (St Vitus dance).

- Sydenham chorea is one of the major clinical manifestations of acute rheumatic fever and the most common form of acquired chorea in childhood.
- Chorea usually develops 1–8 months after the group A streptococcal (GAS) infection, whereas carditis and arthritis usually develop within the first month.

Pathology

- Autoimmune response following GAS infection.
- Antibodies directed against the streptococcal bacteria cross-react with neurons in the basal ganglia, particularly the caudate and subthalamic nuclei leading to chorea.

Clinical Features

- It usually affects children between 5 and 13 years of age.
- More frequent in girls than boys.
- Can occur weeks to months after the initial strep infection. The onset usually is insidious but may be sudden.
- The chorea typically begins in the hands, and later involves face and feet also. The movements are rapid, irregular jerks that are continuous while the patient is awake but improve with sleep. The chorea usually is generalized but may be more prominent on one side. Some may have unilateral chorea.

Diagnosis

- The diagnosis is made by clinical features as there is no specific laboratory test.

Treatment

- Sydenham chorea usually improves in 3–4 months.
- Underlying rheumatic fever should be treated with penicillin for at least 10 days followed by antibiotic prophylaxis.
- Chorea can be reduced by many drugs such as valproic acid, phenobarbital, haloperidol, chlorpromazine, and carbamazepine.

Q. Athetosis.

- Athetosis is a type of involuntary movement disorder characterized by slow, continuous, writhing movements.

Pathophysiology

- Athetosis arises from dysfunction of the basal ganglia, especially the striatum (putamen).
- Often results from damage to the indirect pathway, leading to excessive movement.

Causes of Athetosis

- Perinatal and early childhood brain injury (kernicterus, due to neonatal jaundice leading to basal ganglia damage).
- Genetic disorders: Wilson's disease, Huntington's disease (often presents with choreoathetosis).
- Stroke: Involving the basal ganglia, especially in the putamen or thalamus.
- Drug-induced: Antipsychotics, levodopa (less common).
- Metabolic/toxic: Hypoxic injury, bilirubin encephalopathy, heavy metal poisoning.

Clinical Features

- Athetosis is characterized by slow, coarse, writhing, purposeless movements. These movements are typically slower, more sustained, and larger in amplitude compared to chorea.
- Athetosis usually affects the distal parts of the extremities, such as the fingers, hands, and toes, as well as the face, neck, and trunk. The movements can include any combination of flexion, extension, abduction, pronation, and supination, often alternating and in varying degrees. The movements flow randomly from one body part to another, with the direction of movement changing randomly. The affected limbs are in constant motion ("athetosis" means "without fixed position"). Hyperextension of the fingers and wrist and pronation of the forearm may alternate with full flexion of the fingers and wrist and supination of the forearm. Facial grimacing often accompanies these movements. The movements can often be elicited or intensified by voluntary activity of another body part, a phenomenon known as overflow.
- Increases with voluntary movements and stress, and disappears during sleep.
- Voluntary movements are impaired, making coordinated actions difficult or impossible.
- Athetosis is usually unilateral; when it affects both sides, it is called double athetosis.
- Pseudoathetosis (sensory athetosis) is a term used to describe undulating and writhing movements of the extremities resembling athetosis due to loss of proprioception and joint position sense as a result of parietal lobe lesion, tabes dorsalis, and peripheral neuropathies. Movements are more marked when the eyes are closed due to removal of visual cues which compensates for loss of proprioception.
- Choreoathetosis refers to movements that is a combination of chorea and athetosis.

Investigations

- MRI or CT may reveal basal ganglia abnormalities (e.g. in kernicterus, Wilson's disease).
- Blood tests for metabolic, infectious, or genetic conditions.

Treatment

- Address the underlying cause (e.g. chelation for Wilson's disease, bilirubin management in neonates).
- Medications for symptom control:
  - Anticholinergics (e.g. trihexyphenidyl)
  - Dopamine-depleting agents (tetrabenazine)
  - Benzodiazepines or baclofen.
- Botulinum toxin for focal cases.
- Physical and occupational therapy to improve function.

Q. Huntington's chorea (chronic progressive chorea; hereditary chorea; Huntington's disease).

- Huntington's chorea, also known as Huntington's disease (HD), is a chronic, progressive, inherited neurodegenerative disorder characterized by a combination of motor dysfunction (chorea), psychiatric symptoms, and cognitive decline. It is distinct from Sydenham's chorea in that it is genetic, progressive, and fatal.

Etiology and Genetics

- Huntington disease is an autosomal dominant disorder usually beginning during middle age.
- Huntington disease results from a gene mutation causing abnormal repetition of the DNA sequence CAG, which codes for the amino acid glutamine. The resulting gene product, a large protein called huntingtin, accumulates in the neurons leading to degeneration primarily affecting caudate nucleus and putamen (parts of the basal ganglia). Progressive cortical atrophy leads to dementia and psychiatric symptoms.

Clinical Features

- Symptoms and signs develop insidiously, starting at about age 35–40. The disease is progressive and patients usually die 10–15 years after the onset due to motor dysfunction and dementia. Clinical features are chorea, gait disturbances, emotional disturbances, dementia and postural instability.

Diagnosis

- Is based on the clinical features, family history and genetic testing for CAG repeat expansion.
- Brain MRI/CT: Atrophy of caudate nucleus and frontal cortex.

Treatment

- There is no cure. Treatment is mainly symptomatic and supportive.
- Psychosis may improve with antipsychotics (e.g. olanzapine, risperidone).
- Chorea is treated by tetrabenazine, deutetrabenazine, and haloperidol.
- Anxiolytics and antidepressants may be useful in some patients.
- Genetic counseling is essential for affected families.

Q. Hemiballismus.

- Hemiballismus (hemiballism) is a dramatic neurological syndrome characterized by wild, flinging, and incessant movements on one side of the body (hence the term hemiballismus).

Etiology

- This condition is typically caused by infarction or hemorrhage in the region of the contralateral subthalamic nucleus. This results in disinhibition of the motor thalamus and cortex, causing hyperkinetic movements on the opposite side of the body.
- Other causes are abscess, AV malformation, cerebral trauma, tumor, and multiple sclerosis involving subthalamic nucleus.

Pathophysiology

- The subthalamic nucleus normally provides excitatory input to the globus pallidus internus (GPi) → inhibits the thalamus → suppresses movement.
- Damage to the subthalamic nucleus → ↓ GPi activity → ↓ thalamic output → excessive movement.
- In hemiballismus, this disinhibition leads to contralateral violent flinging movements.

Clinical Features

- The movements in hemiballismus are similar to those seen in chorea but are more pronounced. The distinction between severe hemichorea and hemiballismus can be arbitrary, as both involve involuntary and purposeless movements. However, hemiballistic movements are much more rapid and forceful, often affecting the proximal portions of the extremities.
- In fully developed cases, the affected extremities exhibit continuous, violent, swinging, flinging, rolling, and throwing movements.
- These movements persist during waking hours and stop only during deep sleep.
- They are usually unilateral, affecting one entire side of the body, and can be so intense that they move the entire body. Rarely, they can be bilateral or confined to a single extremity (monoballismus). The movements may spare the face and trunk.

Treatment

- Hemiballismus is challenging to treat, extremely disabling, and can sometimes be fatal due to exhaustion and inanition.
- Drugs used in chorea are useful for hemiballismus, but the disorder usually subsides spontaneously within several weeks.
- Prolonged disabling and medically intractable hemiballismus can be treated with contralateral thalamotomy or pallidectomy.

Q. Myoclonus.

- Myoclonus refers to sudden, brief, involuntary jerks or twitches of a muscle or group of muscles. It is a symptom, not a disease itself, and can range from benign (like hiccups or sleep starts) to indicative of a serious neurological condition.
- Myoclonus can also be a part of epileptic disorders such as myoclonic epilepsy.

Causes

Physiologic

- Sleep
- Infants

Pathologic

- Myoclonic epilepsy
- Wilson's disease
- Encephalitis
- Metabolic encephalopathy
- Post-hypoxic myoclonus
- Drugs: levodopa, tricyclic antidepressants.

Treatment

- Many drugs are helpful to treat myoclonus such as clonazepam, valproate and levetiracetam.

Q. Define tremor. Mention different types of tremors.

- Tremor is defined as involuntary, rhythmic, oscillatory movements of a body part.
- It is caused by alternating contractions of antagonistic muscles. It is the most common movement disorder encountered in clinical practice.

General Features of Tremors

- Tremor is the most common of all movement disorders.
- Tremor may be unilateral or bilateral and most commonly involves distal parts of the extremities — the fingers or hands—but may also affect the arms, feet, legs, tongue, eyelids, jaw, and head and may occasionally involve the entire body.
- The rate may be slow, medium, or fast. Oscillations of 3–5 Hz are considered slow; 10–20 Hz, rapid.
- Amplitude may be fine, coarse, or medium. Tremor may be constant or intermittent.
- Tremor may be normal (physiologic) or pathologic. Physiologic tremor is seen in many people during physical or mental stress.
- The severity of tremor may not be related to the seriousness of the underlying disorder. For example, essential tremor is benign, but symptoms can be disabling.

Pathophysiology

- The pathophysiology of tremor depends on its type, but fundamentally, tremors result from abnormal rhythmic firing activity in neural circuits that control movement. These oscillations can arise due to dysfunction in the basal ganglia, cerebellum, thalamus, or sensorimotor cortex, depending on the tremor type.

Types of Tremors

- Tremors may be broadly classified into two types based on its relationship to rest or activity as rest tremors and action tremors. It is important to remember that some tremors fall into more than one potential classification. For example, even though the tremor due to cerebellar disease is classically described as intention tremor, it can be present at rest also. Similarly, rubral tremor can be present at rest as well as during action.
- Most tremors are accentuated by emotional excitement, and many normal individuals develop tremor with anxiety, apprehension, and fatigue. A shivering type of tremor (rigors) may be brought on by cold, but identical movements can be psychogenic.
- When action tremors are severe, they can be present at rest also.

Rest Tremors

- Resting (static) tremor occurs in a body part that is fully supported, relaxed, and not voluntarily activated (e.g. with the hands in the lap), and attenuate when the part is used. Rest tremor is seen primarily in PD and other parkinsonian syndromes. Other causes of rest tremors are rubral tremor and Wilson's disease.
- Note that rest tremor also usually disappears when the patient totally relaxes or sleeps.

Action Tremors

- Action tremors appear when performing some activity. Action tremors are further divided into three subtypes: (1) postural, (2) kinetic, and (3) isometric tremors.
  1. ***Postural tremor:*** becomes evident when the limbs are maintained in an antigravity position (e.g. arms outstretched). Examples of postural tremor are essential tremor, enhanced physiologic tremor and drug induced tremor.
  2. ***Kinetic tremor:*** appears when making a voluntary movement, and may occur at the beginning, during or at the end of the movement. Kinetic tremors include:
     - Simple kinetic tremor, in which tremor is roughly the same throughout the course of a voluntary movement.
     - Intention tremor, characterized by a crescendo increase in tremor as the affected body part approaches its target. The most common example is an intention (terminal) tremor. Intention tremor is a form of action tremor seen primarily in cerebellar disease. The tremor appears when precision is required to touch a target, as in the finger-nose-finger or toe-to-finger test. It progressively worsens during the movement. Approaching the target causes the limb to shake, usually side-to-side perpendicular to the line of travel, and the amplitude of the oscillation increases toward the end of the movement.
     - Task-specific kinetic tremor, which occurs during a specific task such as writing.
  3. ***Isometric tremor***—occurs during muscle contraction against a stationary object, such as making a fist or squeezing an object.

Q. Essential tremor.

- Essential tremor is the most common movement disorder characterized by kinetic and/or postural tremors of hands.

- Essential tremor is a benign condition. However, it may interfere with feeding, speaking, writing, and other activities of daily living.

Etiology

- The cause of essential tremor is uncertain but may be due to genetic mutation which is inherited as autosomal dominant trait. Environmental factors also play a role. Some reports suggest abnormal rhythmic activity in the cerebello-thalamo-cortical loop. Likely involves the inferior olive, Purkinje cell loss in the cerebellum, and dysregulated thalamic output to the motor cortex.

Clinical Features

- Essential tremor occurs at any age but occurs most frequently in the elderly. Family history can be found in almost 50% of cases.
- The frequency of the tremor is usually 6–12 Hz, and most often affects the hands and arms. It can also affect the head (titubation), voice, chin, trunk, and legs.
- It is bilateral, symmetrical and postural. It develops when the hands adopt a posture, such as holding a glass or a spoon. It is slowly progressive but rarely produces severe disability. Writing is shaky and untidy.
- Anxiety exacerbates the tremor, sometimes dramatically.

Investigations

- MRI/CT of brain: To rule out cerebellar lesion.
- Thyroid function tests: To rule out hyperthyroidism.

Treatment

- Treatment is usually not needed. Patients should be reassured that it is not a serious disease.
- Propranolol and primidone are the most effective and well-studied medications for the treatment of essential tremor.
- Small amounts of alcohol can also reduce the severity of tremor. Sympathomimetics (e.g. salbutamol) worsen the tremor and should be avoided.
- Stereotactic thalamotomy and thalamic stimulation are used in severe cases.

Q. Intention tremor.

- Intention tremor is a subtype of kinetic tremor which worsens as the target is apprached. It is due to lesions of cerebellum and its connections. Other causes of intention tremor include Wilson's disease, hepatocerebral degeneration, and mercury poisoning.
- The tremor typically increases in severity as the hand moves closer to its target. Intention tremors are usually coarse due to involvement of proximal muscles. There may be other cerebellar signs such as ataxia, dysmetria, titubation, and dysdiodochokinesia.
- There is no drug available to treat intention tremor. Physical therapy (e.g. weighting the affected limbs, teaching patients to brace the proximal limb during activity) sometimes helps. Patients with severe tremor can be helped by deep brain stimulation of the thalamus.

Q. Enumerate the indications for use of surgery and botulinum toxin in the treatment of movement disorders.

- Surgery is mainly for advanced and drug-refractory cases.
- Botulinum toxin is the first-line for focal movement disorders.
- Both treatments aim to reduce disability and improve quality of life when medications fail.

Indications for Surgical Treatment (Table 5.38)

TABLE 5.38: Indications for surgical treatment of movement disorders

Condition	When surgery is considered
Parkinson's disease	Advanced disease with severe motor fluctuations or dyskinesias not controlled by medication. Medication-resistant tremor.
Essential tremor	Disabling tremor not responding to medications (e.g. propranolol, primidone).
Dystonia (primary generalized or focal)	Severe disabling dystonia not responsive to botulinum toxin or oral drugs.
Tourette syndrome	Severe, medically refractory tics causing self-injury or major disability.
Hemiballismus (rarely)	Severe, disabling movements unresponsive to medications.

- Main surgical techniques used are deep brain stimulation and ablative surgeries.
- ***Deep brain stimulation (DBS):*** targets like subthalamic nucleus (STN), globus pallidus interna (GPi), or thalamus (VIM nucleus).
- ***Ablative surgeries:*** e.g. thalamotomy, pallidotomy (less common now).

Indications for Botulinum Toxin Treatment (Table 5.39)

TABLE 5.39: Indications for botulinum toxin treatment of movement disorders

Condition	When botulinum toxin is used
Cervical dystonia (spasmodic torticollis)	First-line treatment for focal dystonia.
Blepharospasm (eyelid spasm)	First-line for disabling eyelid closure.
Hemifacial spasm	Unilateral involuntary facial contractions.
Focal limb dystonias (e.g. writer's cramp, musician's dystonia)	Localized muscle overactivity unresponsive to oral agents.
Laryngeal dystonia (spasmodic dysphonia)	Voice tremor due to vocal cord dystonia.
Tremor (essential tremor, Parkinson's tremor-selected cases)	When tremor is disabling and focal (e.g. hand tremor).
Bruxism, oromandibular dystonia	Involuntary jaw/tongue movements.

Q. **Enumerate demyelinating neurological disorders.**

- Demyelinating diseases are conditions where there is breakdown of the myelin sheath with relative preservation of axons. This affects the conduction of signals through nerve fibers.
- Examples of demyelinating diseases are as follows.

Central Nervous System (CNS) Demyelinating Disorders

- Multiple sclerosis (MS)
- Neuromyelitis optica spectrum disorder (NMOSD)
- Acute disseminated encephalomyelitis (ADEM)
- Progressive multifocal leukoencephalopathy (PML)
- Central pontine myelinolysis (CPM)/osmotic demyelination syndrome.
- Leukodystrophies (inherited demyelinating disorders).

Peripheral Nervous System (PNS) Demyelinating Disorders

- Guillain-Barré syndrome (GBS)—demyelinating subtype (AIDP)
- Chronic inflammatory demyelinating polyneuropathy (CIDP)
- Charcot-Marie-Tooth disease type 1 (hereditary demyelinating neuropathy)
- Paraneoplastic demyelinating neuropathies.

Q. **Describe the etiology, clinical features, diagnosis and management of multiple sclerosis.**

- Multiple sclerosis is an autoimmune disorder characterized by multiple demyelinating lesions in the brain and spinal cord.

Epidemiology

- Multiple sclerosis (MS) is common in western countries but rare in India and other countries of Asia and Africa.
- It usually affects young people between 15 and 50 years. Rare in childhood and after 60.
- It is about twice as common in women as men.

Etiology

- The exact cause of MS is unknown. It is probably an autoimmune disorder where T-cells, B cells, and macrophages are activated and destroy the myelin sheath.
- Infection by a latent virus (possibly a human herpes virus such as Epstein-Barr virus) has been suspected to trigger a secondary autoimmune response leading to MS.
- Genetic factors may play a role as suggested by increased incidence among certain families and presence of human leukocyte antigen (HLA) allotypes (HLA-DR2).
- Environmental factors also play a role in the causation of the disease. The disease is more common in temperate climate (European countries) than tropical climate (Asian countries).

Pathology

- There are multiple areas of demyelination with reactive gliosis (hence called multiple sclerosis) scattered in the white matter of brain, spinal cord and in the optic nerves.
- Demyelination is initiated by inflammation due to the entry of activated T lymphocytes through the blood-brain barrier. There is release of cytokines and attraction of macrophages which destroy the myelin sheath. Histologically, the characteristic lesion is a plaque of inflammatory demyelination occurring most commonly in the periventricular regions of the brain, the optic nerves and the subpial regions of the spinal cord. After an acute attack, gliosis occurs, leaving a shrunken grey scar (sclerosis). Myelin damage disrupts saltatory conduction, causing slowed or blocked nerve signals.
- In the later stages there is destruction of axons also which is responsible for the progressive and persistent disability.

Disease Patterns

- The different patterns of multiple sclerosis are as follows **(Fig. 5.30)**:
  - ***Relapsing remitting MS (RRMS):*** This is characterized by relapses with full recovery in between. This is the initial type in most patients. However, most patients will eventually enter a secondary progressive phase.
  - ***Secondary progressive MS (SPMS):*** This is characterized by an initial RRMS followed by progression of the disease with minor remissions.
  - ***Primary progressive MS (PPMS):*** This is characterized by disease progression from the onset with occasional minor improvements but without any acute attacks.
  - ***Progressive relapsing MS (PRMS):*** This is characterized by progressive disease from onset, with acute attacks, with or without full recovery. Progression continues during the periods between disease relapses.

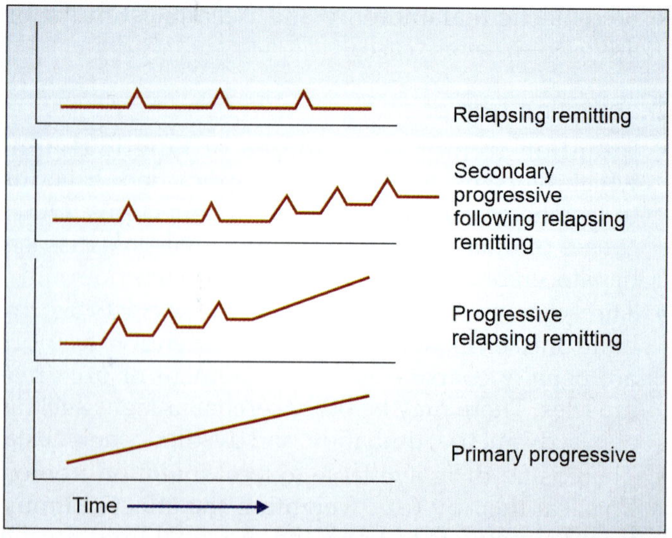

Figure 5.30: Patterns of multiple sclerosis

Clinical Features

- The typical patient presents as a young adult with two or more clinically distinct episodes of CNS dysfunction with at least partial resolution.
- The hallmark of MS is symptomatic episodes that occur months or years apart and affect different anatomic locations (dissemination in time and space).

Cranial Nerves

- Optic neuritis is a common presentation and leads to central scotoma. Trigeminal neuralgia can occur.

Motor System

- Motor symptoms are due to lesions of corticospinal tracts and include upper limb weakness, paraparesis or paraplegia. UMN signs such as spasticity, exaggerated deep tendon reflexes, clonus and extensor plantar responses are usually present.
- Internuclear ophthalmoplegia results if there is a lesion in the medial longitudinal fasciculus connecting the 3rd, 4th, and 6th nerve nuclei.

Sensory System

- Sensory symptoms are also very common feature of MS and are due to demyelinating lesions in spinothalamic, posterior column, or dorsal roots. Sensory symptoms are numbness, tingling, pins-and-needles, tightness, coldness, radicular pains, etc.

Cerebellum

- Lesions in cerebellum and its connections can cause cerebellar signs such as ataxia and incordination.

Spinal Cord

- Spinal cord involvement causes bowel, bladder, and sexual dysfunction leading to urgency, urinary incontinence, constipation or fecal incontinence, erectile dysfunction, etc.
- Neuromyelitis optica (Devic's disease) is a variant of MS characterized by involvement of only optic nerve and spinal cord. Brain lesions are absent. There are symptoms and signs of motor, sensory and sphincter disturbances.
- Lhermitte sign, also called the barber chair phenomenon, is an electric shock like sensation that runs down the back and into the limbs on flexing the neck. It is caused by involvement of the posterior columns of spinal cord.

Other Features

- Heat sensitivity (Uhthoff's phenomenon) is a well-known occurrence in MS; small increases in the body temperature can temporarily worsen current or preexisting signs and symptoms.

Diagnosis

- Multiple sclerosis should be suspected when multiple areas of the CNS are involved at different times. At least two or more different central white matter lesions should occur at different times (i.e. dissemination in place and time).
- MRI of the brain and cervical cord is the investigation of choice. It shows multiple demyelinating lesions. Lesions are often found in the periventricular area. MRI can identify both old and new lesions in different areas.
- Evoked potential recordings (such as visual evoked response) show prolongation and can detect subclinical involvement of the visual, auditory and somatosensory pathways.
- CSF examination may show lymphocytosis or increased protein concentration. CSF electrophoresis shows oligoclonal bands.
- McDonald criteria are standardized diagnostic guidelines used to diagnose multiple sclerosis (MS) based on clinical presentation, MRI findings, and CSF analysis.

Management

- Treatment of multiple sclerosis (MS) focuses on three main goals:
  - Modifying the disease course
  - Managing relapses
  - Alleviating symptoms

Modifying the Disease Course

- Disease-modifying therapies (DMTs) can be used to reduce the frequency and severity of relapses, slow progression, and limit new CNS lesions. DMTs are as follows:
  - Interferon beta-1a and beta-1b: These two are recombinant interferons. Beta interferon therapy reduces the frequency and severity of MS relapses, slows disability progression, reduces the number of new lesions.
  - Glatiramer acetate is a polypeptide consisting of basic amino acids. It is thought to inhibit cellular immune reactions to myelin. It reduces the relapse rates.
  - Immunosuppressive therapy with cyclophosphamide, azathioprine, methotrexate, cladribine, or mitoxantrone may help arrest the course of progressive multiple sclerosis.
  - Fingolimod is an orally administered drug with immunomodulatory effects.
  - Monoclonal antibodies such as natalizumab also reduces relapse rate.

Acute Attacks

- Acute attacks are treated with corticosteroids. A typical course is methylprednisolone, 1 g intravenously for 3 days followed by oral prednisone, 60 or 80 mg per day for 1 week, after which it is tapered over next 2–3 weeks.
- Plasmapheresis and intravenous immunoglobulins have shown benefit in some trials.
- Relapses are also treated with similar course of steroids.

Symptomatic Therapy

- Spasticity—physiotherapy, baclofen, tizanidine, diazepam, injection of botulinum toxin
- Ataxia—isoniazid, clonazepam
- Sensory symptoms—carbamazepine, gabapentin, amitriptyline
- Spastic bladder—anticholinergics like oxybutynin or propantheline
- Fatigue—amantadine, modafinil
- Impotence—sildenafil
- Bowel dysfunction—laxatives, dietary changes
- Depression—antidepressants.

Lifestyle and Supportive Therapies

- Regular exercise and physiotherapy.
- Balanced diet.
- Psychosocial support and counseling.
- Vitamin D supplementation (often low in MS patients).

Q. Describe the anatomy of the spinal cord and enumerate the diseases affecting the spinal cord.

Q. Causes of spinal cord compression (compressive myelopathy).

- The spinal cord extends from the lower border of medulla at the foramen magnum till the lower border of L1 vertebra. The tip of the spinal cord is cone-shaped and is called conus medullaris. In the lumbosacral region, nerve roots from lower cord segments descend vertically within the spinal canal, forming the cauda equina (so called because of resemblance to horse tail).
- The white matter at the cord's periphery contains ascending and descending tracts of myelinated sensory and motor nerve fibers. The central H-shaped gray matter is composed of cell bodies of neurons and nonmyelinated fibers. The anterior (ventral) horns contain lower motor neurons, which receive impulses from the motor cortex via the descending corticospinal tracts **(Fig. 5.31)**. The axons of the lower motor neurons are the efferent fibers of the spinal nerves. The posterior (dorsal) horns contain sensory fibers that originate in cell bodies in the dorsal root ganglia. The gray matter also contains many internuncial neurons that carry motor, sensory, or reflex impulses from dorsal to ventral nerve roots, from one side of the cord to the other, or from one level of the cord to another. The spinothalamic tract transmits pain and temperature sensation contralaterally in the spinal cord; most other tracts transmit information ipsilaterally.

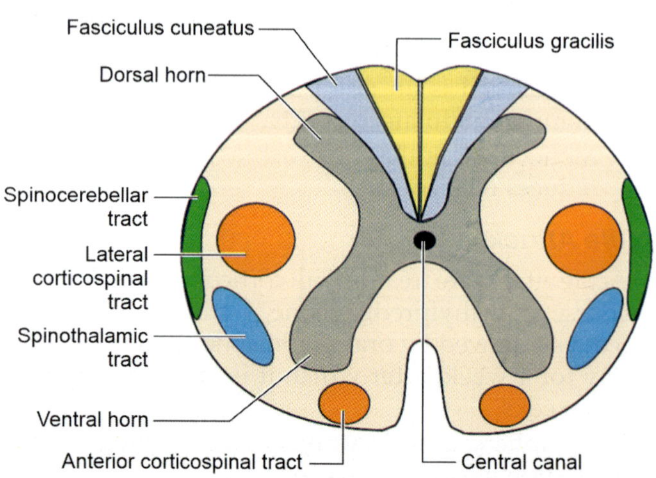

Figure 5.31: Cross section of spinal cord

- On each side of the spinal cord, the anterior and dorsal nerve roots combine to form the spinal nerve as it exits from the vertebral column through the neuroforamina. The cord is divided into 31 functional segments corresponding to the attachments of the 31 pairs of spinal nerve roots.
- The blood supply of the spinal cord consists of one anterior and two posterior spinal arteries. The anterior and posterior spinal arteries arise from the vertebral arteries. The anterior spinal artery supplies the anterior two thirds of the cord and the posterior spinal arteries supply the posterior one third.

Diseases Affecting the Spinal Cord

- Spinal cord problems are generally referred to as myelopathies which are as follows.

Compressive Myelopathy

- ***Extradural:*** TB spine, epidural abscess, epidural tumor, spinal metastases, disc prolapse, spondylosis, lymphomas, extradural AV malformations or hematoma.
- ***Intradural:*** Meningioma, neurofibroma, intradural AV malformations, arachnoiditis.
- ***Intramedullary:*** Syringomyelia, ependymoma, astrocytoma.

Noncompressive Myelopathy

- Transverse myelitis
- Radiation myelopathy
- AIDS myelopathy
- Tropical spastic paraplegia
- Spinal cord infarction
- Multiple sclerosis.

Clinical Features of Spinal Cord Disease

- Spinal cord can be affected both horizontally and vertically to a variable extent. Clinical features depend on how much of the spinal cord is involved horizontally and how much is involved vertically.
- Horizontal lesions of the spinal cord can be grouped into various clinical patterns (syndrome) as follows (*see* the picture).

Complete Spinal Cord Transection (Transverse Myelopathy)

- With complete cord transection, all ascending tracts from below the level of the lesion and all descending tracts from above the level of the lesion are interrupted. Therefore, all motor and sensory functions below the level of spinal cord damage are disturbed. Transverse myelopathy is a general term for diseases causing complete horizontal damage to spinal cord. Transverse myelitis is a type of transverse myelopathy due to inflammation of the cord.

- Examples; transverse myelitis, traumatic injury.

Hemisection of the Spinal Cord (Brown-Séquard syndrome)

- Half of the spinal cord is damaged horizontally. For detailed clinical features, *see* Brown-Séquard syndrome.
- Examples are traumatic injuries, stab injuries.

Central Cord Lesions

- Disease process starts in the center of the spinal cord and extends to the peripheral part of spinal cord. Characteristically, the decussating fibers of the spinothalamic tract anterior to the central canal carrying pain and temperature sensation are affected initially. This results in loss of pain and temperature sensation with the preservation of fine touch and proprioception (dissociation of sensory loss) (*see* syringomyelia for a detailed description of clinical features) **(Fig. 5.32)**.
- Examples, syringomyelia, ependymoma.

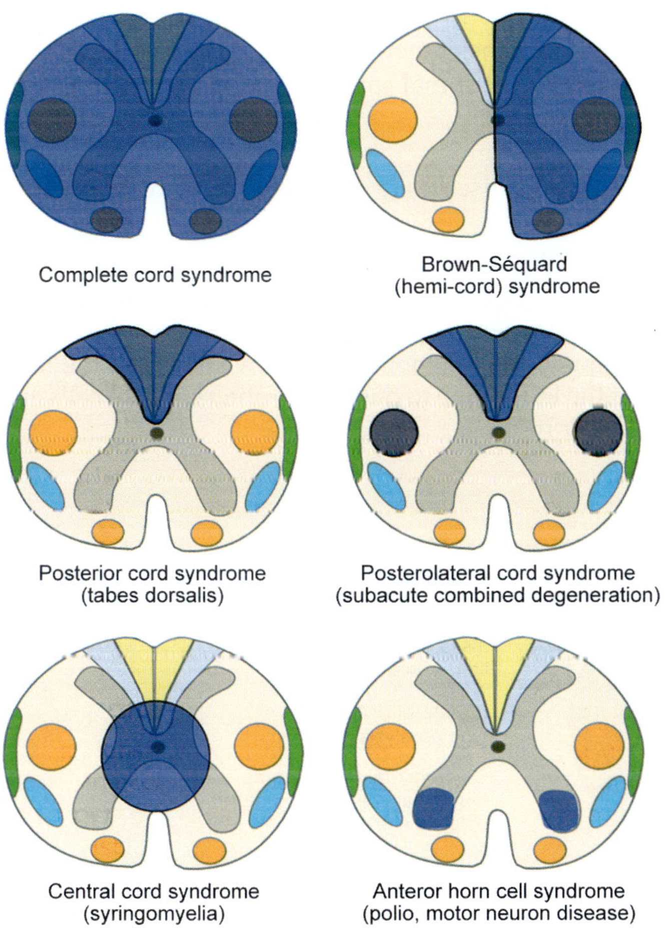

Figure 5.32: Various spinal cord syndromes (indicated by blue-shaded areas)

Based on the Vertical Level of Lesion following Clinical Patterns may be seen

- At or above C5: Respiratory paralysis, quadriplegia.
- At C5–C6: Paralysis of legs, wrists, and hands, weakness of shoulder abduction and elbow flexion, Loss of biceps and brachioradialis reflex.
- Between C6 and C7: Paralysis of legs, wrists, and hands, but shoulder movement and elbow flexion usually possible.
- Between C7 and C8: Loss of triceps jerk reflex, Paralysis of legs and hands.
- At C8 to T1: Horner syndrome (constricted pupil, ptosis, facial anhidrosis), paralysis of legs.
- Between T1 and conus medullaris: Paralysis of legs.

Q. Transverse myelitis.

- Transverse myelitis is a neurological disorder caused by inflammation across the entire width of the spinal cord **(Fig. 5.33)**. It may be infective or noninfective. It is a type of non-compressive myelopathy.

Etiology

- ***Systemic inflammatory disorders:*** SLE, sarcoidosis, Behçet's syndrome, Sjögren's syndrome.
- ***Infectious:*** Herpes zoster, HSV 1 and 2, EBV, CMV, rabies virus, listeria monocytogenes, Lyme's disease, syphilis.
- ***Postinfectious:*** Epstein-Barr virus (EBV), cytomegalovirus (CMV), mycoplasma, influenza, measles, varicella, rubeola, and mumps.
- ***Demyelinating diseases:*** Multiple sclerosis, neuromyelitis optica.
- ***Paraneoplastic:*** Paraneoplastic myelopathy associated with cancer
- ***Idiopathic.***

Clinical Features

- The onset of symptoms may be acute or subacute. Thoracic region is most often involved. Common presenting symptoms are loss of all functions (motor, sensory, autonomic) below the level of lesion.

Motor Disturbances

- All motor functions are lost below the level of lesion. At the level of lesion there are lower motor neuron signs (paresis, atrophy, fasciculations, and areflexia) and below the level of lesion there are UMN type paralysis. Initially, especially with acute lesions, the paralysis is flaccid and areflexic because of spinal shock, but later spastic paraplegia develops.
- There is loss of tendon reflexes in the acute stage due to spinal shock. Subsequently, tendon reflexes become exaggerated and plantar response becomes extensor.
- Abdominal reflexes are absent below the level of lesion.

Sensory Disturbances

- All sensory modalities (soft touch, position sense, vibration, temperature, and pain) are impaired below the level of the lesion. A sensory level is present.

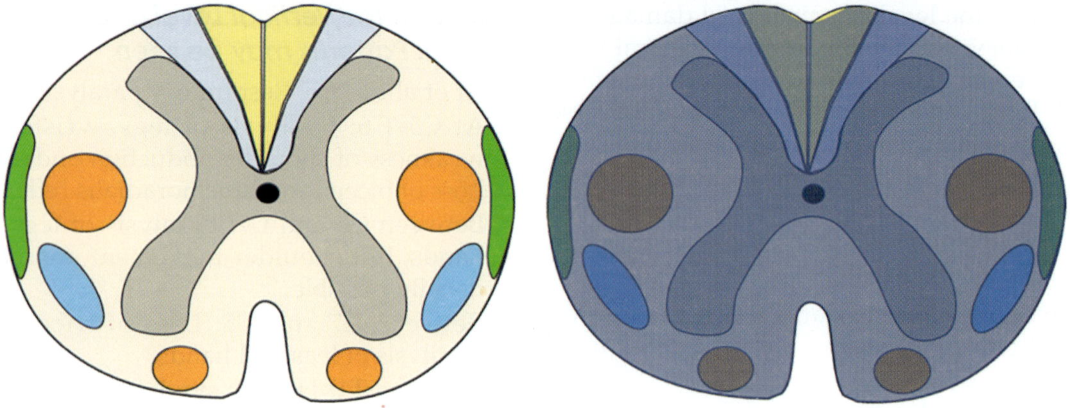

Figure 5.33: Normal spinal cord (left) and transverse myelitis (right, area involved indicated by blue tinge)

Autonomic Disturbances

- Bowel and bladder sphincter dysfunction with incontinence can occur with transverse myelitis. Urgency of micturition is the usual bladder symptom, with urinary retention a later problem. Incontinence of urine is a very late feature. Constipation is the most common bowel symptom. Initially, atonic and, later, spastic rectal and bladder sphincter dysfunction occur with lesions at any spinal level.
- Orthostatic hypotension, loss of sweating, trophic skin changes, impaired temperature control, sexual dysfunction (especially impotence) are other features of autonomic dysfunction.

Investigations

- MRI of spinal cord should be done to rule out any alternate pathology (abscess, mass, etc.).
- CSF cell count and pressure is usually normal but there is increase in its protein content.
- Blood tests: Check for autoimmune markers, infections, and NMO/MOG antibodies.

Treatment

- Care of skin, bladder and bowels, and physiotherapy.
- Treatment of choice for idiopathic transverse myelitis is intravenous administration of methylprednisolone.
- If a cause is identified, treatment should be directed towards that.

Q. Brown-Séquard syndrome.

- Brown-Séquard syndrome results from a lesion involving only one side of the spinal cord **(Fig. 5.34)**. It is usually produced by extramedullary lesions.

Etiology

- Road traffic accidents
- Industrial and sports accidents
- Disc herniation
- Direct injury to the cord with high-velocity missiles or a sharp instrument
- Infarction of spinal cord
- Spinal tumors.
- Multiple sclerosis
- Infectious diseases (e.g. TB, herpes zoster)

Clinical Features (Fig. 5.35)

- Ipsilateral UMN (spastic) weakness due to interruption of the descending corticospinal tract below the level of damage. Lower motor neuron weakness at the level of the lesion due to damage to anterior horn cells and motor root.

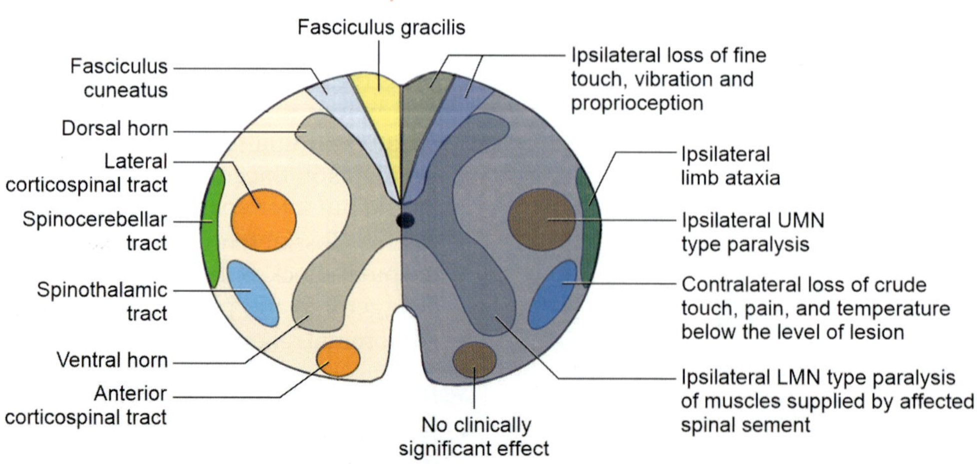

Figure 5.34: Brown-Séquard syndrome (affected structures and their effect on right side)

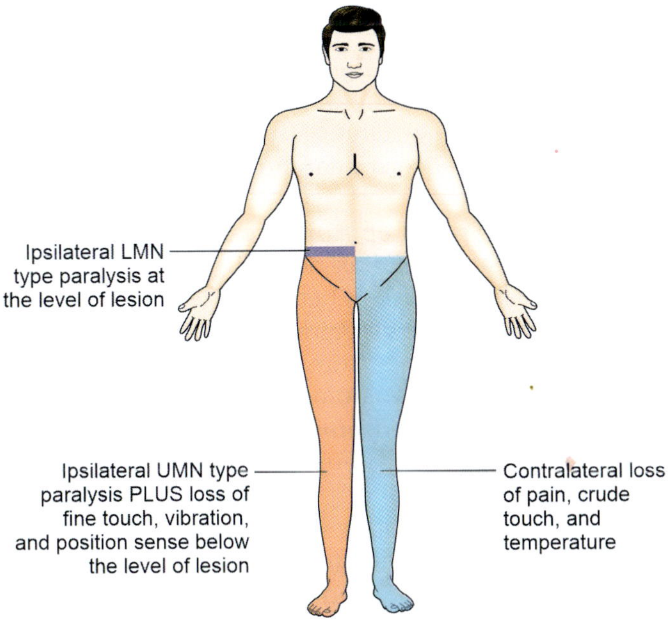

Figure 5.35: Clinical features of Brown-Séquard syndrome

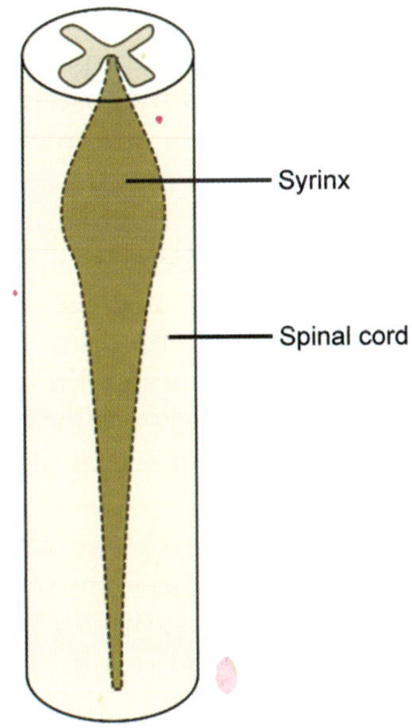

Figure 5.36: Syringomyelia in the spinal cord

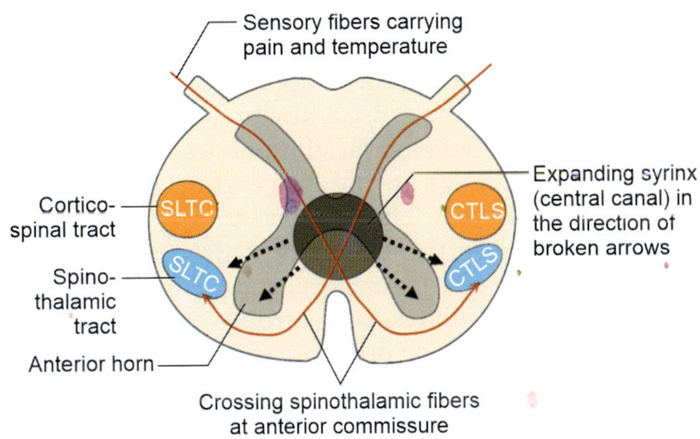

Figure 5.37: Syringomyelia (C: cervical fibers; T = thoracic fibers; L: lumbar; S: sacral)

- Ipsilateral loss of proprioception and vibration below the level of the lesion due to interruption of the ascending fibers in the posterior columns.
- Contralateral loss of pain and temperature sensation due to interruption of the crossed spinothalamic tract. This sensory level is usually one or two segments below the level of the lesion.
- Ipsilateral limb ataxia due to involvement of spinocerebellar tract.

Q. Discuss the etiology, clinical features, diagnosis and management of syringomyelia.

Q. Dissociated sensory loss.

- Syringomyelia refers to fluid-filled cavities within the spinal cord. The cavity is called syrinx and is usually found within the cervical or thoracic spinal cord.
- Syringobulbia means a cavity in the brainstem.

Etiology and Pathology

- Syrinxes usually result from lesions that partially obstruct CSF flow which are as follows:
  - Congenital abnormalities of the craniocervical junction (Chiari type 1 malformation), brain (e.g. encephalocele) or spinal cord (e.g. myelomeningocele).
  - Scarring due to spinal cord trauma, myelitis, chronic arachnoiditis due to tuberculosis and other etiologies, necrotic spinal cord tumors.

Clinical Features

- Clinical features depend on the location of the cavity. Symptoms usually start on one side and then the other side gets involved.
- The syrinx is most commonly encountered in the lower cervical region, extending into the central gray matter and anterior commissure. The cyst interrupts the decussating spinothalamic fibers which carry pain and temperature sensation. This results in classic

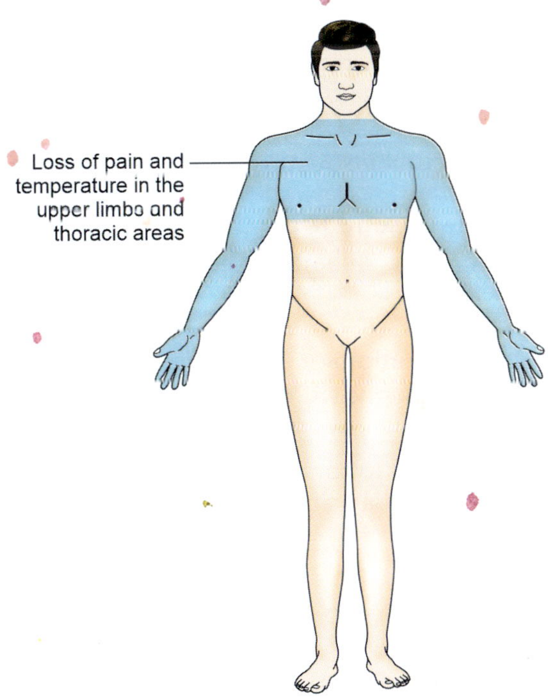

Figure 5.38: Initial distribution of loss of pain and temperature in syringomyelia

dissociated sensory loss where there is loss of pain and temperature sensation with sparing of touch and vibration which are carried by posterior column.

- With anterolateral extension, the spinothalamic tract is affected, producing loss of pain and temperature below the spinal level of the lesion. Because the upper limb and thoracic fibers are situated medially in the spinothalamic tract, and the disease process starts from the center of the spinal cord there is sensory loss affecting the upper limbs and thoracic regions initially. Sacral fibers are located laterally in the spinothalamic tract and sacral fibers are spared initially.
- Extension of the cavity to the anterior horns produces LMN type weakness, muscle atrophy and areflexia involving areas supplied by the affected segments. Lateral extension results in an ipsilateral Horner's syndrome (owing to the involvement of the sympathetic system). As the lesion enlarges, corticospinal tract gets involved and UMN type of weakness (spasticity, weakness of limbs below the lesion, bladder and bowel dysfunction) develop.
- Dorsal extension disrupts dorsal column function (ipsilateral position sense and vibratory loss), and
- Some patients develop facial numbness and sensory loss from damage to the descending tract of the trigeminal nerve (C2 level or above).
- If the syrinx extends into the brainstem (syringobulbia), there is dysphagia, pharyngeal and palatal weakness, asymmetric weakness and atrophy of the tongue, sensory loss involving primarily pain and temperature sense in the distribution of the trigeminal nerve, and nystagmus.
- Thoracic kyphoscoliosis is usually present due to weakness of paraspinal muscles.

Investigations

- MRI—can demonstrate the syrinx cavity.

Treatment

- There is no curative treatment. Treatment depends on the cause.
- If the syrinx cavity is large, decompression of the cavity by syrinx-subarachnoid shunt may produce some benefit.

Q. Describe the etiology, clinical features, differential diagnosis, complications and management of paraplegia.

- Paraplegia refers to paralysis of both lower limbs. Paraparesis refers to partial weakness of both lower limbs.

Etiology

UMN Type Paraplegia

Cerebral causes

- Anterior cerebral artery (ACA), stroke, bilateral ACA infarction or unpaired ACA occlusion.
- Parasagittal meningioma.
- Superior sagittal sinus thrombosis.
- Cerebral palsy.

Spinal cord diseases

- ***Trauma:*** Spinal cord injury (fracture/dislocation).
- ***Vascular:*** Spinal cord infarction (e.g. anterior spinal artery syndrome).
- ***Infectious:*** Spinal epidural abscess, tuberculosis (Pott's disease), HIV-associated myelopathy, viral infections (e.g. HTLV-1, herpes zoster).
- ***Neoplastic (tumors):*** Primary spinal cord tumors (ependymoma, astrocytoma), metastasis to vertebrae or spinal cord, meningiomas, neurofibromas.
- ***Inflammatory/autoimmune:*** Multiple sclerosis, transverse myelitis, neuromyelitis optica (NMO), sarcoidosis.
- ***Degenerative:*** Hereditary spastic paraplegia, subacute combined degeneration (e.g. vitamin B_{12} deficiency).
- ***Spine diseases***: Herniated intervertebral disc, spinal stenosis.
- ***Toxic/metabolic***: Lead poisoning, copper or B_{12} deficiency, adrenomyeloneuropathy.

LMN Type Paraplegia

- Anterior horn cell diseases
- Cauda equina syndromes
- Peripheral neuropathies
- Guillaine-Barré syndrome
- Hypokalemic and hyperkalemic periodic paralysis.

Clinical features

- Acute spinal cord lesions produce flaccid paraplegia initially due to spinal shock. However, later it becomes spastic. Lesions of peripheral nerves (peripheral neuropathy, GB syndrome) result in flaccid paraplegia.
- Paraplegia in extension is seen when only corticospinal tract is involved, because extrapyramidal system takes over resulting in excess tone of antigravity muscles.
- Paraplegia in flexion is seen when both corticospinal and extrapyramidal tracts (reticulospinal tract) are involved, because of increase in tone of flexors.
- Paraplegia in extension and paraplegia in flexion occur only after the spinal shock has ceased.
- A paraplegia in extension can become paraplegia in flexion at later stages as the compression of spinal cord continues and involves entire spinal cord so that both pyramidal and extrapyramidal tracts are involved.
- Bowel and bladder disturbances and sensory symptoms are common in spinal cord lesions.
- Additional clinical features may be present depending on the underlying cause.

Investigations

- Plain X-ray of spine: can detect degenerative changes of spine (spondylosis), vertebral fractures and any other vertebral disease.
- MRI spine: can visualize in detail the spinal cord and its coverings, spine and disc pathology.
- Appropriate tests to rule out underlying cause.

Complications

- Bed sore.
- Limb contracture.
- Deep vein thrombosis and pulmonary embolism due to immobility.
- Osteoporosis due to immobility.
- Fecal impaction with intestinal obstruction due to autonomic dysfunction.
- Urinary tract infection due to bladder dysfunction.

Management of Paraplegia

General Measures

- Patient needs both physical and mental support. Good nutritious diet should be provided. Any intercurrent infection is potentially dangerous and should be treated early.

Bladder Care

- Continuous indwelling catheter is required initially. However intermittent catheterization is better to prevent infection. Once the patient learns the technique of catheterization he can do it himself. Many develop reflex bladder emptying, helped by abdominal pressure. Free urinary drainage is essential to avoid stasis, subsequent infection and calculi formation.

Bowel Care

- Constipation and fecal impaction are common in paraplegics. These should be avoided by stool softeners, laxatives or regular enemas. Digital evacuation may be necessary if stools are hard and impacted. Reflex rectal emptying develops later and patient can pass stools himself.

Skin Care

- Since a paraplegic patient is bedridden most of the time, there is risk of developing pressure sores. Pressure sores (bed sore) are common over pressure points such as sacrum, iliac crests, greater trochanters, heels and malleoli. They can be prevented by maintaining cleanliness and turning the patient every 2 hours. Ripple mattresses and water beds are very useful to prevent pressure sores. If pressure sores develop, plastic surgical repair should be considered. Pressure palsies (e.g. ulnar nerves and common peroneal) must be avoided.

Lower Limbs

- Paralyzed lower limbs are prone to develop contractures and deep vein thrombosis which should be prevented by physiotherapy. Severe spasticity, with flexor or extensor spasms, maybe helped by baclofen, diazepam, dantrolene, tizanidine or botulinum toxin injections.

Treatment of the Underlying Cause

- Underlying cause should be identified and treated.

Rehabilitation

- Many patients with paraplegia can become partially or fully independent. Specialist advice from a rehabilitation unit is necessary.

Q. Describe the nerve supply of urinary bladder. Describe various types of bladder dysfunction.

- The bladder is a hollow bag made of a syncytium of smooth muscle with stretch receptors. There is an internal urethral sphincter made of smooth muscle and an external urethral sphincter which is made of striated muscle.

Nerve Supply of Urinary Bladder

- The nerve supply of the bladder involves autonomic (sympathetic and parasympathetic) as well as somatic innervation, all of which coordinate storage and voiding of urine **(Fig. 5.39)**.

Parasympathetic Supply (pelvic nerves)

- Origin: S2, S3 and S4 spinal segments.
- Nerve Pathway: Pelvic splanchnic nerves → inferior hypogastric plexus. Innervate detrusor muscle and internal sphincter.
- Function: Contracts detrusor muscle and relaxes internal sphincter → **promotes bladder emptying**. This is the main motor supply to the bladder for micturition.

Sympathetic Supply (hypogastric nerves)

- Origin: T11–L2 (thoracolumbar spinal cord)
- Nerve Pathway: Via hypogastric nerve → inferior hypogastric plexus
- Innervate detrusor muscle and internal sphincter.
- Function: Relaxes detrusor muscle and contracts internal urethral sphincter → **promotes bladder filling**.

Somatic (pudendal nerve)

- Origin: S2–S4
- Function: Innervates external urethral sphincter → voluntary control of urination. Also supplies perineum and pelvic floor muscles

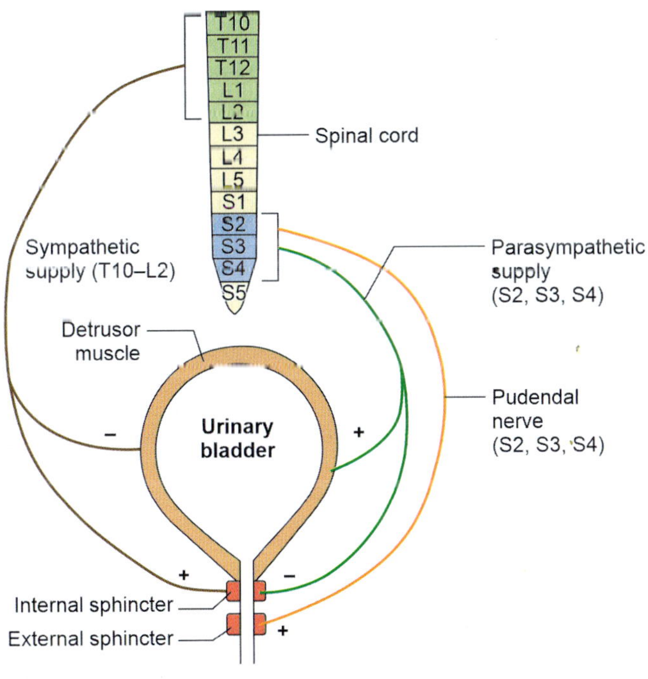

Figure 5.39: Nerve supply of urinary bladder

- Damage leads to loss of continence (inability to hold urine).

Sensory Innervation

- Arise from the stretch receptors in the bladder wall and internal sphincter
- Travel via pelvic (parasympathetic) and hypogastric (sympathetic) afferents
- Send signals to spinal cord and brain about bladder fullness.

Control Centers in the CNS

Region	Role
Frontal cortex	Voluntary control over micturition
Pontine micturition center	Coordinates bladder and sphincter activity
Sacral spinal cord (S2–S4)	Reflex center for parasympathetic control

Various Types of Bladder Dysfunction

- Any condition that impairs bladder afferent and efferent nerve supply can cause neurogenic bladder. Causes may involve the CNS (e.g. stroke, spinal cord injury), peripheral nerves (e.g. diabetic peripheral neuropathy, vitamin B_{12} deficiency), or both (e.g. Parkinson disease, multiple sclerosis, syphilis).
- Mainly there are three types of bladder dysfunction due to the above causes. These are upper motor neuron (UMN), lower motor neuron (LMN), and cortical types, each with distinct clinical features.

Spastic (reflex) Bladder – UMN Type Bladder (also known as automatic bladder)

- Automatic bladder develops when the spinal cord is damaged above the sacral segments, leading to loss of voluntary control but preserved reflex detrusor activity. Bladder emptying occurs reflexively (automatically) in response to filling, without cortical involvement. This results in reflex bladder contractions, often causing involuntary urination.

Lesion location

- Above the sacral micturition center (i.e. above S2–S4, typically cervical or thoracic spinal cord).

Common causes

- Spinal cord injury (above conus medullaris).
- Multiple sclerosis.
- Transverse myelitis.

Pathophysiology

- Loss of inhibitory control from higher centers → uninhibited bladder contractions.
- Reflex arc between bladder and spinal cord remains intact.

Clinical features

- Urgency, frequency
- Incontinence (urge)
- Small bladder capacity
- Detrusor overactivity
- Increased tone of external sphincter → risk of detrusor-sphincter dyssynergia (DSD). Bladder contraction and external urinary sphincter relaxation are typically uncoordinated (detrusor-sphincter dyssynergia) resulting in failure of external sphincter to relax when bladder is contracting which leads to incomplete emptying.

Flaccid (areflexic) Bladder—LMN Type Bladder (also known as autonomous bladder)

- Autonomous bladder (also called atonic bladder) occurs when both the afferent and efferent pathways of the bladder reflex arc are disrupted—typically due to lesions involving the conus medullaris, cauda equina, or peripheral nerves. As a result, both voluntary and reflex bladder contractions are absent. The bladder becomes flaccid and overdistended, leading to urinary retention and overflow incontinence.

Lesion location

- At or below the S2–S4 segments (conus medullaris or cauda equina). It also occurs in the initial stages (stage of spinal shock) of acute cord damage.

Common causes

- Cauda equina syndrome.
- Conus medullaris syndrome.
- Peripheral neuropathies (e.g. diabetes, Guillain-Barré).

Pathophysiology

- Damage to parasympathetic innervation to detrusor muscle.
- Loss of both voluntary and reflexive control.

Clinical features

- Urinary retention.
- Large bladder capacity.
- No urge to void.
- Overflow incontinence (dribbling): This occurs when the bladder filling capacity is exceeded. Bladder pressure increases when the bladder capacity is exceeded which opens the sphincters and incontinence occurs. Urine continuously dribbles as the bladder is unable to contract. Examination reveals a full bladder.
- Absent perineal reflexes (e.g. bulbocavernosus, anal wink).

Cortical (frontal) Bladder—Suprapontine Lesion (also known as uninhibited bladder)

- A cortical or suprapontine bladder dysfunction results from damage above the pontine micturition center (usually in the frontal lobe), where voluntary control over urination is lost, but the reflex arc remains intact.

Lesion location

- Frontal micturition center in frontal lobe or basal ganglia.

Common causes

- Stroke (especially ACA territory)
- Normal pressure hydrocephalus
- Parkinson's disease
- Dementia
- Frontal lobe tumors.

Pathophysiology

- Loss of inhibitory cortical input to the pontine micturition center → pontine micturition center intact → bladder empties reflexively.

Clinical features

- Urinary urgency due to reflex contractions of bladder
- Urge incontinence due to inability to suppress urge to void
- Frequent small voids due to overactivity
- Bladder sensation may be preserved
- Associated cognitive or gait disturbances, especially in NPH, parkinsonism, or frontal lobe lesions.

Summary (Table 5.40)

TABLE 5.40: Comparison of different types of neurogenic bladder

Feature	Spastic (UMN) bladder	Flaccid (LMN) bladder	Cortical bladder
Lesion site	Above S2–S4 (e.g. spinal cord)	At/below S2–S4 (e.g. cauda)	Cortex or basal ganglia
Bladder tone	Increased	Decreased	Variable
Detrusor activity	Overactive	Underactive	Reflex emptying preserved
Sphincter tone	High (→ DSD risk)	Low	Often normal
Incontinence type	Urge	Overflow	Urge
Sensation	Often reduced	Absent	Usually preserved

Investigations

- Micturition can be studied by urodynamic studies which involves constant recording of intravesical and intraurethral pressure, and perineal floor EMG, with fluoroscopic monitoring. These urodynamic studies facilitate the diagnosis of neurogenic bladder dysfunction.
- MRI of the spinal cord can show any spinal cord lesions.

Treatment

- In flaccid bladder (LMN bladder) which causes urinary retention, bladder drainage by continuous indwelling catheter may be necessary. Since, continuous indwelling catheter can cause infection if kept for a long time, intermittent catheterization may be necessary to prevent infection. Prophylactic antibiotics may be necessary. Parasympathomimetic drugs like carbachol and bethenocol cause contraction of the detrusor and are useful in flaccid paralysis of the bladder. Timed voiding, Crede's maneuver (manual bladder expression) should be taught to patient.
- In spastic bladder (UMN bladder), antimuscarinics (e.g. oxybutynin, tolterodine) and beta-3 agonists (mirabegron) may be tried. These drugs decrease detrusor overactivity. Detrusor sphincter dyssynergia can be reduced by alpha-blockers (e.g. tamsulosin) or sphincterotomy.
- Cortical (frontal) bladder is treated in a similar way as spastic bladder. Treat any underlying cause (e.g. NPH).
- Surgery is a last resort. It is indicated in patients who cannot use continuous or intermittent bladder drainage. Sphincterotomy (for men) converts the bladder into an open draining conduit. Sacral (S3 and S4) rhizotomy converts a spastic into a flaccid bladder. Urinary diversion may involve an ileal conduit or ureterostomy.

Q. Mention the various forms of neurosyphilis.

Q. Describe the clinical features and management of meningovascular syphilis.

Q. General paresis of the insane.

Q. Tabes dorsalis.

- The term "neurosyphilis" refers to infection of the central nervous system (CNS) by *Treponema pallidum* (*T. pallidum*). Many patients are able to clear the infection spontaneously or due to antibiotic therapy. Nowadays neurosyphilis is mainly seen in HIV patients who are not able to clear the infection. Neurosyphilis can occur at any time after initial infection.
- Various forms of neurosyphilis are,

Early Forms

- Meningitis—involvement of the cerebrospinal fluid (CSF) and meninges.
- Meningovascular syphilis—involvement of meninges and vasculature.

Late Forms

- General paresis of the insane—involvement of brain parenchyma.
- Tabes dorsalis—involvement of spinal cord parenchyma.

Meningovascular Syphilis

- Just like any other bacterial meningitis, syphilitic meningitis can cause an infectious arteritis of any vessel in the subarachnoid space which results in thrombosis of the vessel leading to ischemia, and infarction of the brain.

- Patients may present as ischemic stroke. Clinical features depend on the vessel involved. Less commonly, anterior spinal artery can get involved leading to spinal cord infarction. The middle cerebral artery and its branches are most commonly affected. Meningovascular syphilis may develop in the first few months or years after the syphilis infection. Associated meningitis may manifest as headache, dizziness, or personality changes.
- CSF analysis shows increased cells with predominant lymphocytes and increased protein concentration. CSF-VDRL is usually but not always reactive. Angiography can demonstrate the narrowed or blocked vessels and neuroimaging shows one or more areas of infarction.

General Paresis (general paralysis of the insane; paretic neurosyphilis; dementia paralytica)

- This is a progressive dementing illness due to involvement of the brain parenchyma by syphilis.
- General paresis usually develops 10–25 years after infection, but it can occur much earlier also.
- In the early stage, patients have forgetfulness and personality change. There is progressive decline in memory and judgment leading to severe dementia. There may be psychiatric symptoms such as depression, mania, or psychosis.
- Neurologic finding include dysarthria, facial and limb hypotonia, intention tremors of the face, tongue, and hands, and reflex abnormalities.
- CSF examination shows increased lymphocytes and protein. The CSF-VDRL is reactive in virtually all patients, and neuroimaging usually shows brain atrophy.

Tabes Dorsalis

- Tabes dorsalis (also called locomotor ataxia) is a disease of the posterior columns of the spinal cord and of the dorsal roots. It has the longest latent period between primary infection and onset (average of about 20 years). It is rare now due to availability of antibiotic therapy.
- Patient presents with sensory ataxia and sensory symptoms such as lancinating pains and paraesthesias. There may be depressed lower limb reflexes, impaired vibratory and position sensation, impaired touch and pain, and optic atrophy.
- Sometimes gastric crises, characterized by recurrent attacks of severe epigastric pain, nausea, and vomiting may be seen.
- Pupillary irregularities are common and include Argyll-Robertson pupil (accommodation reflex present, light reflex absent).
- Other findings seen with tabes dorsalis include absent lower extremity reflexes.

Treatment of Neurosyphilis

- All forms of neurosyphilis are treated as follows.

Drugs of Choice

- Penicillin G 3–4 million units IV every four hours or 24 million units per day continuous IV infusion for 10–14 days.

Alternatives

- Drug of choice for neurosyphilis is aqueous penicillin 3–4 million units IV q 4 h (best penetrates the CNS but may be impractical) or procaine penicillin G 2.4 million units IM once/day plus 500 mg probenecid po qid is recommended; both drugs are given for 10–14 days, followed by benzathine penicillin 2.4 million units IM once a week for 3 weeks. Alternative is ceftriaxone 2 g IV once daily for 10–14 days.
- Because *Treponema pallidum* cannot be cultured in the laboratory, success of neurosyphilis treatment should be monitored by resolution of clinical features and CSF abnormalities. CSF should be examined at three to 6 months after treatment and every 6 months thereafter until CSF white blood cell (WBC) count is normal and CSF-VDRL is nonreactive. The CSF WBC count should decline at 6 months after successful treatment, and all CSF abnormalities should resolve by 2 years after treatment. Failure to meet these criteria should prompt retreatment.

Q. Charcot's joint (neuropathic arthropathy).

- Charcot's joint is chronic, progressive, destructive arthropathy due to loss of sensation of a joint.
- It is seen in tabes dorsalis, syringomyelia, diabetic neuropathy and other sensory polyneuropathies.
- Hips, knees and ankles are most commonly involved.

Pathophysiology

- Lack of proprioception and pain sensation in the joints results in ligamentous laxity, increased range of joint movement, instability, and damage by minor trauma. Pain is minimal even though there may be extensive joint destruction.

Diagnosis

- Clinical suspicion in neuropathic patients
- X-ray: Radiological Features include 6 D's. These are as follows:
    - Destruction of joint surfaces
    - Dislocation or subluxation
    - Debris (intra-articular loose bodies)
    - Density increase (sclerosis)
    - Distension (joint effusion)
    - Disorganization of the joint architecture
- MRI: helpful for early diagnosis or to rule out osteomyelitis.
- Bone scan: can differentiate infection from Charcot changes.

Treatment

- Involves rest to the joint and avoidance of weight bearing in early stages.

- Biphosphnates such as pamidronate and aledronate have been shown to be helpful in the treatment of Charcot's joints.
- In late stages when there is loss of joint architecture and deformities, surgery and orthotic support may help.
- Underlying cause should be tackled.

Q. What are the diseases affecting posterior columns?

Q. What are the sensations carried by posterior columns? Mention the physical signs of posterior column lesion.

Diseases affecting Posterior Columns

Tabes dorsalis

- Late manifestation of neurosyphilis.
- Characterized by demyelination of posterior columns and dorsal roots.

Subacute combined degeneration (SCD)

- Due to vitamin B_{12} deficiency.
- Affects posterior columns and lateral corticospinal tracts.

Multiple sclerosis (MS)

- Demyelinating disease that can involve posterior columns.

Friedreich's ataxia

- Hereditary neurodegenerative disorder involving the posterior columns and spinocerebellar tracts.

Copper deficiency myelopathy

- Mimics subacute combined degeneration.

Trauma or compressive myelopathy

- Spinal cord injury or compression (e.g. from tumors or herniated discs).

Ischemia of posterior spinal artery

- Rare but can cause selective posterior column damage.
- Subacute combined degeneration.
- Tabes dorsalis.
- Compressive and noncompressive myelopathies.

Sensations Carried by Posterior Columns

- Vibration
- Joint position sense (proprioception)
- Fine touch.

Physical Signs of Posterior Column Lesion

- Sensory ataxia
- Positive Romberg sign
- Impaired fine touch, vibration and joint position sense.
- Lhermitte's sign: Electric-shock sensation down the spine on neck flexion (can occur in posterior column disorders like MS or SCD).

Q. Romberg sign.

- The Romberg sign is a clinical test used to assess proprioception—the body's sense of position—which is mediated by the posterior columns of the spinal cord.
- Romberg sign is positive in sensory ataxias. It is not a test to assess the cerebellar function.

How to elicit Romberg sign?

- Ask the patient to stand with the feet together. Then ask the patient to close both the eyes. If the patient shows swaying or loses balance, then Romberg's sign is positive. (*Note*: If the patient cannot stand with the feet together and eyes open, then a cerebellar lesion is present and Romberg's test is not applicable.)

Physiological Basis of Romberg Sign

- To maintain equilibrium, a person requires intact joint position sense, intact vision, and intact vestibular and cerebellar systems. The absence of one can be compensated by the other. In posterior column lesions, joint position sense is lost, but the person maintains balance by visual compensation. When the eyes are closed, visual cue is removed and the person sways or loses balance.

Common Causes of Positive Romberg Test

- Vitamin B_{12} deficiency—subacute combined degeneration of the cord
- Diabetic peripheral large fiber neuropathy
- Friedrich's ataxia
- Tabes dorsalis.

Q. Discuss the etiology, clinical features, diagnosis and management of subacute combined degeneration.

- Subacute combined degeneration is a nutritional disorder of the CNS due to vitamin B_{12} deficiency. There is degeneration of the dorsal and lateral spinal (corticospinal) columns, hence called combined degeneration. Degeneration is due to a defect in myelin formation of unknown mechanism.

Pathophysiology

- B_{12} is essential for myelin formation.
- Deficiency leads to demyelination, especially in:
    - Posterior columns → loss of proprioception and vibration sense.
    - Lateral corticospinal tracts → motor weakness and spasticity.

Clinical Features

- It is subacute in onset.
- Posterior column degeneration produces paresthesias (tingling, "pins and needles" in feet/hands) and ataxia associated with loss of vibration and position sense. Romberg's sign is positive.
- Corticospinal tract degeneration produces weakness, spasticity, extensor plantar response, clonus, paraplegia, and even fecal and urinary incontinence.
- Ankle jerk may be absent due to associated peripheral neuropathy but knee jerk is brisk.

- Other neurologic findings include memory loss, irritability, and dementia due to vitamin B_{12} deficiency.
- There may be macrocytic anemia due to vitamin B_{12} deficiency.

Investigations

- Serum vitamin B_{12} level will be low.
- ↑ Methylmalonic acid and ↑ homocysteine (more sensitive indicators).
- CBC usually shows megaloblastic anemia.
- MRI of the spinal cord shows T2 hyperintensity in posterior and lateral columns of cervical/thoracic spinal cord ("inverted V" sign).

Treatment

- Inj vitamin B_{12} (intramuscular) 1 mg (1000 µg) every day for one week, followed by 1 mg every week for four weeks and then, 1 mg every month for the remainder of the patient's life.
- Ensure adequate intake of B_{12} (animal products or fortified foods).

Q. Discuss the classification, etiology, clinical features, diagnosis and management of motor neuron disease (MND).

Q. Amyotrophic lateral sclerosis (ALS).

- Motor neurone diseases (MND) are a group of degenerative disorders selectively affecting upper or lower motor neurons, or both. The condition is progressive and has a fatal outcome.
- Symptoms vary in severity and include muscle weakness and atrophy, fasciculations, emotional lability, and respiratory muscle weakness.
- MND has worldwide distribution. Males are affected more commonly and generally it starts between 45–60 years.

Types of Motor Neuron Diseases

- **Amyotrophic lateral sclerosis (ALS):** Combination of upper and lower motor neuron signs.
- **Primary lateral sclerosis (PLS):** Predominantly upper motor neuron signs.
- **Progressive muscular atrophy:** Predominantly lower motor neuron signs.
- **Progressive bulbar palsy:** Affects cranial nerves. Signs limited to bulbar muscles.
- **Spinal muscular atrophy (SMA):** Affects lower motor neurons and usually pediatric age group.
- **Kennedy's disease:** Affects lower motor neurons. X-linked; bulbar and limb weakness.

- ALS is the commonest type of MND, affecting the anterior horn cells (responsible for LMN signs) and the corticospinal tract (responsible for UMN signs). Other motor neuron diseases involve only particular subsets of motor neurons. Thus, progressive bulbar palsy and spinal muscular atrophy (SMA) involve the lower motor neurons of brainstem and spinal cord respectively. Primary lateral sclerosis (PLS) affects only upper motor neurons innervating the brainstem and spinal cord. The death of the motor neurons leads to atrophy of the muscles innervated by them.
- In motor neuron disease, sensory system, cerebellum and other areas of the brain are not affected. Motor neurons supplying eye muscles are also not affected.

Amyotrophic Lateral Sclerosis (ALS)

Etiology

- Amyotrophic lateral sclerosis (ALS) is the classical prototype and the commonest type of MND. Most of the ALS cases are sporadic. Some are familial. Even sporadic cases may have some genetic influence. Following are risk factors for the development of ALS. Males and whites are affected more commonly.

- Genetic factors
- Smoking
- Old age
- Toxins: Lead, tin and mercury
- Electric shock
- Radiation exposure
- Excess glutamate activity

Pathology

- Degeneration of **UMNs** in the motor cortex and **LMNs** in the brainstem and anterior horn of the spinal cord. This leads to a combination of both UMN and LMN features in patients.
- Degeneration of UMNs in the motor cortex → UMN type weakness associated with spasticity, hyperreflexia.
- Degeneration of LMNs in the brainstem and anterior horn of the spinal cord → LMN type weakness associated with wasting and fasciculations.

Clinical Features

- Initial symptom is usually insidious onset of weakness and clumsiness of one hand for skilled activity which progresses and gross activity also becomes difficult.
- Slowly the opposite hand is involved and whole of both upper limbs may be affected.
- LMN signs such as wasting, flaccidity, loss of tendon reflexes and fasciculations are seen along with UMN signs such as spasticity and exaggerated reflexes.
- Lower limb involvement may precede or follow upper limb involvement. There is difficulty in walking with spastic gait and pyramidal signs. The knee and ankle jerks are exaggerated. Plantar response is extensor bilaterally.
- Involvement of cranial nerve nuclei (mainly IX, X, XI and XII nerve nuclei) causes difficulty in swallowing, nasal regurgitation and slurred speech. Tongue shows atrophy and fasciculations. UMN involvement results in pseudobulbar palsy with exaggerated jaw jerk.
- There is no sensory loss but subjective sensations like numbness, cramps, neuralgic pain may be complained of. Impotence occurs early in the disease. There is no loss of sphincter control.

- The progression of the disease is variable. It can be rapid and result in death within a year or it may be slow over many years. Death occurs due to respiratory failure.

Investigations

- EMG/NCS: Widespread denervation and reinnervation.
- MRI: to exclude structural or other causes.
- Blood tests: B_{12}, HIV, syphilis, autoimmune markers.
- Genetic testing: in familial cases.

Treatment

- So far, there is no effective drug for the treatment of MND.
- The drug riluzole has been approved for ALS because it produces a modest lengthening of survival. Riluzole blocks release of glutamic acid and may slow the progression of disease by disrupting glutamate-mediated neurotoxicity. There are many drugs currently under trial for MND.
- Edaravone is a free radical scavenger that is thought to reduce oxidative stress and has proven to be beneficial in early-stage ALS.
- Stem cell therapy and immunomodulation therapies are under trial.
- In the absence of specific therapy for MND, rehabilitation measures are helpful. Foot-drop splints facilitate walking and finger extension splints can potentiate grip. If there is difficulty in chewing and swallowing, gastrostomy is helpful for restoring nutrition and hydration.

Q. Discuss the classification, etiology, clinical features, diagnosis and management of peripheral neuropathy.

Q. Mention the causes of polyneuropathies. Discuss the clinical features, diagnosis and management of polyneuropathies.

- The peripheral nervous system extends from the anterior horn cell or the sensory ganglion up to the neuromuscular junction or the receptors.
- Peripheral neuropathy is a general term and refers to any disorder affecting peripheral nervous system.
- Polyneuropathy is a specific term which refers to a generalized, symmetrical process affecting many peripheral nerves, with the distal nerves affected more prominently. Polyneuropathy is a type of peripheral neuropathy.

Classification of Peripheral Neuropathies

See **Table 5.41.**

TABLE 5.41: Classification of peripheral neuropathies

Type	Features	Examples
Mononeuropathy	Pathological process affecting a single nerve	Trauma, tumor, carpal tunnel syndrome affecting median nerve, Saturday night palsy (radial nerve), Bell's palsy
Mononeuritis multiplex(multiple mononeuropathy, or multifocal neuropathy)	Affects 2 or more discrete nerves in separate areas	Leprosy, diabetes, sarcoidosis, HIV, Polyarteritis nodosa
Polyneuropathy	Refers to diffuse, symmetrical disease, usually beginning peripherally. They are classified broadly into demyelinating and axonal types. The polymeuropathies can be acute or chronic, motor or sensory or sensorimotor (i.e. mixed) and autonomic	Guillaine-Barré syndrome, diabetic peripheral neuropathy, vitamin B_{12} deficiency
Monoradiculopathy	Single spinal root is affected	Disc prolapse, trauma, tumor
Polyradiculopathy	Many spinal roots are affected	Spondylosis, arachnoiditis, GB syndrome
Plexopathy	Brachial or lumbosacral plexus are affected	Diabetes, trauma, tumors

Polyneuropathy

Causes of Polyneuropathy

- **Metabolic:** Diabetes mellitus, amyloidosis, porphyria, paraproteinemia, hypothyroidism
- **Toxic:** Alcohol, lead, arsenic, thallium
- **Drugs:** Vincristine, INH, hydralazine, dapsone, amiodarone.
- **Infections:** Leprosy, diphtheria, HIV, Lyme disease.
- **Collagen disorders:** SLE, polyarteritis nodosa, rheumatoid arthritis.
- **Vitamin deficiencies:** B_1, B_6, B_{12}
- **Paraneoplastic:** Carcinoma bronchus
- **Genetic:** Charcot-Marie-Tooth disease
- **Autoimmune:** Guillane barre syndrome (AIDP), vasculitis
- **Idiopathic**

Clinical Features

- In polyneuropathy, Injury tends to be related to axon length; thus, longer axons are affected first, resulting in symptoms that begin in the feet of lower limbs. Sensory symptoms usually precede motor symptoms.
- Since peripheral nerves carry motor, sensory and autonomic fibers, all these components are affected to a variable extent.
- ***Sensory symptoms*:** Patients present with slowly progressive sensory loss and dysesthesias such as tingling, numbness, and burning sensation in the feet,

and mild gait abnormalities (due to proprioceptive loss). As the disease progresses, sensory symptoms also progressively ascend upwards to involve legs and then thigh. When sensory symptoms reach up to the level of knees, hands of upper limbs also start getting involved. Involvement of both lower limbs and upper limbs thus results in classic "glove and stocking" distribution of sensory symptoms **(Fig. 5.40)**. Sensory symptoms may continue to extend proximally in severe cases, affecting the intercostal nerves.

- *Motor symptoms:* As the polyneuropathy progresses, mild weakness of the distal parts of lower limbs (feet) and upper limbs (hands) may begin. This may result in foot drop and wrist drop. There may be distal muscle wasting and loss of distal reflexes.
- *Autonomic symptoms:* these include orthostatic hypotension, bowel and bladder dysfunction, erectile dysfunction, and anhidrosis or hyperhidrosis.

Investigations

- *Electrodiagnostic testing:* Electromyography/nerve conduction studies (EMG/NCS) can determine whether it is axonal or demyelinating in character. Demyelinating disorders are characterized by slow nerve conduction velocity whereas axonal neuropathies are characterized by reduced amplitude of action potentials with relative preservation of the nerve conduction velocity.
- *Nerve biopsy:* Nerve biopsy is occasionally useful for diagnosing the underlying etiology of polyneuropathy such as amyloid. The sural nerve at the ankle is the preferred site for cutaneous nerve biopsy.

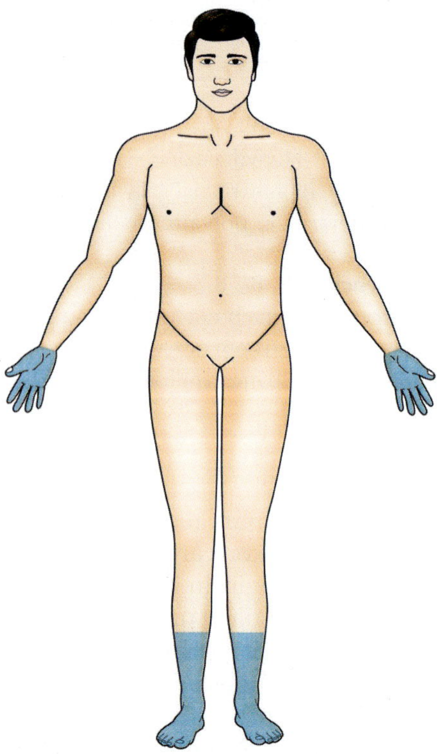

Figure 5.40: Glove and stocking type sensory loss (blue-shaded areas)

- *Other tests:* A standard laboratory "screen" in patients with polyneuropathy includes a complete blood count, ESR, TSH, serum protein electrophoresis, blood glucose, vitamin B_{12} concentration, antinuclear antibody, and urinalysis. Additional testing may include lumbar puncture, genetic testing, and muscle or nerve biopsy.

Treatment

- The aim of treatment is correcting the underlying cause and control of symptoms.
- *Treatment of the underlying cause:* Proper control of diabetes, reducing exposures to toxins, withdrawing the causative drug, etc.
- *Treatment of symptoms and prevention of complications:* Amitriptyline, duloxetine, gabapentin, pregabalin, and carbamazepine can be used to control neuropathic symptoms such as pricking pain and burning sensation. Physiotherapy, use of ankle-foot orthoses, splints, and walking assistance devices can significantly improve lifestyle in the face of significant disability. Proper foot and nail care is important to prevent ulcer formation.

Q. Describe the etiology, clinical features, diagnosis and management of Guillain-Barre syndrome (acute inflammatory demyelinating polyneuropathy-AIDP).

- Guillain-Barré syndrome is an **acute, immune-mediated polyradiculoneuropathy** characterized by rapidly progressive, symmetrical weakness and areflexia.
- AIDP is the most common subtype of GBS, characterized by demyelination of peripheral nerves.

Etiology and Pathogenesis

- Guillain-Barré syndrome (GBS) results from an immune response to a preceding infection that cross-reacts with peripheral nerve components because of molecular mimicry.
- The immune response can be directed towards the myelin or the axon of peripheral nerve, resulting in demyelinating and axonal forms of GBS.
- Many infections can trigger GBS. Commonly implicated infections are *Campylobacter jejuni* infection, cytomegalovirus, Epstein-Barr virus, and human immunodeficiency virus (HIV). Other triggering events are immunization (influenza, meningococcal, etc.), surgery, trauma, and bone-marrow transplantation.
- Nerve damage is due to activated T cells and circulating antibodies such as antimyelin antibodies.

Subtypes of Guillain-Barré Syndrome (GBS)

Acute Inflammatory Demyelinating Polyneuropathy (AIDP)

Demyelinating type. Recovery is rapid.

Acute Motor Axonal Neuropathy (AMAN)

- Axonal type. There is no sensory nerve involvement and no peripheral nerve demyelination. Recovery is rapid.

Acute Motor Sensory Axonal Neuropathy (AMSAN)

- Axonal type. Both sensory and motor fibers are affected and recovery is slow.

Miller Fisher Syndrome (MFS)

- Rare variant of GBS. Demyelinating type. Classically presents as a triad of ataxia, areflexia, and ophthalmoplegia. Patients may also have mild limb weakness, ptosis, facial palsy, or bulbar palsy.

Clinical Features

- The cardinal features of GBS are progressive, symmetric LMN type muscle weakness (flaccid paralysis) and areflexia (absent deep tendon reflexes).
- Weakness usually starts in the lower limbs, and then ascends up to involve trunk and upper limbs (ascending paralysis). Weakness can vary from mild weakness of legs to complete paralysis of all extremity, facial, respiratory, and bulbar muscles. However, in some patients weakness can begin in the arms or facial muscles and then descend down to involve trunk and lower limbs (descending paralysis).
- Severe respiratory muscle weakness may lead to respiratory failure and requires ventilator support.
- Facial (LMN type) and oculomotor nerve involvement occur in some patients. Bilateral facial palsy also can occur.
- Sensory symptoms such as paresthesias occur in the hands and feet in most of the patients, but usually there are no objective sensory deficits. There is often prominent severe pain in the lower back.
- Autonomic neuropathy occurs in majority of patients and manifests as tachycardia, urinary retention, fluctuating BP, orthostatic hypotension, bradycardia, arrhythmias, ileus, and loss of sweating.
- GBS usually progresses over a period of about two weeks and recovery starts after about a month.

Investigations

- *Nerve conduction studies (NCS):* This is used to confirm the diagnosis and also to know the type of GBS. Abnormalities in NCS that are consistent with demyelination are delayed distal latencies, slowed nerve conduction velocities, conduction block etc. In case of axonal damage, needle EMG will show decreased recruitment and rapid firing motor units in weak muscles.
- *CSF analysis (after 1st week):* Protein is elevated with a normal WBC count. This is known as albuminocytologic dissociation, and is present in most patients one week after the onset of symptoms. However, cell count may be increased in patients with HIV infection.
- *Antibodies:* Against nerve components can be detected in the blood of GBS patients. However, antibody testing is not routinely used.

Treatment

- *Plasmapheresis:* Removes the circulating antibodies and helps in fast recovery. 4–6 exchanges over 1–2 weeks are recommended.
- *Intravenous immune globulin (IVIG):* Probably acts by neutralizing circulating antibodies and immunomodulation. IVIG is given in a dose of 0.4 g/kg per day for 5 days.
- Both plasmapheresis and IV immunoglobulins have equal efficacy and combining both of them is not better than any one given alone.
- *Steroids:* Studies have shown that steroids do not provide any benefit in GBS.
- *Supportive therapy:* Bowel and bladder care, adequate nutrition, monitoring for respiratory failure and providing ventilatory support if required, cardiac monitoring, and physiotherapy are all important.

Q. Differentiation between demyelinating and axonal neuropathy (Table 5.42).

TABLE 5.42: Differentiation between demyelinating and axonal neuropathy

Features	Demyelinating neuropathy	Axonal neuropathy
Primary site of damage	Myelin sheath	Axon (nerve fiber)
Part of nerve fiber affected first	Length independent (can affect any part of nerve fiber)	Length dependent (affect the distal most part of longest nerve fibers first
Pattern of involvement	Involve both proximal and distal areas of limbs	Usually affects distal part of limbs (glove and stocking distribution)
Onset	Usually acute	Insidious
Sensory loss	Minimal	Significant (glove and stocking type)
Muscle wasting	No	Yes
Fasciculations	No	Yes
Reflexes	Loss of all deep tendon reflexes	Loss of only distal reflexes such as ankle
Recovery	Rapid and usually complete	Slow with residual deficit
CSF protein	Raised	Normal
Nerve conduction velocity	Very slow	Normal or slightly slow
Amplitude of action potential	Normal	Reduced
Examples	Guillain-Barré syndrome (AIDP)	Diabetic neuropathy Toxic neuropathy

Q. Enumerate the causes of peripheral neuropathies with significant autonomic neuropathy.

- Diabetes mellitus
- Hansen's disease
- Acute intermittent porphyria
- Alcoholism
- Guillain-Barré syndrome
- Amyloidosis
- Inherited: Riley-Day syndrome, Refsum's disease
- Toxic neuropathies: Thallium, acrylamide

Q. Enumerate the causes of peripheral neuropathies with predominant motor weakness (minimal or absent sensory impairment).

- Multifocal motor neuropathy
- Guillain-Barré syndrome
- CIDP
- Lead intoxication
- Acute porphyria
- Diptheria
- Hereditary motor sensory neuropathy (Charcot-Marie-Tooth disease)
- Hereditary motor neuropathy
- Toxic exposure related to dapsone amiodarone, and vincristine.

Q. Carpal tunnel syndrome.

- Carpal tunnel syndrome is a compression neuropathy of the median nerve as it passes through the carpal tunnel in the wrist. This is the most common nerve entrapment disorder.

Pathophysiology of Carpal Tunnel Syndrome

- Carpal tunnel syndrome results from compression of the median nerve within the carpal tunnel, leading to ischemia and impaired nerve function.
- Normally, the carpal tunnel is a fixed space bounded by carpal bones and the flexor retinaculum.
- Any condition that reduces the space or increases contents (e.g. tendon swelling, fluid retention) leads to increased intracarpal pressure leading to compression of median nerve.
- Compression reduces epineural blood flow, causing nerve ischemia. Sustained compression causes segmental demyelination of the median nerve fibers.
- This results in slowed nerve conduction (seen in NCS). Axonal degeneration can occur due to long-standing or severe compression. Axonal loss leads to thenar muscle atrophy and persistent sensory deficits.

Causes

- Idiopathic
- Colles' fracture or other wrist trauma
- Hypothyroidism
- Diabetes mellitus
- Pregnancy (third trimester)
- Obesity
- Rheumatoid arthritis (with wrist involvement)
- Acromegaly
- Amyloidosis
- Renal dialysis patients
- Repetitive wrist motion (typing, tools)
- Use of vibrating tools

Clinical Features

- Pain and paresthesia in the thumb, first two fingers, and the radial-half of the ring finger (the distribution of the median nerve, **Fig. 5.41**). Pain may radiate proximally into the forearm. Many patients experience pain at night and are awakened by abnormal sensations.
- Physical examination may reveal weakness of thenar muscles and flattening of the thenar eminence. There may be sensory loss in the palm and radial three-and-a-half fingers.
- Tinel's sign and Phalen's tests are often positive. Tinel's sign is elicited by tapping the flexor aspect of the wrist: This causes tingling and pain. In a positive Phalen's test, symptoms are reproduced on maximal wrist flexion for 1 minute.
- Nerve conduction studies (NCS) can show delayed conduction through median nerve at the wrist.

Investigations

- Nerve conduction study (NCS): Decreased conduction velocity or block in median nerve across wrist.
- Electromyography (EMG): Denervation in median nerve-innervated muscles.
- Ultrasound/MRI of wrist (optional): Median nerve swelling, tunnel narrowing (supportive).

Treatment

- For mild cases, conservative measures such as, wrist splint at night, oral or local steroid injection, physiotherapy, and yoga can give relief. In pregnancy (fluid retention), it is often self-limiting.
- Surgical decompression of the carpel tunnel is required for severe cases.

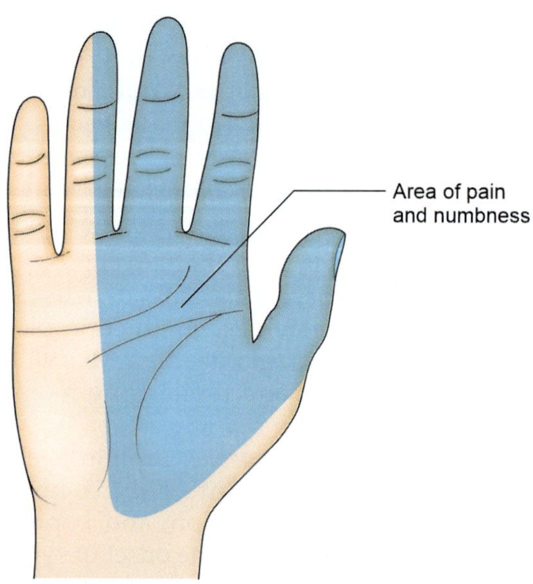

Figure 5.41: Distribution of pain in carpal tunnel syndrome

Q. Meralgia paresthetica.

- Meralgia paresthetica is a mononeuropathy caused by compression of the lateral femoral cutaneous nerve (LFCN) as it passes under the inguinal ligament, leading to purely sensory symptoms in the outer thigh.

Etiology

- Entrapment and compression of the lateral femoral cutaneous nerve can occur due to following reasons.

- Obesity
- Tight garments around the waist
- Scar tissue near the lateral aspect of the inguinal ligament
- Pregnancy
- Diabetes
- Seat belt injuries
- Surgical causes (e.g. pelvic/hip surgery)

Clinical Features

- Tingling, numbness and burning pain over the anterolateral thigh is the classic presentation.
- The discomfort is often worsened by activities which increase intra-abdominal pressure such as coughing and Valsalva maneuvers. Symptoms also worsen with walking, standing, hip extension and improve with sitting or hip flexion.
- There may be sensory loss in the area of lateral femoral cutaneous nerve.

Treatment

- Meralgia paresthetica is a self-limited, benign condition. Reassure the patient that it is not a serious problem. Advice the patient to lose weight if obese and to avoid tight garments and belt.
- In patients with persistent pain in spite of all these measures, drugs like carbamazepine or phenytoin, or gabapentin can be helpful in reducing neuropathic pain.
- Local corticosteroid plus anesthetic injections can be used occasionally to control symptoms. This is both diagnostic + therapeutic.
- Rarely, surgery is necessary. Decompression of the nerve (sectioning the inferior slip of the attachment of the inguinal ligament to the anterior superior iliac spine) or neurectomy may provide long lasting relief in some.

Q. Mention the diseases affecting neuromuscular junction.

Diseases affecting neuromuscular junction are:

Autoimmune
- Myasthenia gravis
- Eaton-Lambert syndrome

Toxic
- Botulism
- Snake venom neurotoxins
- Organophosphate poisoning

Congenital
- Congenital myasthenic syndrome
- Familial limb girdle myasthenia

Q. Describe the etiology, pathophysiology, clinical features, investigations and management of myasthenia gravis.

Q. Cholinergic crisis.

Q. Myasthenic crisis.

- Myasthenia gravis is an immunologically mediated disorder affecting neuromuscular transmission. It is characterized by fluctuating muscle weakness worsened by repetitive use, and improved by resting.
- It is the most common disorder affecting the neuromuscular junction (NMJ) of the skeletal muscles.

Etiology and Pathology

- The basic abnormality in myasthenia gravis is at the neuro-muscular junction. Muscle weakness is due to an antibody-mediated, T-cell dependent immunological attack directed at postsynaptic acetylcholine receptors. Antibodies bind to acetylcholine receptors and prevent acetylcholine action leading to weakness **(Fig. 5.42)**.
- There is a strong association between HLA B8 antigen and myasthenia gravis.
- Thymus plays an unknown role in the pathogenesis. There is an increased incidence of myasthenia gravis in patients with thymoma.

Clinical Features

- The disease occurs at all ages. Usually it starts between 10 and 70 years of age. Onset may be sudden or gradual.
- It is two times more common in women.
- The characteristic feature of weakness in myasthenia gravis is its fluctuation. Muscle strength decreases with activity and improves with rest. Patients complain of easy fatigability. This can be demonstrated by asking the patient to look up without closing the eyes for a minute, count loudly from 1 to 100, and hold the arms in a horizontal position for a minute. Muscle wasting does not occur. Tendon reflexes are preserved. Smooth muscles are not involved.
- The extraocular muscles get involved first in most cases because of which patient complains of diplopia. Weakness of levator palpebrae superioris leads to ptosis.
- Involvement of facial muscles results in difficulty in eye closure, inability to whistle and a distorted smile. There is difficulty in chewing tough foods. Weakness of the pterygoids results in difficulty in closing the mouth, and the jaw may hang. Weakness of bulbar muscles results in difficulty in swallowing (dysphagia) and speaking (dysarthria). Voice becomes low and fades away as the patient continues to speak.
- In the limbs proximal muscles are commonly involved than distal ones. This results in difficulty in raising the arms above the shoulders, difficulty in getting up from squatting position or climbing stairs.
- Involvement of intercostal muscles and diaphragm leads to respiratory difficulty.
- Sensory symptoms are absent.

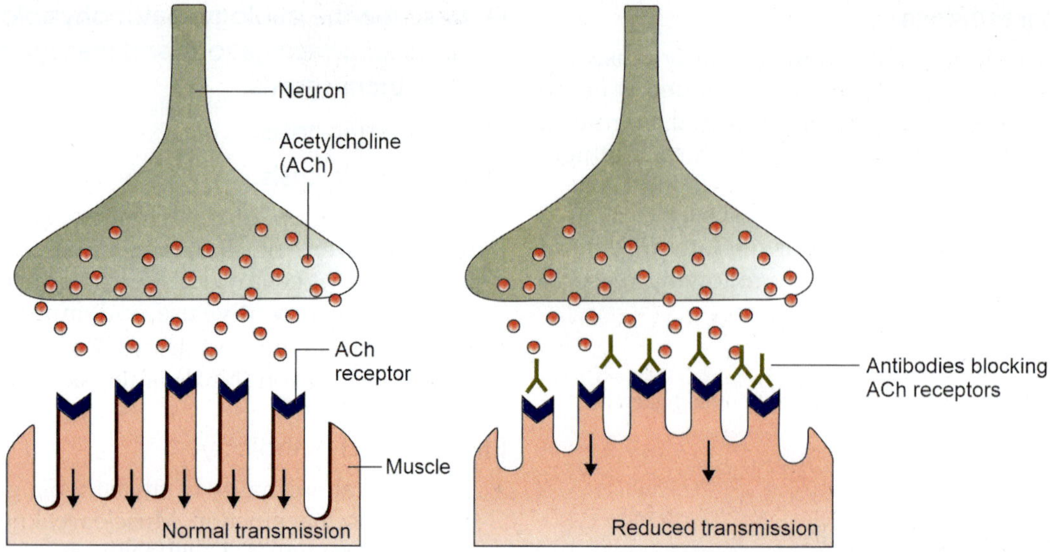

Figure 5.42: Normal NMJ (left) and abnormal NMJ in myasthenia gravis (right)

- There may be other autoimmune diseases such as, rheumatoid arthritis, pernicious anemia, systemic lupus erythematosus, etc.

Diagnosis

- Fluctuating weakness is characteristic of myasthenia gravis. Weakness increases on exertion and improves on resting. The combination of ptosis, ophthalmoplegia with weakness of orbicularis oculi and normal pupils is virtually diagnostic.

Anticholinesterase Tests

- Drugs which inhibit acetylcholinesterase can increase the levels of acetylcholine at the neuromuscular junction and improve muscle weakness. Such drugs include edrophonium and neostigmine.
- ***Neostigmine test*:** 1 mg of neostigmine is given intramuscularly or subcutaneously. Muscle weakness improves in 15–20 minutes and reaches its peak in 30 minutes. 1 ampoule atropine (0.6 mg) can be given before injecting neostigmine to prevent muscarinic side-effects and cardiac complications of neostigmine.
- ***Edrophonium (Tensilon) test:*** Edrophonium is a short-acting anticholinesterase drug. 10 mg is drawn into a syringe. Initially 2 mg is injected IV and if there are no side-effects the balance 8 mg is given after 30 seconds. Muscle weakness improves within a minute and the effect lasts for 5–10 minutes. Atropine can be given before injecting edrophonium to prevent side effects.

Electromyography

- Supramaximal stimulation of a motor nerve at 2–3 Hz results in decrement of the amplitude of the evoked muscle action potential from the first to the fifth response. The test is positive in nearly all patients. The abnormality, i.e. decremental response, is reversed by neostigmine.

Serologic Tests

- The demonstration of antibodies against ACh receptors is a sensitive diagnostic test. Patients with pure ocular myasthenia may not have ACh receptor antibodies.

Other Tests

- A chest X-ray should be taken to rule out any associated thymoma. Thymic tumor would be seen as an anterior mediastinal mass. CT-scan is more sensitive for detecting thymic enlargements.
- Thyroid function tests should be done as 10% of cases have associated hyperthyroidism.

Treatment

Augmentation of Neuromuscular Transmission

- Anticholinesterases are the most commonly used drugs. These are pyridostigmine and neostigmine. Pyridostigmine has fewer muscarinic side effects and is therefore more widely used. In patients who do not respond adequately to anticholinesterases, other forms of therapy should be added.

Immune Suppression

- Prednisolone induces remission or significantly improves the disease (dose 1 mg/kg body weight). After the improvement reaches a plateau, the dose must be lowered gradually over several months to establish the minimum maintenance dose.
- Azathioprine in doses of 2–3 mg/kg/day also induces remissions or provides improvement. Azathioprine along with prednisolone reduces the dose of prednisone and is associated with fewer treatment failures, longer remissions, and fewer side effects than either drug alone. Cyclosporine or mycophenolate mofetil can be used in patients who are refractory to prednisolone and azathioprine.

Other Treatments

- Plasmapheresis is indicated in severe generalized or fulminating myasthenia gravis that is refractory to other forms of treatment. Intravenous immunoglobulin therapy is also useful in severe myasthenia gravis.
- Thymectomy increases the remission rate and improves the clinical course of myasthenia gravis.

Cholinergic and Myasthenic Crisis

- *Cholinergic crisis* is due to overtreatment with anticholinesterase drugs (pyridostigmine and neostigmine). There is increased availability of ACh leading to persistent depolarization of neuromuscular junction and hence weakness. Typically, weakness worsens despite giving increasing amounts of anticholinesterase drugs. Cholinergic crises are associated with muscarinic effects, such as abdominal cramps, nausea, vomiting, diarrhea, miosis, lacrimation, increase in bronchial secretions, diaphoresis, and bradycardia.
- *Myasthenic crisis* is due to severe worsening of myasthenia gravis. There are no muscarinic symptoms. Injection of 2 mg edrophonium (tensilon) given intravenously improves weakness in myesthenic crisis whereas weakness worsens if it is cholinergic crisis. However, in practice, the two types of crises may be difficult to distinguish. Both types of crisis have difficulty with respiration, feeding, or handling of secretions and are best treated by drug withdrawal, endotracheal intubation or tracheostomy, ventilator support and IV fluids.

Q. Eaton-Lambert myasthenic syndrome.

- Eaton-Lambert myasthenic syndrome is a rare autoimmune disorder of the presynaptic neuromuscular junction, characterized by impaired ACh release, leading to proximal muscle weakness.

Pathology

- It is an autoimmune disease where antibodies destroy calcium channels at the motor nerve terminal. This leads to decreased presynaptic release of acetylcholine at the neuromuscular junction causing muscle weakness.
- It is usually associated with small cell carcinoma of the lung.

Clinical Features

- It is more common in males and commonly occurs after the age of 50 years.
- Patient complains of weakness and fatigability more often in the legs with relative sparing of extraocular and bulbar muscles. Weakness may improve after a few seconds of activity (opposite of myasthenia gravis which worsens after activity).
- Autonomic symptoms (dry mouth, constipation, erectile dysfunction, blurred vision) may occur.
- Deep tendon reflexes are depressed or absent.
- EMG shows incremental response to repetitive stimulation.

Treatment

- Consists of removal of tumor if detected, immunosuppression, and enhancement of neuromuscular transmission by guanidine and 3, 4 diaminopyridine (amifampridine).

Q. What is myopathy? Classify myopathies.

- The term *myopathy* refers to muscle diseases in which there is a primary structural or functional impairment of muscle.
- Myopathies therefore do not include diseases of the central nervous system (CNS), lower motor neurons (motor neuron disease), peripheral nerves, or neuromuscular junction which have secondary effects on muscles.

Classification of Myopathies

Hereditary

- Muscular dystrophies
- Congenital myopathies
- Channelopathies (periodic paralysis)
- Metabolic myopathies
- Mitochondrial myopathies

Acquired

- Autoimmune or inflammatory myopathies (dermatomyositis, polymyositis)
- Infectious myopathies (HIV, influenza, coxsackie, trichinosis)
- Endocrine myopathies (thyroid, Cushing's)
- Myopathies due to systemic illness
- Drug induced/toxic myopathies (statins, steroids, alcohol)
- Vitamin D deficiency

Q. What are muscular dystrophies? Enumerate muscular dystrophies. Describe the etiology, clinical features and management of Duchenne's muscular dystrophy.

- Muscular dystrophies are inherited myopathies characterized by progressive muscle weakness and degeneration with subsequent replacement by fibrous and fatty tissue.

Types of Muscular Dystrophies

X-linked muscular dystrophy

- Duchenne
- Becker
- Emery-Dreifuss

Autosomal dominant

- Facioscapulohumeral
- Oculopharyngeal
- Myotonic

Autosomal dominant/recessive

- Limb-girdle

Sporadic

- Congenital

Duchenne Muscular Dystrophy

- Duchenne-type muscular dystrophy is an X-linked recessive disorder resulting from mutations of dystrophin gene located at Xp21.
- The incidence of Duchenne-type muscular dystrophy is 1 in 3500 male births.

Pathogenesis

- Dystrophin is a subsarcolemmal cytoskeletal protein which provides support to the muscle membrane during contraction.
- Dystrophin deficiency weakens the sarcolemma, permitting the influx of calcium-rich extracellular fluid, which then activates intracellular proteases and complement, leading to fiber necrosis.

Clinical Features

- Duchenne dystrophy presents as early as age 2 to 3 years.
- Proximal muscles are affected more severely (limb-girdle pattern).
- The affected child has difficulty running, jumping, and walking up steps. When arising from the floor, affected boys may use hand support to push themselves to an upright position (Gower's sign).
- Calf muscles may appear hypertrophied due to replacement of muscle fibers by fat (pseudohypertrophy).
- The disease is progressive and the child is usually wheelchair bound by the age of 12.
- Paraspinal muscle weakness leads to progressive kyphoscoliosis.
- Respiratory function gradually declines. Most patients die of respiratory complications in their 20s.
- Cardiac muscle is also affected leading to dilated cardiomyopathy and conduction defects.
- The smooth muscle of the gastrointestinal tract is also involved, and intestinal pseudo-obstruction occurs.
- Children also frequently have varying degrees of mental retardation.

Investigations

- Dystrophin gene defect can be detected by DNA analysis. Muscle biopsy can show dystrophin deficiency, muscle fiber degeneration and replacement with connective tissue and fat.
- Serum creatine kinase (CK) levels may be elevated but decrease when there is severe loss of muscle mass.
- Electromyogram (EMG) shows fibrillation potentials and myopathic motor units.

Treatment

- Corticosteroids are the mainstay of treatment for Duchenne-type muscular dystrophy. Prednisolone 0.75 mg/kg/day can improve muscle strength and delay the progression into a wheelchair bound state. Prednisone also delays respiratory compromise, but it cannot prevent deterioration and death.
- Gene therapy for muscular dystrophies is currently under evaluation.
- Stem cell therapy is also under investigation.
- Genetic Counseling: For family planning, carrier detection, prenatal diagnosis.

Becker Muscular Dystrophy

- The pathogenesis, investigations and treatment of Becker muscular dystrophy is same as that of Duchenne muscular dystrophy. Becker muscular dystrophy is a mild form compared to Duchenne and typically becomes symptomatic much later. Ambulation is usually preserved until at least age 15, and many children remain ambulatory into adulthood. Most affected children survive into their 30s and 40s.

Q. Causes of wasting of small muscles of hand.

- Wasting (atrophy) of the small (intrinsic) muscles of the hand typically suggests lower motor neuron (LMN) or muscle pathology. The small muscles include the thenar, hypothenar, interossei, and lumbricals.

Causes

- ***Spinal cord lesions:*** Motor neuron disease, syringomyelia, intramedullary tumors, C8, T1 leisons (cervical spondylosis, trauma).
- ***Medial cord lesions of brachial plexus*:** Pancoast tumor, metastases, trauma, thoracic outlet syndrome.
- ***Median nerve lesions:*** Trauma, carpal tunnel syndrome, vasculitis.
- ***Ulnar nerve lesions:*** Trauma, entrapment, leprosy, vasculitis.
- ***Muscle disease:*** Focal amyotrophy.

Q. Wernicke's encephalopathy.

- Wernicke's encephalopathy is an acute neuropsychiatric syndrome caused by thiamine (vitamin B_1) deficiency.
- It is a medical emergency and is potentially reversible if treated promptly.

Etiology

- Wernicke's encephalopathy usually occurs in chronic alcoholics. Excessive alcohol intake interferes with thiamine absorption from the GI tract and hepatic storage of thiamine.
- Wernicke's encephalopathy may also result from other conditions that cause prolonged undernutrition or vitamin deficiency (e.g. recurrent dialysis, hyperemesis, starvation, gastric plication, cancer, AIDS).
- Loading carbohydrates in patients with thiamin deficiency (i.e. refeeding after starvation or giving IV dextrose-containing solutions to high-risk patients) can trigger Wernicke's encephalopathy because remaining thiamine gets used up for carbohydrate metabolism and acute deficiency is precipitated.

Pathophysiology

- Thiamine is a cofactor for enzymes involved in glucose metabolism. Deficiency impairs cerebral energy metabolism → neuronal injury and death.
- Pathologically there is loss of neuronal processes, gliosis, and petechial hemorrhages in the mammillary bodies, medial thalamus and hypothalamus, midbrain periaqueductal gray matter, floor of the fourth ventricle and cerebellum.

Clinical Features

- Clinical features start suddenly.
- It is manifested by a clinical **triad of encephalopathy, oculomotor dysfunction, and ataxia**.
- Encephalopathy manifests as disorientation, indifference, inattention, drowsiness, or stupor. If patients are not treated, stupor may progress to coma and death.
- Oculomotor dysfunction causes horizontal and vertical nystagmus and partial ophthalmoplegias (e.g. lateral rectus palsy, conjugate gaze palsies).
- Ataxia results from vestibular disturbance and cerebellar dysfunction. Gait is wide-based and slow, with short steps.
- May progress to Korsakoff's syndrome (chronic, irreversible amnesia with confabulation).

Diagnosis

- Diagnosis is clinical and should be suspected in chronic alcoholics and malnourished patients.
- There is decreased level of erythrocyte transketolase. Thiamin levels may be low, but diagnosis is clinical.
- MRI brain may show hyperintensities in mammillary bodies, thalamus, periaqueductal gray mater. MRI is also useful to rule out alternative pathologies.
- Other tests such as CSF studies and blood investigations are helpful to rule out other causes of similar presentation.

Treatment

- If Wernicke's encephalopathy is suspected, it should be treated immediately with IV thiamine 500 mg TID for 2–3 days → then 250 mg daily for 5 days. Give thiamine BEFORE glucose, as glucose can worsen symptoms in deficiency.
- Supportive treatment includes hydration, correction of electrolyte imbalances, and general nutritional therapy, including multivitamins.

Q. Korsakoff psychosis.

- Korsakoff psychosis is a **chronic neuropsychiatric syndrome** characterized by memory deficits, confusion, and behavioral changes.
- It usually follows untreated or inadequately treated Wernicke's encephalopathy. Almost 80% of untreated patients with Wernicke's encephalopathy develop Korsakoff's psychosis.
- Causes are same as that of Wernicke's encephalopathy (Korsakoff's is its chronic sequel).

Pathophysiology

- Neuronal loss, gliosis, and hemorrhage in areas involved in memory and learning: Mammillary bodies, medial thalamus, hippocampus, fornix, prefrontal cortex.
- These changes result from prolonged thiamine deficiency and oxidative stress.

Clinical Features

- Immediate memory is severely affected; retrograde and anterograde amnesia occurs in varying degrees. Remote memory is less affected.
- Disorientation to time and place is common.
- Emotional changes are common; they include apathy, blandness, or mild euphoria with little or no response to events, even frightening ones. Spontaneity and initiative may be decreased.
- Confabulation is often a striking feature. Patients unintentionally fabricate information to fill in memory gaps.
- Features of both Wernicke's encephalopathy and Korsakoff's psychosis can coexist and is called Wernicke-Korsakoff's syndrome.

Diagnosis

- Diagnosis is based on typical symptoms in patients with a history of alcohol abuse. Other causes of symptoms (e.g. CNS injury or infection) must be ruled out by appropriate investigations such as brain imaging and CSF studies.
- MRI brain may show atrophy of mammillary bodies, thalamus.
- Neuropsychological tests: Marked memory and learning deficits.

Treatment

- Treatment consists of thiamine and adequate nutrition (same as that of Wernicke's encephalopathy).

Q. Define dementia. Enumerate the causes of dementia.

Q. Discuss the etiology, clinical features, investigations and management of dementia.

OR

Q. Discuss the etiology, clinical features, investigations and management of Alzheimer's disease.

- Dementia is defined as an acquired deterioration in cognitive abilities that impairs the performance of activities of daily living. Memory is the most common cognitive ability affected.

Causes of Dementia

Degenerative diseases

- Alzheimer's disease (most common cause)
- Dementia with Lewy bodies
- Frontotemporal dementia
- Huntington's disease
- Parkinson's disease

Structural brain problems

- Multi-infarct dementia
- Cerebral vasculitis
- Subdural hematoma
- Normal pressure hydrocephalus

- Binswanger's disease (subcortical ischemic leukoencephalopathy)
- Brain tumors

Metabolic
- Uremia
- Liver failure

Toxic
- Alcohol
- Lead, mercury poisoning

Vitamin deficiency
- B_{12} deficiency, thiamine deficiency, niacin deficiency (pellagra)

Traumatic
- Punch drunk syndrome (boxers)

Infections
- Creutzfeldt-Jacob disease
- HIV infection
- Neurosyphilis

Endocrine
- Hypothyroidism
- Hyperparathyroidsm

- Degenerative diseases such as Alzheimer's disease cause progressive irreversible dementia.
- Some causes of dementias are reversible (**reversible dementias**). These are vitamin B_{12} deficiency, thiamine deficiency, niacin deficiency (pellagra), hypothyroidism, chronic brain infections (syphilis, HIV), normal-pressure hydrocephalus, subdural hematoma, etc.

Alzheimer's Disease

- Alzheimer's disease is a progressive neurologic disorder which results in global cognitive impairment, personality changes, and functional impairments. It was first recognized by German psychiatrist Alois Alzheimer.
- Alzheimer's disease is the most common cause of dementia in the elderly. It accounts for 60–80% of dementias in the elderly. The disease is twice as common among women as among men, partly because women have a longer life expectancy.

Etiology and Pathogenesis

- Most cases are sporadic, with late onset (≥65 years) and unclear etiology. However, about 5–15% of cases are familial (related to specific genetic mutations) and can have an early (presenile) onset (<65 years). At least 5 distinct genetic loci, located on chromosomes 1, 12, 14, 19, and 21, influence initiation and progression of Alzheimer disease.
- Healthy neurons have an internal support structure partly made up of structures called microtubules. These microtubules transport nutrients and molecules from the neuronal body to the ends of the axon and back. A special kind of protein, tau, binds to the microtubules and stabilizes them.
- Neurofibrillary tangles: In Alzheimer's disease, tau is changed chemically. It begins to pair with other threads of tau, to form neurofibrillary tangles. When this happens, the microtubules disintegrate, collapsing the neuron's transport system resulting in impaired communication between neurons and later death of the cells.
- Amyloid plaques: Mutations in genes for the amyloid precursor protein causes impaired processing of amyloid precursor protein, leading to deposition of β-amyloid. β-Amyloid may lead to neuronal death and formation of neurofibrillary tangles and senile plaques, which consist of degenerated axonal or dendritic processes, astrocytes, and glial cells around an amyloid core.
- The cholinergic system is involved in memory function, and cholinergic deficiency has been implicated in the cognitive decline and behavioral changes of Alzheimer disease.
- Brain atrophy is common especially in hippocampus, temporal and parietal lobes.

Clinical Features

- Patient presents with progressive memory loss and decline of other higher mental functions.
- Decline in language function manifests as difficulty in naming and understanding what others are speaking.
- Patient may also have apraxia (inability to carry out skilled motor activities), inability to recognize objects, places or people.
- There may be behavioral changes such as agitation, aggression, wandering and persecutory delusions, loss of insight and depression. Loss of inhibition may lead to inappropriate social behavior.
- In advanced stages, patients cannot walk, feed themselves, or do any other activities of daily living; they may become incontinent. Recent and remote memory is completely lost. Patients may be unable to swallow. They are at risk of undernutrition, pneumonia (especially due to aspiration), and pressure ulcers. At this stage, they are completely dependent on others and placement in a long-term care facility may be required. Additional clinical features may be present depending on the underlying cause.
- Mini-mental status examination (MMSE) helps to confirm the presence of cognitive impairment and to follow the progression of dementia. Neuropsychologic testing should be done when history and bedside mental status testing are not conclusive.
- In advanced stages, the person is mute, lies on bed and succumbs to intercurrent infections.

Investigations

- **Blood tests:** Full blood count, ESR, urea and electrolytes, blood glucose, liver function tests, serum calcium, vitamin B_{12}, folate, thyroid function tests, HIV serology.
- **Imaging:** CT/MRI brain.
- **Others:** EEG, CSF examination.

Management of Dementia

- Management is mainly supportive. Physical, mental and moral support should be provided to the patient by family members and care givers. The burden of illness falls frequently on family members.
- Treatment with antioxidants (mainly vitamin E) may help slow the decline of cognitive functions.
- The cholinesterase inhibitors donepezil, rivastigmine, and galantamine are somewhat effective in improving cognitive function. These drugs inhibit acetylcholinesterase, increasing the acetylcholine level in the brain.
- Memantine, an NMDA (N -methyl-d-aspartate) antagonist, may help slow the loss of cognitive function in patients with moderate to severe dementia and may be synergistic when used with a cholinesterase inhibitor. Ginkgo biloba, a plant extract has also been shown to be useful.
- Other drugs (e.g. antipsychotics) have been used to control behavior disorders. Patients with dementia and signs of depression should be treated with nonanticholinergic antidepressants, preferably SSRIs.
- Treatment of underlying cause.

Q. Creutzfeldt-Jakob disease (CJD).

- Creutzfeldt–Jakob disease (CJD) is a rare, fatal, rapidly progressive neurodegenerative disorder caused by abnormally folded prion proteins.
- A prion (short for proteinaceous infectious particle) is a misfolded protein that can cause infectious and fatal neurodegenerative diseases by inducing normal proteins in the brain to also misfold. It is an abnormal form of a normal cellular protein (PrP^c).
- Creutzfeldt–Jakob disease (CJD) is the most common prion disease in human beings. Other diseases caused by prions are kuru, fatal familial insomnia, scrapie (sheep), and bovine spongiform encephalopathy ("mad cow disease").

Etiology

- Most cases of CJD are sporadic, and are due to spontaneous misfolding of prion protein into abnormal misfolded prion protein. Older age is a risk factor for sporadic cases. Abnormally folded prion proteins then induce a chain reaction of misfolding in normal prion proteins leading to neurodegeneration.
- Other cases may be familial or are acquired by eating meat from cattle with bovine spongiform encephalopathy (mad cow disease) or inoculation (e.g. after cadaveric corneal or dural transplants, use of stereotactic intracerebral electrodes, or use of growth hormone prepared from human pituitary glands). It usually affects middle-aged to elderly people.

Pathology

- Pathologically, there is spongiform change, neuronal loss, and accumulation of the abnormal prion protein in the brain.

Clinical Features

- CJD is diagnosed when there is **rapidly progressive dementia** associated with any two of the following features:
  - Myoclonus
  - Akinetic mutism
  - Pyramidal/extrapyramidal signs
  - Visual disturbance/cerebellar signs
- Death occurs after a mean of 6–12 months.

Diagnosis

- CJD should be suspected in elderly patients with rapidly progressive dementia, especially if accompanied by myoclonus or ataxia.
- MRI can show hyperintensities in basal ganglia and cortical ribboning, which strongly suggest CJD.
- RT-QuIC test (real-time quaking-induced conversion): This is a highly specific for prion disease. A sample (e.g. CSF) suspected to contain abnormal prion proteins is incubated with normal recombinant prion proteins. The misfolded prion (if present) acts as a seed, converting normal proteins into abnormal ones. This conversion is amplified by shaking ("quaking") cycles. The increase in abnormal prion protein can be measured by an appropriate fluorescent dye.
- CSF analysis shows presence of proteins 14-3-3, brain-specific enolase, and tau.
- EEG shows characteristic periodic sharp waves in advanced disease.

Treatment

- There is no known treatment.
- Supportive care:
  - Physical therapy
  - Symptom control (e.g. spasticity, seizures)
  - Genetic counseling for family.

Q. Define hydrocephalus. Discuss the etiology, pathogenesis, investigations and management of hydrocephalus.

- Hydrocephalus is accumulation of excessive amounts of CSF, causing cerebral ventricular enlargement and increased intracranial pressure.
- The increased pressure distinguishes hydrocephalus from atrophy, where there is dilatation of ventricular system due to loss of brain tissue without increased CSF pressure.
- It can be either congenital or acquired from events during or after birth.

Etiology

Hydrocephalus can result from:

- Obstruction of CSF flow (obstructive hydrocephalus).
- Impaired resorption of CSF in the subarachnoid space (communicating hydrocephalus).

Causes of Hydrocephalus

Obstruction
- Chiari-2 type malformation
- Aqueductal stenosis
- Dandy-Walker malformation
- Tumors
- Colloid cyst
- Cerebellar abscess
- Cerebellar or brainstem hematoma

Impaired resorption
- Bacterial meningitis (especially tuberculosis)
- Sarcoidosis
- Subarachnoid hemorrhage
- Normal pressure hydrocephalus (NPH)

Clinical Features

- The signs and symptoms of hydrocephalus are due to raised intracranial pressure (ICP) and dilatation of the ventricles.
- Small children may have increased head circumference.
- Affected patients may have changes in their personality and behavior such as irritability, indifference, and loss of interest.
- Headache, nausea, vomiting, bradycardia, and hypertension may be present due to raised ICP. Compression of the third or sixth cranial nerve may result in extraocular muscle paresis leading to diplopia.
- Fundoscopic examination may reveal papilledema.

Investigations

CT or MRI Scan Head

- Shows dilated ventricles and any associated CNS malformations or tumors.

Lumbar Puncture

- Useful to rule out an infection causing adhesive arachnoiditis or ependymitis. However, it is contraindicated if there is a space-occupying lesion such as an intracranial tumor or a brain abscess, because of the risk of cerebral herniation.

Treatment

Medical Therapy

- Includes the use of diuretics (furosemide and acetazolamide) and serial lumbar punctures. These are less effective than surgical therapy.

Surgical Therapy

- Diversion of the CSF by means of a shunt procedure between the ventricular system and the peritoneal cavity or right atrium may result in prompt relief of symptoms in obstructive or communicating hydrocephalus.

Q. Normal pressure hydrocephalus (NPH).

- Normal pressure hydrocephalus (NPH) is a form of communicating hydrocephalus characterized by ventricular enlargement with normal or slightly elevated cerebrospinal fluid (CSF) pressure, typically seen in older adults.
- It is thought to result from a defect in CSF resorption in arachnoid granulations.

Pathophysiology

- Impaired reabsorption of CSF at the arachnoid granulations leads to gradual CSF accumulation in ventricles.
- Ventricular enlargement occurs without significant increase in pressure.
- Results in compression of periventricular white matter, particularly affecting motor pathways and bladder control.

Clinical Features

- NPH is associated with a classic triad of gait disturbance, dementia, and urinary incontinence. Gait disturbance is the earliest and most prominent feature; characterized by magnetic, wide-based, shuffling gait (resembling Parkinson gait).
- It is most common in adults over the age of 60 years and affects both sexes equally.
- It improves after removing some CSF by lumbar puncture.

Investigations

- MRI/CT brain: Enlarged ventricles (ventriculomegaly), with minimal cortical atrophy.
- CSF tap test: Removal of 30–50 ml CSF via lumbar puncture may improve symptoms temporarily (predicts shunt responsiveness).
- ICP monitoring: Normal or slightly elevated pressure.
- Neuropsychological tests: To assess cognitive function.

Treatment

- Treatment involves repeated lumbar puncture to remove CSF or ventriculoperitoneal shunt operation.

Q. Acute confusional state (delirium).

- Delirium is an acute, transient, usually reversible, fluctuating **disturbance in consciousness and cognition**.
- Delirium is sometimes called acute confusional state or toxic or metabolic encephalopathy.
- Causes of delirium include almost any disorder or drug.

Causes

See **Table 5.43.**

Pathophysiology

- Exact mechanism of delirium is not fully understood but may involve impairment of cerebral oxidative metabolism, neurotransmitter abnormalities, and generation of cytokines. Stress of any kind increases sympathetic activity and decreases parasympathetic activity, impairing cholinergic function and thus contributing to delirium. The elderly are particularly

TABLE 5.43: Causes of delirium

1. Neurological disorders	**5. Systemic organ failure**
• Stroke	• Cardiac failure
• Seizures	• Liver failure: acute, chronic
• Head injury	• Respiratory failure (hypercarbia and hypoxemia)
• CNS infections (meningitis, encephalitis)	• Renal failure: acute, chronic
• Subdural hematoma	**6. Toxins**
• Subarachnoid hemorrhage	• Alcohol intoxication/withdrawal
• Cerebral venous thrombosis	• Carbon monoxide
2. Infections	• Methanol
• Pneumonia	• Insecticides
• Urinary tract infection	**7. Drugs**
• Septicemia	• Narcotics
3. Endocrine disorders	• Cocaine
• Hypo-/hyperthyroidism	• Anticholinergics
• Adrenal disease	**8. Physical disorders**
• Hyper-/hypoglycemia	• Burns
4. Electrolyte imbalance	• Electrocution
• Hyper-/hypocalcemia	• Hyperthermia
• Hyponatremia	• Hypothermia

vulnerable to reduced cholinergic transmission, increasing their risk of delirium. Regardless of the cause, the cerebral hemispheres or arousal mechanisms of the thalamus and brain stem reticular activating system become impaired.

Clinical Features

- Delirium may occur at any age but is more common among the elderly. Most cases of delirium occur during hospitalization. When delirium occurs in younger people, it is usually due to drug use or a life-threatening systemic disorder.
- Delirium is characterized primarily by clouding of consciousness, and difficulty maintaining or shifting attention (inattention). Consciousness level fluctuates; patients are disoriented to time and sometimes to place or person. There may be illusions, hallucinations and delusions. Speech is often disordered, with prominent slurring, rapidity, neologisms, and aphasic errors.
- Symptoms fluctuate over minutes to hours; they may lessen during the day and worsen at night.
- Patients may become irritable, agitated, hyperactive, and hyperalert, or they may become quiet, withdrawn, and lethargic. Elderly people with delirium tend to become quiet and withdrawn which may be mistaken for depression. Some patients alternate between the two. Other symptoms and signs depend on the cause.

Investigations

- Full blood count, ESR
- Urea, creatinine
- Electrolytes
- Glucose
- Calcium, magnesium
- Liver function tests
- Brain imaging (CT and/or MRI)
- Lumbar puncture and CSF analysis
- EEG
- Arterial blood gases
- ECG
- Infection screen (blood cultures, chest X-ray, urine culture).

Management

- Identify and correct the underlying cause.
- Confused patients should be nursed in a well-lit room.
- Maintain adequate hydration and nutrition, treat pain, discomfort, prevent bed sores and minimize the risk of aspiration pneumonitis.
- Low-dose haloperidol (0.5–1.0 mg orally, intravenously or intramuscularly) can be used to control agitation or psychotic symptoms.
- Newer antipsychotic agents, quetiapine, risperidone, and olanzapine have similar efficacy to haloperidol with fewer extrapyramidal side effects.
- Benzodiazepines (e.g. lorazepam 0.5–1.0 mg) can be used in delirium due to withdrawal of sedative drug and alcohol. Benzodiazepines are likely to worsen confusion if used in delirium due to other causes.

Q. Enumerate the causes of intracranial space-occupying lesions. Discuss the clinical features, investigations and their management.

- Intracranial space-occupying lesions refer to any abnormal mass within the cranial cavity that occupies space, potentially causing raised intracranial pressure and focal neurological deficits. These lesions may be neoplastic, infectious, vascular, or other structural abnormalities.

Causes of Intracranial Space-occupying Lesions (SOL)

- ***Neoplastic:*** Meningioma, astrocytoma, glioma, ependymoma, medulloblastoma, metastatic brain tumors.
- ***Infectious:*** Brain abscess, tuberculoma (commonest SOL in developing countries), neurocysticercosis, toxoplasma, echinococcosis (hydatid cysts).
- ***Vascular:*** Subdural hematoma, extradural hematoma, intracerebral hematoma, large aneurysms, hemangiomas.
- ***Inflammatory:*** Sarcoid mass.
- ***Others:*** Embryonic dysplastic lesions (e.g. craniopharyngiomas, hamartomas), arachnoid cyst, colloid cyst (in the ventricles).

Clinical Features

- Signs and symptoms depend on the site of the lesion, its nature and its rate of expansion.
- Frontal lobe lesion causes personality change, urinary incontinence, impaired smell, contralateral hemiparesis and frontal release signs. Non-dominant parietal lobe lesion causes contralateral cortical sensory loss, and hemiparesis. Dominant parietal lobe lesion causes similar signs plus motor aphasia. Temporal lesion causes sensory aphasia (only dominant side), impaired verbal memory, contralateral homonymous upper quadrantanopia, and complex hallucinations (smell, sound, etc.). Occipital lobe lesion causes visual inattention, visual loss, and homonymous hemianopia (with macular sparing).
- Cerebellopontine angle lesions can cause deafness, tinnitus, vertigo and facial palsy.
- Seizures occur in supratentorial lesions.
- Raised intracranial pressure due to lesion causes headache, impairment of conscious level, papilledema, vomiting, bradycardia, and hypertension. Rapidly growing mass lesions are more likely to produce these effects.
- The rise in intracranial pressure may not be uniform and cause displacement of parts of the brain between its various compartments. Temporal lobes herniation through the tentorium due to a large hemisphere mass may cause 'temporal coning' which stretches the 3rd and/or 6th cranial nerves leading to ipsilateral pupillary dilatation and lateral rectus palsy. Pressure on the contralateral cerebral peduncle may cause hemiparesis. Herniation of cerebellar tonsils through the foramen magnum may compress the brainstem and lead to decerebrate posturing and death.

Investigations

- ***CT scan:*** It shows the site, size, nature and effects of the mass lesion. The nature of the lesion can be made out by CT scan most of the time.
- ***Magnetic resonance imaging (MRI):*** More sensitive in picking up early gliomas and posterior fossa lesions than CT-scan.
- ***CT or MR angiography:*** Can pick up aneurysms and AV malformations.
- ***PET scan:*** Can differentiate malignant from benign lesions.
- ***Brain biopsy:*** Stereotactic brain biopsy is the gold standard to determine the nature of lesions. However, biopsy may not be possible with lesions in certain locations.

Management

General Measures

- Control of raised ICP (mannitol, diuretics).
- Seizure prophylaxis (phenytoin, carbamazepine).

Specific Measures

- Surgical removal of nonmalignant lesions.
- Surgical removal, chemotherapy and radiotherapy for malignant lesions.
- Appropriate antimicrobial therapy for infective lesions.

Q. Classify brain tumors. What are the clinical features, investigations and management of brain tumors?

Classification of Brain Tumors

Primary Brain Tumors

- These tumors arise in the brain itself. These are further classified as,
- Gliomas: Astrocytoma, glioblastoma, ependymoma, oligodendroglioma.
- Meningeal tumors: Meningioma
- Pituitary tumors: Pituitary adenoma, craniopharyngioma.
- Embryonal tumors: Medulloblastoma.
- Meningiomas.

Secondary (metastatic) Brain Tumors

- These tumors arise somewhere else and involve brain as a metastatic site. These are the most common type of brain tumors.

Clinical Presentation

- Symptoms due to increased intracranial tension (ICT): Headache (diffuse or localized), nausea and vomiting. Vomiting may be projectile. Headache is usually worse in the early morning due to rise in ICT. If a patient wakes early morning due to headache repeatedly, think of brain tumor. Sometimes loss of consciousness can occur due to sudden raise in ICT which may cut off the brain blood supply.
- Seizures: Either focal or focal with secondary generalized.
- Cognitive dysfunction (memory problems and mood or personality change).
- Focal neurological deficits such as motor weakness (UMN type), sensory loss (cortical sensory deficits), aphasia, visual spatial dysfunction, etc. depending on the location of tumor.

Investigations

- CT scan
- MRI scan
- Perfusion MR Imaging
- PET scan
- Biopsy of the tumor.

Treatment

- Surgical resection is an option for peripherally situated tumors such as meningioma and acoustic neuroma.
- If there is obstructive hydrocephalus causing significant symptoms surgical shunting procedures help.
- Radiation therapy or combined radiation plus chemotherapy is helpful in malignant gliomas.
- Corticosteroids and mannitol help reduce cerebral edema and are usually started before surgery.
- Anticonvulsants (phenytoin, sodium valproate, carbamazepine, levetiracetam) are prescribed to prevent any seizure attacks.
- Palliative care should be given to those with incurable disease.

Q. Cerebellopontine angle tumors.

OR

Q. Acoustic neuroma.

- Cerebellopontine angle (CP angle) is a shallow triangle lying between the cerebellum, the lateral pons and the petrous bone.

Tumors found in CP angle

- Vestibular schwannoma (acoustic neuroma) (most common CP angle tumor)
- Meningioma
- Cholesteatoma
- Hemangioblastoma
- Metastatic tumors
- Pontine glioma
- Medulloblastomas
- Astrocytoma
- 5th, 7th, and 9th nerve neuromas
- lipomas
- Nasopharyngeal carcinoma invasion
- Lymphoma
- Arachnoid cysts
- Aneurysms

Acoustic Neuromas (vestibular schwannomas)

- These tumors arise from the Schwann cells of 8th cranial nerve. They account for approximately 80–90% of CP angle tumors.
- The median age at diagnosis is 50.
- Risk factors for development of acoustic neuroma are loud noise, neurofibromatosis type 1 and 2, and radiofrequency energy due to cell phone (controversial).

Clinical Features of CP Angle Tumors

- Involvement of 5th, 7th, 8th, with or without ipsilateral cerebellar signs is the classical presentation of CP angle tumor.
- ***Symptoms due to 5th nerve involvement:*** Facial numbness or paresthesia, jaw weakness (masseter muscle), and decreased corneal reflex.
- ***Symptoms due to 7th nerve involvement:*** Facial weakness or paralysis, loss of taste (anterior 2/3rd of tongue), decreased lacrimation or salivation.
- ***Symptoms due to 8th nerve involvement:*** Sensorineural hearing loss (most common presenting symptom), tinnitus, vertigo or unsteadiness.
- ***Symptoms due to cerebellar involvement:*** Ataxia (limb or gait), dysmetria or intention tremor, dysdiadochokinesia.
- ***Symptoms due to brain stem compression:*** Very large tumor can press on the brainstem, obstruct CSF flow and lead to raised ICT and hydrocephalus. Lower cranial nerves (9, 10, 11, 12) can get involved and lead to dysarthria, dysphagia, aspiration, hoarseness and dysarthria.
- ***Symptoms due to raised ICT:*** Headache, papilledema, nausea and vomiting, blurred vision.

Investigations

- Contrast CT or MRI scan.
- Audiometry: Shows sensorineural hearing loss.

Treatment

- Surgical resection.
- Stereotactic radiosurgery (gamma knife)—utilizes multiple convergent beams to deliver a high single dose of radiation to a lesion minimizing injury to adjacent structures.
- Proton beam therapy—provides maximal local tumor control with minimal cranial nerve injuries.

Chapter 6

Diseases of Blood

Q. What are the common presenting symptoms/signs of a hematological disorder?

- Blood is a specialized body fluid that performs vital functions in the human body, including transport, regulation, and defense. It circulates through the cardiovascular system, delivering oxygen and nutrients to tissues and removing waste products.

General Signs and Symptoms

- ***Fatigue, malaise, and lassitude*** are seen in patients with moderate to severe anemia. Can also be seen in hematologic malignancies.
- ***Weight loss*** is seen in hematological malignancies. Also seen with other malignancies, HIV and tuberculosis which can also cause anemia.
- ***Fever*** is seen in aggressive lymphomas or acute leukemias.

Hematological Manifestations (often detected on routine blood tests)

- Anemia (↓ RBCs)
- Polycythemia (↑ RBCs)
- Leukocytosis/leukemia (↑ or abnormal white cells)
- Leukopenia/neutropenia (↓ white cells): Increased susceptibility to infections.
- Thrombocytopenia (↓ platelets): Skin and mucosal bleeding.
- Thrombocytosis (↑ platelets): Leads to thrombosis (DVT, stroke, MI)
- Coagulation Disorders (e.g. hemophilia, DIC): Causes hemarthrosis, muscle hematomas, excessive surgical bleeding.
- Bicytopenia (decrease in two cell lines)
- Pancytopenia (decrease in all cell).

Nervous System Complaints

- ***Headache*** is seen in severe anemia or polycythemia. Invasion or compression of the brain by leukemia or lymphoma may also cause headache. Hemorrhage into the brain or subarachnoid space in patients with thrombocytopenia or other bleeding disorders may cause sudden, severe headache.
- ***Paresthesias*** may occur because of peripheral neuropathy in pernicious anemia or secondary to hematologic malignancy or amyloidosis.
- ***Confusion*** may occur with severe anemia, hypercalcemia (e.g. myeloma), and vitamin B_{12} deficiency.
- ***Impairment of consciousness*** may be a result of increased intracranial pressure secondary to hemorrhage (due to coagulopathy) or leukemia or lymphoma in the central nervous system.

Eyes

- ***Pallor:*** Anemia.
- ***Conjunctival plethora*** is seen in polycythemia.
- ***Blindness*** may result from retinal hemorrhages secondary to severe anemia and thrombocytopenia.

ENT

- ***Vertigo, tinnitus, and "roaring"*** in the ears may occur with marked anemia and polycythemia.
- ***Epistaxis*** may occur in patients with thrombocytopenia and von Willebrand's disease.

Oral Cavity

- ***Pale and bald tongue*** in anemia, ***red beefy tongue*** in vitamin B_{12} deficiency.
- ***Macroglossia*** occurs in amyloidosis.
- ***Petechiae and bleeding gums*** may occur with bleeding disorders.
- ***Gum hypertrophy*** due to infiltration of the gingiva with leukemic cells is seen in acute monocytic leukemia (AML).

Lymph Nodes

- ***Lymphadenopathy*** is seen in lymphoma, blast crisis of CML and CLL.

Chest and Heart

- ***Exertional dyspnea and palpitations*** are seen in anemia.
- ***Congestive heart failure*** can occur in severe anemia.
- ***Chest pain*** may arise from involvement of the ribs or sternum with lymphoma or multiple myeloma.

- *Tenderness of the sternum* may be seen in chronic myelogenous or acute leukemia.

Gastrointestinal System

- *Dysphagia* may occur due to iron deficiency (Plummer–Vinson syndrome).
- *Abdominal fullness, premature satiety, belching,* or *discomfort* may occur because of massive splenomegaly.
- *Abdominal pain* may occur in abdominal crises of sickle cell disease, or acute intermittent porphyria.
- *Gastrointestinal bleeding* related to thrombocytopenia or other bleeding disorder may be occult but often is manifest as *hematemesis* or *melena.*

Genitourinary and Reproductive Systems

- *Priapism* (painful penile erection) may occur in leukemia or sickle cell disease.
- *Hematuria* may be a manifestation of hemophilia A or B. *Red urine* may also occur with intravascular hemolysis (hemoglobinuria), myoglobinuria, or porphyrinuria.
- *Menorrhagia* is seen in thrombocytopenia and other bleeding disorders.

Musculoskeletal System

- *Back pain* is seen in hemolytic transfusion reactions, involvement of bone or the nervous system in acute leukemia or lymphoma and myeloma.
- *Arthritis* or *arthralgia* may occur with gout secondary to increased uric acid production.
- *Bone pain* may occur with bone involvement by the hematologic malignancies, sickle cell anemia, and myelofibrosis. In patients with Hodgkin's lymphoma, ingestion of alcohol may induce pain at the site of any lesion, including those in bone.
- *Muscle and joint hematomas* are seen in hemophilia.

Skin and Nails

- *Pallor* is seen in anemia.
- *Platynychia* (flat nails) and *koilonychia* (spoon shaped nails) are seen in iron deficiency anemia.
- *Hyperpigmented knuckles* are seen in vitamin B_{12} deficiency.
- *Jaundice* may be present in pernicious anemia or hemolytic anemia. Jaundice may also occur in patients with hematologic malignancies as a result of liver involvement or biliary tract obstruction.
- *Cyanosis* occurs with methemoglobinemia, sulfhemo globinemia and polycythemia.
- *Itching* may occur in Hodgkin's lymphoma and polycythemia vera.
- *Petechiae* and *ecchymoses* are seen in patients with thrombocytopenia, platelet function abnormalities and von Willebrand disease.
- *Infiltrative lesions* may occur in the leukemias (leukemia cutis) and lymphomas (lymphoma cutis) and are sometimes the presenting complaint.
- *Leg ulcers* are common in sickle cell anemia.

Q. Describe and discuss the meaning and utility of various components of the hemogram (complete blood count—CBC).

- A hemogram or CBC (complete blood count) is a routine, essential blood test that provides detailed information about the three main types of blood cells:
  - Red blood cells.
  - White blood cells.
  - Platelets.

Components of a Hemogram and their Significance (Table 6.1)

TABLE 6.1: Components of a hemogram and their significance

Parameter	Normal range (approx.)	Clinical relevance
Hemoglobin (Hb)	Males: 13–17 g/dl, females: 12–15 g/dl	↓ in anemia, ↑ in polycythemia
RBC count	4.5–6 million/μl	↓ in anemia, ↑ in polycythemia vera
Hematocrit (Hct/PCV)	40–50%	% of blood volume made up of RBCs
MCV	80–100 fl	↓ = microcytic, ↑ = macrocytic anemia
MCH	27–33 pg	↓ in hypochromic anemias
MCHC	32–36%	↓ in iron deficiency, ↑ in spherocytosis
Red cell distribution width (RDW)	11.5–14.5%	Indicates variation in RBC size. Higher the RDW, greater is the variation in RBC size. ↑ in mixed or early deficiency states
WBC count	4,000–11,000/μl	↑ in infection, ↓ in bone marrow suppression
Differential count	Neutrophils, lymphocytes, monocytes, eosinophils, basophils	Helps diagnose infection, allergy, leukemia
Platelet count	150,000–450,000/μl	↓ in thrombocytopenia, ↑ in inflammation or myeloproliferative disorders

Q. Describe the various abnormalities that can be seen in peripheral blood smear.

Q. Importance of blood smear examination.

- Examination of the peripheral blood smear is an inexpensive but powerful diagnostic tool. It provides important clues in the diagnosis of anemias and various disorders of leukocytes and platelets.

RBC Abnormalities (Fig. 6.1)

Size

Microcytosis

- Reduced RBC size, MCV <76 fl. Seen in iron deficiency, thalassemia and sideroblastic anemia.

Macrocytosis

- Increased RBC size, MCV >100 fl. Seen in vitamin B_{12}/folate deficiency, liver disease, alcohol intake, hypothyroidism and drugs (e.g. zidovudine).

Shape (Poikilocytosis)

Target cells

- Central area of hemoglobinization, surrounded by a ring of pallor and an outer area of hemoglobin.
- Seen in liver disease, thalassemia, postsplenectomy and hemoglobin C disease.

Spherocytes

- These are spherical shaped RBCs with no area of central pallor.
- Seen in hereditary spherocytosis, autoimmune hemolysis, and postsplenectomy.

Fragmented RBCs (schistocytes, helmet cells)

- These are seen in disseminated intravascular coagulation (DIC), hemolytic-uremic syndrome (HUS)/ thrombotic thrombocytopenic purpura (TTP).

Sickle cells

- Sickle cell anemia.

Teardrop cells

- Myelofibrosis.

Ovalocytes/Elliptocytes

- Hereditary elliptocytosis, megaloblastic anemia.

Burr cells (Echinocytes)

- Uremia.

Spur cells (Acanthocytes)

- Liver disease.

Inclusions

Nucleated red blood cells

- These are immature RBCs prematurely released into the circulation. Seen in marrow infiltration, severe hemolysis, myelofibrosis and acute hemorrhage.

Howell-Jolly bodies

- These are small round nuclear remnants which are normally removed by the spleen.
- Seen in hyposplenism and postsplenectomy.

Heinz bodies

- Heinz bodies are aggregates of denatured hemoglobin and are not normally found red cells.
- They are found in glucose-6-phosphate dehydrogenase deficiency and thalassemias.
- Heinz bodies are not visible on routine staining, but become visible on a supravital dye such as crystal violet.

Polychromasia

- This refers to the presence of young RBCs and reticulocytes which are prematurely released into the circulation.
- Seen in hemolysis, acute hemorrhage, and increased red cell turnover.

Basophilic stippling

- This refers to the presence of blue granules in the cytoplasm of RBCs, which represent ribosomal precipitates.
- They are most often seen in the thalassemias, alcohol abuse, lead and heavy metal poisoning.

WBC Abnormalities

- Leukocytosis: Infection, leukemia.
- Leukopenia: Aplastic anemia, drug toxicity.
- Cytoplasmic vacuolization of granulocytes is seen in patients with bacteremia or other severe infections. Toxic granulation is found in infections and metabolic derangements.
- Hypersegmented neutrophils are seen in vitamin B_{12} or folic acid deficiency.
- A high percentage of reactive lymphocytes may be seen in viral illnesses such as infectious mononucleosis, viral hepatitis, cytomegalovirus infection, HIV infection, etc.
- Blasts, which are immature cells with large nuclei, nucleoli, and a scant rim of dark blue cytoplasm are found in leukemias.

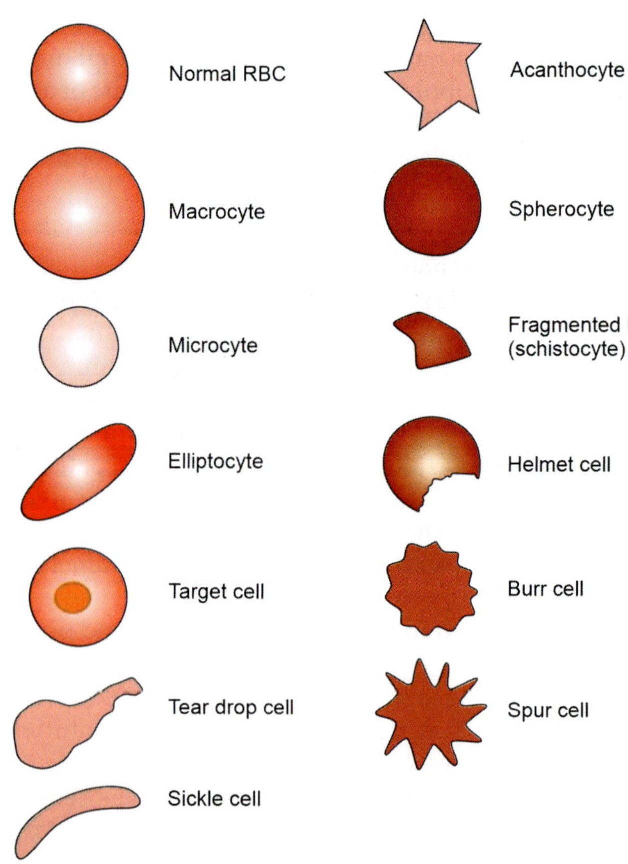

Figure 6.1: Different types of RBC morphology

- Cells with Auer rods (a rod-like conglomeration of granules in the cytoplasm) within a blast cell are pathognomonic of acute myelogenous leukemia (AML).
- Small lymphoid cells with cleaved nuclei may be seen in patients with follicular lymphoma.
- Lymphoid cells with "hairy" cytoplasm may be seen in hairy cell leukemia.
- Lymphoid cells with hyperlobulated nuclei may be seen in patients with adult T-cell leukemia/lymphoma.
- Atypical lymphoid cells with "cerebriform" nuclei (Sezary cells) may be seen in patients with cutaneous T-cell lymphoma.

Platelet Abnormalities

- Giant platelets are seen in ITP, disseminated intravascular coagulation, myeloproliferative disorders, and megaloblastic anemias. Micro thrombocytes are found in the Wiskott–Aldrich syndrome.

Q. Define anemia.

Q. Enumerate the causes and classification of anemia.

- Anemia is defined as a reduction in the number of circulating RBCs.
- Anemia can be classified based on the underlying cause or morphology of RBCs **(Table 6.2)**.

WHO Criteria for Anemia

- Men: Hb <13.0 g/dl.
- Women: Hb <12.0 g/dl.
- Pregnant women: Hb <11.0 g/dl.

TABLE 6.2: Classification of anemia

I. Based on underlying process
Decreased RBC production
• Iron, B_{12}, or folate deficiency
• Bone marrow disorders (e.g. aplastic anemia, pure RBC aplasia, myelodysplasia, tumor infiltration)
• Bone marrow suppression (e.g. drugs, chemotherapy, irradiation)
• Low levels of trophic hormones which stimulate RBC production, such as erythropoietin (e.g. chronic renal failure), thyroid hormone (e.g. hypothyroidism), and androgens (e.g. hypogonadism).
• Anemia of chronic disease/inflammation
Increased RBC destruction
• Inherited hemolytic anemias (e.g. hereditary spherocytosis, sickle cell disease, thalassemia major, PNH)
• Acquired hemolytic anemias (e.g. Coombs'-positive autoimmune hemolytic anemia, hemolytic uremic syndrome, malaria, hypersplenism)
Blood loss
• Acute blood loss (e.g. trauma, hematemesis, hemoptysis).
• Chronic blood loss (e.g. slowly bleeding ulcer or carcinoma).
• Induced bleeding (e.g. repeated diagnostic testing, hemodialysis losses, excessive blood donation).
(Contd.)
(Contd.)
II. Based on the morphology of RBC
Microcytic anemia (MCV below 80 fl)
• Iron deficiency
• Anemia of chronic disease
• Thalassemia
• Copper, vitamin C, and pyridoxine deficiency
Macrocytic anemia (MCV above 100 fl)
• Vitamin B_{12} and folate deficiency
• Drugs interfering with nucleic acid synthesis (zidovudine and hydroxyurea)
• Abnormal RBC maturation (e.g. myelodysplastic syndrome, acute leukemia, LGL leukemia, alcohol abuse, liver disease, and hypothyroidism)
Normocytic anemia (MCV normal. i.e. between 80 and 100 fl)
• Acute blood loss
III. Classification based on reticulocyte response
• Low reticulocyte count: Hypoproliferative (↓ production)
• High reticulocyte count: Hyperproliferative (↑ loss or destruction)

Q. Iron metabolism in the body (Fig. 6.2).

- Iron is vital for all living organisms because it is essential for multiple metabolic processes, including oxygen transport, DNA synthesis, and electron transport. Iron (Fe) is an important component of hemoglobin, myoglobin, and many enzymes in the body.

Normal Iron Requirements

- Daily requirement of iron ranges from 1 to 3 mg, and is more during periods of growth, menstruation, pregnancy and lactation.

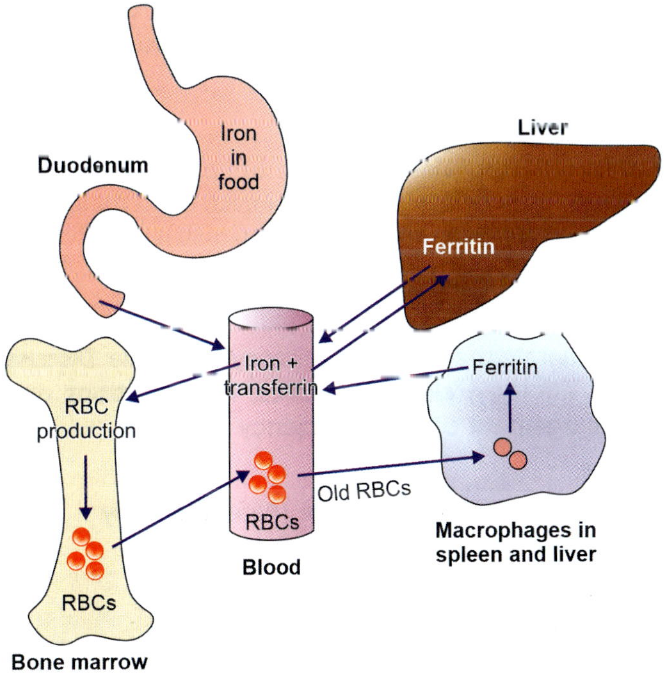

Figure 6.2: Iron metabolism

Iron Intake and Absorption

- Red meat, liver, egg yolk, blood and bone marrow are rich sources of iron. For a vegetarian, sources of iron are green leafy vegetables, dry fruits and jaggery. Milk is a poor source of iron (0.8 mg/L). Iron is present in the outer layers of cereals and hence, polished rice contains less iron than unpolished rice. Cooking utensils of iron may contribute to the iron content of food.
- Nonvegetarian diets contain heme iron which is absorbed better because it is not affected by various intraluminal factors which affect the bioavailability of iron. Iron in egg is complexed with phosphates and is poorly absorbed. In vegetarian food, iron is in the ferric form and is converted into ferrous form before absorption.
- Gastric acid and ascorbic acid (vitamin C) help in this process by maintaining iron in reduced and soluble form. Phytates, phosphates and oxalates interfere with iron absorption by forming insoluble complexes with iron.
- Iron absorption mainly occurs in duodenum. Iron absorption is increased with decreased iron stores and during pregnancy. Plasma iron is bound to transferrin.

Distribution of Iron in the Body

- An average adult male has about 4 g and an adult female about 3 g of iron in the body. 70% of this is in the form of hemoglobin. Iron is stored in the cells of the reticuloendothelial system mainly in the liver, spleen and bone marrow.
- Storage iron is mainly in the form of ferritin. Iron in ferritin is in the form of ferric hydroxyphosphate. Storage of iron as hemosiderin occurs only when there is iron overload exceeding the capacity of storage as ferritin.
- When hemoglobin formation exceeds its destruction, iron is mobilized from the stores, whereas when hemoglobin production is less than the destruction or when iron is absorbed in excess of requirement, iron is deposited in the stores.

Iron Excretion

- Iron is lost by desquamation of epithelium of gut, genito-urinary tract and the skin. An adult male loses 1 mg of iron daily this way. A menstruating female loses about 2 mg of iron daily. A small amount of iron is lost in the milk during lactation.

Q. Enumerate the causes of microcytic anemia. Discuss the etiology, clinical features, investigations and management of iron deficiency anemia.

Q. Pica.

Q. Plummer-Vinson syndrome (Paterson-Kelly syndrome).

Q. Oral iron therapy.

Q. Parenteral iron therapy.

- Microcytic anemia is defined by a mean corpuscular volume (MCV) < 80 fl. Common causes are as follows:

- Iron deficiency
- Anemia of chronic disease
- Sideroblastic anemia
- Thalassemias
- Copper, vitamin C, and pyridoxine deficiency

Iron-deficiency Anemia

- Iron deficiency is the most common cause of microcytic anemia. Other than hemoglobin, iron is also a part of many enzymes in the body which are vital for tissue respiration and organ function.
- Iron is the commonest deficiency disease all over the world. It is widely prevalent in India and is more common in pregnant women.

Causes of Iron Deficiency (Table 6.3)

TABLE 6.3: Causes of iron deficiency

Group	Examples
Blood loss (iron is lost along with blood)	GI bleeding (ulcers, malignancy), menstruation, trauma, surgery
Increased demand	Pregnancy, growth spurts, infancy
Decreased intake	Malnutrition, poor diet
Decreased absorption	Celiac disease, postgastrectomy, achlorhydria
Parasitic infections	Hookworm infestation, especially in developing countries

Clinical Features

- Clinical features include those due to anemia and those due to underlying disease causing iron deficiency.

Symptoms

- Insidious onset of fatigue and exertional dyspnea.
- Palpitations, tinnitus and headache due to hyperdynamic circulation.
- Dysphagia which is more for solids than for liquids due to formation of mucosal webs at the pharyngo-esophageal junction (Plummer-Vinson syndrome).
- Amenorrhea or menorrhagia, excess hair loss and Pica (*see* below) due to iron deficiency.
- Geophagia is common in children and pregnant women. Pagophagia (excessive eating of ice) may be seen, especially in women. All forms of pica are relieved by iron therapy even before the anemia is corrected.
- Iron deficiency also causes functional impairment of various tissues such as the myocardium, peripheral nerves, jejunum, cerebral cortex, kidneys and liver.

Signs

- Glossitis and angular stomatitis may be present. Papillary atrophy of the tongue makes it appear smooth and pale (bald tongue).
- Flattening and concavity of the nails are called platynychia and koilonychia **(Fig. 6.3)** respectively, and are seen earlier in toe nails than in finger nails.

- Mild hepatosplenomegaly may be present.
- The triad of dysphagia due to esophageal webs, koilonychia and splenomegaly in a patient with iron deficiency anemia is known as the ***Plummer-Vinson*** or ***Patterson-Kelly syndrome***. Webs and dysphagia do not respond to iron therapy. Dysphagia is treated by passage of bougie and dilatation. These webs are premalignant.

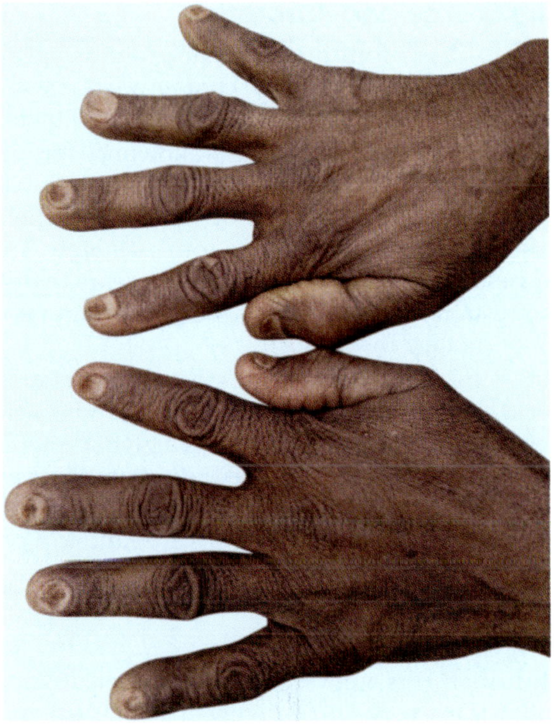

Figure 6.3: Koilonychia

Investigations

- Investigations are required to confirm the diagnosis of iron deficiency and to determine its cause.
- Complete blood picture–RBC count, hemoglobin, hematocrit, MCV, MCH and MCHC are all decreased in iron deficiency anemia.
- Peripheral blood smear–shows microcytic hypochromic RBCs **(Fig. 6.4)**. There may be other morphological abnormalities such as poikilocytosis and presence of target cells. Reticulocyte count is normal unless the patient had a recent acute blood loss, or has received hematinics.
- Iron studies **(Table 6.4)**.

TABLE 6.4: Serum iron profile in IDA

Test	Findings in IDA	Utility
Serum iron	↓	Measures circulating iron
TIBC	↑	Capacity of transferrin to bind iron
Transferrin saturation	↓	% of transferrin bound to iron
Serum ferritin	↓ (most specific)	Reflects iron stores

- Bone marrow—shows micronormoblasts. Iron stores are absent or markedly reduced.

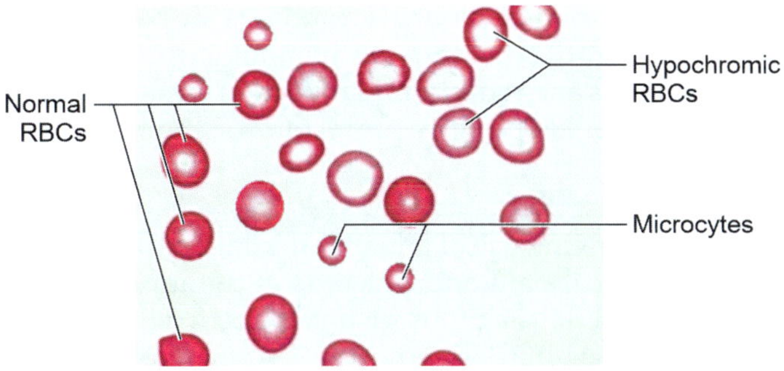

Figure 6.4: Peripheral smear in iron deficiency

- Investigations to identify the cause of iron deficiency–stool for occult blood and helminthiasis, upper GI scopy to rule out peptic ulcer or malignancy, etc. depending on the clinical presentation.

Treatment

- Treatment involves replacement of iron and correction of the cause of iron deficiency. Iron can be given orally or parenterally.

Oral Iron Therapy

- Oral iron therapy is safer and cheaper than parenteral, and is preferred.
- Iron is best given as a single dose at bedtime.
- There are many iron salts available such as ferrous fumarate, ferrous sulfate and ferrous gluconate. There is no significant difference in the absorption of these salts. Oral iron is better tolerated if given after food, but may be absorbed less efficiently.
- Iron is better absorbed in the ferrous form than in the ferric. Iron absorption is increased by simultaneous administration of ascorbic acid and decreased by antacids, certain antibiotics (e.g. quinolones, tetracycline), dietary fiber, tea, coffee, eggs, or milk.
- Hemoglobin level will normalize in about 6–8 weeks of iron therapy. However, iron therapy has to be continued for a total of 6 months to ensure repletion of the body iron stores.
- Adverse effects of oral iron include nausea, vomiting, epigastric discomfort, constipation or diarrhea. They are dose-related, and can be reduced by gradually increasing the dose and giving it after meals.

Parenteral Iron Therapy

- Indications: It is indicated in patients who cannot tolerate oral iron and in pregnant women who present with severe anemia very late in pregnancy. Patients with gastrointestinal diseases such as peptic ulcer and ulcerative colitis are likely to be aggravated by oral iron and need parenteral iron.
- Parenteral preparations: There are iron sucrose, and ferric carboxymaltose. Injection should be given after a test dose because there is a small risk of anaphylaxis. These are all given as IV infusion.
- Iron can be given as single dose IV infusion. For giving total dose iron therapy, the dose of iron can be calculated by the formula [(2.38 × W × D) + 1000],

where W is body weight in kg and D is the hemoglobin deficit in g/dl (15 - patient's hemoglobin). The value obtained is the required quantity of iron in mg. The addition of 1000 mg is provision for the body iron stores.

- Side effects: Both local and systemic side effects can occur following use of parenteral iron. Local reactions include local pain and phlebitis at the infusion test. Anaphylactic reactions also can occur with all the preparations but less with ferric gluconate complex and iron sucrose than iron dextran. Other systemic effects include fever, urticaria, joint pains, nausea, vomiting, diarrhea, abdominal pain, backache, body ache, chest pain, angioneurotic edema, and hypotension.

Treatment of Cause of Iron Deficiency

- For example, treatment of hook worm infestation, piles, peptic ulcer disease and any other bleeding lesions.

Q. Enumerate the causes of macrocytosis/Macrocytic anemia.

- Macrocytosis refers to an increased mean corpuscular volume (MCV > 100 fl), indicating enlarged red blood cells. It can be classified into megaloblastic and non-megaloblastic causes.
- Megaloblastic macrocytosis: Due to defective DNA synthesis (commonly B_{12}/folate deficiency). Characterized by megaloblastic changes in marrow and hypersegmented neutrophils.
- Nonmegaloblastic macrocytosis: Caused by non-DNA-related issues like alcohol use, hypothyroidism, or liver disease, without megaloblastic marrow changes **(Table 6.5)**.

TABLE 6.5: Causes of macrocytic anemia
Abnormal nucleic acid metabolism of erythroid precursors
• Vitamin B_{12} (cobalamin) deficiency
• Folate deficiency
• Drugs (hydroxyurea, zidovudine, methotrexate, azathioprine)
Abnormal RBC maturation
• Myelodysplastic syndrome
• Aplastic anemia
• LGL leukemia
• Multiple myeloma and other plasma cell disorders
Conditions causing reticulocytosis (reticulocytes are larger than mature RBCs)
• Erythropoietin therapy
• Acute blood loss
Others
• Alcohol abuse
• Liver disease
• Hypothyroidism

Q. Enumerate the causes of macrocytic anemia. Discuss the etiology, clinical features, diagnosis and management of vitamin B_{12} (cyanocobalamin) deficiency.

Q. Bone marrow picture in megaloblastic anemia.

- RBCs with MCV more than 100 fl (femtoliters) are called macrocytes (megaloblasts).

Causes of Macrocytic Anemia

See **Table 6.5**.

Vitamin B_{12}

Dietary Source and Absorption

- Vitamin B_{12} is found in animal proteins and dairy products. Vegan diets do not contain adequate vitamin B_{12}. Vegetarians get their B_{12} by dairy products.
- Normal recommended dietary allowance for vitamin B_{12} is 2 microgram/day. Total body stores of vitamin B_{12} is 2–5 milligrams, half of which is in the liver. These stores are enough for approximately 3 years, and hence, it takes approximately 3 years to develop manifestations of vitamin B_{12} deficiency after absorption of dietary B_{12} ceases.
- Dietary B_{12} is liberated in the stomach in the presence of acid and pepsin in the stomach and binds to gastric-derived intrinsic factor (IF). IF is a glycoprotein with very high affinity for B_{12}. The IF-B_{12} complex binds to a specific receptor in the ileum, and is absorbed by an active process. In the plasma, B_{12} is bound to a protein called transcobalamin **(Fig 6.5)**.

Physiological Role of B_{12}

- Vitamin B_{12} is very important for nucleic acid synthesis in every cell. Actively growing and dividing cells, which synthesize DNA rapidly, e.g. mucosal cells and hemopoietic cells, are likely to be particularly affected in B_{12} deficiency. It is also important for the normal integrity of nervous system.
- Thymine (a purine) is important for DNA synthesis. Synthesis of thymine requires tetrahydrofolate (THF). Vitamin B_{12} is required for conversion of methyl THF to THF. Thus lack of vitamin B_{12} causes impaired DNA synthesis and cell division. RNA synthesis continues, resulting in a large cell with a large nucleus. All cell lines have dyspoiesis, in which cytoplasmic maturity is greater than nuclear maturity; this dyspoiesis produces megaloblasts in the marrow before they appear in the peripheral blood. Dyspoiesis results in intramedullary cell death (intramedullary hemolysis), making erythropoiesis ineffective and causing indirect hyperbilirubinemia and hyperuricemia. Because dyspoiesis affects all cell lines, pancytopenia develops in advanced stages of vitamin B_{12} deficiency. Hypersegmentation of neutrophils is common, the mechanism of which is unknown **(Fig 6.6)**.

Etiology of Vitamin B_{12} Deficiency

Inadequate intake

- Strict vegetarians
- Malnutrition (elderly, alcoholics, poverty)

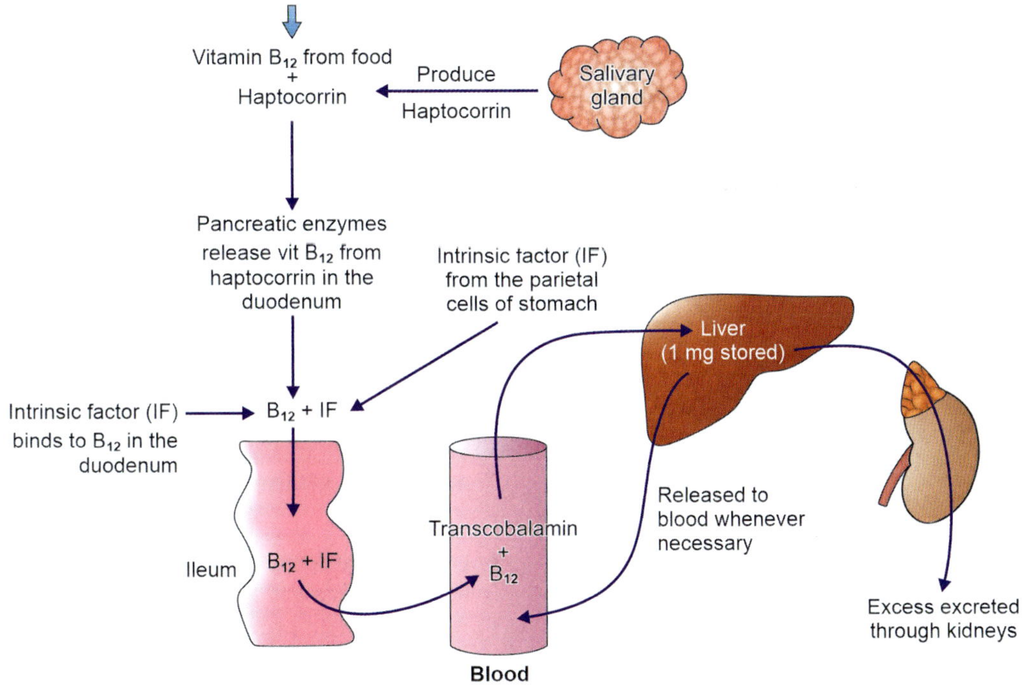

Figure 6.5: Absorption of vitamin B_{12}

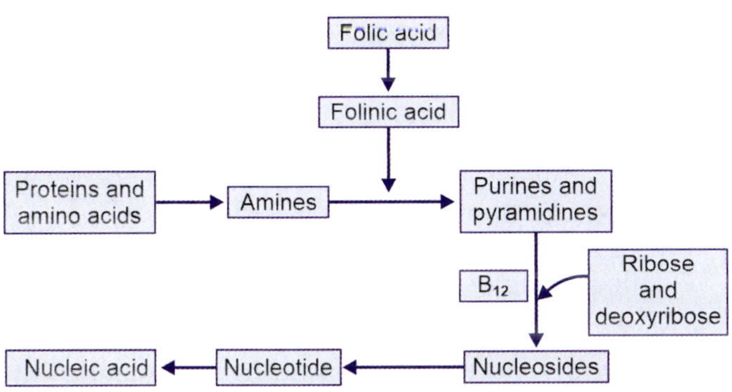

Figure 6.6: Role of vitamin B_{12} and folic acid in the synthesis of nucleic acid

Intrinsic factor deficiency
- Pernicious anemia
- Gastrectomy
- Atrophic gastritis

Decreased absorption
- Malabsorption syndromes
- Ileal resection or bypass
- Crohn's disease
- Blind loops
- Fish tape worm infestation
- Pancreatitis

Increased requirement
- Pregnancy
- Hyperthyroidism
- Chronic hemolytic anemia

Agents that block absorption
- Neomycin
- Biguanides (e.g. metformin)
- Proton pump inhibitors (e.g. omeprazole)

Clinical Features

- Symptoms related to anemia such as easy fatigability, weakness, dyspnea, and effort intolerance.
- Hyperdynamic circulation due to anemia may lead to palpitations, tinnitus and headache.
- Knuckle hyperpigmentation may be present **(Fig. 6.7)**.
- Vitamin B_{12} deficiency causes atrophic glossitis due to which tongue may appear beefy red **(Fig. 6.8)**.
- Vitamin B_{12} deficiency causes symmetrical peripheral neuropathy (with paresthesias, ataxia, loss of vibration and position sense). In severe deficiency, subacute combined degeneration (SCD) of the spinal cord may develop. In SCD, there is involvement of posterior columns and corticospinal tract. Manifestations of SCD are paresthesias, ataxia, loss of vibration and position sense due to posterior column involvement and weakness, spasticity, clonus, and paraplegia due to corticospinal tract involvement.

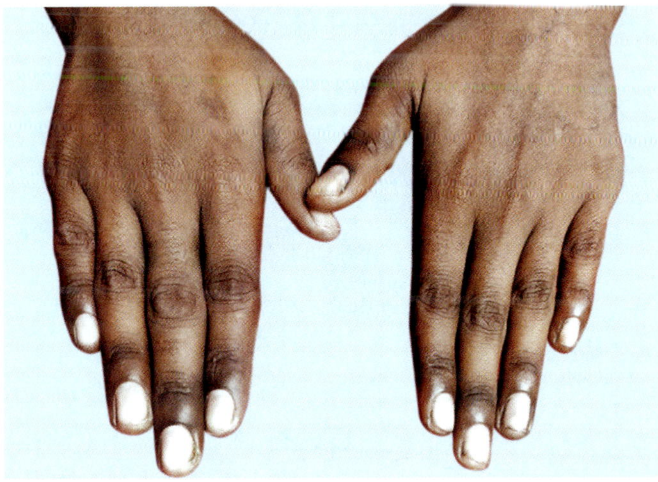

Figure 6.7: Knuckle hyperpigmentation in B_{12} deficiency

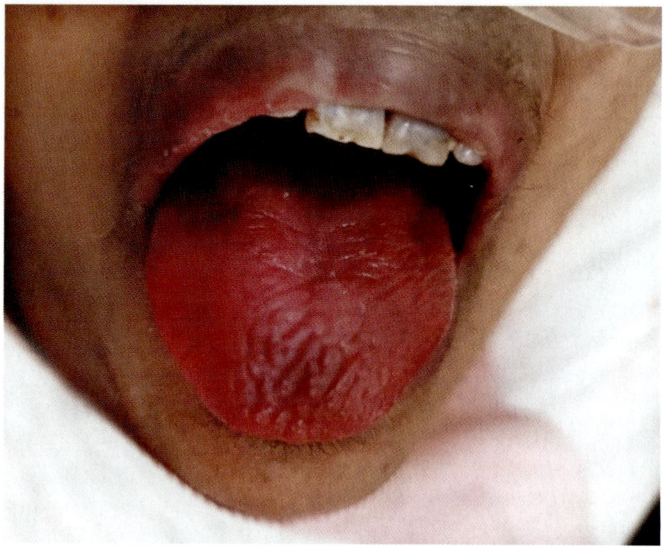

Figure 6.8: Red beefy tongue in B_{12} deficiency

- Other neurologic symptoms of vitamin B_{12} deficiency include memory loss, irritability, and dementia.

Investigations

Complete Blood count

- Hemoglobin level is low.
- Mean corpuscular volume (MCV) is over 100 fl (normal 80–100).
- Mean corpuscular hemoglobin (MCH) and mean corpuscular hemoglobin concentration (MCHC) are usually normal.
- There may be pancytopenia since B_{12} is required for the synthesis of all cell lines including WBCs and platelets.
- Reticulocyte count is low or normal (due to ineffective erythropoiesis).

Peripheral blood smear **(Fig. 6.9)**

- Shows oval macrocytes, few myelocytes and occasional normoblasts. There is anisocytosis and poikilocytosis. Reticulocyte count is low in relation to degree of anemia. Hypersegmented neutrophils are common. When the anemia is severe, there may be leukopenia and thrombocytopenia (pancytopenia) and megaloblasts may be seen in the peripheral blood smear.

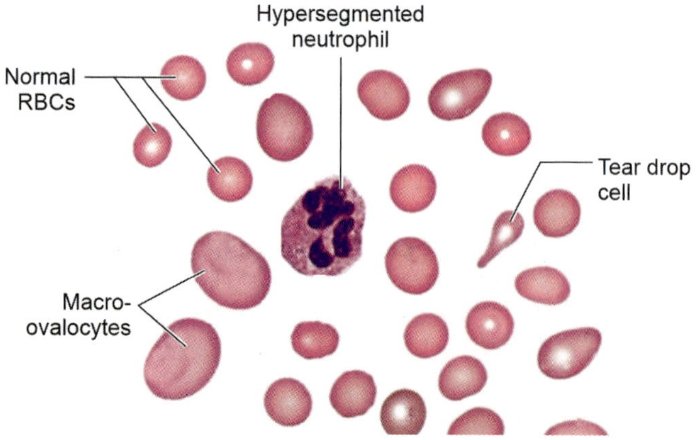

Figure 6.9: Peripheral smear in vitamin B_{12} deficiency

Bone marrow

- Bone marrow test is not routinely indicated for confirmed case of vitamin B_{12} deficiency.
- Bone marrow is hypercellular with frequent mitoses and increased myeloid: erythroid ratio. There is abundant iron store. The characteristic features are: presence of megaloblasts, giant bands and giant metamyelocytes.
- Megakaryocytes are decreased with basophilic agranular cytoplasm and hyper-segmented nucleus.

Vitamin B_{12} and folic acid levels

- The normal vitamin B_{12} level is 300–900 pg/ml; values <200 pg/ml indicate clinically significant deficiency. Serum homocysteine and methylmalonic acid levels are high in vitamin B_{12} deficiency.

Other tests

- LFT: There is mild increase in indirect bilirubin due to ineffective erythropoiesis and hemolysis.
- Anti-intrinsic factor antibodies are positive in pernicious anemia (high specificity).
- Upper GI scopy is useful in cases of pernicious anemia.
- Jejunal biopsy is useful in malabsorption disorders.
- Schilling test can be done to diagnose the cause of vitamin B_{12} deficiency (but not used now).

Treatment

General management

- This is similar to other cases of anemia. For severe symptomatic anemia (Hb <7 g/dl), packed red cell transfusion is given. Before transfusion it is necessary to collect samples for B_{12} and folic acid estimation.

Vitamin B_{12} replacement

- Vitamin B_{12} should be replaced by parenteral route since malabsorption is the cause most of the time.
- *Regimen*:
  - 1000 µg (1 mg) cyanocobalamin IM weekly for 4 weeks. If there are neurological symptoms. If there are symptoms of anemia and/or neurologic symptoms, 1000 µg can be administered daily for three doses or every other day for a week.
  - Then monthly for life (if irreversible cause like pernicious anemia).
- Oral replacement therapy with 2 mg vitamin B_{12} per day is also effective if malabsorption is not the cause of deficiency.
- Patient will experience increase in strength and well-being even before hematological response. Marrow morphology begins to revert to normal within a few hours after treatment is initiated. Reticulocytosis begins 4–5 days after therapy is started and peaks at about day 7, with subsequent remission of the anemia over the next several weeks.
- Any underlying cause of vitamin B_{12} deficiency should be treated (e.g. antibiotics for intestinal bacterial overgrowth, deworming for tape worm infestation).
- Dietary advice: Encourage intake of B_{12}-rich foods (meat, liver, fish, dairy products, eggs). Consider fortified foods or supplements in vegans or vegetarians.

Q. Pernicious anemia.

- Pernicious anemia (PA) is a megaloblastic anemia caused by autoimmune destruction of gastric parietal cells, leading to intrinsic factor deficiency and impaired vitamin B_{12} absorption.
- The disease was given its common name because it was fatal (pernicious) prior to the discovery of treatment, similar to leukemia at that time.
- It is common in whites, and rare in Asians. Females are affected more often than males. It is a disease of the elderly, the average patient presenting near age 60; it is rare under age 30. Patients are likely to be having blood group A.

Pathogenesis

- Intrinsic factor is important for the absorption of B_{12}. Intrinsic factor deficiency causes less absorption of B_{12} and its deficiency.
- Pernicious anemia may be associated with other autoimmune diseases such as thyroid disorders, Addison's disease, hypoparathyroidism, diabetes mellitus, and rheumatoid arthritis.
- Ninety percent of patients have parietal cell antibody in serum and 50% have antibody to intrinsic factor which inhibits binding of B_{12} to intrinsic factor.

Clinical Features

Clinical features are similar to B_{12} deficiency anemia.

Investigations

- In addition to tests done for vitamin B_{12} deficiency, antibodies to parietal cell and antibodies to intrinsic factor may be demonstrated in serum and gastric juice. Serum gastrin levels are elevated.
- Histamine or pentagastrin test: acid secretion does not increase even after injection of histamine or pentagastrin.
- Upper GI scopy and mucosal biopsy: shows atrophic gastritis.

Treatment

- Treatment is similar to B_{12} deficiency anemia. Lifelong therapy with B_{12} is required for pernicious anemia.

Q. Schilling test (Vitamin B_{12} absorption test)

- This is a historical test (not used now) used to determine the cause of vitamin B_{12} malabsorption. This test is now largely obsolete due to improved antibody testing (anti-IF, anti-parietal cell), widespread availability of endoscopy, and practical limitations (use of radiolabeled B_{12}). Additionally, Schilling test takes 2 to 3 weeks to complete, which itself is not feasible.
- Causes of vitamin B_{12} malabsorption are intrinsic factor deficiency, atrophic gastritis, small intestinal bacterial overgrowth, exocrine pancreatic insufficiency, and ileal disease.

Stage I

- Schilling test is performed by administering 1 µg of radiolabeled vitamin B_{12} orally, followed by an intramuscular injection of 1000 µg of vitamin B_{12} simultaneously to saturate vitamin B_{12} binding sites so that absorbed radiolabeled B_{12} is excreted in the urine.
- A 24-hour urine is then collected for determination of the percent excretion of the oral dose. Normally at least 10% of the radiolabeled vitamin B_{12} is excreted in the urine. In patients with pernicious anemia or with deficiency due to impaired absorption, less than 10% of the radiolabeled vitamin B_{12} is excreted.

Stage II

- If absorption is low in Stage I, the test is repeated with intrinsic factor added to the oral radiolabeled B_{12}.
- Improved excretion (>10%) indicates pernicious anemia (due to intrinsic factor deficiency).
- No improvement suggests malabsorption from other causes (e.g. ileal disease).

Stage III

- If urinary excretion of vitamin B_{12} is still less than 10% after adding intrinsic factor, then the test is repeated after a course of antibiotics. Improved absorption suggests small intestinal bacterial overgrowth.

Stage IV

- If the absorption is abnormal even after addition of intrinsic factor and antibiotic course, test is repeated after giving pancreatic enzymes. Improved absorption suggests pancreatic cause.
- If there is no improvement even after all the above stages, ileal disease where the B_{12} gets absorbed should be suspected.

Q. Discuss the etiology, clinical features, diagnosis and management of anemia due to folic acid deficiency.

Physiological Role

- Folate is very important for DNA synthesis and cell division in every cell. Actively growing and dividing cells, which synthesize DNA rapidly, e.g. mucosal cells and hemopoietic cells, are likely to be particularly affected by folate deficiency.
- Its deficiency causes megaloblastic anemia, similar in morphology to vitamin B_{12} deficiency but without neurological symptoms.

Sources of Folic Acid

- Folic acid (folate) occurs in animal products and green leafy vegetables in the polyglutamate form. High amounts are present in liver, kidney, spinach, cabbage, yeast, nuts and fruits. Milk and eggs are poor in folate. It is easily destroyed by cooking.
- Normal daily folate requirement for adults is 1–2 mg/day.

Metabolism

- Polyglutamates in food are cleaved to monoglutamate in the jejunum where it is absorbed. Folates enter plasma and are taken up by liver and other cells.

- Folate is mainly stored in liver. These stores are enough for approximately 3 months and hence, manifestations of deficiency appear after 3 months of deficient diet.

Causes of Folic Acid Deficiency

Inadequate intake
- Alcoholics
- Poor dietary intake
- Overcooked foods

Increased requirements
- Pregnancy
- Rapid growth (infants, adolescents)
- Malignancy (because of rapid cell multiplication)
- Increased hematopoiesis (chronic hemolytic anemias)
- Exfoliative skin disorders (rapid cell turnover)

Malabsorption
- Tropical and nontropical sprue
- Inflammatory bowel disease
- Short bowel syndrome

Drugs
- Methotrexate (folate antagonist)
- Trimethoprim
- Pyrimethamine
- Phenytoin

Clinical Features

- Macrocytic anemia.
- Folate deficiency does not cause neurologic symptoms (unlike vitamin B_{12} deficiency). Only depression, irritability, poor judgment, forgetfulness and sleep deprivation have been seen in some patients.
- Glossitis is less common than in vitamin B_{12} deficiency.
- Mild jaundice (due to ineffective erythropoiesis).
- Anorexia and occasional diarrhea may be present.

Investigations

- Low serum folate levels (normal 6–20 ng/ml; values ≤4 ng/ml are diagnostic of folate deficiency).
- Peripheral blood smear shows macrocytes.
- Bone marrow shows megaloblastic picture.
- Elevated serum homocysteine levels and normal methylmalonic acid levels.

Management

- Correct the underlying cause.
- Oral folic acid supplementation (1–5 mg/day) should be given in deficiency states.
- It should be given prophylactically (400–600 µg/day) to all pregnant women, premature babies, patients receiving dialysis, and in severe and chronic hemolytic states.
- Patients receiving folic acid antagonists such as methotrexate should be given folic acid supplements.
- In the presence of vitamin B_{12} deficiency, folate therapy can aggravate neurological symptoms. Hence, care should be taken to replace vitamin B_{12} before folate therapy.

Q. What are the causes of blood loss anemia? How do you manage it?

Causes of Blood Loss Anemia

Acute blood loss
- Trauma
- GI bleed
- Hemoptysis
- Rupture of ectopic pregnancy
- Postpartum hemorrhage
- Ruptured aneurysm

Chronic blood loss
- Slowly bleeding peptic ulcer
- Use of anticoagulants or antiplatelet agents (e.g. warfarin, aspirin)
- GI malignancy
- Menorrhagia
- Hookworm infestation

Induced bleeding
- Repeated diagnostic testing
- Hemodialysis losses
- Excessive blood donation

Clinical Features

- Anemia due to acute blood loss is symptomatic if severe. Losses of up to 20% of the blood volume can be asymptomatic. Blood loss more than this can cause anxiety, hypotension, syncope, tachycardia, breathlessness, and shock. Hemoglobin level immediately after the bleed may be normal as it takes some time for hemodilution to occur.
- Chronic blood loss as happens in hook worm infestation, peptic ulcer, etc. can produce severe anemia which can be asymptomatic. Symptoms will not appear until severe anemia develops.

Treatment

- In acute blood loss, volume replacement either by blood transfusion, or IV fluids is very important.
- In chronic blood loss anemia, if the patient is severely anemic, packed RBC should be transfused.
- Underlying cause of blood loss should be treated in both acute and chronic blood loss.

Q. Anemia of chronic disease (anemia of chronic inflammation).

- Anemia of chronic disease (ACD) also known as anemia of chronic inflammation, is a common form of anemia associated with chronic infections, inflammatory disorders, or malignancies.

Pathophysiology

- Three pathophysiologic mechanisms have been identified in ACD: (1) Shortened RBC survival due to unknown mechanisms, (2) Impaired erythropoiesis due to decreases in both erythropoietin (EPO) production and marrow responsiveness to EPO and (3) Impaired intracellular iron metabolism.
- Reticuloendothelial cells retain iron from senescent RBCs, making iron unavailable for Hb synthesis.

There is thus a failure to compensate for the anemia with increased RBC production. Macrophage-derived cytokines (e.g. IL-1, TNF, interferon) contribute to the decrease in EPO production and the impaired iron metabolism.

Clinical Features

- Most patients have mild anemia that produces no symptoms. Signs and symptoms of underlying disease may be present.

Investigations

- The anemia is normocytic-normochromic and rarely microcytic-hypochromic.
- Reticulocyte count, leukocyte count and platelet counts are normal.
- The serum iron concentration and transferrin level (also measured as total iron binding capacity, TIBC) are both low and the percent saturation of transferrin is usually normal, which should distinguish ACD from iron deficiency anemia, in which transferrin saturation is low.

Treatment

- Correction of the underlying disorder (best and most effective approach).
- Iron therapy is usually not helpful, as iron is sequestered.
- Administration of recombinant human erythropoietin if anemia is severe.

Q. Discuss the classification, clinical features, diagnosis and management of hemolytic anemias.

- Anemia resulting from increased red cells destruction is called hemolytic anemia. Hemolysis can be defined as a shortening of RBC survival to less than 100 days (normal 120 days).
- Normal marrow has tremendous capacity to compensate for hemolysis, hence anemia occurs only when compensation is not adequate.
- Hemolysis may be an extravascular or an intravascular phenomenon. Autoimmune hemolytic anemia (AIHA) and hereditary spherocytosis are examples of extravascular hemolysis because the RBCs are destroyed in the spleen and other reticuloendothelial tissues. Others are due to intravascular hemolysis.

Classification of Hemolytic Anemias

Hereditary

- Membrane defects: spherocytosis, elliptocytosis, spur cell anemia
- Enzyme defects: G6PD-deficiency, pyruvate kinase deficiency
- Hemoglobin defects: thalassemia, sickle cell anemia

Acquired

- Paroxysmal nocturnal hemoglobinuria (PNH)
- Autoimmune hemolytic anemia (AIHA)
- Mechanical: Prosthetic heart valves, march hemoglobinuria, Microangiopathic hemolytic anemia
- Drugs: dapsone, primaquine
- Infections: malaria, mycoplasma

Clinical Features

History

- Patient may complain of fatigue and other symptoms of anemia.
- Mild jaundice (lemon yellow) due to hemolysis.
- H/o passing red-brown urine (due to hemoglobinuria).
- Left hypochondrial pain due to splenomegaly.
- Right hypochondrial pain due to cholelithiasis. Pigment stones occur due to increased production of bilirubin from hemolysis.
- Family history may be present in hereditary hemolytic anemia.
- Drug history may be positive.
- Symptoms of any underlying disease responsible for hemolysis.

Physical Findings

- Anemia
- Mild jaundice
- Splenomegaly
- Hemolytic facies due to marrow hyperplasia in skull bones and other bones.
- Ankle ulcers (seen in sickle cell anemia)
- Signs of any underlying disease responsible for hemolysis.

Investigations

Evidence of Increased RBC Destruction

- Indirect hyperbilirubinemia, usually less than 5 mg/dl.
- Increased urobilinogen excretion in urine.
- Decreased plasma haptoglobin and hemopexin.
- Increased plasma lactate dehydrogenase (LDH).
- Shortened RBC survival as demonstrated by chromium-51 labeled RBCs.

Evidence of Increased RBC Production to Compensate Destruction

- Increased reticulocyte count (reticulocytosis).
- Finding premature RBCs in peripheral smear (macrocytes, polychromasia, nucleated RBCs).
- Erythroid hyperplasia of bone marrow.

Additional Findings in Intravascular Hemolysis

- Hemoglobinuria.
- Hemosiderinuria.

Tests to Diagnose Underlying Cause of Hemolysis

- Peripheral blood smear examination.
- Coombs' test (to detect antibodies causing hemolysis).
- Hemoglobin electrophoresis (for thalassemia).
- Osmotic fragility, sucrose lysis and hams test (for membrane defects).
- Measurement of enzyme activity (G6PD, pyruvate kinase).
- Other tests are done depending on the suspected underlying cause.

Treatment

Supportive Therapy

- Blood transfusion for severe anemia
- Replacement of vitamins due to increased erythropoiesis (iron, folic acid)
- Treatment of infections
- Treatment of ankle ulcers
- Splenectomy in selected cases.

Specific Therapy

- This depends on the underlying cause—steroids for immune hemolytic anemia, splenectomy in sickle cell anemia and hereditary spherocytosis, withdrawal of offending drug, etc.

Q. Classify immune hemolytic anemias.

- Hemolysis secondary to antibodies against red cell antigens is called immune hemolysis.
- It can be broadly divided into autoimmune and alloimmune hemolytic anemias. In autoimmune hemolytic anemia, antibodies are directed against person's own RBCs. In alloimmune hemolytic anemia, antibodies are directed against transfused RBCs.

Etiology and Classification of Immune Hemolytic Anemias

Autoimmune hemolytic anemia (AIHA)

Warm AIHA

- Idiopathic
- Chronic lymphocytic leukemia
- Hodgkin's lymphoma
- Systemic lupus erythematosus
- Drugs

Cold AIHA (Cold agglutinin disease)

- Idiopathic
- Mycoplasma pneumoniae
- Infectious mononucleosis
- virus infection

Mixed type AIHA

- Dual temp reactivity

Paroxysmal cold hemoglobinuria (PCH)

- Idiopathic
- Viral infections
- Syphilis

Alloimmune hemolytic anemia

- Hemolytic transfusion reactions
- Hemolytic disease of newborn

Q. Discuss the clinical features, diagnosis and management of warm antibody autoimmune hemolytic anemia (AIHA).

- In warm antibody AIHA, antibodies react with RBC antigens at body temperature, hence called warm antibody autoimmune hemolysis. Hemolysis occurs primarily in the spleen. Antibodies are of IgG type.
- The disease is common in adults above the age of 40 years; more common in females.

Etiology

- Many conditions can induce warm antibody formation, which are as follows:

- Idiopathic (commonest cause)
- Connective tissue diseases (e.g. systemic lupus erythematosus)
- Malignancies of the immune system (non-Hodgkin's lymphoma, chronic lymphocytic leukemia)
- Previous blood transfusion or hematopoietic cell transplantation
- Drugs (alpha-methyldopa, sulfonamides, NSAIDs, methotrexate)

Clinical Features

- Onset is insidious.
- Symptoms of anemia—fatigue, palpitations.
- Symptoms of hemolysis—mild jaundice, dark urine.
- Splenomegaly.

Diagnosis

- Features of hemolysis with spherocytosis.
- Positive direct antiglobulin test.

Treatment

- *Blood transfusion*: For significant anemia.
- *Corticosteroids*: Any significant hemolysis is treated with 60 mg of prednisolone daily for 3–4 weeks and then tapered; many need maintenance therapy. Parenteral methyl prednisolone is often used in acutely ill patients.
- *Splenectomy*: Patients who do not respond to steroids and/or require large maintenance dosage are candidates for splenectomy.
- *Immunosuppressive drugs*-like azathioprine or cyclophosphamide are used if significant hemolysis continues despite splenectomy. Intravenous gamma globulin, danazol, cyclosporine and rituximab are used in occasional refractory cases.
- *Folic acid supplements* should be given to all patients with hemolysis because of increased requirements due to increased erythropoiesis.
- *Treatment of underlying cause.*

Q. Cold antibody autoimmune hemolysis (cold hemagglutinin disease; paroxysmal cold hemoglobinuria).

- Here the antibodies causing hemolysis react best at temperatures below 37°C.
- Two forms are recognized: 1. cold hemagglutinin disease (cold AIHA) and 2. paroxysmal cold hemoglobinuria (PCH). They are relatively rare.

Cold Hemagglutinin Disease (cold AIHA)

- It is a disorder where red cells are agglutinated at low temperature. It is a chronic insidious disease most common in adults over 50 years.

Etiology

- ***Primary***: Idiopathic (commonly in elderly).
- ***Secondary***: Triggered by infections (e.g. *Mycoplasma pneumoniae*, Epstein-Barr virus), lymphomas.

Pathophysiology

- Caused by IgM autoantibodies that bind to red blood cells (RBCs) at low temperatures (typically 0–4°C).
- The IgM antibody fixes complement, leading to complement-mediated hemolysis—usually extravascular, occurring primarily in the liver.

Clinical Features

- Patients have symptoms related to both anemia and RBC agglutination.
- Symptoms of anemia include easy fatigability, palpitations, etc.
- Symptoms related to RBC agglutination are dark, purple to gray discoloration of the skin of acral parts (acrocyanosis) (finger tips, toes, nose, and ears) on exposure to cold. The color disappears upon warming of the part.

Diagnosis

- Positive direct Coombs' test (specifically for complement C3d).
- Cold agglutinin titers elevated.
- Peripheral smear: RBC agglutination.

Treatment

- The single most useful therapy in cold agglutinin disease is avoidance of cold. Protective clothing during cold weather, use of leather gloves and stocking, or moving to a warm climate is all that is needed.
- Cytotoxic agents, particularly cyclophosphamide and chlorambucil, are sometimes used to reduce the production of antibody in severe cases. Rituximab has been shown to be useful in severe hemolysis not responding to conventional therapy.
- Steroids are not helpful and splenectomy is also not helpful since spleen is not the site of hemolysis (liver is the site of hemolysis).
- Transfusions are rarely necessary. Blood must be warmed before transfusion.
- Plasmapheresis helps in severe cases.

Paroxysmal Cold Hemoglobinuria (PCH)

- PCH is a rare disease caused by a **biphasic IgG autoantibody** (Donath–Landsteiner antibody) that binds to RBCs in the cold and triggers complement-mediated **intravascular hemolysis** when warmed to body temperature.

Etiology

- Infections (tertiary syphilis, viral infections, mycoplasma pneumoniae and *Haemophilus influenzae*).
- Idiopathic.

Clinical Features

- It occurs mainly in children. Historically associated with syphilis in adults (now rare).
- Hemolysis is precipitated by exposure to cold and is characterized by hemoglobinuria, pallor, jaundice and splenomegaly. The adult form is usually chronic, lasting several years.

Diagnosis

- Donath–Landsteiner test (demonstrates biphasic hemolysin).
- Direct Coombs' test positive.

Treatment

- In children, PCH usually resolves spontaneously in a few weeks. Patient should be kept in a very warm environment.
- If severe hemolysis is present transfusion may be needed.
- Prednisolone (1–2 mg/kg per day) is also helpful to reduce hemolysis. In adults not responding to prednisolone, cyclophosphamide or azathioprine can be tried.
- Splenectomy is not helpful as spleen does not play any role in hemolysis.

Q. Paroxysmal nocturnal hemoglobinuria (PNH).

- This is a rare disorder secondary to an acquired defect in the red cell membrane which makes it sensitive to lysis by complement.
- It is characterized by hemolytic anemia, venous thrombosis, and bone marrow failure.

Pathophysiology

- Caused by a somatic mutation in the PIGA gene in hematopoietic stem cells. This leads to a deficiency of membrane proteins such as CD55, and CD59. These proteins protect RBCs from complement. Their absence makes RBCs vulnerable to complement-mediated lysis, especially at night (due to mild acidosis during sleep).
- Hemolysis is intravascular. Due to ongoing hemolysis, there is free hemoglobin in the circulation which binds to and depletes nitric oxide. Nitric oxide depletion leads to smooth muscle spasm which causes abdominal pain, dysphagia, pulmonary hypertension etc. It also contributes to thrombosis formation by enhancing platelet aggregation.
- PNH is also associated with bone marrow dysfunction, likely due to immunologic attack on hematopoietic stem cells, often leading to leukopenia and thrombocytopenia.

Clinical Features

- PNH affects mainly adults and both sexes.
- Three main features of PNH are hemolytic anemia, venous thrombosis, and bone marrow failure.
- Hemolysis manifests as anemia, mild jaundice and hemoglobinuria. Its nocturnal paroxysmal nature accounts for the name of this disorder. Patients usually complain of dark urine at night ("cola-colored urine") with partial clearing during the day. Hemolysis may be precipitated by infection, iron use, vaccination, or menstruation.

- Venous thrombosis is a frequent complication and can occur in intra-abdominal, cerebral and peripheral veins.
- Bone marrow failure leads to cytopenias or aplastic anemia.
- Smooth muscle spasm leads to dysphagia, abdominal pain, pulmonary HTN, erectile dysfunction (due to nitric oxide depletion by free hemoglobin).

Laboratory Features

- ***Flow cytometry (gold standard test):*** Detects absence or deficiency of CD55 and CD59 on RBCs, which is diagnostic of PNH.
- Evidence of hemolysis includes anemia and raised indirect bilirubin. Urine may be positive for hemoglobinuria.
- Associated leukopenia, thrombocytopenia, and iron deficiency may be present.
- Leukocyte alkaline phosphatase (LAP) score is decreased.
- Coombs' test: Negative (distinguishes from autoimmune hemolysis).
- Bone marrow may be hypercellular or aplastic with depleted or normal iron store.
- HAM test (acidified serum lysis test first described by Dr HAM) and sucrose lysis test are positive. These two tests are historical and obsolete now due to low sensitivity and specificity.
- ***Fluorescent aerolysin assay***: this test uses fluorescently labeled bacterial toxin aerolysin to detect PNH cells. It is more sensitive than flow cytometry.

Treatment

- Management is mainly supportive, consisting of blood transfusions, folic acid supplements and iron replacement.
- Recently, eculizumab a monoclonal antibody that binds to the C5 component of complement and inhibits complement activation has been shown to reduce hemolysis and transfusion requirements in patients with PNH.
- Androgens, steroids and antithrombotic drugs are used occasionally.
- Antiplatelets and anticoagulants may be required to prevent thrombosis.
- Allogeneic stem cell transplant: only curative option; reserved for severe bone marrow failure or transformation.

Prognosis

- The mean survival is 10 years, but with good medical care many survive for longer period.
- PNH may progress into myelodysplasia or acute leukemia.
- Common causes of death include visceral thrombosis (cerebral, hepatic, portal veins), severe anemia, infection, hemorrhage or postoperative complications. Rarely, spontaneous remissions are described.

Q. Coombs' test (antiglobulin test).

- ***Coombs' test*** is used to check whether the blood contains certain antibodies which cause hemolysis.
- There are two types of Coombs' tests: ***direct Coombs' test*** (also known as direct antiglobulin test), and the ***indirect Coombs' test*** (also known as indirect antiglobulin test) **(Table 6.6)**.

Direct Coombs' Test (Fig. 6.10)

- This is used to detect antibodies (IgG) or complement (C3) that are already attached to the surface of patient's RBCs.
- Direct Coombs' test is used to test for autoimmune hemolytic anemia, hemolytic disease of the newborn (HDN), hemolytic transfusion reactions, and drug-induced hemolysis.

TABLE 6.6: Comparison of direct and indirect Coombs' test

Test	Detects	Clinical uses	Sample used
Direct Coombs'	Antibodies/ complement on RBCs	AIHA, HDN, transfusion reaction	Patient's RBCs
Indirect Coombs'	Antibodies in serum	Antibody screen, crossmatch, Rh incompatibility	Patient's serum

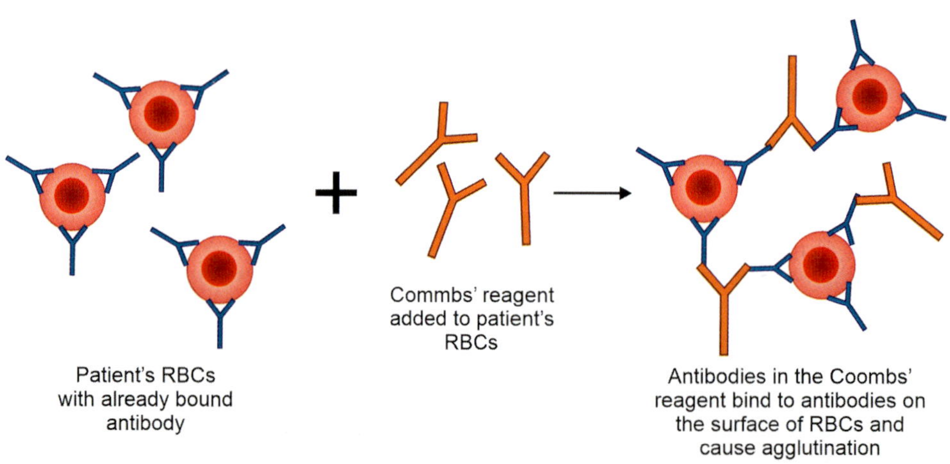

Figure 6.10: Direct Coombs' test

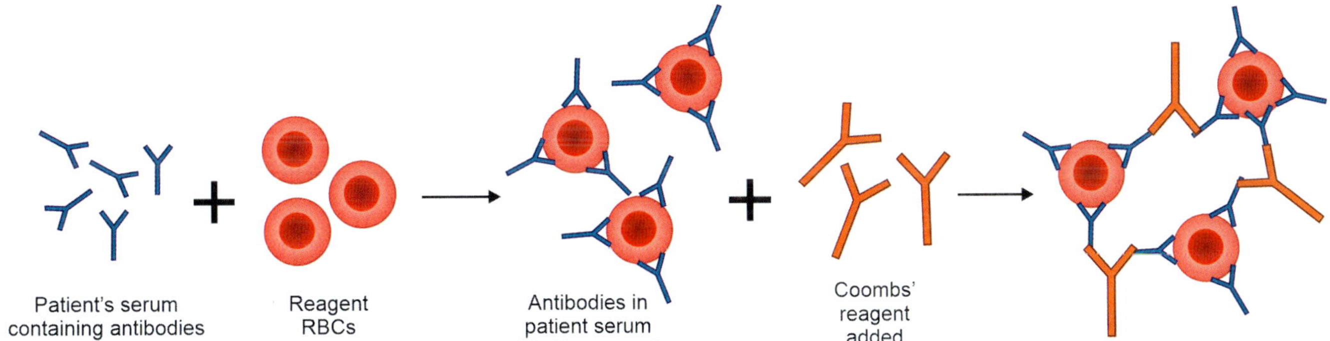

Figure 6.11: Indirect Coombs' test

- Patient's RBCs are washed and mixed with Coombs' reagent (antihuman globulin). If antibodies or complement are bound to RBCs → agglutination occurs (positive test). Negative test rules out significant antibody/complement coating of RBCs.

Indirect Coombs' Test (Fig. 6.11)

- This is used to detect free-floating antibodies (usually IgG) in the patient's serum that could bind to RBCs.
- Used in pretransfusion compatibility testing (cross-matching), antibody screening in pregnancy (Rh incompatibility), and detection of alloantibodies (e.g. anti-D, anti-K).
- Patient's serum is incubated with reagent RBCs → then Coombs' reagent is added. If antibodies are present → they will bind to RBCs → agglutination (positive test).

Q. Define aplastic anemia. Discuss the etiology, classification, clinical features, investigations and management of aplastic anemia.

- Aplastic anemia is defined as pancytopenia with an empty (hypoplastic or aplastic) bone marrow.
- The term "aplastic anemia" is a misnomer because there is not only anemia but also thrombocytopenia and leukopenia (pancytopenia).

Etiology and Classification of Aplastic Anemia

Acquired

- Idiopathic (no identifiable cause, most common cause)
- Cytotoxic drugs
- Radiation
- Idiosyncratic drug reaction (chloramphenicol, gold, NSAIDs, sulfonamides)
- Toxic chemicals (benzene, lindane, glue vapors)
- Viral infections (parvovirus B_{19}, HIV infection, Epstein-Barr virus)
- Autoimmune disorders (eosinophilic fasciitis, SLE, graft versus host disease)
- Paroxysmal nocturnal hemoglobinuria (PNH)
- Thymoma
- Pregnancy (rare, reversible postpartum in some cases)

Inherited

- Fanconi's anemia
- Dyskeratosis congenita
- Shwachman-Diamond syndrome

Pathogenesis

- In idiopathic cases, there is no identifiable cause but in all such cases there is a stem cell defect, (diminished numbers, impaired maturation, proliferation and differentiation). In all other cases, there is damage to bone marrow which may be dose-related or idiosyncratic reaction to radiation, drugs, chemicals or infectious agents.

Clinical Features

- The onset is insidious and symptoms and signs are due to anemia, leukopenia and thrombocytopenia (pancytopenia).
- Anemia causes easy fatigability, exertional dyspnea and pallor.
- Leukopenia causes recurrent infections (pneumonia, urinary tract infections, fungal infections, septicemia).
- Thrombocytopenia causes bleeding manifestations (mucosal hemorrhages, menorrhagia, and petechiae).
- Splenomegaly and lymphadenopathy are not a feature of aplastic anemia. If these are present, suspect some other disease.

Investigations

- Hemoglobin is low.
- There is pancytopenia.
- Reticulocyte count is low in relation to the degree of anemia.
- ESR is elevated.
- Peripheral blood smear shows pancytopenia and normochromic-normocytic RBCs. No abnormal cells are seen in peripheral blood.
- Bone marrow examination shows profoundly hypocellular marrow with a decrease in all cell elements. The marrow space is composed mostly of fat cells and marrow stroma. The residual hematopoietic cells

are morphologically normal. Malignant infiltrates or fibrosis are absent. The bone marrow iron store is normal or increased.

- Additional tests (to determine cause);
  - Viral serologies: Hepatitis, HIV, EBV, CMV
  - Flow cytometry: To screen for PNH clone
  - DNA studies for inherited aplastic anemia.

Treatment

Supportive Therapy

- Involves treatment of infection, correction of anemia with blood transfusion, correction of thrombocytopenia by platelet transfusion.
- Antifibrinolytic agents (tranexamic acid or epsilon-amino caproic acid) are also useful to control bleeding in severe cases.
- Blood and platelet transfusions should be used sparingly in patients who are candidates for hematopoietic stem cell transplantation to avoid sensitization.

Definitive Therapy

- Hematopoietic stem cell transplantation (HSCT): Bone marrow transplantation—This is the treatment of choice in patients below 40 years if an HLA-matched donor is available. It is curative in aplastic anemia, but is limited by the availability of an HLA-matched donor as well as graft versus host disease.
- Immunosuppressive regimens are recommended for those above 40 years. They are not curative, but improve survival. A combination of antithymocyte globulin, cyclosporine, and corticosteroids with or without granulocyte-colony stimulating factor (G-CSF) can be used for immunosuppression.
- Treatment of the underlying cause or agent.

Prognosis

- Prognosis depends upon two factors, disease severity and patient age. Severe aplastic anemia is associated with reduced survival rate and there is a strong inverse relation between patient age and 5-year survival.

Q. Fanconi anemia.

- Fanconi anemia is the most common form of inherited aplastic anemia.
- Random breaks of chromosomes are seen due to defect in DNA repair.
- It is an autosomal recessive disorder characterized by several congenital anomalies, progressive bone marrow failure, and an increased incidence of malignancies.
- It usually presents within the first decade of life. There are skeletal (hypoplastic or absent thumb, radii) cardiac, neurologic (microcephaly, microphthalmia and mental retardation) and renal malformations with hyperpigmentation (patchy) of skin.
- Treatment involves hematopoietic stem cell transplantation, androgens and corticosteroid therapy.

Q. Describe the national programs for anemia prevention.

Anemia Mukt Bharat (AMB)–"Intensified National Iron Plus Initiative (I-NIPI)"

- Launched: 2018 under the POSHAN abhiyaan (nutrition mission).
  Goal: Reduce anemia across all age groups by 3% per year until 2022 and beyond.
- This program uses 6 × 6 × 6 strategy (6 target groups, 6 interventions, and 6 institutional mechanisms for implementation and monitoring).

6 Target Groups (Table 6.7)

TABLE 6.7: Iron supplementation to 6 target groups

Group	Supplementation
6–59 months children	1 ml Iron and folic acid (IFA) syrup biweekly
5–9 years children	45 mg elemental iron + 400 μg folic acid weekly
10–19 years adolescents (in and out of school)	60 mg iron + 500 μg folic acid weekly
Women of reproductive age	60 mg iron + 500 μg folic acid weekly
Pregnant women	Daily IFA (60 mg iron + 500 μg folic acid) starting early
Lactating women	Daily IFA for 6 months postpartum

6 Interventions

- IFA supplementation
- Deworming
- Behavior change communication (BCC)
- Testing and treatment of anemia
- Use of digital hemoglobinometers
- Addressing non-nutritional causes (malaria, hemoglobinopathies, etc.).

6 Institutional Mechanisms for Implementation and Monitoring

- National Anemia Mukt Bharat Unit (NAMBU)
- National Centre of Excellence and Advanced Research on Anemia Control (NCEAR-A)
- State Anemia Mukt Bharat Unit (SAMBU)
- District Anemia Mukt Bharat Unit (DAMBU)
- Anemia Mukt Bharat dashboard
- Convergence with line ministries and departments

Weekly Iron and Folic Acid Supplementation (WIFS) Program

- Launched: 2012.
- Target: School-going adolescents (10–19 years).
- *Components*:
  - Weekly supervised IFA tablet distribution in schools
  - Biannual deworming
  - Nutrition and health education sessions
  - Out-of-school adolescents covered via Anganwadi centers.

Reproductive, Maternal, Newborn, Child and Adolescent Health (RMNCH+A)

- IFA (iron folic acid) supplementation during antenatal and postnatal periods.
- Deworming, anemia screening, and management.
- Institutional delivery to prevent hemorrhage-related anemia.

Integrated Child Development Services (ICDS) Scheme

- Nutritional supplementation and IFA syrup to children (½–6 years) and pregnant/lactating women.
- Growth monitoring and health checkups.

Mid-day Meal (MDM) Scheme

- Provides nutritionally balanced meals in schools
- Supports overall iron intake
- Synergistic with WIFS and AMB

National Health Mission (NHM)/National Nutrition Mission

Integrates anemia control across programs via:
- Health and wellness centers
- POSHAN tracker and monitoring tools
- Community outreach (ASHA, ANM, Anganwadi workers).

Monitoring and Evaluation

- POSHAN dashboard
- Anemia testing using digital hemoglobinometers
- Village Health and Nutrition Days (VHNDs) for outreach.

Q. Erythropoietin.

Q. Ectopic sources of erythropoietin.

- Erythropoietin (EPO) is a glycoprotein growth factor which stimulates erythropoiesis, and RBC maturation.
- Erythropoietin is produced by the kidney and a small amount (<10%) by the liver. In the kidney interstitial fibroblasts are thought to produce erythropoietin and studies have shown that proximal tubular cells also produce erythropoietin. Hypoxia is the main stimulus for erythropoietin release which in turn stimulates RBC production.
- In patients with chronic renal failure, anemia is common due to reduced erythropoietin production. Injection of erythropoietin in chronic renal failure patients restores normal number of RBCs and corrects anemia.
- Ectopic sources of erythropoietin include cerebellar hemangioma, uterine leiomyoma, pheochromocytoma, and hepatoma.

Recombinant Erythropoietin

- This is a synthetic (recombinant) erythropoietin available in the market. Darbepoetin alfa is a synthetic erythropoietin analogue which has longer half-life and hence can be given less frequently.

Indications for Erythropoietin Therapy

- Anemia of chronic kidney disease (most common indication).
- Less common indications are anemia of chronic disease. and anemia associated with cancer chemotherapy.

Side Effects of Erythropoietin Therapy

- Hypertension
- Headache
- Influenza-like syndrome.

Q. Define neutrophilia. Enumerate the causes of neutrophilia.

- Neutrophilia is defined as an absolute increase in the number of neutrophils in the peripheral blood, typically >7,500 cells/µl (in adults).

Causes of Neutrophilia

- Infections—bacterial, fungal, sometimes viral
- Drug-induced—glucocorticoids, lithium
- Inflammation—thermal injury, tissue necrosis, myocardial and pulmonary infarction, hypersensitivity states, collagen vascular diseases
- Myeloproliferative diseases—myelocytic leukemia, myeloid metaplasia, polycythemia vera
- Stress, excitement, vigorous exercise
- Metabolic disorders—diabetic ketoacidosis, acute renal failure, eclampsia, acute poisoning
- Others—metastatic carcinoma, acute hemorrhage or hemolysis.

Q. Define neutropenia and agranulocytosis. Describe the etiology, clinical features and management of neutropenia/agranulocytosis (febrile neutropenia).

- Neutropenia is defined as an absolute neutrophil count (ANC) of less than 1500/µl.
- Agranulocytosis refers to ANC less than 200/µl.
- The risk of infection begins to increase at an ANC below 1000/µl.

Etiology

Decreased production

- Drug induced (chemotherapeutic agents, methotrexate, chloramphenicol, clozapine, carbimazole)
- Hematologic diseases—idiopathic, cyclic neutropenia, Chédiak-Higashi syndrome, aplastic anemia.
- Tumor invasion of bone marrow (myeloma, leukemias, myelofibrosis)
- Nutritional deficiency—vitamin B_{12}, folate (especially alcoholics)
- Infections—tuberculosis, typhoid fever, brucellosis, tularemia, measles, infectious mononucleosis, malaria, viral hepatitis, leishmaniasis, AIDS
- Radiation therapy

Peripheral destruction

- Hypersplenism
- Antineutrophil antibodies
- Autoimmune disorders—Felty's syndrome, SLE

Peripheral pooling (transient neutropenia)

- Overwhelming bacterial infection (acute endotoxemia)
- Hemodialysis
- Cardiopulmonary bypass

Clinical Features

- Can be asymptomatic.
- Increased risk of recurrent infections and sepsis. Common infective organisms include *Staphylococcus aureus*, gram-negative organisms and fungi.
- Common sites of infection include the oral cavity and mucous membranes, skin, perirectal and genital areas.
- Classic presentation is sore throat and fever.
- Ulcers in the throat and mouth.
- Toxemia and sepsis can lead to death.

Investigations

- Total WBC count is low.
- Neutrophil count is low.
- Peripheral smear shows absence of neutrophil and band forms.
- Bone marrow examination shows myeloid aplasia or hypoplasia or myeloid maturation arrest.
- Blood culture may grow the infective organism.
- Imaging studies such as chest X-ray, X-ray of paranasal sinuses, CT scan of the abdomen, etc. may be done based on history and examination findings to identify the focus of infection.

Treatment

- Treatment depends upon the cause and degree of the neutropenia.
- Patients with bone marrow hypoplasia and/or severe infections should receive aggressive antibacterial therapy for fever, even in the absence of signs of infection. Broad spectrum antibiotics to coverage both gram-positive and gram-negative bacteria should be used. Patients with an ANC less than 500/µl and marrow aplasia should always be treated on an inpatient basis with parenteral antibiotics.
- G-CSF (granulocyte colony stimulating factor) should be given to patients with inadequate response to antibiotics.

Q. Define pancytopenia. Enumerate the causes of pancytopenia.

- Pancytopenia refers to reduction of all three cells of blood, i.e. RBCs, WBCs and platelets. If only two types of cells are low, the term bicytopenia is used.
- It is not a diagnosis but a clinical manifestation of an underlying disorder affecting bone marrow function or peripheral destruction/sequestration.

Causes of Pancytopenia

Decreased bone marrow production

- Aplastic anemia
- Vitamin B_{12}, iron and folic acid deficiency
- Myelodysplastic syndrome
- Bone marrow infiltration by carcinoma, leukemia, lymphoma, multiple myeloma, myelofibrosis, Niemann-Pick disease
- Osteopetrosis (marble bone disease)
- Paroxysmal nocturnal hemoglobinuria
- Disseminated tuberculosis
- Overwhelming infections
- Anticancer drugs
- Radiotherapy

Peripheral destruction/sequestration

- Hypersplenism
- Systemic lupus erythematosus

Q. Define eosinophilia. Enumerate the causes of eosinophilia.

- Eosinophilia is defined as absolute eosinophil counts above 500 eosinophils/µl in peripheral blood.
- It is classified as:
  - Mild 500–1500
  - Moderate 1500–5000
  - Severe (hypereosinophilia) >5000

Causes of Eosinophilia

Allergic diseases

- Atopic and related diseases (Hay fever, asthma, eczema, serum sickness, and pemphigus)
- Drug allergy

Infectious diseases

- Parasitic infections (worm infestation, filariasis, Loeffler's syndrome, tropical pulmonary eosinophilia)
- Some fungal infections

Malignancies

- Leukemia
- Lymphomas
- Carcinoma lung, stomach, pancreas, ovary, and uterus
- Mastocytosis

Collagen vascular diseases

- Rheumatoid arthritis
- Eosinophilic fasciitis
- Churg-Strauss syndrome (Eosinophilic granulomatosis with polyangiitis)

Endocrine

- Addison's disease (due to cortisol deficiency)
- Hypopituitarism

Drugs

- Sulfonamides
- Aspirin
- Nitrofurantoin
- Penicillins

Hypereosinophilic syndromes

- Primary (myeloproliferative)
- Secondary (reactive)
- Idiopathic

Q. Sideroblastic anemias.

- Sideroblastic anemias are a group of disorders characterized by:
  - Ineffective erythropoiesis
  - Presence of ring sideroblasts in the bone marrow.
- Ring sideroblasts are erythroblasts with iron-loaded mitochondria forming a ring around the nucleus (seen on Prussian blue stain).

- Sideroblastic anemias are due to deranged synthesis of heme within red cell precursors. Deranged heme synthesis leads to impaired hemoglobin production with the formation of hypochromic, microcytic and other misshaped RBCs.
- Iron cannot be utilized which accumulates inside RBCs leading to ring sideroblasts. Iron overload is also a constant feature of most sideroblastic anemias.
- Sideroblastic anemias are characterized by the presence of sideroblasts in the bone marrow and peripheral blood.
- Sideroblastic anemias are part of a myelodysplastic syndrome but may be hereditary or may occur secondary to drugs or toxins.

Classification

Hereditary
- X-linked (most common)
- Autosomal
- Mitochondrial DNA mutations (e.g. Pearson syndrome)

Acquired
- Pure sideroblastic anemia
- Refractory anemia with ring sideroblasts (RARS)
- Alcoholism
- Drugs (isoniazid, chloramphenicol)
- Copper deficiency
- Hypothermia

Clinical Features

- Symptoms of anemia (fatigue, pallor, weakness).
- Hepatosplenomegaly may be present due to iron overload.

Diagnosis

- Microcytic hypochromic RBCs.
- Iron overload (↑ serum iron, ↑ ferritin, ↓ TIBC, ↑ transferrin saturation).
- Characteristic ring sideroblasts in the bone marrow. The iron laden mitochondria surround the nucleus and appear as the pathognomonic rings with Prussian blue staining **(Fig. 6.12)**.

Treatment

- Anemia in X-linked sideroblastic anemia and due to isoniazid responds to pyridoxine (200 mg daily for 2–3 months).
- Blood transfusions can be given for severe anemia.
- Iron overload can be treated by periodic phlebotomies and desferrioxamine.
- Recombinant human erythropoietin and GM-CSF (granulocyte-monocyte colony-stimulating factor) are helpful in selected cases.
- Luspatercept is a newer agent approved for MDS with ring sideroblasts. It enhances erythroid maturation.
- Bone marrow transplantation can be done in severe transfusion-dependent patients.

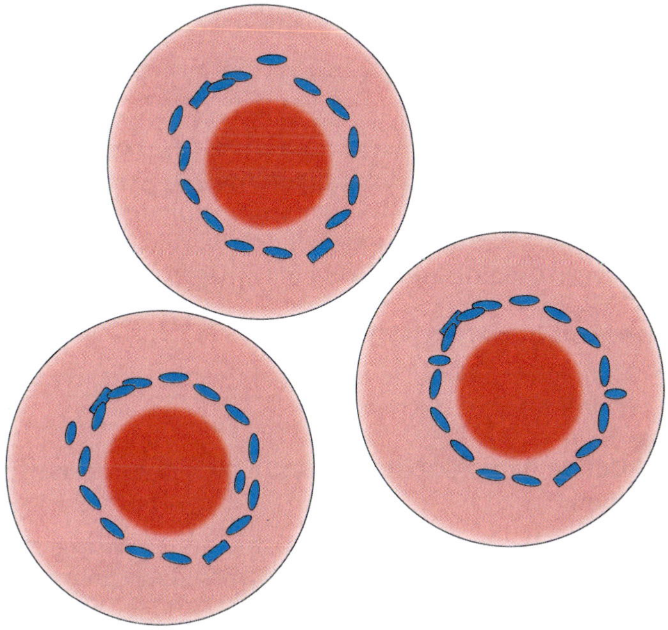

Figure 6.12: Ring sideroblasts in bone marrow

Q. Describe the structure and function of normal hemoglobin.

Q. Normal hemoglobins.

Hemoglobin Structure (Fig. 6.13)

- Hemoglobin (Hb) is a tetramer consisting of four polypeptide chains: two alpha chains and two beta chains. Alpha chain contains 141 amino acids and beta chain 146 amino acids.
- Different hemoglobins are produced during embryonic, fetal, and adult life. The major adult hemoglobin, HbA, has 2 alpha chains and 2 beta chains ($\alpha_2\beta_2$). HbF predominates during fetal life and contains 2 alpha chains and 2 gamma chains ($\alpha_2\gamma_2$). HbA_2 is found in little concentration in adults and contains 2 alpha chains and 2 delta chains ($\alpha_2\delta_2$).
- Each globin chain contains a single heme molecule, consisting of a protoporphyrin IX ring complexed with a single iron atom in the ferrous state (Fe^{2+}). Each heme molecule can bind a single oxygen molecule. Since there are four heme molecules in every molecule

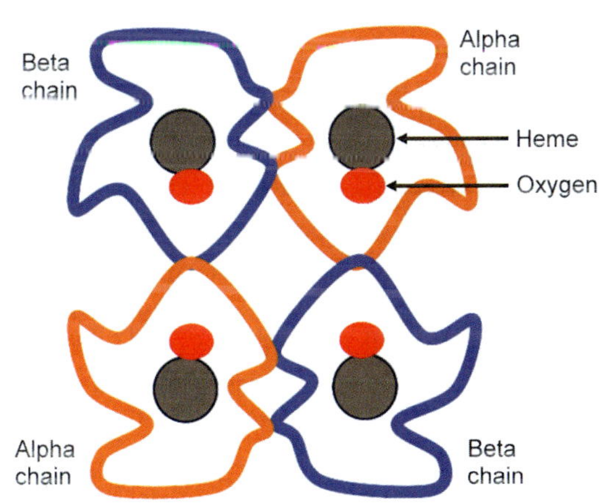

Figure 6.13: Hemoglobin structure

of hemoglobin, it can transport up to four oxygen molecules.

- The exterior surface of globin chain is hydrophilic and soluble whereas the interior forms a hydrophobic pocket into which heme is inserted. The hemoglobin tetramer is highly soluble but individual globin chains are insoluble. Unpaired globin precipitates, forming inclusions that damage the cell. Solubility and reversible oxygen binding are affected in hemoglobinopathies.

Function of Hemoglobin

- Hemoglobin binds to oxygen at the alveolus, retains it, and releases it to tissues.

Q. Define hemoglobinopathies. How do you classify them?

- Hemoglobinopathies are disorders affecting the structure, function, or production of hemoglobin.

Classification

Hereditary Hemoglobinopathies

- **Qualitative abnormality** of hemoglobin: Here the amino acid sequences in globin chains are defective which lead to altered physical or chemical properties of hemoglobin, e.g. HbS, HbC.
- **Quantitative abnormality** of hemoglobin: Here the amino acid sequence is normal, but one or more globin chains are absent, e.g. thalassemias.

Acquired Hemoglobinopathies

- Methemoglobin
- Sulfhemoglobin
- Carboxyhemoglobin.

Q. Discuss the etiology, pathogenesis, clinical features, investigations and management of sickle cell anemia.

Q. Hemoglobin-S (Hb-S).

Q. Sickle cell crisis and its management.

Q. Splenic sequestration syndrome.

- Sickle cell anemia is a hereditary hemoglobinopathy caused by a mutation in the β-globin gene leading to the production of abnormal hemoglobin S (HbS).
- The sickle cell anemia is characterized by the presence of HbS caused by a mutation in the β-globin gene that changes the sixth amino acid from glutamic acid to valine (glutamic acid goes).
- If both genes encoding for beta chain are abnormal, it is called sickle cell disease. It is more severe and is inherited as autosomal recessive manner.
- If only one gene is abnormal, and other gene is normal, it is called sickle cell trait. These patients have mild disease and can be asymptomatic.

Pathophysiology

- RBCs containing HbS turn into sickle-shaped cells on deoxygenation. Other factors leading to sickling are fever, sluggish blood flow, and acidosis. Sickling happens due to polymerization of HbS which distort the shape of RBC **(Fig. 6.14)**.

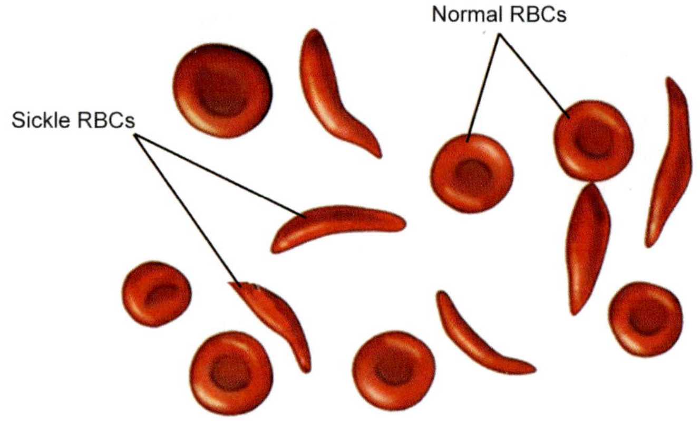

Figure 6.14: Sickle cell anemia

- Sickling of RBCs leads to hemolysis causing anemia. Sickled RBCs cannot negotiate through small vasculature leading to vaso-occlusive complications such as organ damage.

Clinical Manifestations

- Clinical manifestations include anemia (due to hemolysis), pain (due to vascular occlusion causing ischemia), infections (due to damage to spleen), and damage to organ systems.
- Growth retardation and psychosocial problems are common.
- Splenic infarcts result in frequent life-threatening episodes of septicemia. Many types of crisis such as painful crisis, splenic sequestration crisis and aplastic crisis can occur which are life threatening unless treated promptly.
- Vaso-occlusion can cause organ damage (particularly heart and kidney in adults and brain in children).
- Presence of high amount of Hb-F may decrease the symptoms of sickle cell disease because Hb-F interferes with polymerization of HbS.

Painful Crisis (sickle cell crisis)

- Vascular-occlusion can lead to ischemic pain in many areas of the body. Pain is the most common cause of debility in Hb-S disease. Acute episode of severe pain is called painful crisis or sickle cell crisis. Acute pain is the first symptom of disease in many patients and is the most frequent symptom after the age of two years. Acute pain is also the complication for which patients with sickle cell disease commonly seek medical attention.
- Pain may be precipitated by events such as weather conditions (e.g. high wind speed/low humidity), dehydration, infection, stress, menses, alcohol consumption, and nocturnal hypoxemia. However, the majority of painful episodes have no identifiable cause.
- Pain can affect any area of the body, but common in the back, chest, extremities, and abdomen. Dactylitis

(acute pain in the hands and/or feet) is common in children.

- Pain can vary from mild to excruciating. Pain may be accompanied by systemic symptoms such as fever, tachypnea, hypertension, nausea, and vomiting.
- Painful episodes last for two to seven days.
- Frequent pain may lead to psychosocial problems, depression and interfere with daily life.

Splenic Sequestration Crisis

- Vaso-occlusion can occur within the spleen and RBCs can get trapped in the spleen. Most of the circulating red cell mass is sequestrated in the spleen and the spleen rapidly enlarges (within hours). There is marked fall in hemoglobin concentration. There is a risk of hypovolemic shock.
- The patients who are susceptible to this syndrome are those whose spleens have not yet undergone fibrosis. Splenic sequestration crisis is associated with a 10–15% mortality rate, occurring before transfusions can be given.
- Sequestration can be recurrent in survivors and hence, splenectomy is recommended after the first attack. Milder cases can be managed with transfusion and careful observation.

Aplastic Crisis

- In aplastic crisis, there is transient arrest of erythropoiesis, leading to sudden decrease in hemoglobin, and reticulocytes. Bone marrow shows decrease in red cell precursors.
- Most cases of aplastic crisis are precipitated by infections such as parvovirus B_{19}, *Streptococcus pneumoniae*, *Salmonella*, streptococci, and Epstein-Barr virus. Parvovirus B_{19} is the most important of these.
- Affected patients require blood transfusion. Patients usually recover within a few days.

Hyperhemolytic Crisis

- Hyperhemolytic crisis refers to the sudden exacerbation of hemolysis with worsening anemia.
- The causes and mechanisms of hyperhemolytic crisis are multifactorial and are thought to include: blood transfusion, infections, and drug exposure, especially with concomitant glucose-6-phosphate dehydrogenase (G6PD) deficiency.
- Patients may present with acute drop in hemoglobin and markers of increased hemolysis such as jaundice.

Infections

- Sickle cell patients are prone to a variety of infections. Absent splenic function (autosplenectomy due to splenic infarcts) leads to infections with the encapsulated organisms, e.g. strep pneumonia and *H. influenza*. Pneumococcal infections can result in death within hours.
- Urinary tract infections (due to *E. coli*) and osteomyelitis are also common. Salmonella Typhimurium is another common infecting organism.

Specific Organ Systems Complications

- ***CVS:*** Anemia and vaso-occlusive phenomenon can lead to myocardial ischemia and infarction. Repeated blood transfusions can lead to iron overload and restrictive cardiomyopathy.
- ***RS:*** Pneumonia or pulmonary infarction. Acute chest syndrome is due to occlusion of pulmonary vasculature by sickled RBCs. Patients present with chest pain, hypoxia, fever, pulmonary infiltrates. It is one of the leading cause of death in sickle cell disease.
- ***CNS:*** Transient ischemic attacks, strokes and cerebral hemorrhage.
- ***Hepatobiliary system:*** Gallstones (pigmented gallstones due to ongoing hemolysis), recurrent abdominal pain due to vaso-occlusive crisis, hepatomegaly and hepatic dysfunction.
- ***Obstetric and gynecologic system:*** Placental infarcts can lead to intrauterine growth retardation and low-birth-weight babies. The frequency of spontaneous abortion is high.
- ***Genitourinary system:*** Hematuria, urinary tract infection, hyperuricemia and gout are common. Renal failure is common in elderly people. Priapism (painful erection of penis) can occur.
- ***Ocular complications:*** Proliferative retinopathy.
- ***Orthopedic system:*** avascular necrosis of the hip and osteomyelitis.
- ***Skin:*** Ulcers around the ankle.

Investigations

- Features of hemolysis: Mild-to-moderate anemia, reticulocytosis, unconjugated hyperbilirubinemia, elevated serum LDH and low serum haptoglobin.
- Peripheral blood smear reveals sickled RBCs **(Fig. 6.14)**, polychromasia indicative of reticulocytosis, and Howell-Jolly bodies reflecting hyposplenia. RBCs are normochromic.
- Sickle test: Sickling of RBCs occurs when mixed with a solution of sodium metabisulphite.
- Hemoglobin electrophoresis allows the definitive diagnosis of sickle cell disease. Most of the hemoglobin is HbS.
- Genetic analysis can show the specific mutation.

Management

General Measures

- Avoidance of dehydration, cold weather and hypoxia.
- Psychosocial support.
- Dietary advice (adequate calorie intake, folic acid, vitamin C, vitamin E and zinc).

Specific Measures

- ***Infection prevention:*** Infections can be prevented by prophylactic penicillin (till age 5) and immunizations. Pneumococcal and *H. influenza* vaccination should be given to all patients with sickle cell anemia. Hepatitis B vaccination is also necessary. Febrile episodes should be investigated appropriately and treated with early antibiotic therapy.
- ***Pain management:*** Pain should be controlled by aggressive use of analgesics. Most of the time opioid

analgesics such as morphine, fentanyl or tramadol are required. Dehydration should be prevented.

- ***Blood transfusions:*** Transfusions can be used to correct anemia and also in emergencies such as splenic sequestration syndrome. Blood transfusion also decreases the level of HbS by dilution. However hemoglobin should not be raised above 10 g/dl because of increases in viscosity and the risk of vaso-occlusive episodes. Blood transfusions are associated with problems like transmission of viral diseases, iron overload and alloimmunization.
- ***Hydroxyurea:*** Hydroxyurea induces the synthesis of fetal hemoglobin. High levels of fetal hemoglobin (HbF) decrease the severity of crisis and prolong survival in sickle cell patients. Coadministration of hematopoietic agents such as erythropoietin along with hydroxyurea may also be useful.
- ***Voxelotor:*** Inhibits HbS polymerization.
- ***Bone marrow transplantation*** offers the only chance of cure at present.
- Gene therapy is under research.

Prognosis

- Patients now survive up to 6th or 7th decade. Common causes of death include organ failure (predominantly renal) and sickle cell crisis. A high level of HbF predicts prolonged survival.

Q. What are thalassemias? Classify thalassemias.

- Thalassemias are a group of inherited hemoglobin disorders caused by reduced or absent synthesis of one or more globin chains (α or β).
- Thalassemia is common in the Mediterranean region especially amongst Italians and Greeks. The thalassemia belt extends to India and south East Asia. In India, it is found in Punjab, Gujarat, Maharashtra, Karnataka, Bengal and Assam. It is relatively less common in the southern states. On an average, 3% of Indians carry the thalassemia gene (chiefly beta thalassemia). The highest incidence is found in Lohanas and Sindhis.

Classification

- Thalassemias are named according to globin chain deficiency, e.g. in beta thalassemia, there is deficiency of beta chain, and in alpha thalassemia, there is deficiency of alpha chain.

Alpha Thalassemias

- Caused by deletions of one or more of the four α-globin genes **(Table 6.8)**.

TABLE 6.8: Alpha thalassemias

Clinical syndrome	Gene deletions	Features
Silent carrier	1 gene	Asymptomatic
α-thalassemia trait (minor)	2 genes	Mild anemia
Hemoglobin H disease	3 genes	Moderate-to-severe anemia, splenomegaly
Hydrops fetalis (Hb Barts)	4 genes	Usually fatal *in utero* or shortly after birth

Beta Thalassemias

- Caused by mutations in the β-globin gene. There are two genes coding for beta chain (for alpha chain there are four genes) **(Table 6.9)**.

TABLE 6.9: Beta thalassemias

Clinical syndrome	Gene mutation	Features
β-thalassemia trait (minor)	1 defective gene	Mild microcytic anemia
β-thalassemia intermedia	2 partially functional genes	Moderate anemia, not transfusion-dependent
β-thalassemia major	2 defective genes	Severe anemia, transfusion-dependent, growth retardation, skeletal deformities, iron overload

Q. Discuss the etiology, pathogenesis, clinical features, investigations and management of beta thalassemia major (Cooley's anemia).

Etiology

- Beta-thalassemias are genetic disorder of hemoglobin synthesis caused by mutations in the β-globin gene on chromosome 11.
- In β-thalassemia major, both β-globin genes are defective, leading to absent or severely reduced β-globin chain production.
- It is also called Colley's anemia because it was first described by Dr Cooley, an American pediatrician and hematologist.
- Autosomal recessive inheritance.

Pathophysiology

- Since both β-globin genes are defective, there is absent or severely reduced β-globin chain production. This leads to decreased production of hemoglobin causing hypochromia and microcytosis. There is accumulation of unaffected alpha globin chains since their production proceeds at a normal rate. Excess alpha chains are unstable and precipitate, leading to damage of red blood cell membranes. This leads to intramedullary (in the bone marrow) and peripheral hemolysis causing anemia.
- Anemia leads to bone marrow hyperplasia and ineffective erythropoiesis resulting from the intramedullary destruction of the developing erythroid cells.
- Marked expansion of the bone marrow may cause severe bony deformities, osteopenia, and pathologic fractures.
- Iron overload occurs due to increased gastrointestinal iron absorption, repeated blood transfusions. This leads to secondary hemochromatosis, affecting heart, liver, and endocrine organs.

Clinical Features

- Symptoms start late in the first year of life when fetal hemoglobin levels decline.
- Anemia causes pallor, fatigue, irritability, and growth retardation.

- Hemolysis leads to hepatosplenomegaly (due to extramedullary hematopoiesis) and jaundice.
- Anemia and hemolysis stimulate erythropoiesis leading to extensive marrow expansion leading to characteristic chipmunk facies (frontal bossing and prominent check bones).
- 80% of untreated children die within the first 5 years of life as a result of severe anemia, high output heart failure, and infections.
- Repeated blood transfusions can lead to iron overload. Many patients die secondary to iron overload-related cardiomyopathy or arrhythmias.
- Various endocrinological abnormalities such as delayed puberty, diabetes mellitus, hypoparathyroidism and hypothyroidism can occur due to iron overload.
- Repeated blood transfusions can lead to transmission of viruses (HBV, HCV, and HIV).

Differences between Beta Thalassemia Major and Minor (Table 6.10)

TABLE 6.10: Differences between β thalassemia major and minor

Features	Thalassemia major	Thalassemia minor
Symptoms	Symptomatic	Asymptomatic
Genes resposnsible for globin chain synthesis	Both defective	One is normal, one is defective
Anemia	Severe	Mild
Peripheral smear	Severe hypochromasia, microcytosis and erythroblastosis	Mild hypochromasia and microcytosis, few target cells and punctate basophilia
Hb electrophoresis	Hb F elevated Hb A reduced/absent	Hb A_2 elevated
Parents	Both having thalassemia minor	One parent having thalassemia minor

Investigations

- Signs of hemolysis such as anemia, increased indirect (unconjugated) bilirubin, increased LDH and reduced haptoglobin levels.
- HbA is markedly reduced and HbF is raised.
- Peripheral smear shows hypochromia, microcytosis, anisopoikilocytosis, tear drop cells and target cells. Nucleated red cells are abundant but reticulocyte count is low due to ineffective erythropoiesis. RBCs show clumped inclusion bodies representing precipitates of alpha globin cahins within the red cell. These precipitates (Heinz bodies) can be stained with methyl violet or other supravital stains. WBC and platelet counts are normal unless hypersplenism develops.
- Bone marrow shows marked hypercellularity.
- Serum iron and transferrin saturation are increased due to high red cell turnover.
- The osmotic fragility test is significantly reduced.
- Skull X-ray shows widened diploic space and hair-on-end appearance (**Fig. 6.15**). Compression fractures of the vertebrae and marked osteoporosis are common.

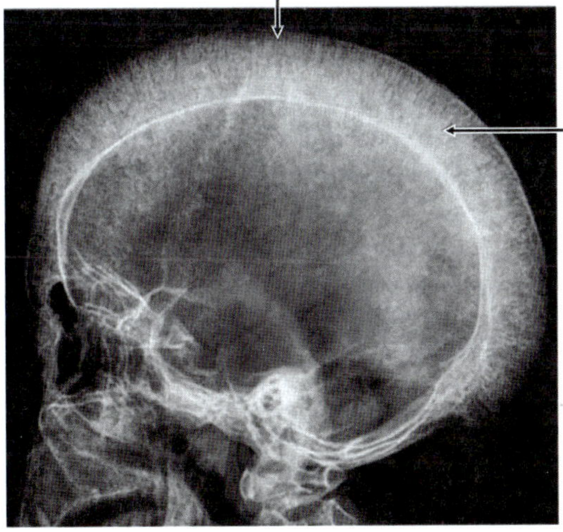

Figure 6.15: Skull X-ray showing hair on end appearance

Management

- Beta thalassemia major requires regular blood transfusion to maintain hemoglobin at >10 g/dl. Correction of anemia leads to normal growth and development.
- Repeated blood transfusions lead to iron overload. Hence, iron chelation therapy should be given (desferrioxamine infusion or oral iron chelator deferiprone).
- Folic acid supplements should be given to all patients because of increased requirements due to increased red cell turnover.
- Splenectomy for gross symptomatic splenomegaly or hypersplenism.
- Endocrine and cardiac management: Regular screening and hormone replacement if needed. Cardiac MRI and echocardiography for early detection of iron overload effects.
- Allogeneic bone marrow transplantation is the treatment of choice for β-thalassemia major and can cure it.
- Gene therapy is under research.
- Genetic counseling and prenatal diagnosis should be offered to affected parents.
- Thalassemia minor requires no treatment except genetic counseling, avoidance of inappropriate iron therapy and close monitoring during pregnancy.

Q. Hereditary spherocytosis.

- Hereditary spherocytosis (HS) is a genetic hemolytic anemia characterized by the presence of spherocytes in the peripheral blood.
- It is usually inherited as an autosomal dominant condition, although 25% of cases have no family history and represent new mutations.

Pathology

- It is due to a defective structural protein (spectrin) of the red cell membrane. Other defective membrane proteins are ankyrin and band 3 protein. All these protein defects lead to reduced surface area of RBCs which lose their biconcave shape and become spherical. The morphologic hallmark of HS is the microspherocyte, which is caused by loss of RBC membrane surface area and has abnormal osmotic fragility *in vitro*. As the spherical cells are unable to pass through the splenic microcirculation, they are trapped and destroyed in the spleen → extravascular hemolysis.

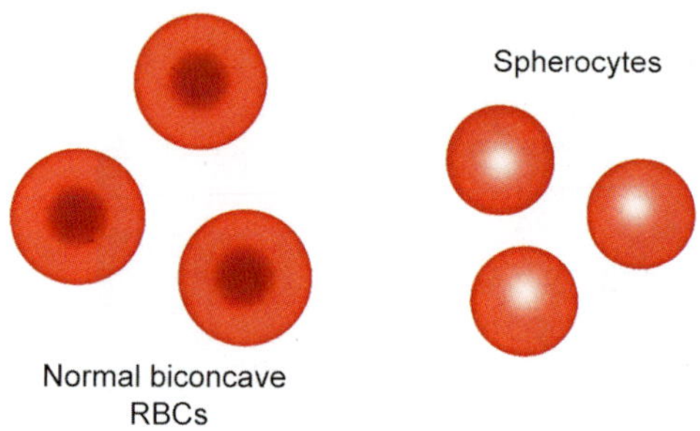

Figure 6.16: Hereditary spherocytosis

Clinical Features

- Signs and symptoms of hereditary spherocytosis (HS) include mild pallor, intermittent jaundice, and splenomegaly.
- Most cases are associated with an asymptomatic compensated chronic hemolytic state.
- A hemolytic crisis can occur when the severity of hemolysis increases; this is seen in association with infection.
- A megaloblastic crisis can occur due to folate deficiency which is common during pregnancy.
- An aplastic crisis occurs in association with parvovirus B_{19} infection.
- Pigment gallstones are present in up to 50% of patients and may cause symptomatic cholecystitis.

Investigations

- Anemia
- Reticulocytosis
- Peripheral smear shows spherocytes **(Fig. 6.16)**.
- LFT shows rise in indirect bilirubin.
- Serum LDH level is raised.
- Direct Coombs' test is negative excluding immune hemolysis.
- Osmotic fragility test shows increased sensitivity to lysis in hypotonic saline solutions.

Management

- Folic acid prophylaxis, 5 mg once weekly, should be given for life.
- Splenectomy may be considered in severe hemolysis.
- Acute, severe hemolytic crises require blood transfusions.

Q. Glucose-6-phosphate dehydrogenase deficiency.

- Glucose-6-phosphate dehydrogenase (G6PD) deficiency is the most common enzyme defect associated with hereditary hemolytic anemia. It is an X-linked disorder, hence seen mostly in males. Females are protected because of two X-chromosomes one of which can carry normal gene.

Pathogenesis

- G6PD is the first enzyme in the pentose phosphate pathway which generates NADPH. NADPH is required to keep the glutathione in reduced state in RBCs.
- Depletion of cellular glutathione results in damage to RBCs by oxidizing agents and various drugs leading to hemolysis.

Precipitating Causes of Hemolysis in G6PD Deficiency

- Drugs: Primaquine, quinine, sulfonamides, dapsone
- Severe stress or illness
- Fava beans
- Infections.

Clinical Features

- Hemolysis usually occurs only under oxidant stress.
- Hemolysis is usually precipitated by infections due to liberation of oxidant molecules by granulocytes and mononuclear phagocytes and oxidant drugs. Ingestion of fava beans (Italian broad beans) can also cause hemolysis in some patients due to the presence of high levels of oxidant pyrimidine analogs in the beans.
- Hemolysis leads to anemia, reticulocytosis, hemoglobinuria, hyperbilirubinemia, and jaundice. Hemoglobinuria can cause renal tubular necrosis and renal failure.
- Many neonates with G6PD deficiency manifest jaundice at 1–4 days of age which usually responds to phototherapy.

Investigations

- Evidence of intravascular hemolysis after infections and certain drugs.
- Estimation of G6PD activity in the RBC.

Treatment

- Asymptomatic individuals require no treatment.
- Mild hemolytic episodes are treated by withdrawing the offending drug, or treatment of the concurrent infection.
- Severe hemolytic episodes may require red cell transfusions to correct anemia and measures to prevent renal failure due to hemoglobinuria.

Q. Methemoglobinemia.

- Methemoglobin is an altered state of hemoglobin in which the ferrous (Fe^{2+}) ions of heme are oxidized to ferric (Fe^{3+}) state. Methemoglobin is unable to bind oxygen. Hence, oxygen delivery to the tissues is impaired.

- Normally a small amount of methemoglobin is formed daily which is reduced back to normal hemoglobin by cytochrome b5 reductase and glucose-6-phosphate dehydrogenase (G6PD).

Causes

- Methemoglobinemia can occur due to congenital or acquired causes.
- Most cases are acquired, due to increased methemoglobin formation by various agents such as dapsone, benzocaine, etc.
- Hereditary methemoglobinemia is due to deficiency of reducing enzymes such as cytochrome b5 reductase. Another congenital cause of methemoglobinemia is hemoglobin M disease.

Clinical Features

- Chronic methemoglobinemia is asymptomatic most of the time. Some may complain of headache and easy fatigability. The main complaint is "cyanosis" or slate-blue color of the skin and mucous membranes. Cyanosis is present when the methemoglobin concentration exceeds 1.5 g/dl.
- Patients with acute methemoglobinemia are usually symptomatic due to acutely impaired oxygen delivery to tissues. Symptoms include headache, fatigue, dyspnea, and lethargy. At higher methemoglobin levels, respiratory depression, altered consciousness, shock, seizures, and death may occur.
- Blood is chocolate colored.

Diagnosis

- Methemoglobinemia should be suspected when there is "cyanosis" in the presence of normal PaO_2 as obtained by arterial blood gases. Levels of methemoglobin should be measured in lab.
- Cyanosis + chocolate-brown blood + low pulse oximetry despite normal PaO_2 = Think of methemoglobinemia.

Treatment

- All patients with hereditary methemoglobinemia should avoid exposure to aniline derivatives, nitrates, and other agents which can induce methemoglobinemia. Methylene blue or ascorbic acid orally may be useful in cytochrome b5 reductase deficiency. Riboflavin has also been shown to be useful.
- In acquired methemoglobinemia any offending agent should be discontinued. In severe methemoglobinemia blood transfusion or exchange transfusion and intravenous methylene blue are helpful. However, methylene blue is not helpful in patients with G6PD deficiency, since the reduction of methemoglobin by methylene blue is dependent upon NADPH generated by G6PD.

Q. Kernicterus.

- Kernicterus refers to brain damage caused by unconjugated bilirubin deposition in basal ganglia and brain stem nuclei, caused by either acute or chronic hyperbilirubinemia. It occurs in neonates due to hyperbilirubinemia of various reasons. Neurologic sequelae develop during the first year after birth.
- The major features of kernicterus include: choreoathetoid cerebral palsy (chorea, ballismus, tremor), sensorineural hearing loss, gaze abnormalities (especially limitation of upward gaze), dental-enamel dysplasia. Cognitive function is usually spared.
- There is no treatment for established kernicterus. It should be prevented by early recognition and treatment of hyperbilirubinemia.

Q. Etiology of leukemia.

- Leukemia is a type of hematological malignancy that originates in the bone marrow and leads to the uncontrolled proliferation of abnormal white blood cells.

Etiology

Idiopathic
- Majority of cases are idiopathic

Ionizing radiation
- Atomic bombing
- X-ray exposure
- Radiotherapy

Viruses
- Human T-cell lymphotropic virus type I (HTLV-I) (can cause adult T-cell leukemia)
- HTLV-II (causes a syndrome resembling hairy cell leukemia).
- Epstein Barr virus

Immunodeficiency state
- Immune deficiency states (e.g. HIV and hypogammaglobulinemia) are associated with an increase in hematological malignancy

Genetics factors
- Trisomy 21 (Down syndrome)
- Trisomy 13 (Patau)
- XXY (Klinefelter syndrome)
- Disorders causing chromosomal instability (Bloom syndrome, Fanconi's anemia, and ataxia-telangiectasia)
- Philadelphia chromosome causing CML)

Chemicals and drugs
- Exposure to benzene and benzene-containing compounds.
- Exposure to tobacco, chemotherapeutic agents (especially cyclophosphamide, melphalan, other alkylating agents, and etoposide).

Q. Classification of leukemias.

Q. Acute *vs.* chronic leukemia.

Classification of Leukemias

Acute leukemias
- Acute lymphoblastic leukemia (ALL)
- Acute myeloid leukemia (AML)

Chronic leukemias
- Chronic lymphocytic leukemia (CLL)
- Chronic myeloid leukemia (CML)

Acute *vs.* Chronic Leukemia

- Acute leukemia is a malignant hematologic disorder characterized by the rapid proliferation of immature blood cells (blasts) in the bone marrow. These blasts replace the healthy cells in the bone marrow, causing the rapid onset of symptoms. Blasts normally make up 1–5% of marrow cells, and having more than 20% blasts in the bone marrow is diagnostic of acute leukemia.
- Chronic leukemias develop slowly and produce symptoms slowly. Here, the leukemic cells more mature and functional.

Q. Define acute leukemia. Discuss the etiology, clinical features, investigations and management of acute leukemia.

Q. Discuss the etiology, clinical features, investigations and management of acute myeloblastic leukemia (AML).

Q. Aleukemic leukemia.

- Acute leukemia is defined as a malignant clonal proliferation of lymphoid or myeloid precursor cell which replace the marrow and ultimately spill over to the peripheral blood and infiltrate lymph nodes, spleen, liver or other organs.
- Normally hematopoietic stem cells proliferate and differentiate into various cellular components of blood. In acute leukemia an early hematopoietic precursor fails to differentiate and instead continues to proliferate in an uncontrolled fashion. As a result, immature myeloid (in AML) or lymphoid cells (in ALL), called ***blasts***, rapidly accumulate and progressively replace the bone marrow which in turn results in decreased production of normal red cells, white cells, and platelets (pancytopenia). Eventually leukemic blasts will pour out into the blood and also infiltrate lymph nodes, spleen, and other vital organs. Acute leukemia is rapidly fatal and most patients die within months of diagnosis. However, in many patients it can be controlled or cured with appropriate therapy.

Acute Myeloid Leukemia (AML)

- Acute myeloid leukemia (AML) is a malignant clonal disorder characterized by the accumulation of immature myeloid precursors (myeloblasts) in the bone marrow, leading to bone marrow failure and infiltration of other tissues.
- It is the most common acute leukemia in adults.

Etiology

Primary (De novo) AML

- No identifiable cause
- Occurs in younger adults

Secondary AML

- Following myelodysplastic syndromes (MDS) or myeloproliferative neoplasms.
- Post-chemotherapy or radiotherapy. Alkylating agents, topoisomerase II inhibitors.
- Environmental exposures: Benzene, ionizing radiation.

Genetic predisposition

- Down syndrome (increased risk of AML, especially M7 subtype).
- Fanconi anemia.
- Bloom syndrome.
- Chromosomal abnormalities (e.g. t(15;17) in APL subtype, inv(16), t(8;21)).

Classification of AML

French-American-British (FAB) classification)

- M0: Acute undifferentiated leukemia
- M1: AML with minimal differentiation
- M2: AML with differentiation
- M3: Acute promyelocytic leukemia
- M4: Acute myelomonocytic leukemia
- M5: Acute monocytic leukemia
- M6: Acute erythroleukemia
- M7: Acute megakaryocytic leukemia

World Health Organization (WHO) classification of AML

- AML with recurrent genetic abnormalities
- AML with myelodysplasia-related changes
- Therapy-related myeloid neoplasms
- AML not otherwise specified (NOS)
- Myeloid sarcoma
- Myeloid proliferations related to Down syndrome.

Incidence

- Acute myeloid leukemia (AML) is the most common leukemia among the adult population and accounts for about 80% of all cases. The incidence in the West varies from 3 to 13 per 100,000 per year. The average age at the time of diagnosis is about 65 years. Males are affected commonly than females.

Clinical Features

- Two things happen in leukemia which causes all the signs and symptoms. One is leukemic blasts fill the bone marrow and interfere with its function. Another is leukemic blasts infiltrate normal organs and lead to their dysfunction.
- Decreased bone marrow function leads to deficiency of all three cell lines causing anemia, thrombocytopenia, and granulocytopenia. Anemia is present at diagnosis in most patients and causes fatigue, pallor, and headache and in severe cases angina or heart failure. Thrombocytopenia causes bleeding manifestations in the form of petechiae, ecchymoses, bleeding gums, epistaxis, or hemorrhage. Granulocytopenia results in increased incidence of infections.
- Infiltration of normal organs by leukemic blasts lead to various manifestations as follows:
    - Liver and spleen–hepatosplenomegaly.
    - Bone: Bone pain may be present due to leukemic infiltration of the periosteum or expansion of the medullary cavity.

- Skin: Leukemic cells sometimes infiltrate the skin and result in a raised, nonpruritic rash, a condition termed ***leukemia cutis***.
- CNS: Leukemic cells may infiltrate the leptomeninges and cause leukemic meningitis manifesting as headache and nausea. In advanced cases, cranial nerve palsies, other neurological deficits and seizures may develop.
- Gum hypertrophy is especially with M5 subtype.
- Collections of leukemic blast cells, often referred to as ***chloromas*** or ***myeloblastomas***, can occur in virtually any soft tissue and appear as rubbery, fast-growing masses.

- Certain clinical manifestations are unique to specific subtypes of leukemia. For example, DIC (disseminated intravascular coagulation) is common in promyelocytic leukemia (AML-M3) due to release of tissue thromboplastins by leukemic cells when they die.

Laboratory Findings

- Anemia and thrombocytopenia.
- Total leukocyte count is markedly raised (often as high as 100,000/mm^3).
- Peripheral blood smear shows circulating blasts. However, blasts may not always be seen in peripheral smear ("aleukemic leukemia") **(Fig. 6.17)**.
- Bone marrow is usually hypercellular with the presence of blasts. More than 20% blasts are required to make a diagnosis of acute leukemia.
- Serum LDH, uric acid and alkaline phosphatase levels are elevated due to rapid cell turnover.
- The Auer rod, an eosinophilic needle-like inclusion in the cytoplasm, is pathognomonic of AML.
- Cytogenetic studies reveal many chromosome abnormalities which can also predict the prognosis in acute leukemias.
- Flow cytometry: Immunophenotyping to confirm myeloid origin. Positive markers: CD13, CD33.

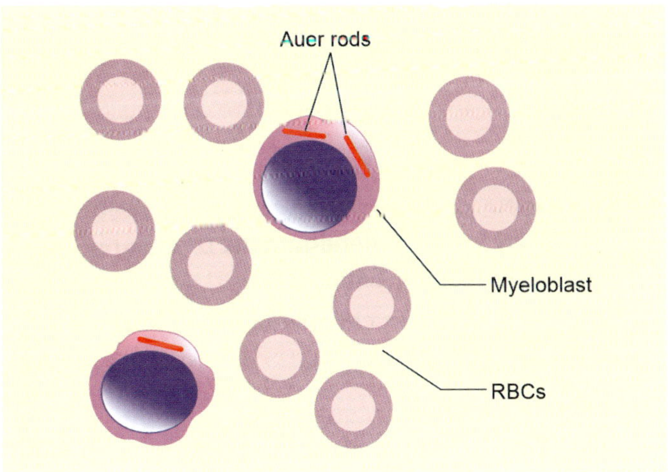

Figure 6.17: Auer rods in AML

Treatment

- Chemotherapy is the mainstay of therapy for acute leukemia. The aim of chemotherapy is to induce remission and maintain it. The type of initial chemotherapy depends on the subtype of leukemia.
- Most patients with AML except acute promyelocytic leukemia are treated with a combination of daunorubicin, cytarabine and etoposide. Acute promyelocytic leukemia is treated with daunorubicin plus tretinoin. Arsenic trioxide has been shown to increase the cure rate of promyelocytic leukemia when added to primary therapy.
- After remission induction, further therapy with curative intent includes standard chemotherapy and autologous or allogeneic bone marrow transplantation. If the leukemia recurs after initial chemotherapy, the prognosis is worse.

Prognosis

- 70–80% of patients under 60 years with AML achieve complete remission. 30–40% of these patients can be cured by high-dose post-remission chemotherapy. The remission and cure rate for older patients is low. Allogeneic bone marrow transplantation is curative in 50–60% cases in young people.

Acute Lymphoid Leukemia (ALL)

- Acute lymphoblastic leukemia (ALL) is a malignant proliferation of immature lymphoid precursors (lymphoblasts) in the bone marrow and peripheral blood.

Incidence

- ALL most commonly affects children and young adults. It is the most common malignancy of childhood. Peak incidence approximately four years age.
- More frequent in boys than in girls.
- Exposure to high-energy radiation in early childhood increases the risk of developing T cell ALL.

Etiology

- Same as AML.

Classification

- B cell ALL (most of the childhood cases).
- T-cell ALL: Frequently presents with mediastinal mass.

Clinical Features

- ALL patients typically present with symptoms of night sweats, easy bruising, skin pallor, unexplained lymphadenopathy, weakness, weight loss, hepatosplenomegaly, or difficulty breathing.
- Pulmonary complications are common in ALL. These include pneumonia, pulmonary leukostasis, malignant pleural effusion and/or pulmonary infiltration and upper airway obstruction.
- The cause of upper airway obstruction can be epiglottitis, enlarged lymph nodes, laryngeal mass comprised of leukemic cells.

- Patients with ALL (especially T cell) may have a mediastinal mass visible on chest radiograph. This mediastinal mass can produce SVC obstruction.
- CNS involvement is common in ALL and can present as meningitis, cranial nerve palsies and seizures.

Laboratory Findings

- Anemia and thrombocytopenia.
- Total leukocyte count is markedly raised (often as high as 100,000/mm^3).
- Peripheral blood smear shows circulating blasts. However, blasts may not always be seen in peripheral smear ("aleukemic leukemia").
- Bone marrow is usually hypercellular with the presence of blasts. More than 20% blasts are required to make a diagnosis of acute leukemia.
- Serum LDH, uric acid and alkaline phosphatase levels are elevated due to rapid cell turnover.
- Patients with ALL (especially T cell) may have a mediastinal mass visible on chest radiograph.
- Cytogenetic studies reveal many chromosome abnormalities which can also predict the prognosis.
- ALL is diagnosed when there is no morphologic or histochemical evidence of myeloid or monocytic lineage. The diagnosis of ALL is confirmed by demonstrating surface markers of primitive lymphoid cells, by flow cytometry and monoclonal antibodies.

Treatment

- ALL is treated with combination chemotherapy, including daunorubicin, vincristine, prednisone, and asparaginase. For patients with Philadelphia chromosome-positive ALL, imatinib (or dasatinib) should be added to initial chemotherapy. As with AML, patients may be treated with either chemotherapy or high-dose chemotherapy plus bone marrow transplantation.
- Recently, chimeric antigen receptor (CAR) T-cell therapy has been approved for ALL.

Q. Differences between AML and ALL (Table 6.11).

TABLE 6.11: Differences between AML and ALL

Features	AML	ALL
Cell linage	Myeloid precursors	Lymphoid precursors
Auer rods	Present	Absent
Age group affected	Commonly adults	Commonly children
Common genetic abnormalities	t(8;21), t(15;17), and inv(16) (p13;q22).	t(9;22) and t(4;11).
Nuclear enzyme, terminal deoxynucleotidyl transferase (Tdt) in leukemic blasts	Rarely present	Present in more than 90%
Lymphadenopathy	Uncommon	Common
Hepatosplenomegaly	Uncommon	Common
CNS involvement	Uncommon	Common
Cytochemical staining (myeloperoxidase, Sudan black B)	Positive	negative

Q. Leukemoid reaction.

- A leukemoid reaction is a marked elevation in white blood cell (WBC) count (usually >50,000/mm^3) that mimics leukemia but is nonmalignant and due to a reactive cause, such as infection or stress.

Causes of Leukemoid Reaction

Infections

- Severe bacterial infections (e.g. pneumonia, sepsis).

Inflammatory Conditions

- Rheumatoid arthritis
- Vasculitis

Drugs and Toxins

- Corticosteroids
- G-CSF administration

Other

- Hemorrhage
- Hemolysis
- Burns

Differentiation from Leukemia

- Counts are usually less than 1 lakh.
- Bone marrow is normal.
- Leukocyte alkaline phosphatase score (LAP) is increased.
- There is left shift as evidenced by presence of myelocytes and metamyelocytes.
- Presence of toxic granules in neutrophils.
- Band forms may be seen.
- Blasts are absent.
- Basophilia and eosinophilia are not seen in leukaemoid reaction.
- Treatment of underlying condition corrects the leukocyte counts.

Q. Discuss the pathophysiology, clinical features, investigations and management of chronic myeloid leukemia (CML).

Q. Peripheral smear in chronic myeloid leukemia.

Q. Philadelphia chromosome.

Q. Imatinib mesylate.

- Chronic myeloid leukemia (CML) is a myeloproliferative disorder characterized by overproduction of myeloid cells.

Pathophysiology

- CML is characterized by a specific chromosomal abnormality, called the Philadelphia chromosome which occurs due to reciprocal translocation between the long arms of chromosomes 9 and 22. The abnormal chromosome 22 is known as Philadelphia chromosome **(Fig. 6.18)**.
- The oncogene ***c-abl***, normally situated in the long arm of chromosome 9, gets translocated to chromosome 22, where a specific gene called ***bcr*** (breakpoint cluster region) is situated. Both ***abl*** and ***bcr*** form a fusion gene, ***abl/bcr***, which is important in the pathogenesis of CML. The fusion gene ***bcr/abl*** produces a protein possessing tyrosine kinase activity. This leads to tumor cell proliferation and inhibition of apoptosis.
- Patients who are Philadelphia chromosome negative tend to be older, mostly male and respond poorly to treatment.

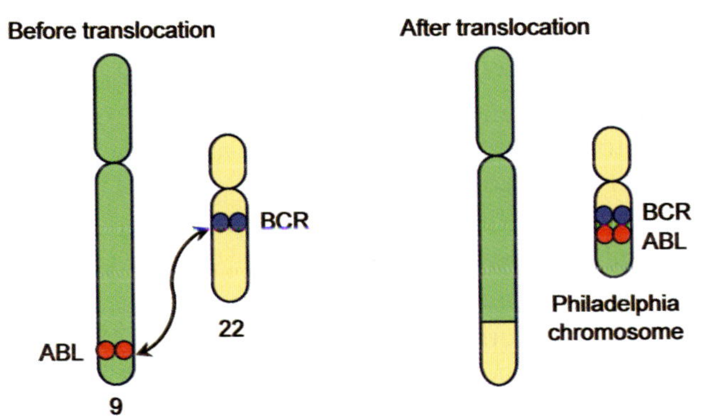

Figure 6.18: Philadelphia chromosome

Natural Course

- The disease has 3 stages: (1) chronic stable phase, (2) accelerated phase and (3) blast crisis.
- The chronic phase is characterized by a large increase in peripheral blood leukocytes. Most patients are in stable phase at presentation. This phase may last months to years.
- In accelerated phase neutrophil differentiation becomes progressively impaired and leukocyte counts are more difficult to control. There is worsening anemia, progressive thrombocytopenia or thrombocytosis, persistent or worsening splenomegaly, clonal evolution, increasing blood basophils, and increasing marrow or blood blasts.
- In blast crisis, myeloid or lymphoid blasts fail to differentiate and large number of blasts is found in peripheral blood. Blast crisis carries very poor prognosis. Blasts in blood or marrow increase to >20%.

Clinical Features

- CML has an annual incidence of 1–2 cases per 100,000, with a slight male predominance. CML is a disorder of middle age (median age at presentation is 50 years).
- The clinical hallmark of CML is the uncontrolled production of maturing granulocytes, predominantly neutrophils, but also eosinophils and basophils.
- Patients usually present with fatigue, weight loss, night sweats, and low-grade fever due to the hypermetabolic state caused by overproduction of white blood cells.
- Bleeding episodes are common due to platelet dysfunction.
- Abdominal fullness, early satiety, left upper quadrant pain, and discomfort may be complained of due to massive splenomegaly.
- Acute gouty arthritis may be present due to overproduction of uric acid.
- Extremely high leukocyte counts may cause symptoms due to hyper-viscosity such as priapism (painful persistent erection), respiratory distress, visual blurring, and altered mental status.
- Examination reveals pallor, massive splenomegaly, and sternal tenderness due to bone marrow hyperplasia. Hepatomegaly may also be present.

Laboratory Findings

- Anemia is usually present.
- Total WBC count is usually above 1 lakh/µl.
- Platelet count is normal or elevated.
- Absolute basophilia and eosinophilia are almost always present.
- LAP score (leukocyte alkaline phosphatase): Low in CML (helps distinguish from leukemoid reaction).
- Peripheral blood smear shows presence of myelocytes and metamyelocytes. RBC morphology is normal.
- Bone marrow aspiration and biopsy in patients with CML in chronic phase shows myeloid hyperplasia, increase in reticulin fibers and vascularity. There is increase in the myeloid-to-erythroid ratio in the bone marrow as well as a marked increase in the number of megakaryocytes and the number of more immature forms. Blast crisis is diagnosed when blasts are more than 20% in the bone marrow.
- The diagnosis of CML is established by demonstration of the Philadelphia chromosome or the BCR-ABL fusion gene. BCR-ABL can be detected in the peripheral blood by polymerase chain reaction (PCR) test, which has now supplanted cytogenetics.

Treatment

Tyrosine Kinase Inhibitors (imatinib mesylate, dasatinib, nilotinib)

- The treatment of CML has been revolutionized by the introduction of tyrosine kinase inhibitors such as imatinib mesylate, which inhibit the tyrosine kinase activity of the ***BCR/ABL*** oncogene. Imatinib inhibits proliferation and induces apoptosis in cells positive for ***BCR/ABL***. Tyrosine kinase inhibitors are the first line drugs for chronic and accelerated phase of CML. Imatinib is well tolerated and controls the disease in 98% of chronic phase patients with positive Philadelphia chromosome. In chronic phase of CML, the dose of imatinib is 400 mg orally daily. Side effects are nausea, periorbital swelling, edema, rash, and myalgia. Blood counts normalize and splenomegaly regresses within several weeks, usually within 3 months. Philadelphia chromosome becomes negative within 6 months (maximum 12 months). Dasatinib is another agent which is effective in patients not responding to imatinib. However, tyrosine kinase inhibitors imatinib does not cure the patient. It controls the disease as long as it is given.

Omacetaxine

- Omacetaxine is a new drug introduced for the treatment of CML. It is a protein translation inhibitor that is indicated for chronic- or accelerated-phase CML with resistance and/or intolerance to 2 or more tyrosine kinase inhibitors.

Busulphan or Hydroxyurea

- These agents suppress the bone marrow and reduce the leukocyte count. Conventional treatment of CML in chronic phase has been single agent therapy with busulphan or hydroxyurea. However, due to the availability of newer agents such as imatinib, these agents are being used less commonly now.
- Hydroxyurea is preferred over busulphan. It is given in a dose of 20–30 mg/kg OD orally daily. Blood counts should be monitored and the dose is adjusted as per the counts. WBC counts recover within a short time after discontinuation of the drug.
- Busulphan is given in a dose of 6–8 mg daily orally and reduced as the leukocyte count falls. It should be discontinued when the leukocyte count falls below 20,000/µl and resumed if the count reaches 50,000/µl.

Interferon Therapy

- Alpha IFN inhibits the late progenitors which may be the major phase of CML clonal expansion. Patients with early chronic phase respond better. Reduction of *'bcr-abl'* oncogene expression has been reported after therapy with IFN. Complete hematological response is seen in 35–85% of patients. Side effects include influenza-like symptoms, lethargy, poor memory, and myalgias. However, due to the availability of newer agents such as imatinib, interferon alpha is now used only for refractory cases in combination with other agents.

Allogeneic Bone Marrow Transplantation or Stem Cell Transplantation

- If the patients do not respond to imatinib, this is the 2nd choice of therapy. The best results (80% cure rate) are obtained in patients under 40 years of age if transplanted within 1 year after diagnosis. Bone marrow should be obtained from HLA matched siblings.

Leukapheresis

- Leukapheresis is sometimes used to control the number of WBCs in emergency situations. It is useful in two types of patients: the hyperleukocytic patient in whom rapid cytoreduction can reverse symptoms and signs of leukostasis (e.g. stupor, hypoxia, tinnitus, papilledema, priapism), and in the pregnant patient with CML who can be controlled by leukapheresis treatment without other drugs which can cause damage to the fetus.

Anagrelide

- Anagrelide can be used to decrease very high platelet count not responding to imatinib alone.

Course and Prognosis

- In the past, median survival was 3–4 years. However, after the introduction of imatinib mesylate, 4-year survival and remission is 80%.

Q. Accelerated phase of CML.

- The accelerated phase (AP) of CML is an intermediate stage between the chronic phase and blast crisis. It indicates disease progression and is associated with poorer prognosis and resistance to therapy.

Clinical Features

- Clinical features that signal the conversion of the chronic to the accelerated phase include unexplained fever, bone pain, weakness, night sweats, weight loss, and loss of sense of well-being, arthralgias, or left upper quadrant pain.
- Localized or diffuse lymphadenopathy may develop.
- Increase in spleen size.
- Anemia worsens.
- Increase in leukocyte count with blasts 10–19% in peripheral blood.
- Increase in basophil count (≥20%)
- Poor response to therapy.

Treatment

- Drug of choice for treatment of accelerated phase is one of the tyrosine kinase inhibitors such as imatinib.
- Omacetaxine mepesuccinate is an option for patients resistant to ≥2 tyrosine kinase inhibitors (TKI).
- Allogeneic stem cell transplantation should be considered for eligible patients (especially younger patients or TKI-resistant cases).
- Supportive care: Transfusions for anemia, hydroxyurea for cytoreduction (temporarily), management of infections and bleeding.

Q. Blast crisis in CML.

- Blast crisis (BC) is the terminal phase of chronic myeloid leukemia. It represents transformation of CML into an acute leukemia (myeloblastic). A variety of mutations has been associated with progression to blast crisis. Mutations of the BCR-ABL tyrosine kinase domain have been observed in up to 80% of patients.
- Blast crisis can develop from days to decades after diagnosis of CML.

Clinical Features

- Sudden deterioration in a previously stable CML patient.
- Severe fatigue, pallor, weight loss.
- Fever, infections due to neutropenia.

- Bleeding/bruising due to thrombocytopenia.
- Rapidly enlarging spleen or lymph nodes.

Diagnostic Criteria (WHO)

- CML is said to be in blast crisis when any of the following is present:
  - ≥20% blasts in blood or bone marrow.
  - Presence of large clusters of blasts in bone marrow biopsy.
  - Extramedullary blast proliferation (e.g. in lymph nodes, skin, CNS).

Treatment of Blast Crisis

- Patients in myeloid blast crisis can be treated with acute myeloid leukemia (AML) induction chemotherapy regimens (daunorubicin, cytarabine and etoposide) in combination with a tyrosine kinase inhibitor; some patients can be treated with a TKI alone.
- Stem cell transplantation can also be considered at this phase.

Q. Discuss the types, clinical features, investigations, clinical staging and management of chronic lymphocytic leukemia (CLL).

- Chronic lymphocytic leukemia (CLL) is a clonal malignancy of mature B lymphocytes. It is characterized by a progressive accumulation of functionally incompetent lymphocytes which respond poorly to antigenic stimulation.
- It is the **most common leukemia** in adults, typically affecting individuals >60 years of age.

Pathophysiology

- 98% of cases of CLL are of B-cell origin (CD5+ B type lymphocytes). In 2–3% of cases, malignant lymphocytes can be of T cell origin.
- Malignant lymphocytes multiply and accumulate in the bone marrow initially and subsequently spill over to blood and infiltrate lymph nodes and lymphoid organs leading to lymphadenopathy, hepatomegaly and splenomegaly
- As CLL progresses, abnormal hematopoiesis results in anemia, neutropenia, and thrombocytopenia.
- The abnormal B lymphocytes cannot produce immunoglobulins leading to hypogammaglobulinemia and increased susceptibility to infections.

Clinical Features

- CLL is a disease of older patients, and most cases occur after the age of 50 years. Peak age is around 65 years. It is more common in western countries.
- More in males than females (2:1).
- Many patients are asymptomatic and the diagnosis is suspected when lymphocytosis is noted on routine blood testing. Others present with fatigue or lymphadenopathy.
- On examination, most patients have generalized lymphadenopathy and 50% have splenomegaly.
- Recurrent infections are common due to immunodeficiency.
- CLL usually runs a slow course, but some subtypes may behave aggressively.

Staging

- A staging system (Rai system) has been developed for CLL which is as follows:

Stage 0: Absolute lymphocytosis of >10,000/µl in blood
***Stage I*:** Lymphocytosis plus lymphadenopathy
Stage II: Lymphocytosis plus hepatomegaly or splenomegaly
Stage III: Lymphocytosis plus anemia (Hb <11 g/dl)
Stage IV: Lymphocytosis plus thrombocytopenia (<1 lakh)

Laboratory Findings

- The white blood count is usually greater than 20,000/µl and may be markedly elevated to several hundred thousand.
- The hallmark of CLL is isolated lymphocytosis. Usually more than 75% of the circulating cells are lymphocytes. Lymphocytes resemble normal small lymphocytes, but few large and activated lymphocytes may be seen.
- RBC count and platelet count is usually normal initially but may decrease in advanced disease.
- Bone marrow shows infiltration with lymphocytes.
- Immunophenotyping demonstrates B lymphocyte markers such as CD5+.
- Lymph node biopsy shows well differentiated, small, non-cleaved lymphocytes.
- Hypogammaglobulinemia is present in many patients and becomes more common with advanced disease.

Treatment

- Observation (watch-and-wait) for asymptomatic, early-stage CLL with regular monitoring every 3–6 months.
- For symptomatic patients treatment with a Bruton tyrosine kinase (BTK) inhibitors can be used. BTK inhibitors are targeted agents that block Bruton's tyrosine kinase, a key enzyme in the B-cell receptor (BCR) signaling pathway, which is crucial for B-cell survival, proliferation, and migration. Options are continuous therapy with either acalabrutinib or zanubrutinib or fixed-duration targeted therapy with venetoclax plus obinutuzumab; ibrutinib plus venetoclax; acalabrutinib plus venetoclax; or acalabrutinib plus venetoclax and obinutuzumab.
- Patients with immunosuppression and recurrent bacterial infections may benefit from prophylactic infusions of gamma globulin given every month.

Prognosis

- In the past, median survival was 6 years. However, newer therapies have improved the prognosis. Patients with stage 0 or stage I disease have a median survival of 10–15 years.
- Patients with stage III or stage IV disease have a 2-year survival of greater than 90% with newer therapies.

Q. Hairy Cell Leukemia.

- Hairy cell leukemia (HCL) is an uncommon chronic B-cell lymphoproliferative disorder. The malignant lymphocytes have characteristic hair like cytoplasmic projections on their surface, hence called hairy cell leukemia **(Fig. 6.19)**.

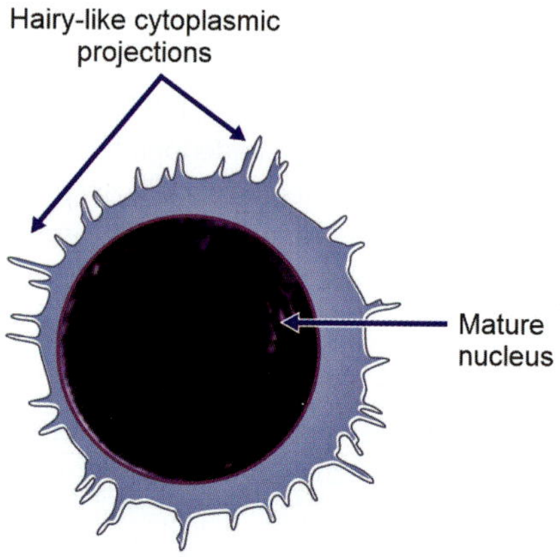

Figure 6.19: Hairy cells with cytoplasmic projections

Etiology

- The etiology of HCL is unknown, although ionizing radiation, Epstein-Barr virus, organic chemicals, woodworking, and farming have been mentioned as possible causes.

Clinical Features

- The median age at onset is 50–55.
- More common in males than females (4:1).
- Patients may present with fatigue, weakness and weight loss.
- Bleeding manifestations due to thrombocytopenia.
- Recurrent infections due to leukopenia.
- Massive splenomegaly.
- Hepatomegaly and lymphadenopathy are uncommon.

Laboratory Findings

- There is anemia, thrombocytopenia and leukopenia (pancytopenia).
- Monocytopenia (decrease in absolute monocyte count) is a distinguishing feature.
- The characteristic "hairy cells" are usually present in small numbers on the peripheral blood smear and have numerous cytoplasmic projections.
- Bone marrow is usually inaspirable (dry tap due to fibrosis), but biopsy shows hypercellular marrow and hairy cell infiltration.
- Flow cytometry shows B cell markers on malignant cells.
- BRAF V600E mutation is found in ~90% of cases. This mutation is a key molecular hallmark of classic hairy cell leukemia. It constitutively activates the BRAF kinase, leading to uncontrolled cell proliferation and survival.

Treatment

- The treatment of choice is cladribine which is a purine analog. It is given at a dose of 0.14 mg/kg daily for 7 days. Cladribine accumulates in lymphoid cells and kills them because they are rich in deoxycytidine kinase. Complete remission is seen in more than 80% of patients. Pentostatin also produces similar results, but is more cumbersome to administer.
- BRAF inhibitors (e.g. vemurafenib) for refractory or relapsed cases with BRAF mutations.
- Rituximab (anti-CD20 monoclonal antibody) used in combination or for relapsed disease.

Course and Prognosis

- With new therapies more than 95% of patients with hairy cell leukemia survive longer than 10 years.

Q. Mention the myeloproliferative disorders.

- Myeloproliferative disorders are **clonal hematopoietic stem cell disorders** characterized by **proliferation of one or more myeloid lineages** (granulocytic, erythroid, megakaryocytic) in the **bone marrow**, often with increased numbers of mature cells in the peripheral blood.
- These conditions may evolve into acute leukemia. For example, CML (also considered as a myeloproliferative disorder) may turn into AML.

Major Myeloproliferative Neoplasms (WHO Classification)

- Polycythemia vera.
- Primary (idiopathic) myelofibrosis.
- Essential thrombocytosis.
- Chronic myeloid leukemia.

Q. Define polycythemia. Enumerate the causes of polycythemia.

- Polycythemia is defined as an increase in circulating red blood cells above normal. Polycythemia is suspected when the hemoglobin is >16 g/dl in women and >16.5 g/dl in men or hematocrit >49% in men, >48% in women.
- Polycythemia may be absolute when the number of cells is actually increased or relative when the plasma volume is decreased without actual increase in absolute number of cells.

Classification and Causes of Polycythemia

Relative Polycythemia

- Definition: Apparent increase in RBCs due to plasma volume loss, not actual increase in red cell mass.
- Causes: Dehydration, burns, stress polycythemia.

Absolute Polycythemia

- Definition: True increase in red cell mass.
- Subdivided into:

Primary polycythemia

- Caused by an intrinsic bone marrow disorder.
- Example: Polycythemia Vera (PV), a myeloproliferative neoplasm, often with JAK2 V617F mutation.

Secondary polycythemia

- Due to increased erythropoietin (EPO) production. Causes are as follows:
- Hypoxia-driven: Heavy smoking, chronic lung disease (COPD), high altitude, cyanotic congenital heart disease, obstructive sleep apnea.
- EPO-producing tumors: Renal cell carcinoma, hepatocellular carcinoma, cerebellar hemangioblastoma, uterine fibroids (rarely).
- Drugs: Anabolic steroids, exogenous erythropoietin.

Q. Discuss the etiology, clinical features, diagnosis and management of polycythemia vera.

- Polycythemia vera (PV) is a myeloproliferative disorder. It is a low-grade neoplastic disorder caused by clonal proliferation of erythroid precursors.
- "Vera" means "true" in Latin, denoting that it is a primary, clonal disorder, not secondary or relative polycythemia.
- The term "polycythemia rubra vera" was earlier used which is now outdated and no longer used in formal classifications. The reason is "rubra" means "red" which indicates involvement of only RBCs, but actually all cell lines (WBCs and platelets) are also involved, hence polycythemia vera is a better term.

Etiology

- Genetic mutation: 95% of cases have the JAK2 V617F mutation. A minority have mutations in JAK2 exon 12.
- Mutation leads to activation of the JAK-STAT pathway, which causes excess cell production, independent of erythropoietin levels.

Pathology

- PV involves increased production of all cell lines, including RBCs, WBCs, and platelets.
- Increase in RBC volume increases the viscosity of the blood. Increased blood viscosity leads to thrombosis and occlusion of microcirculation in many organs.
- Hemorrhages may occur due to damage to the capillaries and also dysfunction of the platelets.
- Hyperuricemia occurs due to increased red cell turnover.
- Bone marrow is hypercellular.
- As the disease progresses, anemia and myelofibrosis develop.
- Extramedullary erythropoiesis takes place in the spleen, liver and other sites.

Clinical Features

- Usually occurs above the age of 20 years and the incidence increases with age.
- Males are affected more often.
- Initial symptoms are vague, such as headache, dizziness, tinnitus, weakness, lassitude, and fatigue.
- Thrombotic manifestations range from digital ischemia to Budd-Chiari syndrome with hepatic vein thrombosis. Abdominal thromboses are particularly common. The cerebral, retinal, cardiac and/or peripheral vessels may be the seat of vascular occlusion.
- Neurologic symptoms such as vertigo and visual disturbances may occur due to hyper viscosity.
- Hypertension is often present.
- Hyperuricemia may lead to secondary gout.
- Severe pruritus, especially after a hot bath, is a common symptom.
- Erythromelalgia (burning pain in the feet or hands accompanied by erythema, pallor, or cyanosis) is common in polycythemia and is due to microvascular thrombotic occlusions.
- Congestion and plethoric appearance of the face with congested conjunctivae.
- Splenomegaly is present in polycythemia vera but absent in secondary polycythemia.
- Fundoscopy reveals congestion of the discs, engorged veins, and hemorrhages.

Investigations

- Examination of blood reveals high Hb (>16.5 g/dl in men) or >16.0 g/dl in women), increased hematocrit and decreased ESR. There is also elevated WBCs and platelets.
- Leukocyte alkaline phosphatase is high.
- The red cell volume can be accurately estimated isotopically using 51Cr labeled erythrocytes.
- Bone marrow shows hypercellularity with normoblastic hyperplasia and prominence of megakaryocytes.
- JAK2 mutation is present in virtually all patients with PV.
- Serum erythropoietin (EPO) level is low.

Complications

- Thrombosis and hemorrhages.
- Transformation into acute myeloid leukemia, myelofibrosis or chronic myeloid leukemia.
- Cardiac failure, hypertension and secondary gout.

Treatment

- Therapy aims at keeping the blood volume normal, with the PCV around 40–45%.

Phlebotomy (first line treatment)

- This is the mainstay of therapy in polycythemia. It is the treatment of choice in women of child-bearing age and in younger patients (age <40 years). Initially about 500 ml of blood is withdrawn on alternate days to bring down the hematocrit to normal. Later on phlebotomy can be done less frequently to maintain hematocrit below 45%.

Antiplatelet Agents

- Low dose aspirin (75–100 mg/day) or clopidogrel should be given to all patients with polycythemia to prevent thrombotic events. Anagrelide also inhibits platelet aggregation and can be used if other drugs are not effective.

Cytotoxic Drugs

- Hydroxyurea is the first line agent to reduce the cell numbers without tumor-producing potential.
- Drugs like busulphan, cyclophosphamide, and chlorambucil are useful in severe cases of polycythemia vera associated with high platelet count (> 6 lakh/mm^3), massive splenomegaly, thrombotic tendency, and elderly patients especially with poor cardiovascular status.

Ruxolitinib

- Ruxolitinib is an inhibitor of JAK2 pathway and is approved for the treatment of patients who do not respond to hydroxyurea.

Allopurinol

- Is useful in patients with symptomatic hyperuricemia.

Q. Differences between primary and secondary polycythemia (Table 6.12).

TABLE 6.12: Differences between polycythemia vera and secondary polycythemia

Features	Polycythemia vera	Secondary polycythemia
Definition	Myeloproliferative disorder (clonal stem cell disorder)	A reactive increase in RBC mass due to elevated erythropoietin (EPO)
Etiology	JAK2 mutation → autonomous RBC production	Secondary to an underlying disorder producing hypoxia or EPO-secreting tumors
Cell lines affected	Increase in all cell lines (RBCs, WBCs and platelets)	Increase of only RBCs
Erythropoietin levels	Normal or decreased	Increased
Oxygen saturation	Normal	Often low in hypoxia related causes
Splenomegaly	Present	Absent
Leukocyte alkaline phosphatase	Increased	Normal
Bone marrow	Panhyperplasia	Erythroid hyperplasia only
Treatment	Phlebotomy, hydroxyurea	Mainly phlebotomy
Risk of transformation	May progress to myelofibrosis or acute leukemia	No malignant transformation risk

Q. What is myelofibrosis? Enumerate the causes of myelofibrosis.

- Myelofibrosis refers to replacement of normal bone marrow by fibrous tissue leading to pancytopenia and extramedullary hematopoiesis.
- Myelofibrosis can be primary (idiopathic) or secondary to other diseases involving bone marrow.

Causes of Myelofibrosis (Table 6.13)

TABLE 6.13: Causes of myelofibrosis

Primary myelofibrosis (idiopathic)

- A chronic myeloproliferative neoplasm
- Caused by clonal proliferation of hematopoietic stem cells

Secondary (reactive) myelofibrosis

Malignancies

- Lymphoma
- Leukemias (particularly chronic myelogenous and hairy cell)
- Multiple myeloma
- Polycythemia vera
- Essential thrombocytosis
- Malignant histiocytosis
- Myelodysplastic syndrome
- Metastatic malignancies (breast cancer, prostate cancer etc. infiltrating marrow)

Toxins

- Benzene
- Thorium dioxide
- Ionizing radiation

Infections

- Tuberculosis
- Leishmaniasis
- Fungal infections (e.g. histoplasmosis)

Autoimmune disorders (rarely)

- SLE
- Systemic sclerosis

Q. Discuss the etiology, clinical features, investigations and management of idiopathic myelofibrosis (primary myelofibrosis; agnogenic myeloid metaplasia).

- Primary myelofibrosis is a chronic myeloproliferative disorder due to genetic mutations and is characterized by fibrosis by fibrous tissue leading to pancytopenia and extramedullary hematopoiesis.
- Fibrosis occurs due to increased secretion of platelet-derived growth factor (PDGF) and other cytokines from atypical megakaryocytes in the bone marrow.
- Since bone marrow failure occurs, compensatory extramedullary hematopoiesis takes place in the liver, spleen, and lymph nodes.

Etiology

- It arises due to genetic mutations JAK2 V617F (~65%), CALR mutation (~20–25%), MPL mutation (~5–10%), and triple-negative (~10%).
- It has also been linked exposure to thorium dioxide, petroleum manufacturing plants (especially toluene and benzene), and ionizing radiation.

Clinical Features

- Usually affects adults over 50 years of age.
- Insidious onset.

- Fatigue and weakness due to anemia.
- Infections due to leukopenia.
- Bleeding manifestations due to thrombocytopenia.
- Weight loss due to hypermetabolic state.
- Abdominal fullness and early satiety due to massive splenomegaly and hepatomegaly. Painful episodes of splenic infarction may occur.
- Extramedullary hematopoiesis in the liver leads to portal hypertension with ascites, and esophageal varices.
- Bone pain due to marrow expansion.
- Gout due to high uric acid from high cell turnover.

Laboratory Findings

- Anemia is usually present.
- Total leukocyte count is variable—increase in early stages and decrease in later stages.
- The platelet count is also variable.
- ***Peripheral blood smear:*** Shows poikilocytosis and teardrop red cells. Nucleated RBCs and WBCs are present. Giant degranulated platelets may be seen. The triad of teardrop poikilocytosis, leukoerythroblastic blood, and giant abnormal platelets is highly suggestive of myelofibrosis.
- ***Bone marrow:*** Usually cannot be aspirated (dry tap). In early stages it is hypercellular with a marked increase in megakaryocytes and reticulin fibers. In later stages, biopsy shows severe fibrosis, with eventual replacement of hematopoietic precursors by collagen.
- Leukocyte alkaline phosphatase (LAP) score is elevated.

Treatment

- Patients with mild disease have excellent survival rate and require no specific therapy other than occasional blood transfusions.
- For younger patients with advanced disease allogeneic stem cell transplantation is the treatment of choice.
- If bone marrow transplantation is not possible, supportive treatment with thalidomide (improves systemic symptoms, anemia, splenomegaly, and refractory cytopenias), blood transfusions and erythropoietin (for anemia), and hydroxyurea (for splenomegaly, thrombocytosis, and leukocytosis) can be used. Etanercept also improves systemic symptoms.
- Splenectomy is indicated for splenic enlargement causing recurrent painful episodes, severe thrombocytopenia, or an unacceptable transfusion requirement.
- Inhibitors of the JAK2 pathway such as ruxolitinib have a significant effect on splenomegaly and symptoms even if there is no JAK2 mutation.

Course and Prognosis

- The median survival from time of diagnosis is approximately 5 years. Newer therapies have improved survival.
- May transform to acute myeloid leukemia (AML) in ~10–20%.

Q. Essential thrombocytosis (Essential thrombocythemia).

- Essential thrombocytosis is a myeloproliferative disorder characterized by marked proliferation of megakaryocytes in the bone marrow leading to increased platelet count.
- It is an uncommon disorder and the cause is unknown.

Clinical Features

- The median age at presentation is 50–60 years, and there is a slightly increased incidence in women.
- Patients may be asymptomatic and the disorder is often suspected when an elevated platelet count is found.
- Patients may present with thrombosis. Venous thrombosis may occur in unusual sites such as the mesenteric, hepatic, or portal vein.
- Microvascular occlusion by platelets causes symptoms such as headache, lightheadedness and erythromelalgia. Erythromelalgia is painful burning of the hands accompanied by erythema which responds to aspirin.
- Paradoxically, bleeding may occur due to qualitative platelet defect.
- Splenomegaly is present in some patients.

Laboratory Findings

- Platelet count is elevated and is usually more than ≥450,000/µl.
- The white blood cell count is often mildly elevated.
- Hemoglobin and RBC morphology is normal.
- Peripheral blood smear shows large and increased platelets.
- Bone marrow biopsy shows megakaryocytic hyperplasia.
- Secondary causes (infection, inflammation, iron deficiency, malignancy) should be excluded.

Treatment

- The risk of thrombosis can be reduced by control of the platelet count, which should be kept below 500,000/µl. The drug of choice to achieve this is ***hydroxyurea. Anagrelide*** is an alternative.
- Vasomotor symptoms such as erythromelalgia and paresthesias can be controlled by aspirin.
- Daily aspirin intake reduces the risk of thrombosis.

Course and Prognosis

- Essential thrombocytosis is an indolent disorder and long-term survival is excellent. There is a small risk of transformation into myelofibrosis or acute leukemia.

Q. Myelodysplastic Syndrome.

- The myelodysplastic syndrome (MDS) is group of disorders characterized by peripheral cytopenias, dysplasia in one or more myeloid precursors, a hypercellular or hypocellular bone marrow, and a high risk of conversion to acute myeloid leukemia.
- They were also called "preleukemia" in the past since they may evolve into AML.

Etiology

- These disorders are usually idiopathic but may arise after radiation exposure and chemotherapy. Some chromosomal abnormalities such as deletions of long arms of chromosomes 5 and 7 may be seen.

Pathology

- MDS is characterized by clonal proliferation of hematopoietic cells, including erythroid, myeloid, and megakaryocytic forms. The bone marrow is normal or hypercellular, but ineffective hematopoiesis causes anemia (most common), neutropenia, and thrombocytopenia. Ineffective hematopoiesis is also associated with morphologic cellular abnormalities in bone marrow and blood. Extramedullary hematopoiesis may occur, leading to hepatomegaly and splenomegaly.
- MDS can lead to myelofibrosis or may progress to AML.

Classification

- The classification of MDS by WHO (2022) is as follows:

MDS with defining genetic abnormalities
- MDS with isolated del(5q)
- MDS with mutated SF3B1
- MDS with biallelic TP53 inactivation

MDS, morphologically defined
- MDS with low blasts
- MDS with increased blasts

MDS/AML (Myelodysplastic/myeloproliferative overlap)
- For cases with 10–19% blasts but not meeting AML criteria.

Clinical Features

- Patients are usually over 60 years of age.
- Many patients are asymptomatic, and the condition is first suspected because of abnormal blood counts.
- Patients usually present with fatigue (due to anemia), infection (due to leukopenia), or bleeding (due to thrombocytopenia) related to bone marrow failure. The course may be indolent, and the disease may present as a wasting illness with fever, weight loss, and general debility.
- Examination reveals pallor, bleeding, and signs of infection. Splenomegaly may be present.

Laboratory Findings

- Anemia may be severe and require blood transfusion.
- *Peripheral smear:* White cell count is usually normal or reduced, and neutropenia is common. The neutrophils may exhibit morphologic abnormalities, including deficient numbers of granules or a bilobed nucleus (Pelger–Huet anomaly). Promyelocytes or blasts may be seen. The platelet count is normal or reduced.
- *Bone marrow:* Is characteristically hypercellular. Erythroid hyperplasia is common. Prussian blue stain may demonstrate ringed sideroblasts. The myeloid series is often left-shifted, with increased blasts (<20%) (≥20% = AML).

Treatment

- Anemia is treated by red blood cell transfusions. Erythropoietin injection given weekly subcutaneously reduces the red cell transfusion requirement. Lenalidomide, a thalidomide derivative, improves anemia and reduces the need for blood transfusion.
- Myeloid growth factors such as G-CSF (granulocyte colony stimulating factor) help patients with severe neutropenia.
- Azacitidine (5-azacytidine) relieves symptoms, decreases the rate of transformation to leukemia and the need for transfusions, and improves survival.
- Allogeneic stem cell transplantation is the only curative therapy for myelodysplasia.

Course and Prognosis

- Myelodysplasia is an ultimately fatal disease, and patients most commonly succumb to infections or bleeding.
- Patients with excess blasts have short survivals (usually < 2 years) and have a higher risk of developing acute leukemia.

Q. Define lymphomas.

Q. Discuss the etiology, classification, clinical features, clinical staging, investigations and management of Hodgkin's lymphoma.

- Lymphomas are malignant transformations of lymphoid cells.
- They are divided into two major types: non-Hodgkin's lymphoma (NHL) and Hodgkin's lymphoma (HL). NHL is the most common type of lymphoma.

Hodgkin's Lymphoma (HL)

- Hodgkin's lymphoma (HL) is named after the British physician who first described it. The cancer cells in Hodgkin's lymphoma are known as Reed-Sternberg cells (named after the physicians who discovered them) which are derived from B lymphocytes.

Etiology

- Exact cause is unknown, but multiple genetic, environmental, infectious, and immunological factors are believed to contribute to its development.

Infectious Agents

- Epstein–Barr virus (EBV): Found in ~40–60% of HL cases.

Genetic and Molecular Factors

- Many genetic alterations and chromosomal abnormalities are known to increase the risk of HL.
- First-degree relatives of HL patients have a higher risk.
- Concordance in monozygotic twins suggests a genetic predisposition.

Immunodeficiency

- Increased risk in individuals with HIV/AIDS, post-transplant immunosuppression, and congenital immunodeficiency syndromes.

Environmental and Lifestyle Factors

- Occupational exposures (e.g. wood dust, organic solvents) and smoking increase the risk of developing HL.

Pathological Classification

- Pathologically Hodgkin's lymphoma is divided into 4 subtypes **(Table 6.14)**.

TABLE 6.14: Classification of Hodgkin's lymphoma

Type		Incidence	Prognosis
Lymphocytic predominant	All these are types of classical Hodgkin Lymphomas, characterized by Reed-Sternberg (RS) cells	5%	Very good
Mixed cellularity		20%	Good
Nodular sclerosis		70%	Fair
Lymphocyte depleted		Rare	Poor
Nodular lymphocyte predominant Hodgkin's lymphoma (NLPHL)	This is a rare type of HL characterized by "popcorn" cells (variant RS cells)	Rare	Very good

- Nodular sclerosis is the most common type and lymphocyte depleted is the least common type.

Clinical Features

- Hodgkin's lymphoma has bimodal age distribution, with one peak in the 20s and a second over age 50 years.
- More common in males.
- The majority of patients present with overt disease, most often as an asymptomatic enlarged lymph node or a mass on chest X-ray.
- Lymphadenopathy is most often found in neck. Other sites of lymph node involvement are cervical, supraclavicular, axillary, inguinal, mediastinal and intrabdominal nodes. Involved lymph nodes are painless and non-tender with a rubbery consistency.
- Constitutional symptoms such as fever in excess of 38°C, drenching night sweats, and weight loss exceeding 10% of baseline body weight over 6 months are designated as B symptoms and indicate advanced disease. Fever is usually of low grade and irregular. Rarely, a cyclic pattern of high fevers for 1–2 weeks alternating with afebrile periods of similar duration is present at diagnosis. This fever pattern is called ***Pel-Ebstein fever*** and is virtually diagnostic of Hodgkin's lymphoma.
- Compression of various structures by tumor masses can produce many signs and symptoms. These are jaundice due to bile duct obstruction, leg swelling due to lymphatic obstruction in the pelvis or groin, dyspnea due to tracheobronchial compression, paraplegia due to compression of the spinal cord, Horner syndrome due to compression of cervical sympathetic chain by enlarged lymph nodes, hoarseness of voice due to compression of recurrent laryngeal nerves, radicular pain due to compression of nerve roots, superior vena cava obstruction due to compression by enlarged mediastinal lymph nodes, etc.
- Hepatosplenomegaly may be present.
- An unusual symptom of Hodgkin's disease is pain in an involved lymph node following alcohol ingestion (rare but characteristic).
- Patients may have a variety of nonspecific symptoms reflecting organ involvement or paraneoplastic syndromes.
- Skin manifestations such as ichthyosis, urticaria, erythema multiforme, and skin infiltration may be seen.

Staging of Hodgkin Lymphoma

- The Lugano classification **(Table 6.15)** is the current staging used for both Hodgkin's and non-Hodgkin's lymphoma. It is based on Ann Arbor classification with integration of PET-CT information to determine the extent of disease.

TABLE 6.15: Lugano classification (based on Ann Arbor classification)

Stage	Criteria
I	1 lymph region only *or* single extranodal site
II	≥2 lymph node regions on the same side of the diaphragm ± localized extralymphatic site (IIE)
III	Lymph node involvement on both sides of the diaphragm, which may include spleen or localized extranodal involvement
IV	Disseminated involvement of one or more extralymphatic organs (e.g. liver, bone marrow), with or without lymph node involvement

- In addition, patients are designated as stage A if they lack constitutional symptoms and stage B if they have constitutional symptoms (>10% weight loss over 6 months, fever, or night sweats are present).

Investigations

- Complete blood count shows normocytic normochromic anemia, normal WBC count and elevated ESR. Lymphopenia, if present is a bad prognostic factor.
- ALP may be elevated due to liver or bone involvement.
- LDH levels may be raised and indicate bad prognosis.
- Liver function tests may be abnormal due to hepatic infiltration. An obstructive pattern may be caused by enlarged nodes at the porta hepatis.
- Chest X-ray: Can show mediastinal widening due to involvement of mediastinum and lymph nodes. It can also show pericardial effusion.
- CT scan of the thorax, abdomen, and pelvis: This is used to establish the extent of disease.

- Whole-body positron emission tomography (PET scan)—is more sensitive imaging technique than CT scan to find out the extent and staging of disease. PET scan can differentiate malignant from non-malignant lesions.
- Lymph node biopsy—can establish the diagnosis of lymphoma. Presence of Reed-Sternberg cells is characteristic of Hodgkin's lymphoma.
- Bone marrow biopsy is required sometimes, if infiltration to bone marrow is suspected.
- Staging laparotomy is less commonly done now due to the availability of PET scan.

Treatment

Radiotherapy

- Radiotherapy is used as initial treatment only for patients with low-risk stage IA and IIA disease. Radiotherapy is also indicated for lesions causing serious pressure problems.

Chemotherapy

- Limited chemotherapy can be given for some patients treated with radiotherapy.
- Most patients with Hodgkin's disease (including stage III-B and IV disease) are best treated with combination chemotherapy using doxorubicin (adriamycin), bleomycin, vincristine, and dacarbazine (ABVD). Another regimen includes cyclophosphamide, vincristine, procarbazine, and prednisolone (COPP). These drugs are given every 3–4 weeks for a total of 6–8 cycles. Treatment response is assessed clinically and by repeat CT.

Autologous Stem Cell Transplantation

- Should be considered for patients who relapse after initial chemotherapy.

Combined Modality Treatment

- Radiotherapy is given after chemotherapy to sites where there was originally bulk disease.

Prognosis

- The prognosis of patients with stage IA or IIA is excellent, with 10-year survival rates in excess of 80%. Patients with disseminated disease (IIIB, IV) have poorer prognosis.

Q. Reed-Sternberg cells.

- Reed–Sternberg (RS) cells are the pathognomonic cells of classical Hodgkin lymphoma. The presence of these cells differentiates Hodgkin's from non-Hodgkin's lymphoma.
- These are large malignant lymphoid cells of B-cell origin with paired, mirror imaged nuclei (binucleate) with large nucleoli. There is a characteristic clear area around the nucleoli giving an "owl's eyes" appearance to the nuclei **(Fig. 6.20)**. They are found in affected lymph nodes.
- They are often only present in small numbers but are surrounded by large numbers of reactive normal T cells, plasma cells and eosinophils.

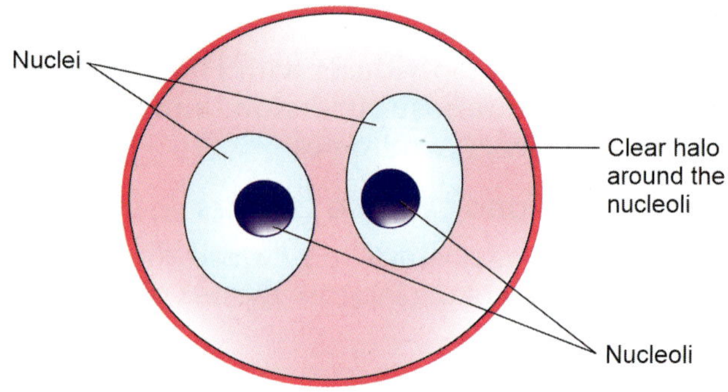

Figure 6.20: Reed-Sternberg cells

Q. Discuss the classification, clinical features, clinical staging, investigations and management of non-Hodgkin's lymphoma (NHL).

- The non-Hodgkin's lymphomas (NHL) are a heterogeneous group of cancers of lymphocytes. NHL is more common than Hodgkin's lymphoma.

Classification

WHO Classification of the Non-Hodgkin's Lymphomas

B-cell NHLs (~85%)

Aggressive (High-grade):

- Diffuse large B-cell lymphoma (DLBCL)–most common
- Burkitt lymphoma
- Primary mediastinal B-cell lymphoma

Indolent (Low-grade):

- Follicular lymphoma
- Marginal zone lymphoma
- Small lymphocytic lymphoma (SLL)
- Lymphoplasmacytic lymphoma (Waldenström's)

T-cell and NK-cell NHLs (~15%)

- Peripheral T-cell lymphoma
- Cutaneous T-cell lymphoma (e.g. Mycosis fungoides)
- Anaplastic large cell lymphoma
- Extranodal NK/T-cell lymphoma, nasal type

Etiology

- The exact etiology is unknown in most of the cases. Many risk factors have been identified which are as follows:

Immune deficiency states

- AIDS
- Ataxia telangiectasia
- Immunosuppressive therapy

Occupational and environmental exposure

- Organic solvents
- Hair dyes
- Ultraviolet rays

Infectious agents

- EBV
- HTLV-1
- HHV-8
- Hepatitis-C
- *H. pylori* (gastric lymphoma)

Pathology

- Most (80–85%) NHL arise from B cells; the remainder arise from T cells or natural killer cells. Either precursor or mature cells may be involved.
- In most cases of NHL, activation of proto-oncogenes is the major abnormality. In some cases, there may be deletion of tumor suppressor genes. For example, in Burkitt's lymphoma, there is translocation between the long arms of chromosomes 8 and 14 which causes overexpression of protooncogene c-*myc* which in turn leads to malignant transformation of lymphocytes. In the follicular lymphomas, the t(14,18) translocation results in overexpression of ***bcl-2***, resulting in decreased apoptosis and malignant transformation.

Clinical Features

- NHL is more common in men than women.
- Its incidence increases with age and is higher in whites than in other ethnic groups. Median age 65–70 years.
- Clinical presentation can be indolent to aggressive. Patients with indolent lymphomas usually present with painless enlargement in one or more of the lymph nodes, particularly in the neck, axilla, or inguinal areas. Lymph nodes in the thorax, abdomen and pelvis can be involved. Even the indolent lymphomas are usually disseminated at the time of diagnosis, and bone marrow involvement is common.
- Patients with intermediate and high-grade lymphomas may have constitutional symptoms such as fever, drenching night sweats, or weight loss (B-symptoms). Patients with Burkitt's lymphoma may complain of abdominal pain or fullness due to frequent involvement of nodes in the abdomen.
- Extranodal involvement is common in NHL and can involve any organ in the body, and there may be clinical features relating to that organ dysfunction. Examples are neurological symptoms with CNS lymphoma, breathlessness with MALT lymphomas in the lung, epigastric pain and vomiting with gastric MALT or diffuse large B-cell lymphomas, bowel obstruction with small bowel lymphomas, testicular masses with testicular lymphoma, and skin lesions with cutaneous lymphomas. SVC obstruction can occur due to mediastinal lymphadenopathy. Bone marrow involvement leads to bone marrow failure manifesting as recurrent infections, bleeding, and anemia.
- Examination reveals lymphadenopathy which is rubbery and nontender. Hepatosplenomegaly may be present.

Investigations

- Anemia is usually present.
- ESR is raised.
- Serum LDH is usually elevated.
- Chest X-ray may show a mediastinal mass due to lymph node enlargement.
- CT scan of the chest, abdomen, and pelvis, blood tests, bone marrow biopsy, and PET scan.
- Peripheral smear is usually normal.
- Bone marrow aspiration and biopsy.
- CSF cytology if CNS involvement is suspected.
- **Lymph node or tissue biopsy** is the **gold standard test** to confirm the diagnosis.
- Immunophenotyping of surface antigens to distinguish T- and B-cell tumors. This may be done on blood, marrow or nodal material.
- Genetic studies will help to find the molecular abnormality.

Lugano Staging of Non-Hodgkin's Lymphoma

- This is same as that of Hodgkin's lymphoma (*see* under Hodgkin's lymphoma).

Treatment

- Treatment depends on whether the behavior of many of these neoplasms is indolent or aggressive, localized or disseminated and the patient condition. Some lymphomas can be managed initially with observation, whereas other situations, such as spinal cord compression require emergency treatment.

Radiotherapy

- Local radiotherapy can be used for localized low grade lymphomas either alone or in combination with chemotherapy. Radiotherapy is also used as palliative therapy to treat symptomatic sites of relapse.

Chemotherapy

- Most patients require chemotherapy, either single or combinations of drugs. Common chemotherapy regimens are as follows;
  - R-CHOP = Rituximab + Cyclophosphamide + Hydroxydaunorubicin (Doxorubicin) + Oncovin (Vincristine) + Prednisone
  - BR regimen = Bendamustine + Rituximab.
- Combination chemotherapy is especially helpful in intermediate and high-grade lymphomas.

Autologous Stem Cell Transplantation

- Individuals with very high-risk lymphoma are best treated with stem cell transplantation.

Splenectomy

- Can improve cytopenias
- Palliative therapy for symptomatic splenomegaly.

Q. Enumerate the differences between Hodgkin and non-Hodgkin's lymphoma (Table 6.16).

TABLE 6.16: Differences between HL and NHL

Feature	Hodgkin's lymphoma	Non-Hodgkin's lymphoma
Peak incidence	Bimodal peak, one peak in the 20s and another peak over age 50 years.	65–70 years
Reed-Sternberg cells	Present and pathognomonic	Absent

(Contd.)

TABLE 6.16: Differences between HL and NHL *(Contd.)*

Feature	Hodgkin's lymphoma	Non-Hodgkin's lymphoma
B-symptoms	More common	Less common
Alcohol induced pain in involved lymph nodes	Yes	No
Dissemination at presentation	Well localized	Widespread
Origin	B lymphocytes and unifocal	B or T cells and multifocal
Extranodal involvement	Late	Early
Involvement of Waldeyer's ring	Uncommon	Common
Involvement of epitrochlear node	Uncommon	Common
Involvement of mediastinum	Common (especially nodular sclerosis subtype)	Uncommon
Involvement of bone marrow	Late	Early

Q. Burkitt's lymphoma.

- Burkitt's lymphoma is a highly aggressive B-cell non-Hodgkin's lymphoma (NHL).
- It often presents with extranodal disease and occurs most often in children and immunocompromised hosts.
- Epstein-Barr virus (EBV) has been implicated in the causation of disease.

Pathology

- Most cases are associated with t(8:14), translocation between chromosomes 8 and 14.
- Burkitt's lymphoma is the most rapidly growing human tumor, and pathology reveals a high mitotic rate, a monoclonal proliferation of B cells, and a "starry-sky" pattern of benign macrophages that have engulfed apoptotic malignant lymphocytes.

Clinical Features

- Three clinical forms of Burkitt's lymphoma can be recognized: endemic, sporadic, and immunodeficiency-associated.
- The endemic form presents as a jaw or facial bone tumor that spreads to extranodal sites.
- The nonendemic form has an abdominal presentation, with massive disease and ascites.
- Immunodeficiency-related cases more often involve lymph nodes.

Investigations

- Histology shows tumor cells, frequent mitotic figures and starry sky appearance.
- Chromosome analysis may show 8/14 translocation.
- Antibodies against EBV may be detected.

Treatment

- Treatment should be initiated within 48 hours of diagnosis.
- Combination chemotherapy CHOP (cyclophosphamide, hydroxydoxorubicin, oncovin, and prednisolone) or CODOX-M/IVAC (cyclophosphamide, oncovin, doxorubicin, methotrexate and ifosfamide, etoposide, VP-16 or etoposide, cytarabine).
- Intrathecal methotrexate or cytarabine for CNS prophylaxis.

Q. Mycosis fungoides.

- Mycosis fungoides is type of non-Hodgkin's lymphoma of T-cell origin with primary involvement of the skin.

Clinical Features

- It presents as a cutaneous eruption with erythematous scaly patches or plaques, often resembling eczema or psoriasis. As the disease progresses, patches may evolve into infiltrated plaques with a more generalized distribution.

Diagnosis

- Skin biopsy
- Peripheral blood smear may show atypical lymphocytes with cerebriform nuclei (Sezary cells).
- For staging, bone marrow biopsy and CT of chest, abdomen, and pelvis.

Treatment

- Topical application of steroid, retinoid, or chemotherapeutic agents (nitrogen mustard). Other skin-directed therapies include phototherapy (UVB or PUVA, *see* below), or radiation therapy (localized electron beam therapy).

Q. Hematopoietic stem cell transplantation (bone marrow transplantation).

Q. Indications and complications of hematopoietic stem cell transplantation.

- Hematopoietic stem cells (HSCs) are multipotent, self-renewing stem cells responsible for the continuous production of all blood cell lineages throughout life. They reside primarily in the bone marrow.

Sources of Hematopoietic Stem Cells

- ***Bone marrow:*** Marrow is the original source of stem cells. They are removed by bone marrow puncture.
- ***Peripheral blood:*** This has become a preferred alternative to marrow to obtain stem cells. Stem cells have to be mobilized into the peripheral blood by injecting granulocyte-macrophage colony-stimulating factor (GM-CSF).
- ***Placental blood:*** T lymphocytes in placental blood appear to be less alloreactive than T cells from adults and hence less likely to produce GVHD. Placental blood is obtained from the umbilical cord after birth.

Hematopoietic Stem Cell Transplantation (HSCT)

- HSCT is a medical procedure where hematopoietic stem cells are infused into a patient to restore bone marrow function after bone marrow has been damaged or destroyed, typically by high-dose chemotherapy or radiation.
- Hematopoietic stem cell has remarkable regenerative capacity, and can settle in the marrow space following intravenous injection.
- Transplantation of a few percent of a donor's bone marrow volume results in complete replacement of the recipient's entire lymphohematopoietic system, including red cells, granulocytes, B and T lymphocytes, and platelets, as well as cells comprising the fixed macrophage population, including Kupffer cells of the liver, pulmonary alveolar macrophages, osteoclasts, Langerhans' cells of the skin, and brain microglial cells.

Types of Bone Marrow Transplantation

Syngeneic transplantation

- Here the donor is identical twin. Advantages are there is no risk of graft-versus-host disease (GVHD) and there is no risk of contamination with tumor cells as in autologous transplantation.

Allogeneic transplantation

- Here the donor and recipient are not immunologically identical. Here the immune cells developing from the donor marrow can react against the recipient causing graft vs host disease (GVHD). Sometimes immunocompetent cells of the patient can reject the transplant. Hence both donor and recipient should be HLA matched.

Autologous transplantation

- Here patient's own stem cells are removed and stored for subsequent reinfusion after the patient receives high-dose myeloablative therapy. Unlike allogeneic transplantation, there is no risk of GVHD or graft rejection. However, autologous transplantation lacks a graft-versus-tumor (GVT) effect, and the autologous stem cell product can be contaminated with tumor cells which can lead to relapse.

Method of transplantation

- Marrow is usually collected from the donor's posterior and sometimes anterior iliac crests with the donor under general or spinal anesthesia. Hematopoietic stem cells can also be obtained from peripheral blood after giving the donor hematopoietic growth factors for 4–5 days. Umbilical cord blood contains a high concentration of hematopoietic progenitor cells, and can be used for transplantation.
- The recipient should be prepared before transplantation which involves eradication of patient's underlying disease and, immunosuppressing the patient adequately to prevent rejection of the transplanted marrow. However, if the donor is a histocompatible sibling, no treatment is required because no host cells require eradication. Eradication of host immune cells involves various regimens of busulfan, cyclophosphamide, melphalan, thiotepa, carmustine, etoposide, and total-body irradiation in various combinations.
- Typically, 10–15 ml/kg of marrow is aspirated, placed in heparinized media, and filtered to remove fat and bony spicules. Then, this marrow is infused through a large-bore central venous catheter. Cells produced by transplanted stem cells begin to appear after a week in the peripheral blood.

Indications for Stem Cell Transplantation

Malignant diseases

- Leukemias
- Lymphoma
- Myelodysplastic syndrome (MDS)
- Multiple myeloma

Nonmalignant diseases

- Immunodeficiency disorders (severe combined immunodeficiency, Wiskott-Aldrich syndrome, and Chédiak-Higashi syndrome).
- Aplastic Anemia
- Thalassemia major
- Sickle cell anemia
- Storage diseases caused by enzymatic deficiencies (Gaucher's disease, Hurler's syndrome

Complications of Bone Marrow Transplantation

- ***Due to preparatory regimens***: Infections due to immunosuppression (herpes simplex virus, cytomegalovirus, varicella-zoster virus); cardiotoxicity; hemorrhagic cystitis if high dose cyclophosphamide is used; hair loss; and pancytopena.
- GVHD (graft-versus-host disease)
- Veno-occlusive disease of the liver
- Graft failure
- Secondary malignancies.

Q. Graft-versus-host disease (GVHD).

- This is seen in allogenic bone marrow transplantation. It arises when the donor's immune cells (graft) recognize the recipient's body (host) as foreign and mount an immune response against it.

Acute GVHD

- GVHD developing within the first 100 days after transplantation is termed acute GVHD.
- Acute GVHD is characterized mainly by skin, GIT, and liver involvement. Skin manifestations include erythematous maculopapular rash; GIT involvement manifests as persistent anorexia or diarrhea, or both; and liver involvement with elevated bilirubin and liver enzymes.
- Since many conditions can mimic acute GVHD, diagnosis usually requires skin, liver, or endoscopic biopsy for confirmation. In all these organs, endothelial damage and lymphocytic infiltrates are seen. The incidence of acute GVHD is higher in recipients of stem cells from mismatched or unrelated donors and in older patients.

Chronic GVHD

- GVHD developing 100 days after transplantation is termed chronic GVHD.
- Chronic GVHD resembles an autoimmune disorder affecting multiple organs. It presents with malar rash, dry eyes, dry mouth (sicca syndrome), arthritis, restrictive lung disease, GI involvement, and bile duct degeneration and cholestasis.

Management of GVHD

- GVHD can be prevented by HLA matching and immunosuppressive prophylaxis (e.g. methotrexate, cyclosporine, tacrolimus).
- GVHD can be treated with glucocorticoids, anti-thymocyte globulin, mycophenolate, or monoclonal antibodies targeted against T cells.

Q. What are plasma cell disorders? Enumerate the plasma cell disorders.

- Plasma cell disorders are a group of diseases characterized by the abnormal proliferation of plasma cells which are immune cells derived from B lymphocytes.
- In these disorders, plasma cells produce monoclonal immunoglobulins (M-protein or paraprotein), leading to various clinical manifestations including bone lesions, renal dysfunction, anemia, and immunodeficiency.

Classification of Plasma Cell Disorders

- Monoclonal gammopathies of undetermined significance (MGUS)
- Smoldering multiple myeloma (SMM)
- Multiple myeloma
- Plasmacytoma
- Light chain (AL) amyloidosis
- Waldenstrom's macroglobulinemia
- POEMS syndrome
- Heavy-Chain diseases

Q. Discuss the etiology, clinical features, investigations and management of multiple myeloma.

- Multiple myeloma is a malignancy of plasma cells.
- It is characterized by neoplastic proliferation of a single clone of plasma cells in the bone marrow resulting in extensive skeletal destruction with osteolytic lesions, osteopenia, and/or pathologic fractures.

Risk Factors

- *Age*: Most common in adults >60 years.
- *Gender*: Slightly more common in males.
- *Race*: Higher incidence in African descent.
- *Genetic factors*: Family history, chromosomal abnormalities.
- *Environmental*: Radiation, exposure to benzene or herbicides.

Clinical Features

- Myeloma is a disease of older adults (median age at presentation, 65 years).
- Myeloma causes clinical symptoms and signs through a variety of mechanisms.
- Replacement of the bone marrow by malignant plasma cells leads to anemia initially and later pancytopenia.
- Anemia causes fatigue, exertional dyspnea, and exertional palpitations.
- Neutropenia may lead to recurrent infections.
- Low platelet count may lead to bleeding tendency.
- Bone involvement causes bone pain, osteoporosis, lytic lesions, pathologic fractures, and hypercalcemia. Bone pain is most common in the back or ribs.
- The paraproteins secreted by the malignant plasma cells (either IgG or IgA) may cause hyperviscosity manifesting as vertigo, nausea, visual disturbances, and alterations in mental status.
- The light chain component of the immunoglobulin may cause renal failure. Light chain components may be deposited in various organs as amyloid causing variety of symptoms due to organ damage.
- Examination may reveal pallor, bone tenderness, and soft tissue masses. Fever may be present due to infection. Neurologic signs related to neuropathy and spinal cord compression may be present. Features of amyloidosis such as enlarged tongue, neuropathy, congestive heart failure, or hepatomegaly may be present.
- Key clinical features can be remembered by the mnemonic **CRAB**. C = Calcium increase due to bone destruction, R = Renal dysfunction, A = Anemia, B = Bone lytic lesions.

Laboratory Features

- Normocytic normochromic anemia.
- Leukocyte count and platelet counts are usually normal initially but may be low with advanced disease.
- ESR is elevated due to increased rouleaux formation.
- Hypercalcemia, high uric acid and renal failure.
- The hallmark of myeloma is the finding of a paraprotein on serum protein electrophoresis. A M-band is typically seen in myeloma. In sporadic cases, no paraprotein is present ("nonsecretory myeloma").
- X-rays of bones may show multiple punched out (lytic) lesions. Such lesions are commonly seen in the axial skeleton: skull **(Fig. 6.21)**, spine, proximal long bones, and ribs. Sometimes only generalized osteoporosis may be seen.
- Positron emission tomography (PET) scans are useful for staging of myeloma.
- Beta-2 microglobulin level has prognostic significance in myeloma. Beta-2 microglobulin level of >4 mg/L is associated with poor prognosis.
- Bone marrow biopsy shows infiltration by morphologically abnormal plasma cells (>10% clonal plasma cells is definitive for diagnosis).
- Bone marrow cytogenetic characteristics also have prognostic significance. Deletions of chromosome 13q and the translocation t(4,14) are associated with a poor outcome.

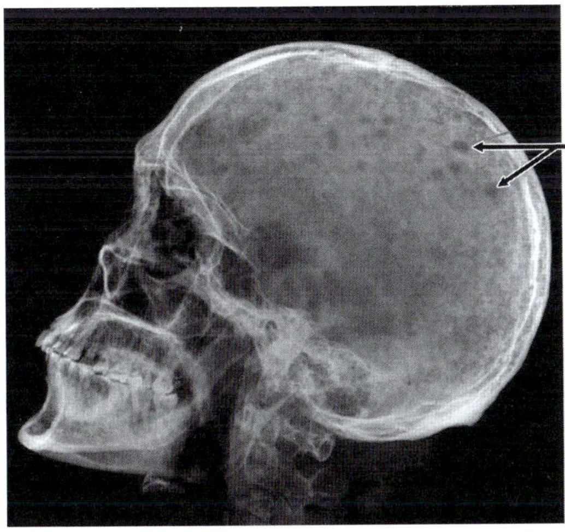

Figure 6.21: Lytic lesions in multiple myeloma

Treatment

- Asymptomatic patients with minimal disease can be observed without treatment since there is no advantage to early treatment of asymptomatic myeloma.
- Symptomatic patients may be treated with an initial triple regimen **Bortezomib + Lenalidomide + Dexamethasone (BLD).** Alternative triple regimen with less toxicity is **Daratumumab + Lenalidomide + Dexamethasone (DLD)**, preferred for transplant ineligible patients).
- Autologous stem cell transplant is offered to patients <70–75 years. Lenalidomide is commonly used post-transplant for maintenance therapy.
- Localized radiotherapy can reduce bone pain and eradicate the tumor at the site of pathologic fracture.
- Hypercalcemia can be treated with mobilization and hydration. The bisphosphonates (pamidronate 90 mg or zoledronic acid 4 mg intravenously monthly) reduce hypercalcemia and pathologic fractures.
- Blood transfusion for anemia.

Indicators of Poor Prognosis in Multiple Myeloma

- Low serum albumin
- Presence of renal failure
- Thrombocytopenia
- Age ≥70 years
- Advanced lytic bone lesions
- Beta-2-microglobulin >4 mg/L
- Hypercalcemia
- Low hemoglobin
- Bone marrow plasma cell percentage ≥50%

Q. Causes of renal failure in multiple myeloma.

- Myeloma cast nephropathy (myeloma kidney) (most common cause)
- Development of renal amyloidosis
- Renal tubular dysfunction
- Urate nephropathy due to high uric acid levels
- Recurrent urinary tract infections
- Hypercalcemia, with or without nephrocalcinosis
- Tubulointerstitial nephritis
- Plasma cell infiltration of the kidneys
- Hyperviscosity syndrome

Q. Discuss the mechanism of coagulation (hemostasis).

Q. Coagulation cascade.

Normal Hemostasis

- Hemostasis is the physiological process that stops bleeding at the site of vascular injury. It involves a complex interplay between the vascular endothelium, platelets, and the coagulation cascade. The mechanism of hemostasis occurs in three main sequential but overlapping phases:
  - Vascular phase (vasoconstriction).
  - Platelet phase (primary hemostasis).
  - Coagulation phase (secondary hemostasis).

Vascular Phase (vasoconstriction)

- Initiated immediately after injury to the blood vessel.
- Endothelial cells release endothelin, a potent vaso-constrictor → smooth muscle contraction leads to vasoconstriction, reducing blood flow to the affected area.
- Temporary reflex to minimize blood loss while other mechanisms activate.

Platelet Phase (primary hemostasis)

- Exposure of subendothelial collagen and von Willebrand factor (vWF) triggers platelet adhesion.
- Platelets adhere to collagen via vWF and glycoprotein Ib (GpIb) receptors.
- This activates platelets, causing them to change shape and release granules (e.g. ADP, thromboxane A_2) → recruit more platelets to the site → formation of the platelet plug to temporarily block the vessel breach.
- The normal hemostatic process can be divided into primary and secondary components.

Coagulation Phase (secondary hemostasis)

- Involves the coagulation cascade, a series of enzymatic reactions resulting in the formation of fibrin, which stabilizes the platelet plug. Secondary hemostasis requires several minutes for completion and is important to prevent bleeding in larger vessels and late bleeding occurring hours or days after the injury.
- The cascade is divided into:
  - Intrinsic pathway (activated by contact with sub-endothelial surfaces),
  - Extrinsic pathway (triggered by tissue factor released from damaged tissue),
  - Common pathway (where both pathways converge).

Coagulation Cascade (Fig. 6.22)

- Coagulation cascade (secondary hemostasis) involves a number of steps. Each step leads to activation of a molecule which in turn activates next molecule.

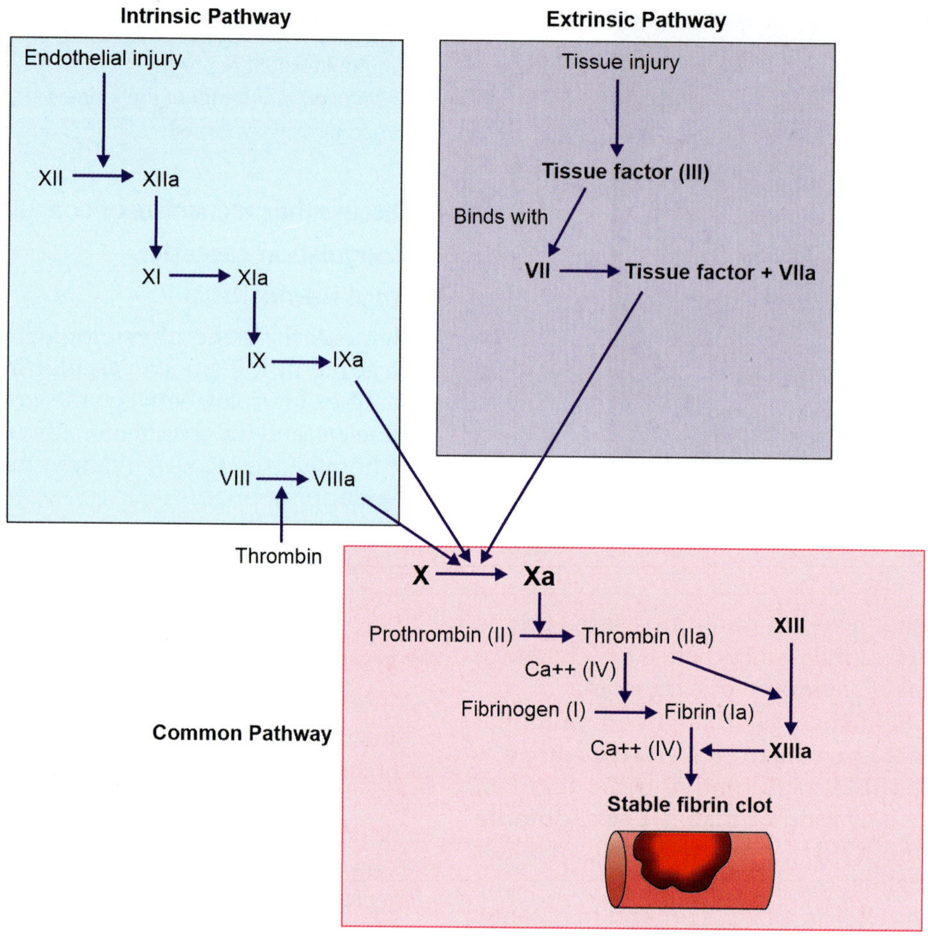

Figure 6.22: Coagulation cascade

Coagulation cascade can start by two independent activation pathways, the intrinsic pathway and extrinsic pathway (tissue factor–mediated). Both pathways merge at the point of factor X activation and subsequent steps are same for both.

Intrinsic Pathway (contact activation pathway)

- Triggered by endothelial damage which exposes blood to subendothelial collagen and negatively charged surfaces (e.g. basement membrane, phospholipids). The intrinsic pathway is called "intrinsic" because all necessary factors are present within the blood.
- Key steps:
  1. Factor XII → XIIa (activated by contact with subendothelial collagen)
  2. XIIa activates XI → XIa
  3. XIa activates IX → IXa
  4. IXa + cofactor VIIIa + Ca^{2+} + phospholipids → activate Factor X → Xa

Extrinsic Pathway (tissue factor pathway)

- Extrinsic pathway is activated by external trauma (extravascular tissue damage) due to the release of tissue factor (TF) (also called factor III). The extrinsic pathway is quick and efficient, immediately triggered by tissue injury and involves factor VII and tissue factor, which is not normally in contact with circulating blood.
- *Key steps*:
  1. Tissue factor (TF) binds with factor VII → VIIa
  2. TF-VIIa complex activates factor X → Xa

Common Pathway

- Common pathway of the coagulation cascade is the final phase shared by both the intrinsic and extrinsic pathways. It begins with the activation of Factor X and ends with the formation of a fibrin clot.
- *Key steps*:
  1. Factor X → Xa
     - Activated by either the intrinsic (via IXa + VIIIa) or extrinsic (via TF + VIIa) pathways.
  2. Factor Xa + Factor V → Prothrombinase complex
     - Calcium (Factor IV) and phospholipids are required.
     - This complex converts prothrombin (Factor II) → Thrombin (Factor IIa).
  3. Thrombin (IIa) then acts on:
     - Fibrinogen (Factor I) → Fibrin (Factor Ia)
     - Activates Factor XIII → XIIIa, which cross-links fibrin strands to stabilize the clot.

Q. Discuss the evaluation of a patient with a bleeding disorder.

OR

Q. Discuss the approach to hemorrhagic disorders.

OR

Q. How will you investigate a case of bleeding disorder?

Q. Differences between bleeding and clotting disorders.

- Bleeding disorders can result from vascular, platelet, coagulation, or fibrinolytic defects (excessive fibrinolysis). A systematic approach is essential to identify the underlying cause and initiate appropriate management.

History

The following points should be elicited from the history:

- ***Site of bleeds:*** Superficial bleeds (skin and mucous membranes) such as petechiae, purpura, gum bleeding, epistaxis, gastrointestinal hemorrhage or menorrhagia indicates a platelet disorder, thrombocytopenia, or von Willebrand disease. Deep seated bleeding such as bleed into muscle, joint, or retroperitoneum indicates a coagulation defect. Recurrent bleed at the same site indicates a local structural abnormality.
- ***Duration of history:*** Onset in childhood may suggest a coagulation defect such as hemophilia. It also suggests inherited hemostatic disorder. Recent onset suggests an acquired disorder.
- ***Precipitating causes:*** Bleeding arising spontaneously indicates a more severe defect than bleeding that occurs only after trauma.
- ***Surgery or trauma:*** Ask about all past surgeries or trauma. Bleeding from a platelet disorder usually occurs immediately after trauma or surgery, and is easily controlled by local measures (such as local pressure). Bleeding due to coagulation defects (e.g. hemophilia) occurs hours or days after injury, and cannot be controlled by local measures.
- ***Family history:*** A family history of bleeding suggests an inherited hemostatic disorder such as hemophilia. However, about one-third of cases of hemophilia arise in individuals without a family history.
- ***Systemic illnesses:*** Enquire about the presence of liver disease, renal failure, paraproteinemia or a connective tissue disease (vasculitis) which can cause bleeding.
- ***Drugs:*** Many drugs can cause bleeding either by bone marrow suppression or by inhibiting vitamin K dependent clotting factors and platelets. Examples are aspirin, clopidogrel, warfarin, etc.

Physical Examination

- Examination should note the presence of any bleeding in the skin and mucous membranes such as petechiae, ecchymoses and hematomas.
- Bleeding into body cavities, the retroperitoneum, or joints is common in coagulation disorders such as hemophilia.
- Joint deformities may be present in coagulation disorders due to recurrent bleeding.
- Hematomas can also compress nerves and lead to neurological deficits. For example, retroperitoneal hematoma can compress femoral nerve. Intracerebral bleed can lead to stroke and altered sensorium. Intracerebral bleed is the leading cause of death in hemostatic disorders.
- Look for evidence of liver disease; splenomegaly may cause thrombocytopenia due to hypersplenism.

Investigations (Table 6.17)

TABLE 6.17: Investigations done in bleeding and clotting disorders

Investigation	Normal value	Significance
Platelet count	1.5–4.5 lakh	Low in many disorders. Low count causes prolongation of bleeding time whereas PT remains normal.
Bleeding time	<8 min	Prolonged in thrombocytopenia, abnormal platelet function, and deficiency of von Willebrand factor.
Prothrombin time (PT)	12–15 seconds	PT screens the extrinsic or tissue factor–dependent pathway. PT is prolonged in deficiencies of factors II, V, VII, and X, vitamin K deficiency, and warfarin use
Activated partial thromboplastin time (APTT)	30–40 seconds	Screens the intrinsic limb of the coagulation system. APTT is prolonged in deficiencies of factors II, V, VIII, IX, X, XI, XII, heparin antibodies against clotting factors and presence of lupus anticoagulant
Fibrinogen level	1.5–4.0 g/L	Low levels found in DIC and liver disease
Thrombin time	3–5 seconds	Tests the conversion of fibrinogen to fibrin.

Differences between Primary (bleeding) and Secondary (clotting) Hemostatic Disorders (Table 6.18)

TABLE 6.18: Differences between primary and secondary clotting disorders

Features	Primary hemostatic disorder (bleeding disorder, e.g. platelet defects)	Secondary hemostatic disorder (coagulation disorder, e.g. hemophilia)
Onset of bleeding after trauma	Immediate	Delayed—hours or days
Age of onset	Late	Childhood
Sites of bleeding	Superficial: skin and mucous membranes	Deep: joints, muscle, retroperitoneum

(Contd.)

TABLE 6.18: Differences between primary and secondary clotting disorders *(Contd.)*

Features	Primary hemostatic disorder (bleeding disorder, e.g. platelet defects)	Secondary hemostatic disorder (coagulation disorder, e.g. hemophilia)
Physical findings	Petechiae, ecchymoses	Hematomas, hemarthroses
Family history	Usually absent	Usually present
Inheritance	Autosomal dominant	Autosomal or X-linked recessive
Local measures	Can control bleeding	Cannot control bleeding
PT/aPTT	Usually normal	Often prolonged (depending on the pathway affected)
Bleeding time	Prolonged	Normal

Q. Define thrombocytopenia. Discuss the causes, clinical features, investigations and management of thrombocytopenia.

Q. Tourniquet test (capillary resistance test; Hess test).

- Thrombocytopenia is defined as a platelet count less than 150,000/µl (normal 150,000–450,000).

Causes of Thrombocytopenia

Decreased production

- Aplastic anemia
- Marrow infiltration: Leukemia, lymphoma, myeloma, metastasis, myelofibrosis, osteopetrosis
- Myelodysplasia
- Nutritional: Vitamin B_{12} and folic acid deficiency
- Chronic alcoholism
- Infections : HIV, hepatitis B/C, EBV, parvovirus
- Drugs : Anticancer drugs, antimetabolites

Increased destruction

- Idiopathic thrombocytopenic purpura (ITP)
- HELLP syndrome (hemolytic anemia, elevated liver function tests, and low platelet count) in pregnant women
- Secondary (CLL, SLE)
- Hypersplenism
- Disseminated intravascular coagulation (DIC)
- Thrombotic thrombocytopenic purpura
- Hemolytic-uremic syndrome
- Sepsis
- Infections (dengue, HIV)
- Drugs (heparin, quinine, sulfonamides)

Dilutional

After massive blood transfusion

Clinical Features

- Bleeding manifestations may not occur until the platelet count falls below 10,000/µl.
- Patients present with bleeding manifestations from cutaneous and mucus membranes.
- Cutaneous bleeding manifestations include petechiae, purpura, ecchymosis, epistaxis, and gum bleeding.
- Mucosal bleeding presents with epistaxis, GI bleed (hematemesis and melena), genitourinary bleeding. Women may present with menorrhagia.
- Intracranial bleeding can occur in severe thrombocytopenia and cause death.
- ***Tourniquet test (Hess test):*** A sphygmomanometer cuff is tied around the arm and inflated above diastolic blood pressure but below systolic pressure. Cuff is deflated after 5 minutes. In thrombocytopenia, petechial spots appear in the forearm. More than 10 petechial spots in a square inch area is considered positive Hess test. It is due to the increased capillary fragility in thrombocytopenia.

Investigations

- Low platelet counts
- Anemia may be present due to blood loss
- Prolonged bleeding time
- Peripheral smear: This gives information on morphology of cells, presence or absence of platelet clumping, etc. Peripheral smear can also diagnose diseases such as leukemia.
- Bone marrow examination: This may show aplasia, an infiltrative disease, or increased number of megakaryocytes in excessive peripheral destruction (e.g. in ITP).
- Other tests: should be directed at the suspected cause. HIV serology, liver function tests, ultrasound abdomen to look for splenomegaly, etc. are helpful.

Management

- Treat the underlying cause.
- Avoid drugs that impair platelet function (NSAIDs, aspirin).
- Platelet transfusion is required in the following situations:
  - Active bleeding with platelet count <50,000/µl
  - Platelet count <10,000/µl without bleeding (to prevent spontaneous hemorrhage)
  - Before invasive procedures/surgery if <50,000/µl.

Q. Heparin-induced thrombocytopenia (HIT).

- Heparin-induced thrombocytopenia (HIT) is a serious, immune-mediated adverse reaction to heparin therapy, characterized by thrombocytopenia and a prothrombotic state (paradoxically, increased risk of thrombosis despite low platelets). HIT is the most common type of drug-induced thrombocytopenia.

Types of HIT

- There are two types of HIT. Type 1 and type 2 HIT.
- Type 1 HIT presents within the first 2 days after exposure to heparin, and the platelet count normalizes even with continued heparin therapy. Type 1 HIT

is non-immune mediated reaction and is due to the direct effect of heparin on platelet activation.

- Type 2 HIT is an immune-mediated disorder that typically occurs 4–10 days after exposure to heparin. It is caused by an IgG autoantibody that reacts with platelet factor 4 (PF4) on the platelet surface, usually in a complex with heparin. The interaction of the antibody with PF4 is prothrombotic due to the release of platelet microparticles into the circulation. Because of prothrombotic state, arterial and venous thrombosis may occur. In general medical practice, the term HIT refers to type 2 HIT.
- The risk of HIT is higher with unfractionated heparin than with low-molecular-weight heparin. It is seen usually after 5–10 days of heparin use and often the first finding is asymptomatic thrombocytopenia.

Diagnosis

- HIT should be suspected in any patient who develops thrombocytopenia while receiving heparin. Finding HIT antibodies confirms the diagnosis.

Treatment

- Heparin should be immediately stopped and alternative anticoagulants should be started.
- Fondaparinux does not cause HIT and can be used instead of heparin. The direct thrombin inhibitors (such as argatroban and bivalirudin) or rivaroxaban can also be used as alternatives to heparin.

Q. Describe the etiology, clinical features, diagnosis and management of immune thrombocytopenic purpura (ITP).

- Immune thrombocytopenic purpura (ITP) is an autoimmune disorder characterized by isolated thrombocytopenia due to the presence of an IgG autoantibody against platelets.

Etiology

- ITP is due to development of antibodies to one's own platelets, usually triggered by a preceding infection. Any infection can trigger antibody production but common cause is viral infections. Common causes are as follows.

- Primary ITP: No identifiable cause.
- Infections: HIV, HCV, EBV, Helicobacter pylori
- Lymphoproliferative diseases: Chronic lymphocytic leukemia (CLL), lymphoma
- Autoimmune diseases: SLE, antiphospholipid syndrome
- Drugs: Acetazolamide, aspirin, carbamazepine, phenytoin, methyldopa.

Pathogenesis

- Antibody bound platelets are destroyed in the spleen, where splenic macrophages with Fc receptors bind to antibody-coated platelets. Since the spleen is the major site both of antibody production and platelet destruction, splenectomy is highly effective therapy for ITP.

Clinical Features

- ITP is a disease of young. Peak incidence is between ages 20 and 50 years.
- Females are more commonly affected than males.
- Patients present with mucosal or skin bleeding. Common types of bleeding are epistaxis, oral bleeding, menorrhagia, purpura, and petechiae. Intracerebral bleed can be fatal in these patients.
- On examination, patient appears well. Bleeding manifestations such as petechiae and purpura may be noted. In ITP, usually there is no splenomegaly and presence of splenomegaly should make one suspect an alternative diagnosis.

Laboratory Features

- The hallmark of the disease is thrombocytopenia.
- Bleeding time is prolonged due to low platelets but clotting time is normal.
- Other counts are usually normal except for occasional mild anemia due to bleeding.
- Peripheral smear is normal except reduced platelets.
- Antiplatelet antibodies are usually positive (not routinely useful due to low specificity).
- Bone marrow is normal except increased number of megakaryocytes.
- Tests to rule out any underlying triggering cause such as HIV ELISA, IgG antibodies against *H. pylori*, ANA and anti dsDNA (to rule out SLE).

Differential Diagnosis

- Thrombotic thrombocytopenic purpura (TTP)
- DIC
- Gestational thrombocytopenia
- Drug induced thrombocytopenia
- Infections (e.g. dengue, HIV)
- Hypersplenism
- Myelodysplasia
- Congenital thrombocytopenias
- Acquired pure megakaryocytic aplasia

Treatment

- Few patients may have spontaneous remission, but most will require treatment.

Platelet Transfusions

- Platelet transfusions are given if the platelet count is below 10,000/µl because spontaneous bleeding can occur below this level. However, even these exogenous platelets are destroyed and the effect lasts only a few hours. Platelet transfusion should be reserved for cases of life-threatening bleeding in which even fleeting hemostasis may be of benefit.

Steroids

- Prednisolone 1–2 mg/kg/day acts by decreasing the affinity of splenic macrophages for antibody-coated platelets. It also reduces the production of antibody and binding of antibody to the platelet surface. Platelet count will usually begin to rise within a week, and responses are almost always seen within 3 weeks. Steroids are continued until the platelet count is normal, and the dose should then be gradually tapered. Dexamethasone can also be used.

Immunoglobulin Therapy

- Used for rapid rise in platelet count in emergencies.
- Intravenous immunoglobulin (IVIG), 1 g/day for 3–5 days, is highly effective in raising the platelet count.
- IVIG works by blocking Fc receptors on macrophages, thereby inhibiting phagocytosis. However, this treatment is expensive, and it should be reserved for bleeding emergencies. A less expensive alternative is Rho immunoglobulin (RhIG) which is anti-Rh antibody. Mechanism of action is same as that of IVIG.

H. pylori Eradication

- *H. pylori* infection also has been implicated in many cases of ITP. Testing and eradicating *H. pylori* infection can cure many cases of ITP.

Splenectomy

- Splenectomy is indicated if patients do not respond to other therapies such as steroids or immunoglobulin.

Other Therapies

- These are tried if the patient does not respond to above therapies.
  - Danazol.
  - Immunosuppressive agents (vincristine, azathioprine, cyclosporine, and cyclophosphamide).
  - Rituximab.
  - High-dose immunosuppression and autologous stem cell transplantation.
  - Thrombopoietin receptor agonists, such as romiplostim and eltrombopag stimulate platelet production.

Prognosis

- Prognosis is good and most patients will recover with medical line of management. Patients may die due to intracranial hemorrhage.

Q. Thrombotic thrombocytopenic purpura (TTP).

- Thrombotic thrombocytopenic purpura (TTP) is rare, life threatening disorder characterized by thrombocytopenia, microangiopathic hemolytic anemia, and organ dysfunction due to widespread microvascular thrombosis.

Etiology and Pathogenesis

- TTP is caused by **deficient activity** of the plasma enzyme **ADAMTS13** which cleaves large von Willebrand factor into smaller sizes. Reduced activity of ADAMTS13 enzyme leads to accumulation of unusually large von Willebrand factor (VWF) multimers which cause platelet aggregation and microthrombi formation.
- Deficiency of enzyme ADAMTS13 can be due to hereditary or acquired factors. Most cases are acquired due to an autoantibody against ADAMTS13.
- There is formation of widespread microthrombi which occlude small blood vessels. These microthrombi are mainly made of von Willebrand factor and platelets. When RBCs pass through these occluded blood vessels, they get lysed because of shear forces leading to hemolytic anemia. Occlusion of blood vessels also leads to ischemia and multiple organ dysfunction. Platelet count becomes low as they get used up in microthrombi formation. The brain, heart, and kidneys are particularly likely to be affected.

Clinical Features

- Thrombocytopenia leads to bleeding tendency manifesting as mucosal bleeding as well as petechial or purpuric skin spots.
- Anemia (due to microangiopathic hemolysis) leads to fatigue, pallor, and jaundice.
- Microthrombi cause ischemia and dysfunction of multiple organs. Brain dysfunction can present as headache, stroke, seizures, confusion, and vertigo. Renal involvement presents as hematuria and/or proteinuria and rarely as renal failure. Mesenteric ischemia symptoms include abdominal pain, nausea, vomiting, and diarrhea.
- There may be history suggestive of an infection few days before the onset of above symptoms (such as fever, malaise, body ache, diarrhea).

Diagnosis

- Typical clinical features
- Low plasma ADAMTS13 enzyme level
- Presence of thrombocytopenia and anemia
- Presence of schistocytes in peripheral smear suggesting microangiopathic hemolytic anemia
- Normal clotting tests.

Differential Diagnosis

- Hemolytic uremic syndrome (HUS): This is now considered as a different entity from TTP.
- Immune thrombocytopenia (ITP)
- Disseminated intravascular coagulation (DIC)
- Preeclampsia and eclampsia in pregnant ladies.

Treatment

- Untreated thrombotic thrombocytopenic purpura is usually fatal (up to 90% mortality).
- Daily **plasma exchange**: First-line and **lifesaving treatment.** It removes autoantibodies and replenishes ADAMTS13 levels. May be required for several days to many weeks.
- Corticosteroids can be used with plasma exchange.
- Rituximab is useful when there is recurrence after when plasma exchange is stopped or in patients with relapses.

- Caplacizumab (anti-vWF agent) inhibits the interaction between unusually large von Willebrand factor multimers and platelets and can be considered in patients refractory to plasma exchange and/or corticosteroids.

Q. Hemolytic-uremic syndrome (HUS).

- Hemolytic-uremic syndrome (HUS) is an acute, fulminant disorder characterized by thrombocytopenia, microangiopathic hemolytic anemia, and acute kidney injury.
- HUS usually occurs in children following an infection, typically with Shiga toxin–producing bacteria (e.g. Escherichia coli O157:H7), but may also occur in adults.
- Note that even though most of the clinical features are similar to TTP, HUS and TTP are different entities because their etiology and pathogenesis is different.

Etiology

- Acute hemorrhagic colitis due to shiga toxin–producing bacteria (e.g. *Escherichia coli* O157:H7, or some strains of Shigella dysenteriae) is the most common cause. Occasionally the cause is pneumococcal infection and rarely HIV infection.
- Small minority of cases may be due to dysregulation of the complement system.

Pathophysiology

- HUS typically develops after consuming undercooked beef or unpasteurized milk which is contaminated with causative bacteria. The Shiga toxin formed by the *E. coli* in the intestine is absorbed into the blood stream. The toxin then binds to glycosphingolipid found on different cells of the body. The damage that ensues leads to an increase in thrombin and fibrin levels resulting in microthrombi. These microthrombi lead to platelet consumption, causing thrombocytopenia. Microthrombi present in the blood vessel also lead to mechanical shear stress leading to hemolytic anemia. The Shiga toxin also has a high affinity to glomerular endothelium and tubular cells, and causes acute kidney injury.
- Multiple organs develop damage due to microthrombi in addition to kidneys. These include brain, heart, and intestines.

Clinical Features

- There may be H/o of vomiting, abdominal pain, and bloody diarrhea indicating infection with shiga toxin producing bacteria.
- Brain involvement produces weakness, confusion, and seizures.
- Kidney injury may produce hematuria, decreased urination or anuria, and/or hypertension.
- Gastrointestinal tract ischemia (due to mesenteric ischemia) may cause hemorrhagic colitis, with abdominal pain, nausea, vomiting, and bloody diarrhea. Note that same GI symptoms may also occur even prior to the development of HUS due to Shiga toxin producing bacteria.
- Cardiac involvement may cause arrhythmias.
- Thrombocytopenia may produce bleeding manifestations.

Investigations

- Complete blood count (CBC) shows thrombocytopenia and anemia.
- Peripheral blood smear may show fragmented RBCs (schistocytes) due to microangiopathic hemolysis.
- Direct antiglobulin (Coombs') test is negative and excludes autoimmune hemolytic anemia.
- LDH is elevated.
- Prothrombin time (PT), and aPTT are normal (these will be elevated in DIC).
- Plasma ADAMTS13 enzyme activity is helpful to exclude TTP (low levels are found in TTP).
- Renal function tests (urea, creatinine) may show evidence of kidney injury.
- Liver function tests (LFT) show raised indirect bilirubin due to hemolysis.
- Stool testing for Shiga toxin and stool culture for *E. coli* O157:H7.

Treatment

- Hemodialysis for renal failure
- Blood transfusion for anemia
- Platelet transfusion only if there is active b bleeding.
- Antibiotics are usually not required as the disease is self-limiting.
- In patients with HUS due to complement dysregulation, complement inhibition with eculizumab or ravulizumab can help.

Q. Discuss the etiology, clinical manifestations, investigations and management of von-Willebrand's disease.

Q. von-Willebrand's factor.

- von Willebrand's disease is the most common inherited bleeding disorder caused by quantitative or qualitative defects in von Willebrand's factor (vWF).
- It is transmitted in an autosomal dominant pattern. Rarely it can be acquired also.

Etiology

- von Willebrand's disease is due to deficient or defective von Willebrand factor (VWF).
- VWF is important for platelet adhesion to subendothelium. VWF is synthesized by megakaryocytes and endothelial cells. The gene for von Willebrand's factor is located on chromosome 12.
- VWF also acts as a carrier for factor VIII in the circulation, increasing the half-life of factor VIII. Hence, in von Willebrand's disease, there may be secondary coagulation disturbance due to decreased levels of factor VIII.

Clinical Features

- von Willebrand's disease affects both men and women.
- Most cases are mild.
- Patients present with mucocutaneous bleeding; Easy bruising, epistaxis, gingival bleeding, menorrhagia.
- Severe disease may present with hemarthroses and deep muscle hematomas (like in hemophilia).
- Some patients may come to attention because of excessive bleeding after surgical incisions or dental extractions. Bleeding tendency is exacerbated by aspirin.
- Characteristically, bleeding decreases during pregnancy or estrogen use.

Investigations

- Bleeding time is prolonged in the presence of normal platelet count.
- Defective or absent platelet aggregation.
- Levels of von Willebrand's factor in plasma are reduced.
- Ristocetin cofactor test is the most specific and shows decreased biological activity of VVF.
- Factor VIII levels are often reduced in vWD.

Management

- Since the bleeding is mild, no treatment is necessary except before surgery or dental procedures.
- Desmopressin acetate (DDAVP) can increase the vWF levels by two to threefold by releasing stored vWF from endothelial cells. It can be given before surgery or dental procedures.
- The antifibrinolytic agent epsilon amino caproic acid (EACA) is useful as adjunctive therapy during dental procedures. It is given after DDAVP.
- Avoid aspirin/NSAIDs.

Q. Discuss the etiology, clinical features, investigations and management of Hemophilia-A.

- Hemophilia-A (classic hemophilia) is a hereditary bleeding disorder due to deficiency of coagulation factor VIII.
- Most of the cases are due to quantitative reduction of factor VIII. However a small number of cases are due to qualitative defect in factor VIII.
- Antenatal diagnosis can be made by chorionic villous sampling or amniocentesis.

Pathogenesis

- ***Factor VIII (antihemophilic factor)*** is a large (265-kDa) single-chain protein that regulates the activation of factor X by proteases generated in the intrinsic pathway. Hence deficiency of factor VIII leads to defective coagulation and bleeding.
- Factor VIII is synthesized in liver and circulates in the blood. von Willebrand's factor (vWF) factor acts as a carrier of factor VIII in blood.
- Hemophilia is caused by mutations in F8 gene on X chromosome which codes for factor VIII. Since hemophilia is an X-linked recessive disease, males are usually affected. One in 10,000 males is born with deficiency or dysfunction of the factor VIII molecule. However, rarely, female carriers can be affected if their normal X chromosome is also disproportionately inactivated. Females may also become affected if their father is a hemophiliac and mother is a carrier.
- Hemophilia is classified as mild, moderate and severe based on the residual factor VIII activity in the blood.
  - **Severe** (<1% activity): Spontaneous bleeding into joints, muscles, and internal organs.
  - **Moderate** (1–5%): Bleeding after minor trauma.
  - **Mild** (6–40%): Bleeding after major trauma or surgery.

Clinical Features

- Hemophilia-A is the second most common hereditary hemostatic disorder after von Willebrand's disease. It is a severe clotting disorder.
- Family history of hemophilia is usually positive.
- The bleeding tendency is related to factor VIII levels. Patients with mild hemophilia bleed only after major trauma or surgery, those with moderately severe hemophilia bleed with mild trauma or surgery, and those with severe disease bleed spontaneously.
- Bleeding can occur anywhere but commonly occurs in deep tissues such as joints (knees, ankles, elbows), muscles, and from GIT.
- Bleeding into joints (hemarthrosis) is common in hemophilia-A and is almost diagnostic of the disorder. Recurrent bleeding into joints leads to joint destruction and joint deformities.
- Intracranial hemorrhage can occur in severe cases.
- Earlier when HIV screening of donor blood was not widely adopted, many hemophiliacs got infected with HIV due to factor VIII transfusion and many of these have already developed AIDS. However this is uncommon now due to universal screening of donor blood.

Investigations

- Activated partial thromboplastin time (aPTT) is prolonged.
- Normal prothrombin time (PT), bleeding time, and platelet count.
- Factor VIII levels are reduced.
- Genetic testing for F8 gene mutations (for diagnosis and carrier detection).

Treatment

- Treatment of hemophilia-A involves infusion of factor VIII concentrates, either recombinant or heat treated.
- In minor bleeding, it is enough if the factor VIII levels are raised to 25% of normal. For moderate bleeding, levels should be kept above 25% of normal. When major surgery is to be performed, factor VIII level should be raised to 100% and then maintained above 50% for 10–14 days.
- For mild hemophilia, DDAVP (desmopressin) is enough for minor surgeries. It causes release of stored factor VIII and will raise the factor VIII levels two- to threefold for several hours.

- EACA (epsilon amino caproic acid) may be added if bleeding persists after treating with factor VIII and desmopressin.
- Fresh frozen plasma can be used if factor VII concentrate is not available.
- Emicizumab is a monoclonal antibody that mimics factor VIII function, and may be an effective treatment for hemophilia-A.
- Gene therapy is currently in the developmental phase.
- Avoid the use of aspirin in these patients.
- Patients with hemophilia should be vaccinated against hepatitis B.

Prognosis

- Prognosis is good now because of the availability of factor VIII concentrates. Intracerebral hemorrhage is the usual cause of death but uncommon.

Q. Factor VIII (antihemophilic factor).

- Factor VIII also known as antihemophilic factor A is a crucial blood-clotting protein, which plays a key role in the intrinsic pathway of the coagulation cascade.

Function

- Acts as a cofactor for factor IXa, which, in the presence of calcium and phospholipids, activates factor X to Xa–a critical step in the formation of a stable fibrin clot.

Physiology of Factor VIII

- Factor VIII is produced primarily in the liver sinusoidal endothelial cells (not hepatocytes).
- Circulates in plasma bound to von Willebrand factor (vWF), which protects it from degradation.
- It is activated by thrombin (factor IIa) during coagulation. After activation, it dissociates from vWF and participates in the formation of the tenase complex (VIIIa-IXa complex).
- Half-life is approximately 8–12 hours, but varies depending on the formulation in replacement therapy.

Deficiency of Factor VIII

- Causes hemophilia A, a clotting disorder with varying severity depending on the residual activity level of factor VIII: severe <1%, moderate: 1–5%, mild 6–40%.

Therapeutic use of Factor VIII

- Replacement therapy: Recombinant or plasma-derived factor VIII concentrates are used for treatment and prophylaxis of bleeding episodes in hemophilia A.

Q. Discuss the etiology, clinical features, investigations and management of hemophilia B (Christmas disease).

- Hemophilia B (Christmas disease) is a hereditary bleeding disorder due to deficiency of coagulation factor IX. It is sometimes called Christmas disease, named after Stephen Christmas, the first patient diagnosed with this disease. Inheritance is same as hemophilia-A (X-linked recessive). Caused by mutations in the F9 gene, located on the X chromosome.
- Most cases are due to reduced levels of factor IX but some cases may be due to qualitative defect in factor IX.
- Factor IX deficiency is less common than factor VIII deficiency but is otherwise clinically and genetically identical.

Clinical Features

- Same as hemophilia-A, but less severe.

Investigations

- Factor IX levels are reduced.
- Other laboratory features are same as factor VIII deficiency.

Treatment

- Transfusion of factor IX concentrates. Recombinant factor IX is available now.
- Fresh frozen plasma can be used in emergencies if factor IX concentrate is not available.
- DDAVP is not useful in this disorder.
- Aspirin should be avoided.

Prognosis

- Slightly better prognosis than hemophilia A, but the difference is not dramatic.

Q. Anticoagulants (coagulation inhibitors).

Q. Indications of anticoagulation

- Anticoagulants are medications that prevent or reduce blood coagulation, thereby decreasing the risk of thrombosis (formation of abnormal blood clots). They are widely used in clinical practice for preventing and treating thromboembolic disorders.

Anticoagulants (Table 6.19)

TABLE 6.19: Anticogulants

Class	Examples	Mechanism of action
Heparins	Heparin, LMWH (low molecular weight heparins)	Activate antithrombin III; inhibit thrombin and Xa
Vitamin K antagonists	Warfarin	Inhibit synthesis of Factors II, VII, IX, X (vitamin K–dependent)
Direct thrombin inhibitors	Dabigatran	Directly inhibit thrombin (Factor IIa)
Direct factor Xa inhibitors	Rivaroxaban, Apixaban	Inhibit activated Factor X
Indirect factor Xa inhibitor	Fondaparinux	Indirect Factor Xa inhibitor via antithrombin
Thrombolytics (fibrinolytics)	Alteplase, Streptokinase	Not true anticoagulants; dissolve fibrin clots

Indications of Anticoagulation

- Prophylaxis and treatment of deep vein thrombosis.
- Pulmonary embolism.
- Acute coronary syndrome.
- Atrial fibrillation (to prevent cardioembolic stroke).
- Patients with prosthetic heart valves.
- Procoagulant states.
- Prevention of clotting during dialysis, ECMO, etc.

Monitoring (Table 6.20)

TABLE 6.20: Monitoring of anticoagulation

Drug	Monitoring required	Test
Heparin (UFH)	Yes	aPTT
LMWH	No (except in renal impairment/ pregnancy)	Anti-Xa assay
Warfarin	Yes	PT/INR
DOACs	No routine monitoring (may need in emergencies)	Specific drug-level assays or anti-Xa

Adverse Effects

- Bleeding (most common and serious)
- HIT (heparin induced thrombocytopenia with unfractionated heparin)
- Osteoporosis (with long-term heparin)
- Hypersensitivity reactions.

Reversal Agents

Anticoagulant	Reversal agent
Warfarin	Vitamin K, FFP, PCC
Heparin	Protamine sulfate
LMWH	Partial reversal with protamine
Dabigatran	Idarucizumab
Rivaroxaban, Apixaban	Andexanet alfa, PCC

Q. Newer oral anticoagulants (NOACs).

- Also called direct oral anticoagulants (DOACs), these agents directly inhibit specific clotting factors and have transformed the management of thromboembolic disorders. These are as follows.

Classification of NOACs

Class	Drugs
Direct thrombin inhibitor	Dabigatran
Direct factor Xa inhibitors (Note that the names of these drugs contain 'xa' and 'ban' which means they block the action of Xa)	Rivaroxaban Apixaban Edoxaban Betrixaban

Advantages Over Warfarin

- Fixed dosing (no need for routine monitoring).
- Rapid onset and offset of action.
- Fewer food and drug interactions.
- Lower risk of intracranial hemorrhage.
- No need for bridging with heparin in most cases.

Clinical Uses

- Non-valvular atrial fibrillation (for stroke prevention).
- Treatment and prevention of DVT/pulmonary embolism.
- Postoperative thromboprophylaxis (e.g. after hip/ knee surgery).
- Some are being investigated for use in coronary artery disease and cancer-associated thrombosis.

Limitations

- Not suitable for patients with mechanical heart valves or severe mitral stenosis.
- Caution in renal impairment, especially with dabigatran.
- Short half-life: Non-adherence increases thrombotic risk quickly.
- Cost: Higher than warfarin.
- Limited options for monitoring in case of bleeding or surgery (though assays are being developed).

Q. Low-molecular weight heparins (LMWHs).

- Low-molecular weight heparins (LMWHs) are anticoagulants derived from standard (unfractionated) heparin by depolymerization, resulting in shorter chains. They inhibit clot formation mainly by inhibiting factor Xa, with less effect on thrombin (factor IIa).
- Common LMWH agents: Enoxaparin, dalteparin, tinzaparin

Mechanism of Action

- LMWHs bind to antithrombin (AT) and enhance its activity.
- This inhibits factor Xa (primary action) and factor IIa (thrombin) (minor action).
- Unlike unfractionated heparin (UFH), LMWHs have a higher anti-Xa:anti-IIa ratio (about 3–5:1).

Advantages of LMWHs over Unfractionated Heparin

- LMWHs have more predictable anticoagulant effect due to better bioavailability.
- Allows for fixed dosing without the need for continuous aPTT monitoring in most patients.
- Longer half-life allows for once or twice daily dosing, compared to the continuous IV infusion or frequent injections required for UFH. This improves convenience, especially in outpatient or home settings. patients.
- Lower risk of heparin-induced thrombocytopenia (HIT).
- LMWHs are associated with less risk of osteoporosis in long-term use compared to UFH.

Disadvantages of LMWHs Compared to Unfractionated Heparin

- LMWH is renally excreted, hence it accumulates in renal impairment. UFH is safer in patients with severe renal dysfunction as it is cleared by the reticulo-endothelial system.

- Protamine sulfate only partially reverses the effect of LMWH (60–70%), whereas UFH effect can be fully reversed by protamine.
- Due to longer half-life and fixed dosing, LMWH cannot be easily adjusted once given, whereas UFH allows rapid titration and quick cessation (important in procedures or bleeding events).

Clinical Uses

- Prevention and treatment of venous thromboembolism (VTE):
  - Deep vein thrombosis (DVT)
  - Pulmonary embolism (PE)
- Acute coronary syndromes (e.g. NSTEMI, unstable angina)
- Bridging anticoagulation during perioperative warfarin interruption
- Anticoagulation in pregnancy
- Cancer-associated thrombosis

Dosing

- Enoxaparin example: for DVT prophylaxis → 40 mg SC once daily. For DVT treatment or acute coronary syndrome 1 mg/kg SC every 12 hours.

Monitoring

- Routine monitoring not required in most cases.

Side Effects

- Bleeding (most common)
- Thrombocytopenia (rare, but possible in HIT)
- Injection site hematoma or pain
- Osteoporosis (long-term use)
- Renal accumulation in impaired function.

Contraindications

- Active bleeding
- History of heparin-induced thrombocytopenia (HIT)
- Severe renal failure (use with caution)
- Major bleeding risk (e.g. recent hemorrhagic stroke).

Reversal of Effect

- No specific antidote with complete reversal
- Protamine sulfate partially reverses LMWH (about 60–70% efficacy)
- Severe bleeding: Stop LMWH, consider protamine, supportive care, and transfusion.

Q. Discuss the etiology, clinical features, investigations and management of disseminated intravascular coagulation (DIC; comsumptive coagulopathy)

- Disseminated intravascular coagulation (DIC) is a life threatening condition characterized by widespread intravascular coagulation associated with increased consumption of platelet and clotting factors.
- DIC involves abnormal, excessive generation of thrombin and fibrin in the circulating blood. During the process, increased platelet aggregation and consumption of coagulation factors occur resulting in **simultaneous risks of thrombosis and severe bleeding**.
- DIC produces both thrombosis and hemorrhage. DIC that evolves slowly (over weeks or months) causes primarily venous thrombotic and embolic manifestations; DIC that evolves rapidly (over hours or days) causes primarily bleeding.

Etiology of DIC

- DIC usually results from exposure of tissue factor to blood, initiating the coagulation cascade. DIC most often occurs in the following circumstances.

- Sepsis (especially gram-negative infections)
- Severe tissue injury (trauma, burns, head injury)
- Cancer (particularly carcinomas of the pancreas, prostate, and acute promyelocytic leukemia)
- Obstetric complications (amniotic fluid embolism, HELLP syndrome, eclampsia, retained fetal products, septic abortion)
- Abdominal aortic aneurysm
- Hemolytic transfusion reaction (ABO incompatibility)
- Snake bite
- Fulminant hepatic failure

Pathogenesis of DIC (Fig. 6.23)

- Normally coagulation is mediated by thrombin and kept confined to a localized area by a combination of blood flow and coagulation inhibitors especially antithrombin III. When these mechanisms are overwhelmed by the markedly increased production of thrombin, thrombin may circulate and lead to disseminated intravascular coagulation.
- There is widespread deposition of fibrin leading to blocked blood vessels and tissue ischemia, consumption of platelets and clotting factors. Consumption of clotting factors and platelets → leads to bleeding.
- The major stimulus to thrombin activation in DIC comes from the tissue factor.

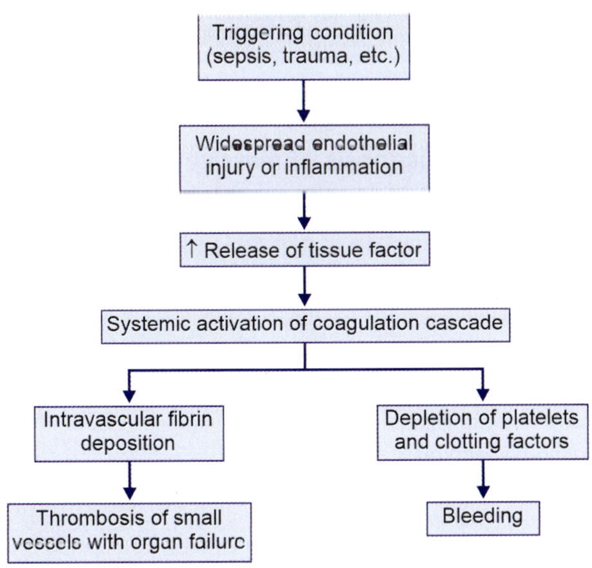

Figure 6.23: Pathophysiology of DIC

Clinical Features

- DIC leads to both bleeding and thrombosis. Bleeding is more common than thrombosis.
- Bleeding may occur at any site, but spontaneous bleeding and oozing at venipuncture sites or wounds are important clues to the diagnosis.
- Thrombosis is most commonly manifested by digital ischemia and gangrene.
- Other manifestations include dysfunction of liver, kidney, lungs, and central nervous system. DIC also causes microangiopathic hemolytic anemia.

Laboratory Findings

- Hypofibrinogenemia, thrombocytopenia, and elevated fibrin degradation products. D-dimer is the most sensitive fibrin degradation product.
- ↑ PT and aPTT.
- Peripheral smear shows schistocytes (fragmented RBCs) due to microangiopathic hemolytic anemia.
- Antithrombin III levels may be markedly reduced.

Treatment of DIC

- Underlying cause of DIC should be treated.
- ***Replacement therapy:*** platelets should be transfused to maintain a platelet count greater than 30,000/µl. Fibrinogen is replaced with cryoprecipitate. Coagulation factor deficiency may require replacement with fresh-frozen plasma. When there is excessive fibrinolysis, EACA 1 g intravenously per hour may be tried in combination with heparin. EACA should not be used without heparin in DIC because of the risk of thrombosis. Antithrombin III replacement has not been shown to reduce mortality rate of severe sepsis with DIC. However, one trial has shown benefit by the use of activated protein C.
- Heparin may be used in cases with predominant thrombosis (controversial). Heparin is not effective if antithrombin III levels are markedly reduced. If antithrombin III levels are very low, it can be raised by giving fresh-frozen plasma or antithrombin III concentrates.

Q. Causes of splenomegaly.

Q. Differential diagnosis of massive splenomegaly.

Causes of Splenomegaly

Mild splenomegaly

Acute infections: typhoid, malaria, septicemia, sub-acute bacterial endocarditis

Moderate splenomegaly

- Leukemia, lymphomas
- Polycythemia vera
- Hemolytic anemias
- Cirrhosis of liver
- Hemochromatosis
- Tumors and cysts
- Tuberculosis

Massive splenomegaly

- Chronic myeloid leukemia (CML)
- Myelofibrosis
- Gaucher's disease
- Chronic lymphocytic leukemia (CLL)
- Hairy cell leukemia
- Kala-azar (visceral leishmaniasis)
- Tropical splenomegaly syndrome (hyperreactive malarial splenomegaly syndrome)
- Thalassemia major
- AIDS with disseminated *Mycobacterium avium* complex infection.

Differential Diagnosis of Massive Splenomegaly

Chronic Myeloid Leukemia (CML)

Clinical features

- Median age at presentation is around 50 years.
- Patients may have systemic symptoms such as fatigue (due to anemia), malaise, weight loss, excessive sweating).
- Abdominal fullness and left hyphochondrial pain due to massive splenomegaly.
- Bleeding episodes due to platelet dysfunction.
- Moderate to massive splenomegaly with hepatomegaly.
- Pallor due to anemia.

Laboratory findings

- Normocytic normochromic anemia.
- WBC count is markedly raised (usually >100,000).
- Platelet count may be raised, but in advanced disease falls.
- Peripheral smear shows presence of myelocytes and metamyelocytes.
- Philadelphia chromosome is positive in > 95% cases.
- Leukocyte alkaline phosphatase (LAP) score is very low.

Myelofibrosis

Clinical features

- The median age at presentation is 67 years.
- The most common presenting complaint is severe fatigue.
- Hepatomegaly.

Laboratory findings

- Anemia.
- WBC count is variable and thrombocytopenia is often present.
- Leukocyte alkaline phosphatase (LAP) score is increased.
- Peripheral smear shows teardrop-shaped RBCs, nucleated RBCs and granulocyte precursors (myelocytes, metamyelocytes, and blasts).
- Bone marrow is often difficult to aspirate, usually yielding a "dry" tap. Bone marrow biopsy shows extensive replacement of the marrow by fibrosis, which is the hallmark of the disease.

Gaucher's Disease

Clinical features

- It is an autosomal recessive disorder.
- Hepatosplenomegaly, anemia, thrombocytopenia, and bone disease.
- Bone manifestations include fractures, infarctions, and vertebral collapse.

Laboratory findings

- Thrombocytopenia and anemia.
- Liver enzymes may be mildly elevated.
- Acid phosphatase is elevated in patients with active bone disease.
- Reduced glucocerebrosidase activity in leukocytes.

Chronic Lymphocytic Leukemia (CLL)

Clinical features

- Painless lymphadenopathy
- Weight loss, fever and night sweats without evidence of infection
- Easy fatigability
- Hepatomegaly may be present.

Laboratory findings

- Anemia
- Increased WBC count
- Thrombocytopenia.

Hairy Cell Leukemia

Clinical features

- The median age of presentation is approximately 55 years, with a male predominance.
- Symptoms include abdominal fullness, fatigue, weakness, weight loss, and bleeding tendency.
- Lymphadenopathy is unusual.

Laboratory features

- Pancytopenia
- Peripheral smear shows malignant cells with cytoplasmic projections ("hairy cells")
- Bone marrow shows presence of hyper cellularity and hairy cells.

Kala-azar (visceral leishmaniasis)

Clinmical features

- Visceral leishmaniasis is a parasitic disease caused by the obligate intracellular protozoa **Leishmania**.
- It is also known as kala-azar (Hindi for black sickness or fever) and is a systemic disease that can be life-threatening.
- The 90% of cases occur in Bangladesh, northeastern India, Nepal, Sudan, and northeastern Brazil.
- Clinical features are organomegaly, fever and cachexia.

Laboratory features

- Pancytopenia due to massive splenomegaly and bone marrow involvement.
- Hypergammaglobulinemia
- Abnormal liver function tests, hypoalbuminemia and hyperbilirubinemia.
- Antibodies against Leishmania positive.
- A skin or bone marrow aspirate usually shows amastigotes.

Tropical Splenomegaly Syndrome (hyperreactive malarial splenomegaly syndrome)

Clinical features

- Patient is from malaria endemic area.
- Recurrent attacks of malaria in the past.

Laboratory features

- Pancytopenia.
- Peripheral smear may demonstrate malarial parasite.

Thalassemia Major

Clinical features

- Thalassemia is common in the Mediterranean region especially amongst Italians and Greeks. The thalassemia belt extends to India and south East Asia.
- Symptoms start late in the first year of life when fetal hemoglobin levels decline.
- Pallor, irritability, growth retardation, hepatosplenomegaly and jaundice develop due to severe hemolytic anemia.
- Characteristic chipmunk facies (frontal bossing and prominent cheek bones) due to bone marrow expansion.
- An 80% of untreated children die within the first 5 years of life, as a result of severe anemia, high output heart failure, and infections.

Laboratory features

- Signs of hemolysis such as anemia, increased indirect (unconjugated) bilirubin, increased LDH and reduced haptoglobin levels.
- Hemoglobin electrophoresis shows markedly reduced HbA and raised HbF.
- Peripheral smear shows hypochromia, microcytosis, anisopoikilocytosis, tear drop cells and target cells. WBC and platelet counts are normal unless hypersplenism develops.
- Bone marrow shows marked hypercellularity.
- The osmotic fragility test is significantly reduced.
- Skull X-ray shows widened diploic space and hair-on-end appearance. Compression fractures of the vertebrae and marked osteoporosis are common.

AIDS with Mycobacterium avium Complex

Clinical features

- Intermittent or persistent fever, fatigue, malaise, anorexia, and weight loss.
- Lymphadenopathy and hepatomegaly may be present.

Laboratory features

- HIV serology is positive.
- Anemia and neutropenia from bone marrow involvement.

- Elevated liver enzymes due to liver involvement.
- Blood culture is positive for nontuberculous mycobacteria.

Q. Hypersplenism.

- Hypersplenism is a clinical syndrome characterized by an overactive spleen, which leads to excessive destruction (sequestration) of blood cells.
- It is associated with splenomegaly, pancytopenia or a reduction in the number of one or more types of blood cells, hyperplasia of the precursor cells in the marrow, and decreased RBC/platelet survival.

Causes of Hypersplenism

- Any disease which produces splenic enlargement can produce hypersplenism.

Pathophysiology

- Spleen is the major organ of the monocyte/macrophage system.
- As the blood passes through the white and red pulp, old and defective blood cells are removed by the spleen. The macrophages in the spleen hold, retard, modify ("pitting"), or remove ("culling") old and senescent RBCs. The normal pitting function of the spleen removes nuclear residua (Howell-Jolly bodies) and the normal culling function of the spleen removes senescent RBCs.
- All these normal activities of the spleen can be markedly accentuated in a large spleen leading to pancytopenia (anemia, neutropenia and thrombocytopenia). This is called hypersplenism.

Clinical Features

- Hypersplenism is suspected when there is cytopenia along with splenomegaly.

Treatment of Hypersplenism

- Underlying causes should be treated.
- Splenectomy or splenic ablation by radiation therapy may be considered if cytopenia is very severe.

Q. Enumerate the causes of generalized lymphadenopathy.

Q. Differential diagnosis of generalized lymphadenopathy in an adult.

- Lymphadenopathy is classified as localized when it involves only one region and generalized when it involves two or more noncontiguous lymph node regions. It typically indicates a systemic disorder. Non-contiguous lymph node regions mean separate anatomical areas that are not directly next to each other (i.e. not in the same group or chain).

Causes of Generalized Lymphadenopathy

- ***Infections:*** Disseminated tuberculosis, cat scratch disease, secondary syphilis, HIV, infectious mononucleosis, histoplasmosis, coccidioidomycosis, cryptococcosis, toxoplasmosis, leshmaniasis.
- ***Malignancy:*** Metastatic Ca, lymphoma, leukemia.
- ***Connective tissue diseases:*** Rheumatoid arthritis, SLE, sarcoidosis.
- ***Endocrine disorders:*** Hypothyroidism, Addison disease.
- ***Drugs:*** Allopurinol, hydralazine, phenytoin.

Differential Diagnosis of Important Causes

HIV Infection

Clinical features

- Common in persons with high risk sexual behavior and intravenous drug addicts.
- Fever, weight loss, and chronic diarrhea may be present.
- Nontender lymphadenopathy primarily involving the axillary, cervical, and occipital nodes.

Lab features

- HIV-ELISA test positive.
- Western blot test confirms the diagnosis.

Disseminated Tuberculosis

Clinical features

- Nodes are typically nontender, enlarge over weeks to months without prominent systemic symptoms, and can progress to matting and fluctuation.
- Fever, weight loss, night sweats.
- Hepatosplenomegaly.

Lab features

- Montoux test may be positive.
- Chest X-ray may show military mottling.
- Lymph node or liver biopsy may show caseating granulomas.

Infectious Mononucleosis

Clinical features

- Triad of fever, pharyngitis, and lymphadenopathy
- Maculopapular rash may be present
- Lymphadenopathy is typically symmetric and involves the posterior cervical nodes more than the anterior group.
- Lymphadenopathy may also be present in the axillary and inguinal areas, which distinguishes infectious mononucleosis from other causes of pharyngitis.

Lab features

- Atypical lymphocytosis in the peripheral blood.
- Paul-bunnel test and monospot test may be positive.

Systemic Lupus Erythematosus

- Nodes are soft, nontender, and discrete.
- Cervical, axillary, and inguinal areas are usually involved.
- Lymphadenopathy is more frequently noted at the onset of disease or in association with an exacerbation.
- Other features such as joint pain and rash (especially malar rash) may be present
- ANA and anti dsDNA may be positive.

Brucellosis

Clinical features

- Fever, polyarthritis, hepatosplenomegaly
- Common in veterinary staff and slaughter house personnel.

Lab features

- Positive blood culture.
- Positive Brucella agglutination test.

Lymphomas (Hodgkin's and non-Hodgkin's)

Clinical features

- Constitutional symptoms like fever and weight loss.
- Painless rubbery lymphadenopathy, usually in the neck or supraclavicular fossae.
- Dry cough, breathlessness and dysphagia may occur due to mediastinal lymphadenopathy.
- Hepatosplenomegaly may be present.

Lab features

- Normochromic, normocytic anemia.
- LDH may be raised.
- Lymph node biopsy confirms the disease. Characteristic Reed-Sternberg cells are found in Hodgkin's lymphoma.

Chronic Lymphocytic Leukemia (CLL)

Clinical features

- More common in elderly males
- Recurrent infections are common due to immunodeficiency.
- Hepatosplenomegaly.

Lab features

- WBC count is usually greater than 20,000/µl.
- The hallmark of CLL is isolated lymphocytosis. Usually more than 75% of the circulating cells are lymphocytes.
- Bone marrow shows infiltration with lymphocytes.
- Lymph node biopsy shows well differentiated, small, non-cleaved lymphocytes

CML in Blast Crisis

Clinical features

- Fever, hemorrhage, generalized lymphadenopathy, bone pain and sternal tenderness.
- Abrupt increase in spleen size.

Lab features

- Peripheral smear and bone marrow show more than 20% blasts.
- Philadelphia chromosome is positive in most cases.

Drugs

- Many drugs can cause serum sickness characterized by fever, arthralgias, rash, and generalized lymphadenopathy. Phenytoin can cause generalized lymphadenopathy in the absence of a serum sickness reaction.
- There is temporal correlation between drug intake and the onset of lymphadenopathy. Withdrawal of offending drug leads to resolution of lymphadenopathy.

Q. Describe the indications for blood transfusion and the appropriate use of blood components.

Q. Precautions before blood transfusion.

Q. Complications of blood transfusion.

- Blood transfusion is the process of transferring blood or blood components from a donor into the bloodstream of a recipient through an intravenous (IV) line.

Packed Red Blood Cells Transfusion (PRBCs)

- A packed red blood cells (PRBCs) involves transfusion of only the red blood cells from a donor's blood to the recipient, rather than whole blood.
- Each unit of PRBC is ~250–300 ml and contains concentrated red cells with minimal plasma and white blood cells. 1 unit transfusion raises hemoglobin by ~1 g/dl.

Indications

- Acute blood loss (>30% blood volume)
- Symptomatic anemia (e.g. dyspnea, tachycardia, angina)
- Hemoglobin (Hb) <7 g/dl in stable patients
- Hb <8 g/dl in patients with cardiovascular disease or post-op.

Advantages of PRBC Transfusion over Whole Blood Transfusion

- Since PRBCs are concentrated red cells with minimal plasma, volume overload is minimized compared to whole blood transfusions — beneficial in patients with heart failure or renal insufficiency.
- PRBCs can be stored longer (35–42 days with additive solutions).
- By removing most plasma and white blood cells, PRBCs lower the risk of febrile nonhemolytic reactions and immunologic complications compared to whole blood.

Platelet Transfusion

- Used to prevent or treat bleeding due to thrombocytopenia or platelet dysfunction.

Indications

- Platelet count <10,000/µl (prophylactic).
- Platelet count <50,000/µl with bleeding or invasive procedures.
- Platelet count <100,000/µl in neurosurgery or ocular surgery.
- Platelet dysfunction (e.g. antiplatelet drug use) with active bleeding.

Types of Platelet Products

Random donor platelets (RDP)

- Collected from multiple donors
- One unit increases platelet count by ~5,000–10,000/μl.

Single donor platelets (SDP/Apheresis)

- Collected via apheresis from a single donor.
- One unit ≈ 6 RDPs, raises count by ~30,000–60,000/μl.
- Preferred for HLA-matched or repeated transfusions.

Fresh Frozen Plasma

- Fresh frozen plasma (FFP) is prepared from single units of whole blood or from plasma collected by apheresis techniques. It is frozen at minus 18 to minus 30°C within eight hours of collection and can be stored up to one year.
- FFP contains all of the coagulation factors present in the blood.
- Contains albumin.
- ABO compatibility is required before transfusion, but Rh typing is not required.
- A dose of 10–15 ml/kg (3–5 units) will correct coagulation abnormality.

Indications

- Bleeding due to excess warfarin, vitamin K deficiency, or deficiency of multiple coagulation factors (e.g. DIC, liver disease, dilutional coagulopathy).
- Treatment of TTP.
- Hemophilia.

Cryoprecipitate

- **Cryoprecipitate** is made from FFP which is frozen and repeatedly thawed in a laboratory.
- It contains high concentration of certain clotting factors such as Factor VIII, von Willebrand factor and fibrinogen. Unlike FFP, cryoprecipitate does not contain all the clotting factors (factor IX and X). cryoprecipitate does not contain albumin also.

Indications

- Fibrinogen deficiency.
- von Willebrand disease and hemophilia-A if recombinant products are not available.

Compatibility Testing

- Before transfusion, the recipient's and the donor's blood are cross-matched to avoid hemolytic transfusion reactions. Although many antigen systems are present on red blood cells, only the ABO and Rh systems are specifically tested prior to all transfusions.
- Incompatible blood transfusion can lead to severe blood transfusion reactions.

Precautions before Blood Transfusion

- Proper precautions before starting a blood transfusion are critical to ensure patient safety and prevent transfusion reactions or complications.

Confirm Transfusion Order

Check the physician's written order for:

- Type of component (e.g. PRBCs, platelets)
- Volume/dose
- Indication
- Rate of transfusion.

Verify Patient Identity (crucial)

- Match the patient's full name and identification number with the blood product and request form.
- Use two identifiers (e.g. name, date of birth, medical record number).
- Perform bedside check with another qualified healthcare professional (double-check protocol).

Check Blood Product Label

- Match blood group and Rh type
- Check expiration date
- Confirm compatibility (crossmatch)
- Ensure the product is visually normal (no clots, discoloration, or leaks).

Take Informed Consent

- Ensure patient (or legal representative) has given informed consent after understanding:
  - The need for transfusion
  - Benefits
  - Potential risks and alternatives

Baseline Assessment

- Record baseline vital signs (temperature, BP, HR, RR, O_2 saturation)
- Assess for signs of preexisting fever, infection, or allergic reaction.
- Review previous transfusion history and any prior reactions.

Premedications (only if required)

- Antihistamines (e.g. diphenhydramine) or antipyretics (e.g. paracetamol) may be given if there is a history of mild transfusion reactions.

Keep Emergency Medicines Ready

- Epinephrine antihistamines, corticosteroids. Useful in case of allergic and anaphylactic reactions.
- Ensure resuscitation equipment (e.g. oxygen, suction, defibrillator) is nearby.

Complications of Blood Transfusion

- Transfusion reactions (hemolytic, nonhemolytic)
- Transmission of infections (hepatitis B, HIV, hepatitis C, malaria, syphilis)

- Circulatory overload
- Hypocalcemia (due to citrate binding to calcium in stored blood)
- Hyperkalemia (due to potassium coming out of RBCs in stored blood)
- Hypothermia (due to massive blood transfusion of fridge stored blood)
- Thrombocytopenia (seen in massive blood transfusion because platelets do not survive for long in stored blood)
- Iron overload (seen in thalassemia due to recurrent blood transfusion)

Q. Blood transfusion reactions (Fig. 6.24).

- Although blood transfusion is a common procedure in medical settings, it can lead to serious transfusion reactions.
- Transfusion reactions are defined as adverse events following a blood transfusion, with the severity ranging from minor to life-threatening. In a clinical setting, any new symptom or change in vital signs occurring within 24 hours of a blood transfusion should be considered a transfusion reaction until proven otherwise.

Management of any Suspected Transfusion Reaction

- Stop the transfusion immediately.
- Keep IV access open with normal saline.
- Check the patient's identity and verify the blood unit label.
- Notify the blood bank and attending physician.
- Monitor vital signs continuously.
- Send investigations:
  - Repeat blood typing and crossmatch.
  - Direct antiglobulin test (Coombs' test).
  - Hemolysis labs: LDH, bilirubin, haptoglobin, plasma free hemoglobin.
  - Urine for hemoglobinuria.
  - Blood cultures (if febrile or suspected sepsis).
  - Chest X-ray (if respiratory symptoms).

Q. Hemolytic transfusion reactions.

- Severe hemolytic reactions occur if ABO incompatible blood is transfused. Most of these cases are due to clinical or laboratory errors or mislabeled specimens.
- Here, the donor RBCs are destroyed by the recipient's immune system due to incompatibility.
- There are two types: (1) Acute hemolytic transfusion reaction (AHTR), and (2) Delayed hemolytic transfusion reaction (DHTR).

Acute Hemolytic Transfusion Reaction (AHTR)

- Onset: Within minutes to hours of transfusion.
- Severity: Life-threatening, especially with ABO mismatch.

Pathophysiology

- Mechanism: Intravascular hemolysis due to preformed recipient antibodies, most commonly anti-A or anti-B (ABO incompatibility).
- Complement activation → hemolysis → cytokine storm.
- Free hemoglobin → renal injury → acute kidney failure.
- DIC may develop due to widespread endothelial damage.

Clinical Features

- Fever and chills
- Flank or back pain
- Hypotension, shock
- Hemoglobinuria (cola-colored urine)
- Chest tightness, dyspnea
- Bleeding (DIC)
- Acute renal failure.

Delayed Hemolytic Transfusion Reaction (DHTR)

- Onset: 3–14 days posttransfusion.
- Mechanism: Extravascular hemolysis due to secondary (anamnestic) immune response against minor RBC antigens (e.g. Kidd, Duffy, Kell).
- Often occurs in patients previously sensitized (e.g. from prior transfusion or pregnancy).

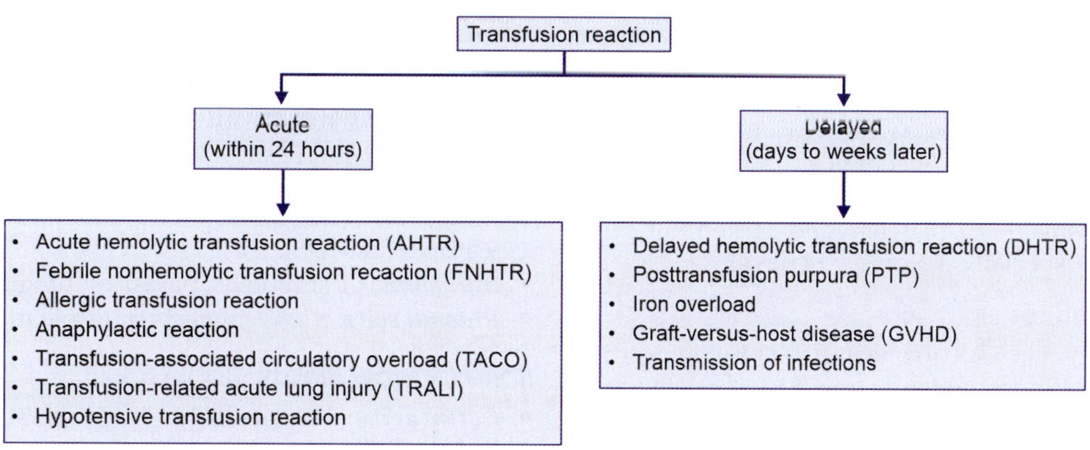

Figure 6.24: Transfusion reactions

Clinical Features

- There may be low-grade fever, jaundice, unexplained fall in hemoglobin, mild fatigue or malaise.
- May be asymptomatic and detected only by lab tests.

Laboratory Findings

- Decrease in hemoglobin
- Increased LDH due to hemolysis
- Indirect bilirubin may be elevated due to hemolysis
- Evidence of renal failure and DIC
- Plasma appears pink due to hemoglobinuria
- Direct antiglobulin test (Coombs') is positive
- Urine may show hemoglobinuria.

Treatment

- If a hemolytic transfusion reaction is suspected, blood transfusion must be immediately stopped.
- Identification of the recipient and of the blood should be checked. The donor transfusion bag and infusion set should be returned to the blood bank, along with a fresh blood sample of the patient for retyping and repeat cross-matching.
- Patient should be hydrated well to prevent renal failure due to hemoglobinuria. Forced alkaline diuresis may help prevent renal damage.

Q. Transfusion-related acute lung injury (TRALI).

- Transfusion-related acute lung injury (TRALI) is a syndrome characterized by acute respiratory distress following transfusion. It is a non-cardiogenic pulmonary edema caused by immune-mediated injury to the lungs, and is one of the leading causes of transfusion-related mortality.

Definition

TRALI is defined as:

- Acute lung injury (ALI) developing during or within 6 hours of transfusion.
- Hypoxemia ($PaO_2/FiO_2 \leq 300$ mm Hg or oxygen saturation <90% on room air).
- Bilateral pulmonary infiltrates on chest X-ray.
- No evidence of circulatory overload or cardiac failure.

Pathophysiology

- Donor plasma contains antibodies against recipient leukocyte antigens (HLA class I/II).
- These antibodies activate neutrophils in the pulmonary microvasculature → capillary leakage → non-cardiogenic pulmonary edema.
- Blood components commonly implicated are fresh frozen plasma (FFP), platelets, and packed RBCs (less common, especially if stored >14 days).

Clinical Features

- Incidence is 1 in 5,000 to one in 10,000, but many cases are mild. Mild-to-moderate transfusion-related acute lung injury probably is commonly missed.
- Symptoms of TRALI typically develop within 6 hours of a transfusion. Patients develop breathlessness. There may be associated fever, cyanosis, and hypotension. Examination reveals bilateral crepitations. Chest X-ray shows evidence of bilateral pulmonary edema (non-cardiogenic pulmonary edema or ARDS).

Treatment

- Stop the transfusion immediately.
- Maintain airway and oxygenation. Administer high-flow oxygen. Intubation and mechanical ventilation if needed.
- Majority of patients recover within 72–96 hours.

Q. Bone Marrow aspiration and biopsy: indications and interpretation.

- Bone marrow aspiration and biopsy are diagnostic procedures used to evaluate the structure and cellularity of the bone marrow.
- **Aspiration:** Withdraws liquid marrow to examine individual cell morphology and for flow cytometry/cytogenetics.
- **Biopsy:** Obtains a solid core of marrow to assess architecture, cellularity, and fibrosis.

Indications for Bone Marrow Examination (Table 6.21)

TABLE 6.21: Indications for bone marrow examination

Hematologic disorders • Unexplained cytopenias (anemia, leukopenia, thrombocytopenia) • Unexplained pancytopenia • Aplastic anemia • Myelodysplastic syndromes (MDS) • Leukemias (acute/chronic) • Lymphomas (staging or diagnosis) • Plasma cell disorders (e.g. multiple myeloma)
Nonhematologic conditions • Fever of unknown origin (FUO) • Metastatic cancers (to evaluate marrow involvement) • Diagnosis of infections (e.g. tuberculosis, histoplasmosis in immunocompromised patients) • Storage diseases (e.g. Gaucher disease)
Monitoring or staging • Response to chemotherapy or bone marrow transplantation • Staging of lymphomas or certain solid tumors

Interpretation of Results

Bone Marrow Aspiration Smear

- ***Cell morphology***: Evaluate precursors of red cells, white cells, and platelets.
- ***Myeloid:erythroid (M:E) ratio***: Normal is 2:1 to 4:1.
- ***Abnormal cells***: Blasts (↑ in leukemia), dysplastic features (in MDS).
- ***Infections***: Granulomas, parasites, fungi.
- ***Plasma cells***: >10% suggests multiple myeloma.

Bone Marrow Biopsy (Table 6.22)

- ***Cellularity***: Hypocellular (e.g. aplastic anemia), hypercellular (e.g. leukemia).
- ***Architecture***: Disruption can indicate malignancy.

- *Fibrosis:* Seen in myelofibrosis, can be graded (reticulin stain).
- *Infiltrates*: Malignant cells (e.g. metastatic cancer), granulomas, amyloid.
- *Examples of diagnostic patterns* **(Table 6.22)***:*

TABLE 6.22: Examples of diagnostic patterns in bone marrow biopsy

Condition	Key findings
Acute leukemia	Hypercellular marrow, ↑ blasts (>20%)
Aplastic anemia	Hypocellular marrow with fatty replacement
Myelodysplastic syndrome	Dysplastic changes in one or more lineages
Multiple myeloma	↑ Plasma cells (>10%), abnormal morphology
Lymphoma infiltration	Nodular or diffuse lymphoid aggregates
Myelofibrosis	↑ Reticulin/collagen fibrosis, "dry tap" on aspiration

Q. Conditions requiring hematologist consultation.

- Blasts on peripheral smear → possible acute leukemia.
- Rapidly worsening cytopenias.
- Severe thrombocytopenia with bleeding risk.
- Hemophilia, von Willebrand disease, or other inherited bleeding disorders.
- Suspected aplastic anemia or bone marrow failure.
- Autoimmune hemolytic anemia, G6PD deficiency, sickle cell disease, or thalassemia.
- Hyperviscosity symptoms in conditions like Waldenström's macroglobulinemia.

Chapter 7

Diseases of Liver and Biliary System

Q. Enumerate the functions of liver.

- Liver is a vital organ responsible for metabolism, detoxification, synthesis, storage, and immune functions. It performs over 500 functions. Main functions are listed below.

Metabolism
- Carbohydrate
- Protein
- Lipids
- Drugs and alcohol
- Hormones

Synthesis
- Albumin
- Coagulation factors
- Complement factors
- Haptoglobin
- Ceruloplasmin
- Transferrin
- Bile acids

Excretion
- Bile salts
- Bilirubin

Storage
- Iron
- Copper
- Vitamins A, D and B_{12}

Detoxification
- Metabolizes and detoxifies drugs, alcohol, and toxins.
- Converts ammonia (toxic) into urea (nontoxic).

Q. What are the signs and symptoms of liver disease?

Signs and Symptoms of Liver Disease

- Jaundice (acute hepatitis, decompensated cirrhosis, liver abscess, liver metastases, obstructive jaundice).
- Easy fatigability and malaise
- Altered mental status (due to hepatic encephalopathy)
- Pruritus (in obstructive jaundice)
- Abdominal distension (ascites, hepatomegaly)
- Light-colored stools (in obstructive jaundice)
- Bleeding tendency (due to reduced synthesis of clotting factors).
- Peripheral edema (cirrhosis with portal HTN)
- Gynecomastia (chronic liver disease)
- Spider angioma (acute or chronic liver disease)
- Palmar erythema (chronic liver disease)
- Flapping tremors (hepatic encephalopathy)
- Right upper quadrant tenderness (acute hepatitis, fatty liver, congested liver, hepatic abscess)
- Hepatomegaly (fatty liver, acute hepatitis, hepatoma, liver metastases, liver abscess, congestive hepatomegaly in CCF).

Q. Liver function tests (LFT) and their interpretation.

Q. Diagnostic tests for the evaluation of liver disease.

- Liver function tests are (LFTs) are a group of blood tests used to assess liver integrity, synthetic function, excretory function, and cholestasis. They help evaluate liver disease, monitor progression, and detect drug or alcohol toxicity.

Categories of LFTs (Table 7.1)

TABLE 7.1: Categories of LFT

Category	Test	Purpose
Hepatocellular injury	ALT, AST	Detect hepatocyte damage
Cholestasis markers	ALP, GGT, Bilirubin	Assess bile flow obstruction
Synthetic function	Albumin, PT/INR	Evaluate protein synthesis and coagulation
Excretory function	Bilirubin (direct/ total)	Evaluate bile excretion and conjugation

Tests for Liver Injury

Aminotransferases (transaminases): AST and ALT

- Normal circulating liver enzyme levels are due to enzymes released during normal hepatocyte turnover. These liver enzymes are increased during liver cell injury or death.

- Normal serum levels of AST and ALT are 5–40 IU/L.
- Serum AST and ALT level increases in acute hepatocyte injury due to infections (viral hepatitis, dengue, leptospirosis, etc.), autoimmune hepatitis, toxins (alcohol, drugs) and ischemia (ischemic hepatitis). Elevated ALT is more specific for liver injury. AST is also present in the heart, skeletal muscle, kidneys, and pancreas, and hence elevated AST may reflect rhabdomyolysis or injury to one of these organs.
- The magnitude of AST and ALT elevations varies depending on the cause of the hepatocellular injury. The following are typical AST and ALT patterns in various diseases (**Table 7.2**).

TABLE 7.2: Magnitude of AST, ALT elevation in various liver diseases

Disease	Magnitude of AST and ALT elevation
Acute viral hepatitis or toxin-related hepatitis	>25 times the upper limit of normal. Usually ALT is more than AST
Chronic hepatitis B and C	Normal to <2 times the upper limit of normal
Ischemic hepatitis	>50 times the upper limit of normal
Alcoholic liver disease	<8 times the upper limit of normal; AST: ALT ratio > 2:1

- Aminotransferase levels may be low in massive hepatic necrosis because liver injury is so extensive that little enzyme activity remains.
- Aminotransferase levels can be used to monitor activity of chronic liver disease such as chronic hepatitis-B or C.
- In most liver diseases, the ratio of AST to ALT is usually less than or equal to 1. However, ratios are usually 2 or more in alcoholic fatty liver and alcoholic hepatitis, reflecting increased synthesis as well as secretion of mitochondrial AST into plasma and selective loss of ALT activity due to pyridoxine deficiency seen in alcoholism. An elevated AST/ALT ratio can also be found in in fulminant hepatitis due to Wilson's disease.

Tests for Cholestasis

Alkaline Phosphatase

- Alkaline phosphatases can be found in many organs (liver, bile ducts, intestine, bone, kidney, placenta, and leukocytes). Serum alkaline phosphatase mainly comes from liver and bone.
- The normal level in adults is 40–130 U/L. Alkaline phosphatase levels are elevated in cholestatic hepatobiliary diseases. Modest increases (up to 3 times normal) occur in many hepatic parenchymal disorders, such as hepatitis and cirrhosis. Larger increases (3–10 times normal) are seen in biliary obstruction. Major elevations also occur with intrahepatic cholestasis and with infiltrative or mass lesions (malignancy, lymphoma, leukemia). It is also elevated in bone disorders (Paget's disease, osteomalacia, bone metastases), during rapid bone growth in children, pregnancy, and chronic renal failure.
- To know whether elevated ALP is due to hepatobiliary disease, levels of 5′-nucleotidase can be measured. If 5′-nucleotidase levels are also elevated along with ALP, it means ALP elevation is due to hepatobiliary disease.

5′-nucleotidase

- 5′-nucleotidase are also elevated in cholestasis. Its major use is to confirm whether an elevated serum alkaline phosphatase is hepatic in origin. It can be increased in late pregnancy.

Gamma-glutamyl transpeptidase (GGT)

- The normal range is 9–48 units per liter (U/L).
- GGT is present in many tissues. Its level is increased in hepatobiliary diseases, but is not specific to hepatobiliary diseases. It can also be elevated in myocardial infarction, neuromuscular diseases, pancreatic disease, pulmonary disease, and diabetes. Its levels are especially elevated in alcoholic liver disease. Hence, it is sometimes used for monitoring abstinence from alcohol. GGT levels parallel those of ALP; hence, it can be used to confirm whether ALP elevation is due to hepatobiliary disease.

Tests to Assess Metabolic Function

- Bilirubin, ammonia and various drugs are metabolized or detoxified in the liver. Serum levels of these metabolites can be a sensitive indicator of liver disease.

Bilirubin

- Normally, total bilirubin is mostly unconjugated, with values of <1.2 mg/dl.
- Direct hyperbilirubinemia is seen in cholestatic hepatobiliary diseases and Dubin-Johnoson disease.
- Indirect hyperbilirubinemia is found in Gilbert's syndrome, Crigler Najjar syndromes, and hemolysis.
- High bilirubin levels correlate with a poorer prognosis in alcoholic hepatitis, primary biliary cirrhosis, and fulminant hepatic failure.

Ammonia

- Ammonia is a byproduct of amino acid metabolism and is removed from blood by the liver, converted to urea in Krebs cycle, and excreted by the kidneys. Normal serum level is 15–45 micrograms per deciliter (μg/dl).
- Ammonia levels are elevated in liver dysfunction and portosystemic shunting. Measurements of blood ammonia are used to confirm a diagnosis of hepatic encephalopathy and to monitor the success of therapy.
- Elevated ammonia levels also occur when ammonia production is increased by intestinal flora (e.g. after a high-protein meal or gastrointestinal bleeding),

by the kidney (in response to metabolic alkalosis or hypokalemia), or in rare genetic diseases that affect urea cycle.

Tests for Hepatic Synthetic Function

Prothrombin Time

- Prothrombin time (PT) reflects the plasma concentrations of factors VII, X, and V, prothrombin, and fibrinogen.
- Normal value is 11–13.5 seconds, or INR (international normalized ratio) of 0.8–1.1.
- Since clotting factors are synthesized in liver, a prolonged PT occurs in liver diseases. Prolonged PT can also occur due to vitamin K deficiency, one cause of which is malabsorption from cholestatic liver disease since bile juice is important for the absorption of this fat-soluble vitamin.

Serum Albumin Level

- The normal range is 3.5–5 grams per deciliter (g/dl). Albumin is produced solely by the liver. Hence albumin levels can be decreased in liver dysfunction and there will be reversal of albumin globulin ratio (normal 2:1).
- Other causes of low albumin are nephrotic syndrome, protein-losing enteropathy, severe burns, exfoliative dermatitis, and major gastrointestinal bleeding.

Common Patterns in LFTs

Hepatocellular Injury Pattern

- ALT and AST ↑↑ (often >10× normal).
- ALP and bilirubin normal or mildly increased.
- Key point is disproportionate elevation in ALT and AST compared with the ALP.
- *Examples*: Viral hepatitis, drug-induced liver injury.

Cholestatic Pattern

- ALP and GGT ↑↑.
- Direct bilirubin ↑.
- ALT/AST mildly elevated.
- Key point is disproportionate elevation of ALP compared with the ALT/AST.
- *Examples*: Bile duct obstruction, PBC, PSC.

Mixed Pattern

- All enzymes elevated.
- Seen in: Drug injury, alcoholic hepatitis, tumor infiltration.

Other Tests Used in Liver Disease (not included under liver function tests)

Examination of Urine and Stool

- Bilirubinuria indicates increase in plasma conjugated bilirubin levels. Stool occult blood may be positive due to portal gastropathy, portal hypertension and GI malignancy which might have metastasized to liver.

Hematologic Tests in Liver Disease

- Anemia can occur due to bleeding esophageal varices, hypersplenism or bone marrow suppression by alcohol. Pancytopenia can occur due to hypersplenism or bone marrow suppression by alcohol.
- Target cells (erythrocytes with an expanded cell membrane) may be found in chronic liver disease due to abnormalities in serum lipids. Spur cells (acanthocytes) can occur in advanced alcoholic cirrhosis.

Tests for Specific Liver Diseases

- Specific tests for viral antigens, nucleic acids, and antibodies are available for the hepatitis viruses (hepatitis A, B, C, D, E) as well as Epstein-Barr virus, cytomegalovirus and herpesviruses.
- Antimitochondrial antibodies are virtually diagnostic of primary biliary cirrhosis. Antinuclear, anti–smooth muscle and anti–liver microsomal antibodies are present in autoimmune hepatitis.
- Iron studies may help to rule out hemochromatosis. Serum copper and ceruloplasmin levels may help to rule out Wilson's disease.

Liver Biopsy

- Liver biopsy is useful in the diagnosis of diffuse or localized parenchymal diseases, including chronic hepatitis, cirrhosis, and malignancy.
- Liver biopsy for diffuse disease can be done blindly. However localized disease such as tumors requires biopsy under ultrasound or CT guidance. Liver biopsy can also be done under direct visualization during laparoscopy or laparotomy.
- Contraindications include coagulopathy, high-grade biliary obstruction, and biliary sepsis.

Q. Describe the liver function tests in acute hepatitis and obstructive jaundice.

LFTs in Acute Hepatitis (e.g. viral hepatitis, drug-induced liver injury)

- Acute hepatitis is characterized by hepatocellular injury, leading to leakage of enzymes from damaged hepatocytes into the blood.

Aminotransferases (ALT and AST, previously called SGPT and SGOT)

- Markedly elevated (often >10× normal).
- ALT > AST, especially in viral hepatitis.
- In alcoholic hepatitis AST is at least 2 times more than ALT.
- AST and ALT levels can exceed 1000 IU/L.

Alkaline Phosphatase (ALP)

- Normal or only mildly elevated.

Bilirubin (total and direct)

- Both direct (conjugated) and indirect (unconjugated) bilirubin are elevated due to impaired conjugation and excretion.

- Bilirubin level in acute hepatitis ranges from 5 to 20 mg/dl. Jaundice is usually visible in the sclera or skin when the serum bilirubin is more than 2.5 mg/dl.

Serum Albumin

- Is usually normal in acute hepatitis; may decrease in prolonged or severe cases. Globulin level may be mildly elevated.

Prothrombin time (PT)

- PT may be prolonged and reflects a severe hepatic synthetic defect, signifies extensive hepatocellular necrosis, and indicates a worse prognosis.

LFTs in Obstructive Jaundice

Aminotransferases (ALT and AST)

- Mild-to-moderate elevation.
- Typically, not as high as in acute hepatitis.

Alkaline Phosphatase (ALP)

- Serum alkaline phosphatase is markedly elevated (>3–10 times normal). 5′ nucleotidase and gama glutamyl transferase are also elevated and usually parallel that of alkaline phosphatase.

Bilirubin (total and direct)

- Conjugated bilirubin is more than unconjugated bilirubin.
- Levels can be markedly elevated.

Serum Albumin

- Serum albumin and globulin levels are usually normal.

Prothrombin Time (PT)

- Prothrombin time (PT) may be prolonged secondary to vitamin K malabsorption because bile juice is required for the absorption of this fat-soluble vitamin.

Q. Endoscopic retrograde cholangiopancreatography (ERCP).

- ERCP is a technique that combines the use of endoscopy and fluoroscopy to diagnose and treat certain problems of the biliary or pancreatic ductal systems.

ERCP Procedure

- Patient is put under sedation and lied on his left side A side-viewing duodenoscopy is passed through the pylorus and into the second part of duodenum to visualize ampulla of Vater, and it is then cannulated. By adjusting the angle of the endoscope it can be either cannulated into the common bile duct or into the pancreatic duct which is then visualized with a fluoroscopy.
- ERCP is a technically demanding procedure, and there is risk of serious complications (e.g. pancreatitis).

Indications for ERCP

- Removal of stones from CBD or pancreatic duct.
- Endoscopic therapy of postoperative biliary leaks and strictures.
- Identifying and treating underlying cause in patients with recurrent acute pancreatitis.
- Treatment of symptomatic strictures in chronic pancreatitis.
- Treatment of pancreatic-duct disruptions or leaks by placement of bridging or transpapillary pancreatic stents.
- Draining symptomatic pancreatic pseudocysts.
- Palliation of biliary obstruction in patients with pancreatic or biliary cancer.
- Tissue sampling in patients with pancreatic, biliary and ampullary cancers.
- Biliary pancreatitis.
- Patients with type I sphincter of Oddi dysfunction (SOD) respond to ERCP guided sphincterotomy.

Complications for ERCP

- Pancreatitis
- Bleeding
- Sepsis
- Perforation.

Q. Magnetic resonance cholangiopancreatography (MRCP).

- MRCP is a noninvasive imaging technique that uses magnetic resonance imaging (MRI) to visualize the biliary and pancreatic ducts without the need for contrast injection or endoscopy.
- It is a digital reconstruction technique based on an abdominal MRI scan, and has excellent sensitivity and specificity. Unlike ERCP, MRCP does not require contrast material to be administered into the ductal system. However, MRCP does not allow any intervention to be performed, such as stone extraction, stent insertion, or biopsy.

Indications

- Because of its relative safety, it is useful for screening patients with a low likelihood of disease. In those with a higher probability, ERCP is still the procedure of choice because of its therapeutic options.
- MRCP is mainly used for diagnosis of hepatobiliary and pancreatic conditions which are as follows:
    - Choledocholithiasis (common bile duct stones)
    - Biliary obstruction (due to strictures or tumors)
    - Bile duct anomalies (e.g. choledochal cysts)
    - Postoperative biliary complications (e.g. strictures, leaks).
    - Pancreatic duct strictures or stones
    - Pancreatic divisum
    - Assessment of pancreatic tumors.

Advantages

- Noninvasive (no need for endoscope or contrast dye).
- No radiation exposure (as MRI is used).

- Good visualization of ductal anatomy and surrounding tissues.
- Safer in patients with coagulopathy or high risk for ERCP.

Limitations

- Cannot perform therapeutic interventions (e.g. stone removal, stenting).
- MRCP has lower resolution than conventional direct cholangiography and can miss small stones (<4 mm), small ampullary lesions, primary sclerosing cholangitis, and strictures of the ducts. MRCP also has difficulty visualizing small stones in the pancreatic duct.
- Not suitable for patients with MRI contraindications (e.g. pacemakers, metal implants).
- Patient must remain still, and breath-holding may be required.

Q. Percutaneous transhepatic cholangiography (PTC).

- PTC is an interventional radiological procedure used to visualize the biliary tree by injecting contrast dye directly into the intrahepatic bile ducts through the skin (percutaneous route) using a needle passed through the liver (transhepatic).
- It is done under local anesthesia. PTC is more accurate than ultrasonography or CT scan for identifying the cause and site of biliary tract obstruction. However, PTC is technically more difficult and has more complications.
- Complications include bacteremia, and hemobilia.

Indications

- Evaluation of obstructive jaundice when ERCP or MRCP is inconclusive or not possible.
- Visualization of biliary strictures, stones, or tumors.
- Assessment of post-surgical bile duct injuries.
- PTC can also be used for therapeutic interventions like drainage of infected bile in cholangitis, extraction of biliary tract stones, dilation of benign biliary strictures, or placement of a stent across a malignant stricture.

Q. Endoscopic ultrasound (EUS).

- Endoscopic ultrasound (EUS) is a technique where an ultrasound transducer is attached to the tip of an endoscope and passes into the upper GI tract to obtain echo images. EUS examination resembles standard endoscopy of the upper gastrointestinal tract.
- It provides good resolution images of the gut wall and the surrounding organs and blood vessels.
- It is useful to evaluate pancreas, bile ducts, for obtaining FNAC, etc.

Q. Indications and contraindications of liver biopsy.

- Liver biopsy is a medical procedure in which a small sample of liver tissue is removed for microscopic examination.
- Liver biopsy can be done by many methods: percutaneous, transjugular, or laparoscopic routes.
- Percutaneous liver biopsy is the simplest and most commonly performed approach.
- It can be done under ultrasound or CT guidance which is especially useful when there is focal pathology of liver (such as tumor).

Indications for Liver Biopsy

- Diagnosis, grading and staging of liver diseases, such as chronic hepatitis B or C, primary biliary cirrhosis, primary sclerosing cholangitis, autoimmune hepatitis, non-alcoholic steatohepatitis (NASH), hemochromatosis or Wilson's disease.
- Unexplained liver disease or abnormal liver function tests
- Monitoring the liver following a liver transplant
- Diagnosis of a liver mass
- Pyrexia of unknown origin.

Contraindications for Liver Biopsy

- Significant blood clotting abnormalities
- Severe obstructive jaundice
- Severe ascites
- Local skin infection at the biopsy site
- Suspected hemangioma or vascular tumor
- Uncooperative patient.

Q. Discuss the metabolism of bilirubin.

Q. Physiological and biochemical basis of jaundice.

- Bilirubin is a yellow pigment formed from the breakdown of heme, primarily from senescent red blood cells. Its metabolism involves several key steps in the reticuloendothelial system, liver, and intestines.
- Normal adults produce about 4 mg bilirubin per kg body weight per day. A 70–90% of bilirubin comes from degradation of hemoglobin and the remainder comes from the degradation of nonhemoglobin hemoproteins such as myoglobin, the P-450 cytochromes, catalase, and peroxidase.

Formation of Bilirubin (hemoglobin breakdown)

- Occurs mainly in the spleen and reticuloendothelial cells.
- Hemoglobin is broken down into heme and globin.
- Heme is converted to biliverdin (green pigment) by ***heme oxygenase***. Biliverdin is nontoxic and water-soluble.
- Biliverdin is converted to bilirubin by ***biliverdin reductase***.

Transportation in Blood

- Bilirubin is bound to albumin in plasma and transported to liver.
- The total plasma bilirubin concentration in normal adults is less than 1.5 mg/dl. Most of the plasma bilirubin is unconjugated and only a small fraction is conjugated. Unconjugated bilirubin is also called

indirect bilirubin because it does not react directly with diazo reagent used to estimate the amount of bilirubin in plasma using van den Bergh reaction, and requires the addition of agents like ethanol. Conjugated bilirubin is water soluble and is also called direct bilirubin because it reacts directly with diazo reagent without the addition of agents such as ethanol or urea. The indirect bilirubin is calculated by subtracting the direct bilirubin from the total.

Hepatic Uptake, Conjugation, and Excretion into Bile

- In the liver, uptake of unconjugated bilirubin from plasma happens by a facilitated transport process and to a lesser extent by diffusion. Liver converts unconjugated bilirubin into conjugated bilirubin mono- and diglucuronides by a specific UDP-glucuronyl transferase. These bilirubin mono- and diglucuronides are water soluble and are secreted into bile canaliculi, then into the bile ducts, and finally into the intestine.
- Conjugated bilirubin is loosely bound to albumin and can be excreted by the kidneys. Hence, bilirubinuria is found in obstructive or cholestatic jaundice. Newborn infants have decreased capacity to conjugate bilirubin which leads to unconjugated hyperbilirubinemia (physiologic jaundice of the newborn). If severe, this can lead to CNS damage (kernicterus). Exposure to blue light (phototherapy) converts bilirubin to water-soluble photoisomers which are easily excreted in bile, thereby decreasing CNS damage.

Intestinal Metabolism

- Following canalicular secretion, conjugated bilirubin enters the biliary tree, reaches the duodenum, and passes down the gastrointestinal tract. In the gut (ileum and colon), most of the conjugated bilirubin is converted into urobilinogen by bacteria. Some urobilinogen is reabsorbed by the intestine, returns to the liver through the portal circulation, and is re-excreted into bile (enterohepatic recirculation). A portion is oxidized to stercobilin (gives stool its brown color). A small fraction of urobilinogen is excreted in urine as urobilin, giving urine its yellow color.
- Urine urobilinogen is increased in hemolysis, which increases the load of bilirubin entering the gut and therefore the amount of urobilinogen formed and reabsorbed, and in liver disease due to reduced extraction of urobilinogen by the liver leading to increased excretion by the kidneys. In obstructive jaundice, conjugated bilirubin does not enter the gut; hence there is no formation of urobilinogen leading to reduced excretion of urobilinogen in the urine.

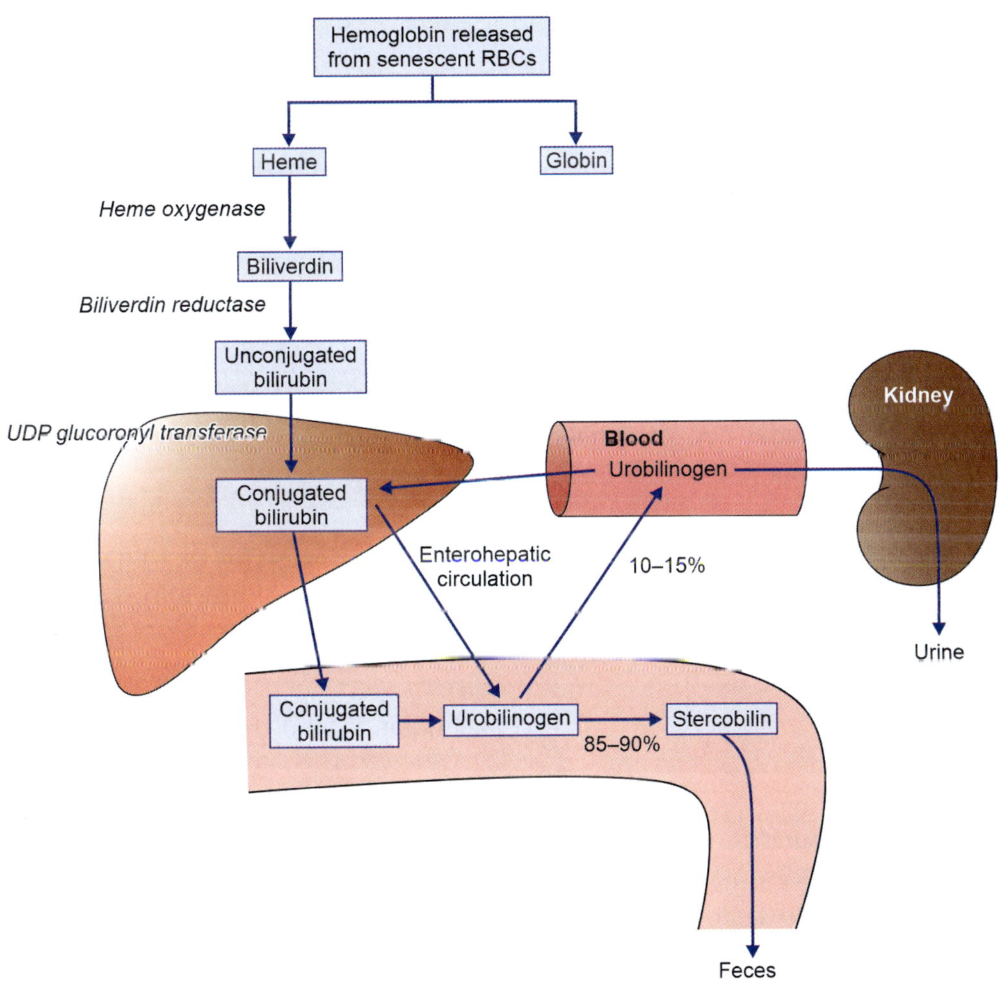

Figure 7.1: Bilirubin metabolism

- Gilbert's syndrome and Crigler-Najjar syndrome types 1 and 2 are characterized by unconjugated hyperbilirubinemia due to genetic defects in bilirubin conjugation. In contrast, Dubin-Johnson syndrome is characterized by conjugated or mixed hyperbilirubinemia due to defects in excretion of conjugated bilirubin into the bile.

Q. van den Bergh reaction.

- van den Bergh reaction is a chemical test used to differentiate types of bilirubin in the blood—primarily direct (conjugated) and indirect (unconjugated) bilirubin.
- This test involves the reaction of bilirubin with a diazo compound (diazotized sulfanilic acid), producing azobilirubin which can be quantified by spectrophotometry. Conjugated bilirubin reacts directly with diazo compound without the addition of alcohol hence it is also called direct bilirubin. Unconjugated bilirubin requires the addition of alcohol and hence called indirect bilirubin.
- The indirect and direct bilirubin can be distinguished based upon their rate of production in the presence or absence of alcohol. The fraction produced within one minute without the addition of alcohol represents the concentration of direct bilirubin. Fast reaction of direct bilirubin is due to the absence of internal hydrogen bonding and water solubility. Total bilirubin is that amount that reacts in 30 minutes after the addition of alcohol. Indirect bilirubin is calculated by subtracting direct bilirubin from total bilirubin. Total bilirubin concentration by this technique is usually below 1 mg/dl.
- van den Bergh reaction slightly overestimates direct bilirubin because a fraction of unconjugated bilirubin also gives a direct reaction. Endogenous substances, such as plasma lipids, and drugs, such as propranolol, can interfere with the diazo reaction and produce unreliable results. Bilirubin complexed to albumin (delta bilirubin) also may give a direct reaction.

Q. Enumerate the causes of tender hepatomegaly.

- Viral hepatitis
- Acute alcoholic hepatitis
- Liver abscess (pyogenic, amebic)
- Acute fatty liver
- Congestive cardiac failure
- Budd-Chiari syndrome
- Hepatocellular Ca
- Actinomycosis of the liver
- Wiel's disease (leptospirosis)

Q. Enumerate the causes of jaundice. How do you approach a case of jaundice?

- Jaundice is defined as yellowish discoloration of skin, mucous membranes and sclera due to hyperbilirubinemia. Hyperbilirubinemia may be due to abnormalities in the formation, transport, metabolism, and excretion of bilirubin. Total serum bilirubin is normally 0.3–1 mg/dl. Jaundice is clinically detectable when levels are more than 2.5 mg/dl.

Causes of Jaundice

Prehepatic (hemolytic) causes

Due to increased unconjugated bilirubin from excess red cell breakdown

- Hemolytic anemia (e.g. hereditary spherocytosis, autoimmune hemolytic anemia, G6PD deficiency)
- Malaria
- Transfusion reactions
- Ineffective erythropoiesis (e.g. megaloblastic anemia)

Hepatic (hepatocellular) causes

Due to impaired uptake, conjugation, or excretion by hepatocytes. May cause mixed (conjugated + unconjugated) hyperbilirubinemia

- Acute viral hepatitis (HAV, HBV, HCV, HEV)
- Alcoholic hepatitis
- Drug-induced liver injury (e.g. paracetamol overdose, anti-TB drugs)
- Autoimmune hepatitis
- Wilson's disease
- Hemochromatosis
- Cirrhosis
- Leptospirosis
- Liver tumors (primary or metastatic)
- Gilbert's syndrome
- Crigler-Najjar syndrome
- Dubin-Johnson syndrome
- Rotor syndrome

Posthepatic (obstructive) causes

Due to obstruction of bile flow (increased conjugated bilirubin)

- Choledocholithiasis
- Biliary atresia (in neonates)
- Carcinoma of bile duct
- Sclerosing cholangitis
- Choledochal cyst
- External pressure on common duct
- Pancreatitis
- Ca head of pancreas
- Periampullary carcinoma.

Approach to a Case of Jaundice

- The cause of jaundice in majority of cases can be diagnosed by careful history and physical examination.

History

- Enquire about the onset and duration of jaundice. Patients often notice darkening of urine even before the onset of jaundice which indicates the actual time of onset of problem more accurately than onset of jaundice. Jaundice appearing over a few days to a week implies acute hepatitis (viral, toxins, leptospirosis, etc.). Jaundice appearing over the course of weeks implies a subacute hepatitis or extrahepatic obstruction due to malignancy, gallstone, chronic pancreatitis, or stricture of common bile duct. Intermittent jaundice may indicate gallstones, ampullary carcinoma, or drug induced hepatitis.

- History of constitutional symptoms such as fever, nausea, vomiting, myalgia, malaise, etc. suggests viral hepatitis or liver abscess as the cause of jaundice. Also enquire about changes in stool color, pruritus, steatorrhea, and abdominal pain (including location, severity, duration, and radiation). Clay colored stools, pruritus, and pain abdomen are classically seen in obstructive jaundice. Right hypochondrial pain can also be present in acute hepatitis, liver abscess, and hepatocellular carcinoma.
- A past history of jaundice may implicate chronic hepatitis, cirrhosis, or a genetic hyperbilirubinemia (i.e. Gilbert's or Dubin–Johnson syndrome) as the cause.
- H/o coagulopathy (e.g. easy bruising or bleeding, tarry or bloody stools) indicates severe liver disease. H/o melena and hematemesis may be present in cirrhosis of liver with portal hypertension.
- Arthritis or urticaria may sometimes precede the onset of jaundice in hepatitis-B infection. Arthritis may also accompany or precede autoimmune hepatitis.
- Drug history should be obtained in detail as many drugs are known to produce hepatic dysfunction and jaundice (e.g. isoniazid, rifampicin, estrogens, antiepileptics, etc.)
- H/o contact with others with jaundice, recent transfusions, needle or narcotic use indicates potential exposure to hepatitis viruses. Recent foreign travel to areas of poor sanitation carries a risk of exposure to hepatitis A or E virus or *Entamoeba histolytica*. Farmers, sewage workers, and workers at slaughterhouses are at risk of getting leptospirosis.
- Any H/o of surgery either recent or remote may have implications in a case of jaundice. Type of anesthesia (certain anesthetic agents can cause hepatitis), hypotension during surgery (ischemic hepatitis), injury to bile duct during surgery can present with jaundice. Surgery on biliary tract in remote past can present with jaundice due to biliary stricture.
- A family history of jaundice or liver disease may suggest hereditary hyperbilirubinemias (i.e. Crigler–Najjar, Gilbert's, Dubin–Johnson, or Rotor's syndromes), Wilson's disease, hemochromatosis, and alpha-1 antitrypsin deficiency. Family h/o anemia with jaundice may suggest hereditary spherocytosis.
- Personal history should include questions about risk factors for hepatitis such as amount and duration of alcohol use, injection drug use, and high-risk sexual behavior.

General Examination

- Weight loss is usually present in hepatocellular carcinoma, liver metastases, or cirrhosis.
- Look for the presence of stigmata of chronic liver disease which includes spider nevi, palmar erythema, gynecomastia, decreased body hair, caput medusae, Dupuytren contractures, parotid gland enlargement, and testicular atrophy.
- Purpura and ecchymotic patches on the skin indicate significant liver impairment.
- Lymph node enlargement especially left supraclavicular and periumbilical indicates the possibility of hepatocellular carcinoma.
- Raised JVP can indicate right-sided heart failure, which can cause hepatic congestion and cirrhosis (cardiac cirrhosis).
- Pedal edema is common in cirrhosis of liver with portal HTN.

Systemic Examination

- ***Abdomen***: Look for the presence of hepatosplenomegaly, or ascites. Jaundice with ascites indicates either cirrhosis or malignancy with peritoneal spread. Splenomegaly is also common in cirrhosis of liver with portal HTN. Right upper quadrant tenderness with palpable gallbladder (Courvoisier sign) suggests obstruction of the cystic duct due to malignancy.
- ***CVS examination***: To rule out cardiac failure especially right heart failure because it can cause congestive hepatitis and cardiac cirrhosis.
- ***RS examination***: Lung malignancy can metastasize to liver. Tuberculosis from lungs can involve liver. Pleural effusion can be present in cirrhosis with portal HTN.
- ***Nervous system examination***: Hepatic encephalopathy can occur due to liver failure. Wilson disease can involve both CNS and liver.

Investigations

- Complete blood count: Anemia and reticulocytosis is seen in hemolytic jaundice. Leukocytosis and neutrophilia are common in cholangitis and alcoholic hepatitis. Eosinophilia plus jaundice is suspicious for toxic hepatitis.
- Liver function tests: Helpful to confirm the presence of liver impairment and also to diagnose the type of jaundice **(Fig. 7.2)**.
- Blood urea, creatinine: can be elevated.
- Blood sugar level: Hypoglycemia can occur in severe liver disease due to reduced gluconeogenesis.
- Serum electrolytes.
- Urine examination: Normally bile pigments are absent in the urine. A jaundiced patient with absent urinary bilirubin indicates hemolytic jaundice or a hepatic defect in bilirubin uptake or conjugation.
- Ultrasound abdomen: Helpful to diagnose liver abscess, malignancies, cirrhosis, bile duct obstruction, ascites, and pancreatic pathologies.
- Hepatocellular workup: Viral serologies, autoimmune antibodies, serum ceruloplasmin, ferritin.
- Cholestatic workup: In addition to ultrasound, CT, magnetic resonance cholangiopancreatography (MRCP), endoscopic retrograde cholangiopancreatography (ERCP), percutaneous transhepatic cholangiography (PTC), endoscopic ultrasound (EUS) are helpful.
- Liver biopsy if indicated.

Treatment

- The underlying cause of jaundice and any complications should be treated.
- Jaundice itself requires no treatment in adults (unlike in neonates).
- Severe itching may be relieved with cholestyramine which is a bile salt binding compound.

Flowchart to diagnose the cause of jaundice (Fig. 7.2).

Q. Discuss briefly the congenital hyperbilrubinemic disorders.

- Congenital hyperbilirubinemic disorders are inherited conditions affecting bilirubin metabolism, leading to either unconjugated or conjugated hyperbilirubinemia, often presenting with chronic or intermittent jaundice **(Table 7.3)**.

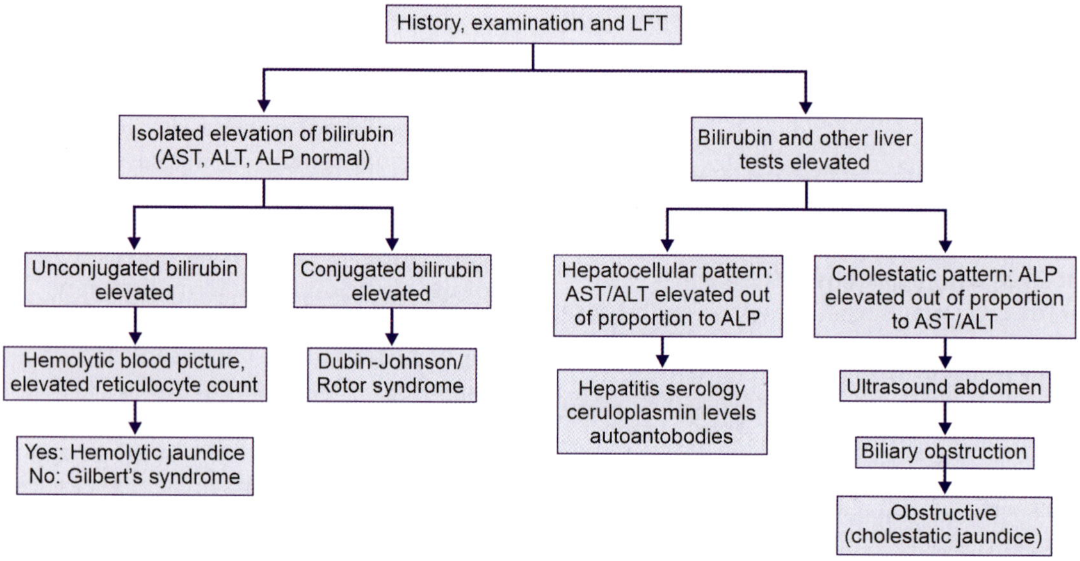

Figure 7.2: Approach to a case of jaundice

TABLE 7.3: Congenital hyperbilrubinemic disorders

	Inheritance	Defect	Type of hyperbilirubinemia	Key features
Gilbert's syndrome	Autosomal recessive	Mild deficiency of UDP-glucuronyl transferase	Unconjugated	Benign, asymptomatic jaundice. More common in males. Urobilinogen in the urine is increased but there is no bilirubinuria. Peripheral blood smear, reticulocyte count and haptoglobin are normal (suggesting absence of hemolysis). Hyperbilirubinemia increases after fasting. No treatment required (Phenobarbital can increase the activity of UDP-glucoronyl transferase). Prognosis is excellent.
Crigler-Najjar syndrome type I	Autosomal recessive	Complete absence of UDP-glucoronyl transferase	Unconjugated	Seen in infants. Bilirubin is very high (20–25 mg/dl, can be as high as 50 mg/dl). Stool color is normal, but fecal urobilinogen excretion is diminished due to the marked reduction in the conjugation of bilirubin. Peripheral blood smear, reticulocyte count and haptoglobin are normal (suggesting absence of hemolysis). Prognosis poor. Death occurs due to kernicterus , unless vigorously treated.
Crigler-Najjar syndrome type II	Autosomal dominant	↓ UDP-glucuronyl transferase	Unconjugated	Usually benign, kernicterus occurs rarely. Hyperbilirubinemia can be reduced by treatment with phenobarbital.
Dubin–Johnson syndrome	Autosomal recessive	Reduced ability to transport conjugated bilirubin into biliary canaliculi	Conjugated	Benign, asymptomatic jaundice. Gallbladder not visualized on oral cholecystography. BSP (bromsulphalein) test shows reduced clearance. Liver darkly pigmented on gross examination (black liver). Biopsy shows centrilobular brown pigment. No treatment required. Prognosis excellent.
Rotor's syndrome	Autosomal recessive	Faulty excretory function of hepatocytes	Conjugated	Similar to Dubin–Johnson syndrome, but liver is not pigmented and the gallbladder is visualized on oral cholecystography. Prognosis excellent.

Q. Discuss the clinical and laboratory differentiation of different types of jaundice.

See **Table 7.4.**

Q. Describe the etiology, epidemiology, clinical features, laboratory features and treatment of hepatitis A. Add a note on its prevention.

Many viruses can cause viral hepatitis. These are as follows:

- ***Hepatitis viruses***: Hepatitis A, B, C, D, E.
- ***Other viruses***: Cytomegalovirus, Epstein Barr virus, herpes simplex virus, yellow fever virus.

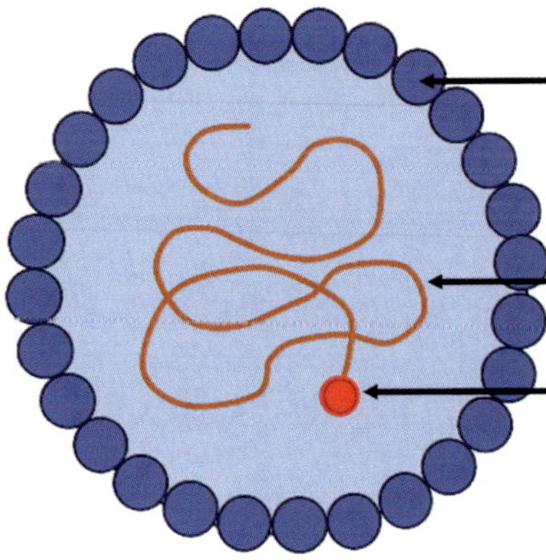

Figure 7.3: Hepatitis A virus

Hepatitis A

- Hepatitis A is a viral liver disease caused by the hepatitis A virus (HAV). It is an acute, self-limiting condition that does not result in chronic liver disease and is preventable by vaccination.

Etiology

- Hepatitis A is caused by hepatitis A virus which is a single stranded RNA virus that belongs to the family of Picornaviridae **(Fig. 7.3)**.
- It is resistant to freezing, detergents and acids. It can be inactivated by heat (>85°C), formalin and chlorine.
- Replication occurs in the liver. The virus is secreted into the bile and found in stool. Highest titers are found in stool during the incubation period and early symptomatic phase of illness.

Epidemiology

- It is transmitted almost exclusively by the fecal-oral route through ingestion of contaminated food or water. Consumption of shellfish from contaminated waterways is a rare source of hepatitis A infection. Very rarely through blood transfusion.
- People at risk of acquiring hepatitis A include travelers to developing countries, children in day care centers, men who have sex with men, injection drug users, hemophiliacs given plasma products, and persons in institutions.

TABLE 7.4: Clinical and laboratory differentiation of different types of jaundice

Clinical features	Hemolytic	Hepatocellular	Obstructive
Color of jaundice	Lemon yellow	Orange yellow	Greenish yellow
Depth of jaundice	Mild	Moderate	Deep
Pruritus	Absent	Sometimes	Present
Bleeding tendency	Absent	Present	Present (late)
Bradycardia	Absent	Absent	Present
Pallor	Present	Absent	Absent
Splenomegaly	Present	Sometimes	Absent
Features of liver cell failure	Absent	Present	Present (late)
Stool color	Normal	Normal	Light color (clay color)
Urine color	Normal	Dark	Dark
Laboratory features			
Bilirubin	Predominantly unconjugated	Mixed	Predominantly conjugated
ALT, AST	Normal	Markedly increased	Minimally Increased
Alkaline phosphatase	Normal	Increased	Markedly increased
Serum albumin	Unchanged	Decreased	Unchanged
Prothrombin time	Normal	Prolonged and does not respond to parenteral vitamin K	Prolonged in late stages and responds to parenteral vitamin K
Urine bilirubin	None	Increased	Increased
Urine urobilinogen	Increased	Increased	Absent

Note: Hemolytic jaundice is also known as acholuric jaundice because bilirubin is absent in the urine. The reason is, in hemolytic jaundice there is rise in indirect bilirubin which is insoluble in water, bound to albumin and hence not excreted through the kidneys. Hence, in typical hemolytic jaundice, urine stays normal or slightly darker from urobilinogen, but never from bilirubin. Another point to note is cola-colored urine in intravascular hemolysis which is due to hemoglobinuria and not due to bilirubin.

- It is more prevalent in low socioeconomic groups in which a lack of adequate sanitation and poor hygienic practices facilitate spread of the infection.

Clinical Features

- Incubation period is 15–50 days (mean 30 days).
- HAV infection usually results in an acute, self-limited illness and only rarely leads to fulminant hepatic failure. Fulminant hepatic failure is likely to occur when hepatitis-A infection is superimposed on preexisting chronic hepatitis-B or hepatitis-C.
- Symptomatic infection is more common in adults than children. Jaundice occurs in 70% of adults infected with HAV but in smaller proportions of children.

Prodromal phase

- Illness begins with the abrupt onset of prodromal symptoms including, fatigue, malaise, nausea, vomiting, anorexia, fever, and right upper quadrant pain.

Icteric phase

- Jaundice, dark urine, and pruritus develop in a few days. Prodromal symptoms decrease as the jaundice appears.
- Physical examination shows jaundice and hepatomegaly. There may be splenomegaly, and cervical lymphadenopathy.

Recovery phase

- Gradual resolution of jaundice over 1–2 months
- Fatigue may persist for weeks.
- Hepatitis A does not lead to chronic infection, chronic hepatitis, cirrhosis or carrier state.

Extrahepatic manifestations

- There can be extrahepatic manifestations such as vasculitis, arthritis, optic neuritis, transverse myelitis, thrombocytopenia, aplastic anemia, and red cell aplasia.

Laboratory Findings

- Serum aminotransferases are markedly elevated (often >1000 IU/L). ALT (SGPT) is more elevated than AST (SGOT). Aminotransferase elevations precede the bilirubin elevation. Total bilirubin is elevated (upto 30mg/dl) and consist of both conjugated and unconjugated fractions. ALP is normal or mildly elevated. Other laboratory abnormalities are increased CRP, ESR and immunoglobulins.
- Prothrombin time (PT) may be prolonged and signifies extensive hepatocellular necrosis and worse prognosis.
- IgM-anti-HAV antibody appears early in the disease and persists for 4–12 months. It can be used for the diagnosis of acute hepatitis A. IgG antibodies also appear early in the course and persists for life. Other viral markers such as HbsAg, anti-HCV and anti-HEV should be done to rule out other causes of viral hepatitis.
- Imaging studies such as ultrasound abdomen are done if there is possibility of an alternative diagnosis. It may show hepatomegaly in acute hepatitis.

Treatment

- There is no specific antiviral therapy for HAV.
- The disease is usually self-limited, and treatment is mainly supportive with hydration, vitamins and antipyretics.
- Prognosis is excellent in most cases. Fulminant hepatic failure is rare but may occur, Liver transplantation should be considered for patients who develop fulminant liver failure.

Prevention of Hepatitis A

- Improvement of sanitation, hand washing before eating, heating foods appropriately, and avoidance of water and foods from endemic areas prevent the transmission of virus. Chlorination and household bleach (1:100 dilution) inactivate the virus.
- ***Vaccine:*** A safe and effective HAV vaccine is available (example: HAVRIX by GlaxoSmithKline). It is given as two injections 6 months apart (1.0 ml intramuscular). It is recommended for patients at high risk of acquiring hepatitis A such as travelers to endemic areas, children in communities with high rates of infection, men who have sex with men, injection drug users, patients with chronic liver disease and recipients of pooled plasma products, such as hemophiliacs.
- ***Post exposure prophylaxis:*** Vaccine is not effective for post exposure prophylaxis because antibodies take few days to develop. Immune globulin is recommended for post exposure prophylaxis of household and intimate contacts of persons with acute hepatitis A. The dose is 2 ml given intramuscularly within 2 weeks of exposure. Concurrent HAV vaccination is also appropriate.

Q. Describe the etiology, epidemiology, pathogenesis, clinical features, laboratory features and treatment of hepatitis B.

Q. Prevention of hepatitis B.

- Hepatitis B is a viral infection of the liver caused by the hepatitis B virus (HBV).
- It can present as an acute or chronic disease and may lead to liver inflammation, fibrosis, cirrhosis, or hepatocellular carcinoma.

Etiology

- Hepatitis B is caused by the hepatitis B virus (HBV) which is a DNA virus **(Fig. 7.4)** belonging to the family of Hepadnaviridae. Hepatitis B virus contains:
    - Outer envelope with hepatitis B surface antigen (HBsAg)
    - Core containing hepatitis B core antigen (HBcAg) and e antigen (HBeAg)
    - Partially double-stranded DNA genome
    - DNA polymerase with reverse transcriptase activity.

Epidemiology

- Incubation period is about 90 days (30–180 days).
- The virus infects only humans and higher apes.

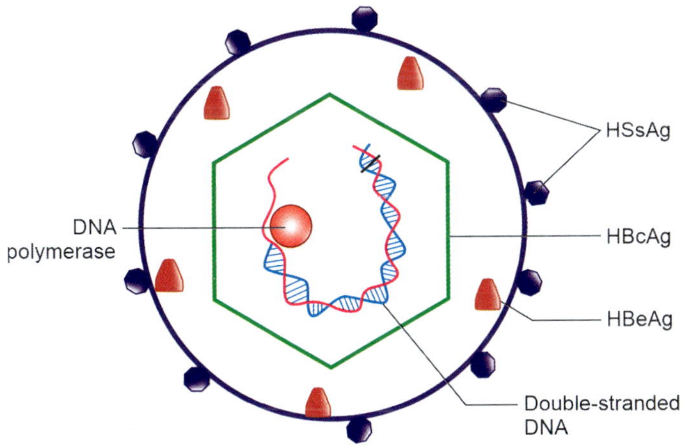

Figure 7.4: Structure of hepatitis B virus

- It is transmitted by parenteral (blood transfusion, needle sharing), perinatal (mother to child during delivery), and sexual routes.
- Persons at risk of developing infection include; spouse of an acutely infected person, unprotected sex with multiple partners (especially men who have sex with men), health care workers, injection drug users, recipients of repeated transfusions, especially with pooled blood concentrates (e.g. hemophiliacs), dentists, prisoners, family members of chronically infected persons, persons on hemodialysis, being born to an infected mother.
- Prevalence is high in sub-Saharan Africa and Southeast Asia, Down syndrome, lepromatous leprosy, leukemia, Hodgkin's disease, polyarteritis nodosa, patients receiving hemodialysis, injection drug users, lower socioeconomic groups, and older age groups.

Pathogenesis

- The pathogenesis of HBV-related liver disease is largely due to immune-mediated mechanisms resulting in destruction of HBV-infected hepatocytes by cytotoxic T cells. Rarely HBV can cause direct cytotoxic liver injury. Outcomes depend on age at infection and host immune response. Possible outcomes are as follows:
  - Acute self-limited hepatitis (in 90–95% of immunocompetent adults).
  - Fulminant hepatitis (rare.)
  - Chronic hepatitis B (defined as persistence of HBsAg >6 months. Risk is higher if infected perinatally).
  - Cirrhosis.
  - Hepatocellular carcinoma (HCC).

Clinical Features

Acute Hepatitis-B

- Clinical features are similar to hepatitis-A.
- About 70% of patients with acute hepatitis B have subclinical or anicteric hepatitis, while 30% develop icteric hepatitis. The disease is more severe in patients with underlying liver disease.

Chronic Hepatitis B

- Defined as persistence of HBsAg >6 months
- May be asymptomatic (inactive carrier) or symptomatic with progressive liver damage → cirrhosis, HCC.

Extrahepatic Manifestations

- These are common in chronic hepatitis B, but rarely can occur in acute hepatitis B also. They are:
  - Polyarteritis nodosa (PAN)
  - Glomerulonephritis
  - Rash, arthralgia.

Laboratory Findings

- Liver function tests are same as described in hepatitis A.
- Laboratory features specific to hepatitis B are as follows **(Table 7.5)**.

TABLE 7.5: Hepatitis B viral markers

Test	Interpretation
HBsAg	Active infection (acute or chronic). Confirms the diagnosis of hepatitis-B infection
Anti-HBs antibody	Immunity (recovery or vaccination)
HBeAg	High infectivity
Anti-HBe	Lower infectivity
Anti-HBc IgM	Acute infection
Anti-HBc IgG	Past or chronic infection
HBV DNA (PCR)	Viral load; assesses replication and treatment need

Treatment

- For acute hepatitis B treatment is mainly supportive which is same as that of acute hepatitis A. Most of the acute hepatitis B cases resolve within 6 months without any specific antiviral therapy. However if the virus is not cleared within 6 months (chronic hepatitis), then treatment is required.
- For fulminant acute hepatitis, antivirals or liver transplantation may be considered.
- For chronic hepatitis B (persistence of HBsAg for more than 6 months) many treatment options with antiviral drugs are available. The antiviral drugs effective against hepatitis B are entecavir, tenofovir, telbivudine, alfa-interferon, lamivudine, and adefovir. These drugs can be used in combination also.
- Tenofovir and entecavir are first-line treatment. They are more potent with low resistance. Older drugs like lamivudine and adefovir have more resistance.

Complications

- Serum sickness-like syndrome
- Glomerulonephritis with nephrotic syndrome
- Polyarteritis nodosa-like systemic vasculitis
- Fulminant hepatitis (massive hepatic necrosis)
- Chronic hepatitis B (persistence of HBeAg beyond 3 months or HBsAg beyond 6 months). Chronic

hepatitis B can lead to cirrhosis of liver and hepatocellular carcinoma.
- Aplastic anemia
- Transverse myelitis.

Prognosis

- 95–99% of patients recover completely.
- Fulminant hepatitis: 0.1–1%
- Chronic hepatitis: 1–10%
- Carrier state: 0.1–30%

Prevention

Preexposure Prophylaxis

- Recombinant hepatitis B vaccine (e. g. Engerix B), 1 ml (20 µg) given IM at 0, 1, and 6 months.
- Alternative schedules have been approved, including accelerated schedules of 0, 1, 2, and 12 months and of 0, 7, and 21 days plus 12 months. Vaccine should be given to deltoid and not gluteal region. A booster dose is required after 5 years. Half the dose is given for children.
- Vaccination is indicated for high risk groups. But now a days hepatitis B vaccination is being given to all.
- Standard vaccination schedule (for adults) is as follows:

Dose	Timing
1st dose	Any choosen date
2nd dose	1 month after 1st dose
3rd dose	6 months after 1st dose
Booster dose	5 years later

Post-exposure Prophylaxis

- Hepatitis B immune globulin: 0.06 ml/kg IM should be given within 1 week after exposure, followed by a complete course of hepatitis B vaccine started within the first week. After sexual exposure immunoglobulin can be given upto 14 days.
- For perinatal exposure of infants born to an HBsAg-positive mother, a single 0.5-ml IM dose of immunoglobulin should be given immediately after birth in combination with a complete course of 3 injections of hepatitis B vaccine to be started within the first 12 hours of life.

Q. Discuss the clinical features, investigations and management of chronic hepatitis B.

- Hepatitis B is considered chronic when HBsAg persists for more than 6 months after initial infection.
- Liver injury and pathogenesis of chronic hepatitis B are immunologically mediated. Antigen-specific cytotoxic T cells mediate the cell injury in hepatitis B and also account for ultimate viral clearance. The progression of acute to chronic hepatitis B is attributed to lack of a vigorous cytotoxic T-cell response to hepatitis B antigens.

Epidemiology

- Chronic hepatitis B afflicts 400 million people worldwide. Persons at high risk of chronic hepatitis B include men who have sex with men, persons with multiple sexual partners, hemophiliacs, oncology and renal dialysis patients, and health care workers.
- Most patients with chronic hepatitis B eventually recover. But some may progress to cirrhosis and end-stage liver disease. Some patients may go into an inactive carrier state with no symptoms, normal serum aminotransferase levels, and inactive liver disease on liver biopsy.

Clinical Features

- Chronic hepatitis B can range from an asymptomatic carrier state to progressive liver disease.

Asymptomatic Phase (carrier state)

- No symptoms.
- Normal liver enzymes.
- Detected incidentally on screening.

Symptomatic Phase (active disease)

- Symptomatic patients may present with constitutional symptoms such as fatigue, malaise, low-grade fever, anorexia and jaundice which is persistent or intermittent.
- Stigmata of chronic liver disease such as ascites, hepatomegaly, palmar erythema, gynecomastia, and spider angioma may be present.
- Complications include hepatocellular carcinoma (HCC) and liver failure.
- The extrahepatic manifestations of chronic hepatitis B include mucocutaneous vasculitis, glomerulonephritis, and polyarteritis nodosa.

Investigations

- HBsAg, HBeAg, and HBV DNA persist, generally at high levels. There are two general forms of chronic hepatitis B. HBeAg-positive chronic hepatitis B, in which there are high levels of HBV DNA, and less commonly HBeAg-negative form, where there are moderate levels of HBV DNA in serum.
- Aminotransferases (ALT, AST) remain elevated. But one-third of patients may have normal or near-normal aminotransferases.
- Alkaline phosphatase level is normal or marginally elevated.
- Serum bilirubin level is normal to moderately elevated.
- Hypoalbuminemia is present.
- Prothrombin time is prolonged.
- Alpha-Fetoprotein (AFP): Marker for hepatocellular carcinoma. Done if HCC is suspected.
- Ultrasound abdomen or CT scan are useful to rule out cirrhosis or hepatocellular carcinoma and to guide liver biopsy.
- Liver biopsy may be indicated to assess severity of disease, predict response to therapy, or rule out hepatocellular carcinoma.

Treatment of Chronic Hepatitis-B

Goals of Treatment

- Suppress HBV replication.
- Prevent progression to cirrhosis, liver failure, and hepatocellular carcinoma (HCC).
- Achieve HBsAg loss and seroconversion (rare, but ideal).
- Improve liver histology and prolong survival.

Indications to Start Antiviral Therapy

- Acute liver failure or decompensated or compensated cirrhosis regardless of viral load or ALT or HBeAg status.
- HBV DNA > 2000 IU/ml and ALT elevated and/or liver biopsy/fibroScan shows significant fibrosis.
- HBV DNA > 20,000 IU/ml + ALT >2 times the upper limit (especially in HBeAg+).
- Immunosuppressed or undergoing chemotherapy.
- Co-infection with HIV or HCV.

Entecavir

- It is considered a first-line treatment for HBV infection.
- Entecavir is a nucleoside analogue and inhibits HBV DNA polymerase. It has a high antiviral potency, and resistance to it is uncommon.
- Adverse effects include exacerbations of hepatitis B virus infection after discontinuation, lactic acidosis and severe hepatomegaly with steatosis.

Tenofovir

- Tenofovir has replaced adefovir (an older nucleotide analog) as a first-line treatment. It is a nucleotide analogue (adenosine monophosphate) reverse transcriptase and hepatitis B virus (HBV) polymerase inhibitor. Tenofovir is the most potent oral antiviral for hepatitis B; resistance to it is minimal.
- It has few adverse effects. Its main side effects are lactic acidosis and severe hepatomegaly with steatosis. The dose is one 300 mg once daily orally.

Pegylated Interferon Alpha

- This is effective in patients with a low viral load and elevated serum transaminases. However, it is not the first choice treatment. It acts by augmenting the native immune response. Interferon therapy is not recommended in patients with normal or near-normal serum aminotransferase levels (even if HBeAg is present) because it is usually ineffective in this situation. Interferon has to be given by subcutaneous injection.
- It is given for 4–6 months in HBeAg-positive chronic hepatitis in whom the response is good. Response rates are lower in HBeAg-negative chronic hepatitis, even with longer duration of therapy.
- Longer-acting pegylated interferons which can be given once weekly have been developed and are effective in both HBeAg-positive and HBeAg-negative chronic hepatitis.
- Interferon is contraindicated in the presence of decompensated cirrhosis (e.g. ascites, jaundice, coagulopathy, encephalopathy). In such patients it can precipitate liver failure.

General Measures

- All household and sexual contacts of patient should be vaccinated.
- Vaccination against hepatitis A also is recommended.
- Patients with hepatitis B should avoid all but the most necessary use of immunosuppressive medications. Severe flares of hepatitis B and even deaths have followed short courses of corticosteroids or cancer chemotherapy.

Q. HBsAg; hepatitis B surface antigen.

- Hepatitis B surface antigen (HBsAg) historically known as the Australia antigen, is a protein on the surface of the hepatitis B virus (HBV). It is the earliest marker of HBV infection and indicates that a person is infected with hepatitis B.
- It was first discovered Baruch Blumberg in the serum of an Australian aboriginal individual—hence the name "Australia antigen". This discovery led to the development of the hepatitis B vaccine, and Blumberg later won the Nobel Prize.
- It is the serologic hallmark of HBV infection. It can be detected by radioimmunoassay (RIA) or enzyme immunoassay (EIA).
- HBsAg appears in serum 1–10 weeks after an acute exposure to HBV, before the onset of symptoms.
- In patients who recover, HBsAg usually becomes negative after 3–6 months. Persistence of HBsAg for more than 6 months indicates chronic hepatitis-B. Usually less than 1% of patients progress to chronic hepatitis B.
- The disappearance of HBsAg is followed by the appearance of anti-HBsAg antibodies indicates recovery from hepatitis-B infection.
- Since antibodies against HBsAg are protective against hepatitis-B, HBsAg is used in the manufacturing of hepatitis-B vaccines.

Q. Chronic hepatitis B carrier.

Q. Conditions associated with hepatitis B carrier state.

- A hepatitis B carrier is a person who is chronically infected with hepatitis B virus (HBV) but has: no symptoms, normal liver enzymes, and Low or undetectable viral load.
- After hepatitis-B infection, HBsAg disappears from the blood in 3–6 months in 90% of adults. But in 10% the virus persists for more than 6 months; these persons are called chronic carriers.
- The difference between chronic hepatitis and chronic carrier state can be made by the presence or absence of liver injury as evidenced by elevated liver enzymes (ALT, AST). If HBsAg is positive without liver enzyme elevation then it is carrier state. If HBsAg is positive

along with elevated liver enzymes, then it is chronic hepatitis.

- The prevalence of chronic carrier state is low in low endemicity countries (1% in America, Europe, Australia), 1–6% in intermediate-endemicity countries (India, Middle East, Russia) and 7–30% in high-endemicity countries (Africa, China, Taiwan).
- The carrier state usually lasts indefinitely but HBsAg occasionally disappears spontaneously (1% per year). About 10–20% of chronic carriers are HBeAg-positive and highly infectious.
- Liver biopsy in the majority (80%) of chronic carriers is nearly normal (asymptomatic carriers) but in about 20% changes of chronic hepatitis are present.
- LFT (ALT) should be monitored in carriers every 6–12 months.
- Risks associated with carrier state are as follows:
  - Small risk of developing hepatocellular carcinoma (HCC), develop in HCC.
  - Reactivation of HBV (especially during immuno-suppression).
  - Extrahepatic immune-mediated disorders (poly-arteritis nodosa, membranous glomerulonephritis cryoglobulinemia, and aplastic anemia (rare)
  - Transmission risk to close contacts.

Conditions Associated with Hepatitis B Carrier State (risk factors for chronic carrier status)

- Neonates and infants (after perinatal transmission).
- Young children.
- Immunocompromised individuals (HIV-positive, transplant recipients, cancer patients on chemotherapy, patients on steroids).
- Impaired cell-mediated immunity (e.g. chronic uremia, malignancy, lepromatous leprosy, Down syndrome).

Q. Describe the etiology, epidemiology, clinical features, laboratory features and treatment of hepatitis C.

- Hepatitis C is an infection caused by the hepatitis C virus (HCV) which primarily affects the liver. It was previously called non-A, non-B hepatitis.

Etiology

- Hepatitis C is caused by hepatitis C virus which is a single stranded RNA virus belonging to Flaviviridae family.

Epidemiology

- Frequency is higher among African Americans and Mexican Americans than white persons.
- Most frequent in persons 30–50 years of age
- More frequent in men than women
- Transmitted by parenetral, perinatal, and sexual routes (just like hepatitis B)
- Persons at risk of acquiring infection are same as those in hepatitis B.
- Breast feeding does not increase risk.
- Unlike hepatitis B, **most people with acute hepatitis C cannot clear the virus** and either become chronic carriers or develop chronic hepatitis.

Clinical Features

- Incubation period is 15–150 days (mean, 50 days).

Acute Hepatitis C

- Often **asymptomatic**.
- If present: fatigue, nausea, mild jaundice, abdominal discomfort.
- Only ~15–25% of cases clear the virus spontaneously.

Chronic Hepatitis C (develops in ~75–85%)

- May remain asymptomatic for years.
- Nonspecific symptoms: fatigue, malaise, right upper quadrant pain.
- In advanced stages: Cirrhosis, portal hypertension, HCC.

Extrahepatic Manifestations

- Mixed cryoglobulinemia, glomerulonephritis, lichen planus, Sjögren's syndrome, thyroid dysfunction, and insulin resistance/diabetes.

Investigations

- LFTs are similar to other viral hepatitis.
- Diagnosis of hepatitis C can be made by demonstrating the presence of serum anti-HCV antibody. Diagnosis is confirmed with HCV RNA testing which is the gold standard for establishing the diagnosis of hepatitis C.
- Hepatitis A and hepatitis B should be ruled out by appropriate tests (*see* above).
- In patients with significant cholestasis, ultrasound abdomen and imaging of the biliary tree may be indicated to rule out obstruction from stone or neoplasm.
- Liver biopsy is rarely necessary.

Treatment

- Treatment should be started for almost all the patients whether it is acute infection or chronic infection. There are a number of new, highly effective direct-acting antiviral drugs (DAAs) for hepatitis C which are basically many types of protease inhibitors. The availability of protease inhibitors has changed the prognosis of hepatitis C infection.
- Common regimens
  - Sofosbuvir + Velpatasvir
  - Glecaprevir + Pibrentasvir
  - Sofosbuvir + Ledipasvir (for some genotypes)
- Current recommendation is to follow patients for 3 to 4 months to allow spontaneous HCV clearance and then treat those who have persistent viremia (i.e. chronic hepatitis C).
- Liver transplantation is indicated for patients with fulminant hepatic failure and severe encephalopathy.

Prevention

- No active or passive immunization available for hepatitis C.
- Universal precautions should be adhered to while handling patients.
- Other general preventive measures include safe sexual practices, using disposable needles, etc.

Q. Chronic Hepatitis C.

- Chronic hepatitis C is diagnosed when hepatic inflammation and necrosis continue for ≥6 months.
- Mild chronic hepatitis C is nonprogressive or only slowly progressive. Severe chronic hepatitis C is can lead to cirrhosis, liver failure, or hepatocellular carcinoma.

Epidemiology

- Chronic hepatitis C develops in up to 85% of patients with acute hepatitis C. It may be the most common cause of chronic hepatitis. It is the most frequent indication for liver transplantation.
- Most frequent in persons 30–50 years of age.
- More frequent in men than women.

Clinical Features

- Are same as chronic hepatitis B.

Investigations

- Serologic markers of HCV (anti-HCV) infection remain positive even after 6 months. HCV RNA also remains detectable.
- Aminotransferases (ALT, AST) remain elevated. But one-third of patients may have normal or near-normal aminotransferases.
- Alkaline phosphatase level is normal or marginally elevated.
- Serum bilirubin level is normal to moderately elevated.
- Hypoalbuminemia may be present.
- Prothrombin time may be prolonged.
- Autoantibodies such as rheumatoid factor can be present and needs to be differentiated from rheumatoid arthritis in patients with arthralgias.
- Ultrasound abdomen or CT scan is useful to rule out hepatocellular carcinoma and to guide liver biopsy.
- Liver biopsy may be indicated to assess severity of disease, predict response to therapy, or rule out hepatocellular carcinoma.

Treatment

- Same as that described under acute hepatitis C.

Q. Hepatitis D (delta hepatitis).

- Delta hepatitis is an infection caused by hepatitis D virus (HDV) which primarily affects the liver.

Etiology

- Delta hepatitis is caused by HDV which is a defective RNA virus (delta agent) belonging to the genus delta virus. It requires hepatitis B virus (HBV) (specifically HBsAg) to replicate. It causes the most severe form of viral hepatitis.
- HDV requires the helper function of HBV (or other hepadnaviruses) for its replication and expression. It can infect a person simultaneously with HBV (co-infection) or superinfect a person already infected with HBV (superinfection).

Epidemiology

- About 10 million people are infected worldwide. Incidence is decreasing now.
- HDV infection is endemic among persons with hepatitis B. 5–8% of hepatitis B chronic carriers have anti-HDV.
- It is endemic in Mediterranean countries (northern Africa, southern Europe, the Middle East).
- HDV infection is common in persons exposed frequently to blood and blood products (injection drug users and hemophiliac persons).

Risk Factors

- Persons infected with hepatitis B.
- Close personal contact with people with HDV.
- Frequent exposure to blood or blood products.

Clinical Features

- Incubation period: 30–180 days.
- Because HDV relies absolutely on HBV, the duration of HDV infection is determined by the duration of HBV infection.
- HDV increases the severity of HBV infection and accelerates the progression of chronic hepatitis to cirrhosis.
- Other clinical features are similar to hepatitis B.

Investigations

- Presence of HDV infection can be identified by anti-HDV seroconversion (an increase in titer of anti-HDV or *de novo* appearance of anti-HDV). It may take 30–40 days for anti-HDV to appear in acute infection.
- Tests for the presence of HDV RNA are useful for determining the presence of ongoing HDV replication and relative infectivity.
- Demonstration of intrahepatic HDV antigen in liver biopsy.
- Other tests are similar to other viral hepatitis.

Treatment

- Treatment of coexistent hepatitis B.
- The only approved treatment for hepatitis D is pegylated interferon and bulevirtide (in some countries).

Prevention

- In HBV-negative persons, hepatitis B vaccine can prevent hepatitis D infection.
- In HBV-positive persons, there is no product to prevent HDV superinfection. Avoidance of percutaneous exposures and limitation of intimate contact with persons who have HDV infection are recommended.

Q. Hepatitis E.

- Hepatitis E is an acute infection caused by hepatitis E virus (HEV) which primarily affects the liver.

Etiology

- Hepatitis E virus is a non-enveloped single-stranded RNA virus.
- Transmitted by fecal-oral route by eating or drinking contaminated food or water.
- HEV is excreted in the stool during the late incubation period.

Epidemiology

- Highest incidence of HEV infection is in Asia, Africa, Middle East, and Central America
- Most epidemics in developing countries are due to contaminated drinking water (e.g. after monsoon flooding).
- Several reports suggest a zoonotic reservoir for HEV in swine.

Clinical Features

- Highest attack rate is between 15–40 years of age.
- Incubation period: 15–60 days.
- Fulminant hepatic failure occurs more frequently during pregnancy, resulting in high mortality rate especially in the third trimester. Reasons for this are unknown.
- Other clinical features are similar to viral hepatitis-A.

Investigations

- Diagnosis is established by detection of the HEV genome in serum or feces by PCR or by the detection of IgM antibodies to HEV.
- LFT results are same as that of acute hepatitis-B.

Treatment

- Same as acute hepatitis A.

Prevention

- A vaccine is available in China which is 95% effective in preventing the infection..
- Travelers to endemic areas should avoid drinking water of unknown purity, uncooked shellfish, and uncooked fruits or vegetables.

Q. Define chronic hepatitis.

Q. Discuss the causes, pathology, clinical features, investigations and management of chronic hepatitis.

Definition

- Chronic hepatitis is defined as persistent inflammation of the liver lasting for more than 6 months, characterized by elevated liver enzymes, histological evidence of liver cell injury, and variable degrees of fibrosis.

Etiology

- Viral hepatitis: hepatitis B, C, D.
- Autoimmune hepatitis
- Drugs: Isoniazid, amiodarone, methotrexate.
- Alcoholic steatohepatitis.
- Nonalcoholic fatty liver disease (NAFLD).
- Metabolic causes (Wilson disease, hemochromatosis, alpha-1 antitrypsin deficiency, primary biliary cirrhosis, sclerosing cholangitis).

Pathology

- Chronic hepatitis is characterized by: Interface hepatitis (piecemeal necrosis), lobular inflammation, portal inflammation, and fibrosis (may progress to bridging fibrosis or cirrhosis).

Clinical Features

- Many patients are asymptomatic.
- Some may have malaise, anorexia, fatigue, low-grade fever and nonspecific upper abdominal discomfort.
- Jaundice is usually absent. Signs of chronic liver disease (e.g. splenomegaly, spider nevi, palmar erythema) or complications of cirrhosis (e.g. portal hypertension, ascites, encephalopathy) may be present in advanced cases.

Investigations

- Liver function tests show elevation of liver enzymes such as AST and ALT.
- Viral serologic tests.
- Autoantibodies, immunoglobulins, α_1-antitrypsin level, and other tests.
- Liver biopsy.

Treatment

- Supportive care.
- Treatment of cause (e.g. corticosteroids for autoimmune hepatitis, antivirals for HBV and HCV infection, withdrawal of offending drug in drug induced chronic hepatitis).
- Corticosteroids and immunosuppressants should be avoided in chronic hepatitis B and C because these drugs enhance viral replication.

Prognosis

- Drug induced chronic hepatitis often regresses completely when the causative drug is withdrawn. Untreated chronic viral hepatitis can lead to cirrhosis or development of hepatocellular carcinoma.

Q. Drug-induced liver injury (hepatitis).

- Drug-induced hepatotoxicity is defined as any degree of liver injury caused by a drug or a toxic substance.
- Many therapeutic agents can cause hepatic injury. Drug-induced liver disease can mimic viral hepatitis, biliary tract obstruction, or other types of liver disease.
- Mechanism of hepatocellular injury may be divided into two broad groups: ***(1) Intrinsic (predictable) hepatotoxicity, (2) Idiosyncratic reactions (immune-mediated hypersensitivity).***

Intrinsic (predictable) Hepatotoxicity

- Here the hepatotoxicity is predictable, dose dependent, and can affect all individuals if a high dose is taken. Examples are isoniazid, rifampicin, paracetamol, valproic acid, and vitamin A.

Idiosyncratic Reactions (immune-mediated hypersensitivity)

- Here the hepatotoxicity is not predictable, sporadic, and not related to dose. Occasionally it is associated with features of allergic reaction, such as fever and eosinophilia. In some patients, liver damage is from a metabolite that is produced only in certain individuals on a genetic basis. Examples are amiodarone, disulfiram, halothane, pyrazinamide, and streptomycin.

Types of Hepatotoxicity

Hepatocellular (elevated ALT)

- Paracetamol
- Halothane
- Isoniazid
- Rifampicin
- Pyrazinamide
- Alcohol
- Estrogens
- Anabolic steroids
- Erythromycin
- Chlorpromazine

Cholestatic (elevated alkaline phosphatase and total bilirubin)

- Amoxicillin/clavulanate
- Anabolic steroids
- Chlorpromazine
- Clopidogrel
- Oral contraceptives
- Erythromycins
- Estrogens
- Phenothiazines

Mixed (elevated alkaline phosphatase and ALT)

- Amitriptyline
- Azathioprine
- Carbamazepine
- Phenytoin
- Sulfonamides

Pathogenesis

- Direct toxicity (paracetamol overdose)
- Metabolic activation to reactive intermediates
- Immune-mediated (hypersensitivity)
- Mitochondrial injury or oxidative stress
- Disruption of bile formation or secretion (cholestasis).

Clinical Features

- Asymptomatic LFT abnormalities (most common)
- Nausea, vomiting, fatigue
- Right upper quadrant pain
- Jaundice
- Pruritus (if cholestatic)
- Hepatomegaly.
- Acute liver failure (in severe cases): encephalopathy, coagulopathy.

Investigations (Table 7.6)

TABLE 7.6: Investigations in drug induced liver injury

Test	Findings
LFTs	ALT/AST ↑ (hepatocellular), ALP/GGT ↑ (cholestatic), ↑bilirubin
PT/INR	Elevated in severe liver failure
Serum albumin	May be decreased in chronic or severe injury
Eosinophilia	May be present in hypersensitivity reactions
Liver biopsy	Helps confirm pattern of injury (if needed)

Diagnosis

- Clinical suspicion based on history of drug/toxin exposure.
- Exclude other causes (viral hepatitis, autoimmune hepatitis, metabolic liver disease).

Treatment

- Main treatment is withdrawal of the offending drug.
- N-acetylcysteine is useful in paracetamol toxicity.
- Supportive therapy for the specific type of liver injury.
- Liver transplant in cases of fulminant hepatic failure.

Q. Define acute liver failure (fulminant hepatic failure). Discuss the causes, pathology, clinical features, investigations and management of acute liver failure.

Definition

- Acute liver failure also known as fulminant hepatic failure is rapid deterioration of liver function resulting in coagulopathy and encephalopathy in a patient without preexisting liver disease, typically within 8 weeks of symptom onset.

Etiology

- ***Viral hepatitis:*** Hepatitis A, B, and E, Epstein-Barr virus, CMV, herpes simplex virus
- ***Autoimmune hepatitis:*** Idiopathic or known autoimmune liver disease
- ***Drugs and toxins:*** Paracetamol overdose, phosphorus poisoning, ***Amanita phalloides*** mushroom toxin
- ***Vascular causes:*** Portal vein thrombosis, Budd-Chiari syndrome, ischemic hepatitis
- ***Metabolic causes:*** Wilson disease, Reye's syndrome
- ***Pregnancy-related:*** Acute fatty liver of pregnancy
- ***Miscellaneous:*** Malignant infiltration of the liver, sepsis, and autoimmune hepatitis.

Remember the mnemonic

A: Acetaminophen, hepatitis A, autoimmune hepatitis
B: Hepatitis B, Budd-Chiari syndrome
C: Cryptogenic, hepatitis C, cytomegalovirus
D: Hepatitis D, drugs
E: Esoteric causes—Wilson's disease, Budd-Chiari syndrome
F: Fatty Infiltration—Fatty liver of pregnancy, Reye's syndrome

Pathology

- Massive hepatocyte necrosis.
- Disruption of hepatic architecture.
- Impaired detoxification → ↑ ammonia → hepatic encephalopathy.
- Impaired synthesis of clotting factors → coagulopathy.
- Multi-organ failure may occur.

Clinical Features

- Jaundice is often present.
- Liver may be enlarged and tender especially in acute hepatitis. An enlarged liver may be also be seen with congestive heart failure and Budd-Chiari syndrome. Liver size may decrease when there is significant loss of volume due to hepatic necrosis.
- Ascites may be present.
- Hepatic encephalopathy: This may range from mild alteration of consciousness to deep coma. Recognition of hepatic encephalopathy is central to the diagnosis of fulminant hepatic failure. Hepatic encephalopathy is mainly due to development of cerebral edema.
- Coagulopathy: Since the synthesis of most of the clotting factors occurs in the liver, liver failure leads to development of coagulopathy. Patient may have bleeding from any site but upper GI bleed is common presenting as hematemesis and melena.
- Renal failure is common due to development of hepatorenal syndrome.
- Systemic inflammatory response syndrome with DIC and multiple organ dysfunction is common. This may occur with or without an underlying infection. ARDS and respiratory failure contribute to high mortality in fulminant hepatic failure.
- Hypotension and hyperdynamic circulation are usually present due to peripheral vasodilatation. Adrenal insufficiency is common in liver failure and may contribute to hypotension.

Investigations

- Complete blood count: There may be evidence of infection or DIC.
- LFTs: AST, ALT (markedly ↑), bilirubin ↑
- PT/INR: Prolonged
- Serum ammonia level ↑
- Serum electrolytes
- Blood sugar level: Often decreased (hypoglycemia)
- ABG: Usually shows metabolic acidosis
- Blood urea and creatinine level: Elevated
- Serum copper, ceruloplasmin level (if suspecting Wilson disease).
- Blood cultures: For patients with suspected infection
- Viral serologies (to rule out acute viral hepatitis)
- Drug or toxicology screening (if drug or toxin ingestion is suspected)
- Autoimmune markers (for autoimmune hepatitis diagnosis): Antinuclear antibody (ANA) and anti-smooth muscle antibody (ASMA)
- Ultrasound/Doppler: To assess liver size, flow (rule out Budd–Chiari)
- CT brain: If encephalopathy to rule out cerebral edema or other causes.

Treatment

- Treatment of underlying cause is most important.
- Maintenance of proper fluid and electrolyte balance.
- Support of nutrition (through Ryle's tube), respiratory and hemodynamic function.
- Prophylactic use of proton pump inhibitors because of the high risk of gastrointestinal bleeding.
- Management of encephalopathy: Cerebral edema is the most common cause of death in acute liver failure. Intracranial pressure can be monitored by an epidural catheter. Cerebral edema can be decreased by hyperventilation and mannitol (0.5–1 mg/kg body weight 8th hourly). If there is no response to above measures, pentobarbital coma should be induced using a bolus of 3–5 mg/kg intravenously. Since there is evidence that ammonia plays major role in the development of hepatic encephalopathy, elevated ammonia levels should be reduced with enteral administration of lactulose. Bowel wash can reduce intestinal bacterial load and decrease the production of ammonia. Administration of antibiotics such as neomycin or rifaximin orally can sterilize the bowel and decrease ammonia production by bacteria. Sedatives should be avoided if possible.
- Sedatives should be avoided unless needed in the intubated patient because these agents can aggravate or precipitate encephalopathy
- Management of renal failure: Hemodialysis should be considered for renal failure.
- Management of coagulopathy: If there is active bleeding clotting factors should be replaced by transfusion of fresh frozen plasma (FFP). Vitamin K should be given parenterally to help in the synthesis of clotting factors. Recombinant factor VIIa may be used intravenously in patients who do not respond to FFP.
- Liver transplantation is the definitive treatment in liver failure. It should be considered in all patients with fulminant hepatic failure.

Prognosis

- Prognosis is poor and mortality can be as high as 80%.

Q. Reye's syndrome.

- Reye's syndrome is a rare form of acute encephalopathy with hepatic dysfunction that tends to occur after some acute viral infections, particularly when aspirin is used.

Etiology and Pathogenesis

- The exact cause is unknown, but usually follows chickenpox or influenza infection. Use of salicylates (aspirin) during the above infections is a major precipitating factor for the development of Reye's syndrome.

- Pathologically fatty degeneration of liver, astrocyte edema and loss of neurons in the brain, and edema and fatty degeneration of the kidneys is seen. Hepatic mitochondrial dysfunction results in hyperammonemia, which is thought to induce astrocyte edema, resulting in cerebral edema and increased intracranial pressure (ICP).

Clinical Features

- It is usually seen in children <18 years. Acute encephalopathy with cerebral edema develops. Clinical features include nausea, vomiting, headache, excitability, delirium, and combativeness with frequent progression to coma.
- Incidence has now decreased as aspirin use in patients with varicella or influenza has decreased.

Investigations

- LFT is altered and findings are similar to acute viral hepatitis.
- Prothrombin time (PT) is prolonged
- Serum ammonia is markedly elevated.

Treatment

- Treatment is mainly supportive and includes intravenous hydration, infusions fresh-frozen plasma, and intravenous mannitol to reduce cerebral edema.
- Anti-encephalopathy measures.

Prognosis

- The mortality rate in Reye's syndrome is approximately 30%.

Q. Discuss fatty liver (hepatic steatosis) and its causes.

Q. Nonalcoholic fatty liver disease (NAFLD).

Q. Nonalcoholic steatohepatitis (NASH).

- Accumulation of excess fat (mainly triglycerides) in the liver is called fatty liver or hepatic steatosis.
- When fatty liver is due to alcohol consumption, it is known as alcoholic fatty liver.
- When fatty liver is not due to alcohol, it is known as nonalcoholic fatty liver disease (NAFLD). NAFLD is subdivided into nonalcoholic fatty liver (NAFL) and nonalcoholic steatohepatitis (NASH). In NAFL, hepatic steatosis is present without inflammation, whereas in NASH, hepatic steatosis is associated with hepatic inflammation.
- Fatty liver is a benign disease and carries good prognosis. However, if the underlying cause is not treated (e.g. alcohol) it may progress and result in significant fibrosis and even cirrhosis.

Nonalcoholic Fatty Liver Disease (NAFLD) and NASH

- NAFLD is a spectrum of liver conditions occurring in individuals who consume little to no alcohol, and is characterized by hepatic steatosis in more than 5% of hepatocytes, as seen on imaging or histology.
- The following discussion applies to both NAFLD and NASH.

Causes of NAFLD

- Obesity (most common)
- Type 2 diabetes mellitus
- Hyperlipidemia (elevated triglycerides and cholesterol).
- Metabolic syndrome
- Rapid weight loss or malnutrition
- Certain medications (e.g. corticosteroids, methotrexate, tamoxifen, amiodarone)
- Total parenteral nutrition (TPN)
- Viral hepatitis (especially hepatitis C, genotype 3)
- Polycystic ovary syndrome (PCOS)
- Sedentary lifestyle
- Genetic factors.

Spectrum of NAFLD

Simple Steatosis (NAFL)

- Fat accumulation without significant inflammation or fibrosis. Generally benign, but may progress in some cases.

Nonalcoholic Steatohepatitis (NASH)

- Steatosis with inflammation and hepatocyte injury (ballooning), with or without fibrosis. Can progress to cirrhosis, hepatocellular carcinoma (HCC), and liver failure.

Pathogenesis of NAFLD (the "multiple-hit hypothesis")

- The "multiple-hit hypothesis" is the currently accepted model explaining the development and progression of nonalcoholic fatty liver disease (NAFLD). It suggests that multiple concurrent and sequential factors (or "hits") act together on a genetically predisposed individual, leading from simple steatosis to nonalcoholic steatohepatitis (NASH), fibrosis, and eventually cirrhosis.
- ***Insulin resistance:*** This is the central mechanism leading to increased free fatty acid flux to the liver and increased lipogenesis in the liver.
- Fat-laden hepatocytes are vulnerable to oxidative stress from mitochondrial dysfunction and reactive oxygen species (ROS). ROS also damage stored fats forming toxic lipid intermediates. All these processes trigger Kupffer cell activation → proinflammatory cytokines (e.g. TNF-α, IL-6), hepatocyte apoptosis or necrosis, and influx of inflammatory cells.
- Chronic inflammation stimulates stellate cell activation → collagen deposition → fibrosis. Over time, fibrosis progresses to cirrhosis and possibly hepatocellular carcinoma (HCC).

Clinical Features

- The signs and symptoms of fatty liver depend on the severity and the underlying cause. Many patients are asymptomatic.

- General symptoms (nonspecific) include fatigue, malaise, right upper quadrant (RUQ) discomfort or vague abdominal pain, and bloating or feeling of fullness. Liver is enlarged, firm and usually nontender. However, mild tenderness may be present in some patients.
- Rapid accumulation of fat (example, total parenteral nutrition, hepatotoxins) may lead to marked liver tenderness, due to stretching of Glisson's capsule.
- Advanced disease (NASH with fibrosis or cirrhosis) may present with splenomegaly (if portal hypertension develops), spider angioma, palmar erythema, ascites, jaundice, and encephalopathy (late-stage cirrhosis).

Investigations

- Liver function tests are usually normal or show mild elevations of alkaline phosphatase or aminotransferases.
- Fatty liver can be detected by CT, MRI, or ultrasound.
- Transient elastography (FibroScan): Assesses liver stiffness (fibrosis).
- If there is doubt about the diagnosis, liver biopsy will show increased fat content, presence of any fibrosis, and possibly the underlying primary disorder.

Treatment

- Lifestyle changes are recommended for all patients with NAFLD (such as regular exercise, diet control).
- Underlying cause should be treated (e.g. control of diabetes, weight loss in obesity, etc.).
- Pharmacologic therapy (in select patients): Vitamin E, pioglitazone, GLP-1 agonists
- Regular monitoring for development of cirrhosis.

Q. Alcoholic liver disease (ALD).

- Alcoholic liver disease (ALD) refers to a spectrum of liver damage caused by chronic excessive alcohol consumption. The spectrum of ALD includes: (1) alcoholic fatty liver, (2) alcoholic hepatitis, and (3) alcoholic cirrhosis.
- Alcoholic fatty liver or steatosis: At this stage, fat accumulates in the liver parenchyma. Earliest and most common stage and reversible with abstinence. Usually asymptomatic or presents with hepatomegaly.
- Alcoholic hepatitis: Here, there is inflammation of liver parenchyma. It can be acute or chronic. Presents with jaundice, fever, RUQ pain, and liver dysfunction. Appropriate treatment along with alcohol abstinence can reverse this stage. Recurrent episodes can occur and are often associated with binge alcohol intake. More severe cases may end up in liver failure.
- Alcoholic cirrhosis: Liver damage at this stage is irreversible and leads to complications of cirrhosis and portal hypertension.

Pathogenesis

- Alcohol is a major hepatotoxin. Liver tolerates mild alcohol consumption, but as the consumption of alcohol increases, it interferes with the metabolic functions of liver leading to slowly accumulating damage. Quantity and duration of alcohol intake are the highest risk factors for the development of the liver disease. Women are more susceptible than men. Concurrent infection with hepatitis B or hepatitis C increases the chances of liver damage. Alcohol induced liver damage mainly occurs by following 3 mechanisms:
  1. ***Acetaldehyde formation:*** Alcohol is converted into the acetaldehyde by alcohol dehydrogenase. Acetaldehyde is then detoxified to acetate by aldehyde dehydrogenase. Acetaldehyde is the main toxic metabolite of alcohol which produces liver damage. When excess acetaldehyde is produced due to excess alcohol consumption, then it accumulates and produces liver damage by following mechanisms:
     - Forms protein adducts, DNA adducts → impairs cellular function.
     - Promotes inflammation and immune activation.
     - Causes mitochondrial dysfunction.
     - Stimulates collagen production → contributes to fibrosis.
  2. ***CYP2E1 and oxidative stress*:** Chronic alcohol intake induces CYP2E1 which in turn produces reactive oxygen species (ROS). ROS also damage liver by various mechanisms.
  3. ***NADH/NAD$^+$ imbalance*:** Ethanol metabolism by ADH produces excess NADH. Excess NADH inhibits fatty acid oxidation, promotes lipogenesis, leads to steatosis (fatty liver), and inhibits gluconeogenesis → risk of hypoglycemia.
- All the above mechanisms produce liver inflammation which causes alcoholic hepatitis. Continued inflammation leads to cell necrosis and apoptosis resulting in hepatocyte loss. Subsequent attempts at regeneration result in fibrosis and nodules leading to cirrhosis. Stellate (Ito) cells which are present in liver sinusoids get activated and produce excessive amount of fibrous tissue which contributed to fibrosis seen in cirrhosis.
- The pathological progression generally follows this sequence: Steatosis → Alcoholic Hepatitis → Fibrosis → Cirrhosis.

Clinical Features

- Patients develop problems during their 30s or 40s.
- Alcoholic fatty liver is often asymptomatic. Liver may be enlarged and smooth, but is not usually tender.
- Alcoholic hepatitis presents with fatigue, fever, jaundice, right upper quadrant pain, tender hepatomegaly, and sometimes a hepatic bruit. Severe alcoholic hepatitis may present with features of liver failure such as ascites, encephalopathy, variceal bleeding, and hypoglycemia.
- Cirrhosis, if compensated, may be asymptomatic. If it is decompensated features of liver cell failure and portal hypertension are present which include hepatic encephalopathy, coagulopathy, ascites, variceal bleeding, and splenomegaly.

Investigations

- Liver function tests: Alterations depend on the stage of liver disease. In alcoholic hepatitis, elevations of liver enzymes is moderate (<300 IU/L). The ratio of aspartate aminotransferase (AST) to alanine aminotransferase (ALT) is ≥2. The basis for low ALT is a dietary deficiency of pyridoxal phosphate (vitamin B6), which is needed for ALT to function.
- Complete blood count (CBC).
- Ultrasound abdomen: Shows fatty infiltration, nodular liver in cirrhosis.

Treatment

- Abstinence from alcohol (most crucial step). Improves survival and can reverse early disease.
- Supportive care.
- Corticosteroids or pentoxifylline for severe alcoholic hepatitis.
- Rarely liver transplantation.

Q. Discuss the etiology, pathogenesis, clinical features, investigations, complications and management of cirrhosis of liver.

Q. Child-Turcotte-Pugh scoring system.

- Cirrhosis refers to a late stage of chronic liver disease characterized by fibrosis, distortion of the hepatic architecture and the formation of regenerative nodules.
- It represents the final common pathway of many types of chronic liver injury.

Causes of Cirrhosis

- Alcoholic liver disease
- Chronic viral hepatitis (HBV, HCV)
- Nonalcoholic fatty liver disease (NAFLD/NASH)
- Autoimmune hepatitis
- Inherited and metabolic diseases:
  - Hemochromatosis
  - Wilson's disease
  - Alpha-1 antitrypsin deficiency
- Biliary causes:
  - Primary biliary cholangitis
  - Primary sclerosing cholangitis
- Drug/toxin-induced (e.g. methotrexate, amiodarone, isoniazid)
- Chronic right heart failure (cardiac cirrhosis)
- Cryptogenic cirrhosis (no identifiable cause)

Epidemiology

- Alcoholic cirrhosis is the most common type of cirrhosis seen all over the world. Posthepatitis cirrhosis especially due to hepatitis B or C is the second most common cause of cirrhosis.
- Cirrhosis is more common in males but primary biliary cirrhosis is more common in females.
- Cirrhosis is the most common indication for liver transplantation.

Pathophysiology

- Cirrhosis is the final common pathway of many types of chronic liver injury.
- The pathogenesis of liver cirrhosis involves a chronic cycle of injury, inflammation, fibrogenesis, and regeneration that ultimately leads to disruption of normal liver architecture and function.

Chronic Liver Injury

- Caused by factors like alcohol, viruses (HBV, HCV), metabolic disorders, or autoimmune attacks. This leads to repeated hepatocellular damage and necrosis.

Inflammatory Response

- Damaged hepatocytes release damage-associated molecular patterns (DAMPs).
- These activate Kupffer cells (liver macrophages), which release proinflammatory cytokines (TNF-α, IL-1, IL-6), TGF-β, PDGF and reactive oxygen species (ROS). These cytokines and ROS lead to recruitment of inflammatory cells (neutrophils, lymphocytes).

Activation of Hepatic Stellate Cells

- This is the key event in fibrogenesis. Stellate cells, which are normally quiescent (store vitamin A), get activated by cytokines (e.g. TGF-β, PDGF), ROS and endotoxins.
- Activated stellate cells transform into myofibroblast-like cells and produce excess collagen and other extracellular matrix proteins.

Fibrosis Formation

- Collagen and extracellular matrix proteins accumulate in space of Disse, disrupting sinusoidal blood flow, hepatocyte nutrition and oxygenation. Bridging fibrosis forms between portal tracts and central veins which leads to formation of fibrous septa.

Nodular Regeneration

- Surviving hepatocytes undergo regeneration in response to injury. However, regenerative nodules are surrounded by fibrous tissue, not organized within normal lobular structure, and result in distorted architecture and loss of functional liver units.

Vascular Remodelling and Portal Hypertension

- Fibrous bands and nodules compress intrahepatic vasculature leading to increased resistance to portal blood flow → development of portal hypertension and formation of portosystemic collaterals.

Hepatocellular Dysfunction

- Finally, due to all the above changes, there is loss of functional hepatocyte mass leading to impaired synthetic and metabolic capacity which results in **jaundice, coagulopathy, hypoalbuminemia, and encephalopathy**.

- Chronic Injury → Inflammation → Stellate cell activation → Fibrosis → Nodular regeneration → Architectural distortion → Portal hypertension + Liver failure.

Role of Nitric Oxide (NO) in the Pathogenesis of Cirrhosis and Portal HTN

- Sinusoidal endothelial cells normally synthesize both nitric oxide (NO) and endothelin-1 which act on stellate cells causing relaxation or contraction of the sinusoids, and thus regulate sinusoidal blood flow. In patients with cirrhosis, there is increase in endothelin-1 production and decrease in NO production. This leads to increased intrahepatic vasoconstriction. Both hepatic fibrosis and intrahepatic vasoconstriction lead to portal hypertension.
- In systemic and splanchnic circulation, the opposite effect happens, with an increase in the production of NO leading to systemic and splanchnic vasodilation and hyperdynamic circulation. This activates renin-angiotensin-aldosterone system (RAAS), leading to sodium and water retention. Thus, in cirrhosis with portal hypertension, there is depletion of NO intrahepatically but an excess of NO extrahepatically in the splanchnic and systemic circulation, which lead to sinusoidal vasoconstriction and splanchnic (systemic) vasodilation.
- Splanchnic vasodilation leads to decreased perfusion pressure in kidneys, which activates RAAS system, leading to retention of sodium and water and renal vascular constriction. Renal hypoperfusion leads to renal failure which is called hepatorenal syndrome.

Gross Appearance (Fig. 7.5)

- Cirrhosis can be classified histologically into two types: (1) Micronodular cirrhosis is characterized by small nodules less than 3 mm in diameter (seen in alcoholic cirrhosis), (2) Macronodular cirrhosis is characterized by larger nodules which are more than 3 mm in diameter (seen with posthepatitis cirrhosis). Differentiation between these morphologic types of cirrhosis has limited clinical value.

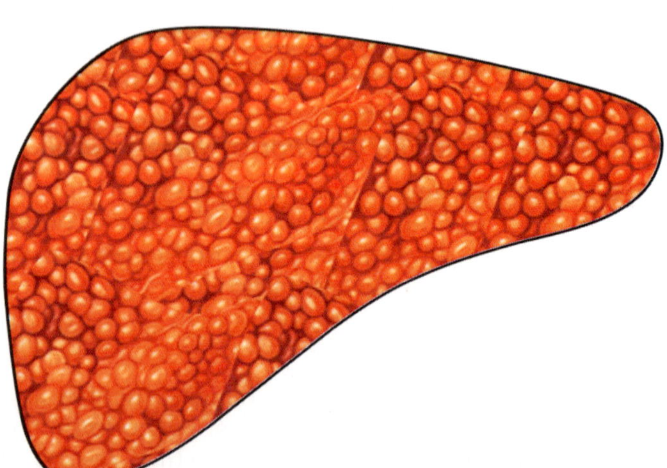

Figure 7.5: Nodular and shrunken liver in cirrhosis

Clinical Features (Fig. 7.6)

- Clinical features of cirrhosis can be divided into general symptoms, signs of liver cell failure, and complications due to portal hypertension or hepatocellular dysfunction.

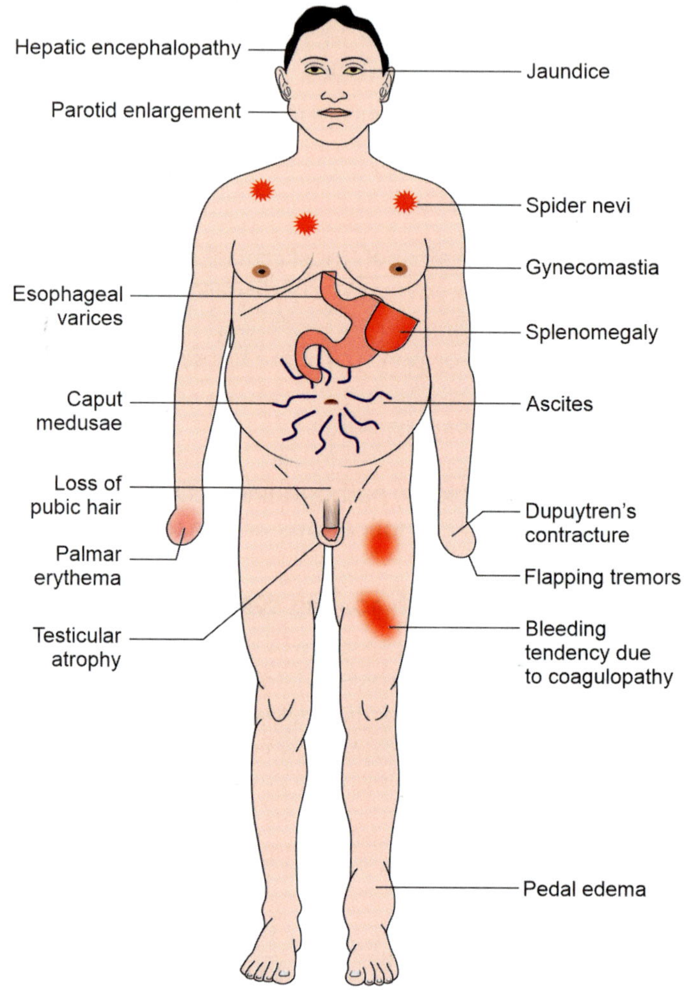

Figure 7.6: Clinical features of cirrhosis of the liver

General Symptoms

- Fatigue
- Anorexia and weight loss
- Weakness
- Nausea and vomiting
- Right upper quadrant abdominal discomfort
- Pruritus (due to bile salt accumulation)
- Jaundice (especially in decompensated cirrhosis)

General Examination

- Muscle wasting
- Pallor due to GI blood loss
- Jaundice
- Spider naevi (especially over the chest and upper back)
- Bleeding manifestations such as purpura and ecchymosis
- Palmar erythema
- Pruritus
- Decreased body hair

- Gynecomastia
- Testicular atrophy
- Flapping tremors (in hepatic enecephalopathy)
- Parotid gland enlargement
- Edema
- Clubbing may be present in primary biliary cirrhosis.
- Signs of virilization in women
- Melanosis: Gradual darkening of the exposed areas of the skin
- There is increased estrogen level in cirrhosis due to liver dysfunction which leads to formation of spider nevi and palmer erythema. Hyperestrogenemia also contributes to gynecomastia in males.
- Hypogonadism can develop in cirrhosis leading to decreased libido and impotence in males with loss of secondary sexual characteristics and feminization. Women can develop amenorrhea and irregular menstrual bleeding as well as infertility.

Abdomen

- Liver is shrunken, firm and nodular.
- Splenomegaly may be present.
- Ascites as evidenced by bulging flanks, shifting dullness and fluid thrill.
- Caput medusa (dilated veins around the umbilicus).

CVS

- Look for evidence of right heart failure (cardiac cirrhosis) such as raised JVP, right sided S3, S4, dilated heart, etc.

RS

- Pleural effusion (especially right sided) may develop in severe ascites.

NS

- Patient can be in altered sensorium due to hepatic encephalopathy, electrolyte imbalance, hypoglycemia, etc.

Clues to Specific Etiology (Table 7.7)

TABLE 7.7: Clues to specific etiology of cirrhosis

Type of cirrhosis	Clue
Alcoholic cirrhosis	History of prolonged and excessive alcohol consumption. Rule out other causes of cirrhosis since only 10–15% of individuals with excessive alcohol intake develop cirrhosis.
Primary biliary cirrhosis (PBC)	Middle-aged women with unexplained pruritus or elevated ALP. Positive serum antimitochondrial antibody Liver biopsy should be performed to confirm diagnosis.
Secondary biliary cirrhosis	History of previous biliary tract surgery or gallstones H/o recurrent bouts of ascending cholangitis H/o right upper quadrant pain Clinical and laboratory evidence of prolonged obstruction to bile flow. Ultrasound abdomen and cholangiography may demonstrate the underlying pathologic process.
Posthepatitis cirrhosis	Positive viral serology.
Cryptogenic cirrhosis	No identifiable cause of cirrhosis Liver biopsy also rules out any specific cause
Cardiac cirrhosis	Signs and symptoms of heart failure usually overshadow liver disease Presence of firm, enlarged liver with signs of chronic liver disease in patients with valvular heart disease, constrictive pericarditis, or cor pulmonale of long duration (>10 years) should suggest cardiac cirrhosis
Metabolic, hereditary, drug-related, and other types of cirrhosis	Specific history, clinical and lab features may be present Specific lab tests and liver biopsy required to confirm the diagnosis

Investigations

Complete Blood Count

- Anemia may be present due to blood loss, folate deficiency and hypersplenism. Pancytopenia due to hypersplenism.

Liver Function Tests

- Hypoalbuminemia and increased globulin levels (reversal of A:G ratio). Bilirubin level and aminotranseferases may be mildly elevated. ALP is mildly elevated. Prothrombin time (PT) may be prolonged.

Urea, Creatinine, Serum Electrolytes

- Urea and creatinine are usually normal unless there is development of hepatorenal syndrome.
- Metabolic disturbances such as hyponatremia, hypokalemia and hypoglycemia may be present. Hypoglycemia is due to impaired gluconeogenesis by the liver.

Investigations to Identify the Underlying Cause

- Hepatitis serologies (HBsAg, anti-HCV).
- Iron, total iron-binding capacity and ferritin if hemochromatosis is suspected.
- Antimitochondrial antibody (AMA) if primary biliary cirrhosis is suspected.

- Antinuclear antibody, anti-smooth-muscle antibody if autoimmune etiology is suspected.
- Serum copper and ceruloplasmin levels if Wilson disease is suspected.
- Alpha-1-antitrypsin levels if deficiency is suspected.

Imaging

- Abdominal ultrasound with Doppler may show nodular liver, splenomegaly and dilated portal vein with collateral vessels.
- CT or MRI is rarely required.

Liver Biopsy

- This is the test for definitive diagnosis of cirrhosis but not routinely required except in cases of doubt about diagnosis and etiology. It shows regenerating nodules and fibrosis.

Treatment

Supportive Treatment

- *Diet*: Should provide adequate calories and protein (1–1.5 g/kg/day). Reduce protein intake to 60–80 g/day if there is hepatic encephalopathy. Restrict sodium if there is fluid retention. Benefit of branched-chain amino acids to prevent or treat hepatic encephalopathy is uncertain. Vitamin supplementation is advisable especially vitamin K.

Treat the Underlying Cause

- Alcoholic liver disease: Complete alcohol cessation is crucial. Counseling, support groups, and medications like naltrexone or acamprosate may help.
- Chronic hepatitis B or C: Antiviral therapy (e.g. tenofovir, entecavir for HBV; direct-acting antivirals for HCV).
- Nonalcoholic fatty liver disease (NAFLD/NASH): Weight loss, diabetes control, and exercise. Manage dyslipidemia and metabolic syndrome.
- Autoimmune hepatitis: Immunosuppressants like prednisone and azathioprine.
- Hemochromatosis: Phlebotomy and iron chelation.
- Wilson's disease: Copper chelators (e.g. penicillamine, trientine) and zinc.

Manage Complications

- ***Portal hypertension and variceal bleeding***: Portal hypertension can be reduced by nonselective beta blockers such as propranolol or nadolol. Nitrates can be used for patients in whom betablockers are contraindicated. Esophageal varices should be treated by endoscopic varicieal ligation. TIPS (transjugular intrahepatic portosystemic shunt) is considered for refractory cases.
- ***Ascites:*** Salt restriction, diuretics (spironolactone ± furosemide). Paracentesis for large-volume ascites. TIPS in refractory cases.
- ***Spontaneous bacterial peritonitis*** **(SBP):** Treated with antibiotics (e.g. cefotaxime).
- ***Hepatic encephalopathy:*** Lactulose (1st line). Lactulose syrup is used daily (15 ml at night) to prevent hepatic encephalopathy. Rifaximin is also used as an adjunct to reduce bacterial load in gut which produce ammonia.
- ***Hepatorenal syndrome***: Vasoconstrictors (e.g. terlipressin), albumin, and liver transplant evaluation.

Prevent Further Damage

- Vaccinations: Hepatitis A and B, influenza, pneumococcal.
- Avoid hepatotoxic drugs and alcohol.
- Regular monitoring for hepatocellular carcinoma (HCC) with ultrasound ± alpha-fetoprotein (AFP) every 6 months.

Liver Transplantation

- Indicated for decompensated cirrhosis in suitable patients.

Prognosis

- The overall prognosis in cirrhosis is poor. Only 25% of patients survive 5 years from diagnosis. Prognosis is more favorable if the underlying cause can be corrected, such as alcohol abuse. Complications such as variceal bleed can cause unexpected death.
- ***Indicators of poor prognosis in cirrhosis:*** presence of jaundice, ascites, encephalopathy, renal impairement, hyponatremia (<130 mEq/L), elevated hepatic venous pressure gradient, albumin <3 g/dl, bilirubin >3 mg/dl, cachexia, upper gastrointestinal bleeding.
- The Child-Pugh score is a validated tool to assess prognosis in cirrhosis.

Child-Turcotte-Pugh Scoring System to Assess the Severity of Liver Disease (Table 7.8)

TABLE 7.8: Child-Turcotte-Pugh scoring system

Parameter	Points assigned		
	1	2	3
Ascites	Absent	Slight	Moderate
Bilirubin, mg/dl	<2	2–3	>3
Albumin, g/dl	>3.5	2.8–3.5	<2.8
Prothrombin time			
Seconds over control	<4	4–6	>6
OR INR	<1.7	1.7–2.3	>2.3
Encephalopathy	None	Grade 1–2	Grade 3–4

- A total score of 5–6 is considered grade A (well-compensated disease).
- Score 7–9 is grade B (significant functional compromise).
- Score 10–15 is grade C (decompensated disease).
- These grades correlate with one- and two-year patient survival—grade A: 100 and 85%; grade B: 80 and 60%; and grade C: 45 and 35%.

Complications

- Variceal bleeding
- Spontaneous bacterial peritonitis
- Hepatic encephalopathy

- Hepatorenal syndrome
- Hepatopulmonary syndrome
- Hepatocellular carcinoma.

Q. What is biliary cirrhosis? Discuss the etiology, pathology, clinical features, investigations, and management of primary biliary cirrhosis.

Q. Secondary biliary cirrhosis.

- Biliary cirrhosis is cirrhosis of liver due to injury or prolonged obstruction of intrahepatic or extrahepatic biliary system.
- It is associated with impaired biliary excretion, destruction of liver parenchyma, and progressive fibrosis.
- Biliary cirrhosis can be divided into 2 types.
  - ***Primary biliary cirrhosis (PBC):*** It now called primary biliary cholangitis. Here, cirrhosis is due to chronic inflammation and fibrous obliteration of intrahepatic bile ductules.
  - ***Secondary biliary cirrhosis (SBC):*** Here cirrhosis is due to prolonged obstruction of extrahepatic bile ducts.
- Although PBC and SBC are separate entities, many clinical features are similar.

Primary Biliary Cirrhosis (primary biliary cholangitis)

- Primary biliary cirrhosis (PBC) is liver cirrhosis due to chronic inflammation and fibrous obliteration of intrahepatic bile ductules.

Epidemiology

- PBC is common in Europe and America but is rare in Africa and Asia.
- Female are affected more commonly (female-to-male ratio 9:1).
- It is also more common amongst cigarette smokers.

Etiology and Pathology

- Its cause is unknown but probably an autoimmune disorder.
- It can be associated with other autoimmune disorders such as sicca syndrome, autoimmune thyroiditis, type 1 diabetes, etc.
- Genetic predisposition and environmental factors (smoking) also play a role.
- The condition is strongly associated with the presence of antimitochondrial antibodies (AMA), which are diagnostic. Antinuclear antibodies (ANA) are also positive in these cases.
- The main pathology is chronic granulomatous inflammation of the portal tracts, which destroys small and middle-sized intrahepatic bile ducts. This in turn leads to fibrosis and cirrhosis of the liver.

Clinical Features

- Most patients are women.
- Many patients are asymptomatic for years.
- The condition typically presents with an insidious onset of itching and/or tiredness. Itching may precede jaundice by months or years. Over a period of months to years, itching and jaundice worsen.
- As cirrhosis develops, signs of hepatocellular failure and portal hypertension develop and ascites appears.
- Steatorrhea can occur due to impaired fat absorption due to impaired bile excretion into the duodenum. There is malabsorption of fat-soluble vitamins such as vit-D leading to osteomalacia or osteoporosis causing bone pain or fractures (hepatic osteodystrophy).
- Impaired excretion of cholesterol through bile leads to elevation of serum cholesterol and subcutaneous lipid deposition around the eyes (xanthelasmas) and over joints and tendons (xanthomas).
- Physical examination may reveal scratch marks on the skin due to itching, hyperpigmentation, xanthelasmas and xanthomas, hepatomegaly, splenomegaly, and clubbing of the fingers.

Investigations

- LFTs show a cholestatic pattern. There is elevation of the serum ALP (alkaline phosphatase). Serum 5′-nucleotidase activity and γ-glutamyl transpeptidase levels are also elevated. Serum bilirubin is usually normal and aminotransferase levels are minimally increased.
- Hypercholesterolemia is common.
- Antimitochondrial antibody (AMA) is present in most patients.
- Ultrasound abdomen shows normal extrahepatic biliary ducts.
- Liver biopsy confirms diagnosis.

Treatment

- There is no specific treatment for PBC.
- Ursodeoxycholic acid (UDCA) has been shown to improve biochemical markers of cholestasis and jaundice. It also slows disease progression but does not change the final outcome. The hydrophilic UDCA improves bile flow, replaces toxic hydrophobic bile acids in the bile acid pool, and reduces apoptosis of the biliary epithelium. UDCA should be given in doses of 13–15 mg/kg per day.
- Immunosuppressants such as corticosteroids, azathioprine, penicillamine and ciclosporin have all been tried in PBC but none is effective.
- Relief of symptoms: itching can be controlled by UDCA and cholestyramine (an oral bile salt–sequestering resin). Other drugs helpful for itching are rifampicin, opiate antagonists (naloxone or naltrexone), ondansetron, and ultraviolet light. Steatorrhea can be reduced by a low-fat diet and substituting medium-chain triglycerides for dietary long-chain triglycerides. Fat-soluble vitamins A, D, E, and K should be supplemented. Patients should be screened periodically for osteoporosis and osteomalacia by bone densitometry and treated as needed with calcium supplements, vitamin D

and/or bisphosphonate agents (e.g. alendronate) if osteoporosis is present.

- Liver transplantation is the only treatment which offers a cure for PBC. It should be considered in liver failure and intractable pruritus. Recurrence of PBC after liver transplantation is rare.

Secondary Biliary Cirrhosis

- This is cirrhosis of liver due to prolonged obstruction of extrahepatic bile ducts.
- Obstruction may be due to gallstones, benign bile duct strictures or sclerosing cholangitis. Carcinomas rarely cause secondary biliary cirrhosis because patients die before cirrhosis develops.
- Clinical features and biochemical findings are same as primary biliary cirrhosis. In addition there may be recurrent episodes of cholangitis associated with fever and right upper quadrant pain. Cholangitis requires treatment with antibiotics, which can be given continuously if attacks recur frequently.
- Ultrasound abdomen and cholangiography (PTC or ERCP) can identify the site and cause of obstruction.
- Treatment involves relief of obstruction to bile flow, by either endoscopic or surgical means. Antibiotics should be given for episodes of cholangitis.

Q. Cardiac cirrhosis.

Definition

- Cardiac cirrhosis is cirrhosis of liver due to prolonged, severe right-sided heart failure. Other cardiac disorders which can produce cirrhosis are valvular heart disease and constrictive pericarditis.

Pathogenesis

- Right-sided heart failure leads to retrograde transmission of elevated venous pressure and congestion of the liver. Hepatic sinusoids become dilated and the liver becomes tensely swollen.
- Prolonged passive congestion and ischemia from reduced cardiac output leads to necrosis of centrilobular hepatocytes and fibrosis. Ultimately extensive fibrosis leads to cirrhosis.
- Gross examination of the liver shows alternating red (congested) and pale (fibrotic) areas, a pattern referred to as "nutmeg liver."

Clinical Features

- Features of heart failure are more prominent than cirrhosis. Patients complain of dyspnea, orthopnea, and PND. Signs of congestive cardiac failure such as raised JVP, lung crepitations, S3 gallop, tricuspid regurgitation murmur, peripheral edema and enlarged heart are usually present.
- Hepatomegaly is common. Other features of cirrhosis may be present.

Investigations

- LFTs are similar to other causes of cirrhosis.
- ECG and echocardiogram show features of right heart failure or other cardiac disease.

Treatment

- Underlying cardiac disorder must be treated. Mainstay of treatment is diuretics. Loop diuretics (furosemide) or spironolactone can be used.
- Treatment of cirrhosis is same as other types of cirrhosis (*see* cirrhosis).

Q. Describe the anatomy of the portal venous system. How do you define and classify portal hypertension?

Q. Discuss the etiology, pathology, clinical features, investigations, complications and management of portal hypertension.

Definition of Portal Hypertension

- Portal hypertension is chronic elevation of the portal venous pressure ≥10–12 mm Hg (normal, 5–8 mm Hg).

Anatomy of the Portal Venous System

- The portal venous system is a vascular network that drains blood from the entire gastrointestinal (GI) tract starting from the esophago-gastric junction down to the upper one-third of the rectum, spleen and pancreas. The veins of the portal system are valveless.
- The portal vein is formed by the union of the superior mesenteric vein and the splenic vein **(Fig. 7.7)**.
- Portal vein divides into right and left branches at the hepatic hilum which further divide into segmental branches. These end up into hepatic sinusoids. From sinusoids, blood drains into hepatic veins (right, left and middle) and then into the inferior vena cava (IVC).

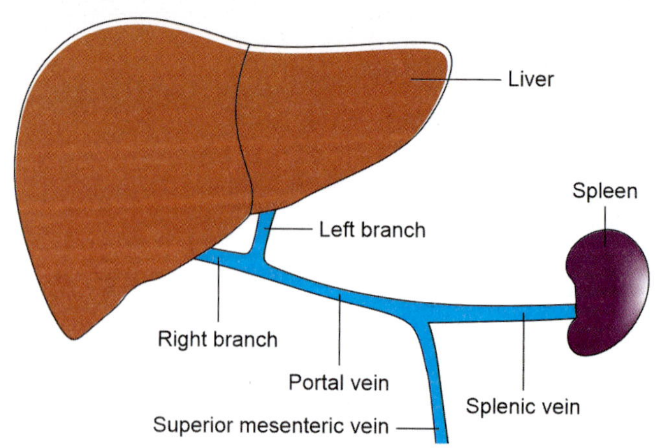

Figure 7.7: Anatomy of the portal venous system

Etiology of Portal HTN

Prehepatic

- Portal vein obstruction (e.g. portal vein thrombosis).
- Increased blood flow through portal vein (splanchnic arterio-venous fistula, massive splenomegaly).

Intrahepatic (most common type)

- Cirrhosis
- Drug toxicity (e.g. vinyl chloride, arsenic, vitamin A, 6-mercaptopurine)
- Malignant or metastatic hepatic diseases
- Myeloproliferative diseases
- Nodular regenerative hyperplasia
- Sarcoidosis
- Schistosomiasis
- Wilson's disease

Posthepatic

- Hepatic vein thrombosis (Budd-Chiari syndrome)
- Cardiac disease (e.g. constrictive pericarditis, right heart failure)
- Inferior vena cava obstruction.

Pathology

- Portal venous pressure depends on portal blood flow and portal vascular resistance. Increased vascular resistance is the main cause of portal hypertension.
- Increased portal vascular resistance leads to decreased portal blood flow to the liver and development of collateral vessels, allowing portal blood to bypass the liver and enter the systemic circulation directly (portosystemic shunting).
- Collateral vessels are seen in the esophagus, stomach, rectum, anterior abdominal wall, and in the renal, lumbar, ovarian and testicular vasculature. As collateral vessel formation progresses, more and more portosystemic shunting takes place.
- Dilatation of collateral vessels in the lower end of esophagus leads to varices.
- Increased portal pressure leads to congestion of the spleen and splenomegaly.
- Rarely increased blood flow through portal vein can cause portal HTN (example massive splenomegaly from which there is high blood flow into the portal vein).

Clinical Features

- The clinical features of portal hypertension result mainly from portal venous congestion and collateral vessel formation.
- Splenomegaly is present usually (mild-to-moderate). If splenomegaly is absent, diagnosis of portal hypertension is unlikely. Splenomegaly results in hypersplenism which can cause thrombocytopenia or even pancytopenia.
- Dilated veins may be seen on the anterior abdominal wall. Dilated veins radiating from the umbilicus are called caput medusae. Venous hum may be heard over a large umbilical collateral vein (Cruveilhier-Baumgarten syndrome).
- Dilated veins in the esophagus and stomach (gastroesophageal varices) can bleed and cause hematemesis and melena.
- Rectal varices can also cause bleeding and are often mistaken for hemorrhoids.
- Fetor hepaticus results from portosystemic shunting of blood, which allows mercaptans to pass directly to the lungs.
- Severe portal HTN can lead to ascites.

Investigations

- ***Blood tests:*** Anemia may be present due to hypersplenism and bleeding varices. Liver function tests are usually normal in patients with non-cirrhotic portal hypertension but may be altered in cirrhosis.
- ***Endoscopy***: Upper GI endoscopy shows gastroesophageal varices.
- ***Ultrasonography***: Ultrasonography (USG) of the liver and portal venous system helps to establish the diagnosis of portal HTN. It shows dilated collaterals around the gastroesophageal junction and splenic hilum, splenomegaly, and dilated portal vein and splenic vein. It can also help in diagnosing the cause of portal HTN such as cirrhosis, portal vein thrombosis, etc. Doppler USG can assess the direction and velocity of blood flow in the portal vein.
- ***Liver biopsy***: is indicated in selected cases to diagnose the cause of portal HTN.
- ***Portal venography:*** Demonstrates the site and often the cause of portal venous obstruction and is performed prior to surgical intervention.

Complications of Portal Hypertension

- Variceal bleeding
- Congestive gastropathy
- Hypersplenism
- Ascites
- Renal failure
- Hepatic encephalopathy.

Treatment

Reduction of Portal Pressure

- Nonselective beta-blockers such as propranolol or nadolol reduce portal pressure through splanchnic vasoconstriction and reduced cardiac output. Drugs should be titrated to a target pulse rate of 60/min or reduction of resting pulse by 25%. Nitrates (isosorbide mononitrate and dinitrate can be used if beta-blockers are contraindicated.
- Portosystemic shunt surgeries such as protocaval shunt, splenorenal shunt, etc. are done less commonly now with the availability of TIPS.
- TIPS (transjugular intrahepatic portosystemic shunt): Here, a portal-systemic shunt is placed through internal jugular vein percutaneously. It decompresses the portal circulation.
- Wherever possible, underlying cause of portal HTN should be treated.
- Liver transplantation is helpful in selected patients.

Treatment of Complications

- Complications such as variceal bleed, encephalopathy, ascites, etc. should be treated as per standard guidelines.

Q. Discuss the etiology, clinical features, diagnosis, differential diagnosis, investigations, and management of acute variceal bleeding.

Q. Transjugular intrahepatic portosystemic stent (TIPS).

- Acute variceal bleeding (AVB) is a life-threatening complication of portal hypertension, typically due to liver cirrhosis.
- Variceal bleeding occurs from esophageal varices that are usually located within 3–5 cm of the esophago-gastric junction, or from gastric varices **(Fig. 7.8)**.
- Higher grade of varices (grade 3 and 4), red spots and red stripes, high portal pressure and liver failure, aspirin and other nonsteroidal anti-inflammatory drugs (NSAIDs) are associated with increased risk of variceal bleeding.
- Variceal bleeding can be severe and mortality from bleeding esophageal varices is high (up to 50% in those with advanced liver disease).

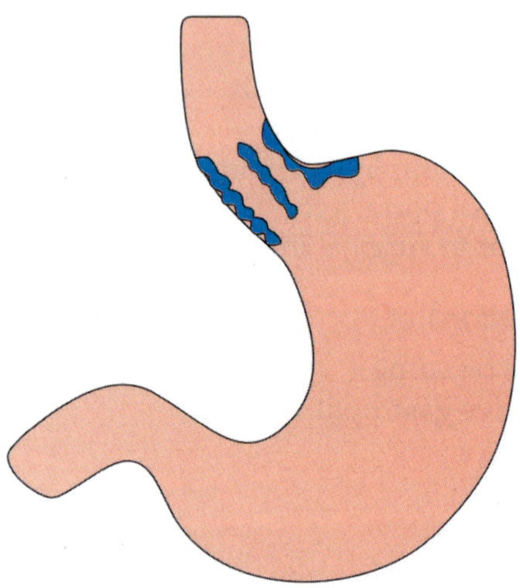

Figure 7.8: Esophageal varices

Etiology

- Cirrhosis (most common)
- Noncirrhotic portal hypertension (e.g. schistosomiasis, portal vein thrombosis).

Clinical Features

- Hematemesis: vomiting of fresh or altered blood ("coffee grounds" appearance). Any hematemesis in a patient with cirrhosis with portal HTN should be assumed as variceal bleed until proven otherwise.
- Melena: Altered (black) blood passed by rectum.
- Hemodynamic changes: Significant variceal bleed may lead pallor, tachypnea, tachycardia, and hypotension.
- Features of chronic liver disease: Ascites, jaundice, spider angiomata. Encephalopathy (in severe cases).
- Nasogastric tube lavage reveals fresh or altered blood in the stomach.
- Upper GI scopy can confirm the diagnosis.

Differential Diagnosis of Variceal Bleed

- Peptic ulcer.
- Mallory–Weiss tears.
- Gastroduodenal erosions
- Erosive esophagitis
- Cancer
- Aortoenteric fistulae
- Vascular lesions.

Investigations

- CBC: Anemia, thrombocytopenia.
- Coagulation profile: Prolonged PT/INR.
- LFTs: Assess severity of liver dysfunction.
- Renal function: Urea, creatinine (risk of hepatorenal syndrome).
- Endoscopy: Gold standard investigation to confirm source of bleeding (esophageal or gastric varices). Also allows for therapeutic intervention.
- Abdominal ultrasound with Doppler: To look for cirrhosis with portal hypertension.

Management of Acute Variceal Bleeding

- Variceal bleeding is a life-threatening emergency. Patients should be admitted to an intensive care unit. Blood pressure, pulse rate, urine output, and mental status should be monitored.
- Intravascular volume replacement should be done with IV fluids and blood transfusion.
- Replacement of clotting factors with fresh-frozen plasma is important in patients with coagulopathy.
- The measures used to control acute variceal bleeding include endoscopic therapy (banding or sclerotherapy), balloon tamponade, esophageal transection, TIPS and sphlanchnic vasoconstrictors.

Variceal Banding

- This is the treatment of choice in acute variceal bleeding. It stops variceal bleeding in 80% of patients and can be repeated if bleeding recurs. This is a technique in which varices are sucked into an endoscope accessory, and occluded with a tight rubber band. The occluded varix subsequently sloughs with variceal obliteration. It should be repeated at regular intervals to obliterate all varices. Banding is more effective than sclerotherapy, with fewer side effects and is the treatment of choice.

Sclerotherapy

- In this technique, varices are injected with a sclerosing agent to obliterate them. It is less preferred now because of the availability of band ligation. Sclerotherapy can cause transient dysphagia, chest pain, esophageal perforation and esophageal strictures.

Splanchnic Vasoconstrictors

- Terlipressin and octreotide reduce the portal pressure and can stop variceal bleeding. Terlipressin dose is 2 mg IV 6-hourly until bleeding stops and then 1 mg 6-hourly for a further 24 hours.
- Octreotide is given as 50 μg IV bolus followed by an infusion of 50 μg per hour.

Balloon Tamponade

- This is used less commonly nowadays due to the availability of endoscopic therapies.
- This technique employs a Sengstaken-Blakemore tube with two balloons which exert pressure in the fundus of the stomach and in the lower esophagus respectively when inflated.
- The tube is passed through the mouth into the stomach and gastric balloon is inflated with 200–250 ml of air, which controls gastric variceal bleed. Then esophageal balloon is inflated to compress the esophageal varices.
- Pressure in the esophageal balloon should be monitored with a sphygmomanometer and should not exceed 40 mm Hg.
- Balloon tamponade will almost always stop esophageal and gastric fundal variceal bleeding, but this is only a temporary measure. Definitive therapy such as banding or sclerotherapy should be arranged as early as possible.

Transjugular Intrahepatic Portosystemic Stent (TIPS)

- TIPS can be used for acute bleeding not responding to sclerotherapy or banding.
- This technique involves placing a stent between portal and hepatic vein in the liver to reduce portal pressure. It is done under radiological guidance via the internal jugular vein. Patency of the portal vein must be confirmed before the procedure by angiography. Any coagulation defect should be corrected by fresh frozen plasma, and prophylactic antibiotics are given. Successful shunt placement stops and prevents variceal bleeding.
- Shunt narrowing or occlusion can happen which can cause rebleeding from varices. It can be corrected by angioplasty.
- Although TIPS is better than endoscopic therapy in preventing rebleeding, survival is not improved. There is a higher risk of hepatic encephalopathy with TIPS since the portal blood is shunted directly into systemic circulation.

Prevention of Recurrent Bleeding

- Recurrent bleeding happens in almost all the patients who have bled previously. Hence, following preventive measures are needed.
- Band ligation
- Sclerotherapy
- Portosystemic shunt surgery
- Beta-adrenoceptor antagonists: Propranolol or nadolol reduce portal venous pressure and prevent recurrent variceal bleeding.

Q. List the drugs used to reduce portal venous pressure.

Splanchnic vasoconstrictors
- Vasopressin
- Terlipressin
- Somatostatin
- Octreotide

Nonselective beta blockers
- Propranolol
- Nadolol
- carvedilol

Nitrates

Isosorbide mononitrate and dinitrate.

Q. Define hepatic encephalopathy (portosystemic encephalopathy or hepatic coma). Discuss the etiology, pathogenesis, clinical features, investigations, and treatment of hepatic encephalopathy.

- Hepatic encephalopathy (HE) is a reversible neuropsychiatric syndrome occurring in patients with advanced liver failure.
- Its severity ranges from inversion of sleep rhythm and mild intellectual impairment to coma.

Etiology

Chronic Liver Disease (more common)

- Cirrhosis with or without portosystemic shunts
- Precipitating factors often present

Acute Liver Failure (ALF)

- Viral hepatitis (e.g. hepatitis A, B)
- Drug toxicity (e.g. paracetamol overdose)
- Acute ischemic or toxic liver injury

Precipitating Factors in Chronic Liver Disease (Table 7.9)

TABLE 7.9: Precipitating factors in chronic liver disease

Factor	Examples
Increased nitrogen load	GI bleeding, high-protein diet, constipation
Electrolyte imbalance	Hypokalemia, hyponatremia
Infections	Spontaneous bacterial peritonitis, UTI, pneumonia
Drugs	Sedatives, benzodiazepines, narcotics
Hypovolemia	Diarrhea, overdiuresis, paracentesis without albumin
TIPS procedure	Portosystemic shunting can precipitate HE

Pathophysiology (Fig. 7.9)

- Hepatic encephalopathy results from the accumulation of neurotoxic substances (ammonia, gaba aminobutyric acid, mercaptans and manganese), particularly ammonia, due to liver dysfunction and/or portosystemic shunting. This leads to altered neurotransmission, astrocyte dysfunction, and cerebral edema, manifesting as cognitive and motor disturbances.

- Normally, ammonia is produced in the gut by bacterial breakdown of nitrogenous substances (e.g. proteins, blood) and is detoxified by the healthy liver. In the presence of liver failure and portosystemic shunting ammonia enters systemic circulation and brain. Ammonia has multiple neurotoxic effects. It can alter the transit of amino acids, water, and electrolytes across astrocytes and neurons. It can impair amino acid metabolism and energy utilization in the brain. Ammonia can also inhibit the generation of excitatory and inhibitory postsynaptic potentials.
- In the brain, astrocytes convert ammonia to glutamine (via glutamine synthetase). Excess glutamine accumulates in astrocytes → osmotic swelling → cerebral edema. This mechanism is especially significant in acute liver failure.
- Neurotransmitter imbalance: Ammonia also causes neurotransmitter imbalance in the brain. There is accumulation of inhibitor neurotransmitters like GABA-like substances and reduced excitatory neurotransmission → CNS depression.

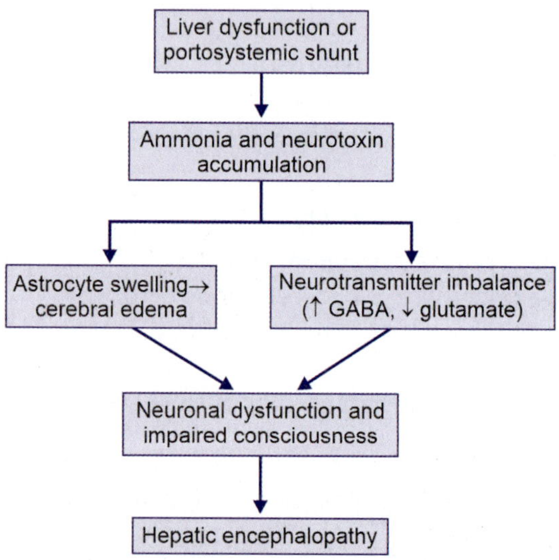

Figure 7.9: Pathogenesis of hepatic encephalopathy

Clinical Features

- Early hepatic encephalopathy may not be clinically recognizable except for mild cognitive, psychomotor, and attention deficit on standardized tests.
- Alteration of sleep cycle characterized by day time sleepiness and nighttime insomnia is an early symptom (inversion of sleep rhythm).
- As the severity of hepatic encephalopathy increases, it leads to confusion, restlessness, drowsiness, disorientation, stupor, and finally coma. Convulsions can sometimes occur.
- Examination usually shows a flapping tremor (asterixis), inability to perform simple mental arithmetic calculations and draw objects such as a star (constructional apraxia). As the condition progresses, hyperreflexia and bilateral extensor plantar responses may be seen.
- Focal neurological signs may be rarely present in hepatic encephalopathy. However, other causes such as stroke should be ruled out in such patients.
- Signs of liver cell failure such as fetor hepaticus (sweet musty odour to the breath due to the presence of mercaptans), jaundice, spider naevi, coagulation defects may be present.

Clinical grading of hepatic encephalopathy

Grade 1: Euphoria or depression, mild confusion, slurred speech, disordered sleep rhythm

Grade 2: Lethargy, moderate confusion

Grade 3: Marked confusion, incoherent speech, sleeping but arousable

Grade 4: Coma; initially responsive to noxious stimuli, later unresponsive

Flaps are present in grade 2 and 3, and absent in grade 1 and 4 hepatic encephalopathy.

Differential Diagnosis of Hepatic Encephalopathy

- Subdural hematoma
- Drug or alcohol intoxication
- Delirium tremens
- Wernicke's encephalopathy
- Primary psychiatric disorders
- Hypoglycemia
- Neurological problems
- Wilson's disease.

Investigations

- Diagnosis is made by clinical features. However, following tests may be helpful in doubtful situations.
- Serum ammonia level is increased. But the severity of hepatic encephalopathy does not correlate with ammonia level.
- Complete blood count: hemoglobin may be low due to variceal bleeding. WBC may be elevated due to infection. Thrombocytopenia may be present.
- LFTs: Elevated bilirubin, ALT/AST, low albumin.
- Coagulation profile: ↑ PT/INR.
- Serum electrolytes, urea, creatinine, glucose, etc. should be done to rule out other causes of altered sensorium.
- Electroencephalogram (EEG) shows diffuse slowing of the normal alpha waves with eventual development of delta waves.
- Brain imaging (CT or MRI) to rule out structural brain lesions which can cause altered sensorium such as subdural hematoma, stroke.

Treatment

- Lactulose is given orally, initially at a dose of 30 ml three or four times daily. The dose should then be titrated so that two or three soft stools per day are produced. Lactulose is a non-absorbable synthetic disaccharide. It is digested by bacteria in the colon to short-chain fatty acids, resulting in acidification of colon contents. This acidification favors the formation of ammonium ion (NH_4^+) from ammonia. Ammonium is not absorbable, and excreted in the stools. Lactulose also inhibits intestinal bacteria by formation of acidic environment which decreases ammonia production by bacteria. Lactulose can also be given rectally as retention enema.

- Rifaximin 400 mg three times daily controls ammonia-producing intestinal bacteria. Alternative antibiotics are metronidazole, neomycin and vancomycin.
- Opioids and sedatives should be avoided. Oxazepam can be given to control agitation as it is not metabolized by the liver.
- L-ornithine L-aspartate (LOLA) enhances ammonia detoxification in liver and muscle.
- Dietary protein should be restricted. Vegetable protein is better tolerated than meat protein. Gastrointestinal bleeding should be controlled and blood should be purged from the gastrointestinal tract. This can be done by nasogastric aspiration and by giving lactulose to induce diarrhea.
- Chronic or refractory hepatic encephalopathy requires liver transplantation.

Q. Hepatorenal syndrome.

Definition

- Hepatorenal syndrome (HRS) is a functional renal failure that occurs in patients with advanced liver disease (usually cirrhosis), in the absence of intrinsic kidney pathology.
- Hepatorenal syndrome is diagnosed only when other causes of renal failure (including prerenal azotemia and acute tubular necrosis) have been excluded.

Pathogenesis

- The exact cause of this syndrome is not clear, but altered renal hemodynamics appears to be involved. There is intense renal vasoconstriction, perhaps in response to systemic and splanchnic vasodilation accompanying cirrhosis. Persistent renal vasoconstriction leads to decreased GFR and renal failure. Kidneys are structurally normal. If these kidneys are transplanted to people without liver disease, they function normally.

Types of Hepatorenal Syndrome

- Type 1 (HRS-AKI): Rapidly progressive renal failure (doubling of serum creatinine to >2.5 mg/dl in <2 weeks).
- Type 2 (HRS-CKD): Slowly progressive renal failure, often associated with refractory ascites.

Clinical Features

- Features of decompensated cirrhosis (jaundice, ascites, encephalopathy)
- Worsening azotemia
- Hyponatremia
- Progressive oliguria
- Hypotension
- It is often precipitated by severe gastrointestinal bleeding, sepsis, or vigorous diuresis or paracentesis.

Diagnostic Criteria for HRS

- Cirrhosis with ascites
- Diagnosis of **AKI** per KDIGO (↑ serum creatinine ≥0.3 mg/dl in 48 hours or ≥50% increase from baseline in 7 days).
- **No response** after 2 days of diuretic withdrawal and albumin infusion (1 g/kg/day up to 100 g/day).
- **No shock**, nephrotoxic drugs, or structural kidney disease.
- Urinary findings: low sodium (<10 mEq/L), bland sediment, low proteinuria.

Treatment

- There is no effective treatment for hepatorenal syndrome so far.
- Intravenous albumin infusion may help in some cases.
- Splanchnic vasoconstrictors such as terlipressin, and octreotide can be tried and have shown benefit. Terlipressin is the preferred vasoconstrictor. Combination of midodrine and octreotide are used if terlipressin is not available. Noradrenaline infusion which causes splanchnic vasoconstriction has also shown benefit.
- TIPS has been reported to improve renal function in some patients but its use cannot be universally recommended.
- Liver transplantation is the treatment of choice for hepatorenal syndrome.

Q. Define ascites. Discuss the causes and approach to a case of ascites.

Q. Discuss the etiology, clinical features, investigations and management of a case of ascites.

Q. Puddle sign.

- Ascites refers to the accumulation of excess fluid in the peritoneal cavity.

Causes of Ascites

- Cirrhosis with portal HTN
- Cardiac failure
- Renal failure
- Hypoproteinemia (nephrotic syndrome, protein-losing enteropathy, malnutrition)
- Intra-abdominal malignancy
- Pancreatitis
- Abdominal tuberculosis
- Hepatic venous occlusion (Budd-Chiari syndrome, veno-occlusive disease)
- Rare causes (Meigs' syndrome, chylous ascites, vasculitis, hypothyroidism)

Clinical Features

Symptoms

- Abdominal distension
- Dyspnea and orthopnea due to pushed up diaphragm
- Epigastric and retrosternal burning sensation due to gastroesophageal reflux due to increased intra-abdominal pressure.

- Low-grade fever and weight loss suggests tuberculous etiology.
- Presence of exertional dyspnea, orthopnea and PND suggests heart failure.

Signs

- Presence of jaundice and dilated veins over the abdomen **(Fig. 7.10)** indicate cirrhosis of liver with portal HTN. Other stigmata of live disease such as spider naevi, palmar eryrthema, gynecomastia, etc. may be present.
- Diffuse abdominal distension with fullness in the flanks. Skin appears shiny **(Fig. 7.11)**.
- Umbilicus is flush with the skin or everted.
- Shifting dullness present on percussion. Horse shoe shaped dullness is present in supine position.
- Fluid thrill is present in tense ascites.
- ***Puddle sign*:** This is useful to detect even minimal ascites (as low as 120 ml). Patient is put in prone position for 5 minutes. Then he is put in knee elbow position. Diaphragm of stethoscope is applied to the most dependent part of the abdomen. One flank is flicked with a finger repeatedly while auscultating. Move the diaphragm gradually to opposite flank. A change in percussion note indicates presence of fluid.

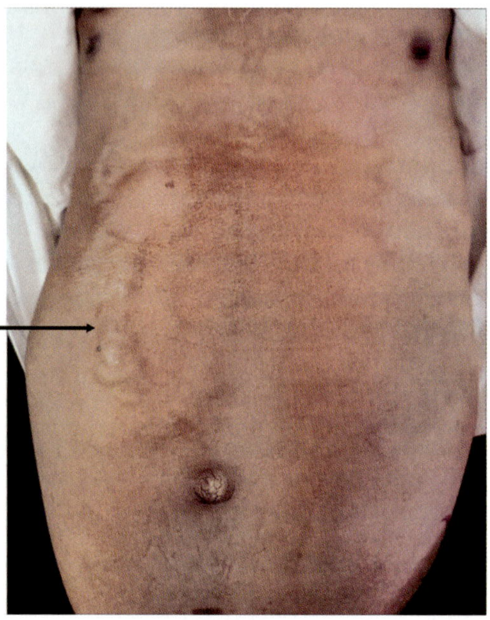

Figure 7.10: Dilated veins on abdomen in portal HTN

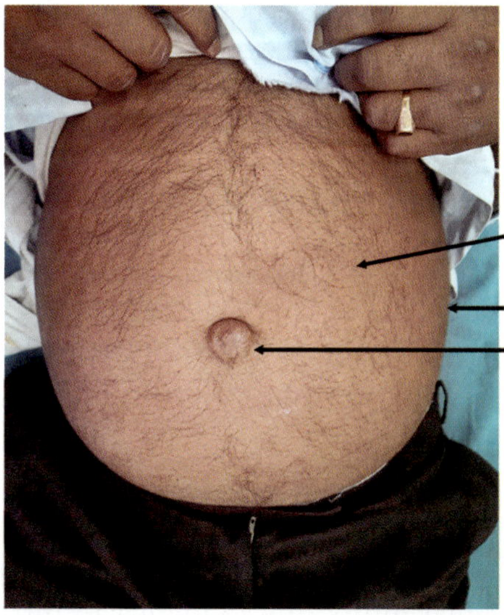

Figure 7.11: Ascites

- Tenderness may be present in the abdomen and points towards an infectious etiology such as tuberculosis or peritonitis.
- Herniae, abdominal striae, divarication of the recti and scrotal edema may be present.
- Pleural effusion may be present in some patients usually on the right side.
- In cases of ascites due to heart failure, signs of heart congestive heart failure such as raised JVP, basal lung crepitations and third heart sound may be present.
- In cases of malignant ascites, sometimes a mass may be palpable per abdomen.

Investigations

Ultrasound Abdomen

- This is the easiest and most sensitive test to detect ascites. It can also show the underlying cause of ascites in many cases such as cirrhosis of liver, intra-abdominal malignancy, portal HTN, etc.

Ascitic Fluid Analysis

- *Appearance:* Clear or straw colored in case of transudates. Turbid appearance is seen in infections and malignancy. White color appearance is seen in chylous ascites. Dark brown color indicates biliary tract perforation. Black fluid may indicate the presence of pancreatic necrosis or metastatic melanoma.
- *Cell count:* Normal ascitic fluid contains fewer than 500 WBCs/µl and fewer than 250 polymorphonuclear leukocytes (PMNs)/µl. High WBC count is found in infections. A PMN count of greater than 250 cells/µl is highly suggestive of bacterial peritonitis. Presence of high percentage of lymphocytes indicates tuberculous etiology.
- *Serum-ascites albumin gradient (SAAG):* The SAAG is the best single test for classifying ascites into transudative (SAAG >1.1 g/dl) and exudative (SAAG <1.1 g/dl) causes. SAAG >1.1 g/dl is typical of cirrhosis of liver with portal HTN. SAAG is calculated by subtracting the ascitic fluid albumin value from the serum albumin value.
- *Total protein:* Total ascitic fluid protein greater than or equal to 2.5 g/dl indicates exudative ascites. An elevated SAAG and a high protein level are observed in most cases of ascites due to hepatic congestion. The combination of a low SAAG and a high protein level is characteristic of malignant ascites.
- *Culture/Gram stain/AFB stain:* are useful to identify the infecting organism in cases of ascites due to intra-abdominal infections.
- *Malignant cytology:* useful in cases of suspected malignant ascites.

- ***Ascitic fluid amylase:*** is typically >1000 mg/dl in pancreatic ascites.
- ***Adenosine deaminase (ADA):*** is usually more than 40U/L in tuberculous ascites.
- CB-NAAT too rule out TB.

Chest X-ray

- Pleural effusion may be present in cases of massive ascites.

CT Abdomen

- Useful to diagnose or rule out cirrhosis, malignancy, tuberculosis, etc.

ECG/Echocardiogram

- To rule out congestive cardiac failure.

Treatment

- Treat the underlying cause.
- Diuretics are helpful in reducing ascites especially in portal HTN. Spironolactone or furosemide can be used.
- Sodium intake should be restricted to 20–30 mEq/day.
- Therapeutic paracentesis may be performed in patients who require rapid symptomatic relief for refractory or tense ascites.
- The transjugular intrahepatic portosystemic shunt (TIPS) is useful in cirrhotic patients with refractory ascites.

Q. Discuss the pathogenesis and management of ascites in cirrhosis.

- Ascites is the accumulation of fluid in the peritoneal cavity and is a hallmark complication of decompensated liver cirrhosis. Its pathogenesis is multifactorial, involving hemodynamic, hormonal, and renal mechanisms:

Pathogenesis of Ascites in Cirrhosis

Portal HTN

- Cirrhosis leads to architectural distortion and increased resistance to portal blood flow.
- This causes portal hypertension, increasing hydrostatic pressure within the splanchnic circulation, promoting fluid transudation into the peritoneal cavity.

Renal Retention of Sodium and Water

- Cirrhosis of liver leads to accumulation of nitric oxide which causes splanchnic and peripheral arterial dilatation leading to a decrease in effective circulating blood volume. This apparent decrease in intravascular volume (underfilling) is sensed by the kidney, leading to activation of renin-angiotensin system with secondary hyperaldosteronism, increased sympathetic activity, and increased antidiuretic hormone (ADH) release. All these changes lead to salt and water retention.

Hypoalbuminemia

- Decreased serum albumin in cirrhosis leads to decreased oncotic pressure in the splanchnic circulation and ascites formation.

Investigations

Ascitic Fluid Analysis

- Ascitic fluid is clear or straw colored in cirrhosis. It is usually transudate unless complicated by SBP. Cell count is less than 250.
- The ascites protein concentration and the serum-ascites albumin gradient (SAAG ratio) is used to distinguish ascites due to transudation from ascites due to exudation. Cirrhotic patients usually have transudate with a SAAG ratio of >1.1.

Ultrasound Abdomen

- It confirms the diagnosis especially when small amounts are present.
- Ultrasound abdomen can also point towards the underlying cause of ascites such as cirrhosis, pancreatitis, etc.

Treatment

- ***Salt restriction:*** <2 g per day.
- ***Fluid restriction:*** 1 liter/day.
- ***Diuretics:*** Spironolactone is the initial drug of choice (50–400 mg/day). Furosemide (40–160 mg/day) can be added if not responding to spironolactone alone. Spironolactone can cause painful gynaecomastia and hyperkalemia. Diuresis is improved if patients are rested in bed while the diuretics are acting, perhaps because renal blood flow increases in the horizontal position.
- ***Paracentesis:*** Therapeutic paracentesis is done in severe ascites. Albumin infusion should be given during large volume paracentesis. This should be followed by maintenance diuretic therapy and sodium restriction.
- ***Shunts:*** Portacaval shunt, peritoneo-venous shunt and TIPS can reduce ascites but do not improve life expectancy.

Q. Refractory ascites.

- Patients who do not respond to doses of 400 mg spironolactone and 160 mg furosemide are considered to have refractory or diuretic-resistant ascites.

Pathophysiology

Refractory ascites occurs due to:

- Severe portal hypertension
- Profound splanchnic vasodilation, leading to decreased effective arterial blood volume
- Renal vasoconstriction and activation of RAAS, causing intense sodium and water retention
- Progressive hepatorenal dysfunction.

Differential Diagnosis of Refractory Ascites

- Malignant ascites
- Nephrogenic ascites (end stage renal disease)
- Budd-Chiari syndrome (hepatic vein thrombosis).

Treatment Options

- Liver transplantation
- Serial therapeutic paracentesis
- Colloid replacement
- Extracorporeal ultrafiltration and reinfusion
- Transjugular intrahepatic portosystemic stent-shunt (TIPS)
- Peritoneovenous shunt
- Surgical portosystemic shunts.

Q. Spontaneous bacterial peritonitis (SBP).

- Spontaneous bacterial peritonitis (SBP) is defined as an ascitic fluid infection without an evident intra-abdominal surgically treatable source. Patients with cirrhosis are very susceptible to infection of ascitic fluid.
- The source of infection cannot usually be determined, but most organisms isolated from ascitic fluid or blood cultures are of enteric origin and *Escherichia coli* is the organism most frequently found. The bacteria are transported from the lumen of intestine into peritoneal cavity due to loss of defense mechanisms which normally contain the bacteria within the lumen.

Clinical Features

- Fever, abdominal pain, rebound tenderness, and absent bowel sounds in a patient with obvious features of cirrhosis and ascites.
- Abdominal signs are mild or absent in about one-third of patients, and in these patients hepatic encephalopathy and fever are the main features.
- Hypotension and hypothermia suggest advanced infection and such patients usually do not survive.

Investigations

- Blood count shows leukocytosis.
- Ascitic fluid analysis: cloudy fluid, total leukocyte counts is >500/mm^3 and neutrophil count is >250/mm^3.
- Ascitic fluid Gram's stain and culture can identify the organism which is usually *E. coli*.
- Finding of multiple organisms on culture should arouse suspicion of a perforated viscus.
- Ultrasound abdomen to rule out other causes of peritonitis such as hollow viscus perforation.

Treatment

- Broad-spectrum antibiotics, such as cefotaxime 2 g IV every eight hours for 5–10 days. Ceftriaxone and ceftazidime have similar efficacy. Intravenous or oral quinolone is an alternative.
- Recurrence of SBP is common in high-risk patients and may be reduced by prophylactic quinolones such as norfloxacin (400 mg daily) or ciprofloxacin (250 mg daily) for 5–7 days.

Q. Discuss the etiology, pathogenesis, clinical features, investigations and management of acute cholangitis.

Q. Charcot's triad.

- Acute cholangitis refers to infection of the bile duct which is characterized by fever, jaundice, and abdominal pain.
- Cholangitis was first described by Charcot.

Etiology

- Acute cholangitis is most often caused by biliary obstruction, and *Escherichia coli* is the most common organism. Causes are as follows:

Biliary tract obstruction
- Gallstones (choledocholithiasis)—most common cause
- Benign biliary strictures (e.g. post-surgical)
- Malignant obstruction (e.g. cholangiocarcinoma, pancreatic cancer)
- Parasites (e.g. ***Clonorchis sinensis***)
- Biliary stents or post-ERCP strictures

Biliary interventions
- Endoscopic retrograde cholangiopancreatography (ERCP).
- Percutaneous transhepatic cholangiography (PTC).

Congenital abnormalities
- Choledochal cysts
- Biliary atresia (in infants)

Pathogenesis

- Acute cholangitis is caused mainly by bacteria.
- Biliary obstruction causes stasis of bile. The organisms ascend from the duodenum and infect the stagnant bile. Hematogenous spread from the portal vein is a rare source of infection.
- High intrabiliary pressure due to obstruction of biliary tree promotes the migration of bacteria from the portal circulation into the biliary tract and subsequent colonization.
- The sphincter of Oddi normally prevents duodenal reflux into the biliary tree and ascending bacterial infection. When there is sphincter of Oddi dysfunction or after endoscopic sphincterotomy, choledochal surgery, or biliary stent insertion, pathogenic bacteria enter the biliary tree and lead to infection.

Clinical Features

- ***Charcot triad:*** Refers to fever, right upper quadrant pain, and jaundice. It occurs in 50–75% of patients with acute cholangitis.
- Reynolds' pentad is ***Charcot triad*** + hypotension + altered mental status. It indicates severe or septic cholangitis, often requiring urgent biliary decompression.
- Confusion and hypotension can occur in severe cholangitis.
- Septic shock in severe cases can lead to multi-organ failure.

Investigations

- Leukocytosis with neutrophilia.
- LFT shows cholestatic pattern with elevation of alkaline phosphatase, and predominantly direct hyperbilirubinemia.

- Serum amylase may be elevated due to associated pancreatitis.
- Blood cultures can sometimes identify the organism.
- Ultrasound abdomen my show common bile duct dilatation and stones.
- Endoscopic retrograde cholangiopancreatography (ERCP): Diagnostic as well as therapeutic (used mainly after stabilization).
- Magnetic resonance cholangiopancreatography (MRCP) is a noninvasive alternative to ERCP to evaluate biliary tree.
- Endoscopic ultrasound is another means to visualize common duct stones.

Treatment

- The mainstays of therapy are antibiotics and establishment of biliary drainage.

General Measures

- Intravenous fluids, antipyretics, correction of coagulopathy, and frequent monitoring of vital signs for evidence of sepsis.

Antibiotics

- Broad spectrum antibiotics to cover gram negative bacteria and anaerobes. Effective antibiotics include: Ceftriaxone + metronidazole or piperacillin-tazobactam. Alternatives: Carbapenems in resistant cases. Antibiotics are adjusted based on culture results.
- Antibiotics should be given for 1–2 weeks.

Biliary Drainage

- If there is no response to antibiotic therapy, biliary drainage should be considered. Biliary drainage can be achieved by ERCP, a direct percutaneous approach, or open surgical decompression. Endoscopic sphincterotomy with stone extraction and/or stent insertion is now the treatment of choice for establishing biliary drainage in acute cholangitis.

Q. Discuss the etiology, pathology, clinical features, investigations, and management of Budd-Chiari syndrome.

- Budd-Chiari syndrome refers to obstruction of hepatic venous outflow. Obstruction can be anywhere from the small hepatic veins inside the liver to the inferior vena cava.
- Most common cause is thrombosis of the hepatic veins and/or the intrahepatic or suprahepatic inferior vena cava.
- Regardless of the cause, patients with Budd-Chiari syndrome develop post sinusoidal portal hypertension, which leads to complications similar to those observed in patients with cirrhosis.

Etiology

- Hypercoagulable states
  - Myeloproliferative diseases
  - Factor V Leiden mutation
  - Antiphospholipid antibody syndrome
  - Antithrombin III deficiency
  - Protein C deficiency
  - Protein S deficiency
  - Paroxysmal nocturnal hemoglobinuria
  - Oral contraceptives
  - Pregnancy
- Mechanical obstruction: Hepatocellular carcinoma, hydatid cysts, abscesses, trauma or surgery involving hepatic veins or IVC.
- Membranous webs of the inferior vena cava and/or the hepatic veins.
- Idiopathic.

Pathology

- Obstruction of hepatic venous outflow → centrilobular congestion and hepatocyte necrosis.
- Leads to sinusoidal hypertension, hepatomegaly, ascites, and liver failure.
- Chronic cases show fibrosis, nodular regeneration, and eventual cirrhosis.

Clinical Manifestations

- Budd-Chiari syndrome is more common in women, and usually presents in the third or fourth decade.
- Presentation can be categorized as acute or chronic.
- In acute form, patients usually present with severe right upper quadrant pain, tender hepatomegaly, jaundice and ascites. Fulminant hepatic failure can also occur.
- More gradual occlusion causes gross ascites and often upper abdominal discomfort.
- Peripheral edema occurs when there is inferior vena cava obstruction.
- Cirrhosis and portal hypertension develop in chronic form.

Investigations

- LFT: In acute Budd-Chiari, LFT shows acute hepatitis pattern with AST and ALT elevation.
- Ascitic fluid analysis: Usually shows exudative pattern.
- Doppler ultrasound: Show occlusion of the hepatic veins and reversed flow or associated thrombosis in the portal vein. Enlarged caudate lobe (drains into IVC directly).
- CT scan and MRI may also demonstrate occlusion of the hepatic veins and inferior vena cava.
- Liver biopsy: Shows centrilobular congestion with fibrosis depending upon the duration of the illness.
- Venography: This is the gold standard for diagnosis. However, since it is invasive, it is done if CT and MRI are unable to show hepatic venous occlusion.
- Hypercoagulable profile: Protein C/S, antithrombin III, JAK2 mutation, antiphospholipid antibodies.

Treatment

- Treat the underlying cause.
- Medical management involves thrombolysis if thrombosis is of recent origin, and anticoagulation.

For anticoagulation, heparin is given initially followed by oral anticoagulation. Ascites is treated with diuretics.

- TIPS (trans jugular intrahepatic portosystemic shunt) followed by anticoagulation: this creates an alternative venous outflow tract. Can be used in extensive hepatic vein occlusion.
- For caval webs or hepatic venous stenosis, decompression via percutaneous transluminal balloon angioplasty with intraluminal stents can maintain hepatic outflow.
- Surgical shunts, such as portacaval shunts, are less commonly performed now that TIPS is available.
- Liver transplantation and lifelong anticoagulation should be considered for progressive liver failure.

Q. Enumerate the tumors of liver.

Q. Discuss the etiology, pathology, clinical features, investigations, and management of hepatocellular carcinoma (hepatoma).

Tumors of liver

Benign

- Hemangioma
- Hepatic adenoma
- Focal nodular hyperplasia
- Lipoma, angiomyolipoma

Malignant

- ***Primary***
  - Hepatocellular carcinoma (most common primary malignant liver tumor)
  - Fibrolamellar carcinoma (variant of HCC, seen in young adults).
  - Cholangiocarcinoma (bile duct cancer)
  - Angiosarcoma
- ***Secondaries (most common overall liver malignancies)***
  - From colon, breast, lung, pancreas, stomach, etc.

Hepatocellular Carcinoma

This is the most common primary liver tumor.

Risk Factors

- Chronic hepatitis B and C infection
- Cirrhosis due to any etiology
- Environmental toxins (aflatoxin)
- Hemochromatosis
- Tobacco and alcohol abuse
- Nonalcoholic steatohepatitis (NASH)

Pathology

- HCC usually develops in a cirrhotic liver.
- Macroscopically, the tumor appears as a single mass or multiple nodules. Blood supply is from hepatic artery and it tends to spread by invasion into the portal vein and its radicles. Lymph node metastases are common but lung and bone metastases are rare.
- Microscopically, hepatocellular carcinoma can be divided into 3 types: Well-differentiated, moderately differentiated, and poorly differentiated. Tumor cells resemble hepatocytes when well differentiated.
- Integration of the hepatitis B virus genome into the host genome is the primary mechanism of cancer development in hepatitis-B infection.

Clinical Features

- Many patients are asymptomatic and detected through screening programs.
- Weight loss, anorexia and abdominal pain.
- Variceal hemorrhage can occur due to underlying cirrhosis.
- Examination may reveal ascites, jaundice, hepatomegaly or a right hypochondrial mass. A bruit may be heard over the tumor due to increased blood supply.

Screening

- Screening for hepatocellular carcinoma, by ultrasound scanning at 3–6 month intervals, is useful in high-risk patients. This may identify tumor at early stage which may be curable by surgical resection, local ablative therapy or transplantation.

Investigations

Blood tests

- Alpha-fetoprotein (AFP) level is increased in hepatocellular carcinoma (>400 ng/ml suggestive). However, it may also increase in active hepatitis due to hepatitis B and C, and in acute hepatic necrosis (e.g. due to paracetamol toxicity).
- ALP is usually elevated but other LFTs may be normal.
- Hepatitis serologies (HBV, HCV).

Ultrasound

- This will detect lesions as small as 2–3 cm. It may also show other underlying pathologies like cirrhosis.

CT

- On CT, hepatocellular carcinoma appears hypervascular. It can define the extent and spread of tumors to other organs.

Liver biopsy

- This can confirm the diagnosis of hepatocellular carcinoma and exclude metastatic tumor.

Management

Surgical therapy

- ***Hepatic resection***: Small localized tumors can be removed by resection in patients with good liver function. Patients with cirrhosis are not suitable for resection because of high risk of liver failure. However, it can be considered in some cirrhotic patients with small tumors and good liver function.
- ***Liver transplantation:*** This can be considered in patients with underlying cirrhosis or decompensated liver disease.

Local ablative therapies

- Transcatheter arterial chemoembolization (TACE) is the most commonly offered therapy. TACE is performed by selectively cannulating the feeding artery to the tumor and delivering high local doses of chemotherapy, including doxorubicin, cisplatin, or mitomycin C.

- Another newly developed local treatment is TheraSphere which delivers low-dose brachytherapy to the tumor. TheraSphere uses 20–40 μm glass beads that are loaded with radioactive yttrium and delivered angiographically.
- Radiofrequency ablation: under ultrasound guidance, a conducting needle is placed within the tumor and electric current is given. The electric current leads to agitation of the ions in the tissue, heat generation, and desiccation of the tissues surrounding the probe.

Sorafenib and lenvatinib (multikinase inhibitors)

- These two drugs have been shown to be useful in hepatocellular carcinoma.

Prevention

- Hepatitis B vaccination can prevent cancer due to hepatitis B infection.

Q. Alpha-fetoprotein.

- Alpha fetoprotein (AFP) is a protein produced by the liver and yolk sac of a developing baby during pregnancy. AFP levels go down soon after birth.
- The normal value in males or non-pregnant female is generally less than 10 ng/ml.
- AFP levels can increase in the following conditions.
  - Hepatocellular carcinoma (levels >400 ng/ml are highly suggestive of HCC, especially in cirrhotic patients).
  - Germ cell tumors (non-seminomatous testicular tumors, ovarian germ cell tumors). Used alongside β-hCG for diagnosis and monitoring.
  - Other cancers: malignant teratoma, stomach, pancreas, lung, and colon cancers (occasionally elevated).
- AFP can also be used to monitor tumor recurrence after treatment. Elevation of AFP after remission suggests tumor recurrence. Failure of the AFP value to return to normal by approximately 1 month after surgery suggests the presence of residual tumor.
- Limitations: May be normal in HCC, especially in small tumors or well-differentiated forms. False positives and negatives can occur; must be interpreted in clinical context and alongside imaging (e.g. ultrasound, CT/MRI).

Q. Discuss the etiology, clinical features, investigations, and management of pyogenic liver abscess.

- A pyogenic liver abscess **(Fig. 7.12)** is a collection of pus in the liver parenchyma caused by bacterial infection. Pyogenic liver abscess is curable but fatal if untreated.

Etiology

- Biliary obstruction causing ascending cholangitis and abscess formation (most common cause)

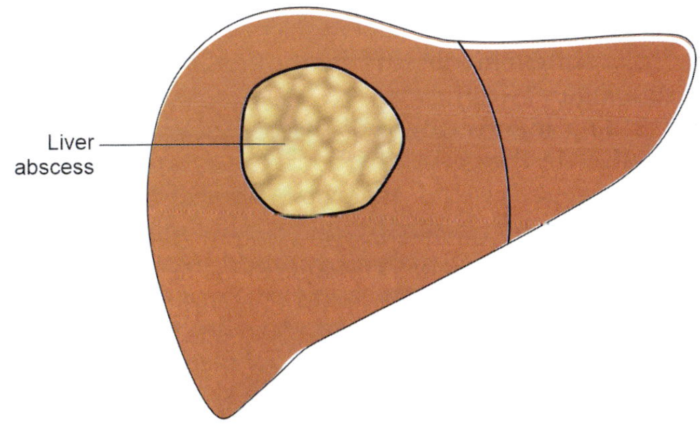

Figure 7.12: Liver abscess

- Infection via portal vein (appendicitis, diverticulitis, inflammatory bowel disease)
- Hematogenous via hepatic artery (infective endocarditis, sepsis)
- Direct extension from adjacent sites (e.g. subphrenic abscess)
- Trauma or post-surgical infections
- Cryptogenic (unknown cause)

Pathogenesis

- Liver abscesses are common in older and immunosuppressed patients.
- Infection can reach the liver in several ways. Commonest route is ascending infection due to biliary obstruction (cholangitis) or direct spread from an empyema of the gallbladder.
- Single abscess is common in the right lobe. Multiple abscesses are usually due to infection secondary to biliary obstruction.
- Common organisms are *E. coli*, streptococci, and Bacteroides. Multiple organisms are present in one-third of patients.

Clinical Features

- Patients appear ill with fever, chills and rigors. There may be weight loss. Liver abscess can present as PUO without any localizing symptoms.
- Abdominal pain is usually present and felt in the right upper quadrant, often radiating to the right shoulder.
- Examination shows tender hepatomegaly. Icterus may be present.

Investigations

- Leukocytosis.
- Bilirubin and alkaline phosphatase are elevated. Serum albumin is often low.
- Blood culture may grow the causative organism.
- Ultrasound or CT abdomen is the most useful investigation and shows 90% or more of symptomatic abscesses.
- Needle aspiration under ultrasound guidance confirms the diagnosis and provides pus for culture.
- Chest X-ray may show a raised right diaphragm and lung collapse or an effusion at the base of the right lung.

Management

- Management involves antibiotic therapy and abscess drainage.
- Pending identification of the organism, empirical antibiotic therapy which covers gram-positive, gram-negative and anaerobes should be started. Combination of third generation cephalosporin such as ceftriaxone (covers gram-positive and gram-negative) and metronidazole (covers anaerobes) can be started. Alternatives are piperacillin-tazobactam or carbapenems (in severe or resistant cases). Antibiotics should be given for at least four to six weeks.
- Needle aspiration or drainage through a catheter is required if the abscess is large (>5 cm) or if it does not respond to antibiotics.
- Surgical drainage is required for chronic persistent abscess.

Complications

- Rupture into peritoneal cavity or pleura.
- Sepsis and septic shock.
- Empyema.
- Hepatic vein or portal vein thrombosis.

Q. Discuss the etiology, clinical features, investigations, and management of amebic liver abscess.

- An amebic liver abscess (ALA) is a focal collection of necrotic liver tissue caused by invasive *Entamoeba histolytica* infection.
- It is the most common extraintestinal manifestation of amebiasis.
- It is more common in men.
- A single abscess is found in the right lobe of the liver in most patients, although multiple abscesses can be present in some.

Etiology

- *Entamoeba histolytica*.

Pathogenesis

- Transmission: Fecal-oral route via ingestion of contaminated food or water.
- Ingested cysts release trophozoites in the intestine.
- Trophozoites invade the colonic mucosa and may enter the portal circulation.
- They travel to the liver, causing necrosis and abscess formation, usually in the right lobe.

Clinical Features

- Fever with chills.
- Abdominal pain in the right upper quadrant.
- Concurrent diarrhea or past history of dysentery may be present.
- Examination shows tender hepatomegaly. Jaundice may be present in some.

Diagnosis

- Leukocytosis.
- Elevated alkaline phosphatase and hepatic transaminases.
- Fecal microscopy may show *Entamoeba histolytica* in some patients.
- Ultrasound abdomen can identify the location, size and number of abscesses.
- CT or MRI are more accurate than ultrasound.
- Serologic testing: Antiamebic antibodies will be positive in most patients with amebic liver abscess.
- Aspiration: This is required if there no response to antibiotic therapy after three to five days, if a cyst appears to be at imminent risk of rupture, or to rule out other diagnoses. Aspiration is done under ultrasound or CT guidance. Amebic liver abscess has "anchovy sauce" appearance (**Fig. 7.13**). Trophozoites may be seen on microscopy of the aspirate.

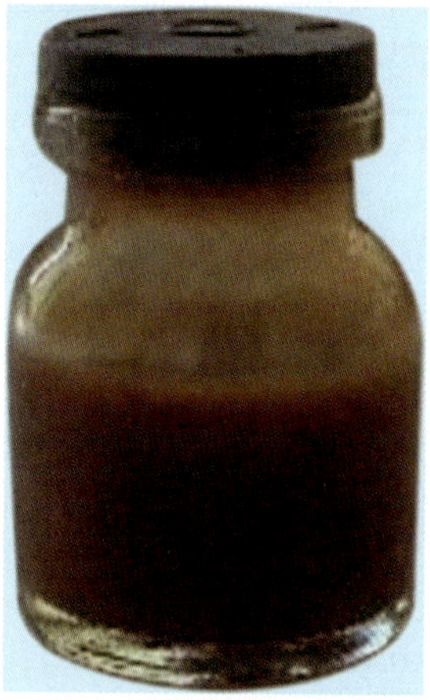

Figure 7.13: Anchovy sauce appearance of liver abscess

Treatment

- Both tissue and luminal agents are used in the treatment of amebic liver abscess.
- The most commonly used tissue agent is metronidazole (500–750 mg orally three times daily for minimum 10 days). Intravenous therapy is not required as it is well absorbed orally. Other alternatives are tinidazole, ornidazole and nitazoxanide. Chloroquine also has amebicidal activity but is rarely used.
- Luminal agents are used to kill intraluminal organisms. These are paromomycin or diloxanide furoate.
- Aspiration may be required if there is no response to medical therapy.

Q. Liver transplantation.

- Liver transplantation is the surgical replacement of a diseased liver with a healthy liver from a donor. It is a lifesaving procedure for patients with end-stage liver disease or acute liver failure.
- The outcome following liver transplantation has improved significantly over the last decade. However, the number of liver transplants is limited by the availability of donors.

Types of Liver Transplantation

Orthotopic Liver Transplantation

- The entire diseased liver is removed and replaced with a whole donor liver in the same anatomical position.

- Donor is typically a brain-dead deceased person.
- Most common type of liver transplantation.

Living Donor Liver Transplantation

- A portion of the liver is donated by a living person (usually a relative). The liver regenerates in both donor and recipient. Often used in countries with a shortage of deceased donors.

Split Liver Transplantation

- A single deceased donor liver is divided into two segments: Larger part (right lobe) for an adult recipient, smaller part (left lobe) for a pediatric recipient.

Indications

- Fulminant hepatic failure
- Metabolic diseases (hemochromatosis, galactosemia)
- Decompensated cirrhosis
- Hepatocellular carcinoma
- Hepatic trauma

Contraindications

- Uncontrolled sepsis
- Extrahepatic malignancy
- Severe cardiopulmonary disease
- Active alcohol or substance abuse
- Advanced age (relative)
- Poor psychosocial support

Procedure

- Liver is obtained either from cadavers or from living donors. Full liver can be transplanted from cadavers. Only a portion of the liver is taken from living donors.
- Patients should be maintained on immunosuppression after transplantation. Less immunosuppression is needed for liver transplantation than for kidney and heart/lung transplantation. Steroids along with tacrolimus or mycophenolate mofetil are used for immunosuppression.

Complications

Early Complications

- Acute rejection.
- Surgical complications (hepatic artery thrombosis, anastomotic biliary strictures).
- Infections (pneumonia, wound infections, CMV hepatitis).

Late Complications

- Recurrence of original disease in the graft
- Complications due to the immunosuppressive therapy such as infections and renal impairment from cyclosporin
- Chronic vascular rejection.

Q. Enumerate the causes of hemochromatosis.

Q. Discuss the etiology, pathology, clinical features, investigations, and management of hereditary (primary) hemochromatosis.

- Hemochromatosis refers to a group of disorders characterized by excessive iron accumulation in the body. Iron is deposited in various organs leading to organ damage.
- It may be hereditary (primary) or secondary.

Causes of Hemochromatosis (iron overload states)

Primary Hemochromatosis (hereditary)

- Caused by genetic mutations affecting iron metabolism (e.g. HFE gene mutations)

Secondary

- Repeated blood transfusion
- Ineffective erythropoeisis (thalassemia, sideroblastic anemia)
- Liver disease
- Dietary iron overload (prolonged oral iron therapy, African iron overload)
- Porphyria cutanea tarda

Hereditary Hemochromatosis

Etiology

- Hereditary hemochromatosis is caused by mutations in the HFE gene or other related genes which cause increased intestinal iron absorption and iron overload. It is inherited as an autosomal recessive disease.

Pathogenesis

- There is increased intestinal iron absorption and progressive iron accumulation in various organs.
- Important organs involved are liver, pancreas, heart, skin, and joints.
- Excess iron is hazardous, because it stimulates reactive oxygen species formation, causing oxidative damage, fibrosis, and organ dysfunction.

Clinical Features

- Males are affected more commonly (90% of patients are male) as iron loss in menstruation and pregnancy protects females.
- Symptomatic disease usually presents in men aged 40 years or over, because it takes many years for iron to accumulate and cause organ damage.
- Many organ systems are involved producing their own clinical manifestations.
- ***Liver involvement***: Hepatomegaly, cirrhosis, hepatocellular carcinoma.
- ***Heart***: Cardiomyopathy, heart failure, conduction defects
- ***Pancreas***: Diabetes mellitus
- ***Joints***: Arthralgia
- ***Skin***: Leaden-gray pigmentation
- ***Testicles:*** Atrophy and impotence
- Skin pigmentation along with diabetes is called 'bronzed diabetes'.

- Hemochromatosis patients are prone to develop hepatocellular ca and other malignancies.

Investigations

- Serum ferritin and iron are increased. TIBC is low.
- MRI of liver/heart can non-invasively quantify iron deposition.
- Liver biopsy: It can confirm the diagnosis. It shows heavy iron deposition and hepatic fibrosis. Iron content of the liver can be measured directly.
- Genetic testing: Mutations involving the HFE gene can be identified. If HFE gene mutation is absent, mutations of other genes should be suspected.

Management

- *Venesection (phlebotomy):* It is the main treatment for hereditary hemochromatosis. It can also be used for secondary hemochromatosis. It is the simplest, cheapest, and most effective way to remove accumulated iron. Weekly removal of 500 ml blood (250 mg iron) is done until the serum iron is normal; this may take 2 years or more. Thereafter, maintenance venesection is continued as required to keep the serum ferritin normal.
- *Chelation therapy:* It is used if phlebotomy is contraindicated (e.g. anemia). Deferoxamine is the drug traditionally used for iron chelation therapy and has to be given subcutaneously. Deferasirox and deferiprone are new agents which can be given orally.
- Diabetes and cirrhosis are treated as per standard guidelines.
- First-degree family members should be screened for hemochromatosis by genetic testing and serum ferritin levels.

Prognosis

- Hemochromatosis patients without cirrhosis have a normal life expectancy. Cirrhosis due to hemochromatosis has better prognosis than other forms of cirrhosis. Development of hepatocellular carcinoma in cirrhotic patients is the main cause of death.

Q. Discuss the etiology, pathology, clinical features, investigations, and management of Wilson disease (hepatolenticular degeneration).

- Wilson disease is a rare autosomal recessive disorder of copper metabolism. Here, total body copper is increased, and excess copper is deposited in various organs causing damage.

Etiology and Pathology

- It is caused by a variety of mutations in the gene ATP7B on chromosome 13. ATP7B gene encodes a copper-transporting ATPase enzyme necessary for incorporation of copper into ceruloplasmin, and excretion of copper into bile. Deficiency of this enzyme leads to copper accumulation in the liver, brain, cornea, and other tissues.
- Normally dietary copper is absorbed from the stomach and proximal small intestine, taken up by the liver, incorporated into ceruloplasmin, and secreted into the blood. Any excess copper is excreted into the bile.
- Cellular damage is due to free copper-induced oxidative stress.

Clinical Features

- Most patients present below the age of 40 years.
- Various organs can get damaged due to excess copper accumulation. Most important organs involved are liver and nervous system.
- Liver disease usually occurs in younger age group. It can manifest in many ways such as acute hepatitis, fulminant liver failure, chronic hepatitis and cirrhosis. Wilson disease should be suspected in any case of recurrent acute or chronic liver disease of unknown cause in a patient under 40 years.
- Neurological damage causes basal ganglion syndromes and dementia. Clinical features include a variety of extrapyramidal features, particularly tremor, chorea, athetosis, dystonia, parkinsonism and dementia.
- Kayser-Fleischer rings are greenish-brown discoloration of the corneal margin usually first seen at the upper margin due to copper deposition in Descemet's membrane. They are best seen by slit lamp examination and disappear with treatment.
- Other manifestations include renal tubular damage and osteoporosis.

Investigations

- Low serum ceruloplasmin and high serum copper level. However, advanced liver failure from any cause can reduce the serum ceruloplasmin, and occasionally it is normal in Wilson disease.
- 24-hour urinary copper excretion: >40 µg/day is highly suggestive of Wilson's disease.
- AST and ALT are usually elevated.
- Kayser-Fleischer rings: Detected by slit-lamp examination.
- Liver biopsy: Copper content is high. There may be fatty infiltration and portal fibrosis.
- MRI brain: May show hyperintensities in basal ganglia, thalamus, midbrain, and pons.
- Genetic testing: This is limited by the presence of multiple mutations.

Management

- Lifelong therapy is required in patients with Wilson's disease and treatment should be given in two phases: removing the tissue copper that has accumulated and then preventing re-accumulation.
- Copper removal is achieved by the administration of potent chelators such as D-penicillamine and trientine. Trientine is preferred because of fewer side effects. Side effects of D-penicillamine include rashes, protein-

losing nephropathy, lupus-like syndrome and bone marrow suppression. Oral zinc is also useful and acts by preventing copper absorption.
- Prevention of reaccumulation during the maintenance phase can be achieved with lower dose of penicillamine or trientine or zinc. Treatment should not be stooped suddenly as it may precipitate liver failure and it should continue even through pregnancy.
- Patients should be advised to avoid copper-rich foods such as liver, kidney, shellfish, nuts, beans, peas, chocolate, and mushrooms.
- First degree relatives should be screened for Wilson disease and treatment should be given to affected individuals, even if they are asymptomatic.
- Liver transplantation is indicated for fulminant hepatic failure and decompensated liver disease that are unresponsive to drug therapy.

Prognosis

- The prognosis is excellent, if treatment is started before there is irreversible damage.

Q. Discuss the etiology, pathology, clinical features, investigations, complications and management of acute cholecystitis.

Etiology

- Acute cholecystitis is an acute inflammation of the gallbladder, usually due to obstruction of the gallbladder neck or cystic duct by a gallstone. Rarely, obstruction may be due to mucus, parasitic worms or a tumor.

Types

- ***Calculous cholecystitis*** (≈90–95%): Caused by gallstone obstruction of the cystic duct.
- ***Acalculous cholecystitis*** (≈5–10%): Occurs without gallstones, often in critically ill patients (trauma, burns, sepsis, TPN).

Risk Factors

- Female sex
- Age >40 years
- Obesity, rapid weight loss
- Pregnancy
- Prolonged fasting
- Total parenteral nutrition (TPN).

Pathology

Calculous Acute Cholecystitis

- Gallstone obstructs the **cystic duct** → bile stasis and increased intraluminal pressure.
- Leads to **chemical irritation** of the gallbladder wall and **inflammation**
- Secondary **bacterial infection** often supervenes (e.g. ***E. coli***, **Klebsiella**, **Enterococcus**, **Bacteroides**). Infection with gas-forming organisms can cause emphysematous cholecystitis in elderly and diabetes patients.
- Mucosal necrosis and wall thickening may occur.
- If untreated, can lead to gangrene or perforation.

Acalculous Cholecystitis

- Usually seen in critically ill or immunocompromised patients
- Due to ischemia, stasis, and infection, not stones

Clinical Features

- Patients complain of abdominal pain in the right upper quadrant or epigastrium. Pain may radiate to the right shoulder or back. Pain is steady and severe.
- There may be nausea, vomiting, and anorexia.
- There is often a history of fatty food ingestion before the onset of pain.
- Examination shows a febrile, sick looking patient with tachycardia and tachypnea.
- There is right hypochondrial tenderness, and occasionally a gallbladder mass is palpable.
- There may be guarding in the right hypochondrial area.
- Murphy's sign: while palpating gallbladder just below the liver edge, patient is asked to take deep inspiration, causing the gallbladder to descend toward the examining fingers. Patients with acute cholecystitis experience increased pain and may have an inspiratory arrest.

Investigations

- Leukocytosis.
- AST, ALT and amylase may be mildly elevated
- Plain X-ray of the abdomen and chest: It may show radiopaque gallstones, and rarely gas in the gallbladder due to emphysematous cholecystitis or gallbladder perforation. Chest X-ray is also useful to rule out right lower lobe pneumonia which can produce referred pain in the right hypochondrium and mimic acute cholecystitis
- Ultrasound abdomen: This is the most useful investigation and detects gallstones and gallbladder thickening due to cholecystitis.
- Cholescintigraphy (also known as HIDA scan: Hepatic iminodiacetic acid scan) is indicated if the diagnosis is not sure even after ultrasonography. It involves IV injection of technetium labeled HIDA, which is selectively taken up by hepatocytes and excreted into bile. If the cystic duct is patent, this agent will enter the gallbladder, leading to its visualization. The test is positive if the gallbladder does not visualize, which is invariably due to cystic duct obstruction, usually from edema associated with acute cholecystitis or an obstructing stone.
- CT scan abdomen: It can easily demonstrate gallbladder wall edema associated with acute cholecystitis. CT is useful when complications of acute cholecystitis (such as emphysematous cholecystitis or gallbladder perforation) are suspected or when other diagnoses are considered.

Complications

- Gangrene
- Perforation
- Cholecystoenteric fistula
- Gallstone ileus
- Emphysematous cholecystitis.

Management

Medical

- Bed rest, analgesics, intravenous hydration.
- Keep the patient NBM (nil by mouth). Nasogastric aspiration through a Ryle's tube is needed if there is persistent vomiting.
- Antibiotics: a cephalosporin (such as cefuroxime) plus metronidazole are given intravenously.

Surgical

- Surgery is required if cholecystitis progresses in spite of medical therapy and when complications such as empyema or perforation develop. Laparoscopic cholecystectomy is the procedure of choice.
- Percutaneous cholecystostomy: For critically ill or non-surgical candidates. Involves ultrasound-guided drainage of the gallbladder.

Q. Acute cholangitis.

- Acute cholangitis is caused by bacterial infection of bile ducts. It is usually due to ascending infection from duodenum.
- The most important predisposing factor for acute cholangitis is biliary obstruction and stasis due to biliary calculi, strictures or tumors. It can also occur after ERCP.
- It is characterized by fever, rigors, jaundice, and abdominal pain. Fever, right upper quadrant pain, and jaundice constitute **Charcot's triad (Fig. 7.14)**. Confusion and hypotension can be there in severe cholangitis.
- Investigations show leukocytosis, elevated ALP, and elevated direct bilirubin. Liver enzymes may be mildly elevated. Blood culture may grow the causative organism. Ultrasound abdomen may detect gall bladder or common bile duct stones.

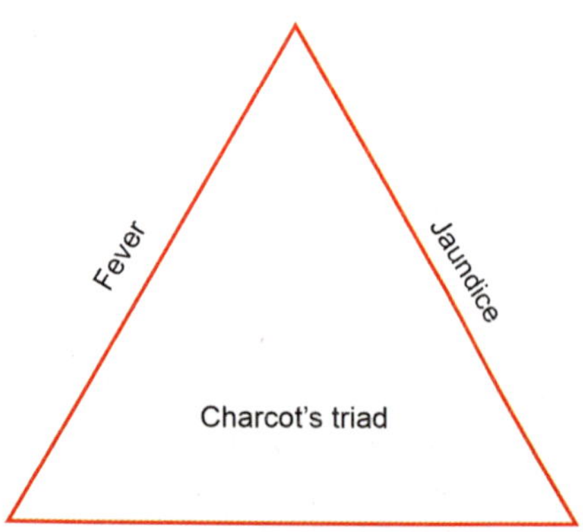

Figure 7.14: Charcot's triad

- Treatment is with antibiotics (metronidazole 500 mg IV every eight hours PLUS a third generation cephalosporin, such as ceftriaxone 1 g IV every 24 hours. Underlying cause should be treated.

Q. Gallstone disease (cholelithiasis).

- Cholelithiasis refers to the formation and presence of stones (gallstones) within the gallbladder **(Fig. 7.15)**. These stones are formed from components of bile and can vary in size and composition.
- Gallstone formation in the gallbladder is a common disorder. Gallstones are the commonest cause of gallbladder disease.

Types of Gallstones

- Gallstones are classified into cholesterol stones, pigment stones, and mixed stones. Mixed stones are the commonest.
- ***Cholesterol stones:*** They are more common in Western countries. Yellow-green in color. Associated with obesity, metabolic syndrome.
- ***Pigment stones:*** More common in developing countries. Black or brown in color. Seen in hemolytic conditions and infection or stasis in the biliary tract.
- Gallstones contain varying quantities of calcium salts, including calcium bilirubinate, carbonate, phosphate and palmitate, which are radiopaque.

Etiology/Risk Factors

- There are many risk factors for development of gallstones. Mainly there are 4 risk factors summarized by the "4 Fs":
  - Female
  - Fat (obesity)
  - Fertile (pregnancy, high estrogen states)
  - Forty (age >40)
- Complete list of risk factors is as follows.

Increased Cholesterol Secretion

- Female gender
- Pregnancy

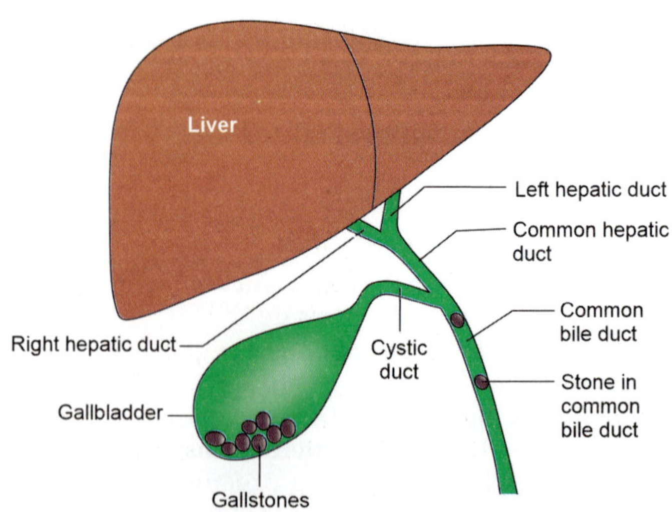

Figure 7.15: Cholelithiasis

Manipal Prep Manual of Medicine

7

- Obesity
- Rapid weight loss

Impaired Gallbladder Emptying

- Pregnancy
- Gallbladder stasis
- Fasting
- Total parenteral nutrition
- Spinal cord injury

Defective Bile Salt Synthesis

- Old age (impaired bile acid synthesis)
- Cirrhosis of liver (impaired bile acid synthesis)

Excessive Intestinal Loss of Bile Salts

- Ileal resection/disease.

Miscellaneous

- Hemolysis (increased bilirubin)
- Infected bile

Pathogenesis

- Cholesterol is held in solution in bile by its association with bile acids and phospholipids in the form of micelles and vesicles. Excess cholesterol, or deficiency of bile acids leads to precipitation of cholesterol and cholesterol stone formation. Similarly excess bilirubin in the bile can precipitate and lead to pigment stone formation.
- 'Biliary sludge' refers to gelatinous bile that contains numerous microspheroliths of calcium bilirubinate granules and cholesterol crystals. It may progress to gallstone formation in many patients.

Clinical Features

- Majority of patients with gallstones are asymptomatic.
- Gallstones can cause epigastric discomfort, fatty food intolerance, dyspepsia and flatulence. Other presentations are biliary colic, acute and chronic cholecystitis.

Complications

- Acute cholecystitis: Inflammation of the gallbladder
- Porcelain gallbladder (due to precipitation of calcium salts in the gallbladder wall).
- Choledocholithiasis
- Cholangitis: Infection of the bile ducts
- Gallstone pancreatitis
- Fistulae between the gallbladder and duodenum or colon
- Cancer of the gallbladder.

Investigations

- Plain X-ray abdomen will show radiopaque gallstones.
- Ultrasonography can demonstrate both radio-opaque and radiolucent gallstones and also other abnormalities.
- Oral cholecystography and CT can also be used.
- Liver function tests (LFTs): May be abnormal if there is biliary obstruction.
- MRCP/ERCP: For evaluating and managing bile duct stones.

Management

- Asymptomatic gallstones usually do not require treatment.
- Symptomatic gallstones are best treated by open or laparoscopic cholecystectomy.
- Endoscopic management: ERCP for common bile duct stones.
- Medical dissolution of gallstones can be achieved by oral administration of the bile acids chenodeoxycholic or ursodeoxycholic acid. Radiolucent gallstones and stones smaller than 15 mm are suitable for medical therapy.

Chapter 8

Diseases of Kidney and Urinary Tract

Q. Describe the structure of a nephron. What are the functions of kidneys?

Structure of a Nephron (Fig. 8.1)

- Nephron is the basic structural and functional unit of the kidney. Each kidney contains ~1 million nephrons.
- Each nephron consists of the glomerulus, proximal convoluted tubule, loop of Henle and distal convoluted tubule. Glomerulus is a tuft of capillaries where blood filtration begins. It receives blood from the afferent arteriole and drains into the efferent arteriole. Bowman's capsule is a double-walled, cup-like structure surrounding the glomerulus. It collects the filtrate from the blood.
- Proximal convoluted tubule (PCT): The first segment after the Bowman's capsule. It reabsorbs water, ions (e.g. Na^+, Cl^-), and nutrients (e.g. glucose, amino acids) back into the blood.
- Loop of Henle: A U-shaped part of the tubule that extends into the medulla. It has:
  - Descending limb: Permeable to water but not to solutes.
  - Ascending limb: Impermeable to water, actively transports salts out.
- Distal convoluted tubule (DCT): Involved in selective reabsorption and secretion of ions, helping in pH and electrolyte balance.
- Collecting duct: Receives filtrate from multiple nephrons; final concentration of urine occurs here under the influence of hormones like ADH (antidiuretic hormone). The collecting ducts of multiple nephrons drain into the renal pelvis and ureter.

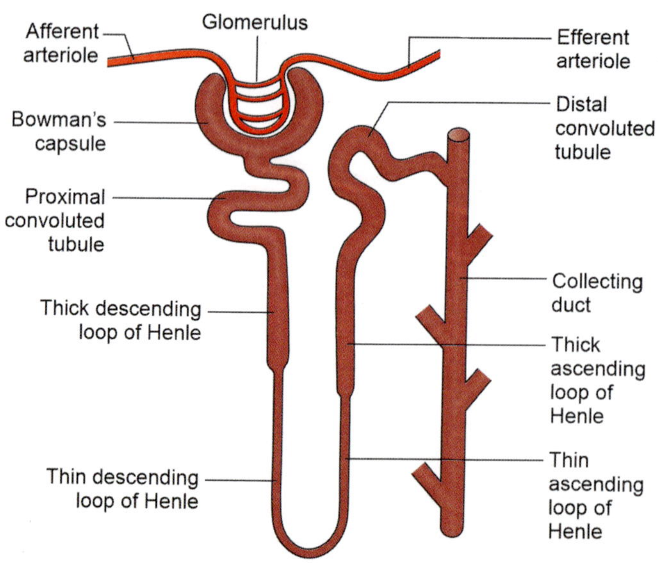

Figure 8.1: Structure of a nephron

Functions of the Kidneys

Homeostasis

- Maintenance of volume and composition of body fluids.
- Maintenance of acid base balance.
- Electrolyte balance.

Excretion of Metabolic Wastes and Toxins

- Excretion of metabolic end products (including ammonia, urea and creatinine from protein, and uric acid from nucleic acids), drugs and toxins.

Endocrine Functions

- Production of erythropoietin, which is important for RBC production.
- Vitamin D metabolism: It hydroxylates 25-hydroxycholecalciferol to 1-25-dihydroxycholecalciferol which is the active form of vitamin-D.
- Secretion of renin from the juxtaglomerular apparatus in response to hypotension and changes in sodium content of fluid in the distal convoluted tubule.

Q. What are the signs and symptoms of kidney and urinary tract disease? How do you approach a suspected case of kidney disease?

- Kidney and urinary tract diseases can present with a wide range of signs and symptoms. These may be local (urinary) or systemic, depending on the cause and stage of the disease. In the initial stages of kidney disease, patients may be asymptomatic.

Common Symptoms

Urinary Symptoms

- Dysuria (painful urination)
- Frequency and urgency
- Hematuria (blood in urine–visible or microscopic)
- Nocturia (frequent urination at night)
- Oliguria (low urine output)
- Anuria (absence of urine output)
- Cloudy or foul-smelling urine.

Systemic Symptoms

- Fatigue and weakness (due to anemia or uremia)
- Edema (swelling, especially around eyes, ankles, and feet)
- Nausea and vomiting (uremic symptoms)
- Loss of appetite
- Hypertension
- Pruritus (itching)
- Confusion or altered mental status (in severe uremia).

Pain

- Flank or lower back pain (suggestive of kidney stones, infections, or obstruction)
- Suprapubic discomfort (bladder involvement).

Approach to a Suspected Case of Kidney Disease

- A structured approach includes history-taking, physical examination, and appropriate investigations.

History

- Fever occurs in urinary tract infection and pyelonephritis.
- Anuria—total absence or <100 ml urine output per day. Suggests renal failure or urinary outflow obstruction.
- Oliguria refers to urine output of less than 500 ml per day. It also suggests renal failure or urinary outflow obstruction.
- Polyuria is urine output exceeding 3 liters per day. It suggests recovering renal failure or some metabolic cause such as hyperglycemia, hypercalcemia, hypokalemia, etc.
- Loin pain suggests pyelonephritis or renal calculi.
- Severe colicky pain radiating from loin to groin suggests ureteric colic due to ureteric calculi.
- Lower limb swelling associated with early morning facial puffiness suggests renal failure or nephrotic syndrome.
- Dysuria, increased frequency, urgency suggest urinary tract infection. Suprapubic pain is seen in cystitis.
- Impaired urinary flow, hesitancy, dribbling of urine, incomplete emptying of bladder suggests bladder outflow obstruction. Urinary retention, incontinence/enuresis suggests sphincter or bladder wall dysfunction.
- Passing red colored urine indicates hematuria which can be seen in glomerulonephritis, ureteric stone, Henoch-Schönlein purpura, renal cell carcinoma, etc.
- Passing turbid and frothy urine suggests proteinuria.
- Passing yellow colored and foul smelling urine suggests urinary tract infection.
- Systemic features (fatigue, nausea, weight loss).
- Past medical history (diabetes, hypertension, recurrent UTI, kidney stones). All these are risk factors for kidney disease.
- Drug history (nephrotoxic drugs like NSAIDs, aminoglycosides).
- Family history of kidney disease (e.g. adult polycystic kidney disease).

Physical Examination

- **Blood pressure:** Hypertension is seen in acute or chronic kidney disease. HTN is a common feature of glomerulonephritis, but it is not a feature of nephrotic syndrome.

General Examination

- Pallor may be seen due to anemia which is due to decreased erythropoietin production in chronic kidney disease.
- JVP may be elevated due to fluid overload state in renal failure.
- Pedal edema and facial puffiness may be seen in nephrotic syndrome and fluid overload due to oliguric or anuric renal failure.
- Petechiae and bleeding tendency may be seen due to platelet dysfunction due to uremia.

Abdomen

- Loin pain tenderness (suggests pyelonephritis).
- Suprapubic tenderness suggests cystitis.
- Abdomen may be distended due to urinary retention.
- Sometimes uremia can present as acute abdomen.

CVS

- Pericardial rub may be seen in uremic pericarditis
- Pericardial effusion is seen in fluid overload state due to renal failure.

RS

- Pulmonary edema and pleural effusion may be seen in cases of acute or chronic renal failure causing fluid overload states.

Nervous System

- Uremia can cause peripheral neuropathy.
- Uremic encephalopathy can occur when there is significant rise in blood urea.
- Electrolyte and fluid imbalances which are common in renal disease can affect nervous system function.

Investigations

- *CBC:* Anemia due to decreased production of erythropoietin.
- *Blood urea and creatinine:* Are elevated in renal disease.

- *Urine analysis:* It can show proteinuria (suggests glomerular disease), hematuria (disease anywhere in the urinary tract), pyuria (seen in glomerulonephritis and UTI), RBC casts (seen in glomerulonephritis). Urine culture if infection is suspected.
- *Urine protein:creatinine ratio or 24-hour protein:* To quantify proteinuria.
- *Serum electrolytes:* Hyponatremia is seen due to fluid overload. Hyperkalemia is common in both acute and chronic renal failure. Hypocalcemia is seen in chronic kidney disease due to reduced synthesis of 1-25-dihydroxycholecalciferol.
- *Other routine tests:* Such as blood sugar, LFT have to be done.
- *Ultrasound abdomen:* It shows any structural abnormalities of kidneys and urinary tract. Size of the kidneys, masses, cysts, stones, etc. can be detected by ultrasound abdomen. Shrunken kidneys are seen chronic kidney disease.
- *CT abdomen:* It can show more details of the findings that are found in ultrasound abdomen. Contrast agent should not be given in renal failure because it is nephrotoxic.
- *Kidney biopsy:* It is required in many types of primary and secondary glomerulonephritis and also in suspected renal cell carcinoma.

Diagnosis of Renal Disease using above Information

- Using the history, clinical examination findings and investigation data, we have to first narrow down the cause of kidney disease into three types: prerenal, intrinsic renal, and postrenal problems **(Table 8.1)**.

TABLE 8.1: Types of renal diseases

	Examples
Prerenal disease	Hypovolemic shock, cardiac failure, hypotension
Intrinsic renal disease	Glomerulonephritis, interstitial nephritis, nephritic syndrome, diabetic nephropathy
Postrenal disease	Renal calculi, prostate hyperplasia, bladder outlet obstruction, urethral stricture

Q. Glomerular filtration rate (GFR).

- Glomerular filtration rate (GFR) is the volume of blood filtered through the kidney per minute. It is expressed in ml/min.
- It is considered the best overall indicator of kidney function. Normal GFR in young, healthy adults is about 90–120 ml/min and declines with age. GFR also decreases due to disease or damage to kidneys.

How GFR is Measured or Estimated

- Measured GFR: The best method for GFR measurement is inulin clearance. Inulin is neither absorbed nor secreted by the renal tubule and therefore it is the ideal for measuring GFR. However, its measurement is cumbersome and therefore it is mostly used in research settings. For this reason, the estimated GFR (eGFR), which represents the best routinely available measurement of kidney function, is usually used.
- Estimated GFR (eGFR) is commonly used in clinical practice and can be calculated by using serum creatinine or cystatin C levels. There are various creatinine and cystatin C based formulas for estimating GFR which can be used bedside. Some of the formulas that are used are chronic kidney disease epidemiology collaboration (CKD-EPI) creatinine equation and modification of diet in renal disease study (MDRD) equation and Cockcroft-Gault formula. Cockcroft-Gault formula is less accurate than CKD-EPI method in estimating GFR.
- The estimated glomerular filtration rate (eGFR) is used to screen for and detect early kidney damage, to help diagnose chronic kidney disease (CKD), and to monitor kidney status.

Clinical Significance of eGFR

- eGFR can be used to diagnose the stage of kidney disease. eGFR of <15 indicates end stage renal disease.
- Many drugs require dose adjustment based on GFR, especially nephrotoxic or renally excreted medications.
- Falling GFR indicates worsening kidney function.
- Dialysis often considered when GFR <15 ml/min/1.73 m² with symptoms.

Q. Define the terms "azotemia, uremia, anuria, oliguria, polyuria, proteinuria and hematuria".

- **Azotemia:** Refers to the biochemical elevation of urea and creatinine in the blood. It is often asymptomatic (lab finding only). It can be due to prerenal, renal and postrenal causes. All types of azotemia are characterized by decrease in GFR.
- **Uremia:** This refers to azotemia plus clinical manifestations of raised urea and creatinine. Uremia is more severe and symptomatic than azotemia.
- **Anuria:** Total absence or <100 ml urine output per day
- **Oliguria:** Urine output of less than 500 ml per day
- **Polyuria:** Urine output exceeding 3 liters per day
- **Proteinuria:** Presence of abnormal amounts of protein in the urine, usually >150 mg/day. Suggests glomerular or tubular damage. Proteinuria of >3.5 g/day indicates nephrotic syndrome (nephrotic-range proteinuria).
- **Hematuria:** Presence of blood (red blood cells) in the urine due to various causes.

Q. Causes of anuria.

Prerenal causes (↓ renal blood flow → ↓ filtration)
- Severe dehydration
- Hypovolemia (e.g. hemorrhage, burns)
- Shock (septic, cardiogenic, hypovolemic)
- Bilateral renal arterial occlusion

Intrinsic (renal) causes (damage to kidney tissue)

- Acute tubular necrosis (ATN)—due to ischemia or toxins
- Severe glomerulonephritis
- Acute cortical necrosis—often irreversible
- Acute interstitial nephritis—commonly drug-induced
- Malignant hypertension
- Hemolytic uremic syndrome (HUS) or thrombotic microangiopathies

Postrenal causes (obstruction of urine outflow)

- Bilateral ureteric obstruction (e.g. tumors, stones)
- Bladder outlet obstruction (e.g. enlarged prostate, urethral stricture)
- Neurogenic bladder (severe)
- Urethral trauma or clot retention

Q. Causes of polyuria.

- Polyuria is defined as excessive urine output, typically >3 liters per day in adults.

- **Osmotic diuresis:** Hyperglycemia, hypercalcemia, administration of mannitol and radiocontrast agents
- **Diabetes insipidus:** Central and nephrogenic diabetes insipidus
- **Excessive intake of water:** Psychogenic polydipsia, hypothalamic disease
- **Renal disorders:** Medullary cystic diseases, resolving ATN or obstruction
- **Drugs:** Diuretics, demeclocycline

Q. Define proteinuria. Enumerate the causes of proteinuria.

- *Proteinuria* is excretion of abnormal amount of protein in the urine.
- Normal protein excretion is less than 150 mg per day. Out of this 150 mg, albumin fraction is less than 30 mg. Albumin excretion between 30 and 300 mg per day is called microalbuminuria. Albumin excretion above 300 mg per day is called macroalbuminuria.
- Nephrotic-range proteinuria: >3.5 g/day.

Causes of Proteinuria

Glomerular proteinuria

- Nephrotic syndrome
- Glomerulonephritis (e.g. IgA nephropathy, lupus nephritis)
- Diabetic nephropathy
- Hypertensive nephrosclerosis
- Preeclampsia

Tubular proteinuria (impaired reabsorption of normally filtered proteins)

- Acute tubular necrosis
- Tubulointerstitial diseases

Overflow proteinuria

- Multiple myeloma

Postrenal causes

- Urinary tract infection (UTI)
- Urinary tract malignancy
- Kidney stones
- Contamination (e.g. vaginal secretions)

Orthostatic proteinuria

- Increase in protein excretion in upright position but normal protein excretion when supine.

Transient proteinuria

- Fever or heavy exercise.

Q. Define hematuria. Enumerate the causes of hematuria. How do you approach a case of hematuria?

- *Hematuria* is defined as ≥3 RBCs per high-power field (HPF). Hematuria may be grossly visible (macroscopic hematuria) or detectable only on urine examination (called microscopic hematuria) **(Fig. 8.2)**.
- Red urine does not always indicate hematuria. Red urine without hematuria is seen in hemoglobinuria, myoglobinuria, beeturia (due to excess beetroot ingestion), rhubarburia, medications (phenazopyridine, methyldopa, senna) and porphyria.

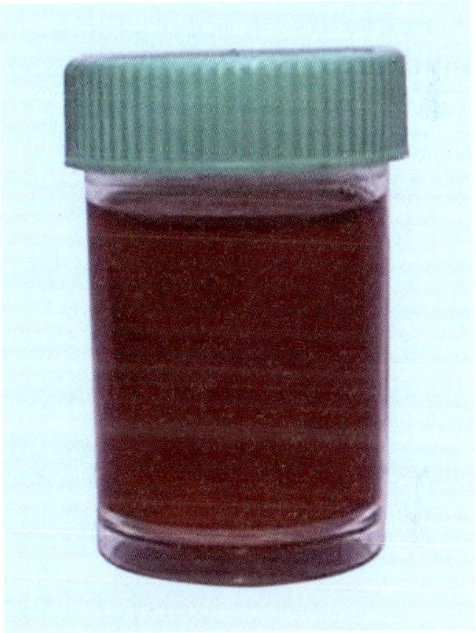

Figure 8.2: Hematuria

Causes of Hematuria

Glomerular causes

- Glomerulonephritis (e.g. IgA nephropathy, post-streptococcal GN)
- Alport's syndrome
- Thin basement membrane disease
- Lupus nephritis
- Vasculitis (e.g. ANCA-associated)

Nonglomerular (postrenal) causes

- Stones
- Cancer of urinary tract (kidney, bladder, prostate)
- Urinary tract infection
- Vigorous exercise
- Sickle cell anemia
- Bleeding disorders
- Trauma
- BPH
- Endometriosis

Approach to a Case of Hematuria

History

- Clues suggesting the site of bleeding.
  - Initial hematuria: Hematuria is seen at the beginning of micturition and later urine becomes clear. Suggests bleeding from urethra.
  - Total hematuria: Blood is present throughout micturition uniformly. Likely source of blood is bladder or above.
  - Terminal hematuria: Hematuria towards the end of micturition. Suggests bleeding from prostate or bladder base.
- Color of urine: Bright red hematuria suggests bleeding from lower urinary tract. Brown or tea-colored suggest glomerular origin (kidneys).
- Concurrent pyuria and dysuria suggest urinary tract infection as a cause of hematuria.
- A recent upper respiratory infection suggests post-infectious glomerulonephritis or IgA nephropathy.
- A positive family history of renal disease suggests hereditary nephritis or polycystic kidney disease, Alport's syndrome, or sickle cell disease.
- Unilateral flank pain, which may radiate to the groin, suggests a stone.
- Presence of hesitancy and dribbling in an old man suggests BPH.
- Recent vigorous exercise or trauma may suggest these as the causes of hematuria.
- History of bleeding from multiple sites suggests a bleeding disorder or excessive anticoagulant therapy.
- Cyclic hematuria in women during menstruation suggests endometriosis of the urinary tract. However, contamination with menstrual blood should be ruled out.
- Painless gross hematuria suggests the possibility of urothelial cancer.
- Drugs: Anticoagulants, cyclophosphamide (hemorrhagic cystitis).

Physical Examination

- *Vitals:* Fever indicates pyelonephritis or UTI. Hypertension indicates glomerulonephritis.
- *General examination*: Pedal edema suggests glomerulonephritis. Presence of joint pain, rash suggests Henoch-Schönlein purpura, connective tissue disease or SLE.
- *CVS*: Presence of a murmur should raise the suspicion of infective endocarditis especially in the presence of fever.
- *RS*: Presence of crepitations and rhonchi can occur in Goodpasture's syndrome.
- *Abdomen*: Look for any mass (cancer, obstruction) and bruit (renal ischemia). Per-rectal examination is done to look for any prostate enlargement.

Lab Tests

- *Urine microscopy*—shows presence of RBCs. The presence of RBC casts suggests bleeding from the kidney most often due to glomerulonephritis. Dysmorphic RBCs (with irregular outer cell membrane) and acanthocytes (RBCs with membrane protrusions representing early form of dysmorphic RBCs) suggest hematuria of glomerular origin. Uniform RBCs or presence of clots suggests nonglomerular hematuria.
- *Urine cytology*—is done if cancer of urinary tract is suspected.
- *Cystoscopy*—is subsequently done if malignant and/or atypical/suspicious cells are identified.
- *Imaging*—includes plain radiograph of KUB region, intravenous pyelography (IVP), retrograde pyelography, ultrasonography, MRI, and CT scan.
- *Renal biopsy*—is required in hematuria of glomerular origin along with the presence of proteinnuria and renal failure.
- *Other tests* that are done are renal function tests, urine for AFB, platelet count, coagulation studies and autoantibodies (ANA, ANCA).

Q. Tamm-Horsfall protein.

Tamm-Horsfall protein, also known as uromodulin, is the most abundant protein excreted in normal human urine. It is secreted by thick ascending limb of loop of Henle. It coats the luminal surface of the cell membrane.

Significance of Tamm-Horsfall Protein

- Tamm-Horsfall protein protects against urinary tract infection by binding to bacteria and viruses, preventing them adhering to uroepithelial cells.
- Inhibits calcium crystal aggregation, thus may reduce stone formation.
- Tamm-Horsfall protein forms the matrix of all urinary casts. The casts may contain only the matrix (hyaline casts) or can include degenerated cells or filtered proteins (granular casts), or intact cells that are present in the tubular fluid (red, white, or epithelial cell casts).
- Tamm-Horsfall protein may coaggregate with light chains in multiple myeloma and cause cast nephropathy, in which dense intratubular casts occlude the flow of urine and cause renal failure.
- Mutations in the gene encoding for Tamm-Horsfall protein cause autosomal dominant tubulointerstitial kidney disease (ADTKD-UMOD), characterized by hyperuricemia, medullary cysts, interstitial nephritis, and progressive renal failure.

Q. Discuss the role of ultrasound in the diagnosis of renal diseases.

- Ultrasound (USG) is a noninvasive, radiation-free, widely available, and cost-effective imaging modality that plays a central role in evaluating renal and urinary tract disorders. Ultrasound is often the first and only method required for renal imaging.
- It can show renal size and position.
- It can identify obstruction in the urinary tract by detecting dilatation of the collecting system.
- It can identify the location and size of renal calculi.
- It can distinguish tumor, abscess and cyst.

- It can show other abdominal, pelvic and retroperitoneal pathology.
- It can image the prostate and bladder, and estimate completeness of emptying in suspected bladder outflow obstruction.
- In chronic renal disease ultrasonographic density of the renal cortex is increased and corticomedullary differentiation is lost.
- Renal biopsy and cyst puncture can be done under ultrasound guidance.
- Doppler ultrasound is used to show blood flow in extrarenal and intrarenal blood vessels.

Q. Discuss the indications, contraindications and complications of kidney biopsy.

- A kidney biopsy involves obtaining a small tissue sample from the kidney (typically via percutaneous needle biopsy) for microscopic examination.
- It is used to establish exact diagnosis, monitor renal diseases, and to judge the prognosis and need for treatment.
- It is done percutaneously under ultrasound guidance.

Indications

It is typically done when noninvasive tests are inconclusive and histologic diagnosis will affect management as given in the following list:

- Unexplained AKI/CKD
- Chronic renal failure with normal-sized kidneys
- Unexplained nephrotic syndrome in adults
- Nephrotic syndrome in children that has atypical features or is not responding to treatment.
- Unexplained nephritic syndrome
- Rapidly progressive GN (suspected crescentic GN, vasculitis)
- Systemic diseases with renal involvement (e.g. SLE, vasculitis, amyloidosis)
- Unexplained hematuria or proteinuria.

Contraindications

- Coagulation abnormalities or thrombocytopenia
- Uncontrolled hypertension
- Small hyperechoic kidneys (indicate chronic irreversible disease)
- Solitary kidney (relative contraindication)
- Hydronephrosis
- Active renal or perirenal infection
- Skin infection over the biopsy site
- Uncooperative patient.

Complications

- Pain at biopsy site
- Hematuria, usually minor but may produce clot colic and obstruction
- Perirenal hematoma
- Arteriovenous fistula
- Injury to adjacent organs (puncture of the liver, pancreas, or spleen).

Q. Define acute kidney injury (acute renal failure). Discuss the causes, clinical features, investigations and management of acute kidney injury.

Definition

- Acute kidney injury (AKI) earlier known as acute renal failure refers to rapid decrease in renal function over hours to days. It results in:
  - Retention of nitrogenous waste (e.g. urea, creatinine),
  - Dysregulation of fluid, electrolyte, and acid-base balance.
- It is usually reversible and accompanied by a reduction in urine volume.

Diagnostic Criteria for AKI

- Increase in serum creatinine by ≥0.3 mg/dl within 48 hours, or
- Increase in serum creatinine to ≥1.5 times baseline, which is known or presumed to have occurred within the prior seven days, or
- Urine volume <0.5 ml/kg/hour for 6 hours.

Causes

Prerenal (due to decreased perfusion of kidneys)

- Volume depletion (hemorrhage, vomiting, diarrhea, pancreatitis, burns)
- Heart failure
- Septic shock
- Hepatorenal syndrome
- Renal artery occlusion/stenosis
- Drugs: ACE inhibitors, NSAIDs

Renal (renal parenchymal damage)

- ***Acute tubular necrosis:*** *Ischemia* (causes are the same as for prerenal ARF, but generally the insult is more severe), *Infection* (acute pyelonephritis), *toxins* (radiocontrast, aminoglycosides, amphotericin etc), hemoglobinuria, myoglobinuria.
- ***Glomerular diseases:*** Acute glomerulonephritis, RPGN.
- ***Acute interstitial nephritis:*** Drugs, infections.
- ***Vascular:*** Vasculitis, malignant hypertension.

Postrenal

Obstruction to urine flow: Stone, tumor, prostate enlargement, urethral stenosis.

Pathogenesis

Glomerular filtration occurs due to the pressure gradient from the glomerulus to the Bowman's space. Glomerular pressure depends on renal blood flow (RBF) and is controlled by the combined resistances of afferent and efferent arterioles. Almost all the causes of AKI cause reduction in renal blood flow which is the common pathologic pathway for decreasing glomerular filtration rate (GFR). The etiology of AKI consists of 3 main mechanisms—prerenal, renal (intrinsic), and postrenal.

- Prerenal causes are the most common cause of acute renal failure. All prerenal causes act through renal hypoperfusion. If hypoperfusion is rapidly reversed, renal parenchymal damage does not occur. If hypoperfusion persists, ischemia can result, causing intrinsic renal failure. ACE inhibitors prevent efferent renal arteriolar constriction out of proportion to the afferent arteriole leading to decrease in GFR. Nonsteroidal anti-inflammatory drugs (NSAIDs) prevent afferent arteriolar vasodilation by inhibiting prostaglandin-mediated signals. Note that NSAIDs can also cause intrinsic renal failure due to acute interstitial nephritis.

- Renal (intrinsic) causes of AKI either damage glomerulus (glomerulonephritis) or tubules (ATN). Myoglobinuria (derived from rhabdomyolysis) and hemoglobinuria (derived from hemolysis) can cause direct damage to tubular cells. Drugs such as NSAIDs, aminoglycosides, contrast agents can cause intrinsic renal failure.
- Postrenal causes are the least common cause of acute renal failure. It occurs when urinary flow from both kidneys, or a single functioning kidney, is obstructed. This leads to elevated intraluminal pressure in the nephron, causing a decrease in GFR. If the obstruction is relieved, this type of renal failure is reversible.

Clinical Features

- Oliguria or anuria may be present. Anuria suggests obstructive cause.
- Signs and symptoms of fluid overload (due to decreased urine output) can occur and include breathlessness, facial and pedal edema, ascites, pleural and pericardial effusions. Pericardial effusions may result in cardiac tamponade.
- Urea accumulation can cause following uremic symptoms/signs:
  - Nausea, vomiting, malaise, and altered sensorium.
  - Neurologic examination may show features of encephalopathy with flapping tremors and confusion. Seizures can occur.
  - Platelet dysfunction can lead to bleeding.
  - Pericardial friction rub can be present.
- In ATN clinical course can be divided into 3 phases—oliguric phase, maintenance phase and diuretic phase.
  - *Oliguric phase:* Characterized by decreased urine output. lasts an average of 10–14 days (can vary from few hours to 4 weeks).
  - *Maintenance phase:* This is characterized by low GFR and low urine output continues during this phase. It may last for days to weeks.
  - *Diuretic phase:* This is characterized by polyuria and is due to defective urine concentrating ability of tubules. Patient may develop dehydration, hyponatremia and hypokalemia during this phase. After diuretic phase kidney function usually recovers.
- Arrhythmias can occur due to electrolyte imbalance such as hyper and hypokalemia.
- The lung examination may show crepitations due to volume overload.
- There may be signs and symptoms of underlying disorder causing renal failure.

Investigations

Complete Blood Count

- Low hemoglobin may be present in prerenal AKI due to hemorrhage. Peripheral blood smear may show schistocytes in conditions such as hemolytic uremic syndrome (HUS) or thrombotic thrombocytopenic purpura (TTP).

Urea and Creatinine

- These are elevated. In prerenal AKI, there is disproportionate elevation of urea in relation to creatinine (urea creatinine ratio is usually >20:1).

Urine Analysis

- Urine is acellular and contains transparent hyaline casts in prerenal AKI.
- Plenty of pus cells in urine suggests UTI as cause of AKI.
- RBC and WBC are present in AKI due to glomerulonephritis. RBC casts **(Fig. 8.3)** indicate glomerular injury or rarely interstitial nephritis.
- WBC casts and nonpigmented granular casts suggest interstitial nephritis, whereas broad granular casts are characteristic of chronic kidney disease and probably reflect interstitial fibrosis and dilatation of tubules.
- Pigmented "muddy brown" granular casts and casts containing tubule epithelial cells are characteristic of ATN. RBC and WBC may also be present in intraluminal obstruction or prostatic disease, but casts are typically absent.
- Eosinophiluria (>5% of urine leukocytes) suggests allergic interstitial nephritis.
- Abundant uric acid crystals suggest acute urate nephropathy.
- Proteinuria of >1 g/d suggests glomerular damage or excretion of myeloma light chains.
- Hemoglobinuria or myoglobinuria should raise the possibility of renal failure due to hemolysis and rhabdomyolyis.

Serum Electrolytes

- Abnormalities include hyperkalemia, hypocalcemia and hyperphosphatemia.

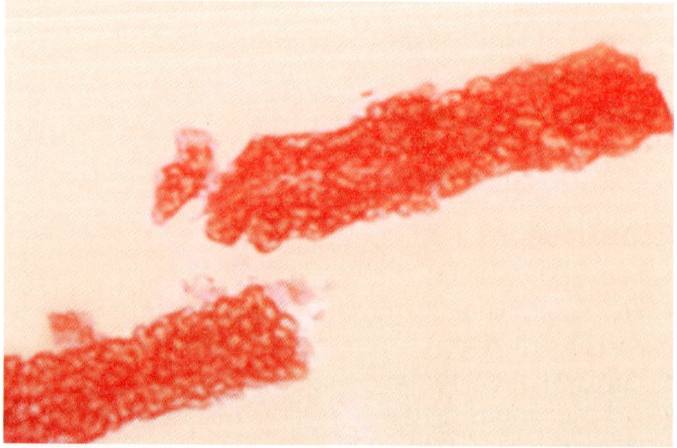

Figure 8.3: RBC casts

ECG

- May reveal changes of hyperkalemia and also any cardiac problems.

Tests to Rule Out Infections

- Antistreptolysin O titer is elevated in post-streptococcal glomerulonephritis.
- Other serology: If clinically suspected, e.g. hepatitis-B, hepatitis-C, leptospirosis, Hantavirus. All these diseases can involve kidneys.

Autoimmune Workup

- If diagnosis is not clear from above investigations consider ANA, ANCA, complement levels, etc. to rule out connective tissue disorder.

Renal Ultrasound and Renal Doppler

- This is done urgently if renal failure due to obstruction is suspected. *Renal Doppler* can identify patency of renal arteries and veins.

Chest X-ray

- May show evidence of pulmonary edema.

Kidney Biopsy

- Kidney biopsy is indicated when renal function does not return for a prolonged period and a prognosis is required to develop long-term management.

Management

- Correct the underlying cause of the AKI.
- Treat fluid and electrolyte abnormalities. Loop diuretics such as frusemide or torsemide can be used if there is fluid overload. On the other hand, fluids should be given if there is hypovolemia causing renal failure. Hyperkalemia should be corrected by anti-hyperkalemia measures such as salbutamol nebulization, potassium binding resins, etc.
- Correct metabolic acidosis with oral or IV bicarbonate
- Nephrotoxic drugs such as NSAIDs, aminoglycosides etc should be avoided.
- Restriction of water (unless there is hypovolemia), Na, phosphate, and K intake, but provision of adequate protein.
- Hemodialysis is required for the following if conservative measures fail.

Indications for Hemodialysis

- Urea >180 mg/dl and creatinine >8 mg/dl
- Refractory fluid overload with pulmonary edema
- Resistant hyperkalemia
- Severe metabolic acidosis (pH <7.1)
- Signs of uremia, such as pericarditis, neuropathy, or altered mental status.

Q. Fractional excretion of sodium (FeNa).

Fractional excretion of sodium (FeNa) is a clinical calculation used primarily to help differentiate between prerenal and intrinsic renal causes of acute kidney injury (AKI).

Formula

$$\text{FeNa} = \frac{\text{Urine Na} \times \text{plasma creatinine (mg/dl)}}{\text{Plasma Na} \times \text{Urine creatinine (mg/dl)}} \times 100$$

Interpretation (Table 8.2)

TABLE 8.2: FeNa interpretation

FeNa (%)	Interpretation	Likely cause
<1%	Kidneys are conserving sodium	Prerenal AKI (e.g. hypovolemia, CHF)
>2%	Kidneys are not conserving sodium	Intrinsic AKI (e.g. acute tubular necrosis)
1–2%	Indeterminate	May require further evaluation

Limitations

- FeNa may be falsely low in early ATN.
- It may not be reliable if the patient is on diuretics, which increase sodium excretion. In such cases, Fractional Excretion of Urea (FeUrea) may be more reliable.

Q. Define chronic kidney disease (CKD) and its stages. Discuss the causes, clinical features, investigations and management of CKD.

- *Chronic kidney disease (CKD)* (earlier known as chronic renal failure) is defined as presence of kidney damage or decreased kidney function for three or more months, irrespective of the cause.
- CKD can be divided into following stages **(Table 8.3)**.

TABLE 8.3: Stages of CKD

Stage 1	Kidney damage with normal or increased GFR (>90 ml/min/1.73 m^2)
Stage 2	Mild ↓ in GFR (60–89 ml/min/1.73 m^2)
Stage 3a	Mild to moderate ↓ in GFR (45–59 ml/min/1.73 m^2)
Stage 3b	Moderate to severe ↓ in GFR (30–44 ml/min/1.73 m^2)
Stage 4	Severe ↓ in GFR (15–29 ml/min/1.73 m^2)
Stage 5	Kidney failure (GFR <15 ml/min/1.73 m^2 or dialysis)

- CKD stage 1 and 2 cannot be diagnosed based on GFR alone as GFR can be normal in these stages. Stage 5 CKD is also known as end-stage renal disease (ESRD).

Etiology of CKD

Primary glomerular diseases

- Focal and segmental glomerulosclerosis (FSGN)
- Membranoproliferative glomerulonephritis (MPGN)
- IgA nephropathy
- Membranous nephropathy

Secondary glomerular diseases

- Diabetic nephropathy
- Hypertension
- Amyloidosis
- Postinfectious glomerulonephritis

- HIV-associated nephropathy
- Collagen-vascular diseases
- Sickle cell nephropathy

Tubulointerstitial nephritis
- Drugs
- Heavy metals
- Analgesic nephropathy
- Reflux/chronic pyelonephritis
- Idiopathic

Obstructive nephropathies
- Prostate enlargement
- Calculus
- Retroperitoneal fibrosis
- Tumor

Vascular diseases
- Renal artery stenosis
- Vasculitis

Hereditary diseases
- Polycystic kidney disease
- Medullary cystic disease
- Alport's syndrome

Clinical Features

- CKD is often asymptomatic in early stages and becomes symptomatic as GFR declines.
- Clinical features result from:
  - Accumulation of nitrogenous waste products (uremia)
  - Fluid and electrolyte imbalances
  - Hormonal and metabolic disturbances
  - Complications in multiple organ systems.

General and Constitutional Symptoms

- Fatigue, weakness (due to anemia, uremia)
- Loss of appetite, nausea, vomiting (due to uremia)
- Pruritus (itching)—due to uremia or high phosphate
- Sleep disturbances, restless legs
- Metallic taste in mouth (dysgeusia)
- Uremic breath (ammonia-like odor)
- Growth failure is common in childhood CKD, and is multifactorial. It is due to metabolic acidosis, decreased caloric intake, renal osteodystrophy, and alterations in growth hormone metabolism.

Fluid and Electrolyte Imbalance

- In most patients with stable CKD, there is retention of sodium and water leading to fluid overload. Fluid overload manifests as facial puffiness, peripheral edema, ascites, pleural and pericardial effusions. It contributes to development of hypertension also. Rarely hyponatremia is seen (dilutional hyponatremia), and responds to water restriction.
- Hyperkalemia is seen in CKD, as potassium excretion is impaired. Rarely hypokalemia is seen as a result of renal potassium wasting in diseases such as Fanconi's syndrome, renal tubular acidosis, or other forms of hereditary or acquired tubulointerstitial disease. However, even in these conditions, as the GFR declines, hyperkalemia becomes common.

Acid-base Disturbance

- Metabolic acidosis is common due to inability to excrete acid load due to less ammonia formation in the kidneys. In severe metabolic acidosis, patient may have deep respiration (Kussmaul's respiration), anorexia, nausea, vomiting, hiccoughs, pruritus, muscular twitching, fits, drowsiness and coma.

Cardiovascular System

- Hypertension: Common and both cause and consequence of CKD.
- Heart failure due to fluid overload and hypertension.
- Uremic pericarditis (in late stages).
- Atherosclerosis: Abnormal lipid metabolism is common in CKD. Typically, triglyceride and cholesterol levels are increased and add to the risk for cardiovascular disease.
- Arrhythmias: Due to electrolyte disturbances (especially hyperkalemia).

Respiratory System

- Dyspnea: From fluid overload or metabolic acidosis
- Pulmonary edema
- Kussmaul respiration: Deep, labored breathing due to acidosis (in advanced CKD)
- Pleural effusion.

Hematologic System

- Anemia: Normocytic, normochromic due to ↓ erythropoietin (EPO).
- Platelet dysfunction: ↑ Bleeding tendency (epistaxis, ecchymosis).
- Leukocyte dysfunction: Impaired immunity → ↑ infection risk.

Musculoskeletal System

- Renal osteodystrophy: Kidney is the site of formation of 1-25-dihydroxycholecalciferol (active vitamin D). Diminished active vitamin D formation in CKD leads to hypocalcemia and hyperphosphatemia (due to phosphate retention). Hypocalcemia and hyperphosphatemia stimulate PTH production. Increased PTH (hyperparathyroidism) stimulates bone turnover and leads to osteitis fibrosa cystica characterized by marrow fibrosis and bone cysts, bone pain, and fractures.
- Osteomalacia due to vitamin D deficiency.
- Muscle weakness and cramps due to hypocalcemia, and electrolyte imbalance.

Nervous System

- Peripheral neuropathy due to uremia.
- Cognitive dysfunction, confusion, asterixis (flapping tremor) in uremic encephalopathy
- Seizures, coma (late stages).

Dermatologic Features

- Pruritus (often severe)
- Dry, flaky skin
- Hyperpigmentation (due to retained urochromes)
- Uremic frost (rare, white crystals of urea on skin in ESRD)

Gastrointestinal System (all manifestations due to uremia)

- Nausea, vomiting
- Anorexia, weight loss
- Gastritis, GI bleeding
- Hiccups.

Endocrine and Reproductive Systems

- Secondary hyperparathyroidism due to hypocalcemia → bone disease (osteitis fibrosa cystica).
- Infertility, decreased libido
- Amenorrhea, erectile dysfunction
- Insulin resistance.

Uremia

- Uremia refers to a constellation of signs and symptoms seen in renal failure. Manifestations of the uremic state include anorexia, nausea, vomiting, growth retardation, peripheral neuropathy, and CNS features such as altered sensorium, seizures, and coma.
- Bleeding may occur due to abnormal platelet adhesion and aggregation due to uremia.
- Pericarditis and pericardial effusion also occur in uremia and is an indication for dialysis.

Investigations

Blood Investigations

- Urea and creatinine are elevated. The level of serum creatinine correlates with the degree of renal impairment.
- Serum electrolytes: hyperkalemia, hypocalcemia, and hyperphosphatemia are seen. Bicarbonate levels are reduced.
- Anemia is seen which is usually normocytic normochromic.
- Hepatitis-B, C and HIV serology if dialysis is needed (vaccination against hepatitis B if no previous infection; isolation of dialysis machine if positive)
- ANA if connective tissue disease is suspected.
- ANCA if vasculitis is suspected.
- Anti-GBM antibodies if Goodpasture's syndrome is suspected.
- Complement levels (C3, C4): Low in lupus, MPGN, post-infectious GN.
- Serum protein electrophoresis if multiple myeloma involving kidney is suspected (light chain nephropathy). It may show M band.

Urine Analysis

- Shows fixed specific gravity of around 1.010 (isosthenuria, because of loss of urine concentrating ability of kidneys) and presence of broad casts.
- WBCs are present in the urine in UTI, papillary necrosis, BPH and renal tuberculosis.
- Eosinophils are present in allergic tubulointerstitial disease.
- RBC casts are seen in glomerulonephritis.
- Urine protein:creatinine ratio (UPCR) quantifies proteinuria in spot sample. 24-hour urine protein is alternative for measuring proteinuria.

Imaging Studies

- Chest X-ray: May show pulmonary edema and pericardial effusion.
- ECG: May show signs of hyperkalemia or cardiac disease.
- Renal artery Doppler: If renal artery stenosis is suspected.
- Ultrasound abdomen: usually shows bilateral small sized kidneys (in advanced stages). Ultrasound can also rule out obstruction, polycystic kidney disease, etc.
- CT/MRI: If needed for further structural evaluation, polycystic kidney, or masses.

Kidney Biopsy

- To establish the diagnosis in selected cases when the cause of CKD is not clear.

Management

Management of CKD involves the following issues:

- Treatment of underlying cause of CKD.
- Preventing or slowing the progression of CKD.
- Treatment of complications of renal failure.
- Renal replacement therapy if needed.

Treatment of Underlying Cause

- Identify the underlying cause of renal failure and institute treatment for that. For example, control of diabetes, hypertension, immunosuppression in glomerulonephritis, etc.
- Some underlying causes for CKD are as follows.

- Hypertension
- Renal artery stenosis
- Cardiac failure
- Urinary tract obstruction
- Urinary tract infection
- Systemic infections
- Nephrotoxic drugs
- Autoimmune diseases like SLE

Slowing the Progression of CKD

- Treatment of the underlying cause itself slows down CKD progression.
- ACE inhibitors have been shown to slow the progression of CKD in diabetics. ACE inhibitors should be used, where tolerated. Monitor creatinine and potassium after starting on ACE inhibitors as there can be worsening of GFR and hyperkalemia. Angiotensin II receptor antagonists also have similar effect.

- Restriction of dietary protein intake also delays the progression of CKD.
- Avoid nephrotoxic drugs (NSAIDs, aminoglycosides, contrast agents).

Treatment of the Complications of Renal Failure

- *Anemia:* Recombinant human erythropoietin is effective in correcting the anemia of CKD. Severe anemia should be corrected by blood transfusion.
- *Volume overload:* should be treated by a combination of dietary sodium restriction and diuretic therapy, usually with a loop diuretic given daily.
- *Hyperkalemia*
    - Avoid potassium rich foods such as coconut water, fruit juices, etc.
    - Loop diuretics such as frusemide to increase urinary potassium losses.
    - Potassium binding agents (Kayexalate 5 grams with each meal).
    - Salbutamol nebulizations.
    - 50% dextrose 100 ml with 10 units of insulin infusion 8th hourly. This will push the potassium into the cells and decreases serum potassium.
    - Bicarbonate infusion or orally will also decrease potassium.
- *Metabolic acidosis:* Sodium bicarbonate (in a daily dose of 0.5–1 mEq/kg per day) should be given to maintain serum bicarbonate concentration above 22 mEq/L. Sodium citrate may be used in patients unable to tolerate sodium bicarbonate.
- *Hyperphosphatemia:* This is treated by oral phosphate binders to maintain serum phosphorus levels less than 5 mg/dl. Calcium carbonate or calcium acetate can be used as phosphate binders, but have the risk of causing hypercalcemia. The nonabsorbable agent sevelamer is a cationic polymer that binds phosphate through ion exchange. Sevelamer controls the serum phosphate concentration without inducing hypercalcemia.
- *Renal osteodystrophy:* This is treated by calcitriol (1, 25-dihydroxyvitamin D) and control of phosphate levels.
- *Hypertension:* is controlled by a combination of antihypertensives and diuretics. ACE inhibitors or angiotensin II receptor blocker can be used initially if creatinine is not high. Other antihypertensives are calcium channel blockers, clonidine, beta blockers and alpha blockers.
- *Abnormal lipids:* Hypercholesterolemia is almost universal in patients with significant proteinuria, and increased triglyceride levels are also common in patients with CKD. This can be controlled with HMG-CoA reductase inhibitors (e.g. atorvastatin, rosuvastatin).
- *Bleeding*: It is due to abnormal platelet function. Dialysis can partially correct the bleeding tendency.

Renal Replacement Therapy

- If conservative measures are inadequate, hemodialysis must be planned.
- Renal transplantation can be considered in suitable patients.

Q. Distinguishing acute kidney injury (AKI) from chronic kidney disease (CKD) (Table 8.4).

TABLE 8.4: Distinguishing acute kidney injury (AKI) from chronic kidney disease (CKD)

Feature	AKI	CKD
Onset	Over hours to days	Over months to years. Persists for 3 months or more
Duration	<3 months	≥3 months
Reversibility	Usually reversible	Often irreversible and progressive
Common cause	Usually prerenal or postrenal	Usually intrinsic renal
Past history of kidney disease	Usually absent	Usually present
Urine volume	Often oliguria or anuria	May have polyuria or nocturia due to concentrating defect (except in advanced stages)
Kidney size on ultrasound	Usually normal size	Small size with loss of corticomedullary differentiation
Dialysis	Required for short period	Required repeatedly
Renal transplantation	Not required	Required
Eye–band keratopathy	Absent	Seen in CKD
Broad waxy casts in urine	Absent	Usually present
Presence of anemia	Absent	Present
Hypocalcemia	Absent	Present
Parathyroid hormone (PTH)	Normal (unless prolonged)	Elevated (secondary hyperparathyroidism due to hypocalcemia)
Urine specific gravity	High	Low or fixed
Renal osteodystrophy	Absent	Present
Peripheral neuropathy	Absent	May be present

Q. Enumerate the causes of CKD with normal or enlarged kidneys.

Usually, CKD is associated with bilateral small contracted kidneys due to chronic scarring. However, some important causes of CKD may present with normal-sized or enlarged kidneys, especially early in the disease course. These are as follows:

- Diabetic nephropathy
- Polycystic kidney disease
- Myeloma

- Rapidly progressive glomerulonephritis
- Infiltrative diseases (lymphoma, leukemia, sarcoidosis)
- Amyloidosis
- HIV-associated nephropathy
- Obstruction.

Q. Renal diet.

- Patients with kidney disease need to modify their diet because their kidneys have limited ability to excrete sodium, potassium, phosphorus, and excess fluid. In addition high protein intake leads to formation of more nitrogenous waste products which accumulate in the body due to kidney disease. Diet should be low in sodium, potassium, phosphorous, and protein. Hence, following modifications in the diet should be done.
- Limit total sodium content to <2,000 mg/day (~<5 g salt/day). Avoid processed, canned, salty foods.
- All fruits are rich in potassium especially bananas. Coconut water and ragi is also rich in potassium. Hence intake of fruits, ragi, and coconut water should be limited to prevent hyperkalemia.
- Intake of phosphorous rich foods such as meat, cheese, canned fish should be limited.
- Protein rich foods include almost all the non-vegetarian foods and should be limited in quantity.
- Calories intake of 30–35 kcal/kg/day to maintain weight and prevent catabolism.
- Fluid intake should be restricted only if oliguria/anuria or fluid overload present.

Q. Describe the pathophysiology, clinical findings, and management of uremia.

- The literal meaning of uremia is "urine in the blood". Uremia is a clinical syndrome resulting from the accumulation of urea and other nitrogenous waste products due to advanced renal failure (typically GFR <10–15 ml/min/1.73 m²). It reflects end-stage kidney dysfunction and affects multiple organ systems.

Etiology

- CKD due to any reason
- Acute kidney injury.

Pathophysiology

- Kidney failure leads to disturbances of acid-base homeostasis, fluid and electrolyte regulation, hormone production and secretion, and waste elimination. All these abnormalities can result in metabolic disturbances and also lead to anemia, hypothyroidism, hypertension, acidemia, hyperkalemia, and malnutrition.
- Anemia in kidney disease is usually due to decreased erythropoietin production by the failing kidneys. Other factors contributing to anemia are iron or vitamin deficiencies, hyperparathyroidism, hypothyroidism, and decreased lifespan of RBCs.
- The buildup of uremic toxins in the blood may lead to platelet dysfunction and development of coagulopathy.
- Metabolic acidosis is a major complication associated with uremia and ESRD because renal tubular cells are the primary regulators of acid-base balance. As kidney failure progresses, there is decreased secretion of hydrogen ions and impaired excretion of ammonium, and eventually buildup of phosphate and additional organic acids (e.g. lactic acid, sulfuric acid, hippuric acid). This increased anion-gap metabolic acidosis leads to hyperventilation, lethargy, anorexia, muscle weakness, and congestive heart failure (due to a decreased cardiac response).
- Hyperkalemia may also occur in the setting of both acute or chronic renal failure. This condition becomes a medical emergency when serum potassium reaches a level greater than 6.5 mEq/L. This level may be exacerbated with excessive potassium intake or use of certain medications (e.g. potassium-sparing diuretics, angiotensin-converting enzymes (ACE) inhibitors, angiotensin-receptor blockers, beta blockers, NSAIDs). Acidosis resulting from renal failure may additionally contribute to the development of hyperkalemia.
- Hypocalcemia, hyperphosphatemia, and elevated parathyroid hormone levels may additionally occur as a result of renal failure. Hypocalcemia occurs due to decreased production of active vitamin D (1,25 dihydroxyvitamin D) which is responsible for gastrointestinal (GI) absorption of calcium and phosphorus and suppression of parathyroid hormone excretion. Hyperphosphatemia occurs because of impaired phosphate excretion in the setting of renal failure. Both hypocalcemia and hyperphosphatemia stimulate hypertrophy of the parathyroid gland and resultant increased production and secretion of parathyroid hormone. Altogether, these changes in calcium metabolism can result in osteodystrophy (renal bone disease) and may lead to calcium deposition throughout the body (i.e. metastatic calcification).
- Declining renal function can result in decreased insulin clearance, necessitating a decrease in dosage of antihyperglycemic medications to avoid hypoglycemia. Uremia may also lead to impotence in men or infertility (e.g. anovulation, amenorrhea) in women as a result of dysfunctional reproductive hormone regulation.
- The buildup of uremic toxins may also contribute to uremic pericarditis, and pericardial effusions leading to abnormalities in cardiac function. Together with metastatic calcification as a result of declining renal function, these may contribute to worsening of underlying valvular dysfunction or suppression of myocardial contractility.

Clinical Features of Uremia

- Symptomatic uremia tends to occur once creatinine clearance decreases below 10 ml/min unless kidney failure develops acutely, in which case, some patients may become symptomatic at higher clearance rates.

- Uremic fetor, ammonia or urine-like odor of the breath may occur in uremic patients.
- Gastrointestinal disturbances include anorexia, nausea, vomiting, and gastrointestinal bleeding.
- Fluid overload leads to facial puffiness, pedal edema, ascites, pleural and pericardial effusion. Pulmonary edema and pleural effusion may cause breathlessness.
- Fatigue is common and is usually due to anemia, fluid and electrolyte disturbances.
- Neuromuscular disturbances are insomnia, flapping tremors, myoclonus, restless leg syndrome, peripheral neuropathy, seizures and coma.
- Fatigue as a result of anemia is considered one of the major components of the uremic syndrome.
- Cardiovascular abnormalities are hypertension, atherosclerosis, valvular stenosis and insufficiency, chronic heart failure, and angina may all develop as a result of a buildup of uremic toxins and metastatic calcification associated with uremia and ESRD.
- Bleeding manifestations may occur due to platelet dysfunction.

Investigations

- Complete hemogram
- Urea, creatinine
- Serum sodium, potassium, calcium, phosphate, parathyroid hormone, albumin, and bicarbonate level
- Urine analysis
- ECG
- Renal ultrasound
- CT brain if patient presents with altered mental status to rule out intracranial pathology such as hemorrhage
- Other investigations based on clinical assessment.

Treatment

- Correct electrolyte imbalances: Treat hyperkalemia (calcium gluconate, insulin, glucose, diuretics, dialysis).
- Control acidosis: Sodium bicarbonate (oral or IV).
- Manage volume overload: Diuretics (if responsive), fluid restriction.
- Dialysis is indicated in severe or symptomatic uremia (e.g. nausea, vomiting, hyperkalemia, metabolic acidosis).
- Renal transplantation may be considered for all patients with CKD.

Q. Describe the pathophysiology, laboratory diagnosis and treatment anemia in CKD.

- Anemia is common in CKD. It starts when GFR drops to below 60. Anemia is rare when the GFR is above 80. As the GFR worsens, the anemia gets more severe.

Causes of Anemia in CKD

- Decreased erythropoietin (EPO) production (main cause of anemia in CKD).
- Iron deficiency: Due to poor dietary intake, blood loss (e.g. hemodialysis), and reduced iron absorption.
- Shortened RBC survival: Uremic toxins shorten RBC survival.
- Vitamin B_{12} and folic acid deficiency: Due to malnutrition in CKD.
- Bone marrow suppression due to uremic toxins.
- Chronic inflammation: Increases hepcidin, blocking iron release and absorption (functional iron deficiency).

Clinical Features

- Clinical features are similar to other causes of anemia.

Investigations

- CBC: Hb is low, MCV normal
- Peripheral blood smear: Normocytic normochromic anemia
- Iron indices (iron, ferritin, TIBC, transferrin saturation)
- Vitamin B_{12} and folate levels
- Serum EPO: Inappropriately low for the degree of anemia.

Treatment

- Treatment is considered when hemoglobin is less than 10 g/dl. In all patients with CKD, the goal of hemoglobin is less than 11.5 g/dl because higher values have shown higher cardiovascular mortality.
- Erythropoietin stimulating agents (ESAs) together with iron supplementation is the treatment of choice in anemia of CKD.
- Recombinant human erythropoietin and darbepoetin alfa are the two ESAs generally used in the management of anemia in CKD. Darbepoetin alfa has longer half-life and allows less frequent dosing.
- Iron supplementation is also very important in CKD. Due to decreased absorption of oral iron, intravenous iron is preferable in hemodialysis patients.

Q. Renal osteodystrophy [CKD-mineral and bone disorder (CKD-MBD)].

- Renal osteodystrophy is a part of the broader term CKD–Mineral and bone disorder (CKD–MBD). It refers specifically to the skeletal complications of chronic kidney disease, while CKD–MBD includes abnormalities of bone, mineral metabolism, and vascular calcification.
- Renal osteodystrophy consists of a mixture of osteomalacia, osteitis fibrosa cystica (due to secondary hyperparathyroidism), osteoporosis and osteosclerosis.

Pathogenesis

- CKD (usually stage 3 or later) leads to diminished conversion of cholecalciferol to its active metabolite, 1-25-dihydroxycholecalciferol in the kidneys. In addition, CKD also leads to increased phosphate level in the blood. Diminished 1-25-dihydroxycholecalciferol leads to hypocalcemia.
- Both hypocalcemia and hyperphosphatemia stimulate parathyroid glands which lead to secondary hyperparathyroidism. Another factor contributing to

hyperparathyroidism in CKD is decreased fibroblast growth factor 23. FGF-23 is responsible for decreasing phosphate levels in the body, and a decrease in FGF-23 can lead to secondary hyperparathyroidism.

- Secondary hyperparathyroidism leads to bone resorption leading to osteitis fibrosa cystica. Osteomalacia is another consequence due to vitamin-D deficiency.
- Vascular calcification especially of coronary arteries is another important feature of CKD-MBD which has been ignored earlier. This can lead to acute coronary events contributing to increased mortality in CKD patients.

Clinical Features

- Can be asymptomatic.
- If symptomatic, signs and symptoms include bone pain, muscle weakness, joint pain, bone deformation and bone fracture.
- Growth retardation in children.
- Calciphylaxis (painful skin necrosis due to vascular calcification).
- Vascular calcification (contributing to cardiovascular morbidity).

Investigations

- Blood tests will show decreased calcium and calcitriol (vitamin D_3) and increased phosphate and parathyroid hormone.
- X-rays will show chondrocalcinosis at the knees and pubic symphysis, osteopenia, osteitis fibrosa cystica **(Fig. 8.4)** and bone fractures.

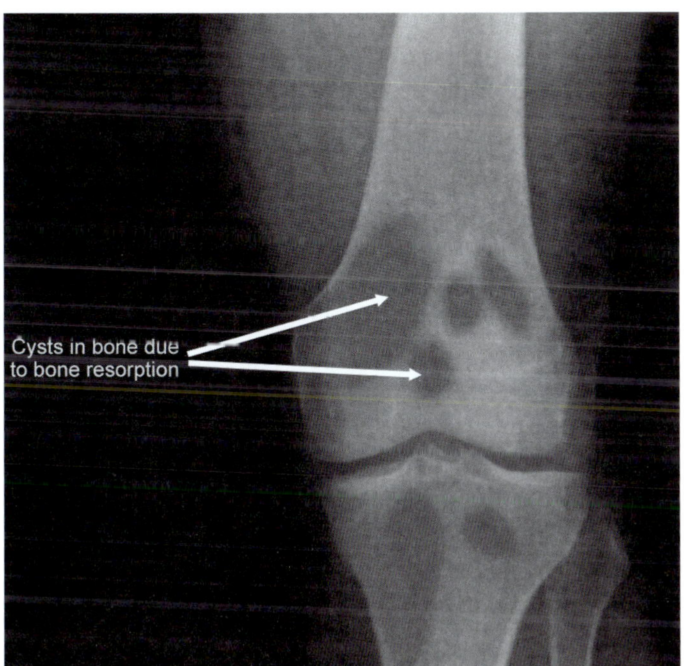

Figure 8.4: Osteitis fibrosa cystica

Management

- Serum calcium and phosphate levels should be kept as near to normal as possible. Hypocalcemia is corrected by giving calcium supplements and active vitamin D_3. Hyperphosphatemia is controlled by avoiding phosphate rich foods (milk, cheese, eggs) and by giving phosphate-binding drugs with food.
- Parathyroidectomy may be needed in severe bone disease with autonomous parathyroid function.
- Regular hemodialysis improves the prognosis of these patients. Kidney transplantation has been shown to reverse the disease process.

Q. Discuss the etiology, clinical features, investigations and management of nephrotic syndrome.

- Nephrotic syndrome is defined as proteinuria of more than 3.5 g/day due to a glomerular disorder accompanied by hypoalbuminemia and edema.

Etiology

Idiopathic or primary nephrotic syndrome

- Minimal change disease
- Focal segmental glomerulosclerosis (FSGS)
- Membranous nephropathy
- Membranoproliferative glomerulonephritis (MPGN)

Secondary nephrotic syndrome

- Diabetes mellitus
- SLE and other collagen diseases
- Amyloidosis
- Vasculitis (Wegener's granulomatosis, Goodpasture's syndrome, etc.)
- Infections (post-streptococcal, hepatitis B, hepatitis C, HIV infection, filariasis)
- Drugs (penicillamine, NSAIDs, lithium, street heroin)
- Malignancy (Hodgkin's lymphoma, leukemia)

Pathophysiology

- Nephrotic syndrome is characterized by proteinuria, hypoalbuminemia and peripheral edema.
- ***Proteinuria*** occurs because of damage to glomerular capillary endothelial cells, the glomerular basement membrane (GBM), or podocytes, which normally filter serum protein selectively by size and charge.
- ***Hypoalbuminemia*** is due to urinary protein loss. Catabolism of filtered albumin by the proximal tubule as well as redistribution of albumin within the body also contribute to hypoalbuminemia.
- ***Edema formation*** is due to salt and water retention which can be explained by two different mechanisms. First mechanism is low plasma oncotic pressure due to hypoalbuminemia which in turn is due to heavy proteinuria. Low-plasma oncotic pressure leads to fluid leakage from the intravascular space into interstitial leading to edema. Intravascular volume depletion leads to under-perfusion of the kidneys which stimulates renin-angiotensin system causing increased renal sodium and water retention further leading to edema formation. Another mechanism may be primary renal sodium retention at a distal nephron site, perhaps due to altered responsiveness to hormones such as atrial natriuretic factor.
- ***Hyperlipidemia*** and ***lipiduria*** is due to increase in the synthesis of lipoprotein by liver to compensate

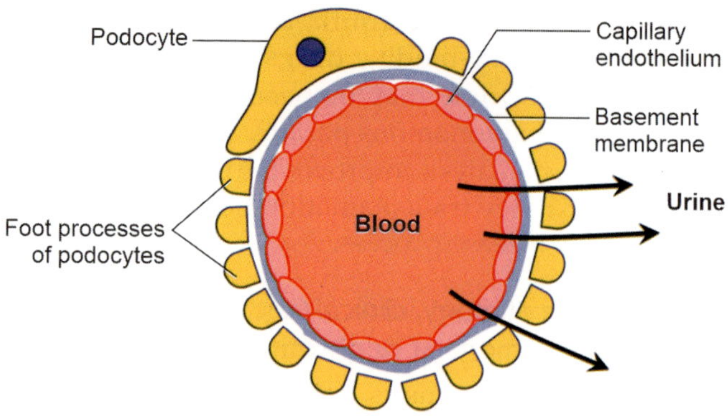

Figure 8.5: Normal glomerulus

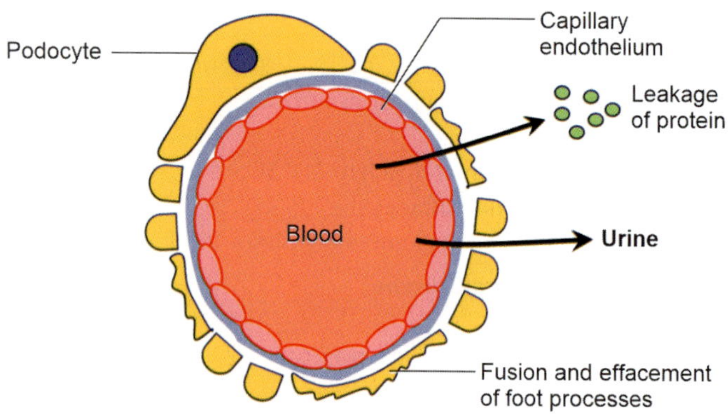

Figure 8.6: Abnormal glomerulus in nephrotic syndrome

for protein loss. This results in ↑ serum cholesterol, triglycerides, LDL, and lipiduria ("fatty casts," "oval fat bodies" in urine).

- ***Hypercoagulability*** is due to loss of anticoagulant factors (antithrombin III, protein C, and protein S) in urine and also due to increased hepatic synthesis of clotting factors.
- ***Increased infection risk*** is due to loss of immunoglobulins in urine.

Clinical Features

- Nephrotic syndrome occurs at any age but is more prevalent in children, mostly between ages 1½ and 4 years.
- Frothy urine due to proteinuria
- Weight gain due to fluid retention
- Peripheral edema is the hallmark of the nephrotic syndrome. Initially it is noted in the dependent areas such as the lower extremities, but later becomes generalized. Early morning facial puffiness is seen in most patients even before the development of generalized edema.
- Patients can experience dyspnea due to pulmonary edema and pleural effusion.
- Ascites may be present.
- Patients are more prone to infection due to loss of immunoglobulins and complements in the urine.
- Patients also have hypercoagulable state due to urinary losses of antithrombin III, protein C, and protein S and increased platelet activation. Patients are prone to renal vein thrombosis and other venous thromboemboli.
- Microcytic hypochromic anemia may result from loss of transferrin in the urine.
- Vitamin D deficiency may result from loss of cholecalciferol binding protein.

Investigations

- Urine analysis shows heavy proteinuria. 24-hour urine protein excretion should be measured and it shows nephrotic range proteinuria (>3.5 g/day). Normal protein excretion is <150 mg/day. Minimal hematuria may also be present.
- Serum albumin is low (<3 g/dl).
- Urea and creatinine may be elevated if there is renal failure.
- Total cholesterol and LDL-cholesterol is elevated in most patients. HDL-cholesterol is normal or decreased.
- Blood sugar and glycosylated hemoglobin tests for diabetes
- Antinuclear antibody (ANA) and ANCA test for collagen vascular disease and vasculitis
- Serum anticoagulants and complement levels are decreased.
- Hepatitis B and C serology, HIV serology
- Renal biopsy if the cause is not clear especially in an adult patient. Pathological changes include effacement and fusion of foot processes of podocytes **(Figs 8.5 and 8.6)**.

Management

Protein Loss

- The daily total dietary protein intake should replace the daily urinary protein losses so as to avoid negative nitrogen balance. Angiotensin converting enzyme (ACE) inhibitors and angiotensin receptor blockers reduce the amount of proteinuria.

Edema

- This can be managed by dietary salt restriction and diuretics. Commonly used diuretics include thiazide and loop diuretics.

Hyperlipidemia

- Dietary modification and exercise should be advised. HMG-CoA reductase inhibitors (statins) can be used in patients not responding to dietary measures.

Hypercoagulable State

- Anticoagulation therapy is given for at least 3–6 months in patients with evidence of thrombosis. Patients with renal vein thrombosis and recurrent thromboemboli require indefinite anticoagulation.

Treatment of the Underlying Cause

- Minimal change disease responds to steroids.
- Steroids are beneficial in only 20–30% cases of focal segmental glomerulosclerosis (FSGS). Cyclophosphamide and cyclosporine are alternatives.

- Membranous nephropathy responds to alternating monthly corticosteroids and monthly oral chlorambucil over 6 months. Recent controlled studies using only corticosteroids for 6 months have shown similar beneficial results. Membranous nephropathy with progressive renal failure may benefit from cyclophosphamide plus corticosteroids.
- Diabetic nephropathy requires optimization of glycemic and BP control.

Q. Minimal change disease (nil disease or lipoid nephrosis).

- Minimal change disease is a primary glomerular disease that accounts for most cases of nephrotic syndrome in children and 10–15% of idiopathic nephrotic syndrome in adults.

Etiology

- Most of the cases are idiopathic (primary).
- Some cases may be secondary to following causes:
  - Infections: Tuberculosis, syphilis, mycoplasma, ehrlichiosis, hepatitis C virus, HIV
  - Malignancies: Leukemia, Hodgkin and non-Hodgkin lymphoma
  - Allergy: Bee sting, cat fur, fungi, poison ivy, ragweed pollen, house dust
  - Drugs: NSAIDs, lithium, antibiotics (ampicillin, cephalosporins), immunizations
  - Autoimmune diseases.

Pathophysiology

- T-cell–mediated immune response → cytokine release → damage to podocytes.
- Loss of negative charge barrier → selective proteinuria (mostly albumin).
- No immune complex deposition (unlike other glomerular diseases).

Clinical features

- Patients typically present with periorbital and peripheral edema. Periorbital edema is noted first.
- Malaise, easy fatiguability and weight gain
- Frothy urine
- Normal blood pressure (typically)
- Preserved renal function.

Investigations

- Urea and creatinine are normal.
- Urine analysis shows nephrotic range proteinuria (>3.5 g/day) and occasionally hematuria. RBC casts are absent.
- Serum albumin is low.
- ↑ Serum cholesterol and triglycerides.
- Serologic workup (including antinuclear antibodies and complements) is normal.
- Kidney biopsy is usually not required in children except in atypical cases. However, kidney biopsy is required in adults. Biopsy shows no glomerular abnormalities on light microscopy. The tubules may show lipid droplet accumulation from absorbed lipoproteins (hence also called lipoid nephrosis). Complement and Ig deposits are absent on immunofluorescence. Electron microscopy shows effacement or "fusion" of the foot processes of epithelial podocytes.

Treatment

- Initial therapy is with steroids, prednisolone 60 mg/m^2 per day (maximum of 60 mg/day). When proteinuria disappears, prednisolone is continued at the same dose for 1 month and then on alternate day (at the same daily dose) for 2 months. Thereafter, the alternate day dose is gradually decreased.
- Complete remission occurs in >80% of patients treated with corticosteroids, and treatment is usually continued for 1–2 years.
- Response may be slower in adults, and they should not be considered steroid-resistant until they have failed to respond to 4 months of treatment.
- Relapses can occur in children and adults. First relapse is treated similarly as the initial episode. Patients who relapse third time or who become steroid dependent may be treated with a 2 month course of an alkylating agent (cyclophosphamide 2 mg/kg/day or chlorambucil). Another alternative is low dose cyclosporine (4–6 mg/kg/day for 4 months), but this carries the risk of nephrotoxicity.
- Mycophenolate mofetil or rituximab may be considered if the above drugs are not effective.

Q. Discuss the etiology, pathogenesis, clinical features, investigations and management of glomerulonephritis (nephritic syndrome).

- Glomerulonephritis (GN) refers to a group of disorders causing inflammation of the glomeruli. Here the glomeruli are damaged due to inflammation.
- Glomerulonephritis classically presents with:
  - Hematuria (often with RBC casts)
  - Oliguria
  - Hypertension
  - Edema
  - Mild to moderate proteinuria

Etiology

Primary glomerular diseases: Diffuse proliferative glomerulonephritis, focal segmental glomerulosclerosis (FSGS), membranous glomerulonephritis, membranoproliferative glomerulonephritis, crescentic glomerulonephritis, IgA nephropathy.

Systemic diseases: SLE, Wegener's granulomatosis, polyarteritis, Henoch-Schönlein purpura, Goodpasture's syndrome, sickle cell nephropathy.

Infections: Post-streptococcal glomerulonephritis, syphilis, subacute bacterial endocarditis, hepatitis B and C, HIV infection, infectious mononucleosis, cytomegalovirus, malaria, schistosomiasis.

Miscellaneous: Malignancy, eclampsia, serum sickness, drugs (penicillamine), malignant hypertension.

Pathogenesis (Figs 8.7 and 8.8)

- Most types of glomerulonephritis are immunologically mediated. Glomerular injury occurs by two main mechanisms, either by deposition of antibody in the glomerular basement membrane or by deposition of immune complexes.
- Immune complexes are formed 'in situ' by antibodies which complex with glomerular antigens, or with other antigens ('planted' antigens, e.g. viral or bacterial ones) that have localized in glomeruli.
- The antibodies and immune complexes trigger injury by complement activation, fibrin deposition, release of cytokines and recruitment of inflammatory cells.
- All these result in structural damage to glomerular capillaries and basement membrane.
- This leads to hematuria, proteinuria, and potential renal failure, depending on the severity and type of GN.

Clinical Features

- Hematuria (tea-or cola-colored urine).
- Oliguria.
- Edema: Edema is found first in body parts with low tissue tension, such as the periorbital and scrotal regions.
- Hypertension.
- Mild proteinuria (<3.5 g/day).

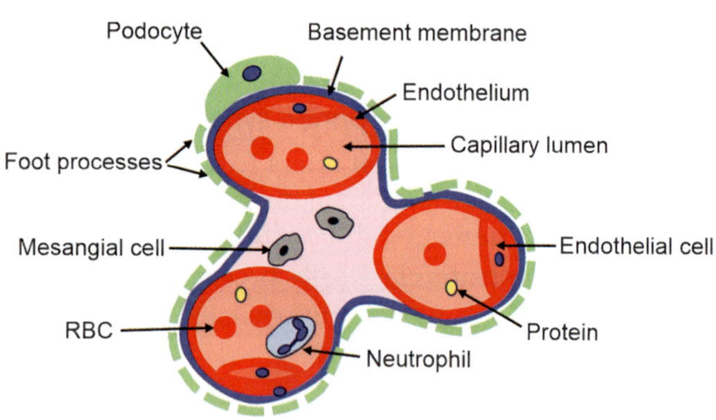

Figure 8.7: Normal glomerulus

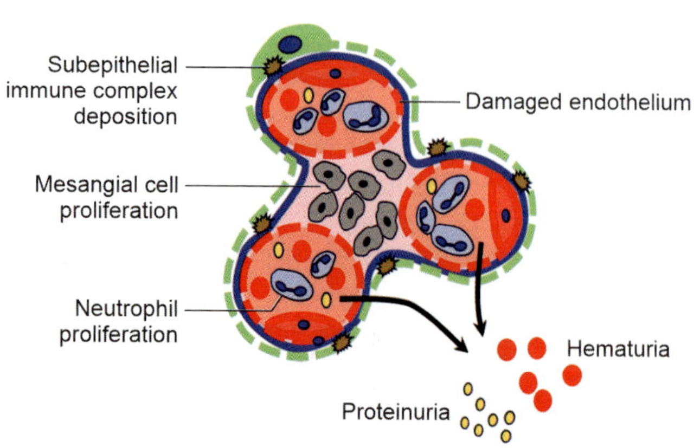

Figure 8.8: Abnormal glomerulus in glomerulonephritis

Investigations

Blood Tests

- CBC, CRP/ESR.
- Elevated urea and creatinine.
- Complement levels (C3, C4) are usually decreased.
- ASO titer and anti-DNase B are increased in post-streptococcal glomerulonephritis.
- Anti-GBM antibody levels are elevated in Goodpasture syndrome.
- ANA and anti-dsDNA are positive in lupus nephritis.
- ANCA is positive in vasculitis.
- Hepatitis serologies.

Urine Analysis

- Hematuria (microscopic or gross) often with RBC casts. RBC casts are diagnostic of glomerulonephritis. Dysmorphic RBCs may also be present.
- Moderate proteinuria (usually <3.5 g/day).

Renal Ultrasound

- To assess kidney size and exclude obstruction.

Renal Biopsy

- Indicated in unclear diagnosis or rapidly progressive disease.
- Confirms histologic subtype and guides treatment.

Treatment

- General supportive measures include control blood pressure, fluid and salt restriction, diuretics for edema, and dialysis if severe renal failure or fluid overload.
- Depending on the nature and severity of disease, treatment may involve high-dose steroids, cyclophosphamide, and rituximab.
- Plasmapheresis can be used in Goodpasture's disease as a temporary measure until chemotherapy takes effect.
- Underlying disease requires specific treatment.

Q. Differentiate between nephrotic and nephritic syndrome (Table 8.5).

TABLE 8.5: Differences between nephrotic and nephritic syndrome

	Nephrotic syndrome	Nephritic syndrome
Primary pathology	Podocyte injury → ↑ permeability to proteins	Glomerular inflammation → capillary wall damage
Proteinuria	Massive (>3.5 g/day)	Moderate (<3.5 g/day)
Hematuria	Minimal	Significant
Oliguria	Less common	Common
Hypertension	Absent	Present
Generalized edema	Severe and generalized	Mild-to-moderate
RBC casts in urine	Absent	Present
Hypoalbuminemia	Present	Rarely
Hyperlipidemia/ hyperlipiduria	Yes	No
Urea and creatinine	Usually normal	Often elevated
Complement levels	Usually normal	May be low

Q. Discuss the etiology, pathogenesis, clinical features, investigations, complications and management of post-streptococcal glomerulonephritis.

- Poststreptococcal glomerulonephritis (PSGN) is acute glomerulonephritis occurring after infection with group A β-hemolytic Streptococcus (GAS).

Etiology

- Group A beta hemolytic streptococci are responsible for poststreptococcal glomerulonephritis. Skin and throat infections with this organism are followed by glomerulonephritis.

Pathogenesis

- Streptococcal antigens (e.g. streptococcal exotoxin B) act as planted antigens in the glomeruli or form circulating immune complexes.
- Immune complex deposition in the glomerular basement membrane and mesangium.
- Complement activation (especially classical pathway) → ↓ serum C3 levels.
- Recruitment of inflammatory cells → damage to glomerular capillary walls.
- Glomerular inflammation → hematuria, reduced GFR, sodium and water retention.

Clinical Features

- It occurs in children between the ages of 5 and 15 years, but can occur in adults also.
- It is more common in males.
- Patients present with oliguria, hematuria (dark/cola-colored urine) and edema.
- Systemic symptoms of headache, malaise, anorexia, and flank pain (due to swelling of the renal capsule) may be present.
- Hypertension and mild-to-moderate proteinuria is usually present.
- Subclinical disease is common and is characterized by asymptomatic microscopic hematuria.

Investigations

- Urine analysis shows hematuria, proteinuria, pyuria, and RBC casts. Proteinuria can sometimes be in the nephrotic range.
- Urea and creatinine may be elevated.
- Serum complement levels are low.
- Streptococcal culture may be positive from the infected site (throat or skin).
- ASO titer, anti-DNAase or antihyaluronidase antibodies are increased.
- Renal biopsy is rarely required. It shows mesangial and endothelial cell proliferation, glomerular infiltration with polymorphonuclear leukocytes, granular subendothelial immune deposits and subepithelial deposits.

Complications

- Pulmonary edema, hypertensive encephalopathy, and permanent renal failure.

Management

- Treatment is mainly supportive.
- The measures are salt restriction, diuretics, anti-hypertensives and dialysis if required.
- Antibiotic treatment for streptococcal infection should be given to all patients and their cohabitants. Antibiotic choices are penicillins (ampicillin, amoxicillin) or cephalosporins or macrolides or clindamycin. Oral penicillin V or amoxicillin are the 1st drugs of choice and are given for 10 days.
- Steroids and cytotoxic drugs are of no value.
- Prognosis is good and permanent renal failure is uncommon.

Q. IgA nephropathy.

- IgA nephropathy is the most common type of primary glomerulonephritis worldwide. It is a nephritic syndrome caused by deposition of IgA immune complexes in the mesangium of the glomeruli.
- It presents as slowly progressive hematuria, proteinuria, and, often, renal insufficiency. Sometimes it can progress rapidly causing rapidly progressive glomerulonephritis (RPGN).

Etiology

- IgA nephropathy is an autoimmune disease. Usually, there is an infectious disease preceding IgA nephropathy which triggers abnormal immune response.

Pathogenesis

- Overproduction of abnormal IgA1 (galactose-deficient IgA1) by mucosal immune system (often after infections).
- Formation of autoantibodies against this aberrant IgA1.
- Immune complexes of IgA1 + antibodies deposit in the mesangium.
- Mesangial proliferation and inflammation → glomerular injury → hematuria, proteinuria.

Clinical Features

- It occurs in all age groups but more common in young adults. Males are more commonly affected.
- Patients present with gross painless hematuria, proteinuria and hypertension within 1–2 days following a mucosal infection (respiratory tract, GI tract). Hematuria is usually recurrent or persistent. There may be acute exacerbations of hematuria in association with respiratory tract infections.

Diagnosis

- IgA nephropathy should be suspected in patients who present with gross hematuria, particularly within 2 days of a febrile mucosal illness or with flank pain.
- Urinalysis
- Renal biopsy shows mesangial deposition of IgA and complement (C3) on immunofluorescent staining. IgA

deposits are not specific for IgA nephropathy because similar IgA deposits are also seen in other diseases such as Henoch-Schönlein purpura (a systemic small-vessel vasculitis with similar IgA deposition).

Treatment

- Patients with mild disease should be monitored at 6–12 month intervals to assess for disease progression.
- Patients with persistent proteinuria should be treated with an ACE inhibitor/ARBs.
- Patients with progressive disease should be treated with corticosteroids, immunosuppressants.

Q. Rapidly progressive glomerulonephritis (crescentic glomerulonephritis).

- Rapidly progressive glomerulonephritis (RPGN) **is a type of** glomerulonephritis characterized by rapid progression to renal failure (within days to weeks) and crescent formation in the glomeruli.
- It is a clinical emergency.

Etiology

Type I (Anti-GBM antibody mediated)
- Autoantibodies against glomerular basement membrane (GBM)
- *Example*: Goodpasture syndrome (kidney + lung involvement)

Type II (Immune complex mediated)
- Deposition of immune complexes
- *Examples*: IgA nephropathy, poststreptococcal glomerulonephritis, lupus nephritis, membranoproliferative glomerulonephritis.

Type III (Pauci-immune)
- No immune deposits; associated with ANCA.
- *Examples*: Granulomatosis with polyangiitis (previously called Wegener granulomatosis), microscopic polyangiitis, eosinophilic granulomatosis with polyangiitis (Churg-Strauss syndrome).

Pathology

- RPGN is characterized by presence of crescents in renal biopsy, hence also called crescentic glomerulonephritis.
- Crescents are formed by the accumulation of proliferating parietal epithelial cells and infiltrating macrophages and fibrin in the Bowman's space, compressing the glomerular tuft.
- RPGN can be classified into 3 types based on pathologic features.
  - *Antiglomerular basement membrane (GBM) antibody disease:* Linear deposits of antibodies on immunofluorescence.
  - *Immune complex RPGN:* Granular deposits of immune complexes on immunofluorescence.
  - *Pauci-immune RPGN:* Few or no immune deposits on immunofluorescence.

Clinical Features

- Manifestations are usually insidious, with weakness, fatigue, fever, nausea, vomiting, anorexia, arthralgia, and abdominal pain.

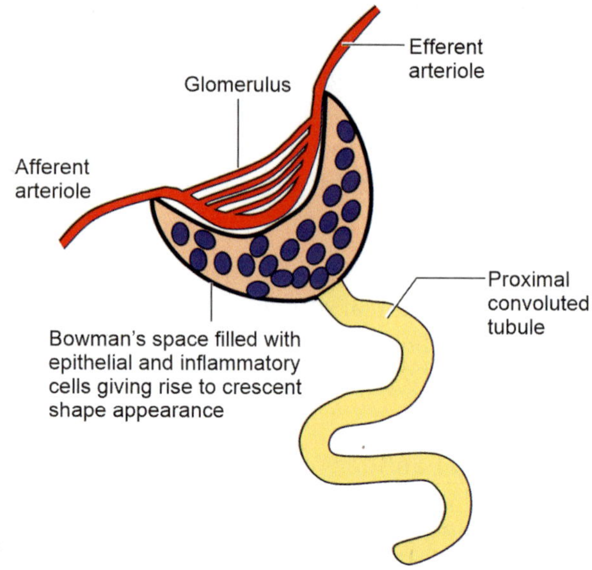

Figure 8.9: Crescent-shaped appearance in RPGN

- Patients with anti-GBM antibody disease (Goodpasture syndrome) may have pulmonary hemorrhage, which can present with hemoptysis.
- Patients also complain of hematuria, oliguria, and generalized edema.

Investigations

- Urea and creatinine are elevated because of renal failure.
- Urine analysis shows nephritic pattern with hematuria, RBC casts, WBCs and proteinuria.
- Oliguria or anuria
- Serologic testing—includes anti-GBM antibodies (present in anti-GBM antibody disease); antistreptolysin O antibodies (post-streptococcal GN), anti-DNA antibodies, or cryoglobulins (immune complex RPGN); and ANCA titers (pauci-immune RPGN).
- Complement level is low in immune complex RPGN.
- Renal ultrasound shows normal sized kidneys.
- Chest X-ray may show infiltrates in Goodpasture syndrome and other vasculitides.
- Kidney biopsy shows presence of crescents **(Fig. 8.9)**.

Treatment

- Supportive therapy involves diuretics, antihypertensives and dialysis if required.
- For immune complex and pauci-immune RPGN, corticosteroids (methylprednisolone 1 g IV daily for 3–5 days followed by prednisone 1 mg/kg orally daily). Cyclophosphamide orally daily is added to prednisolone.
- Plasmapheresis is recommended for anti-GBM antibody disease.
- Kidney transplantation in end stage renal disease.

Prognosis

- An 80–90% of untreated patients progress to end-stage renal disease within 6 months.

Q. Tubulointerstitial nephritis (Interstitial nephritis).

- Tubulointerstitial nephritis refers to inflammatory disease of renal tubules and the surrounding interstitium.

Classification

Acute Tubulointerstitial Nephritis (ATIN)

- Sudden onset
- Often reversible with treatment
- Commonly drug-induced.

Chronic Tubulointerstitial Nephritis (CTIN)

- Long-standing, progressive disease
- Irreversible fibrosis and tubular atrophy
- Associated with chronic exposures or systemic diseases.

Etiology

Drugs (allergic)
- Penicillins, NSAIDs, allopurinol, lithium, proton pump inhibitors

Autoimmune
- Sarcoidosis, Sjögren's syndrome, SLE

Infections
- Pyelonephritis, leptospirosis, tuberculosis, CMV, HIV, EBV

Toxic
- Myeloma light chains, mushrooms, Chinese herbal nephropathy, lead.

Pathophysiology

- Interstitial nephritis is primarily characterized by inflammation of the renal interstitium and tubules, often with minimal glomerular involvement. The inflammation is triggered by drugs or infections or other etiologic factors.
- Inflammatory response in interstitial space → edema, infiltration by lymphocytes, plasma cells, eosinophils (especially in drug-induced cases).
- Tubular cell injury → impaired urine concentration, electrolyte imbalance.
- In chronic cases—fibrosis, tubular atrophy, and permanent nephron loss.

Clinical Features

- Tubulointerstitial nephritis can be acute or chronic. More than 95% of cases of acute ttubulointerstitial nephritis result from infection or an allergic drug reaction. Chronic tubulointerstitial nephritis arises when chronic tubular insults cause gradual interstitial infiltration and fibrosis, tubular atrophy and dysfunction, and a gradual deterioration of renal function, usually over years.
- Acute ttubulointerstitial nephritis may be asymptomatic. Fever, rash, arthralgias may be present in allergic (drug induced) interstitial nephritis. Some patients develop polyuria and nocturia due to a defect in urinary concentration and Na reabsorption.
- Chronic tubulointerstitial nephritis starts insidiously and presents with polyuria and nocturia due to impaired concentrating ability. Progressive renal failure eventually occurs.

Investigations

- Urea and creatinine are elevated.
- Hyperkalemia and acidosis may be present.
- Urine analysis shows proteinuria, sterile pyuria and eosinophils.
- Renal biopsy shows intense inflammation, with polymorphonuclear leukocytes and lymphocytes surrounding tubules and blood vessels and invading tubules (tubulitis), and occasional eosinophils (especially in drug-induced disease).
- Imaging: Small, shrunken kidneys in chronic TIN.

Management

- Underlying cause should be treated such as withdrawal of offending drug.
- Steroids (e.g. prednisolone 1 mg/kg/day) accelerate recovery and may prevent long-term scarring in allergic and autoimmune interstitial nephritis. Steroids should be given for 2–3 months.
- Supportive measures such as dialysis if required.

Q. Polycystic kidney disease (PKD).

- Polycystic kidney disease is a genetic disorder, characterized by the growth of fluid filled cysts in the kidneys **(Fig. 8.10)**.
- It leads to progressive kidney enlargement, tissue destruction, and ultimately chronic kidney disease (CKD) or end-stage renal disease (ESRD).
- Incidence is approximately 1 in every 1000 live births.
- There are 2 types of PKD. Infantile polycystic kidney disease and adult polycystic kidney disease. Infantile PKD is rare, autosomal recessive and usually fatal. Adult PKD is common and is inherited as autosomal dominant trait.

Pathogenesis

- Mutations in PKD1 and PKD2 genes are responsible for this disease. These genes code for proteins responsible for normal tubular structure and cilia function. Loss of these proteins leads to abnormal tubular cell proliferation and cyst formation. There is

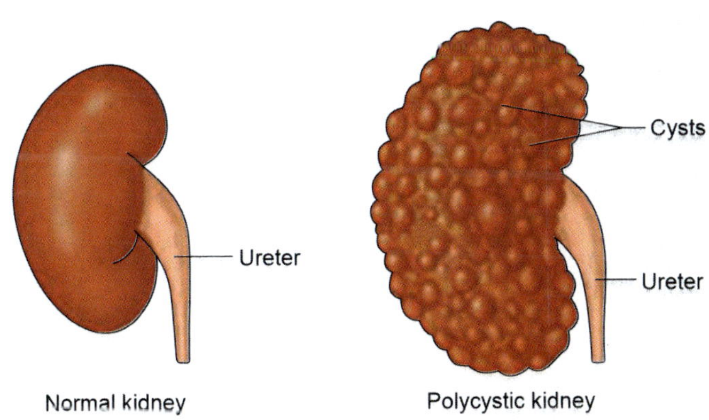

Figure 8.10: Polycystic kidney disease

increased fluid secretion into cysts leading to gradual enlargement and compression of normal kidney tissue leading to kidney failure.

Clinical Features (adult PKD)

- Patients are usually asymptomatic until later life.
- After the age of 20, there is often insidious onset of hypertension.
- Vague discomfort in loin or abdomen due to enlarged kidneys.
- Sometimes acute loin pain or renal colic due to hemorrhage into a cyst.
- One or both kidneys may be palpable and the surface may be nodular.
- Family history is usually positive
- Gradual reduction in renal function
- Some patients may have hepatic cysts, and berry aneurysms in the brain.
- Mitral and aortic regurgitation are also frequent in these patients.

Investigations

- Ultrasound abdomen shows multiple cysts in both kidneys.
- CT/MRI: Better resolution; used to monitor progression or complications.
- Urea and creatinine are elevated.
- Urinalysis: Hematuria, proteinuria.
- Genetic testing: Confirms diagnosis (especially in uncertain cases).

Management

- There is no treatment to alter the rate of progression of renal failure.
- Control of hypertension
- Tolvaptan (vasopressin V2 receptor antagonist) slows cyst growth and renal decline in ADPKD.
- Dialysis if required.
- Kidney transplantation in end stage renal disease.

Q. Discuss the etiology, pathogenesis, clinical features, investigations and management of urinary tract infection.

- Urinary tract infection (UTI) is defined as the bacterial invasion of the urinary tract. It can occur anywhere between the urethra and the kidney. UTI is the commonest of all bacterial infections.
- It is more common in women because of short urethra (4 cm) and up to 50% of women have a UTI at some time. UTI is uncommon in males except in the first year of life and in men over 60 because of prostate hypertrophy causing urinary obstruction.
- Even though most cases of UTI can be treated easily, some cases can lead to renal damage and chronic renal failure.
- UTI can be lower UTI or upper UTI.
  - ***Lower UTI:*** Cystitis and urethritis.
  - ***Upper UTI***: Ureteritis, pyelonephritis.
- UTI can be uncomplicated or complicated.
  - ***Uncomplicated UTI:*** UTI occurring in a healthy host with a normal urinary tract, typically in non-pregnant, premenopausal women without structural or functional abnormalities.
  - ***Complicated UTI***: A UTI associated with increased risk of treatment failure or serious outcomes, due to underlying medical conditions or urinary tract abnormalities. Occurs in men, pregnant women, diabetics, catheterized patients, or with structural abnormalities (stricture urethra, BPH, stone, neurogenic bladder, etc.).
- Some patients, usually females, have symptoms of UTI without any bacteria in the urine. This is called urethral syndrome. This can occur due to infection with difficult to culture organisms (e.g. Chlamydia, certain anaerobes), intermittent or very low-count bacteriuria, reaction to toilet preparations or disinfectants, symptoms related to sexual intercourse, or post-menopausal atrophic vaginitis. Antibiotics are not indicated for urethral syndrome.

Etiology of UTI

- UTIs are primarily caused by the ascent of pathogens from the urethra to the bladder and, in some cases, to the kidneys.

Community organisms causing UTI

- *Escherichia coli* derived from GIT (most common cause, 75% of UTIs)
- *Proteus mirabilis*
- *Enterococcus faecalis*
- *Pseudomonas species*
- Streptococci
- *Staphylococcus saprophyticus*
- Klebsiella

Predisposing Factors for UTI

- Female gender (shorter urethra)
- Sexual activity
- Use of spermicides
- Urinary stasis (e.g. BPH, obstruction, stones, neurogenic bladder)
- Instrumentation (e.g. catheterization)
- Pregnancy
- Diabetes mellitus
- Immunosuppression

Pathogenesis

- Most of the UTI (95%) are due to ascending infection from the urethra to bladder. Remaining are due to hematogenous spread of infection. The first step is colonization of the periurethral area with bacteria.
- Attachment of bacteria to the uroepithelial cells is an active process mediated by bacterial adhesins and receptors on the epithelial cells. Urothelium of susceptible persons may have more receptors to which virulent strains of *E. coli* become adherent. In women, the ascent of organisms into the bladder is easier than

in men because of the relatively short urethra and absence of bactericidal prostatic secretions.

- Sexual intercourse and instrumentation of the bladder may also introduce organisms into the urethra and bladder.
- Multiplication of organism then depends on the size of the inoculum, virulence of the bacteria and host defenses.
- Inflammatory response in the mucosa leading to symptoms of infection.
- In some cases, ascension to kidneys causes pyelonephritis.
- Hematogenous spread is rare, seen with organisms like *Staphylococcus aureus*.

Risk Factors for UTI

Incomplete bladder emptying

- Bladder outflow obstruction (BPH, urethral stricture)
- Neurogenic bladder (e.g. multiple sclerosis, diabetic neuropathy, myelopathy)
- Gynecological abnormalities (e.g. uterine prolapse)
- Vesicoureteric reflux

Foreign bodies

- Urethral catheter or ureteric stent

Loss of host defenses

- Atrophic urethritis and vaginitis in post-menopausal women
- Diabetes mellitus
- Immunosuppression

Females

- Due to short urethra (4 cm)

Others

- Pregnancy
- Sexual activity

Clinical Features

- Increased frequency of micturition
- Pain in the urethra during micturition (dysuria)
- Suprapubic pain during and after voiding (in cystitis)
- Urgency
- Intense desire to pass more urine after micturition due to spasm of the inflamed bladder wall (strangury).
- Passing cloudy urine with unpleasant odor and occasionally hematuria
- Systemic symptoms such as fever and chills may occur. Prominent systemic symptoms with fever and loin pain suggest acute pyelonephritis.

Investigations

- Urine microscopy: Shows presence of WBCs (>5 per high power field is significant) and sometimes RBCs. Bacteria also may be visible.
- Mid-stream urine culture and sensitivity. Growth of $>10^5$/ml organisms is regarded as significant.
- Complete blood count: may show increased leukocyte count.
- Serum creatinine, blood urea and electrolytes may show evidence of renal failure.
- Renal ultrasound or CT to identify obstruction, cysts, or calculi
- Pelvic examination in women with recurrent UTI to exclude cystocele, rectocele and uterovaginal prolapse
- Rectal examination in elderly men to assess prostate
- Intravenous urography for any anatomical/physiological anomalies
- Micturating cystourethrography for vesicoureteric reflux
- Cystoscopy in patients with hematuria or a suspected bladder lesion
- Blood culture in septicemic cases.

Management

- Adequate fluid intake to maintain good urine output.
- Antibiotic therapy. The choice of antibiotic depends on the organism. Since the most common organism is *E. coli*, initial antibiotic therapy should be directed against this organism. Antibiotic choices are cotrimoxazole, amoxicillin, ampicillin, cephalosporins, quinolones and nitrofurantoin. Antibiotic should be modified once urine culture sensitivity reports are available. Duration of therapy is usually 3–5 days.
- Complicated UTI usually requires parenteral antibiotics for 7–14 days.
- Asymptomatic bacteriuria should be treated if the patient is pregnant or immunocompromised.
- Any underlying risk factor predisposing to UTI should be corrected such as BPH, cystocele, stones, etc.
- Alkalization of urine with potassium citrate may help if there is severe dysuria.

Preventive Measures for Recurrent UTI

- Fluid intake of at least 2 liters/day
- Regular complete emptying of bladder
- If vesico-ureteric reflux is present, practice double micturition (empty the bladder then attempt micturition 10–15 minutes later)
- Good perineal hygiene
- Emptying of the bladder before and after sexual intercourse.

Q. Sterile pyuria.

- Sterile pyuria means presence of pus cells (WBCs) in the urine without the growth of organisms on routine urine culture.

Causes

- Partially treated UTI
- Contamination of the urine sample by sterilizing solution
- Contamination of the urine sample with vaginal leukocytes
- Interstitial nephritis
- Calculi in the urinary tract
- Infection with difficult to culture organisms (TB, Chlamydia, Mycoplasma, fungal infections)
- Non-infectious causes (SLE, bladder tumors, chemical cystitis, foreign body)
- Appendicitis

Investigations

- Repeat urine culture, with proper technique.
- Urine PCR or CB-NAAT for Chlamydia, Mycoplasma, Ureaplasma.
- AFB stain and culture, or PCR for tuberculosis.
- Urine cytology (if malignancy suspected).
- Renal imaging (if stones or structural abnormalities are suspected).
- Blood tests: Eosinophilia (suggests interstitial nephritis), ANA (for lupus).

Clinical Relevance

- Sterile pyuria should not be ignored, especially if persistent, symptomatic, or occurring in high-risk patients (e.g. immunocompromised, elderly, or those with a history of TB or stones). It often signals an atypical infection or non-infectious inflammatory condition.

Q. Vesicoureteral reflux.

- Vesicoureteral reflux (VUR) is the retrograde passage of urine from the bladder into the upper urinary tract **(Fig. 8.11)**.
- It is the most common urologic anomaly in children, occurring in approximately 1% of newborns.
- VUR may transport bacteria from the bladder to the kidney leading to pyelonephritis. Recurrent pyelonephritis may lead to renal scarring, renal failure and hypertension.
- Diagnosis of VUR is made by demonstration of reflux of urine from the bladder to the upper urinary tract by either contrast micturating cystourethrogram or radionuclide cystogram.
- Treatment includes medical or surgical therapy. Medical treatment consists of prophylactic antibiotic therapy with trimethoprim-sulfamethoxazole, trimethoprim alone, or nitrofurantoin. Surgical correction includes open surgical repair or endoscopic correction.

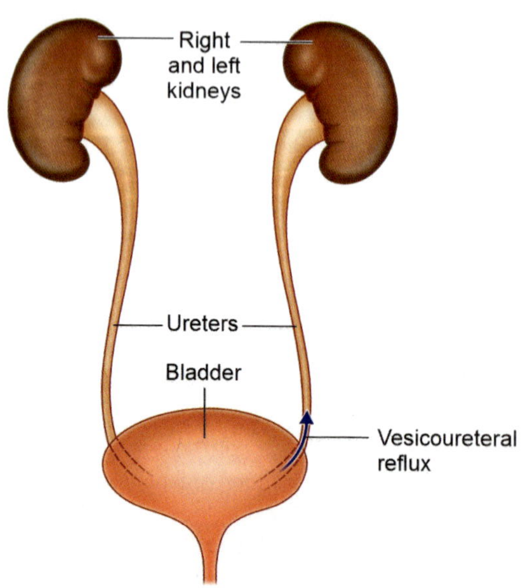

Figure 8.11: Vesicoureteral reflux

Q. Discuss the etiopathogenesis, clinical features, investigations and management of acute pyelonephritis.

- Pyelonephritis refers to infection of the renal parenchyma.
- Pyelonephritis is a serious infection and is less common than lower urinary tract infection (urethritis, cystitis).

Etiopathogenesis

- Pyelonephritis is usually due to ascending infection from the bladder. Rarely, it is due to hematogenous spread due to bacteremia. Common organisms are *E. coli*, *Klebsiella pneumoniae* and Staphylococcus.
- Preexisting renal damage, such as cyst or scarring facilitates infection.
- The renal pelvis is inflamed and small abscesses may be present in the renal parenchyma. Histological examination shows focal infiltration by neutrophils, which can often be seen within the tubules.

Clinical Features

- Acute pyelonephritis presents as a classic triad of costovertebral angle (renal angle) pain, fever and tenderness over the kidneys.
- Costovertebral angle pain is usually acute onset, unilateral or bilateral and may radiate to the iliac fossa and suprapubic area. Costovertebral angle (CVA) tenderness is often present (positive Murphy's punch sign). There may be associated tenderness and guarding in the lumbar region. Vomiting may be present.
- Fever is high grade with chills and rigors.
- Rarely, patients may present with sepsis, multi-organ dysfunction, hypotension, and acute renal failure.

Investigations

- Peripheral blood leukocytosis
- Urine examination shows presence of pus cells (neutrophils), organisms, RBCs and tubular epithelial cells.
- Urine culture and sensitivity.
- Blood culture may sometimes grow the causative organism.
- Renal ultrasound
- CT scan may be required in doubtful cases.

Complications

- *Emphysematous pyelonephritis* commonly occurs in patients with diabetes. It is a severe, necrotizing form of pyelonephritis with gas formation and extension of the infection through the renal capsule.
- Renal and perinephric abscess formation.
- AKI
- Renal scarring and CKD
- Sepsis with multi-organ dysfunction.

Management

- Adequate fluid intake, if necessary by intravenous route.

- *Antibiotic therapy:* For uncomplicated pyelonephritis, initial antibiotic choice can be oral trimethoprim-sulphamethoxazole or a fluoroquinolone. Intravenous ceftriaxone is another option if the patient is not able to take orally. For complicated pyelonephritis, broad-spectrum antibiotics such as piperacillin-tazobactam, cefepime, meropenem or imipenem should be given parenterally. Antibiotics should be modified based on culture sensitivity reports. Antibiotics should be given for 7–14 days.
- *Surgery* may be necessary if there is abscess formation.

Q. Renal replacement therapy.

Q. Hemodialysis.

- Renal replacement therapy (RRT) refers to medical treatments that replace the function of failed kidneys, including removal of waste products, excess fluids, and correction of electrolyte imbalances. It is used in acute kidney injury (AKI) and end-stage renal disease (ESRD).

Types of RRT

Hemodialysis (HD)

- Blood is filtered through a dialyzer (artificial kidney) via a machine. Usually done 3 times a week for ESRD patients.

Peritoneal Dialysis (PD)

- Uses the peritoneal membrane in the abdomen as a filter.
- Can be done at home (e.g. continuous ambulatory peritoneal dialysis—CAPD).

Continuous Renal Replacement Therapy (CRRT)

- Used in **critically ill** patients with AKI, typically in ICUs.
- Slow and continuous (e.g. CVVH, CVVHD).

Kidney Transplantation

- Best long-term solution for ESRD.
- Involves surgical replacement with a donor kidney.

Dialysis

- Dialysis is based on the principle that solutes shift from high concentration compartment to low concentration compartment if separated by a semipermeable membrane. During dialysis, serum solutes (e.g. urea, creatinine) diffuse passively between fluid compartments down a concentration gradient. In the context of dialysis, patient blood forms one compartment (contains high concentration of urea, creatinine) and dialysis fluid forms another compartment separated by a semipermeable membrane. In hemofiltration, serum water passes between compartments down a hydrostatic pressure gradient, dragging solute with it. Both dialysis and hemofiltration can be done intermittently or continuously.
- Dialysis is divided broadly into three types: hemodialysis (HD), peritoneal dialysis (PD), and continuous renal replacement therapy (CRRT).
- Hemodialysis employs an artificial membrane across which the exchange of solutes takes place. Peritoneal dialysis is done by using the peritoneal membrane as the semipermeable membrane. Continuous renal replacement therapy (CRRT) is a slower type of dialysis which is over a period of 24 hours continuously to remove waste products and fluid from the patient. CRRT provides gentler solute (waste) and fluid removal than standard dialysis techniques; hence it is helpful in hemodynamically unstable patients such as patients with hypotension.

Indications for Dialysis

(*Mnemonic*: AEIOU, Table 8.6)

TABLE 8.6: Indications for dialysis or RRT

Indication	Description
Acidosis	Severe metabolic acidosis (pH <7.1)
Electrolyte	Refractory hyperkalemia (K^+ >6.5 mmol/L)
Intoxication	Certain drug/toxin overdoses (e.g. lithium, ethylene glycol)
Overload	Fluid overload unresponsive to diuretics
Uremia	Signs like pericarditis, encephalopathy, bleeding

Hemodialysis

- Hemodialysis (HD) is a process by which blood is filtered outside the body using a dialysis machine and a dialyzer to remove uremic toxins, excess water, and correct electrolyte imbalances.
- Hemodialysis is more efficient than peritoneal dialysis in removing urea and creatinine. In hemodialysis there is diffusion of solutes between plasma and dialysate fluid across a semi-permeable membrane following a concentration gradient.
- Semipermeable membrane is made of cellulose, cellulose acetate or synthetic material (polymethyl methacrylate, polycarbonate).

Technique (Fig. 8.12)

- Blood from the patient is made to flow through the dialysis machine which contains a semipermeable membrane. This semipermeable membrane separates the blood and dialysis fluid. Solutes such as urea, creatinine and potassium shift from high concentration compartment (blood) to low concentration compartment (dialysis fluid) through the semipermeable membrane.
- Fluid is removed by applying negative pressure to the dialysate side (ultrafiltration). After passing through the dialysis machine blood goes back to the patient.
- Heparin is given to prevent clotting of the blood as it passes through the dialysis machine.
- Vascular access can be obtained by placing a catheter into the femoral or internal jugular vein. AV fistula can be created in the forearm for permanent vascular access.
- Initially hemodialysis is done for 1 hour to avoid sudden change in fluid and electrolyte balance in the patient. Subsequently hemodialysis is done for 3–4 hours 3–4 times a week.

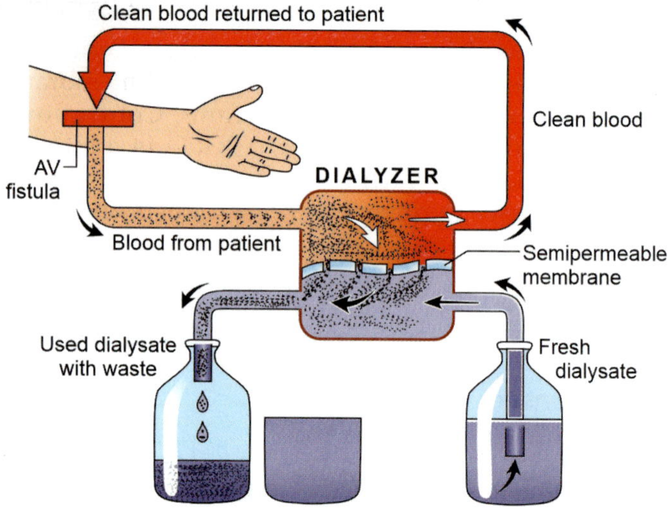

Figure 8.12: Hemodialysis

Indications for Hemodialysis

See **Table 8.6.**

Complications of Hemodialysis

- Nausea, vomiting, and headache.
- Hypotension due to fluid removal and hypovolemia.
- Cardiac arrhythmias due to sudden potassium and acid-base shifts.
- Hemorrhage due to anticoagulation.
- Air embolism due to disconnected or faulty lines and equipment malfunction.
- Allergic reaction to dialysis membrane or sterilant.
- Dialysis disequilibrium syndrome may follow a session of dialysis. It is due to cerebral edema which develops due to rapid decrease in plasma osmolality. It is characterized by nausea, vomiting, restlessness, headache, hypertension, myoclonic jerks and in severe cases seizures and coma.
- Cardiac disease has been found to be higher in patients on long term hemodialysis.
- Dementia is more common in patients on long-term dialysis. Reasons for this may be other comorbid illness and age rather than dialysis itself. Dementia associated with aluminum intoxication in dialysis patients is now uncommon due to adoption of alternatives to aluminum-containing compounds as phosphate binders.

Advantages

- Rapid clearance of toxins.
- Controlled and efficient fluid and electrolyte management.

Disadvantages

- Requires hospital or dialysis center visits
- Vascular access complications
- Dietary and fluid restrictions.

Q. Peritoneal dialysis (PD).

- Peritoneal dialysis is a form of renal replacement therapy in which the peritoneal membrane (lining of the abdominal cavity) is used as a semipermeable membrane to remove waste products, electrolytes, and excess fluid from the blood.
- It is less efficient than hemodialysis, and is rarely used in AKI. It requires an intact peritoneal cavity and is not feasible after recent abdominal surgery.

Technique

- Access to the peritoneal cavity is obtained through a peritoneal catheter made of silicon rubber with numerous side holes at the distal end.
- 1.5–3 L of a dextrose-containing solution is infused into the peritoneal cavity and allowed to dwell for 2–4 hours. Uremic toxins and electrolytes diffuse from the blood vessels in the peritoneum pass into the dialysis fluid during this period which is then removed and fresh dialysis fluid is infused.

Forms of PD

- PD can be done manually or using an automated device. In manual methods dialysis fluid is infused into the peritoneum manually and is drained manually. Automated PD uses an automated device to do multiple nighttime exchanges, sometimes with a daytime dwell.
- *Continuous ambulatory peritoneal dialysis (CAPD)*: Involves multiple exchanges during the day (usually four, but sometimes three or five) with an overnight dwell. The dialysate is infused into the abdomen at bedtime and is drained upon awakening.
- *Automated peritoneal dialysis (APD):* This is an automated form of therapy in which a machine performs exchanges while the patient sleeps often followed by a long daytime dwell.

Complications of Peritoneal Dialysis

Advantages

- Can be done at home also.
- Greater patient independence.
- More stable hemodynamics (no sudden fluid shifts).
- Better preservation of residual renal function.
- Useful in children.

Disadvantages

- Not suitable for everyone (e.g. obese, post-abdominal surgery).
- Peritonitis
- Increased risk of hernias
- Hyperglycemia due to use of dextrose containing fluid as the dialysis fluid
- Weight gain due to glucose absorption from the dialysis fluid
- Protein malnutrition.

Q. Dialysis disequilibrium syndrome.

- Dialysis disequilibrium syndrome refers to an array of neurological manifestations that are seen during or shortly after hemodialysis.

Pathophysiology

- In severe uremia, urea accumulates in both blood and brain tissues.
- During initial dialysis, urea is removed rapidly from blood, but not as quickly from the brain (due to slow diffusion across the blood-brain barrier).
- This creates an osmotic gradient: Water shifts into the brain, causing cerebral edema.
- Dialysis disequilibrium syndrome (DDS) most commonly occurs in first few dialysis sessions and in patients with high predialysis urea.

Clinical Features

- Signs and symptoms of cerebral edema, such as headache, blurred vision due to papilledema, decreased level of consciousness, convulsions, delirium occurring immediately after dialysis should raise the suspicion of DDS.

Investigations

- CT or MRI brain is required to rule out other neurological problems such as stroke, intracranial bleed, etc.
- Serum electrolytes.

Treatment

- Usually self-limited. However, for severe symptoms hemodialysis should be stopped.
- If seizures occur, antiepileptics should be given such as diazepam, and phenytoin.
- Brain edema can be reduced by IV mannitol and glycerol.

Prevention

- Initial sessions of dialysis should be short so as to gradually bring down the blood urea.
- Prophylactic administration of osmotically active agents (mannitol, glucose) and using high sodium dialysate in high-risk patients.

Q. Renal transplantation.

- Renal transplantation is the surgical implantation of a healthy donor kidney into a patient with end-stage renal disease (ESRD) to restore kidney function.
- Kidney transplantation is the most common organ transplantation done.
- It offers the best chance of long-term survival in patients with end-stage renal disease. It can restore normal kidney function and correct all the metabolic abnormalities of CKD.

Indications

- End-stage renal disease (ESRD) due to:
  - Diabetic nephropathy
  - Hypertensive nephrosclerosis
  - Glomerulonephritis
  - Polycystic kidney disease
  - Obstructive uropathy
- GFR <15 ml/min/1.73 m^2 with symptoms or complications.

Procedure

- Kidney grafts are taken from a cadaver or a living donor.
- ABO (blood group) and HLA antigens should be matched between the donor and recipient, otherwise failure of the transplant can occur due to graft rejection. Transplantation usually succeeds if all known class I (HLA-A, B, and C) and class II antigens (HLA-DR) between donor and recipient are matched.
- Patient should be dialyzed before transplantation to achieve a near normal metabolic state.
- Surgical technique: the new kidney is placed in one or the other iliac fossa, in an extraperitoneal position that allows ease of repeated biopsy to detect the cause of graft dysfunction. The renal artery is anastomosed to common iliac artery. Renal vein is anastomosed to common iliac vein. Ureter is implanted into the bladder. Patients own kidneys are left *in situ* **(Fig. 8.13)**.

Management after Transplantation

- Immunosuppressive therapy is given to prevent graft rejection usually life long. A commonly used regimen is a combination of prednisolone, ciclosporin and azathioprine. Use of newer immunosuppressive drugs such as tacrolimus, mycophenolate mofetil and rapamycin is increasing.
- Rejection is treated by short courses of high-dose steroids in the first instance. Antilymphocyte antibodies or plasma exchanges are used in resistant cases.
- All transplant patients require regular lifelong follow-up to monitor renal function and immunosuppression.

Complications

- Graft rejection due to various causes. It can be hyperacute, acute, or chronic.
- Opportunistic infections due to immunosuppression.
- Surgical complications: Vascular thrombosis, urine leak, ureteric stricture.
- Malignancy risk (especially skin, lymphoma) due to immunosuppression.

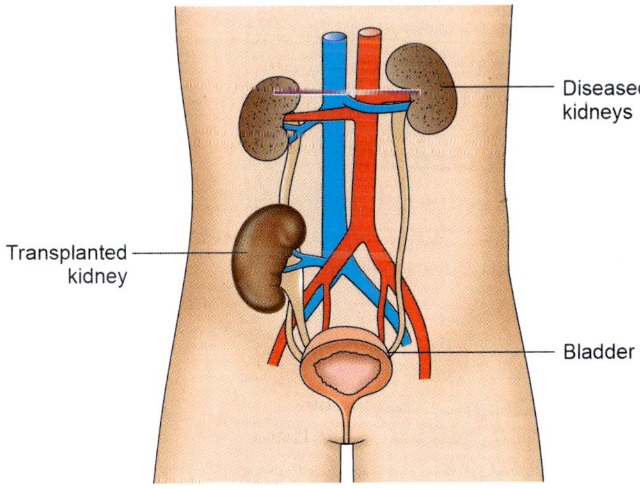

Figure 8.13: Kidney transplantation

Contraindications to Renal Transplantation

Absolute

- Active infection or sepsis
- Active malignancy
- Active vasculitis or anti-GBM disease
- Severe cardiovascular disease
- Severe occlusive aorto-iliac disease
- Persistent substance abuse
- Severe mental retardation
- Severe psychiatric disease.

Relative

- Very young children (<1 year) or older people (>75 years).
- High risk of disease recurrence in the transplant kidney.
- Severe bladder or urethral abnormalities.
- Significant comorbidity.

Advantages over Dialysis

- Improved quality of life
- Better long-term survival
- Freedom from dialysis routine
- Lower dietary and fluid restrictions.

Graft Survival Rates

- 1-year survival: ~90–95%.
- 10-year survival: ~50–60%.

Q. Renal tubular acidosis.

- Renal Tubular Acidosis (RTA) is a group of disorders of the renal tubules in which there is a defect in the ability to maintain acid-base balance, leading to a normal anion gap (hyperchloremic) metabolic acidosis despite normal glomerular function.
- Metabolic acidosis occurs due to a defect in the kidney to reabsorb bicarbonate or to excrete hydrogen ions.
- RTA should be suspected in patients with metabolic acidosis with normal anion gap or with unexplained hyperkalemia or hypokalemia.
- There are four major types of RTA:
  1. Type 1 RTA or distal RTA
  2. Type 2 RTA or proximal RTA
  3. Type 3 RTA is obsolete and is now considered a combination of types 1 and 2
  4. Type 4 RTA or hypoaldosteronism.

Type 1 RTA or distal RTA

- Distal RTA is due to impaired hydrogen ion secretion in the distal tubule due to defect in H^+-ATPase pump or increased back-leak of H^+.

Causes

- Autoimmune: Sjögren's syndrome, SLE
- Drugs: Amphotericin B, lithium
- Hereditary: Mutations in H^+-ATPase
- Obstructive uropathy, hypercalciuria
- Sickle cell disease (tubulointerstitial damage)

Features

- Polyuria and polydipsia due to impaired concentrating ability.
- Hypokalemia is frequently seen in distal RTA and the exact reason for this is unknown. Hypokalemia causes weakness, fatigue, and arrhythmias.
- Chronic acidosis leads to bone demineralization and hypercalciuria. Bone demineralization leads to rickets in children and osteomalacia in adults. Hypercalciuria may lead to nephrolithiasis.
- Urine pH is abnormally high (>5.5) in spite of systemic acidosis.
- ABG shows normal anion gap metabolic acidosis.
- Plasma bicarbonate is usually below 15 mEq/L.

Treatment

- Alkali therapy (usually potassium citrate) improves both calcium and potassium balance, and prevents stones and nephrocalcinosis. Potassium citrate is preferred because it corrects both hypokalemia and acidosis, and reduces stone formation.

Type 2 RTA or proximal RTA

- This is due to failure of proximal tubules to reabsorb filtered bicarbonate from the urine, leading to bicarbonate wasting and acidosis.

Causes

- Fanconi syndrome
- Multiple myeloma
- Drugs (acetazolamide, sulfonamides, ifosfamide, outdated tetracycline)
- Heavy metals (lead, cadmium, mercury)

Features

- ABG shows normal anion gap metabolic acidosis. Since distal segments can reabsorb bicarbonate, plasma bicarbonate concentration is usually between 12 and 20 mEq/L.
- Urine pH is above 7.5 and there is bicarbonaturia when the serum bicarbonate concentration is raised to a normal level.
- Proximal RTA is commonly associated with generalized proximal tubular dysfunction called the Fanconi syndrome. In addition to bicarbonaturia, generalized proximal dysfunction causes glucosuria, phosphaturia, uricosuria, aminoaciduria, and tubular proteinuria. Loss of phosphate may lead to bone demineralization.

Treatment

- Supplementation of bicarbonate.

Type 3 RTA or mixed RTA

- This is due to carbonic anhydrase II deficiency in both proximal and distal tubules. It is extremely rare and has features of both type 1 and type 2 RTA. Additional features are osteopetrosis, cerebral calcification, and mental retardation.

- Treatment is same as that for type 1 and type 2 RTA.

Type 4 RTA (hyperkalemic RTA)

- This is due to either aldosterone deficiency or tubular resistance to the action of aldosterone.
- Aldosterone stimulates the secretion of both hydrogen and potassium in the distal tubules. Hence, hypoaldosteronism causes retention of hydrogen ions leading to acidosis and retention of potassium leading to hyperkalemia.

Causes

Aldosterone deficiency (hypoaldosteronism)
- Primary adrenal insufficiency (Addison's disease)
- Hyporeninemic hypoaldosteronism (especially in diabetic nephropathy)
- Heparin, NSAIDs

Aldosterone resistance
- Potassium-sparing diuretics: Spironolactone, eplerenone, amiloride, triamterene
- Obstructive uropathy
- Tubulointerstitial disease

Clinical Features

- Often asymptomatic
- Fatigue
- Muscle weakness or flaccid paralysis (severe cases) due to hyperkalemia.

Investigations

- Hyperkalemia.
- ABG shows normal anion gap metabolic acidosis.
- Urine pH is appropriate ie, below 5.5 in the presence of acidosis.
- Bicarbonate concentration is decreased.
- Plasma aldosterone ↓ (if primary adrenal or diabetic cause).

Treatment

- Aldosterone deficiency is treated with fludrocortisone.
- Hyperkalemia is controlled by restricting dietary potassium and diuretics.
- Sodium bicarbonate (if metabolic acidosis is symptomatic).

Key differences between types of RTA (Table 8.7)

Q. Renal tuberculosis.

Q. Tuberculosis of urinary tract.

- Tuberculosis of the kidney is secondary to tuberculosis elsewhere due to hematogenous spread.
- Initially, lesions develop in the renal cortex; these may ulcerate into the renal pelvis and involve the ureters, bladder, epididymis, seminal vesicles and prostate.
- Kidney calcification and ureteric stricture are common.

Clinical Features

- Fever, malaise, night sweats, weight loss
- Hematuria (sometimes macroscopic)
- Loin pain
- Symptoms of bladder involvement (frequency, dysuria)
- Chronic renal failure due to urinary tract obstruction or destruction of kidney tissue.

Investigations

- WBCs (pyuria) are present in the urine but routine urine cultures are negative ('sterile pyuria'). Early morning urine specimens should be examined by special techniques of microscopy and culture to detect tuberculous bacilli.
- Cystoscopy to assess bladder involvement.
- Chest X-ray to look for pulmonary tuberculosis.
- Montoux test may be positive.
- Ultrasound and CT abdomen to assess kidneys and bladder.
- IVU (Intravenous urography): To assess distortion of kidneys and ureteric strictures.

Treatment

- Antituberculous therapy as for pulmonary tuberculosis.
- Surgery may be required to relieve urinary tract obstruction or to remove a severely infected kidney.

Q. Renal artery stenosis (RAS).

- Renal artery stenosis refers to narrowing of one or both renal arteries. >70% narrowing is associated with reduction of blood flow to kidneys (**Fig. 8.14**).

TABLE 8.7: Key differences between types of RTA

Feature	Type 1	Type 2	Type 4
Mechanism of acidosis	Impaired H^+ secretion in distal tubule	Impaired HCO_3^- reabsorption in proximal tubule	Hypoaldosteronism or resistance to aldosterone
Site	Distal tubule	Proximal tubule	Collecting duct
Urine pH	>5.5	Initially high, later <5.5	<5.5
Potassium	Low	Low or normal	High
Risk of stones	High	No	No
Fanconi features	No	Yes	No
Treatment	Sodium bicarbonate or potassium citrate	Large doses of bicarbonate, thiazide diuretics	Fludrocortisone (if hypoaldosteronism), dietary K^+ restriction

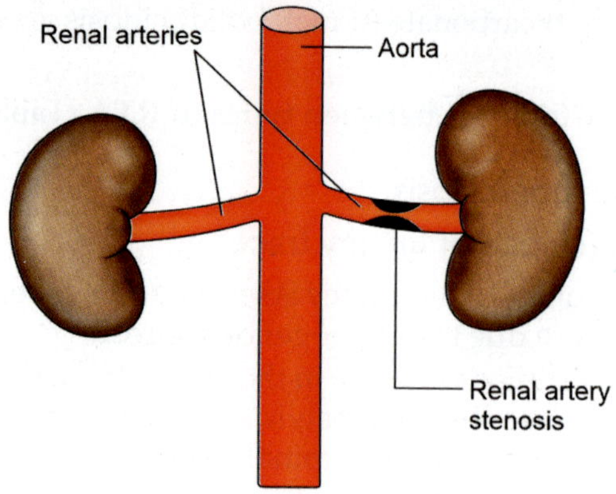

Figure 8.14: Renal artery stenosis

Etiology

- Atherosclerosis (most common cause)
- Fibromuscular dysplasia
- Vasculitis (Takayasu's, PAN).

Clinical Features

- Hypertension is present if RAS is unilateral. Hypertension is due to activation of the renin-angiotensin system in response to renal ischemia. Hypertension is severe, and may be difficult to control.
- Renal failure if RAS is bilateral.
- Evidence of vascular disease elsewhere especially in the legs.
- Deterioration of renal function with ACE inhibitors. This happens because ACE inhibitors or angiotensin II receptor antagonists block efferent arteriolar vasoconstriction which maintains glomerular filtration pressure in ischemic kidney.
- Repeated flash pulmonary edema.

Investigations

- Ultrasound abdomen: shows asymmetry in kidney size in unilateral RAS and bilaterally shrunken kidneys in bilateral RAS.
- Renal artery Doppler can identify significant renal artery stenosis.
- Renal isotope scanning may show delayed uptake of isotope and reduced excretion by the affected kidney, but this is unreliable in the presence of renal impairment.
- Renal arteriography is the definitive test, but is invasive and carries the risk of contrast nephropathy.
- MR angiography and spiral CT angiography are noninvasive are being increasingly used.

Management

- Medical management with antihypertensives, low-dose aspirin and lipid-lowering drugs.
- Angioplasty, with placement of stents.
- Surgical resection of the stenosed segment and re-anastomosis.

Q. Renal cell carcinoma (RCC); renal adenocarcinoma.

- Renal cell carcinoma (RCC) is the most common malignant tumor of the kidney in adults. It is an adenocarcinoma and arises from renal tubules; most commonly from the proximal convoluted tubule.
- It can spread into the renal pelvis, causing hematuria, along the renal vein into the inferior vena cava and to perinephric tissues. Lymphatic spread occurs to para-aortic nodes, and blood-borne metastases can occur to anywhere in the body.

Risk Factors

- Smoking doubles the risk
- Obesity
- Excess use of phenacetin
- Acquired cystic kidney disease in dialysis patients.
- Some familial syndromes, particularly von Hippel–Lindau disease.
- Exposure to certain radiopaque dyes, asbestos, cadmium, and leather tanning and petroleum products.

Clinical Features

- It is twice as common in males as in females. The peak incidence is between 50 and 70 years of age, and it is uncommon before 40.
- Symptoms usually do not appear until late, when the tumor may already be large and metastatic.
- Most common manifestation is gross or microscopic hematuria.
- Weight loss, fever, malaise
- Hypertension (due to renin secretion)
- Polycythemia (due to erythropoietin)
- Loin pain, abdominal mass may be present
- RCC may secrete many substances leading to various paraneoplastic syndromes. These include fever, hypercalcemia, anemia, thrombocytosis, neuropathy, etc.

Investigations

- Ultrasound abdomen: Distinguishes between solid tumor and simple renal cysts.
- CT abdomen and chest: Helps in knowing the extent and staging of tumor.
- Biopsy of the lesion.

Management

- Radical nephrectomy is performed wherever possible. This includes the removal of kidney, perirenal fascial envelope and ipsilateral para-aortic lymph nodes. Radical nephrectomy should be considered even when metastases are present, because this leads to reduction of systemic effects and regression of metastases.
- Advanced/metastatic RCC: Immunotherapy with checkpoint inhibitors (nivolumab, ipilimumab), or tyrosine kinase inhibitors (sunitinib, pazopanib), or mTOR inhibitors (everolimus, temsirolimus) may be considered.
- RCC is resistant to radiotherapy and chemotherapy.

Chapter 9

Endocrinology and Diabetes Mellitus

Q. What is endocrinology? Mention the major endocrine organs and their functions.

- Endocrinology is the branch of medicine that focuses on the endocrine system, its diseases, and the hormones it produces.

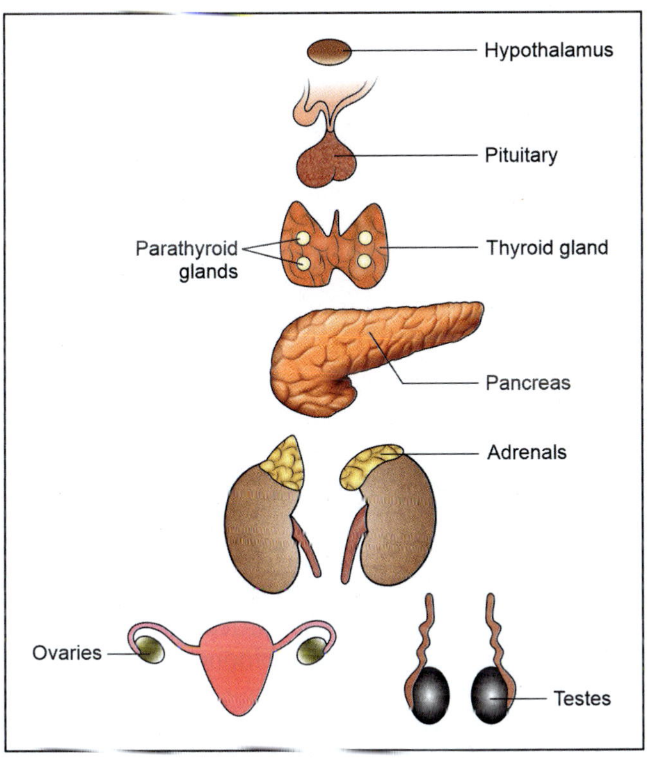

Figure 9.1: Major endocrine glands

Key Endocrine Glands and Hormones

(Fig. 9.1 and Table 9.1)

TABLE 9.1: Key endocrine glands and hormones

Gland	Major hormones	Primary functions
Hypothalamus	TRH, CRH, GnRH, GHRH	Regulates pituitary gland
Pituitary	GH, TSH, ACTH, LH, FSH, PRL, ADH, oxytocin	Controls other endocrine glands (master gland)
Thyroid	T3, T4, calcitonin	Metabolism, growth, calcium regulation
Parathyroid	Parathyroid hormone (PTH)	Increases blood calcium
Adrenal glands	Cortisol, aldosterone, adrenaline	Stress response, blood pressure, electrolyte balance
Pancreas	Insulin, glucagon, somatostatin	Blood sugar regulation
Ovaries	Estrogen, progesterone	Sexual development and reproductive function in females
Testes	Testosterone	Sexual development and reproductive function in females

Q. Enumerate the common presenting complaints of endocrine dysfunction.

Easy fatigability: Hypothyroidism, diabetes mellitus, hyperparathyroidism, hypogonadism, adrenal insufficiency, Cushing's syndrome
Weight gain: Hypothyroidism, Cushing's syndrome
Weight loss: Thyrotoxicosis, adrenal insufficiency, diabetes mellitus
Amenorrhea/oligomenorrhea: Menopause, polycystic ovarian syndrome, hyperprolactinemia, hypothyroidism, thyrotoxicosis, premature ovarian failure, Cushing's syndrome
Precocious puberty: Gonadotrophin excess
Delayed puberty: Hypopituitarism, hypogonadism
Polyuria and polydipsia: Diabetes mellitus, diabetes insipidus, hyperparathyroidism (due to hypercalcemia), Conn's syndrome (due to hypokalemia)
Hypertension: Pheochromocytoma, Cushing's syndrome, hypothyroidism
Hypotension, hypoglycemia: Adrenal insufficiency
Heat intolerance: Thyrotoxicosis, menopause
Palpitations: Thyrotoxicosis, pheochromocytoma
Thyroid enlargement: Goiter, Graves' disease, Hashimoto's thyroiditis
Prominence of eyes: Graves' disease
Hirsutism: Polycystic ovarian syndrome, congenital adrenal hyperplasia, Cushing's syndrome
Alopecia: Cushing's syndrome, hypothyroidism

Galactorrhea: Hyperprolactinemia
Loss of libido: Hypogonadism
Visual dysfunction: Pituitary tumor
Headache: Acromegaly, pituitary tumor, pheochromocytoma
Muscle weakness (usually proximal): Thyrotoxicosis, Cushing's syndrome, hypokalemia (e.g. Conn's syndrome), hyperparathyroidism, hypogonadism
Paresthesiae and tetany: Hypoparathyroidism
Recurrent ureteric colic: Hyperparathyroidism (due to hypercalcemia leading to stones)
Coarsening of features: Acromegaly, hypothyroidism

Q. Discuss briefly the anatomy of pituitary gland, hormones secreted and their functions.

Anatomy (Fig. 9.2)

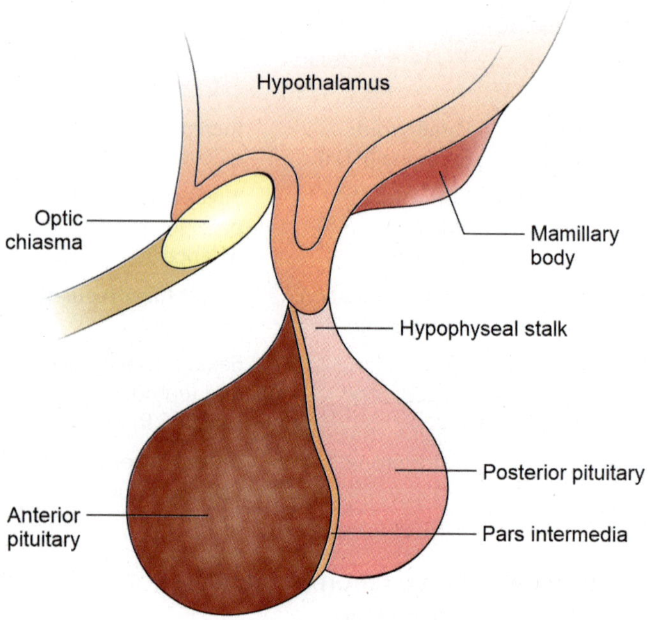

Figure 9.2: Pituitary gland

- Pituitary gland (also called the hypophysis) is a small, pea-sized endocrine gland that lies within the sella turcica of the sphenoid bone and is bridged over by a fold of dura mater.
- It is composed of two predominant lobes, anterior (adenohypophysis) pituitary and posterior (neurohypophysis) pituitary. The intermediate lobe is rudimentary in humans. Anterior pituitary makes up about 75% of the gland.
- Important relations of the gland are sphenoid sinus antero-inferiorly, cavernous sinus (with internal carotid arteries and cranial nerves III, IV, V, and VI) laterally, and optic chiasma anterior to the pituitary stalk.
- The gland is connected to the hypothalamus by the hypophyseal (infundibular) stalk, which has portal vessels carrying blood from the median eminence of the hypothalamus to the anterior lobe and nerve fibers to the posterior lobe.
- Pituitary gland has dual embryologic origin. The anterior pituitary is formed from Rathke's pouch, and posterior pituitary from the floor of the third ventricle.

Hormones Secreted by Pituitary and their Functions (Tables 9.2 and 9.3)

TABLE 9.2: Anterior pituitary hormones

Hormone	Target Organ(s)	Function
Growth Hormone (GH)	Bones, muscles, liver	Stimulates growth, protein synthesis, and fat metabolism
Thyroid-stimulating Hormone (TSH)	Thyroid gland	Stimulates production of thyroid hormones (T3, T4)
Adrenocorticotropic Hormone (ACTH)	Adrenal cortex	Stimulates cortisol production
Follicle-stimulating Hormone (FSH)	Ovaries, testes	Stimulates follicle development and spermatogenesis
Luteinizing Hormone (LH)	Ovaries, testes	Triggers ovulation and testosterone production
Prolactin (PRL)	Mammary glands	Stimulates milk production
Melanocyte-stimulating Hormone (MSH) ***(in humans, minimal role)***	Melanocytes	May influence skin pigmentation slightly

TABLE 9.3: Posterior pituitary hormones ***(produced in the hypothalamus)***

Hormone	Target organ(s)	Function
Antidiuretic Hormone (ADH/ Vasopressin)	Kidneys	Promotes water reabsorption; concentrates urine; raises blood pressure
Oxytocin	Uterus, mammary glands	Stimulates uterine contractions and milk ejection during lactation

Q. Hypopituitarism (panhypopituitarism).

- Hypopituitarism refers to decreased production of hormones by pituitary gland.
- It can result either from diseases of the pituitary gland, or diseases of the hypothalamus leading to deficiency of hypothalamic releasing hormones.
- There may be deficiency of one or more or all the hormones produced by pituitary. When all the anterior pituitary hormones are deficient, it is called panhypopituitarism.

Causes of Hypopituitarism

Pituitary diseases
- Mass lesions-pituitary adenomas, cysts, metastatic cancer
- Trauma (e.g. head injury)
- Postpartum pituitary infarction (Sheehan's syndrome)
- Pituitary surgery
- Pituitary radiation
- Hemorrhage
- Infections (e.g. tuberculosis, syphilis)
- Infiltrative lesions–hemochromatosis, sarcoidosis.

Hypothalamic diseases
Mass lesions, sarcoidosis, surgery, radiotherapy, tuberculosis, hemorrhage.

Clinical Features

- The clinical manifestations of hypopituitarism depend upon the cause as well as the deficiency of each anterior pituitary hormone.
- *Growth hormone deficiency*: It leads to short stature in children. In adults, it may result in diminished muscle mass, increased fat mass and diminished sense of well being.
- *TSH deficiency*: Clinical features are due to accompanying thyroxine deficiency. Features are fatigue, lethargy, cold intolerance, decreased appetite, constipation, facial puffiness, dry skin, bradycardia, delayed relaxation of deep tendon reflexes, and anemia.
- *ACTH deficiency*: Presentation is due to cortisol deficiency. This can be in the form of acute adrenal insufficiency characterized by hypotension. Mild, chronic deficiency causes fatigue, anorexia, weight loss, decreased libido, hypoglycemia, and eosinophilia.
- *Gonadotropin deficiency (FSH and LH)*: It causes hypogonadism in both men and women. Women have ovarian hypofunction resulting in inability to ovulate, infertility, oligomenorrhea or amenorrhea, vaginal dryness and atrophy, and fatigue. Estradiol deficiency causes hot flushes. Men have testicular hypofunction, which results in infertility and decreased testosterone secretion. The latter causes decreased energy and libido and decreased bone mineral density.
- *Prolactin deficiency*: It leads to inability to lactate after delivery.
- Patients with a pituitary or sellar mass may have symptoms related to the mass, such as headache, visual loss, or diplopia.

Investigations

- Serum levels of all the hormones secreted by pituitary gland are low. These are low ACTH, low TSH, low FSH and LH, and low growth hormone. In addition to low levels of these hormones, the corresponding hormones stimulated by these are also low. These include low cortisol, low T3 and T4, low testosterone and low estradiol.
- CT or MRI of the head to identify pituitary pathology.

Treatment

- Treatment of hypopituitarism involves the treatment of each individual target gland hormone deficiencies.
- ACTH deficiency is treated by giving hydrocortisone or other glucocorticoid.
- TSH deficiency, which results in thyroxine deficiency, is treated with L-thyroxine.
- In men with gonadotropin deficiency, testosterone replacement is indicated when fertility is not desired. If fertility is desired, they are treated with gonadotropins. In women with gonadotropin deficiency, estrogen and progesterone replacement is enough if fertility is not desired. If fertility is desired, they should be treated with gonadotropin or pulsatile GnRH therapy to induce ovulation.
- Growth hormone is replaced with recombinant human growth hormone.

Q. Pituitary infarction (Sheehan's syndrome).

- Sheehan's syndrome is a form of ischemic pituitary necrosis that occurs due to severe hypotension or hemorrhagic shock during or after childbirth, leading to anterior pituitary gland failure (hypopituitarism).
- The pituitary gland is physiologically enlarged in pregnancy and is therefore very sensitive to the decreased blood flow caused by massive hemorrhage and hypovolemic shock.
- Typically affects only the anterior lobe; posterior pituitary function (ADH secretion) is usually preserved.
- In developed countries, Sheehan's syndrome is less common due to improved obstetrical care. However, in underdeveloped and developing countries, it remains a common cause of hypopituitarism.

Clinical Features

- Patients often have a history of severe postpartum hemorrhage causing hypotension and requiring blood transfusion.
- Severe hypopituitarism manifests during the first days or weeks after delivery. Less severe hypopituitarism manifests weeks or months after delivery.
- In any postpartum woman with shock, lactation failure, or amenorrhea—always consider Sheehan's syndrome.

Acute Phase (within days)

- Failure to lactate or difficulties with lactation are common initial symptoms of Sheehan's syndrome (due to prolactin deficiency). Hypotension and shock (ACTH deficiency → adrenal insufficiency) may also occur in the acute phase.

Subacute/Chronic Phase (weeks to months/years)

- Many women also report amenorrhea or oligomenorrhea after delivery (due to FSH and LH deficiency). Other features include fatigue, anorexia, weight loss (due to decreased ACTH), and features of hypothyroidism (due to decreased TSH).

Investigations

- Hormone testing: There is deficiency of all the hormones produced by pituitary and also hormones stimulated by pituitary hormones.
  - ↓ ACTH → low cortisol
  - ↓ TSH → low free T4
  - ↓ LH/FSH → low estrogen/progesterone
  - ↓ Prolactin
  - ↓ GH → low IGF-1
- CT scan or MRI show empty sella or pituitary atrophy.

Treatment

- Treatment is same as that for hypopituitarism.

Q. Enumerate the causes of short stature.

- Short stature is defined as a height more than 2 standard deviations below the mean for age and sex (i.e. below the 3rd percentile).

Causes of Short Stature

Normal variants
- Familial short stature
- Constitutional delay of growth and puberty
- Idiopathic short stature

Nutritional
- Malnutrition
- Vitamin or mineral deficiencies (e.g. vitamin D)

Chronic systemic diseases
- Malabsorption syndromes (e.g. celiac disease)
- Inflammatory bowel disease (Crohn's, ulcerative colitis)
- Chronic infections (e.g. tuberculosis, HIV)
- Rheumatologic disease (juvenile rheumatoid arthritis, etc.)
- Renal disease (CKD)
- Pulmonary disease (cystic fibrosis, bronchiectasis)
- Cardiac disease (congenital heart disease)

Endocrine disorders
- Growth hormone deficiency
- Cushing's syndrome
- Hypothyroidism
- Pseudohypoparathyroidism (resistance to parathyroid hormone, short stature, and skeletal abnormalities)
- Precocious puberty (early fusion of epiphyses shortens final height)

Genetic syndromes
- Down syndrome
- Turner syndrome (45,X)–girls only
- Prader-Willi syndrome
- Noonan's syndrome
- Russell-Silver syndrome

Skeletal dysplasias
- Achondroplasia—disproportionate short stature
- Hypochondroplasia

Q. Discuss the etiology, clinical features, investigations, and management of acromegaly/gigantism.

- Acromegaly and gigantism are both caused by excessive secretion of growth hormone (GH).
- Gigantism: GH excess before epiphyseal fusion → abnormal linear growth (tall stature).
- Acromegaly: GH excess after epiphyseal fusion → tissue and bone thickening (not height increase).
- If hypersecretion starts in adolescence and persists into adult life, then the two conditions may be combined.
- The mean age at diagnosis of acromegaly is 40–45 years.

Etiology

- **Pituitary adenoma** (most common cause): Usually a GH-secreting somatotroph adenoma.
- **Pituitary hyperplasia:** Secondary to GHRH excess (e.g. hypothalamic tumor).
- **Ectopic GH or GHRH production:** Example: Pancreatic tumors, small-cell lung carcinoma.
- **McCune-Albright syndrome:** Activating mutations of Gs alpha subunit.
- **Carney complex:** Multiple endocrine tumors, including pituitary.

Clinical Features (Fig. 9.3)

- There is stimulation of growth of many tissues, such as skin, connective tissue, cartilage, bone, viscera, and many epithelial tissues.
- Findings include an enlarged jaw (macrognathia) and enlarged swollen hands and feet. Facial features become coarse, with enlargement of the nose, frontal bones and jaw, and the teeth become spread apart. Macroglossia and enlargement of the soft tissues of the pharynx and larynx lead to obstructive sleep apnea.
- Skin thickness is increased and hyperhidrosis is common. Hair growth increases, and some women have hirsutism.
- Enlargement of synovial tissue and cartilage causes hypertrophic arthropathy of the joints.
- Fatigue and weakness can be prominent symptoms. They may result from sleep apnea, cardiovascular dysfunction, neuropathy, hypogonadism, and hyperglycemia.

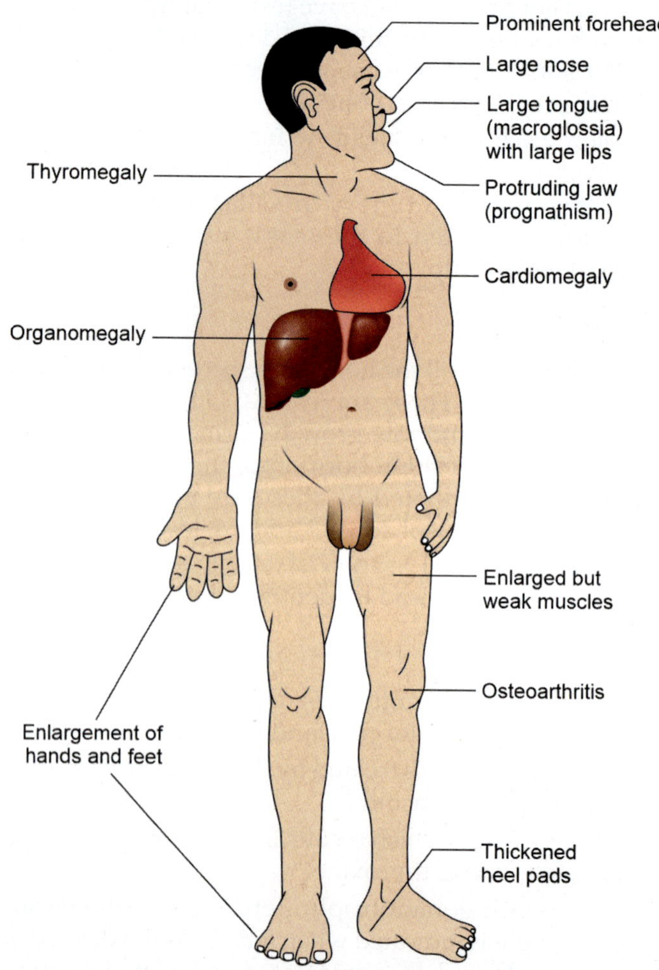

Figure 9.3: Clinical features of acromegaly

- Cardiovascular abnormalities include hypertension, left ventricular hypertrophy, and cardiomyopathy.
- Pituitary adenoma may cause local symptoms such as headache, visual field defects (classically bitemporal hemianopsia due to optic chiasm compression by macroadenoma) and cranial nerve palsies. It may also cause decreased secretion of other pituitary hormones due to its mass effect, most commonly gonadotropins. Many women with acromegaly have menstrual dysfunction, hot flashes and vaginal atrophy due to FSH and LH deficiency.
- There is increased risk of colon cancer and uterine fibroids.
- Mortality is increased in acromegaly due to cardiovascular diseases and cancer.
- Patients with gigantism have tall stature well above age norms.

Investigations

Hormonal Studies

- Insulin-like growth factor-1 (IGF-1) is the mediator of growth hormone actions. Since growth hormone secretion is pulsatile, its measurement is not very reliable and instead IGF-1 measurement can be done as a marker of growth hormone secretion. IGF-I levels are relatively stable and correlate with clinical acromegaly and elevated growth hormone levels. Biochemical diagnosis is made by determining growth hormone and IGF-1 level after OGTT (oral glucose tolerance test) with 75 g glucose. In normal subjects, growth hormone suppresses to below 0.4 µg/L after OGTT. A value greater than 0.4 µg/L of GH after OGTT and high IGF-I levels indicates acromegaly.
- Prolactin concentrations are elevated in about 30% of patients due to cosecretion of prolactin from the pituitary adenoma.

Imaging Studies

- CT or MRI of brain demonstrates pituitary adenoma.
- Skull X-ray may show cortical thickening, enlargement of the frontal sinuses, and enlargement and erosion of the sella turcica. X-rays of the hands show tufting of the terminal phalanges and soft-tissue thickening.

Additional Tests

- Blood glucose levels may be high due to excess growth hormone causing insulin resistance.
- Visual field testing (if tumor near optic chiasm).

Management

Surgical

- Trans-sphenoidal surgery to remove the adenoma is usually the first-line of treatment and may result in cure of GH excess. Surgery is also useful to debulk the tumor followed by second-line therapy.

Medical

- This may be employed in patients in whom surgery is incomplete or contraindicated. Agents which can suppress GH secretion are somatostatin analogs (e.g. octreotide or lanreotide), dopamine agonists (bromocriptine, cabergoline) and GH receptor antagonist (pegvisomant).

Radiotherapy

- Used when surgery and medical treatment fail
- Risk of hypopituitarism.

Q. Growth hormone deficiency.

Causes of Growth Hormone Deficiency

- These are same as the causes listed under hypopituitarism.

Clinical Features

In Children

- Short stature with normal body proportions
- Delayed skeletal maturation
- Increased fat mass (especially abdominal)
- Delayed puberty
- Immature facial features.

In Adults

- Decreased muscle mass and strength
- Increased fat (particularly visceral)
- Reduced bone density (risk of osteoporosis)
- Fatigue
- Dyslipidemia.

Diagnosis

- Reduced serum IGF-1 or growth hormone levels.
- Provocative tests—a subnormal rise in the serum growth hormone concentration after insulin-induced hypoglycemia or after injection of combination of arginine and growth hormone-releasing hormone confirms the diagnosis of growth hormone deficiency.

Treatment

- Recombinant human GH preparations are available. GH is given as subcutaneous injection once a day, usually in the evening.
- All children with GH deficiency should receive recombinant growth hormone to normalize growth and development.
- Growth hormone should also be given to adult patients with severe clinical manifestations and unequivocal biochemical evidence of growth hormone deficiency.
- Dose of GH should be adjusted to maintain serum IGF-1 levels within the normal range.

Q. Hyperprolactinemia; prolactinoma.

Q. Galactorrhea.

- Hyperprolactinemia refers to an abnormally elevated level of prolactin in the blood. Prolactin is a hormone produced by the anterior pituitary gland, primarily responsible for stimulating milk production (lactation) in females.
- Hyperprolactinemia is a common biochemical abnormality.

Causes of Hyperprolactinemia

Physiological
- Stress (e.g. post-seizure)
- Pregnancy
- Lactation
- Nipple stimulation
- Coitus
- Exercise (intense)

Drugs
- Dopamine antagonists (phenothiazines and butyrophenones, antidepressants, metoclopramide, domperidone)
- Dopamine-depleting drugs (reserpine, methyldopa)
- Oral contraceptive pill

Pathological
- Prolactinoma (usually microadenoma)
- Nonfunctioning pituitary adenomas (compressing pituitary stalk)
- Hypothalamic or stalk disorders (tumors, infiltrative diseases, radiation or trauma)
- Polycystic ovarian disease (PCOD)
- Hypothyroidism (via increased TRH stimulating prolactin)
- Renal failure (reduced clearance)
- Ectopic source

Clinical Features

- The cardinal features are galactorrhea and hypogonadism. Galactorrhea refers to lactation without breastfeeding. Prolactin stimulates milk secretion but not breast development, hence galactorrhea is not seen in men, but can occur if there is gynecomastia.
- In women, there is also hypogonadism leading to secondary amenorrhea, anovulation and infertility.
- In men there is decreased libido, reduced shaving frequency and lethargy.
- There may be headache and visual field defects due to mass effect of prolactinoma.

Investigations

- Pregnancy should be excluded by urine pregnancy test and ultrasound in all women of child-bearing age.
- Serum prolactin levels are raised.
- Thyroid function tests to exclude primary hypothyroidism causing TRH-induced prolactin excess.
- MRI or CT scan of head to exclude hypothalamic or pituitary tumor.
- Assessment of other pituitary hormones in patients with a macroadenoma.

Management

- Underlying cause of hyperprolactinemia should be corrected. Examples are stopping offending drugs, correcting primary hypothyroidism, etc.
- Prolactinomas can be treated by the following ways:
  - *Medical*: Dopamine agonist drugs (bromocriptine, cabergoline) are first-line therapy. Dopamine agonists not only lower prolactin levels, but shrink the majority of prolactin-secreting macroadenomas. Cabergoline is the first choice due to more efficacy and lesser side effects.
  - *Surgical*: Surgical removal may be required if the tumor is large and invasive or the patient is unable to tolerate dopamine agonists. Tumor can be removed by trans-sphenoidal surgery.
  - *Radiotherapy*: External irradiation may be required for some macroadenomas to prevent regrowth if dopamine agonists are stopped.

Q. Diabetes insipidus (DI).

- Diabetes insipidus is a condition characterized by excessive excretion of dilute urine (polyuria) and increased thirst (polydipsia) due to either deficiency of antidiuretic hormone (ADH) or renal insensitivity to ADH.
- The posterior lobe of the pituitary is the primary site of ADH storage and release, but ADH is synthesized within the hypothalamus.
- Diabetes insipidus (DI) is of two types: Central DI (now known as arginine vasopressin deficiency), and nephrogenic DI.

Etiology

Central (damage to hypothalamus or posterior pituitary)
- Idiopathic (most common cause)
- Structural hypothalamic or high stalk lesion
- Familial disease (DIDMOAD syndrome-association of diabetes insipidus with diabetes mellitus, optic atrophy, deafness).
- Neurosurgery or trauma
- Cancer (primary brain tumors, metastases)
- Hypoxic encephalopathy
- Infiltrative disorders (histiocytosis, sarcoidosis)

Nephrogenic
- Genetic defects (vasopressin-2 receptor mutation, aquaporin-2 mutation, cystinosis)
- Metabolic abnormality (hypokalemia, hypercalcemia)
- Drugs (lithium, demeclocycline)
- Poisoning (heavy metals)
- Polycystic kidney disease

Clinical Features

- Polyuria and polydipsia: Polyuria has generally been defined as a urine output exceeding 3 L/day in adults. Polyuria leads to excess thirst and polydipsia.
- Nocturia
- Signs of dehydration (if fluid intake is inadequate).

Investigations

- Confirm the presence of polyuria by measuring 24-hour urine volume (>3 liters per day).
- Decide whether polyuria is due to solute diuresis (osmotic diuresis). Examples are hyperglycemia, hypercalcemia, mannitol, etc. Solute diuresis should be suspected when urine osmolality >600 mosmol/kg with a normal serum sodium. In such cases, serum glucose, urea, calcium, potassium, and sodium should be measured.

- Urine osmolality between 300 and 600 mosmol/kg can suggest the possibility of solute diuresis, primary polydipsia, or an arginine vasopressin disorder (central DI). Further testing is needed in such cases as it is difficult to decide the exact cause of polyuria here.
- Polyuric patients with a low urine osmolality of <300 mosmol/kg have either primary polydipsia or an arginine vasopressin disorder. Further testing involves water restriction test to distinguish between polyuria due to psychogenic polydipsia and true DI and, if necessary, administration of desmopressin to distinguish between central and nephrogenic DI.
- *Water restriction test:* This is done to distinguish between polyuria due to psychogenic polydipsia and true DI. Patient is advised not to take any fluids for many hours and his body weight, urine volume, plasma and urine osmolality are monitored hourly. Patients with diabetes insipidus continue to pass large quantity of dilute urine in spite of water deprivation whereas patients with primary polydipsia would pass less amount of concentrated urine. In addition, there is rise in serum osmolality and sodium concentration in diabetes insipidus as there is depletion of plasma volume. When plasma osmolality rises above 300 mOsm/kg, exogenous desmopressin (DDAVP) is given. Central diabetes insipidus is confirmed if urine osmolality rises by at least 50% after DDAVP. Nephrogenic diabetes insipidus is confirmed if desmopressin (DDAVP) does not concentrate the urine.
- *Desmopressin (DDAVP) test:* The test assesses the kidney's response to desmopressin, a synthetic analog of arginine vasopressin (AVP or ADH), which promotes water reabsorption in the kidneys. Desmopressin is given in an initial dose of 10 µg intranasally. Urine osmolality is measured before and after administration (usually at 1–2 hours post-DDAVP). In patients with central diabetes insipidus, there is significant increase (>50%) in urine osmolality. In nephrogenic diabetes insipidus, there is minimal or no increase (<10%) in urine osmolality.
- MRI of the pituitary and hypothalamus to look for mass lesions.

Management

- Treatment of central diabetes insipidus is with desmopressin (DDAVP) which is an ADH analog. Desmopressin is usually administered as a metered dose spray into the nose. In emergencies, desmopressin is given by intramuscular injection. The dose of desmopressin is adjusted to keep the plasma sodium concentrations and/or osmolality in the normal range. The main side effect of desmopressin is excess water retention and hyponatremia.
- Nephrogenic diabetes insipidus is treated by thiazide diuretics (has paradoxical effect of reducing urine volume in diabetes insipidus), amiloride, and NSAIDs (e.g. indomethacin).

Q. Thyroid function tests.

- Thyroid function tests are a group of blood tests used to evaluate how well the thyroid gland is working. These tests help diagnose and monitor hypothyroidism, hyperthyroidism, and other thyroid disorders.
- Thyroid secretes T4 (thyroxine) and T3 (triiodothyronine) which is regulated by pituitary TSH. TSH secretion, in turn, is controlled through negative feedback by thyroid hormones. TSH secretion is regulated by thyroid releasing hormone (TRH) from hypothalamus.
- Thyroid function is assessed by one or more of the following tests **(Table 9.4)**.
    - Serum TSH concentration
    - Serum total T3 and T4 concentration
    - Serum free T3 and T4.

TABLE 9.4: Thyroid function tests

TSH	T3, T4	Interpretation
Normal TSH (0.4–4 mIU/L)	Normal T3 (80–220 ng/dl), T4 (4.5 to 11.5 µg/dl)	Euthyroid
Low TSH	High T3, T4	Primary hyperthyroidism (problem in thyroid gland)
High TSH	Low T3, T4	Primary hypothyroidism (problem in thyroid gland)
High TSH	High T3, T4	TSH-mediated hyperthyroidism (problem in pituitary)
Low TSH	Low T3, T4	Central hypothyroidism (problem in pituitary)

When to use free T3 and free T4 instead of total T3 and T4

- Free T3 and Free T4 are the biologically active forms of thyroid hormones that are not bound to plasma proteins. They provide a more accurate picture of thyroid function in many clinical situations which are as follows.
- ***Pregnancy:*** Increased thyroid-binding globulin (TBG) leads to elevated total T3/T4, but free levels may remain normal.
- ***Use of oral contraceptives or estrogen therapy*:** These increase TBG → falsely elevated total T4/T3. Free levels better reflect true thyroid function.
- ***Liver disease, nephrotic syndrome*:** Lower TBG levels → decreased total T4/T3, but free levels remain normal.
- ***Critical illness or hospitalized patients*:** Total T3/T4 may be low due to nonthyroidal illness (euthyroid sick syndrome). Free hormone levels help differentiate this from true hypothyroidism.
- ***Suspected central (secondary or tertiary) hypothyroidism*:** TSH may be normal or low. In such situation free T4 is more reliable as it is not affected by other factors.
- ***Discordant lab results*:** When TSH is abnormal, but total T3/T4 are normal, measuring free T3/T4 can clarify the diagnosis.

Q. Radionuclide thyroid scanning

- Radionuclide thyroid scanning is a nuclear medicine imaging technique used to evaluate the structure and function of the thyroid gland. It involves the administration of a small amount of radioactive material (radiotracer) that is selectively taken up by thyroid tissue.

Common Radiotracers Used

- Technetium-99 (Tc-99m)—commonly used due to lower radiation exposure and rapid imaging. Technetium-99 is injected intravenously and images of the thyroid are obtained with gamma camera approximately 20 minutes later.
- Iodine-123 (I-123)—preferred for more accurate functional assessment.
- Iodine-131 (I-131)—less commonly used for imaging due to higher radiation; more commonly used for therapy.

Indications

- Evaluation of thyroid nodules (e.g. to differentiate hot *vs.* cold nodules).
- Diagnosis and assessment of hyperthyroidism.
- Investigation of ectopic thyroid tissue (e.g. lingual thyroid).
- Evaluation of goiters.
- Posttreatment monitoring in thyroid cancer (especially with I-131).

Interpretation of Results (Fig. 9.4)

- Uniform tracer uptake throughout the thyroid suggests normal thyroid gland with normal function.
- Increased uniform radionuclide uptake is seen in Graves' disease.

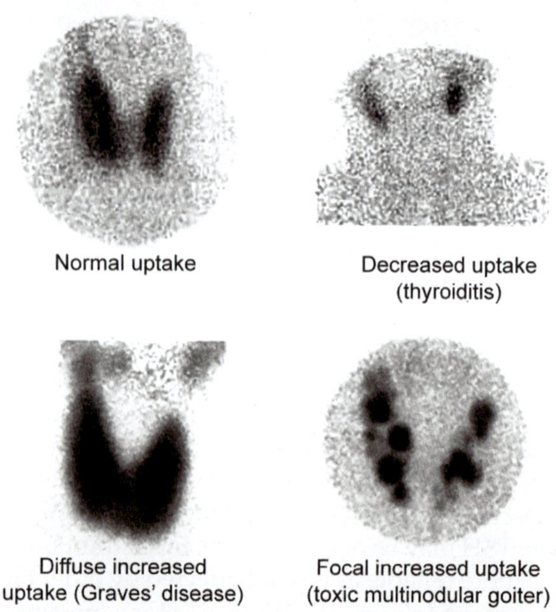

Figure 9.4: Appearance of radioisotope scan in different thyroid diseases

- Toxic adenomas appear as focal areas of increased uptake, with suppressed uptake in the remainder of the gland.
- In toxic multinodular goiter, there are multiple areas of relatively increased or decreased uptake.
- Subacute thyroiditis is associated with very low uptake.
- Thyroid scanning is also used in the follow-up of thyroid cancer. After thyroidectomy and radioablation using radioactive iodine, there is diminished radionuclide uptake in the thyroid gland. Areas of uptake indicate residual or metastatic thyroid cancer tissue.

Contraindication

- Pregnancy and breastfeeding (due to radiation).

Q. Discuss the etiology, clinical features, investigations and management of hyperthyroidism (thyrotoxicosis).

- Hyperthyroidism refers to increased synthesis and secretion of thyroid hormones which leads to the hyper-metabolic state.
- Hyperthyroidism and thyrotoxicosis are closely related but not synonymous. Hyperthyroidism is a condition where the thyroid gland itself produces excess thyroid hormones (T3 and T4). It is a cause of thyrotoxicosis.
- Thyrotoxicosis is a clinical state resulting from excess circulating thyroid hormones, regardless of the source. It includes all causes of excess thyroid hormone in the body, not just from the thyroid gland. For example, excess thyroid hormone supplementation causes thyrotoxicosis but cannot be called as hyperthyroidism. Thyroiditis (e.g. subacute, silent, or postpartum thyroiditis causes hormone leakage without increased synthesis and hence is a cause of thyrotoxicosis but cannot be called hyperthyroidism.

Causes of Hyperthyroidism

Primary hyperthyroidism

- Graves' disease *(most common cause)*—autoimmune stimulation of TSH receptors
- Toxic multinodular goiter (Plummer's disease)—autonomous hormone production from multiple nodules
- Toxic adenoma—single hyperfunctioning thyroid nodule
- Thyroiditis—transient release of hormones (e.g. subacute, silent, postpartum thyroiditis)
- Metastatic follicular thyroid cancer
- Excessive iodine intake *(Jod-Basedow phenomenon)*
- Drug-induced, e.g. amiodarone (can cause both hypothyroidism and hyperthyroidism)

Secondary hyperthyroidism

- TSH-secreting pituitary adenoma *(rare)*
- hCG-producing tumors, e.g. molar pregnancy or choriocarcinoma

Exogenous thyrotoxicosis

- Excessive intake of thyroid hormones (factitious)

Clinical Features

General
- Weight loss despite normal or increased appetite
- Heat intolerance
- Fatigue
- Goiter with bruit
- Single or multiple nodules may be present in the thyroid

GIT
- Diarrhea, hyperdefecation
- Anorexia
- Vomiting

CVS
- Systolic hypertension/increased pulse pressure
- Palpitations
- Sinus tachycardia
- Atrial fibrillation
- High output cardiac failure
- Angina

RS
- Exacerbation of asthma
- Dyspnea on exertion

Hematological
- Lymphadenopathy
- Normochromic normocytic anemia (due to increased plasma volume)

Nervous system
- Tremor
- Muscle weakness
- Periodic paralysis due to hypokalemia caused by increased Na^+/K^+-ATPase activity in skeletal muscles.
- Hyperreflexia
- Ill-sustained clonus
- Proximal myopathy
- Bulbar myopathy

Skin
- Warm, moist skin
- Increased sweating
- Pruritus
- Hair thinning, alopecia
- Palmar erythema
- Pretibial myxedema
- Onycholysis
- Hyperpigmentation
- Vitiligo can occur in association with autoimmune thyroid disorders

Genitourinary system
- Amenorrhea/oligomenorrhea
- Infertility, spontaneous abortion
- Loss of libido, impotence
- Gynecomastia
- Urinary frequency and nocturia

Eyes
- Stare and lid lag
- Gritty feeling or pain in the eyes
- Excessive lacrimation
- Diplopia
- Loss of acuity
- Exophthalmos
- Periorbital and conjuctival edema
- Corneal ulceration
- Ophthalmoplegia
- Papilledema

Bone
- Osteoporosis (fracture, loss of height)

Psychiatric
- Anxiety, irritability, emotional lability, psychosis

- About one-third of elderly patients with hyperthyroidism may be apathetic (apathetic or masked hyperthyroidism), rather than having hyperactivity, tremor, and other symptoms of sympathetic overactivity. Tachycardia may be absent because of coexisting conduction abnormality.

Investigations

- Serum T3 and T4 are elevated.
- Serum TSH is low in primary thyrotoxicosis (problem in thyroid gland) and high in TSH induced thyrotoxicosis (e.g. pituitary adenoma secreting TSH).
- TSH receptor antibodies (TRAb) are elevated in Graves' disease.
- Antithyroid peroxidase (anti-TPO) antibody titers are significantly elevated in Graves' disease, and usually are low or absent in toxic multinodular goiter and toxic adenoma.
- Isotope scanning may show increased or decreased uptake depending on the cause. Increased uptake is seen in Graves' disease. Decreased uptake is seen in thyroiditis. Radioiodine uptake tests have been largely superseded by 99m technetium scintigraphy scans which are quicker to perform with a lower dose of radioactivity, and provide a higher resolution image.
- Thyroid ultrasound can identify nodules and distinguish solid from cystic lesions. Ultrasound-guided FNAC helps in obtaining cytologic material from nodules that are difficult to identify by palpation.

Management

- Definitive treatment of thyrotoxicosis depends on the underlying cause and may include antithyroid drugs, radioactive iodine or surgery.

Antithyroid Drugs

- These drugs decrease the thyroid hormone synthesis and release from thyroid gland. The thionamide derivatives, propylthiouracil (PTU), methimazole and carbimazole are the drugs of first choice in Graves' disease. These drugs interfere with organification and iodotyrosine coupling by inhibiting the peroxidase enzyme.
- These drugs are rapidly absorbed from GIT and concentrated in the thyroid. PTU inhibits peripheral conversion of T4 to T3, contributing 10–20% to the decrease in T3 levels. This effect is not seen

with methimazole and carbimazole. Both PTU and methimazole cross the placenta and can interfere with fetal thyroid function. PTU can cause hepatic failure and hence, used only in first trimester of pregnancy.

- Methimazole is started at a dose of 5–10 mg OD. Improvement of thyrotoxic symptoms usually takes 2–3 weeks. Thyroid hormone values are checked 4 weeks after the start of therapy and if there is no improvement in thyroid function tests, the dose may be increased to 30–40 mg a day. Once thyroid hormone levels normalize, the dose is decreased. Most patients can be maintained on low doses of 2.5–5 mg of methimazole. Methimazole is the preferred drug except in first trimester of pregnancy.
- PTU is given at a dose of 100–150 mg every 8 hours.
- The most important side effect of antithyroid drugs is agranulocytosis. Patients should be told to discontinue their medication and contact their physician when fever occurs or infection develops, especially in the oropharynx. If agranulocytosis develops, antithyroid drugs should be discontinued and broad-spectrum antibiotics should be given. Other treatment modalities such as radioactive iodine should be chosen for further treatment.

Radioactive Iodine

- Radioactive iodine (^{131}I) is used to treat hyperthyroidism in older patients with moderate hyperthyroidism and thyroid enlargement, for patients with a prior allergic or toxic reaction to the antithyroid medication, poor compliance with antithyroid drugs and after antithyroid drugs have failed to induce a long-term euthyroid state.
- Radioiodine treatment is contraindicated during pregnancy and pregnancy should be avoided for 6–12 months after radioiodine treatment.
- Antithyroid drugs should be stopped for 3 or 4 days before radioiodine administration. A dose of 5–10 mCi is usually required. Improvement in thyrotoxicosis occurs after 4–5 weeks, and almost 80% of patients are cured with one dose. The remaining need a second dose, which should be given 6 months after the first dose. After giving radioactive iodine, antithyroid drugs can be added at day 5 to reach a euthyroid state more quickly. Beta-blockers are also used for symptomatic control.
- Rarely radioiodine can induce painful thyroiditis and lead to thyroid storm. Hypothyroidism is a risk and more than 50% of patients become hypothyroid after radioiodine treatment.

Surgical Therapy

- Subtotal thyroidectomy can be used to treat hyperthyroidism in the following situations.
  - Patients with large goiter causing obstructive symptoms.
  - Malignant thyroid nodule.
  - Pregnant women with severe hyperthyroidism, which is difficult to control with antithyroid drugs.
  - Young patients who are difficult to control on antithyroid drugs.
  - Patients with toxic reactions to antithyroid drugs.
  - Patients who are not candidates for antithyroid drugs and refuse radioactive iodine.
- However, hyperthyroidism should be controlled before surgery using PTU or methimazole. Thyroid surgery is contraindicated in severely hyperthyroid patients as it may precipitate thyroid storm.

Symptomatic Treatment

- In all patients with thyrotoxicosis a nonselective β-blocker such as propranolol or nadolol should be used to control symptoms such as tachycardia, palpitations and tremors.

Q. Discuss the etiology, pathogenesis, clinical features, investigations and management of Graves' disease.

- Graves' disease, first described by Robert Graves is an autoimmune disorder and the most common cause of hyperthyroidism.
- It is characterized by the overproduction of thyroid hormones due to stimulation of the thyroid gland by autoantibodies.
- The terms Graves' disease and hyperthyroidism are not synonymous, because some patients with Graves' disease have ophthalmopathy but no hyperthyroidism.

Etiology and Pathogenesis

- Graves' disease is an autoimmune disorder and is caused by autoantibodies to the TSH receptors (TSHR-Ab) that activate the receptor, thereby stimulating thyroid hormone synthesis and secretion as well as thyroid growth (causing goiter). These antibodies are produced by B lymphocytes.
- Infiltrative opthalmopathy and dermopathy are specific to Graves' disease and are due to immunologically mediated activation of fibroblasts in extraocular muscles and skin, with accumulation of glycosaminoglycans leading to water trapping and edema initially, followed by fibrosis later.
- There is a genetic predisposition for Graves' disease as evidenced by strong association of Graves' disease with HLA-B8, DR3 and DR2, and high concordance rate in monozygotic twins. Viral and bacterial infections have been suspected to trigger the development of thyrotoxicosis in genetically susceptible individuals. *Escherichia coli* and *Yersinia enterocolitica* possess cell membrane TSH receptors; antibodies to these microbial antigens may cross-react with the TSH receptors on the host thyroid follicular cell.
- Iodine supplementation in iodine deficient areas can trigger the development of thyrotoxicosis in those with pre-existing subclinical Graves' disease.
- Histologic examination of the thyroid gland shows follicular hyperplasia, and patchy lymphocytic infiltration.

Clinical Features

- Features of hyperthyroidism (discussed under hyperthyroidism).
- Features specific to Graves' disease are ophthalmopathy and infiltrative dermopathy (pretibial myxedema).
- Ophthalmopathy leads to proptosis and lid retraction preventing complete eye closure of the eyes, resulting in exposure keratitis and corneal ulceration. Compression of the optic nerve at the posterior apex by enlarged muscles may lead to blurring and impaired visual acuity, visual field defects, impairment of color vision, and papilledema.
- Treatment of ophthalmopathy involves prevention of drying and infection of the cornea by applying artificial tears and antibiotic drops. Surgical decompression may be required in severe proptosis with optic nerve compression.

Investigations and Treatment

- This is same as that discussed under hyperthyroidism.

Q. Thyroid dermopathy (pretibial myxedema or infiltrative dermopathy).

- Thyroid dermopathy, also known as pretibial myxedema, is a localized skin manifestation most commonly associated with Graves' disease. It represents infiltrative dermopathy due to the accumulation of mucopolysaccharides in the skin.
- The incidence of thyroid dermopathy has declined due to earlier diagnosis and treatment of Graves' disease.

Pathology and Pathogenesis

- Thyroid dermopathy occurs due to the accumulation of glycosaminoglycans, especially hyaluronic acid in the dermis. Characteristic pathologic changes are mucinous edema and the fragmentation of collagen fibers.
- The exact cause of thyroid dermopathy is not proven. These patients have higher serum concentrations of TSH receptor antibodies than patients without dermopathy. TSH receptors have been found in skin fibroblasts. TSH-receptor antibodies probably act on these receptors and stimulate the production of glycosaminoglycans.

Investigations

- Thyroid function tests: Usually show hyperthyroidism (↓TSH, ↑T3/T4).
- Autoantibodies: TRAb (thyrotropin receptor antibodies), TSI (thyroid-stimulating immunoglobulin) often elevated.
- Skin biopsy (not commonly done).

Clinical Features

- Most commonly affected areas are anterior aspects of the lower legs (pretibial region), but can involve feet, upper limbs, or other areas.
- Appearance: Waxy thickened skin, non-pitting edema, reddish-brown or skin-colored plaques or nodules, "peau d'orange" (orange peel) texture, and hair loss over the lesions (**Fig. 9.5**).

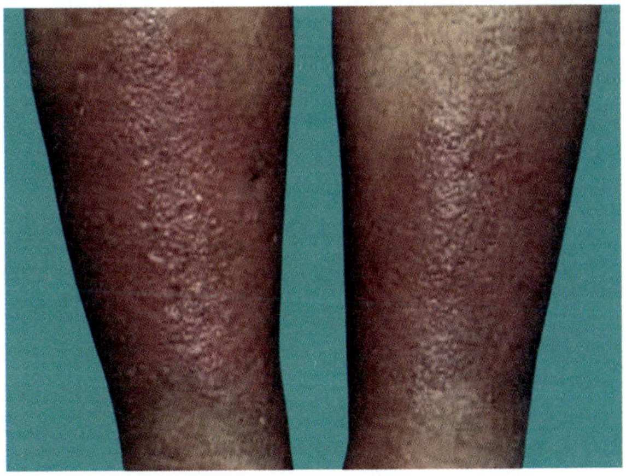

Figure 9.5: Graves' dermopathy

Treatment

- Treat underlying Graves' disease.
- Most patients are asymptomatic and do not require treatment. Indications for treatment are pruritus, local discomfort, or the unsightly appearance.
- The only effective treatment is topical application of a glucocorticoid ointment covered by an occlusive dressing (e.g. 0.02% fluocinolone under plastic wrap) at night. Resistant lesions may require systemic glucocorticoid therapy.

Q. Thyrotoxic crisis ('thyroid storm').

- This is a life-threatening increase in the severity of the clinical features of thyrotoxicosis. It is the most extreme state of thyrotoxicosis and is a medical emergency.
- It is rare and occurs in patients with Graves' disease or toxic multinodular goiter.

Etiology/Precipitating Factors

- Infection
- Trauma to the thyroid gland
- After thyroid or non-thyroid surgery in a patient with poorly controlled hyperthyroidism
- After radioiodine therapy
- Uncontrolled diabetes or ketoacidosis
- Myocardial infarction or stroke.

Clinical Features

- Patients usually present with exaggerated features of hyperthyroidism along with multisystem involvement. Involvement of CNS, CVS, and GI tract is common.
- Hyperpyrexia (often >38.5°C, may exceed 40°C)
- CNS symptoms: Agitation, confusion, psychosis, stupor, or coma
- CVS symptoms. Tachycardia, atrial fibrillation and cardiac failure

- GI symptoms: Severe nausea, vomiting, or diarrhea, and hepatic failure with jaundice.

Investigations

- Elevated T3, T4 and suppressed TSH levels. Rarely TSH may be elevated in instances of excess TSH secretion.
- CBC shows mild leukocytosis, with a shift to the left.
- LFTs show elevated levels of alanine aminotransferase (ALT) and aspartate aminotransferase (AST).
- ECG may show arrhythmias such as atrial fibrillation.

Treatment

Supportive Care

- IV fluids, oxygen, cooloing measures.

Block Peripheral Effects

- Beta-blockers to control symptoms of sympathetic over-activity. Propranolol can be given orally (80 mg 6-hourly) or intravenously (1–5 mg 6-hourly).

Inhibit Hormone Synthesis

- Propylthiouracil 600–1000 mg loading dose followed by 200 mg every four hours inhibits the synthesis of new thyroid hormone. **Propylthiouracil is preferred over methimazole** for treatment of severe thyroid storm because of its early onset of action and capacity to inhibit peripheral conversion of T4 to T3. Methimazole can be used if PTU is not available.
- If the patient is unconscious these drugs can be given through Ryle's tube. Both drugs can also be suspended in liquid for rectal administration. Parenteral preparations of these drugs are not available.

Inhibit Hormone Release (after antithyroid drug)

- Iodine compounds (Lugol iodine or potassium iodide) orally inhibit the peripheral conversion of T4 to T3 and also the release of thyroid hormones. Iodinated radiocontrast such as sodium ipodate can be given intravenously if available and is more effective than potassium iodide or Lugol's solution.
- Given 1 hour after PTU.

Prevent Peripheral Conversion

- Glucocorticoids reduce conversion of T4 to T3. Give hydrocortisone 100 mg IV q8h.

Treat Precipitating Cause

- Antibiotics if infection present, treatment of DKA, etc.

Prognosis

- High mortality (10–30%) even with treatment.
- Early recognition and aggressive therapy are critical.

Q. Enumerate the causes of hypothyroidism.

Q. Discuss the clinical features, diagnosis, and management of primary hypothyroidism.

Etiology of Hypothyroidism

Primary hypothyroidism (problem in the thyroid gland)
- Chronic autoimmune (Hashimoto's) thyroiditis
- Iatrogenic (thyroidectomy, radioiodine therapy or external irradiation)
- Iodine deficiency or excess
- Drugs (thionamides, lithium, amiodarone)
- Infiltrative diseases (Riedel's thyroiditis, hemochromatosis, sarcoidosis, amyloidosis)
- Subacute thyroiditis (deQuervain's)—may result in transient hypothyroidism
- Postpartum thyroiditis.
- Congenital causes (thyroid agenesis, dysgenesis, or defects in hormone synthesis)

Secondary (central) hypothyroidism: TSH deficiency.

Tertiary hypothyroidism: Hypothalamic dysfunction (↓ TRH).

- Primary hypothyroidism refers to hypothyroidism caused by disease of the thyroid gland itself. Decreased secretion of T3 and T4 leads to compensatory increase in TSH secretion. Thus, the combination of a low serum T3, T4 and a high serum TSH concentration indicates primary hypothyroidism.
- Two forms of primary hypothyroidism can be recognized:
  - *Subclinical hypothyroidism*—is defined as a high serum TSH concentration in the presence of normal serum free T4 and T3 concentrations. These patients are usually asymptomatic.
  - *Overt hypothyroidism*—is defined as a high serum TSH concentration in the presence of a low serum free T4 concentration. These patients are usually symptomatic.
- Secondary and tertiary hypothyroidism refers to diseases of pituitary or hypothalamus leading to TSH or TRH deficiency causing hypothyroidism.

Clinical Features

General: Weight gain, fatigue, somnolence, cold intolerance, hoarseness of voice, slurred speech, puffy face and loss of eyebrows

Skin: Dry, cold and pale skin, decreased sweating, nonpitting edema (myxedema), carotenemia, coarse hair and hair loss, xanthelasma

Hematologic: Anemia, macrocytosis

CVS: Bradycardia, diastolic hypertension, reduced cardiac output, angina, pericardial effusion

RS: Hypoventilation, sleep apnea, exertional dyspnea, pleural effusion

GIT: Enlargement of the tongue, constipation (due to decreased gut motility), ileus, decreased taste sensation, ascites

Reproductive system: Oligomenorrhea, amenorrhea or menorrhagia, decreased fertility, increased risk of abortion, decreased libido, erectile dysfunction, delayed ejaculation

Neuropsychiatric: Encephalopathy, myxedema coma, mental retardation in children, carpal tunnel syndrome, cerebellar ataxia, depression, psychosis, myotonia, delayed relaxation of tendon reflexes.

Musculoskeletal: Slow movement, myalgia, arthralgia, aches and stiffness.

Metabolic: Hyperuricemia, hyponatremia hyperlipidemia.

Investigations

- Serum T3, T4 are low and TSH is elevated (>5) in primary hypothyroidism. In secondary hypothyroidism T3, T4 are low and TSH is also low (all three low).
- Thyroid antibodies (if autoimmune suspected): Anti-TPO antibodies and anti-thyroglobulin antibodies are present in Hashimoto's thyroiditis.
- Thyroid ultrasound if nodules or goiter present.
- MRI of pituitary if secondary hypothyroidism suspected.
- Serum cholesterol, triglycerides, lactate dehydrogenase (LDH), creatinine kinase (CK) and AST may be raised.
- Serum sodium levels may be low.
- Chest X-ray may show cardiomegaly.
- ECG may show sinus bradycardia with low voltage complexes and ST segment and T wave abnormalities.

Treatment

- Hypothyroidism is treated with levothyroxine (T4), with doses ranging from 50 to 200 mcg/day. It is given once a day on an empty stomach, preferably in the morning. Most patients require lifelong treatment and periodic evaluations should be done.
- In young healthy adults without coronary artery disease, a starting dose of 75–100 µg/day can be used and then adjusted every 6–8 weeks to reach the final replacement level. In elderly patients and those with coronary artery disease, the initial dose should be 12.5–25 µg/day and increased by 25–50 µg every 6–8 weeks to avoid precipitating angina and heart failure.
- The aim is to achieve a euthyroid status with TSH, T4, and T3 levels in the normal range. TSH is the most sensitive indicator and treatment should be aimed at normalizing TSH level.
- Note that TSH cannot be used to monitor levothyroxine therapy in secondary hypothyroidism. Instead, free T4 (FT4) is the primary test used for monitoring.

Q. Subclinical hypothyroidism.

- Subclinical hypothyroidism is a mild or early form of thyroid failure where serum TSH is mildly elevated (typically 4.5–10 mIU/L), but free T4 and T3 levels are within normal range.
- Patients usually do not have any clinical symptoms (hence called subclinical) and are picked up by routine testing.
- Some evidence suggests that subclinical hypothyroidism is associated with an increased risk of coronary artery disease (CAD) events, congestive heart failure and fatal stroke.

Causes

- Early Hashimoto's thyroiditis (most common)
- Recovery phase after non-thyroidal illness
- Iodine deficiency or excess
- Post-radioiodine or thyroid surgery
- Drugs: Lithium, amiodarone, interferon-α
- Aging.

Clinical Features

- Often asymptomatic
- May have mild hypothyroid symptoms: fatigue, weight gain, cold intolerance.

Evaluation

- The hallmark of subclinical hypothyroidism is an elevated TSH with a normal free T4. Since many non-thyroidal illnesses can cause elevated TSH, it is better to repeat TSH and T4 measurement after 2–3 months.
- Presence of anti-TPO antibodies should be tested since such patients are more likely to progress to overt hypothyroidism and may require treatment.
- Presence of coronary heart disease should be looked for as it influences the treatment decisison in subclinical hypothyroidism.

Treatment

- Treatment with levothyroxine is indicated in following situations
  - Level of TSH is >10 mIU/L.
  - TSH 4.5–10 mIU/L with symptoms, goiter, or positive anti-TPO.
  - Pregnant or planning pregnancy.
  - Presence of cardiovascular risk factors.
- TSH 4.5–10 with no symptoms or risk factors: Observe and monitor TSH periodically.

Q. Myxedema coma.

- Myxedema coma is defined as severe hypothyroidism leading to altered mental status, hypothermia, and multi-organ dysfunction. Myxedema also refers to a dermatologic condition (pretibial myxedema), which occurs in hyperthyroidism and should not be mistaken for myxedema coma.
- Myxedema coma is a medical emergency with a high mortality rate.

Etiology/Precipitating Factors

Occurs in long-standing, untreated hypothyroidism, especially in elderly women. Precipitating factors include:

- Infections (e.g. pneumonia, UTI).
- Cold exposure.
- Sedative or narcotic use.
- Stroke or myocardial infarction.
- Surgery or trauma.

Clinical Presentation

- The hallmarks of myxedema coma are decreased mental status and hypothermia.
- Most patients present with confusion and obtundation. Untreated patients will progress to coma.
- Other features are hypotension, bradycardia, hyponatremia, hypoglycemia, and hypoventilation.

- There may be evidence of a precipitating event such as infection, but fever may be absent in these patients.

Diagnosis

- *Clinical*: High suspicion in an elderly patient with known or suspected hypothyroidism + altered sensorium.
- *Investigations*: ↑ TSH, ↓ Free T4 (if primary hypothyroidism), ↓ cortisol (may co-exist with adrenal insufficiency), Hyponatremia, hypoglycemia, elevated creatinine kinase, hypoxemia, hypercapnia.

Management

- It is a medical emergency. Patient should be admitted to ICU.
- Treatment should be started without waiting for lab reports. Before thyroid hormone is given, however, blood should be drawn for measurements of T3, T4, TSH and cortisol to exclude associated adrenal insufficiency or hypopituitarism.

Thyroid Hormone Replacement

- 300 µg thyroxine is given intravenously over 5–10 minutes initially, followed by 100 µg per day until patient becomes alert and able to take thyroxine orally. If no IV preparation is available same dose may be given through Ryle's tube.

Supportive Measures

- Hydrocortisone, 100 mg IV bolus followed by 100 mg every eight hours till associated adrenal insufficiency is excluded.
- Cover with blankets to correct hypothermia
- Intravenous fluids, electrolytes, and glucose to correct electrolyte abnormalities and hypoglycemia
- Mechanical ventilation if required
- Treat precipitating factors (infection)
- Avoid sedatives and narcotics.

Q. Myxedema madness.

- Myxedema madness refers to psychiatric manifestations of hypothyroidism, typically presenting as psychosis, which may precede other physical symptoms.

Clinical Features

- Delusions, hallucinations (often paranoid)
- Depression, irritability, mania
- Cognitive dysfunction, memory loss
- May occur before diagnosis of hypothyroidism or in long-standing, untreated cases.

Mechanism

- Thought to result from reduced cerebral metabolism due to severe hypothyroidism.

Diagnosis

- Suspect in any patient with new-onset psychosis and signs of hypothyroidism.
- Confirm with thyroid function tests: ↑ TSH, ↓ T3, T4 (in primary hypothyroidism).

Management

- Levothyroxine replacement (oral or IV depending on severity).
- Antipsychotics may be needed short-term, but usually resolve as thyroid function normalizes.
- Psychiatric symptoms often resolve over days to weeks.

Q. Simple goiter.

Simple goiter is an enlargement of the thyroid gland that is not associated with inflammation, cancer, or hyperthyroidism/hypothyroidism.

Types

- ***Endemic goiter:*** Common in areas with iodine-deficient soil (e.g. Himalayas, Alps, Andes).
- ***Sporadic goiter:*** Occurs without a clear environmental cause; may be linked to genetic factors or intake of goitrogens (substances that interfere with thyroid hormone synthesis).

Causes

- Iodine deficiency (most common worldwide).
- Hereditary enzyme defects in thyroid hormone synthesis.
- Goitrogenic foods (e.g. cabbage, cassava).

Clinical Features

- Visible or palpable neck swelling **(Fig. 9.6)**
- Usually nontender
- Euthyroid state (normal thyroid function), but can progress to hypothyroidism or hyperthyroidism in some cases.
- Compression symptoms in large goiters (e.g. difficulty breathing/swallowing).

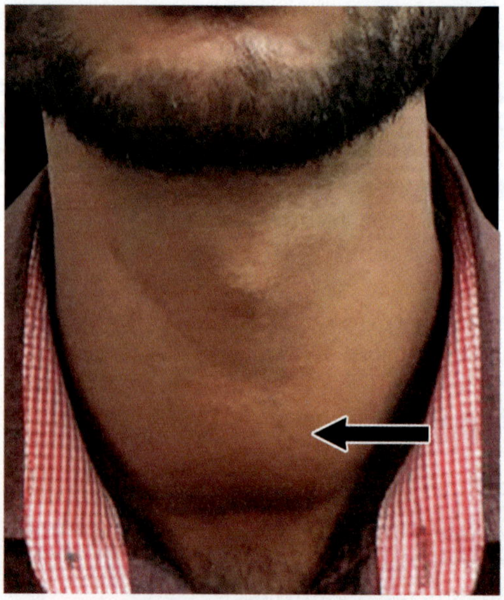

Figure 9.6: Simple goiter (arrow)

Investigations

- Thyroid function tests (T3, T4, TSH)
- Ultrasound of the thyroid
- Radioactive iodine uptake scan (in selected cases).

Treatment

- Iodine supplementation (especially in endemic areas)
- Thyroid hormone replacement (levothyroxine) to reduce TSH stimulation and shrink the gland
- Surgery in cases of large goiter causing compressive symptoms or cosmetic concerns.
- Endemic goiter can be prevented by fortification of common salt with iodine and intramuscular injection of 3–4 ml of iodized oil once in 2 years.

Q. Multinodular goiter.

- Multinodular goiter is an enlargement of the thyroid gland characterized by multiple distinct nodules within the thyroid **(Fig. 9.7)**.
- It can be nontoxic (euthyroid) or toxic (producing excess thyroid hormones).

Causes

- Long-standing simple goiter
- Iodine deficiency (especially chronic)
- Genetic predisposition
- Repeated episodes of thyroid hyperplasia and involution.

Clinical Features

- Irregular, asymmetrical neck swelling
- Multiple palpable nodules
- Usually painless
- Compressive symptoms in large goiters: dysphagia, dyspnea, hoarseness (if recurrent laryngeal nerve involved)
- If toxic, symptoms of hyperthyroidism (weight loss, tremors, palpitations).

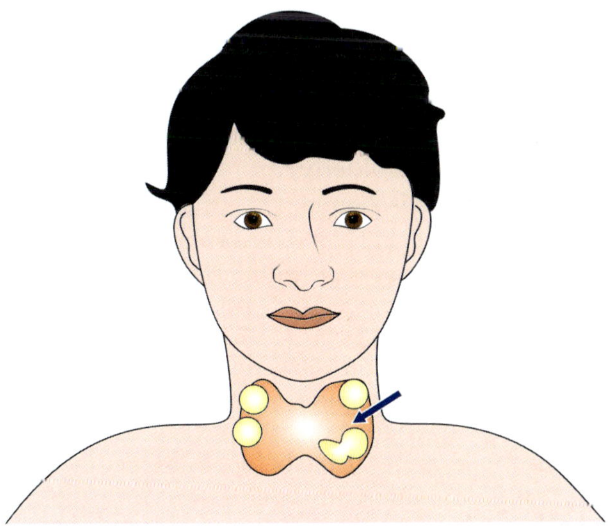

Figure 9.7: Multinodular goiter (arrow)

Investigations

- Thyroid function tests (T3, T4, TSH)
- Ultrasound of the thyroid to assess number, size, and nature of nodules
- Radioisotope thyroid scan
- Chest X-ray and CT or MRI if retrosternal extension or airway compression suspected.
- FNAC is indicated in those with a 'dominant', 'cold' nodule, to exclude thyroid cancer.

Management

- No treatment is required if the goiter is small and patient is euthyroid. However, patients should be followed up yearly as it may progress to toxic multinodular goiter.
- Partial thyroidectomy is indicated for large goiter causing compressive symptoms or for cosmetic reasons.
- Radio-iodine therapy (I-131) is useful in toxic multinodular goiter.

Q. Thyroiditis.

- The term thyroiditis refers to inflammation of thyroid gland.
- Thyroiditis can be divided into three types—acute, subacute, and chronic:
  - Acute thyroiditis is caused by bacterial infection of the gland.
  - Subacute thyroiditis, also known as granulomatous thyroiditis (deQuervain's thyroiditis), is caused by viruses (coxsackie virus, mumps, measles, adenovirus).
  - Chronic thyroiditis includes autoimmune thyroiditis, Hashimoto thyroiditis, postpartum thyroiditis, and drug-induced thyroiditis.

Pathophysiology

- Thyroid inflammation releases thyroid hormones leading to thyrotoxicosis. Initial hyperthyroidism is sometimes followed by a transient period of hypothyroidism. The disease usually resolves spontaneously.

Clinical Features

- Pain in the thyroid, which may radiate to the neck or ears. Thyroid gland is enlarged and tender. Fever, fatigue, malaise, anorexia, and myalgia are common.

Investigations

- ESR is high
- Technicium-99 uptake is low
- Serum thyroglobulin is raised
- Initially hyperthyroidism is seen, followed by euthyroidism, hypothyroidism and ultimately restoration of normal thyroid function.

Treatment

- Anti-inflammatory agents (NSAIDs or steroids) are used to control inflammation.

- Beta-blockers (propranolol) are used to control thyrotoxic symptoms.

Q. Hashimoto's thyroiditis (autoimmune thyroiditis; chronic lymphocytic thyroiditis).

- Hashimoto's thyroiditis is chronic autoimmune inflammation of the thyroid with lymphocytic infiltration. It is the most common cause of hypothyroidism in developed countries.

Etiology

- Autoimmune mechanism: Production of autoantibodies against thyroid components, especially:
  - Antithyroid peroxidase (anti-TPO) antibodies
  - Antithyroglobulin antibodies
- Genetic predisposition: Associated with HLA-DR3, HLA-DR5.
- Environmental factors: High iodine intake, infections, stress.
- Antibodies attack thyroid gland → chronic inflammation → infiltration of the thyroid gland by lymphocytes and plasma cells → destruction of thyroid follicles → decreased hormone production.
- Often coexists with other autoimmune diseases (e.g. type 1 diabetes, celiac disease, vitiligo).

Clinical Features

- More common in women
- Painless, diffuse enlargement of thyroid (goiter) with characteristic firm or rubbery consistency
- Features of hypothyroidism are present
- In some early cases, there may be transient hyperthyroid phase ("Hashitoxicosis") due to leakage of hormones from the inflamed gland.

Investigations

- Thyroid function tests show hypothyroidism (↑ TSH, ↓ T3, T4).
- Anti-TPO (thyroid peroxidase) and anti-Tg (antithyroglobulin) antibodies are present in the serum in >90% of patients with Hashimoto thyroiditis.
- Biopsy shows profuse lymphocytic infiltration, lymphoid germinal centers, destruction of thyroid follicles and fibrosis. May show Hurthle's cell (oncocytic) change in follicular epithelium.

Treatment

- Thyroxine corrects hypothyroidism as well as helps in goiter shrinkage.

Q. Describe the pharmacology, indications, adverse reaction, and interactions of thyroxine.

- Thyroxine (levothyroxine sodium) is a synthetic form of T4 (thyroxine). It is structurally identical to naturally occurring thyroxine produced by the thyroid gland.

Mechanism of Action

- Acts as a prohormone → converted to T3 (triiodothyronine) in peripheral tissues.
- T3 binds to nuclear thyroid hormone receptors (TR) → regulates gene transcription.
- *Effects*:
  - Increases basal metabolic rate
  - Stimulates protein synthesis
  - Enhances lipid and carbohydrate metabolism
  - Promotes growth and development, especially of CNS.

Pharmacokinetics (Table 9.5)

TABLE 9.5: Pharmacokinetics of thyroxine

Parameter	Features
Absorption	70–80% orally absorbed; best on an empty stomach
Distribution	Highly protein bound (>99%)
Conversion	T4 → T3 in liver, kidney, brain
Onset	Slow → clinical effects in 1–2 weeks
Half-life	~7 days
Excretion	Metabolized by deiodination; excreted in urine and bile

Indications

- Replacement therapy in hypothyroidism.
- Suppression therapy: To suppress TSH in thyroid cancer (post-thyroidectomy), benign thyroid nodules, diffuse non-toxic goitre.

Dosage

- Start low, go slow, especially in elderly or cardiac patients.
- Aim for euthyroid state → normalize TSH and Free T4.
- Thyroxine should be taken once daily, in the morning, on an empty stomach (30–60 min before food).
- Young, healthy adults: initial dose 50–100 µg/day.
- Elderly (>60 years) or cardiac disease: 12.5–25 µg/day → increase gradually every 4–6 weeks.
- Check TSH and Free T4 after 6–8 weeks → adjust dose accordingly.
- TSH suppression (e.g. thyroid cancer): Higher doses are used to suppress TSH below normal range ~200–300 µg/day.

Adverse Reactions

- Overdose may cause symptoms of hyperthyroidism.
- Atrial fibrillation (elderly)
- Angina, cardiac ischemia
- Osteoporosis (long-term over-replacement)
- Premature craniosynostosis in children if overdosed.

Drug Interactions

- Thyroxine absorption is decreased by calcium salts, iron salts, cholestyramine, sucralfate, and aluminum hydroxide. Hence, take thyroxine on an empty stomach, at least 30–60 min before meals or other drugs.
- Thyroxine metabolism is increased by phenytoin, carbamazepine, rifampicin, phenobarbital → decreased effectiveness of thyroxine.

- Drugs affecting TBG (thyroxine-binding globulin) levels: estrogens ↑ TBG → ↑ total T4. Androgens and glucocorticoids ↓ TBG → ↓ total T4.
- Thyroxine enhances anticoagulant effect of warfarin → ↑ risk of bleeding.

Q. Describe the pharmacology, indications, adverse reaction, and interactions of antithyroid drugs.

- Antithyroid drugs (also called thionamides) are medications used to inhibit the synthesis of thyroid hormones and are the mainstay of medical management for hyperthyroidism.
- The main drugs are:
  - Propylthiouracil (PTU).
  - Methimazole/Carbimazole (converted to methimazole in vivo).

Pharmacology

Mechanism of Action

- ***Inhibition of thyroid hormone synthesis:*** Both PTU and methimazole inhibit thyroid peroxidase (TPO), an enzyme that catalyzes:
  - Iodination of tyrosine residues in thyroglobulin (organification of iodine)
  - Coupling of iodotyrosines (to form T3 and T4)
- ***Inhibition of peripheral conversion of T4 to T3*** (additional effect of PTU only):
  - PTU inhibits 5′-deiodinase → ↓ T3 production in peripheral tissues.

Pharmacokinetics (Table 9.6)

TABLE 9.6: Pharmacokinetics of antithyroid drugs

Property	Methimazole/ Carbimazole	Propylthiouracil (PTU)
Half-life	6–9 hours	1–2 hours
Dosing	Once daily	Multiple times/day (8 hourly)
Potency	More potent	Less potent
Placental crossing	Crosses placenta	Crosses placenta (more than methimazole)
Protein binding	Low	High (~75%)

Indications

- Graves' disease (most common use)
- Toxic multinodular goiter
- Toxic adenoma
- Preparation of hyperthyroid patients before thyroidectomy (to achieve euthyroidism)
- As adjunct to radioactive iodine therapy (RAI)
- Thyrotoxic crisis (thyroid storm): PTU is preferred because of T4 → T3 inhibition.

Adverse Reactions

Common

- Rash (maculopapular, pruritic)
- Arthralgia
- Fever
- Mild leukopenia (transient)

Serious

- Agranulocytosis (rare but life-threatening).
  - Incidence ~0.1–0.5%.
  - Onset usually within first 3 months.
  - Symptoms: Sore throat, fever → requires immediate cessation of drug and urgent medical attention.
- Hepatotoxicity.
  - PTU → Severe hepatotoxicity, sometimes requiring liver transplantation.
  - Methimazole → Mild hepatotoxicity, cholestatic jaundice.
- Vasculitis (ANCA-positive vasculitis).
- Lupus-like syndrome.

Others

- Taste disturbances
- Myopathy
- Hypothyroidism (due to overtreatment).

Drug Interactions

- Warfarin: Decreased anticoagulant effect due to reduced catabolism of clotting factors.
- β-blockers: Antithyroid drugs enhance the effectiveness of β-blockers in controlling symptoms.
- Theophylline: Thyroid status affects its metabolism.
- Digoxin: ↑ levels as euthyroidism restores.
- Lithium: Additive hypothyroid effect.

Choice of Agent (Table 9.7)

TABLE 9.7: Choice of antithyroid drug

Clinical scenario	Preferred drug
Nonpregnant adults	Methimazole (once daily, better tolerated)
1st trimester of pregnancy	PTU (lower teratogenic risk)
2nd and 3rd trimesters	Methimazole (switch from PTU to avoid hepatotoxicity)
Thyroid storm	PTU (inhibits peripheral T4 to T3 conversion)

Monitoring

- Monitor free T4 and TSH every 4–6 weeks initially.
- CBC (baseline and if symptoms suggest agranulocytosis).
- LFTs (especially for PTU).

Q. Describe the indications of radioiodine therapy and surgery in the management of thyrotoxicosis.

Radioiodine Therapy (Iodine-131)

Mechanism of Action

Oral **I-131** → taken up by thyroid → emits **beta radiation** → **destruction** of overactive thyroid tissue.

Indications for Radioiodine Therapy

- Graves' disease: Adults (>21 years), especially older patients or with comorbidities making surgery risky. Patients with relapse after thionamide therapy.
- Toxic multinodular goiter: Elderly, nonsurgical candidates.
- Toxic adenoma: Single autonomously functioning nodule.

Advantages

- Definitive therapy
- Outpatient procedure
- Cost-effective
- No surgical risk.

Disadvantages

- Risk of permanent hypothyroidism (common in Graves' disease).
- Delayed onset (takes weeks to months to achieve euthyroidism).
- Contraindicated in pregnancy and lactation.
- Worsening of ophthalmopathy in some Graves' patients (use steroids as prophylaxis if needed).

Surgery (Thyroidectomy)

Types

- Total thyroidectomy (most common)
- Near-total thyroidectomy: Removal of entire thyroid gland except for a small remnant typically on one side.
- Subtotal thyroidectomy: Removal of a large portion of both thyroid lobes, leaving bilateral thyroid remnants (rarely used today).

Indications

- Large goiter causing compressive symptoms (dysphagia, dyspnea)
- Suspicion of thyroid malignancy
- Patients with contraindications to radioiodine and antithyroid drugs
- Pregnancy: If patient cannot tolerate drugs (usually done in 2nd trimester if required). Radioiodine is contraindicated.
- Graves' disease: Relapse after medical therapy and radioiodine is unsuitable. Severe ophthalmopathy (avoid radioiodine in this group).
- Toxic multinodular goiter or toxic adenoma: When radioiodine is not feasible or is contraindicated.

Advantages

- Definitive and immediate control of thyrotoxicosis
- Removes suspicious nodules/tumor if present.

Disadvantages

- Requires surgery and hospitalization
- Risks: Hypoparathyroidism, recurrent laryngeal nerve injury, bleeding, hypothyroidism.

Q. Hypothalamic-pituitary-thyroid (HPT) axis.

The HPT axis is a tightly regulated feedback system ensuring appropriate thyroid hormone production **(Fig. 9.8)**.

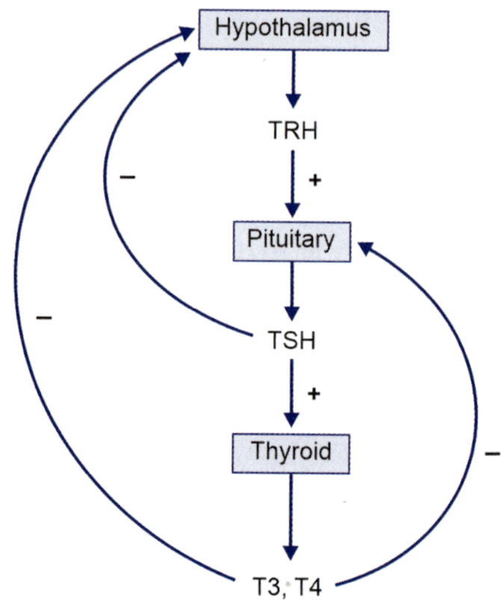

Figure 9.8: Hypothalamic-pituitary-thyroid (HPT) axis

Components and Functions (Table 9.8)

TABLE 9.8: Components of hypothalamic-pituitary-thyroid (HPT) axis

Structure	Hormone	Function
Hypothalamus	**Thyrotropin-releasing hormone (TRH)**	Stimulates anterior pituitary to secrete TSH
Anterior pituitary	**Thyroid-stimulating hormone (TSH)**	• Stimulates thyroid gland to produce T3 and T4 • TSH inhibits hypothalamic secretion of TRH via negative feedback
Thyroid gland	**Triiodothyronine (T3), thyroxine (T4)**	• Regulate metabolism, growth, development • T3 inhibits synthesis and release of TRH from hypothalamus via negative feedback. • T3 inhibits pituitary synthesis and release of TSH via negative feedback

Q. Discuss the iodization programs of the government of India.

- Iodine is an essential micronutrient required for thyroid hormone synthesis.
- Its deficiency leads to a spectrum of disorders called Iodine Deficiency Disorders (IDDs) → including goiter, cretinism, mental retardation, growth retardation, reproductive failure.
- India has long been identified as an iodine-deficient country due to low iodine content in soil in many regions, necessitating a public health intervention.

Iodization Programs of India

National Goitre Control Programme (NGCP)

- Launched in 1962.
- Initial focus → endemic goitre in Himalayan belt.
- Strategy: Supply of iodized salt to endemic areas.

National Iodine Deficiency Disorders Control Programme (NIDDCP)

- Renamed in 1992 → after recognizing the wider spectrum of IDDs.
- Expanded focus: Control of all IDDs, not just goiter.

Objectives of NIDDCP

- Assess the magnitude of IDDs
- Supply **iodized salt** in place of common salt
- Monitor iodine content in salt and urinary iodine excretion
- Health education and communication for awareness
- Periodic surveys to monitor IDD prevalence.

Universal Salt Iodization (USI)

- Key strategy of NIDDCP
- All edible salt must be iodised to at least 30 ppm at production, 15 ppm at consumption
- Compulsory since 1997 (notification under Prevention of Food Adulteration Act).
- Temporary ban on non-iodized salt lifted in 2000; re-imposed in **2005** under the Food Safety and Standards Act.

Key components of iodization program

- **Salt iodization:** Production of iodized salt: coordinated with salt manufacturers. Subsidies and support to small salt producers.
- **Distribution:** Public distribution system (PDS). Open market channels.
- **Quality monitoring:** Salt sample testing at production, retail, and household levels. Urinary iodine excretion surveys → population-level iodine status.
- **Legislation and regulation:** Food safety and standards (prohibition and restriction on sales) regulation mandates sale of iodized salt only for human consumption.
- **Information, education, communication:** Mass media campaigns → raising public awareness about the benefits of iodized salt. School health programs → education of children and teachers.

Achievements of the program

- Household consumption of adequately iodized salt
- Significant reduction in goitre prevalence in several states
- Reduction in neonatal hypothyroidism
- Improved awareness about iodized salt.

Q. Enumerate the causes of hyperparathyroidism.

Causes of Hyperparathyroidism

Primary (caused by autonomous overproduction of parathyroid hormone)

- Parathyroid adenoma (most common cause)
- Parathyroid hyperplasia (can be sporadic or part of MEN syndromes)
- Parathyroid carcinoma (rare)
- Multiple endocrine neoplasia (MEN) syndromes

Secondary (caused by a compensatory increase in PTH due to chronic hypocalcemia)

- Chronic kidney disease (most common cause)
- Vitamin D deficiency
- Malabsorption syndromes (e.g. celiac disease, chronic pancreatitis)
- Hypocalcemia due to pseudohypoparathyroidism
- Hyperphosphatemia (especially in renal failure)

Tertiary: Occurs when secondary hyperparathyroidism becomes autonomous and excessive, typically after long-standing secondary disease. Occurs usually in patients with end-stage renal disease.

Q. Discuss the etiology, clinical features, investigations and management of primary hyperparathyroidism.

Primary Hyperparathyroidism

- Primary hyperparathyroidism is due to a problem in the parathyroid glands themselves. It is characterized by excessive secretion of PTH by one or more parathyroid glands.
- It can be seen at any age but is more frequent in persons over the age of 50 years and is three times more common in women than men.

Etiology

See above.

Clinical Features

- Patients are often asymptomatic and detected incidentally via elevated serum calcium. When symptomatic, the classical features follow the phrase **"Bones, stones, groans, and psychiatric overtones."**

Skeletal Manifestations (Bones)

- Osteopenia or osteoporosis (especially cortical bone loss)
- Severe cases progress to osteitis fibrosa cystica
- Pathologic fractures
- Bone pain and arthralgias.

Renal (stones)

- Polyuria and polydipsia due to hypercalcemia-induced nephrogenic diabetes insipidus
- Kidney stones due to hypercalciuria
- Urinary tract infection due to stone and obstruction may lead to renal failure and uremia.

Gastrointestinal (groans)

- Constipation
- Nausea, vomiting
- Peptic ulcers (increased gastrin secretion due to hypercakcemia)
- Pancreatitis.

Neuropsychiatric (psychiatric overtones)

- Fatigue
- Depression, confusion

- Cognitive dysfunction
- Muscle weakness

Investigations

- Hypercalcemia is the most important finding. Serum calcium is >10.5 mg/dl. Serum phosphate is often low (<2.5 mg/dl).
- Hypercalciuria and hyperphosphaturia are often present.
- Alkaline phosphatase (ALP) is elevated due to high bone turnover.
- Elevated serum levels of PTH confirm the diagnosis of hyperparathyroidism.
- Neck ultrasound or 99mTc-sestamibi scan: For localization of parathyroid adenoma.
- CT and MRI may show subperiosteal bone resorption or renal stones.
- Bone radiographs: It may show demineralization, subperiosteal resorption of bone (especially in the radial aspects of the fingers), mottling of the skull ("salt-and-pepper appearance"), or pathologic fractures. Articular cartilage calcification (chondrocalcinosis) is sometimes found.
- Dual energy X-ray absorptiometry (DEXA) may show reduced bone density.

Treatment

Parathyroidectomy

- Parathyroidectomy is recommended for patients with symptomatic hyperparathyroidism, kidney stones, bone disease, pregnancy and very high serum calcium. During pregnancy, parathyroidectomy is performed in the second trimester.
- Subtotal parathyroidectomy is indicated for parathyroid hyperplasia. Three and one-half glands are usually removed, and a metal clip is left to mark the location of residual parathyroid tissue.
- Parathyroid carcinoma is treated by en bloc resection of the tumor and the ipsilateral thyroid lobe. Adjuvant treatment includes radiation therapy.

Treatment of Hypercalcemia

- Hydration with oral or IV fluids
- Bisphosphonates inhibit bone resorption and decrease serum calcium. Pamidronate 30 mg (in normal saline) or zoledronic acid 4 mg can be given as intravenous infusion. Calcium decreases over several days and the effect may last for weeks to months.
- Calcimimetics: Calcimimetic agents activate the calcium-sensing receptor in the parathyroid gland, thereby inhibiting PTH secretion. Cinacalcet is a calcimimetic agent. It reduces calcium level reducing PTH secretion.

Q. Enumerate the causes of hypercalcemia. Discuss the management of hypercalcemia.

Q. Hypercalcemic crisis.

- Normal calcium level in the body is 8–10 mg/dl. Out of this 4–5.6 mg/dl is ionized calcium and the remaining is bound to albumin. Hence, total calcium concentration may be high with high serum albumin and low with low albumin concentration. This can be corrected by using the formula, Ca = Serum Ca + 0.8 X (Normal albumin–patient albumin).
- Hypercalcemia is defined as a serum total calcium level >10.5 mg/dl.
    - Mild hypercalcemia: 10.5–11.9 mg/dl.
    - Moderate hypercalcemia: 12.0–13.9 mg/dl.
    - Severe hypercalcemia: ≥14 mg/dl.

Etiology of Hypercalcemia

Parathyroid-related causes

- Primary hyperparathyroidism (most common cause)
- Tertiary hyperparathyroidism (in chronic kidney disease)

Malignancy-associated

(Second most common cause)

- Humoral hypercalcemia of malignancy (↑ PTHrP, e.g. squamous cell carcinoma)
- Bone metastases (breast, prostate, myeloma)
- Multiple myeloma (osteolytic lesions)
- Lymphoma (↑ 1,25$(OH)_2$-vitamin D production)

Endocrine causes

- Thyrotoxicosis
- Adrenal insufficiency
- Pheochromocytoma

Drug-induced

- Vitamin D intoxication
- Vitamin A intoxication
- Thiazide diuretics
- Lithium (alters set point of calcium-sensing receptors)
- Theophylline toxicity
- Calcium supplements (especially with milk-alkali syndrome)

Immobilization: Especially in patients with high bone turnover (e.g. adolescents, Paget's disease).

Genetic/miscellaneous

- Familial hypocalciuric hypercalcemia (FHH)
- Parenteral nutrition
- Rhabdomyolysis/tumor lysis syndrome (initial hypocalcemia, later rebound hypercalcemia)
- Granulomatous diseases (e.g. sarcoidosis, TB) → ↑ extrarenal 1α-hydroxylase activity → ↑ calcitriol

Clinical Features

- These are same as that of primary hyperparathyroidism "Bones, stones, groans, and psychiatric overtones." (*see* the previous sections).
- Additionally cardiovascular effects such as shortening of the QT interval, bradycardia, and hypertension can be seen.
- Calcium may precipitate in the corneas ("band keratopathy").

Hypercalcemic Crisis

- Here serum calcium is more than ≥14 mg/dl.
- Most common cause is malignancy related hypercalcemia. Other common causes are primary hyperpara-

thyroidism, vitamin D toxicity, sarcoidosis, and prolonged immobilization (*see* the list of hypercalcemia causes).
- Clinical features are dehydration, hypotension, cardiac arrhythmias (shortened QT interval, bradycardia), abdominal pain, vomiting, muscle weakness, hypotonia, and altered sensorium.

Investigations

- Serum calcium should be corrected for albumin, and an elevated concentration should be confirmed by repeat testing.
- ECG may show shortened QT interval, AV block, bundle branch block, and prolonged PR and QRS.
- Serum PTH level helps to distinguish PTH-mediated from non-PTH-mediated causes of hypercalcemia. In hyperparathyroidism PTH level is elevated.
- Serum concentration of PTH-related protein (PTHrp) is elevated in malignancy related hypercalcemia.
- Serum concentration of the vitamin D metabolites, 25-hydroxyvitamin D (calcidiol) and 1,25-dihydroxyvitamin D (calcitriol), should be measured if there is no obvious malignancy and neither PTH nor PTHrp levels are elevated.
- Serum uric acid and LDH are elevated in malignancy.
- Plasma protein electrophoresis, urine for Bence-Jones protein and bone marrow examination are useful to rule out multiple myeloma.
- Chest X-ray, ultrasound abdomen and CT scan to rule out malignancy.
- Bone scan to rule out bone metastases.

Management

Mild-to-moderate Hypercalcemia

- Patients with mild hypercalcemia do not require immediate treatment. Factors which aggravate hypercalcemia should be avoided. These are drugs such as thiazide diuretics and lithium, volume depletion, prolonged bed rest, and high calcium diet (>1000 mg/day). Adequate hydration is recommended. Symptomatic patients are treated with biphosphonates.

Severe Hypercalcemia (calcium >14 mg/dl; hypercalcemic crisis)

- Rehydration with isotonic saline at an initial rate of 200–300 ml/hour that is then adjusted to maintain the urine output at 100–150 ml/hour.
- Administration of salmon calcitonin 4 IU/kg initially and then every 6–12 hours.
- Biphosphonates: These drugs inhibit osteoclast-mediated bone resorption. Examples are zoledronic acid or pamidronate.
- Calcitonin plus saline reduces calcium concentration within 12–48 hours whereas bisphosphonates will be effective by the second to fourth day.
- Steroids: Prednisolone 5–15 mg 6 hourly or hydrocortisone 100 mg 6 hourly IV. Steroids inhibit vitamin D conversion to calcitriol. They are helpful in vitamin D intoxication, malignancies and granulomatous diseases.
- Hemodialysis should be considered if serum calcium is above 18 mg/dl.

Treatment of the Underlying Cause

Such as malignancy, hyperparathyroidism, etc.

Q. Hypoparathyroidism.

- Hypoparathyroidism is characterized by deficiency of PTH and hypocalcemia.

Causes

- Post-surgical (after thyroidectomy or head and neck surgeries).
- Autoimmune.
- Autosomal dominant hypoparathyroidism.
- Radiotherapy to head and neck area.
- Pseudohypoparathyroidism (resistance to PTH).

Clinical Features

- Most features are due to hypocalcemia are seen (*see* under hypocalcemia below).

Investigations

- Serum calcium: ↓ Decreased
- Serum phosphate: ↑ Increased
- PTH: ↓ Decreased (or inappropriately normal)
- Magnesium: May be low or normal

Treatment

- In acute manifestations of hypocalcemia (such as tetany), intravenous calcium gluconate is given.
- Vitamin D supplementation— Vitamin D (in the form of vitamin D2, or ergocalciferol), or calcitriol (1,25-dihydroxyvitamin D) are given orally daily to maintain normal calcium levels.

Q. Discuss the etiology, clinical features, investigations and management of hypocalcemia.

Q. Enumerate the causes of tetany. Discuss the clinical features and management of tetany.

Q. Trousseaus sign; Chvostek sign.

- Hypocalcemia is defined as serum total calcium <8.5 mg/dl or ionized calcium <4.4 mg/dl.

Etiology of Hypocalcemia (Tetany)

Hypoparathyroidism
- Post-surgical (after parathyroidectomy, thyroidectomy)
- Idiopathic
- Infiltration of the parathyroid gland
- Congenital (e.g. DiGeorge syndrome)

Pseudohypoparathyroidism: Resistance to PTH.

Vitamin D deficiency
- Nutritional deficiency
- Intestinal malabsorption
- CKD
- Vitamin D resistance

Acute pancreatitis: Calcium binds to necrotic fat (saponification).

Drugs: Bisphosphonates, phenytoin, cisplatin, calcitonin.

Miscellaneous

- Hypophosphatemia
- Hypomagnesemia (can cause relative PTH deficiency and end-organ resistance to PTH action.
- Massive blood transfusion (citrate-anticoagulated blood can decrease the concentration of ionized Ca)
- Alkalosis (hyperventilation, excessive vomiting)
- Fluoride intoxication
- Septic shock (due to suppression of PTH release and decreased conversion of 25(OH)D to 1,25$(OH)_2$ D)

Clinical Features

Neuromuscular Irritability

- Tetany: Hypocalcemia leads to neuromuscular irritability leading to tetany. Tetany is uncommon unless the serum ionized calcium concentration falls below 4.3 mg/dl. Other factors that worsen tetany are alkalosis, hypomagnesemia, hypokalemia and serum epinephrine concentrations. Tetany is characterized by both sensory and motor features. Initially sensory symptoms such as circum-oral numbness, paresthesias of the hands and feet are seen. Motor symptoms are stiffness and clumsiness, myalgia, and muscle spasms and cramps. Hand muscle spasm leads to adduction of the thumb, flexion of the metacarpophalangeal (MCP) joints and wrist, and extension of the interphalangeal joints **(Fig. 9.9)** with fingers drawn together and inward ("obstetrician's hand" or "main d'accoucheur" posture).
- Foot (pedal) spasm causes plantar flexion of the foot and toes with toe curling. There may be painful muscle cramps in the foot and calf **(Fig. 9.10)**.
- Latent tetany may be present when signs of overt tetany are lacking. It can be demonstrated by Trousseau's and Chvostek's signs. *Trousseau sign* is the induction of carpal spasm by inflation of a sphygmomanometer above systolic blood pressure for three minutes. It can also be induced by hyperventilation for one to two minutes after release of the cuff. Trousseau's sign is due to the ischemia of the nerve trunk under the cuff which increases excitability. *Chvostek's sign* is contraction of the ipsilateral facial muscles when facial nerve is tapped anterior to the ear. This leads to contraction of corner of the mouth, the nose and the eye.
- Spasm of the respiratory muscles and of the glottis can cause cyanosis.
- Autonomic manifestations include diaphoresis, bronchospasm, and biliary colic.

Psychiatric Manifestations

- Emotional instability, anxiety, depression, confusion, hallucinations, and frank psychosis. All are reversible with treatment.

Dental

- Dental abnormalities occur when hypocalcemia is present during early development. They include dental hypoplasia, failure of tooth eruption, defective enamel and root formation, and abraded carious teeth.

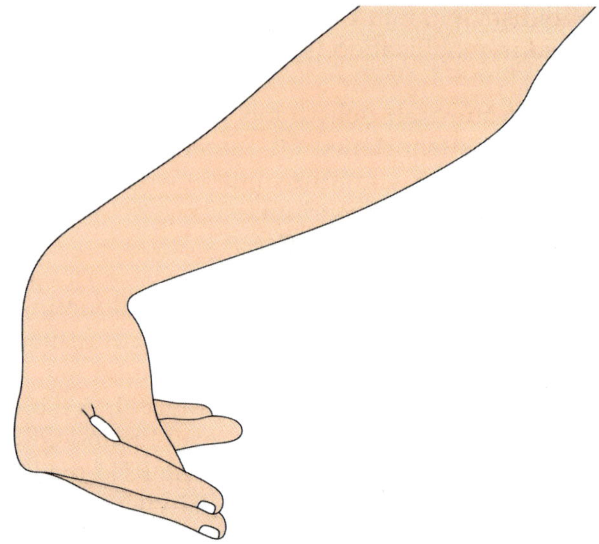

Figure 9.9: Carpal spasm

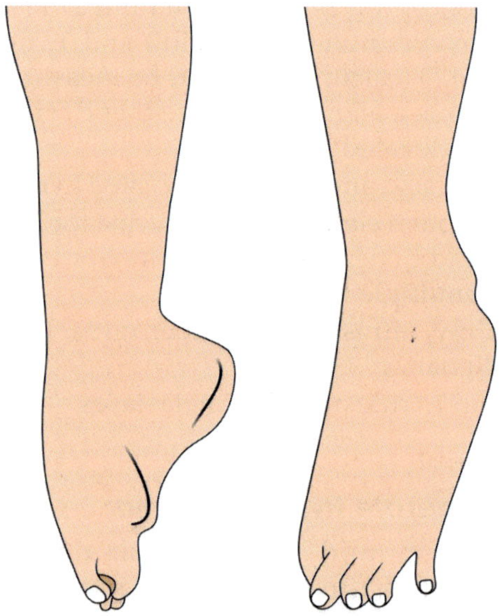

Figure 9.10: Pedal spasm

Cardiovascular

- Hypotension (in acute hypocalcemia), decreased myocardial contractility, and congestive heart failure.

Gastrointestinal

- Steatorrhea due to impaired pancreatic secretion, gastric achlorhydria.

Skeletal

- Hypocalcemia associated with hypophosphatemia, as in vitamin D deficiency, causes rickets in children and osteomalacia in adults.

Other Manifestations

- Skin—Dry skin, hyperpigmentation, dermatitis and eczema, and psoriasis. Hair is brittle and sparse with patchy alopecia.

- Eye—cataracts.
- Endocrine manifestations—impaired insulin release.

Investigations

- Serum calcium level is low.
- Serum PTH level is low in primary hypoparathyroidism and elevated in secondary hyperparathyroidism.
- Serum vitamin D level is low in vitamin D deficiency.
- Serum magnesium level-hypomagnesemia causes hypocalcemia by inducing PTH resistance or deficiency. Serum magnesium should be measured in any patient with hypocalcemia in whom the cause is not clear.
- ECG shows prolonged QT interval.

Management

- Tetany can be treated by rebreathing expired air in a paper bag or administering 5% CO_2 in oxygen. This increases arterial carbon dioxide which increases ionized calcium.
- Injection of 10 ml of a 10% calcium gluconate slow IV raises the serum calcium concentration immediately. An intramuscular injection of 10 ml may be given to obtain a more prolonged effect.
- Intravenous magnesium is given to correct the hypocalcemia associated with hypomagnesemia.
- Persistent hypoparathyroidism and pseudohypoparathyroidism are treated with oral calcium salts and vitamin D.

Q. Give a brief account of hormones secreted by the adrenal gland and their functions. Enumerate the diseases caused by adrenal gland dysfunction.

- Adrenal gland consists of adrenal cortex (90% of the gland) and medulla (10% of the gland). Adrenal cortex is further divided into zona glomerulosa, zona fasciculata, and zona reticularis (remember GFR for glomerulosa, fasciculata and reticularis) **(Fig. 9.11)**.
- Zona glomerulosa consists of small epitheloid cells which secrete aldosterone (mineralocorticoid).
- Zona fasciculata consists of polygonal columnar cells, which secrete cortisol (glucocorticoid).

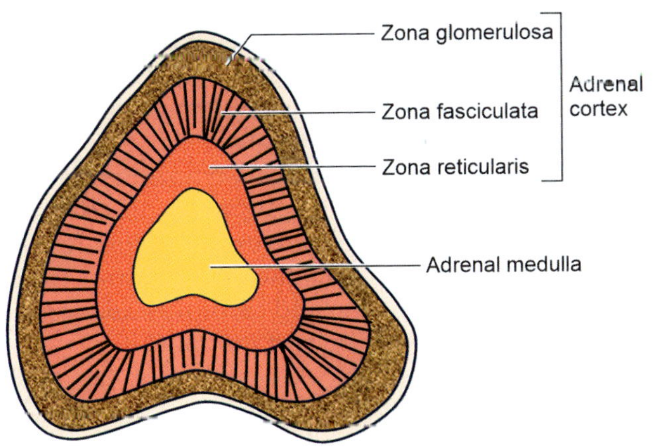

Figure 9.11: Adrenal gland

- Zona reticularis consists of a network of interconnecting cells which secrete adrenal androgens (dehydroepiandrosterone (DHEA)).
- Adrenal medulla consists of chromaffin cells which secrete adrenergic hormones such as epinephrine, norepinephrine and dopamine.

Actions of Adrenal Gland Hormones

Mineralocorticoids (aldosterone): Helps maintain blood volume and blood pressure by retaining sodium and water.

Glucocorticoids (cortisol): Regulation of intermediary metabolism. They counter hypoglycemia, induce protein catabolism and enhance lipolysis. Glucocorticoids also affect the adaptive response to stress and inflammation, immunity, wound healing and muscle and myocardial integrity.

Adrenal androgens: Required for the growth of axillary and pubic hair in both males and females.

Epinephrine (also known as adrenaline) and norepinephrine: These 2 hormones prepare the body for the fight-or-flight response by increasing the heart rate, constricting blood vessels, increasing the metabolic rate, and increasing the respiratory rate.

Diseases Caused by Adrenal Dysfunction

Adrenal hyperfunction

- Glucocorticoid excess—Cushing's syndrome
- Aldosterone excess—hyperaldosteronism (primary aldosteronism-Conn's syndrome, secondary aldosteronism)
- Androgen excess—virilization
- Adrenal medulla—pheochromocytoma

Adrenal hypofunction

- Primary—due to inability of the adrenals to produce hormones (Addison's disease).
- Secondary—due to deficient ACTH secretion by pituitary
- Tertiary—due to deficient CRH production by hypothalamus

Q. Discuss the etiology, clinical features, investigations and management of Cushing's syndrome (glucocorticoid excess).

- Cushing syndrome refers to the clinical state of chronic glucocorticoid excess, regardless of its cause.
- It includes both exogenous (iatrogenic) and endogenous sources of excess cortisol. The most common cause is iatrogenic due to prolonged administration of glucocorticoids such as prednisolone. ACTH-dependent cortisol excess due to a pituitary adenoma is called Cushing's disease.

Etiology

Exogenous (most common cause)

- Prolonged use of glucocorticoids (e.g. prednisone for autoimmune diseases, asthma)

Endogenous

ACTH-dependent Cushing's syndrome

- Pituitary adenoma secreting ACTH (i.e. Cushing's disease)
- Ectopic ACTH syndrome
- Ectopic CRH syndrome

ACTH-independent Cushing's syndrome
- Adrenal adenoma
- Adrenal carcinoma
- Adrenal hyperplasia

Clinical Features (Fig. 9.12)

- The typical patient with Cushing's syndrome is a middle-aged plethoric woman with truncal obesity and hypertension.
- Obesity—the obesity is central (centripetal obesity) with sparing of limbs which gives "lemon on stick appearance" **(Fig. 9.13)**. There is accentuation of normal fat over the upper part of the back, giving a "buffalo hump" appearance. The neck is thick and short. The supraclavicular fat pads are enlarged.
- Skin manifestations—include skin atrophy, easy bruisability, and pink striae in the trunk, breasts, and abdomen **(Fig. 9.14)**. Fungal infections are common. In pituitary tumors secreting ACTH, and in ectopic ACTH syndrome, hyperpigmentation can occur.
- Menstrual irregularities—oligomenorrhea, amenorrhea, etc.

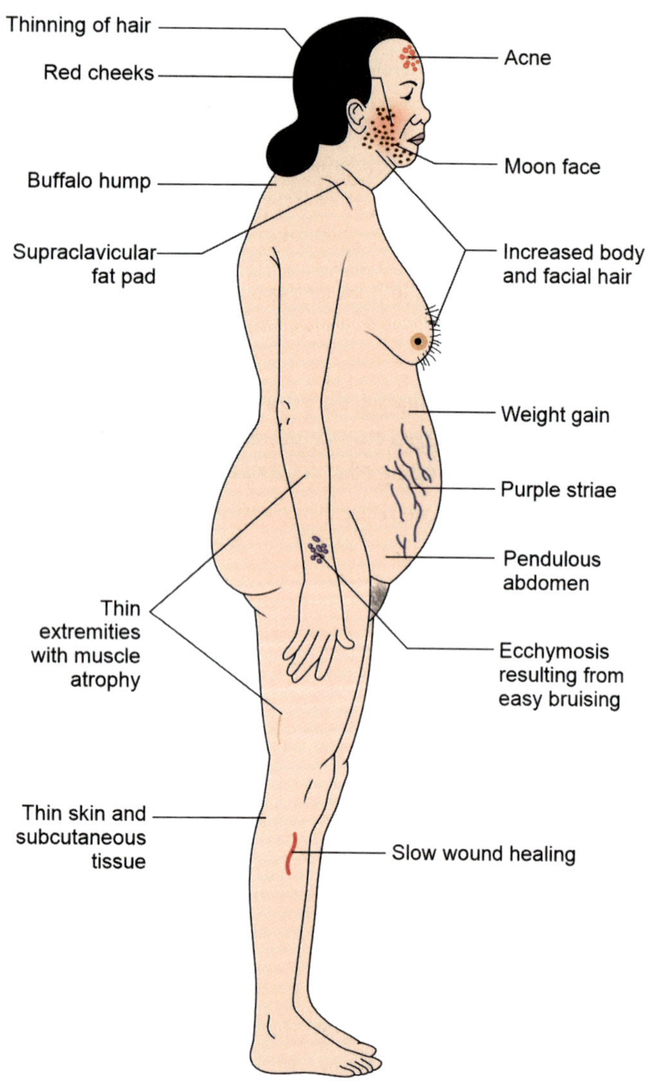

Figure 9.12: Clinical features of Cushing's syndrome

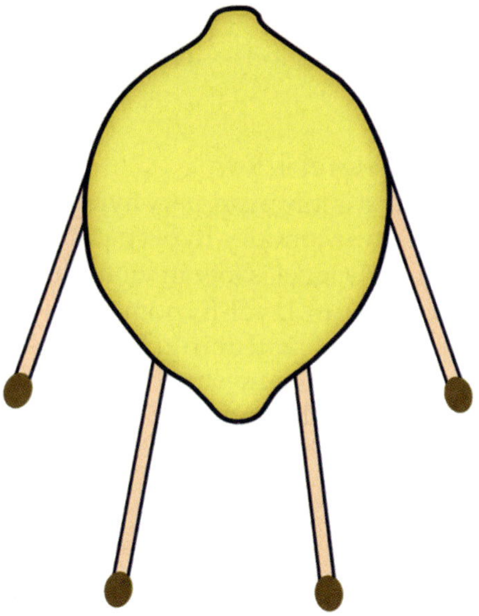

Figure 9.13: Lemon on stick appearance

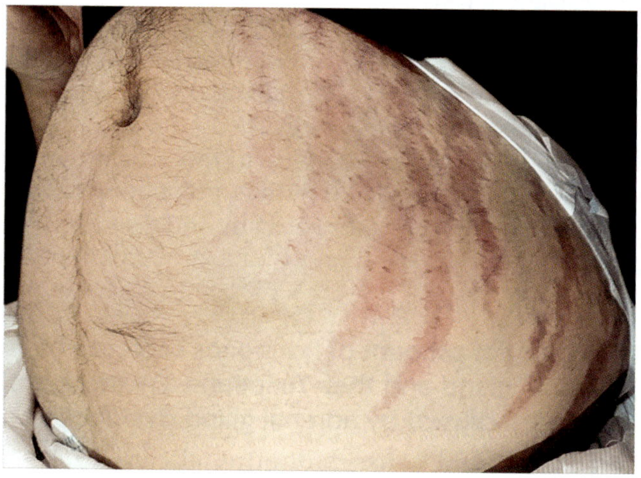

Figure 9.14: Broad, pink striae on the abdomen

- Signs of adrenal androgen excess—women with Cushing's syndrome often have signs of androgen excess. These include hirsutism, thinning of scalp hair, deepening of voice, and clitoral enlargement.
- Musculoskeletal problems—proximal muscle wasting and weakness due to excess steroid hormones. Osteoporosis is common and may lead to pathologic fractures and vertebral collapse. Low back pain is a common presenting feature. Occasionally, patients can present with avascular necrosis of the femoral head. Increased resorption of bones can lead to hypercalciuria and renal calculi.
- Neuropsychiatric symptoms—emotional lability, depression, irritability, anxiety and panic attacks.
- Metabolic—diabetes mellitus may develop due to increased hepatic gluconeogenesis and insulin resistance. Hypertension and cardiovascular risk is a major cause of morbidity and mortality.

Investigations

- Investigations are useful to confirm the diagnosis of Cushing syndrome and to find out the etiology.

Screening Tests (to confirm the presence of Cushing's syndrome)

- For patients with a low index of suspicion, do one of the following first-line tests: Bedtime salivary cortisol (two measurements), 24-hour urinary free cortisol excretion (two measurements), or the overnight 1 mg dexamethasone suppression test. If there is high index of suspicion, then do 2 of the above tests. The diagnosis of Cushing's syndrome is established when at least two different first-line tests are unequivocally abnormal.
- *Bedtime salivary cortisol:* Measurement of salivary cortisol in the late evening before bedtime is based upon the fact that the normal evening nadir in serum cortisol is preserved in patients with physiologic hypercortisolism but not in those with Cushing's syndrome. Saliva collection has many advantages: it is noninvasive and can be easily performed by the patient at home, and cortisol is stable in saliva even at room temperature for several days. It is useful to evaluate at least three samples from different days.
- *Bedtime serum cortisol:* Just like bedtime salivary cortisol, measurement of serum cortisol in the late evening, usually at midnight, is also based upon the fact that the normal nadir in serum cortisol after sleep onset is preserved in patients with physiologic hypercortisolism but not in those with Cushing's syndrome. This test is less convenient than the bedtime salivary cortisol and is therefore not used routinely in clinical practice. However, it is sometimes used at specialized centers. A bedtime serum cortisol >7.5 µg/dl (207 nmol/L) is used to identify Cushing's syndrome.
- *24-hour urinary cortisol excretion:* Collect all urine for 24 hours and measure free cortisol. Cortisol is high in patients with Cushing's syndrome (normal <100 µg/24 hours). The patient can be assumed to have Cushing syndrome if basal urinary cortisol excretion is more than three times the upper limit of normal.
- *Overnight 1 mg dexamethasone suppression test (DST):* 1 mg of dexamethasone is given orally at 11 PM and serum cortisol is measured at 8 AM the next morning. In most normal patients, this drug suppresses morning serum cortisol to ≤1.8 µg/ml. Cortisol >1.8 µg/dl suggests Cushing's syndrome.
- *48-hour low dose dexamethasone suppression test*: This is more sensitive and specific than overnight 1 mg DST. Useful in borderline or equivocal cases. This is a confirmatory test. 0.5 mg dexamethasone is given orally 6th hourly for 2 days starting at 9 AM or noon. Blood sample for serum cortisol is taken at 9 AM on day 3. Normal response is serum cortisol suppressed to <1.8 µg/dl (excludes Cushing's). Cortisol ≥1.8 µg/dl indicates lack of suppression and suggests Cushing's syndrome.

Tests to Determine the Cause of Hypercortisolism: ACTH-dependent vs ACTH-independent

- Once the presence of Cushing's syndrome is confirmed, the next step is to identify whether the cortisol excess is ACTH-dependent (e.g. Cushing's disease, ectopic ACTH) or ACTH-independent (e.g. adrenal tumor). This can be done by measurement of plasma ACTH.
- Increased cortisol level and low ACTH indicate ACTH-independent cortisol excess (e.g. adrenal adenoma/carcinoma). Normal or high ACTH level indicates ACTH dependent cortisol excess and requires further testing.
- *High-dose dexamethasone suppression test:* ACTH dependent cortisol excess can be due to pituitary and ectopic source of ACTH which can be differentiated by the fact that pituitary tumors, but not ectopic tumors, retain some features of normal regulation of ACTH secretion. Thus, pituitary ACTH secretion is suppressed by dexamethasone (although at a higher dose than normal). Hence high dose dexamethasone suppression test can be used to differentiate whether high ACTH is coming from pituitary or from ectopic source.
- *CRH stimulation test:* Further increase in ACTH and cortisol suggests Cushing's disease because pituitary responds to CRH. No increase suggests ectopic ACTH or adrenal tumor.
- *MRI of pituitary* if pituitary adenoma is suspected, and *MRI/CT of adrenal glands* if adrenal cause is likely. *CT chest and abdomen* should be done if ectopic ACTH is suspected.
- Venous catheterization with measurement of inferior petrosal sinus ACTH (i.e. draining directly from the pituitary) is the gold standard test to differentiate Cushing disease *vs* ectopic ACTH. It compares central (pituitary) *vs* peripheral ACTH levels after CRH stimulation. Central >peripheral ACTH (ratio ≥2–3) suggests Cushing disease and both same suggests Ectopic ACTH source. This test is used when MRI is inconclusive or no pituitary tumor is seen.

Additional Tests

- Serum electrolytes (usually high sodium and low potassium), glucose (elevated), glycosylated hemoglobin and bone mineral density measurement.

Management

- Most patients are treated surgically with medical therapy given for a few weeks prior to operation.

Surgery

- In Cushing's disease, trans-sphenoidal surgery with selective removal of the adenoma is the treatment of choice.
- Adrenal adenomas are removed via laparoscopy or a loin incision.
- Ectopic ACTH syndrome-localized tumors (e.g. bronchial carcinoid) should be removed. Unresectable malignancies may be treated by radiotherapy and chemotherapy. Medical therapy can be used for recurrences.

Medical Therapy

- Used for nonsurgical candidates or bridge to surgery. Following drugs can be used.

- Somatostatin analogs: Pasireotide is a somatostatin analog that binds and activates human somatostatin receptors resulting in inhibition of ACTH secretion, which leads to decreased cortisol secretion. It is indicated for treatment of Cushing's disease in which pituitary surgery is not an option or has not been curative.
- Adrenal steroid inhibitors: Metyrapone, ketoconazole, etomidate.
- Glucocorticoid receptor antagonist: Mifepristone.
- Adrenolytic agents: Mitotane. This drug causes adrenal cortical necrosis.

Q. Nelson's syndrome.

- This syndrome occurs in patients who have undergone bilateral adrenalectomy for Cushing's disease.
- It involves rapid enlargement of an existing ACTH-secreting pituitary adenoma due to loss of negative feedback from adrenal glands.
- Clinical features include development of hyperpigmentation (due to high ACTH) within one-or two-years following adrenalectomy, headache and visual disturbances (due to pressure effect of macroadenoma). There may be signs of hypopituitarism due to compression of normal pituitary by the macroadenoma.
- Treatment involves resection of pituitary adenoma and irradiation.

Q. Discuss the etiology, clinical features, diagnosis, and management of mineralocorticoid excess (aldosteronism).

OR

Q. Discuss the etiology, clinical features, diagnosis, and management of primary hyperaldosteronism (Conn's syndrome).

Q. Secondary hyperaldosteronism.

- Hyperaldosteronism is the condition of excessive secretion of aldosterone from the adrenals. Primary hyperaldosteronism occurs due to excessive production of aldosterone within the adrenals. In secondary hyperaldosteronism the stimulus is extra-adrenal.
- Excessive production of aldosterone leads to hypertension, sodium retention, suppression of plasma renin and hypokalemia.

Etiology

Primary hyperaldosteronism (↓ Renin)
- Adrenal adenoma secreting aldosterone (Conn's syndrome)
- Idiopathic bilateral adrenal hyperplasia
- Familial hyperaldosteronism
- Adrenal carcinoma (rare)

Secondary hyperaldosteronism (↑ Renin)
- Pregnancy
- Inadequate renal perfusion, e.g. hypovolemia, cardiac failure, nephrotic syndrome, renal artery stenosis
- Renin-secreting renal tumor (very rare)

Clinical Features

- Sodium retention causes hypertension which is often resistant to treatment.
- Hypokalemia causes muscle weakness or even paralysis.
- Metabolic alkalosis: This is due to increased urinary hydrogen excretion mediated both by hypokalemia and by the direct stimulatory effect of aldosterone on distal acidification.
- There may be nephrogenic diabetes insipidus (excess aldosterone → hypokalemia → renal tubular resistance to ADH → nephrogenic diabetes insipidus).

Investigations

- Serum electrolytes may show hypernatremia, hypokalemia and increased bicarbonate.
- Plasma renin activity and aldosterone levels-renin is low and aldosterone level is high in Conn's syndrome and bilateral adrenal hyperplasia. Aldosterone-to-renin ratio (ARR) of >20–30 with plasma aldosterone >15 ng/dL → is suggestive of primary hyperaldosteronism.
- Abdominal CT-is useful to detect any adrenal tumors.
- If CT is inconclusive, adrenal vein catheterization with measurement of aldosterone or ^{131}iodo-norcholesterol scanning may be helpful.

Management

Primary Hyperaldosteronism

- Treatment for primary hyperaldosteronism includes laparoscopic resection for adenomas.
- For patients who are unable to undergo surgery aldosterone antagonists (spironolactone or eplerenone) can be used to treat both hypokalemia and hypertension. High doses of spironolactone (up to 400 mg/day) may be required but cause gynecomastia.
- Amiloride (10–40 mg/day), which blocks the epithelial sodium channel regulated by aldosterone, or eplerenone can be used if spironolactone is not tolerated due to gynecomastia.

Secondary Hyperaldosteronism

- Underlying cause should be treated.

Q. Pheochromocytoma.

- Pheochromocytoma is catecholamine-secreting tumor that arises from chromaffin cells of the adrenal medulla or the sympathetic ganglia. The catecholamines secreted include norepinephrine, epinephrine, and dopamine.
- 90% of tumors arise in adrenal medulla. There is a useful 'rule of tens' in this condition: 10% are malignant, 10% are extra-adrenal (i.e. in sympathetic ganglia), 10% are bilateral, and 10% are familial.
- Pheochromocytoma may be part of the syndrome of familial multiple endocrine neoplasia (MEN) types 2A and 2B, in which other endocrine tumors (parathyroid or medullary carcinoma of the thyroid) coexist or develop subsequently.

Clinical Features

- Paroxysmal hypertension associated with pallor (occasionally flushing), palpitations, sweating, headache and anxiety (fear of death). Classic triad is considered to be episodic headache, sweating, and palpitations.
- Abdominal pain, vomiting
- Constipation
- Weight loss
- Glucose intolerance
- Panic attacks, anxiety, tremor.

Investigations

- Plasma free metanephrines are elevated. This is the best initial test with high sensitivity (>95%). Metanephrines are metabolites of catecholamines and are continuously produced, making them reliable even between attacks unlike measuring catecholamines directly.
- 24-hour urinary metanephrines → elevated.
- 24-hour urinary catecholamines (epinephrine, norepinephrine, dopamine). This is less sensitive than metanephrines.
- Clonidine suppression test: can be done if results are borderline from above tests. In pheochromocytoma, clonidine fails to suppress catecholamine levels.
- CT or MRI of the abdomen to detect adrenal tumor.
- MIBG scan: Metaiodobenzylguanidine (MIBG) resembles norepinephrine and is taken up by adrenergic tissue. MIBG scan can detect tumors not detected by CT or MRI. Especially useful in extra-adrenal, multiple, metastatic, or occult tumor.
- Positron emission tomography (PET) scan is superior to MIBG in the evaluation of metastatic disease.

Management

- The gold standard treatment of pheochromocytoma is surgical resection of tumor. Preoperative preparation is done with α blocker phenoxybenzamine or labetalol.
- If excision is not possible, medical therapy with alpha and beta blocking drugs (phenoxybenzamine and propranolol, or labetalol) is necessary. Beta blockers should not be given alone, as unopposed alpha action will lead to hypertensive crisis.

Q. Discuss the etiology, clinical features, investigations and management of adrenal insufficiency.

Q. Discuss the etiology, clinical features, investigations and management of Addison disease.

- Adrenal insufficiency refers to inadequate production of glucocorticoids (± mineralocorticoids and androgens) by the adrenal cortex.
- Adrenal insufficiency results from destruction or dysfunction of the entire adrenal cortex.
- It is of two types: Primary (due to destruction or dysfunction of adrenal cortex), secondary (due to pituitary or hypothalamic disease leading to ACTH and CRH deficiency). Primary adrenal insufficiency is also known as Addison's disease.
- Adrenal insufficiency can be acute or chronic. Acute adrenal insufficiency (acute adrenal crisis) is a medical emergency.

Etiology

Primary adrenal insufficiency (Addison's disease)

- **Autoimmune adrenalitis** (most common in developed countries)
- **Infections:** Tuberculosis, HIV, histoplasmosis
- **Carcinoma:** Metastatic carcinoma, lymphoma
- **Infiltrative diseases:** Hemochromatosis, sarcoidosis, amyloidosis
- **Iatrogenic:** Bilateral adrenalectomy, post radiotherapy
- **Adrenal hemorrhage:** Waterhouse-Friedrichsen syndrome following meningococcal septicemia, anticoagulation, trauma
- **Drugs:** Aminoglutethimide, metyrapone, ketoconazole
- **Genetic:** Congenital adrenal hyperplasia, polyglandular syndromes.

Secondary (↓ ACTH from pituitary)

- Pituitary disease
- Withdrawal of glucocorticoid therapy

Tertiary (↓ CRH from hypothalamus)

- Long-term glucocorticoid therapy
- Hypothalamic tumors

Clinical Features (Fig. 9.15)

- Symptoms and signs are due to low glucocorticoid, low mineralocorticoid, low adrenal androgen levels and secondary increase in ACTH (in primary adrenal insufficiency) and renin.
- Glucocorticoid deficiency causes malaise, fatigue, generalized weakness, nausea, vomiting, anorexia,

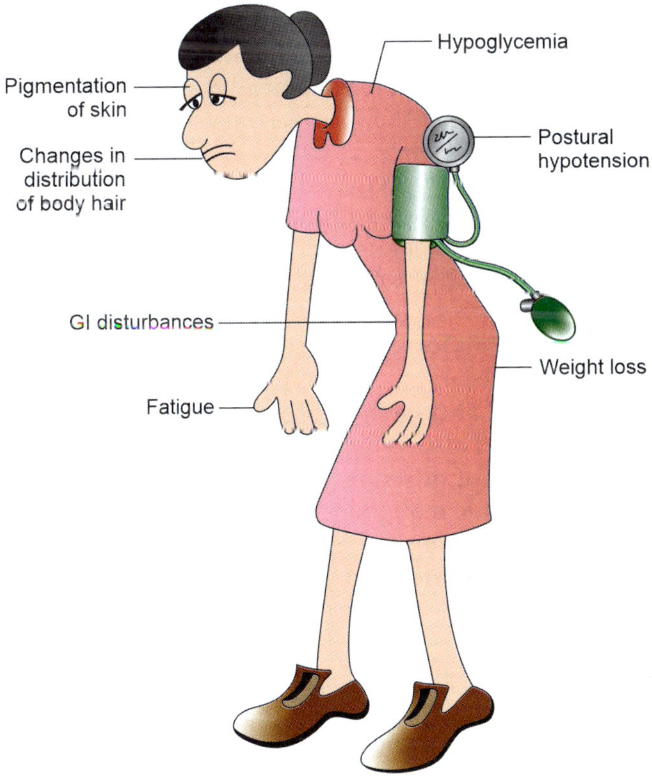

Figure 9.15: Clinical features of adrenal insufficiency

weight loss, postural hypotension with postural drop and hypoglycemia.

- Mineralocorticoid deficiency causes hyponatremia and hyperkalemia. Salt craving, may be present in some patients.
- ACTH excess in primary adrenal deficiency (Addison disease) causes hyperpigmentation. Hyperpigmentation is seen in exposed areas or pressure sites such as knuckles, elbows, knees, palmar creases, nail beds, nipples, tongue, buccal mucosa, gums and conjunctivae. Hyperpigmentation is not seen in secondary adrenal insufficiency as ACTH is low. Vitiligo may be seen especially with autoimmune etiology.

Investigations

- **Serum cortisol level**-an early morning (between 8 and 9 AM) serum cortisol concentration less than 3 µg/dl suggests adrenal insufficiency and a value above 19 µg/dl excludes it.
- **ACTH stimulation test (synacthen test)**–250 µg of ACTH (Synacthen) is given by IM injection at any time of day. Blood samples are drawn at 0, 30, and 60 minutes after injection for plasma cortisol. In normal subjects plasma cortisol is >17 µg/dl either at baseline or at 30 minutes. Cortisol levels fail to increase in primary adrenal insufficiency.
- **Serum ACTH level:** Primary and secondary adrenal insufficiency can be distinguished by measurement of ACTH which is low in ACTH deficiency and high in Addison's disease.
- **Serum electrolytes:** Hyponatremia and hyperkaliemia are seen.
- **HIV test** if risk factors for infection are present.
- **Insulin-induced hypoglycemia test:** This is a gold standard test to assess hypothalamic-pituitary-adrenal (HPA) axis integrity. Specifically used to evaluate secondary (pituitary) or tertiary (hypothalamic) adrenal insufficiency, i.e. where ACTH production is impaired. Hypoglycemia → sensed by hypothalamus → release of CRH → stimulation of ACTH release by pituitary → stimulation of adrenal glands → increased cortisol. Failure of cortisol to rise indicates secondary or tertiary adrenal insufficiency.
- **Plain X-ray abdomen** may show adrenal calcification in tuberculosis.
- **Ultrasound abdomen** is useful to assess the size of adrenals and also to detect any tumors.
- **CT or MRI of adrenals** to look for size of adrenals and metastatic malignancy (better than ultrasound).
- Adrenal and other organ specific antibodies may be present in autoimmune adrenalitis.

Management

- Patients should receive lifelong steroid replacement therapy.
- Cortisol 15 mg in the morning and 5 mg at 6 pm or prednisolone 5 mg in the morning and 2.5 mg in the evening.
- During intercurrent illness the dose of steroid should be doubled. During surgery, oral steroid should be changed to parenteral dose, i.e. hydrocortisone 100 mg 6-hourly for 24 hours, then 50 mg IM 6-hourly until ready to take tablets.
- Patient should carry a steroid card all the time which should give information regarding diagnosis, steroid, dose and doctor. Patients should be encouraged to wear a bracelet engraved with the diagnosis all the time. All these can help in emergencies.
- Underlying cause should be treated.

Q. Acute adrenal crisis (Acute adrenal insufficiency; Addisonian crisis).

- Acute adrenal crisis is a life-threatening emergency resulting from severe deficiency of glucocorticoids (± mineralocorticoids).

Etiology/Precipitating Factors

Acute adrenal crisis can occur in the following situations:

- Serious infection or other major stress in a previously undiagnosed patient with adrenal insufficiency
- Skipping of steroid or failure to increase the dose in a patient with known adrenal insufficiency during major illness or stress
- Bilateral adrenal hemorrhage (Waterhouse-Friederichsen syndrome, anticoagulant therapy)
- Pituitary apoplexy
- Rapid withdrawal of steroids in a patient who is taking them for a long time.

Clinical Features

- Hypotension or shock
- Dehydration
- Nausea, vomiting and abdominal pain. Abdominal rigidity or rebound tenderness may be present mimicking acute abdomen.
- Confusion or disorientation
- Fever may be present due to underlying infection
- Hypoglycemia
- Mnemonic–"5 H's of adrenal crisis": Hypotension, Hyponatremia, Hyperkalemia, Hypoglycemia, Hyperpigmentation (only in primary AI).

Investigations

- There may be hyperkalemia, hypernatremia, hypoglycemia, lymphocytosis and eosinophilia.
- Low serum cortisol
- High ACTH (in primary); low ACTH (in secondary).
- Other tests as described under adrenal insufficiency.

Management

- It is a medical emergency.
- Rapid replacement of steroid, sodium and water deficits are the primary goals of therapy.
- IV fluid (DNS) is started immediately.

- Inj hydrocortisone 100–200 mg is given intravenously and rthen 50 mg IV 6th hourly. 50 mg hydrocortisone can be given IM if there is problem with IV access.
- Once the patient's condition improves, he is put on oral steroids and oral fluids and the dose of steroids is slowly tapered to the maintenance dose.
- The precipitating cause should be identified and treated.

Q. Waterhouse-Friderichsen syndrome.

- This refers to acute adrenal insufficiency due to bilateral adrenal hemorrhage.
- It is caused by severe infection with meningococcus or other bacteria. Rarely, it can be caused by adrenal vein thrombosis leading to venous stasis and hemorrhage.
- Clinical features are same as that of acute adrenal insufficiency. There is development of hypotension with shock. Patient may complain of abdominal pain especially in the flanks. There may be signs of meningococcal infection such as meningitis, cutaneous hemorrhages, etc. In the advanced stages, patient has respiratory failure and slips into coma.
- Treatment is same as that of acute adrenal insufficiency. In addition, appropriate antibiotics should be used to treat meningococcal septicemia (penicillin G) or other bacterial sepsis.

Q. Steroid therapy.

- Steroid therapy refers to the clinical use of corticosteroids, particularly glucocorticoids, to treat a wide range of medical conditions.
- Corticosteroids are synthetic analogs of the natural steroid hormones produced by the adrenal cortex. Corticosteroids are among the most widely used class of drugs.

Types of Corticosteroids

Glucocorticoids

- Examples: Hydrocortisone, prednisone, dexamethasone.
- Effects: Anti-inflammatory, immunosuppressive, metabolic regulation.

Mineralocorticoids

- Example: Fludrocortisone.
- Effects: Sodium and water retention, potassium excretion.

Indications for Steroids

Replacement therapy
- Adrenal insufficiency
- Congenital adrenal hyperplasia

Anti-inflammatory/Immunosuppressive uses
- Anaphylaxis
- Bronchial asthma
- Cerebral edema
- Connective tissue diseases
- Autoimmune diseases
- Nephrotic and nephritic syndrome
- Septic shock
- ARDS
- TB Pericarditis
- Demyelinating diseases
- TB Meningitis
- COVID-19 (in severe cases)

Malignancies
- Leukemia, lymphoma
- In malignancies along with chemotherapy

Other uses
- Preterm labor (to mature fetal lungs–betamethasone)

Contraindications for Steroids

- Active tuberculosis
- Peptic ulcer
- Uncontrolled diabetes
- Uncontrolled hypertension
- Active infection

Side Effects of Steroid Therapy

Metabolic
- Hyperglycemia, insulin resistance
- Weight gain, fat redistribution (Cushingoid features)
- Suppression of hypothalamic-pituitary adrenal (HPA) axis.

Musculoskeletal
- Osteoporosis
- Proximal myopathy
- Growth suppression in children.

Gastrointestinal
- Peptic ulcers
- GI bleeding.

Immunosuppression
- Increased infection risk
- Latent tuberculosis may be reactivated.

Neuropsychiatric
- Mood swings, psychosis
- Insomnia.

Ophthalmic
- Cataracts
- Glaucoma.

Dermatologic
- Skin thinning
- Easy bruising
- Poor wound healing.

Measures to Minimize Side Effects

- Give the minimum effective dose
- Give on alternate day rather than daily
- Give in the morning
- Give for the minimum possible duration
- Monitor blood sugar during therapy
- H_2 blockers or proton pump inhibitors to reduce gastric side effects
- Calcium and vitamin D to prevent osteoporosis.

Withdrawal of Steroid Therapy

- Steroid therapy for more than 3 weeks can cause hypothalamic-pituitary-adrenal axis (HPA) suppression, and if stopped suddenly may cause acute adrenal insufficiency (crisis). Hence, steroid withdrawal must be gradual. All patients must be advised to avoid sudden drug withdrawal.

Q. Congenital adrenal hyperplasia.

Etiology

- Congenital adrenal hyperplasia (CAH) is a group of autosomal recessive disorders characterized by enzyme deficiencies in adrenal steroidogenesis.
- This leads to—cortisol deficiency ± aldosterone deficiency, and excess androgen production.

Pathophysiology

- 21-alpha hydroxylase deficiency causes 90% of all cases of congenital adrenal hyperplasia.
- 21-alpha hydroxylase deficiency causes defective conversion of adrenal precursors to cortisol and, in some cases, to aldosterone. Accumulated hormone precursors (such as 17-OH-progesterone) are shunted into androgen production, causing virilization.
- Cortisol deficiency results in impaired negative feedback and increased ACTH secretion. Increased ACTH causes adrenal hyperplasia and excess production of steroids 'proximal' to the enzyme block.
- All these enzyme defects are inherited as autosomal recessive traits.

Clinical Features

- Cortisol (glucocorticoid) deficiency causes weight loss, hypotension, fatigability, etc.
- Aldosterone deficiency leads to hyponatremia, hypovolemia and hyperkalemia.
- Androgen excess causes ambiguous genitalia in girls, precocious pseudopuberty, amenorrhea and/or hirsutism.
- 17-hydroxylase and 11β-hydroxylase deficiency may produce hypertension due to excess production of 11-deoxycorticosterone, a mineralocorticoid.

Investigations

- High level of plasma 17-hydroxyprogesterone is found in 21-hydroxylase deficiency.
- ↑ ACTH, ↓ cortisol
- ↑ Androgens (testosterone, androstenedione)
- Electrolytes: Hyponatremia, hyperkalemia (salt-wasting).
- Ultrasound or CT abdomen shows adrenal hyperplasia
- Genetic testing in suspected individuals
- Newborn screening: Universal in many countries Dried blood spot for 17-Hydroxyprogesterone on days 2–5.
- In siblings of affected children, antenatal diagnosis can be made by amniocentesis or chorionic villus sampling.

Management

- The aim is to replace deficient corticosteroids, and also suppress ACTH and hence adrenal androgen production.
- This can be achieved by giving a large dose of a long-acting synthetic glucocorticoid (hydrocortisone in children, prednisone in adults) before going to bed to suppress the early morning ACTH peak, and a smaller dose is given in the morning.
- Mineralocorticoid (fludrocortisone) if salt-wasting and hyponatremia is present.
- If hirsutism is the main problem, antiandrogen therapy is given.

Q. Gynecomastia.

- Gynecomastia is defined as a benign proliferation of the glandular tissue of the male breast.
- It presents clinically as the presence of a rubbery or firm mass extending concentrically from the nipple.
- Fat deposition without glandular proliferation is termed pseudogynecomastia. Pseudogynecomastia is seen in obese men.

Causes of Gynecomastia

Physiologic
- Pubertal (transient imbalance of estrogen and testosterone)
- Elderly (due to reduced testosterone production and increased peripheral aromatization of androgens)

Increased estrogen production
- Testicular tumors (Leydig cell tumor, Sertoli cell tumor, hCG-secreting tumors)
- Adrenal tumors
- Estrogen-producing tumors (hepatocellular carcinoma)

Increased peripheral conversion of androgens to estrogens
- Obesity
- Hyperthyroidism
- Liver cirrhosis

Androgen deficiency
- Primary hypogonadism (Klinefelter's syndrome, mumps orchitis)
- Secondary hypogonadism (pituitary/hypothalamic disorders)

Drugs
- Spironolactone
- Cimetidine
- Ketoconazole
- Finasteride
- Digoxin
- Estrogens
- Alcohol

Others
- Chronic renal failure
- HIV infection
- Idiopathic

History

- Ask about the duration of breast enlargement, pain, nipple discharge, whether secondary sexual characteristics are fully developed, and the relationship between onset of gynecomastia and puberty.

- H/o of delayed puberty, decreased libido, and erectile dysfunction suggests hypogonadism.
- H/o chronic alcohol intake, jaundice and ascites suggest cirrhosis of liver. H/o tremor, heat intolerance, and diarrhea suggest hyperthyroidism.
- Enquire about the drug intake which can cause gynecomastia.

Physical Examination

- Look for development of secondary sexual characteristics (e.g. the penis, pubic hair, and axillary hair). Also look for development of mustache and beard. Non-development of these features suggests hypogonadism. Examine the testes for masses or atrophy.
- Examine the breasts for any nipple discharge, consistency, fixation to underlying tissues, and skin changes. Findings which suggest malignancy are eccentric breast swelling, nipple discharge, fixation to the skin, nipple retraction, axillary lymphadenopathy, and hard consistency.
- Look for signs/symptoms of hypogonadism such as absence of pubic hair, testicular atrophy, infantile penis etc.
- Look for symptoms or signs of hyperthyroidism (e.g. tremor, tachycardia, sweating, heat intolerance, weight loss).

Investigations

- Breast ultrasound and mammography is done if breast cancer is suspected.
- If hypogonadism is suspected, serum LH, FSH, testosterone, estradiol, and hCG levels should be measured.
- Further tests are based on the suspicion of underlying disease.

Treatment

- No specific treatment is needed for physiological gynecomastia which usually remits spontaneously.
- Treatment of the underlying cause.
- Drugs causing gynecomastia should be stopped.
- Tamoxifen 10 mg orally bid can be tried if pain and tenderness are very troublesome.
- If cosmetic appearance is unacceptable, surgical removal of excess breast tissue can be done.

Q. Hirsutism.

- Hirsutism is the excessive growth of thick or dark hair in women in locations that are more typical of male hair growth patterns (e.g. mustache, beard, central chest, shoulders, lower abdomen, back, inner thigh). It is due to androgen excess due to many causes.
- Hypertrichosis is a separate condition. It is generalized non–androgen-dependent excessive hair growth.

Etiology

- Idiopathic
- Familial
- Polycystic ovary syndrome (PCOS)
- Congenital adrenal hyperplasia
- Ovarian and adrenal tumors
- Drugs (testosterone, danazol, minoxidil, anabolic steroids)
- Hypothyroidism
- Acromegaly
- ACTH-induced Cushing's disease.

Clinical Features

- Increase in hair is seen on the chin, upper lip, abdomen, and chest.
- Androgen excess also increases sebaceous gland activity, producing acne.
- Menstrual irregularities, anovulation, and amenorrhea are common.
- Defeminization (decrease in breast size, loss of feminine adipose tissue) and virilization (frontal balding, muscularity, clitoromegaly, and deepening of the voice) occur if androgen excess is severe.
- Hypertension is seen in Cushing's syndrome, adrenal 11-hydroxylase deficiency, or cortisol resistance syndrome.

Investigations

- Serum testosterone level is elevated.
- 17-hydroxy progesterone level is elevated in congenital adrenal hyperplasia.
- Ultrasound abdomen to assess adrenals and ovaries.
- Adrenal CT.

Management

- Patients with mild hirsutism can be treated with an oral contraceptive.
- If androgen-secreting tumor is identified → Surgical removal.
- Any drugs causing hirsutism are stopped.
- Antiandrogen therapy—spironolactone, cyproterone acetate, finasteride, and flutamide have antiandrogenic activity and help to decrease hirsutism. These drugs should be used only in nonpregnant women.
- Local treatment—shaving, depilation, waxing, electrolysis, or bleaching are effective measures to remove excess hair. Eflornithine topical cream retards hair growth when applied twice daily to unwanted facial hair. Laser therapy is an effective treatment for facial hirsutism. Alopecia may be treated with minoxidil 2% solution applied twice daily to a dry scalp.

Q. Discuss the classification and pathogenesis of diabetes mellitus.

- Diabetes mellitus is a clinical syndrome characterized by impaired insulin secretion and variable degrees of peripheral insulin resistance leading to hyperglycemia.
- Diabetes occurs world-wide and the incidence of both type 1 and type 2 diabetes is rising. Majority of diabetics have type 2 diabetes. Many factors such as greater longevity, obesity, unsatisfactory diet, sedentary lifestyle and increasing urbanization contribute to development of type 2 diabetes.

- The prevalence of diabetes varies considerably around the world, and is related to differences in genetic and environmental factors. Type 2 diabetes is now being observed in children and adolescents also.
- Type 1 diabetes was previously termed 'insulin-dependent diabetes mellitus' (IDDM) since it is associated with profound insulin deficiency requiring insulin therapy. Type 2 diabetes was previously termed 'non-insulin-dependent diabetes mellitus' (NIDDM) because patients retain the capacity to secrete some insulin but exhibit impaired sensitivity to insulin (insulin resistance) and can usually be treated without insulin replacement. However, in advanced type 2 diabetes there is profound insulin deficiency and it behaves like type 1 diabetes, requiring insulin.

Etiologic Classification of Diabetes Mellitus

I. Type 1 diabetes (beta-cell destruction, leading to absolute insulin deficiency)

- Immune-mediated (autoantibodies present)
- Idiopathic (no autoantibodies).
- Latent autoimmune diabetes in adults (LADA)

II. Type 2 diabetes (associated with insulin resistance)

III. Gestational diabetes mellitus (GDM)

IV. Other specific types of diabetes

- *Monogenic diabetes syndromes*: Such as neonatal diabetes and maturity-onset diabetes of the young.
- *Diseases of the exocrine pancreas*: Pancreatitis, cystic fibrosis.
- *Endocrinopathies*: Acromegaly, Cushing's syndrome, glucagonoma, pheochromocytoma, hyperthyroidism, somatostatinoma.
- *Drug or chemical-induced diabetes*: Glucocorticoids, diazoxide, pentamidine, thiazides, beta-blockers, HIV drugs, etc.)
- *Other genetic syndromes sometimes associated with diabetes:* Down syndrome, Turner's syndrome, Klinefelter's syndrome, and Wolfram syndrome.

Normal Physiology

- In humans, blood glucose is maintained within a narrow range by a balance between factors which increase blood sugar and factors which decrease blood sugar. Factors which increase blood sugar are intestinal absorption of glucose after meals, gluconeogenesis and glycogenolysis by the liver. Factors which decrease blood sugar are glucose uptake by peripheral tissues, particularly skeletal muscles, glycolysis and glycogenesis.
- When blood glucose is high, there is stimulation of insulin secretion from pancreas which facilitates peripheral glucose uptake by liver and skeletal muscles.
- When intestinal glucose absorption declines between meals, hepatic glucose output (gluconeogenesis and glycogenolysis) is increased in response to low insulin levels and increased levels of the counterregulatory hormones (glucagon and adrenaline).

Pathogenesis of Diabetes

Type 1 Diabetes

Genetic predisposition

- Polygenic inheritance; no single gene causes T1DM.
- Strongest association with HLA haplotypes DR3 and DR4. HLA haplotypes account for ~50% of genetic risk.

Autoimmunity

- Type 1 diabetes is a slowly progressive T cell-mediated autoimmune disease. Defective presentation of auto antigens derived from pancreatic islet β cells probably leads to the development of autoimmunity. The pathological picture in type 1 diabetes is characterized by 'insulitis', that is, infiltration of the islets with mononuclear cells (macrophages, T lymphocytes, natural killer cells and B lymphocytes).
- Islet cell antibodies can be detected even before the clinical development of type 1 diabetes.
- Type 1 diabetes may be associated with other autoimmune disorders such as thyroid disease, coeliac disease, Addison's disease, pernicious anemia and vitiligo.

Environmental factors

- Along with genetic factors, environmental factors are important for the expression of type 1 diabetes.
- Reduced exposure to microorganisms in early childhood limits maturation of the immune system and may increase susceptibility to autoimmune disease.
- Some viral infections (mumps, Coxsackie B4, retroviruses, rubella, CMV, EBV) may cause type 1 diabetes as evidenced by isolation of virus particles from the pancreas known to cause cytopathic or autoimmune damage to β cells.
- Dietary factors such as cow's milk, has been implicated in triggering type 1 diabetes. Children who are given cow's milk early in infancy are more likely to develop type 1 diabetes than those who are breastfed. Nitrosamines (found in smoked and cured meats) and coffee have also been proposed as potentially diabetogenic toxins.
- Stress may precipitate type 1 diabetes by increasing counter-regulatory hormones and immunomodulation.

Type 2 Diabetes

- In type 2 diabetes there is a combination of resistance to the action of insulin in liver and muscle, together with impaired pancreatic β-cell function leading to 'relative' insulin deficiency. In the beginning there is increased insulin secretion to counteract insulin resistance. But as the disease progresses, there is progressive beta cell failure and insulin deficiency develops.

Insulin resistance

- Resistance to the action of insulin in the liver and muscle leads to overproduction and underutilization of glucose respectively leading to hyperglycemia. Type 2 diabetes is often associated with central (visceral) obesity, hypertension and dyslipidemia (elevated LDL cholesterol and triglycerides, low HDL cholesterol). Coexistence of this cluster of conditions is called 'insulin resistance syndrome' or 'metabolic syndrome'. Metabolic syndrome predisposes to cardiovascular diseases.

- The exact cause of insulin resistance remains unclear. However, there are many factors which contribute to insulin resistance. Central obesity (especially intra-abdominal fat) causes insulin resistance because large quantities of free fatty acids (FFA) released by adipose tissue compete with glucose to be utilized by peripheral tissues. Adipose tissue also releases many hormones (e.g. cortisol, adipokines) which may decrease the sensitivity of insulin receptors.
- Lack of exercise increases insulin resistance by down-regulation of insulin-sensitive kinases and by the accumulation of FFAs within skeletal muscle. Exercise allows non-insulin-dependent glucose uptake by muscles.

Pancreatic β-cell failure

- There is progressive reduction in beta cell mass. There is deposition of amylin around beta cells which forms insoluble fibrils of amyloid leading to destruction of beta cells.

Genetic predisposition

- Genetic factors are important in the etiology of type 2 diabetes. There is almost 100% concordance rate in monozygotic twins. Many susceptibility genes have been found which increase the risk of developing diabetes.

Obesity

- Overeating increases the risk of type 2 diabetes, especially when combined with obesity and underactivity. The risk of developing type 2 diabetes increases tenfold in people with a body mass index of >30.

Aging

- Type 2 diabetes usually affects middle-aged and elderly. Most of them are over 50 years of age.

Other Specific Types of Diabetes

Most of these types of diabetes have an obvious cause of destruction of pancreatic β cells. Endocrine diseases such as acromegaly or Cushing's syndrome cause diabetes by increasing counter regulatory hormones.

Gestational Diabetes

- The term 'gestational diabetes' refers to hyperglycemia occurring for the first time during pregnancy. Many of these women ultimately develop permanent diabetes.
- During pregnancy, insulin sensitivity is reduced through the action of placental hormones and there is increased insulin demand. Beta cells may be unable to meet this demand which leads to development of gestational diabetes mellitus.

Q. Describe the epidemiology, risk factors, pathogenesis, clinical features, investigations, and treatment type 1 diabetes.

- Type 1 diabetes mellitus is a chronic autoimmune disease characterized by the destruction of insulin-producing β-cells in the pancreas, resulting in absolute insulin deficiency leading to hyperglycemia.
- It was earlier known as insulin dependent diabetes mellitus (IDDM).

Epidemiology

- *Prevalence:* ~5–10% of all diabetes cases worldwide.
- *Age of onset:* Can occur at any age, but two bimodal peaks are observed between age 4–6 years and 10–14 years (puberty-related).
- *Geographic variation*: High incidence in scandinavia (Finland, Sweden) and Sardinia. Low incidence is seen in Asia, South America. In India, regional pediatric prevalence ranges from 3–18/100,000.
- *Gender:* Slight male predominance in some countries; others show equal sex distribution.
- *Incidence trends*: Increasing globally (~3–5% per year). Hypothesized link to environmental factors (hygiene hypothesis, changes in gut microbiome).

Risk Factors

Genetic Susceptibility

- Strongly linked to HLA class II alleles: DR3-DQ2 and DR4-DQ8 (~90% of cases in children).
- Other genes: PTPN22, INS, CTLA4, IL2RA.
- Family history of type 1 diabetes increases the risk.

Environmental Triggers

- Viral infections: Coxsackievirus B, rubella, enteroviruses.
- Early cow's milk introduction.
- Low vitamin D.
- Toxins.
- Gut microbiome alterations.
- Hygiene hypothesis: reduced early microbial exposure may predispose to autoimmune conditions.

Pathogenesis

- Genetic factors and environmental triggers predispose the individual to autoimmune destruction of beta cells. Both cell mediated and antibody mediated immune response play a role in the pathogenesis of type 1 DM (type 1A). Cell-mediated destruction involves chronic insulitis (immune-cell infiltration in islets) involving CD8^{+} T-cells, macrophages, B cells, and dendritic cells.
- Autoantibodies mediating destruction of beta cells are: Insulin (IAA), GAD65, IA-2, ZnT8, islet-cell antibodies (ICA). Multiple and higher-titer autoantibodies confer greater risk
- Stages of disease progression:
  - **Stage 1:** Autoimmunity with ≥2 antibodies, normal glucose.
  - **Stage 2:** Dysglycemia (impaired glucose), still asymptomatic.
  - **Stage 3:** Clinical type 1 DM: Hyperglycemia and symptoms emerge once ~80–90% β-cells are lost.
- A minority (10–30%) have idiopathic, non-autoimmune β-cell destruction (type 1B).

Clinical Features

Asymptomatic

- Many diabetics are asymptomatic and are detected during routine health checkups or when they are seen for some other illness.

Polyuria, Nocturia

- Occurs because of glucose in the urine which acts as an osmotic diuretic.

Polyphagia

- Though there is hyperglycemia, it cannot be used by cells due to lack of insulin or insulin resistance. Hence, a diabetic feels more hungry than usual.

Thirst, Dry Mouth

- This happens because high blood glucose absorbs water from the tissues causing dehydration and thirst. Polyuria also leads to dehydration and increased thirst.

Easy Fatigability

- Inability to properly utilize blood glucose leads to easy fatigability.

Recurrent Infections and Delayed Wound Healing

- Hyperglycemia inhibits inflammatory response, chemotaxis, decreased neutrophil function etc which lead to increased incidence of infections and delayed wound healing. Patients may present with skin sepsis (boils) and genital candidiasis, and complain of pruritus vulvae or balanitis.

Weight Loss

- Since there is loss of calories in the form of glucose in the urine, there is negative energy balance and weight loss. A person loses weight in spite of eating more.

Symptoms of Peripheral Neuropathy

- Such as burning, tingling and numbness occur due to diabetic peripheral neuropathy. Initially these symptoms are felt in feet. Later on, it may involve the legs and hands.

Blurring of Vision

- This is due to the change in refractory power of lens due to hyperglycemia. Diabetic retinopathy is another cause in advanced diabetes.

Presenting as DKA and HHS

- Some patients present for the first time with one of the acute complications of diabetes such as diabetic ketoacidosis (DKA) or HHS (hyperglycemic hyperosmolar syndrome). DKA is common in type-1 diabetes and HHS in type-2 diabetes.

Investigations

Blood Glucose and HbA1c

- Fasting ≥126 mg/dL, or
- Random ≥200 mg/dL with symptoms, or
- 2-hour OGTT ≥200 mg/dL, or
- HbA1c ≥6.5%.

C-peptide

- **Low (<200 pmol/L) or absent C-peptide** indicates β-cell failure typical of type 1 DM. Sample is best taken after glucose ingestion (non-fasting) or post-meal. Preserved levels suggest T2D.

Autoantibodies

- GAD65 autoantibodies—present in ~70–80% of new-onset cases. GAD65 (glutamic acid decarboxylase) is an enzyme in pancreatic β-cells. It is the most sensitive autoantibody test to diagnose type 1 DM.
- Insulin autoantibodies (IAA)—seen in ~50% of children at diagnosis; less common in adults.
- Islet cell antibodies (ICA)—positive in around 60–80%.
- IA-2A (insulinoma-associated-2)—present in ~60% of new cases.
- ZnT8A (zinc transporter 8)—found in ~60%, helps detect LADA as well.

Additional Tests

- Lipid profile
- Renal function tests (serum creatinine, eGFR, urine albumin-creatinine ratio)
- Liver function tests
- Urine examination for proteinuria
- Fundoscopy
- ECG (for cardiovascular risk assessment)
- Neuropathy screening (monofilament, vibration sense).

DKA Work-up

- ABG, electrolytes, serum ketones, urine ketones, serum osmolality.

Screen for Associated Autoimmune Conditions

- TSH, anti-TPO (thyroid), adrenal antibodies, coeliac serology.

Treatment of Type 1 Diabetes

Glycemic Targets

- A1C value of <7%.
- Preprandial glucose 80–130 mg/dl.
- Postprandial peak <180 mg/dl.

Insulin Replacement

- Type 1 DM requires lifelong insulin therapy to achieve glycemic targets. Injection devices include syringes, pens, pumps, and rarely inhaled insulin.
- Many types of insulin regimens are available to achieve the goals which are as follows:

Twice daily insulin

- Twice-daily administration of a mixture of short-acting (**regular insulin, lispro, aspart or glulisine**) and intermediate-acting insulin (**NPH insulin**), given before breakfast and dinner is the commonly used regimen. Many premixed insulin preparations are available containing different proportions of short acting and intermediate acting insulin (30:70 and 50:50).

Basal–bolus regimen

- This requires short-acting insulin (**regular insulin, lispro, aspart or glulisine**) before each meal, and a long-acting insulin (**glargine, detemir or degludec**) injected at bedtime. This regimen mimics the physiological insulin secretion patterns.

Continuous subcutaneous insulin infusion (CSII)

- This makes of insulin pumps worn on the body to deliver continuous basal dose as well as premeal bolus dose. Only rapid acting insulin or analogues are used in the pump. It offers precise dosing and flexibility.

Adjunctive Therapies (these are not routinely recommended)

- Amylinomimetic (pramlintide/symlin)—slows gastric emptying, reduces postprandial glucose.
- Off-label use of GLP-1 agonists (e.g. semaglutide/ozempic)—may reduce insulin doses, aid weight loss, but not FDA-approved for T1 DM
- Other adjuncts (SGLT2 inhibitors, metformin) remain under study and are not routinely used.
- Note that sulphonylureas cannot be used in type 1 DM because these drugs work by stimulating beta cells to release insulin, and in type 1 DM, there is already beta cell failure. Hence, no use of stimulating beta cells.

Islet-cell transplantation and whole-pancreas transplantation

- Can be an option in selected patients with end-stage renal disease or refractory hypoglycemia. It can achieve insulin independence.

Lifestyle and Supportive Care

- **Medical nutrition therapy:** Fiber-rich and low-fat diets.
- **Physical activity:** Improves insulin sensitivity; requires glucose monitoring and insulin adjustments to prevent hypoglycemia.
- **Education and psychosocial support:** Includes self-monitoring of glucose (SMBG), carb counting, hypoglycemia sick-day rules, mental health screening.

Q. Describe the epidemiology, risk factors, pathogenesis, clinical features, investigations, and treatment type 2 diabetes.

- Type 2 diabetes mellitus is a chronic metabolic disorder characterized by hyperglycemia resulting from a combination of:
  - Insulin resistance in peripheral tissues (muscle, liver, adipose tissue), and
  - Progressive beta-cell dysfunction in the pancreas leading to relative insulin deficiency.
- Unlike type 1 diabetes, where there is absolute insulin deficiency due to autoimmune destruction of beta cells, in T2DM, insulin is initially produced but is not used effectively by the body's tissues.
- It was earlier known as insulin dependent diabetes mellitus (IDDM).

Epidemiology

Global Burden

- Over 400 million are affected globally. Projected to reach more than 700 million by 2045.

India

- Over 100 million adults in 2023; major contributor to global diabetes prevalence ("Diabetes capital of the world").

Age

- Typically diagnosed after age 40, but increasing prevalence in younger adults and adolescents in many countries.

Sex

- Affects both sexes equally; slight male preponderance in some populations.

Urban vs Rural

- Higher prevalence in urban populations due to sedentary lifestyle and dietary patterns.

Socioeconomic Impact

- Major cause of morbidity, mortality, and healthcare expenditure worldwide.

Risk Factors

Nonmodifiable

- Age >45 years.
- Sex: Females are 1.2–1.7 times more likely than males to progress from prediabetes and develop T2DM during adolescence.
- Family history of diabetes (first-degree relatives).
- Ethnicity: Higher risk in South Asians, African Americans, Hispanics, Native Americans.
- History of gestational diabetes mellitus (GDM).
- Polycystic ovary syndrome (PCOS).
- Genetic susceptibility.

Modifiable

- Overweight and obesity (especially central/visceral obesity)
- Sedentary lifestyle
- Unhealthy diet (high in refined carbohydrates, fats)
- Smoking
- Excessive alcohol intake
- Low socioeconomic status.

Pathogenesis

- T2DM has a multifactorial etiology, a combination of genetic and environmental factors. The main factors are insulin resistance and progressive beta-cell dysfunction.

Insulin Resistance (main factor initially)

- The presence of insulin resistance explains the strong clinical association of T2DM with obesity and other insulin-resistant states.
- Target tissues (muscle, liver, adipose tissue) become resistant to insulin. Insulin resistance of skeletal muscles is regarded as one of the most important factor in the development of T2DM.
- Reduced glucose uptake by muscles
- Increased hepatic gluconeogenesis
- Lipolysis in adipose tissue → increased free fatty acids → worsening insulin resistance.

Beta-cell Dysfunction (progressive)

- Compensatory hyperinsulinemia initially.
- Progressive loss of beta-cell function and mass → relative insulin deficiency.
- Contributing factors: Glucotoxicity, lipotoxicity, oxidative stress, inflammation, islet amyloid deposition.
- Note that beta cell dysfunction is not mediated by autoantibodies against pancreatic islet cells in type 2 DM unlike in type-1 DM.

Role of Gut Microbiota

- The gut microbiota plays an important and evolving role in the pathogenesis of type 2 diabetes mellitus (T2DM)—an area of active research.
- It influences host metabolism, immune function, and energy homeostasis.
- Dysbiosis (an imbalance in the composition and function of gut microbiota) is associated with insulin resistance and T2DM.

Other Mechanisms

- Altered incretin effect (GLP-1, GIP deficiency or resistance)
- Increased glucagon secretion
- Renal glucose reabsorption (upregulated SGLT2)
- Low-grade systemic inflammation.

Clinical Features

Asymptomatic Phase (common)

- Many diagnosed incidentally during screening.

Classic Symptoms (see under type 1 diabetes for details of clinical features)

- Polyuria
- Polydipsia
- Polyphagia
- Unexplained weight loss
- Fatigue, weakness
- Blurred vision
- Recurrent infections (urinary tract, skin).

Complications (may be the first presentation)

- Microvascular: Retinopathy, nephropathy, neuropathy
- Macrovascular: Coronary artery disease, stroke, peripheral arterial disease
- Other: Non-alcoholic fatty liver disease (NAFLD), depression, infections
- Early type 2 diabetes can be controlled by diet and lifestyle modification alone. Other patients will require drugs or insulin or both.

Treatment of Type 2 Diabetes

Goals of Diabetes Management

- To allow the patient to lead a normal life
- To achieve normal metabolic state
- To prevent long-term complications of diabetes.

Diet (medical nutrition therapy)

- A well-balanced, nutritious diet is important in the management of diabetes.
- The components of the diet should be as follows:
  - Carbohydrates: 45–65% of total daily calories
  - Protein: 10–35%
  - Fat: 25–35% (of which saturated fat is <7%)
- High protein intake may cause progression of renal disease in patients with diabetic nephropathy; for these individuals, protein intake should be restricted to 0.8 g/kg/day.
- Dietary fiber such as cellulose, gum, and pectin are indigestible by humans. Dietary fiber increases intestinal transit and has beneficial effects on colonic function. It slows glucose absorption rate so that hyperglycemia is slightly diminished. Fiber has a favorable effect on blood cholesterol levels also. Diabetics should consume fiber rich foods such as oatmeal, cereals, and beans.
- Artificial and other sweeteners such as aspartame, saccharin, and sucralose can be used instead of sugar by diabetics. They are well tolerated and do not increase blood sugar.
- Patients should avoid sweets and other high calorie foods, reduce fats and oils and increase the intake of green leafy vegetables. Obese patients should consume fewer calories to reduce their weight. Vegetarian food is encouraged and nonvegetarian food is discouraged in diabetics as nonvegetarian food can contribute significantly in terms of calorie and fat content.
- Patients should reduce alcohol consumption and stop smoking.

Exercise

- Regular exercise improves glycemic control and reduces insulin resistance. Exercise facilitates noninsulin dependent glucose entry into the cells.

Oral Antidiabetic Drugs

- Oral drugs are mainly effective in type 2 diabetes because most of them stimulate endogenous insulin secretion which is absent in type 1 diabetes.
- The following are the groups of drugs available to treat diabetes mellitus.

- Sulfonylureas
- Biguanides
- Thiazolidinediones (TZDs)
- Alpha-glucosidase inhibitors
- Meglitinide derivatives
- Glucagonlike peptide–1 (GLP-1) receptor agonists
- Dipeptidyl peptidase 4 (DPP-4) inhibitors
- Selective sodium-glucose transporter-2 (SGLT-2) inhibitors
- Amylinomimetics
- Insulins

Sulphonylureas

Examples

Glibenclamide, gliclazide, glipizide, glimepiride

- Individual sulphonylureas differ in their potency, duration of action and cost. Glibenclamide can cause severe hypoglycemia and should be avoided in the elderly. Gliclazide and glipizide cause few side-effects but are short acting. Glimepiride is long acting, can be given once daily and has less chances of causing hypoglycemia.
- People with type 2 diabetes who fail to respond to initial treatment with sulphonylureas are considered 'primary treatment failures'.
- After many years of diabetes, beta-cell function gradually worsens. When beta cells are completely exhausted, insulin secretion stops and sulphonylureas will not act. This is called 'secondary failure' (i.e. after a period of satisfactory glycemic control). With continuing follow-up, 'secondary failure' affects 3–10% of patients each year.

Mechanism of action

- Sulphonylureas stimulate the release of insulin from the pancreatic β cell (insulin secretagogue). They act through a sulphonylurea receptor which is linked to a K^+ channel on the β-cell surface. K^+ transport triggers insulin secretion.

Indications

- These are used in type 2 diabetes after a trial of diet and exercise fails to control blood sugar. Sulfonylureas are not effective in type 1 diabetes since these drugs require functioning beta cells to produce their effect on blood glucose.

Contraindications

- Severe hepatic or renal impairment.

Side effects

- Hypoglycemia.
- Idiosyncratic reactions: skin rashes, leukopenia, and thrombocytopenia.

Drug interactions

- Drugs that increase sulfonylurea effect → Risk of hypoglycemia' are as follows.
- Ketoconazole, fluconazole, macrolide antibiotics. These drugs decrease the metabolism of sulphonylureas by inhibiting CYP450.
- Sulfonamides (cotrimoxazole) by displacing suphonylureas from plasma proteins, and also ↓ metabolism.
- Monoamine oxidase inhibitors (MAOIs) (selegiline, phenelzine) potentiate hypoglycemia.
- Beta-blockers (propranolol, nadolol) mask hypoglycemia + potentiate effects.
- Alcohol inhibits gluconeogenesis, potentiates hypoglycemia.

Biguanides

Examples

Metformin is the only biguanide available. Phenformin has been withdrawn due to high incidence of lactic acidosis.

Mechanism of action

- It increases insulin sensitivity and peripheral glucose uptake.
- It also impairs glucose absorption by the gut and inhibits hepatic gluconeogenesis.
- It does not stimulate insulin secretion and hence does not cause hypoglycemia.

Indications

- It is not associated with weight gain and hence preferred in obese type 2 diabetes patients.
- It can also be used in type-1 obese diabetic patients as they also have insulin resistance.
- Starting dose is 500 mg BD, can be increased to a maximum of 1 g TID.

Side effects

- Lactic acidosis
- GI intolerance.

Contraindications

- Impaired renal or liver function, severe shock, cardiac failure, peripheral vascular disease. In all these cases, there is tissue hypoxemia (hence, already there is acidosis) which can precipitate lactic acidosis.

Thiazolidinediones (glitazones)

Examples

- Pioglitazone, rosiglitazone.

Mechanism of action

- They stimulate PPAR-γ receptors (peroxisome proliferator-activated receptor-γ). These receptors are present mainly in adipose tissue and enhance the action of insulin. They also release adipokines such as adiponectin and resistin which alter insulin sensitivity in the liver. They do not stimulate insulin secretion and hence, hypoglycemia is not a problem.

Indications

- Usually given along with sulphonylureas in patients intolerant of metformin, or added with both sulphonylurea and metformin.

Side effects

- Increase in body weight
- Hepatotoxicity—troglitazone has been withdrawn because of hepatotoxicity and newer thiazolidinediones should be avoided in patients with liver dysfunction.

- Sodium and fluid retention, hence, must be avoided in cardiac failure.
- Increased risk of bladder cancer has been found in with pioglitazone.

Drug interactions

- Iodinated contrast media → risk of acute kidney injury → ↓ metformin clearance → lactic acidosis risk.
- Diuretics (especially loop diuretics, e.g. furosemide) → volume depletion → AKI → lactic acidosis risk.
- Sulphonylureas and insulin potentiate hypoglycemia when used with metformin.

Alpha-glucosidase Inhibitors

Examples

- Acarbose, voglibose, miglitol

Mechanism of action

- They inhibit alpha-glucosidase enzyme in the intestine which prevents formation of glucose and hence, absorption of glucose. They should be taken with each meal. They only lower postprandial blood glucose. They can be combined with a sulphonylurea.

Side effects

- Since unabsorbed glucose is fermented by intestinal bacteria with production of gas, patients complain of flatulence and abdominal bloating. Unabsorbed glucose acts as an osmotic laxative and produces diarrhea.

Meglitinides and Amino Acid Derivatives

Examples

- Repaglinide, nateglinide.

Mechanism of action

- These drugs are called prandial glucose regulators. These drugs directly stimulate endogenous insulin secretion (similar to sulphonylureas) and are taken immediately before food. Duration of action is less than sulphonylureas and hence, hypoglycemia is also less.

Side effects

- Weight gain.

Drug interactions

- Additive hypoglycemia when combined with sulfonylureas or insulin.
- Digestive enzymes, antibiotics, gut motility agents can affect efficacy.
- When a patient on alpha-glucosidase inhibitors develops hypoglycemia, treat with glucose, not sucrose because these drugs block sucrose breakdown to glucose.

Glucagon Like Peptide–1 Receptor Agonists (GLP-1 Analogs)

Examples

- Exenatide, liraglutide, semaglutide.

Mechanism of action

- Incretins are gut hormones which potentiate glucose-induced insulin secretion. Glucagon-like peptide (GLP-1) is an incretin hormone which stimulates insulin secretion. In addition, GLP-1 suppresses glucagon secretion, delays gastric emptying, reduces appetite and encourages weight loss. GLP-1 is degraded by the enzyme, dipeptidyl peptidase IV (DPP-4).
- GLP-1 analogs mimic GLP-1 action and can be used to treat type 2 diabetes. All these drugs are administered as subcutaneous injection like insulin.

Side effects

- The main side effect is nausea and vomiting. Other side effects are diarrhea and headache.

Drug interactions

- GLP-1 receptor agonists slow gastric emptying → delay absorption of co-administered oral drugs.
- Oral contraceptives: ↓ efficacy possible → advise backup contraception initially.
- Thyroid hormones (levothyroxine): Delayed absorption → monitor TSH more closely.
- Additive risk of hypoglycemia with other antidiabetic drugs.

Dipeptidyl Peptidase IV (DPP-4) Inhibitors

Examples

- Sitagliptin, saxagliptin, linagliptin.

Mechanism of action

- DPP-4 inhibitors prolong the action of incretin hormones GLP-1 and glucose-dependent insulinotropic polypeptide (GIP) by degrading DPP-4. DPP-4 inhibitors can be used as a monotherapy or in combination with metformin or a TZD. They are given once daily and are weight neutral.

Side effects

- The main side effect of DPP-4 inhibitors is nasopharyngitis or upper respiratory tract infection.
- Pancreatitis is another important side effect.

Selective Sodium-glucose Transporter-2 (SGLT-2) Inhibitors

- These are relatively new class of drugs approved recently.
- Examples are dapagliflozin and empagliflozin.

Mechanism of action

- SGLT-2 inhibitors lower the renal glucose threshold. Lowering the renal glucose threshold results in increased urinary glucose excretion thus reducing blood glucose values.

Side effects

- Constipation, diarrhea, nausea, increased urinary frequency (osmotic diuresis due to glucosuria) and genitourinary infections (due to glucosuria).

Drug interactions of SGLT-2 inhibitors

- Additive risk of hypoglycemia with other anti-diabetic drugs.
- Risk of volume depletion when administered with diuretics because both drugs promote osmotic diuresis.

- Inducers of UDP-glucuronosyltransferase (rifampicin, phenobarbital, phenytoin) may decrease the effect of SGLT2 inhibitors.
- Increased risk of UTI when administered with immunosuppressants (steroids, cyclosporine).

Amylinomimetics

- Pramlintide acetate is an amylin analog that mimics the effects of endogenous amylin, which is secreted by pancreatic beta cells. This agent slows gastric emptying, suppresses glucagon, and regulates appetite.

Combination of Oral Agents

- Combining different oral drugs is more effective than either drug used alone. If the blood sugar is not under control with either metformin or sulphonylurea, both can be combined. If blood sugar is still not under control, a glitazone can be added. Finally alpha-glucosidase inhibitors and incretin mimics can be added.
- If blood sugar is still uncontrolled with a combination of all the drugs, then insulin can be added to the oral drugs.

Insulin

- Patients, whose sugar remains uncontrolled even after using a combination of all the oral drugs and newer drugs require insulin.
- Oral drugs can be continued and insulin is added to oral drugs.
- Initially a single dose of intermediate-or long-acting insulin can be started at bedtime. Later on twice daily mixed insulin (short acting plus intermediate acting), or basal bolus type of insulin therapy (short acting insulin before every meal and long-acting insulin as basal insulin) may be used. (*see* under type-1 diabetes for insulin regimens).

Pancreas or Islet Cell Transplantation

- Both these procedures require suitable donors and long-term immunosuppression.
- Pancreas transplantation at the time of renal transplantation is becoming more widely accepted. Solitary pancreatic transplantation in the absence of a need for renal transplantation should be considered only in those patients who fail all other methods of treatment.
- Islet cell transplantation is a minimally invasive procedure, and easier than pancreas transplantation.

Management of Comorbidities

- Hypertension, dyslipidemia, antiplatelet therapy (if indicated), smoking cessation.

Monitoring

- FBS + PPBS: Once every 1–2 weeks at home (self-monitoring), or as advised. More frequent testing if adjusting doses or during illness. In clinic/laboratory: typically, every 1–3 months depending on control.
- HbA1c every 3–6 months.
- Annual screening for complications.

Q. Comparative features of type 1 and type 2 diabetes (Table 9.9).

TABLE 9.9: Comparative features of type 1 and type 2 diabetes

	Type 1	*Type 2*
Etiology	Autoimmune destruction of β-cells	Insulin resistance + β-cell dysfunction
Prevalence	Uncommon (5–10% of diabetes cases)	Common (>80% of diabetes cases)
Typical age at onset	Usually childhood or adolescence	>40 years
Duration of symptoms	Weeks	Months to years
Body weight	Normal or low	Obese
Ketoacidosis tendency	Yes	Rarely
Rapid death without treatment with insulin	Yes	No
Autoantibodies	Yes	No
Diabetic complications at diagnosis	No	25% (because of late presentation)
Family history of diabetes	Uncommon	Common
Insulin levels	Very low or absent	Normal to high initially; may decrease over time
Other autoimmune diseases	Common	Uncommon
HLA-DR3/4	Association	No association
Acanthosis nigricans	No	Common
Management	Mandatory insulin therapy	Lifestyle + oral agents ± insulin

Q. Latent autoimmune diabetes in adults (LADA).

- Latent autoimmune diabetes in adults (LADA) is a slowly progressive form of autoimmune diabetes that clinically resembles type 2 diabetes but is immunologically similar to type 1 diabetes. It typically presents in adults over 30 years and does not initially require insulin at diagnosis.
- Often referred to as "type 1.5 diabetes," LADA combines features of both type 1 and type 2 diabetes.

Pathophysiology

- Autoimmune destruction of pancreatic β-cells due to the presence of autoantibodies (similar to type 1 diabetes).
- Slower progression of β-cell failure compared to classic type 1 diabetes.

- Patients initially respond to oral hypoglycemic agents but progress to insulin dependency within months to a few years.
- Most commonly associated antibodies:
  - GAD65 (glutamic acid decarboxylase) antibodies
  - ICA (islet cell antibodies)
  - IA-2 (insulinoma-associated antigen-2 antibodies)

Diagnostic Criteria

No universally accepted criteria, but the following are often used:

1. Age >30 years at diagnosis
2. Initially non–insulin-requiring (for at least 6 months)
3. Presence of pancreatic autoantibodies, especially GAD antibodies.

Clinical Features

- Presents like type 2 diabetes, often with mild symptoms.
- Lean or normal BMI (unlike typical type 2 diabetics).
- Poor glycemic response to oral hypoglycemics.
- Rapid deterioration of β-cell function over time.
- Increased risk of other autoimmune diseases (e.g. thyroiditis, celiac disease).

Investigations

- Autoantibody testing
  - Anti-GAD65 (most sensitive and specific).
  - ICA, IA-2, ZnT8 antibodies.
- C-peptide levels
  - Initially normal or mildly reduced
  - Decline over time as β-cell destruction progresses.
- Routine diabetes tests
  - FBS, PPBS, HbA1c.

Management

Initial Phase (when insulin is not yet needed)

- Lifestyle modification
- Metformin (use with caution, as sulfonylureas may worsen β-cell loss).
- Avoid sulfonylureas. They may hasten β-cell exhaustion.

Progressive Phase

- Early initiation of insulin therapy is preferred to preserve remaining β-cell function.
- Basal insulin initially, progressing to basal-bolus as needed.

Q. Discuss the diagnosis of diabetes mellitus.

Q. Glucose tolerance test.

Q. Impaired glucose tolerance (IGT).

Q. Impaired fasting glucose (IFG).

- Testing to detect type 2 diabetes and prediabetes in asymptomatic people should be considered in adults of any age who are overweight or obese (BMI ≥25 kg/m^2) and have one or more additional risk factors for diabetes such as physical inactivity, first-degree relative with diabetes, high-risk race/ethnicity (e.g. African American, Latino, Native American, Asian American, Pacific Islander), women who delivered a baby weighing >9 lb or were diagnosed with GDM, hypertension, HDL cholesterol level <35 mg/dl and/or a triglyceride level >250 mg/dl, women with polycystic ovarian syndrome, IGT or IFG on previous testing, other clinical conditions associated with insulin resistance (e.g. severe obesity, acanthosis nigricans), and history of CVD.
- In those without these risk factors, testing should begin at age 45 years.
- If tests are normal, repeat testing at least at 3-year intervals is reasonable.

American Diabetes Association (ADA) criteria for the diagnosis of diabetes

A hemoglobin A1c (HbA1c) level of 6.5% or higher.

or

A fasting plasma glucose (FPG) level of 126 mg/dl or higher; fasting is defined as no caloric intake for at least 8 hours,

or

A 2-hour plasma glucose level of 200 mg/dl or higher during a 75-g oral glucose tolerance test (OGTT),

or

A random plasma glucose of 200 mg/dl or higher in a patient with classic symptoms of hyperglycemia (i.e. polyuria, polydipsia, polyphagia, weight loss) or hyperglycemic crisis.

- Urine glucose tests should never be used alone to diagnose diabetes, since an altered renal threshold for glucose can produce similar findings.

Oral Glucose Tolerance Test (OGTT)

- OGTT is not recommended for routine clinical use but may be required in the evaluation of patients with IFG (impaired fasting glucose) or when diabetes is still suspected despite normal FBS. It is commonly done in the diagnosis of gestational diabetes mellitus.
- OGTT should be performed under controlled conditions to ensure its accuracy. The following should be ensured before doing OGTT.
  - 3 days of unrestricted diet ((>150 g carbohydrates/day) and physical activity.
  - Patient should remain seated and not smoke during the test.
  - OGTT should be done after an overnight fast, using a glucose load containing 75 g of anhydrous glucose dissolved in water; 2 hours post load glucose levels of 200 mg/dl or greater establish the diagnosis of diabetes.
- Factors that decrease the value of OGTT include;
  - Carbohydrate restriction (<150 g for 3 days)
  - Bed rest or severe inactivity
  - Medical or surgical stress
  - Drugs (e.g. thiazides, steroids, β-blockers, phenytoin)
  - Smoking
  - Anxiety from repeated needle sticks.

- Hence, OGTT should not be performed in acutely ill patients.

Interpretation of OGTT Results

	FBS (mg/dl)	Two-hour PPBS (mg/dl)
Normal	<100	<140
IFG	100–125	Normal (<140)
IGT	Normal (<100)	140–199
Diabetes	≥126	≥200 mg/dl

Impaired Glucose Tolerance (IGT) and Impaired Fasting Glucose (IFG)

- 2-hour post load glucose 140–199 mg/dl with FBS being normal is called impaired glucose tolerance (IGT).
- FBS between 100–125 mg/dl with PPBS being normal is called impaired fasting glucose (IFG).
- Both IGT and IFG are now called 'prediabetes' states. People with these pre diabetic states have a relatively high risk of developing diabetes and subsequent vascular disease. All patients with IFG and IGT should be treated with diet and exercise and should be followed up yearly for the progression to diabetes.
- Because individuals with IFG may exhibit severe post prandial hyperglycemia, a 75 g OGTT should be performed in all these patients to rule out diabetes. If 2 hr post load glucose concentration is 200 mg/dl or more, it confirms diabetes; if between 140–199 mg/dl they are defined as having IGT.
- Individuals with HbA1c of 5.7–6.4% are also at increased risk of developing diabetes later and should be counseled about weight reduction (if overweight), diet control and exercise.

Q. Glycated hemoglobin (HbA1c).

- RBCs are freely permeable to glucose. As a result, glucose becomes irreversibly attached to hemoglobin (HbA1c) at a rate dependent upon the prevailing blood glucose. Since HbA1c circulates within RBCs whose life span lasts up to 120 days, its concentration reflects the average blood glucose level in the preceding 120 days (i.e. 3 months).
- Its normal concentration is 4–6%. It is abnormally elevated in diabetic persons with chronic hyperglycemia.
- It should be measured every 3–4 month intervals so that adjustments in therapy can be made to optimize diabetes control.
- The accuracy of HbA1c values can be affected by hemoglobin variants or derivatives; the effect depends on the specific hemoglobin variant or derivative and the specific assay used. Any condition that shortens RBC survival or decreases mean RBC age (e.g. recovery from acute blood loss, hemolytic anemia) will falsely lower HbA1c. Vitamins C and E are reported to falsely lower test results possibly by inhibiting glycation of hemoglobin.

Q. Classify insulin preparations.
Q. Write briefly about different insulin preparations.
Q. Insulin analogues.
Q. Complications of insulin therapy.

- Discovery of insulin was one of the greatest milestones in medicine. It was discovered in 1921 by Banting and Best and they tried this on a patient in 1922. They received Nobel Prize in medicine for this remarkable discovery.

Classification of Insulin Preparations

- Two useful clinical classifications of insulin preparations are as follows.

Based on Duration of Action

Rapid acting
Lispro, aspart, glulisine

Short acting
Regular insulin

Intermediate acting
NPH insulin (**N**eutral **P**rotamine **H**agedron, also called isophane insulin)

Long acting
Glargine, detemir, degludec

Based on Whether the Insulin Provides Prandial Coverage or Basal Coverage

Bolus or Prandial Insulins
Regular or plain insulin, lispro, aspart, glulisine.

Basal Insulins
NPH insulin, glargine, detemir, degludec.

- Regular and NPH insulinare also known as conventional (standard) preparations. They can be derived from beef, pork, or recombinant-DNA technology (human insulin).
- Lispro, aspart, glulisine, glargine, detemir, and degludec are also called insulin analogues or designer insulins. They overcome some of the limitations of conventional insulin preparations. Insulin analogues are molecules that differ from human insulin in amino acid sequence but bind to same insulin receptors and function similarly as human insulin. Advantage of new insulin analogues is that they have better time-action profiles than conventional insulins.

Time-action-profiles of Different Insulin Preparations after Subcutaneous Injection

- Normal physiologic insulin secretion includes both a continuous basal (low-level) insulin secretion and an incremental postprandial secretion associated with meals. However, subcutaneously injected insulin takes sometime to get absorbed into blood stream and start its action. Following is the time action profiles different insulin preparations after subcutaneous injection **(Table 9.10 and Fig. 9.16)**:

TABLE 9.10: Time-action-profiles of different insulin preparations

Insulin formulation	Onset of action	Peak action (hours)	Duration of action (hours)
Lispro aspart glulisine	<15 minutes	1	3–5
Regular (plain)	30–60 minutes	2–4	6–8
NPH	2–4 hours	4–12	10–18
Glargine	2–4 hours	No peak	24
Detemir	Slow	No peak	Up to 24
Degludec	1–2 hours	No peak	Up to to 42

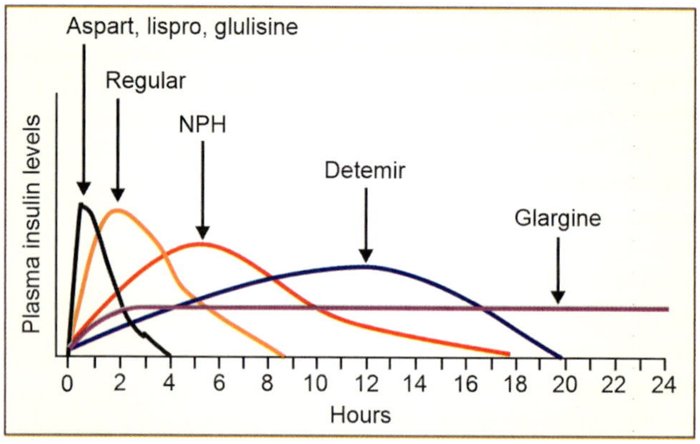

Figure 9.16: Time action profile of different insulins

- Insulin is injected subcutaneously into the anterior abdominal wall, upper arms, outer thighs and buttocks **(Fig. 9.17)**. Accidental intramuscular injection can occur sometimes, but of no consequence except increased risk of hypoglycemia due to rapid absorption.
- Insulin is injected using a syringe with a fine needle (which can be reused several times). Nowadays pen injectors with insulin in cartridge have become popular because they are more convenient and portable.
- Insulin can also be administered through insulin pumps which provide continuous subcutaneous or intravenous infusion of insulin. Insulin pumps can be worn on the body or implanted into the subcutaneous tissue.

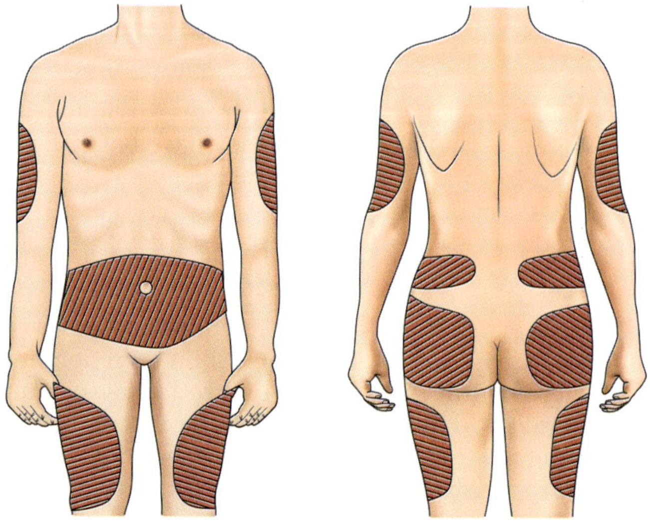

Figure 9.17: Insulin injection sites

- Insulin is given intravenously while treating acute complications of diabetes such as DKA and HHS.

Indications for Insulin

- Type 1 diabetes
- Diabetic ketoacidosis (DKA) or hyperglycemic hyperosmolar syndrome (HHS)
- Presence of serious infection or concurrent illness (e.g. Acute M1, pancreatitis or stroke)
- Major surgery
- Pregnancy: All pregnant women with diabetes mellitus, (whether gestational or previous diabetes) whose disease is not controlled with diet alone should be treated with insulin. All oral agents are contraindicated during pregnancy except metformin which is relatively safe.
- Symptomatic (polydypsia, polyuria, polyphagia and weight loss) uncontrolled diabetes, with persistent elevations of the FBS levels of 300 mg/dl or higher. Intensive insulin therapy with tight glycemic control helps reverse glucose toxicity. Therapy improves both insulin sensitivity and insulin secretion. After 6–8 weeks of good glycemic control, these patients can be switched to an oral agent or can continue insulin therapy.

Insulin Regimens

- Various insulin regimens are used in the treatment of diabetes. Most people require two or more injections of insulin daily. Twice-daily administration of a mixture of short-acting and intermediate-acting insulin, given before breakfast and dinner is the commonly used regimen. Many pre-mixed insulin preparations are available containing different proportions of short acting and intermediate acting insulin (30:70 and 50:50).
- Multiple injection regimens require short-acting insulin before each meal, and a long acting insulin injected at bedtime (basal-bolus regimen).

Regular Insulin or Plain Insulin

- Regular insulin is the natural insulin obtained from animal source or humans. There are only minor differences between human, pork and beef insulins. Animal insulins are more immunogenic than human insulin. Nowadays the use of animal insulin has almost stopped due to the wide availability of recombinant human insulin.

Species	A Chain		B Chain
	8th AA	10th AA	30th AA
Human	Threonine	Isoleucine	Threonine
Pork (porcine)	Threonine	Isoleucine	Alanine
Beef (bovine)	Alanine	Valine	Alanine

- Regular insulin has an onset of action in 15–60 minutes after injection, a peak effect 2–4 hours after injection and duration of action of 5–8 hours.
- Regular insulin has to be injected 20–30 minutes before the meal.

NPH and Lente Insulin

- These two are intermediate acting insulins.
- Neutral protamine hagedron (NPH) insulin is produced by complexing regular insulin with protamine, a protein of fish origin and adding trace amounts of zinc. The protamine insulin complex is poorly soluble at physiologic pH and thus slowly absorbed from the subcutaneous tissue. Hagedron is the name of the scientist who first formulated this preparation.
- Lente insulin is produced by adding zinc to regular insulin which prolongs its action. It dissolves slowly in body fluids and thus exhibits a prolonged duration of action after subcutaneous injection.

Insulin Analogs

- Insulin analogs are molecules that differ from human insulin in amino acid sequence but bind to same insulin receptors and function similarly as human insulin. They overcome some of the limitations of conventional insulin preparations.
- *Short-acting analogues:* lispro, aspart, glulisine.
- *Long-acting analogues:* glargine, detemir.

Insulin Lispro

- Insulin lispro was introduced in 1996. Lispro insulin is produced by interchanging two amino acids on beta chain, i.e. proline at B-28, and lysine at B-29. The first three letters of lysine and proline were combined to name it as LYSPRO. Subsequently LYSPRO was changed to LISPRO since it was planned to release this all over the world and some languages do not contain the letter "Y". Lispro insulin is at least twice as fast acting as regular human insulin.
- After subcutaneous administration, lispro begins acting within 15 min, peaks in activity in 60–90 minutes and has a duration of action of 4–5 hours.
- Because of its fast onset of action, lispro can be given within 15 minutes before meals. It can also be given immediately before or after meals. After taking injection, there is no need to wait for 30 min to take meals (unlike regular insulin), hence lispro is also called no wait insulin.

Advantages of insulin lispro over regular (plain) insulin

- Because of its more rapid onset and peak action, insulin lispro more effectively controls postprandial blood sugar at 1 and 2 hours than regular insulin.
- Lispro is more effective in suppressing hepatic glucose output than regular insulin, because of higher concentrations attained in liver.
- The onset of action of lispro does not vary much with the site of injection as compared to regular insulin.
- Regular insulin has to be injected 20–30 minutes before a meal. However this is not so with lispro insulin which can be injected 0–15 minutes before a meal in all the patients. Hence, it is called "no-wait" insulin. It can even be injected after the meal.
- Because of its shorter duration of action, insulin lispro results in less late post prandial hypolgycemia than regular human insulin. Insulin lispro is superior to regular insulin in the reduction of postprandial hyperglycemia.

Insulin Aspart

- This is a rapidly acting analogue which was introduced after lispro in 2001. In insulin aspart, neutral proline in B-28 position is replaced by the negatively charged aspartic acid resulting in reduced capacity for self association and faster absorption.
- The time-action-profile of aspart is similar to insulin lispro. Its advantages are similar to insulin lispro.

Insulin Glulisine

- Insulin glulisine is a new rapidly acting analogue with a pharmacokinetic profile that is similar to those of insulin lispro and insulin aspart. Trials are being conducted with this molecule.

Insulin Glargine

- Insulin glargine is a long acting human insulin analogue produced by recombinant-DNA technology. It was introduced in 2001. This is the first true basal insulin.
- It differs from human insulin in that glycine replaces asparagine at position 21 of the A-chain, and two arginines are added to the C-terminus of the B-chain. Because of these changes, glargine remains completely soluble in the acidic pH of the vial (pH 4) but precipitates in the neutral pH of subcutaneous tissue after injection. It is then slowly released from these precipitates, prolonging its duration of action without producing any peak. It can be given once a day which provides basal level of insulin throughout the day.
- It is suitable for initial insulin therapy in both type 1 and type 2 diabetes. It is safe for use in children and adolescents. However data are not available about its use in pregnant women.
- Glargine solution is clear and slightly acidic (pH 4) and should not be mixed with any other insulin or solution as this could alter its time-action profile.
- Injection site redness, pain, itching, hives, swelling or inflammation are the most common type of adverse events, probably due to acidic pH of the solution.

Advantages

- Better control of FBS and decreased incidence of nocturnal hypoglycemia compared to NPH insulin.
- There is also more improvement in HbA1C level than with NPH insulin.
- The site of injection does not alter the time action profile of insulin glargine.
- The time of the day at which insulin glargine is injected does not alter glycemic control.
- The plasma levels of insulin glargine do not fluctuate significantly, thus mimicking physiological basal insulin profile.

Disadvantages

- No other insulin can be mixed in the same syringe. It is more acidic (pH 4.0) than other insulins (pH 7.4). If insulin Glargine is mixed with another insulin, both lose activity.

- When using insulin glargine, three or more injections per day of a short-acting insulin may be needed before meals.
- Because it is clear, care must be taken not to confuse it with the short-acting insulin.
- It is also expensive.

Insulin Detemir

- Detemir is another new long-acting insulin analogue. Here, the aminoacid threonine at the B-30 position on the human insulin chain is lacking and a 14-carbon fatty acid (tetradecanoic acid or myristic acid) is attached to lysine at B-29.
- It is a clear solution with a neutral pH. It has a high affinity for serum albumin from which it gets released slowly which accounts for its unique mechanism of prolonged duration of action.
- Insulin detemir acts for nearly 24 hours. Detemir also has prominent action on hepatic glucose output which may be an advantage not seen with other insulins.

Advantages

- Absorption and action of insulin detemir is more predictable, because it is a clear solution and does not require resuspension and it does not precipitate after subcutaneous injection.

Insulin Degludec

- This is a new ultra-long acting insulin analogue. Insulin degludec differs from human insulin in that the amino acid threonine in position B30 has been omitted and a side-chain consisting of glutamic acid and a C16 fatty acid has been attached. These changes allow for the formation of multi-hexamers. When injected subcutaneously, these multi-hexamers form a drug depot store from which monomers are slowly and continuously released accounting for prolonged duration of action of up to 42 hours. Compared to other long acting basal insulins such as glargine and detemir, which have a duration of action of 20–24 hours, insulin degludec provides a consistent level of basal insulin over 42 hours with a low peak:trough ratio. Degludec has low intra-individual variability and plasma concentration is less dependent on the time of injections. Thus it has flexibility in dose timing and predicatbale long duration of action with low risk of hypoglycemia.
- Compared with glargine, degludec is associated with equivalent HbA1c control and significantly lower nocturnal hypoglycemia rates. Degludec is also associated with significantly greater reductions in FPG and lower total doses of insulin versus glargine
- Degludec can be used in chidren aged 1 year and above. Degludec is not recommended during pregnancy due to lack of safety studies. However, some studies have shown no fetal side-effects. Hence if clinically indicated, it can be considered during pregnancy. There is no clinical experience with degludec during breastfeeding. It is unknown whether it is excreted into breast milk.
- Degludec can also be used in renal and hepatic impairment.

Complications of Insulin Therapy

Metabolic

- Hypoglycemia
- Weight gain
- Insulin edema

Local

- Lipoatrophy
- Lipohypertrophy
- Local allergic reactions

Systemic

- Immune insulin resistance
- Anaphylaxis

Q. Enumerate the complications of diabetes. What are the factors associated with increased mortality and morbidity in people with diabetes?

Acute complications

- Diabetic ketoacidosis (DKA)
- Hyperosmolar hyperglycemic state (HHS)
- Hypoglycemia
- Lactic acidosis

Chronic (long-term) complications

Microvascular

- Diabetic retinopathy
- Diabetic neuropathy
- Diabetic nephropathy

Macrovascular

- Coronary artery disease
- Peripheral vascular disease
- Cerebrovascular disease

Others

- Gastrointestinal (gastroparesis, diarrhea)
- Genitourinary (uropathy/sexual dysfunction)
- Dermatological
- Infections
- Cataracts
- Glaucoma
- Periodontal disease

Factors Associated with Increased Mortality and Morbidity in People with Diabetes

- Long duration of diabetes
- Early age at onset of disease
- Uncontrolled blood sugars (as evidenced by high HbA1c)
- Associated hypertension
- Proteinuria; microalbuminuria
- Dyslipidemia (high LDL, low HDL)
- Obesity.

Q. Discuss the pathogenesis, clinical features, investigations, management and complications of diabetic ketoacidosis (DKA).

- DKA is an acute, life-threatening complication of diabetes mellitus, characterized by:
  - Hyperglycemia
  - Ketosis
  - Metabolic acidosis
- Diabetic ketoacidosis (DKA) is a major medical emergency and remains a serious cause of morbidity and mortality in people with diabetes. It is more likely to occur in type 1 diabetes because of complete dependence on insulin.
- Many undiagnosed diabetics may present for the first time with DKA.

Pathogenesis of DKA (Fig. 9.18)

- DKA usually evolves rapidly, over a 24-hour period.
- The cardinal biochemical features of diabetic ketoacidosis are: Hyperglycemia, hyperketonemia and metabolic acidosis.
- Two hormonal abnormalities are largely responsible for the development of hyperglycemia and ketoacidosis in patients with uncontrolled diabetes; insulin deficiency and glucagon excess. However, DKA can develop even without glucagon excess. In addition to these factors, increased catecholamines and cortisol can contribute to the increase in glucose and ketoacid production.
- Hyperglycemia causes osmotic diuresis leading to dehydration and electrolyte loss, particularly of sodium and potassium. Average loss of fluid in DKA is 3–6 liters. Half the deficit is from intracellular compartment leading to cellular dehydration. Remaining half is derived from extracellular fluid compartment which leads to hemoconcentration, hypovolemia, hypotension, decreased renal perfusion and oliguria.
- Ketosis results from insulin deficiency, exacerbated by elevated catecholamines and other stress hormones, resulting in unrestrained lipolysis and supply of free fatty acids for hepatic ketogenesis. Excess accumulation of acidic ketones (β-hydroxy butyric acid and acetoacetate) leads to metabolic acidosis. Metabolic acidosis forces hydrogen ions into the cells, displacing potassium ions, which may be lost in urine or through vomiting leading to hypokalemia.
- There are many precipitating factors which may trigger an attack of DKA due to increased insulin requirements.

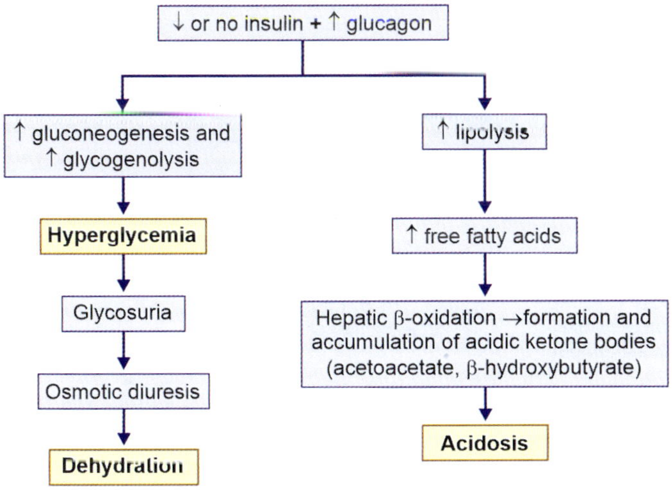

Figure 9.18: Pathogenesis of DKA

Precipitating Factors for DKA

- Inadequate insulin treatment or noncompliance
- Infections (pneumonia, UTI, sepsis, etc.)
- Cerebrovascular accidents
- Myocardial infarction
- Acute pancreatitis
- Drugs (steroids, thiazides, clozapine or olanzapine, cocaine)

Clinical Features

Due to Hyperglycemia

- Polyuria, polydipsia, and weight loss are the initial symptoms. As hyperglycemia worsens, serum osmolality increases leading to neurological signs and symptoms such as lethargy, focal deficits and obtundation which can progress to coma. Blurred vision may occur due to change in the refractory power of lens due to hyperglycemia.

Due to Dehydration

- Loss of skin turgor, dry tongue, cracked lips, sunken eye balls, tachycardia, and hypotension.
- Cold extremities, peripheral cyanosis.

Due to Metabolic Acidosis

- Deep and sighing breathing (Kussmaul breathing). Breath is usually fetid, and acetone smell may be present.
- Nausea, vomiting, and abdominal pain are common in DKA which may be related to acidosis. Abdominal pain is probably due to delayed gastric emptying and ileus induced by metabolic acidosis and electrolyte abnormalities.

Other Features

Signs of underlying precipitating illness may be present such as fever in infections, signs of consolidation in pneumonia, etc.

Investigations

- Blood glucose–is often >250 mg/dl.
- Electrolytes: It sodium level is variable depending on the hydration status. Potassium and bicarbonate are usually low.
- Serum amylase and lipase are elevated in DKA. Sometimes acute pancreatitis can precipitate an attack of DKA in which case amylase and lipase are elevated.
- Blood urea nitrogen (BUN), creatinine: Elevated due to prerenal azotemia.
- Arterial blood gas (ABG) analysis shows presence of metabolic acidosis.

- Plasma ketone bodies are raised.
- Urinalysis: It shows presence of sugar and ketone bodies.
- ECG: It may show changes due to electrolyte abnormalities or MI which might have precipitated DKA.
- Infection screen: Full blood count, blood and urine culture, C-reactive protein, chest X-ray.

Diagnostic Criteria for DKA

- Blood glucose >250 mg/dl
- Arterial pH <7.3
- Serum bicarbonate <15 mEq/L
- Moderate degree of ketonemia and/or ketonuria.

Management of DKA (Fig. 9.19)

Principles of Treatment

- Correction of dehydration, hyperglycemia and electrolyte imbalance
- Identification and treatment of precipitating events
- Frequent patient monitoring.

Quick Initial Assessment

- Check airway and breathing first, especially in patients with altered sensorium. Take focused history and do brief physical examination. Send investigations. Patients with severe DKA require admission in the intensive care unit.

Fluid Replacement

- The average fluid loss is 3–6 liters in DKA. Initially fluid is given at a rate of 1–2 liters of isotonic saline is given rapidly intravenously. Subsequent rate of fluid replacement depends on the hydration status and urine output. Patients who are able to drink can take some or all of their fluid replacement orally.
- Fluid replacement also contributes to correction of hyperglycemia.

Correction of Hyperglycemia

- Unless the episode of DKA is mild, intravenous insulin infusion is the treatment of choice. Initially an intravenous or intramuscular bolus of 0.1 units/kg body wt of regular insulin at is given, followed by a continuous infusion at a dose of 0.1 unit/kg/h (5–7 units/hour in adults).
- Blood glucose should be monitored every hour. It should fall by 50–75 mg/dl per hour. If plasma glucose does not fall by 50 mg/dl from the initial value in the 1st hour, check hydration status; if necessary, the insulin infusion may be doubled every 2 hours until a steady glucose decline between 50 and 75 mg/hour is achieved.
- When the blood glucose reaches 250 mg/dl, it may be possible to decrease the insulin infusion rate to 0.05–0.1 unit/kg/h (3–6 untis/hour), and dextrose (5%) may be started. Dextrose needs to be started along with insulin to facilitate continuation of insulin till the ketone bodies are cleared. This is because ketone bodies take longer time to clear than hyperglycemia.
- During therapy for DKA, blood should be drawn every 2–4 hours for determination of serum electrolytes, glucose and ketone bodies. Typical duration of therapy of DKA is usually 48 hours.
- Criteria for resolution of DKA:
  - Blood glucose <200 mg/dl.
  - Serum beta-hydroxybutyrate <0.6 mmol/L or normalization of the serum anion gap (≤12 mEq/L).
  - Serum bicarbonate ≥18 mEq/L.
  - Venous pH of >7.3.

Potassium Replacement

- **If K^+** is <3.5 mEq, Give KCl (potassium chloride) 10 to 20 mEq/hour, which usually requires 10–20 mEq/L added to each liter of IV fluid. Do not give insulin until K^+ rises to ≥3.5.
- **If K^+** is 3.5–5.0 mEq/L, IV KCl (10–20 mEq) is added to each liter of IV fluid. Adjust potassium replacement

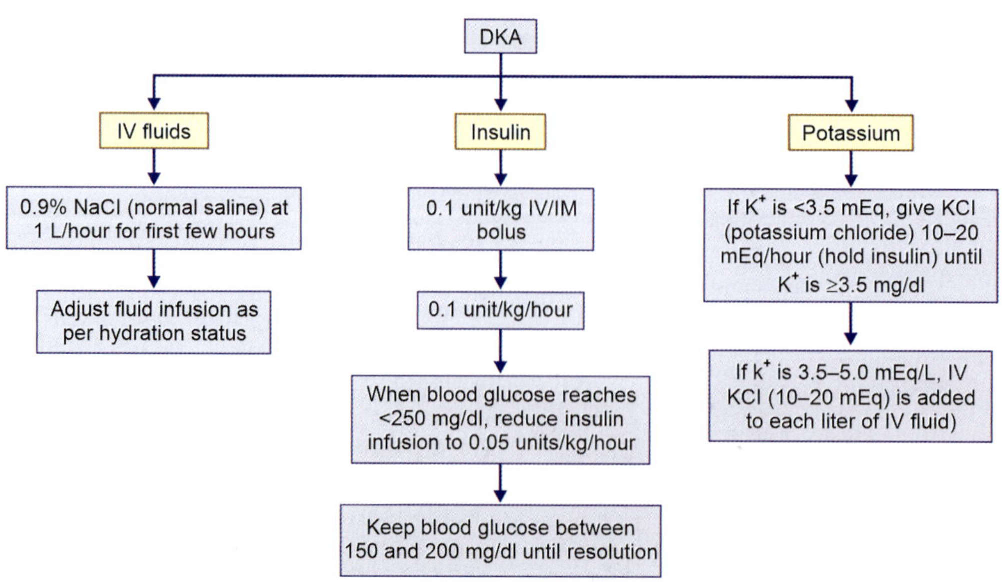

Figure 9.19: Management of DKA

to maintain the serum potassium concentration in the range of 4–5 mEq/L.

- **If K^+** is >5 mEq, do not give any K^+. Monitor hourly.

Bicarbonate Replacement

- If pH is <7, sodium bicarbonate 100 mmol mixed with 400 ml sterile water can be given as IV infusion over 2 hours.

Treatment of the Precipitating Event

- Such as infection should be treated with antibiotics.

Complications of DKA

- Hypoglycemia due to overzealous insulin therapy.
- Hypokalemia due to insulin and bicarbonate therapy.
- Cerebral edema—rare but frequently fatal complication of DKA, most common in children. Cerebral edema most likely happens because of rapid decline in plasma osmolality with treatment. It is minimized by gradual replacement of sodium and water (maximal reduction in osmolality 3 mosm/kgH_2O/hour).
- ARDS
- Mucormycosis (combination of hyperglycemia and acidic pH facilitates fungus growth)
- Myocardial infarction
- Vascular thrombosis due to dehydration and increased viscosity of blood
- Disseminated intravascular coagulation (rare).
- Acute circulatory failure due to dehydration.

Q. Hyperosmolar hyperglycemic state (nonketotic hyperosmolar syndrome).

- Hyperosmolar hyperglycemic state (HHS) is a serious, life-threatening complication of diabetes mellitus, most commonly type 2 diabetes characterized by:
  - Severe hyperglycemia
  - Marked dehydration
  - Increased serum osmolality
  - Minimal or no ketone production.

Precipitating Factors

- These are same as for DKA.

Pathogenesis

- Relative insulin deficiency leads to impaired glucose utilization → hyperglycemia → osmotic diuresis → dehydration.
- Hyperglycemia and dehydration → hyperosmolarity.
- Some amount of insulin is present which is enough to prevent fatty acid oxidation and formation of ketone bodies. Hence, in HHS, significant ketosis and acidosis is absent.

Clinical Features

- Onset may be insidious over a period of days or weeks, with weakness, polyuria, and polydipsia.
- Signs of volume depletion and dehydration are present.
- Acidotic breathing (Kussmaul's respirations) is absent.
- Lethargy and confusion may be present which may progress to convulsions and deep coma.

Investigations

- Severe hyperglycemia is present (usually >600 mg/dl).
- Serum osmolality is markedly raised (>320 mosm/kg).
- Ketosis and acidosis are usually absent or mild.
- Serum bicarbonate >18 mEq/L
- Serum sodium may be low in mild dehydration due to urinary sodium losses. However, as dehydration progresses, serum sodium can exceed 140 mEq/L, contributing to increased serum osmolality.
- Urea and creatinine are usually elevated due to pre-renal azotemia.

Management

- Management of HHS is same as that of DKA with following changes.
- Fluid deficit is more in HHS (average of 6–10 liters) than DKA, hence more fluid is required. IV fluids should be changed to 5% dextrose with 0.45% saline when the blood glucose falls to 300 mg/dl. It is important to maintain serum glucose between 250 and 300 mg/dl till plasma osmolality is ≤315 mosm/kg and patient is mentally alert.
- Insulin infusion is given at a lower dose 0.05 units/kg body weight. No need to give bolus dose.
- There is no role for bicarbonate therapy as pH is not affected in HHS.
- Identify and treat underlying cause (e.g. antibiotics for infection).

Prognosis

- The overall mortality rate of HHS is more than ten times that of DKA. Prognosis is better when it is recognized early and prompt therapy is instituted.

Q. Enumerate the differences between DKA and HHS (Table 9.11).

TABLE 9.11: Differences between DKA and HHS

Features	DKA	HHS
Common in	Type 1 diabetes	Type 2 diabetes
Evolution	Over hours	Over days or weeks
Alteration in sensorium	Variable	Stupor/coma
Acetone smell in breath	Present	Absent
Acidotic breathing (Kussmaul's respirations)	Present	Absent
Abdominal pain, vomiting	May be present	Usually absent
Average fluid deficit	3–6 litres	6–10 liters
Blood glucose	>250 mg/dl	>600 (often >1000)
Arterial pH	<7.3	>7.3
Serum bicarbonate (mEq/L)	<15	>18
Blood/urine ketones	Positive	Absent or trace
Serum osmolality (mosm/kg)	Variable	>320
Mortality	5–10%	20–30%

Q. Lactic acidosis.

- Lactic acidosis is a form of metabolic acidosis characterized by the accumulation of lactate in the body.
- Lactic acidosis is the most common cause of metabolic acidosis in hospitalized patients. It is associated with elevated plasma lactate concentration above 4 mEq/L.

Pathophysiology

- Lactic acid is produced from pyruvate during anaerobic glycolysis. It accumulates when:
  - Tissue hypoxia limits oxidative phosphorylation.
  - Impaired lactate metabolism (e.g. liver failure).

Causes of Lactic Acidosis

Type A lactic acidosis (associated with tissue hypoxia)

- Shock (hypovolemia, cardiogenic, septic)
- Severe hypoxemia
- Cardiac arrest
- Seizures
- Severe anemia

Type B lactic acidosis (Occurs without hypoxia; due to metabolic dysfunction or toxins)

- Liver failure (↓ lactate clearance)
- Renal failure
- Drugs/toxins: Metformin, ethanol, methanol
- Malignancy
- Thiamine deficiency
- Inborn errors of metabolism

Clinical Features

- Nausea, vomiting, abdominal pain
- Hypotension
- Presence of acidotic breathing (Kussmaul's respirations)
- Altered sensorium ranging from stupor to coma.

Investigations

- Plasma bicarbonate and pH are markedly reduced (pH <7.35).
- Anion gap is increased.
- High lactic acid level (>4 mmol/L, normal is <2 mmol/L).

Treatment

- The main treatment in lactic acidosis is correcting the underlying cause such as sepsis, hypovolemia, cardiac failure.
- Use of sodium bicarbonate is contraindicated as it breaks down into carbon dioxide and water in the tissues increasing tissue acidosis. Many other therapies have been tried without much benefit such as sodium dichloroacetate, tromethamine, and thiamine. Hemodialysis is useful in metformin induced lactic acidosis.
- Despite energetic treatment, mortality rate is >50%.

Q. Define hypoglycemia. Discuss the causes, clinical features, diagnosis and management of hypoglycemia.

- Hypoglycemia is a clinical condition characterized by abnormally low plasma glucose levels, typically:
  - Blood glucose <70 mg/dl—biochemical definition
  - Clinically significant hypoglycemia: <54 mg/dl.
  - Severe hypoglycemia: Any glucose level low enough to cause severe neuroglycopenic symptoms requiring assistance.

Causes

In diabetic patients

- Excess insulin (overdose, inappropriate timing)
- Oral hypoglycemic agents (e.g. sulfonylureas, meglitinides)
- Delayed or missed meals
- Excessive physical activity
- Alcohol intake
- Renal or hepatic dysfunction (affects drug metabolism)

In nondiabetic individuals

- Critical illness (sepsis, renal failure, liver failure)
- Hormonal deficiencies (e.g. cortisol, GH)
- Insulinoma or islet cell tumors
- Non-islet cell tumors (produce insulin-like growth factors)
- Severe malnutrition
- Reactive (after gastric surgery–"dumping syndrome")
- Drug-induced: Quinine, pentamidine, salicylates, beta-blockers
- Alcohol-induced: Especially with poor nutrition or fasting
- Malignancies: Sarcomas
- Factitious (deliberately induced)
- Glycogen storage disorders
- Inborn errors of metabolism

Clinical features

Autonomic symptoms (due to acute activation of the autonomic nervous system)

- Sweating
- Tremors
- Palpitations
- Hunger
- Anxiety

Neuroglycopenic symptoms (due to glucose deprivation to the brain)

- Confusion
- Drowsiness
- Speech difficulty
- Visual disturbances
- Inability to concentrate
- Incoordination
- Focal neurological deficits
- Seizures
- Coma in severe cases

Nonspecific

- Nausea
- Tiredness
- Headache

- Whipple's triad: Used to confirm hypoglycemia. Components of this triad are;
  1. Symptoms/signs of hypoglycemia
  2. Low plasma glucose level
  3. Relief of symptoms after glucose correction
- In most instances, patient can recognize the symptoms of hypoglycemia and take appropriate action which includes eating a snack or sugar, etc. However, in certain circumstances (e.g. during sleep, or when distracted by other activities) warning symptoms may not be perceived by the patient, so that appropriate action is not taken and neuroglycopenia with reduced consciousness occurs.
- In diabetic patients who are accustomed to high blood sugar, symptoms of hypoglycemia may occur at higher blood sugar levels. Similarly, patients who have experienced recurrent hypoglycemia attacks may not experience any symptoms even when the blood glucose is well below 50 mg/dl (hypoglycemia unawareness).

Complications of Severe Hypoglycemia

- Impaired cognitive function
- Intellectual decline
- Brain damage
- Coma
- Convulsions
- Focal neurological lesions
- Cardiac arrhythmias
- Myocardial ischemia
- Vitreous hemorrhage
- Hypothermia
- Accidents (including road traffic accidents) with injury

Measures to Prevent Hypoglycemia

- Do not skip meals after taking sulphonylurea or insulin.
- Use the correct dose of insulin and oral antidiabetic agents as prescribed.
- Avoid unaccustomed intense exercise especially on empty stomach.
- Take light snacks in between major meals and also at bedtime.
- Monitor blood sugar frequently.
- Carry supply of fast-acting carbohydrate (sweets, sugar, glucose tablets), and a glucagon injection while going for long travel.

Investigations

- Blood glucose measurement: Fingerstick or plasma glucose level preferably during symptoms.
- 72-hour fasting test (for insulinoma work-up).
- Cortisol and GH levels.
- Imaging (if insulinoma suspected): CT/MRI pancreas, endoscopic ultrasound.

Management of Hypoglycemia

- If the patient is conscious and able to swallow, glucose (50 g) or any other fast acting source of carbohydrate (sweets, honey, etc.) can be given orally.
- If the patient is in altered sensorium and unable to swallow, intravenous glucose (50 ml of 50% dextrose) is given. Inj glucagon (1 mg by intramuscular injection) can also be given if IV access is a problem. As soon as the patient is able to swallow, glucose should be given orally.
- If hypoglycemia has occurred after the use of a long acting insulin or drug such as glibenclamide, above treatment should be followed by an infusion of 10% dextrose for few hours, to prevent recurrence of hypoglycemia.
- If the patient fails to regain consciousness after blood glucose is restored to normal, development of cerebral edema should be suspected. Cerebral edema has high mortality and morbidity, and should be treated with mannitol and high-dose oxygen.
- Identify and eliminate the cause: e.g. adjust insulin and sulfonylurea dose. Patient education about meal timing, carb intake, medication adjustment. Treat underlying tumors or metabolic disorders.

Q. Somogyi phenomenon and dawn phenomenon.

Somogyi Phenomenon

- It is also known as post-hypoglycemic hyperglycemia. It refers to rebound hyperglycemia due to release of counter-regulatory hormones following an episode of hypoglycemia.
- Named after Dr. Michael Somogyi, who proposed that hypoglycemia triggers counter-regulatory hormone responses (like glucagon, cortisol, growth hormone, epinephrine), leading to rebound hyperglycemia.
- It usually happens in the morning after an episode of hypoglycemia at midnight.
- Causes include excess or ill-timed insulin, missed meals or snacks and inadvertent insulin administration.
- It is important to recognize Somogyi phenomenon because control of morning hyperglycemia depends on decreasing the night dose of insulin instead of increasing it.

Diagnosing Somogyi phenomenon

- Somogyi phenomenon should be suspected when morning hyperglycemia worsens or resists treatment with increasing insulin doses. Other clues are normal daytime blood sugar levels, and relatively low HbA1C. The most important thing in the diagnosis of Somogyi phenomenon is considering it in the causes of morning hyperglycemia.
- Documenting nocturnal (3–4 AM) hypoglycemia confirms the diagnosis. Continuous Glucose monitoring (CGM) is the most accurate way to detect night-time trends.

Managing Somogyi Phenomenon

- Reduce night or bedtime insulin.
- Giving night time intermediate acting insulin (NPH/LENTE) at bed time rather than before dinner may help. Substitution of night dose NPH/LENTE with longer acting preparation (glargine, detemir) may also help.

These measures will cause insulin effect to peak in the morning rather than at midnight.

- Substitution of regular insulin with a fast-acting insulin analog, such as lispro, may be of some help.
- Patient should be advised to take a bedtime snack to prevent midnight hypoglycemia.

Dawn Phenomenon

- The Dawn Phenomenon is an early morning rise in blood glucose levels (usually between 4 and 8 AM) without preceding nocturnal hypoglycemia.
- It is due to early morning surge of growth hormone, cortisol, epinephrine, and glucagon. These hormones oppose insulin action and promote hepatic glucose production, leading to hyperglycemia upon waking.
- It can be differentiated from Somogyi phenomenon by documenting the absence of midnight hypoglycemia.
- It is managed by increasing the night dose of insulin.

Q. Discuss the risk factors, pathology, clinical features, diagnosis and management of diabetic nephropathy.

- Diabetic nephropathy (DN) is a progressive kidney disease caused by chronic hyperglycemia, leading to glomerular damage, proteinuria, and eventually chronic kidney disease (CKD) and end-stage renal disease (ESRD) in patients with diabetes mellitus (both type 1 and type 2).
- Diabetic nephropathy is one of the most common causes of end-stage renal disease (ESRD). It is an important cause of morbidity and mortality.
- It is more common in type 1 than in type 2 diabetes.

Risk Factors for Developing Diabetic Nephropathy

- Genetic variables (decreased number of glomeruli)
- Family history of diabetic nephropathy
- Poor control of blood glucose
- Long duration of diabetes (>5 years)
- Ethnicity (e.g. Asian races, African-Americans)
- Presence of hypertension
- Dyslipidemia
- Obesity
- Smoking

Pathology

- There are three major histologic changes in the glomeruli in diabetic nephropathy: Glomerular basement membrane thickening; mesangial proliferation; and glomerular sclerosis.
- The first change to be seen is glomerular basement membrane thickening which is associated with microalbuminuria. Subsequently, nodular deposits (the Kimmelstiel-Wilson lesion) develop, and glomerulosclerosis worsens (heavy proteinuria develops) until glomeruli are progressively lost and renal function deteriorates.
- Renal failure usually takes ≥10 year after the onset of nephropathy to develop.

Clinical Features

- Microalbuminuria (30–300 mg/day)–first clinical sign. Progression to macroalbuminuria (>300 mg/day).
- Passing of foamy urine due to proteinuria.
- Fatigue and foot edema secondary to hypoalbuminemia (if nephrotic range protienuria is present).
- In later stages, patients may develop symptoms and signs of uremia (e.g. nausea, vomiting, anorexia).
- Hypertension is usually present.

Diagnosis

- *Screening for microalbuminuria*: Microalbuminuria is urinary excretion of albumin in a range of 30–300 mg albumin/day. Microalbuminuria can progress to macroalbunuria (excretion of >300 mg albumin per day) or nephrotic range proteinuria (>3 g/day) over many years. All diabetic patients should be screened for albuminuria at the time of diagnosis and yearly thereafter.
- Quantification of albumin excretion can be done by the following methods.
  - Measurement of albumin–to-creatinine ratio on a spot urine test. A ratio of more than 30 mg albumin/g creatinine is abnormal.
  - 24-hour urine albumin excretion->30 mg/24 hours is abnormal.
- *Renal function tests*—urea, creatinine may be elevated in advanced diabetic nephropathy
- Lipid profile, HbA1c, and electrolytes
- Urinalysis—rule out hematuria, casts
- Ultrasound of kidneys is required to know the size of kidneys and any parenchymal changes.
- Kidney biopsy is not routinely necessary unless other kidney diseases are suspected such as glomerulonephritis, etc.

Management

- If there is evidence of nephropathy, further progression can be delayed by strict control of blood glucose (HbA1c <7%) and control of blood pressure.
- ACE inhibitors not only reduce blood pressure but also reduce proteinuria and progression of diabetic nephropathy. Angiotensin II receptor blockers (ARB) and calcium channel blockers such as amlodipine, cilnidipine, and diltiazem also have similar benefits.
- Statins are used to treat dyslipidemia. They also reduce proteinuria.
- Avoid nephrotoxic drugs.
- Renal replacement therapy (dialysis) is required in end stage renal disease.

Q. Diabetic retinopathy.

- Diabetic retinopathy (DR) is a microvascular complication of diabetes mellitus, characterized by progressive retinal damage due to chronic hyperglycemia, leading to vision impairment or blindness if untreated.
- It is the leading cause of preventable blindness in working-age adults globally.

- Diabetic retinopathy (DR) is divided into two major forms: Nonproliferative and proliferative, depending on the absence or presence of abnormal new blood vessels in the retina.

Pathogenesis

- Diabetic retinopathy is primarily caused by chronic hyperglycemia, which leads to progressive microvascular damage in the retina. The pathogenesis involves metabolic, hemodynamic, and inflammatory mechanisms, resulting in capillary leakage, ischemia, and neovascularization.
- There are many mechanisms which can produce retinopathy such as—increased production of sorbitol by polyol pathway, activation of protein kinase C (PKC), increased expression of growth factors such as vascular endothelial growth factor (VEGF) and insulin-like growth factor-1 (IGF-1), hemodynamic changes, formation of advanced glycation endproducts (AGEs), oxidative stress, activation of the renin-angiotensin-aldosterone system (RAAS), and subclinical inflammation and capillary occlusion. Retinal capillary occlusion causes chronic retinal hypoxia and stimulates new vessel formation (neovascularization) and increases vascular permeability (causing retinal leakage and exudation).
- Nonproliferative retinopathy (also called background retinopathy) develops first and causes increased capillary permeability, microaneurysms, hemorrhages, exudates, macular ischemia, and macular edema.
- Proliferative retinopathy develops after nonproliferative retinopathy and is more severe. It is characterized by abnormal new vessel formation (neovascularization) which may rupture and cause retinal and vitreous hemorrhage. Neovascularization is often accompanied by pre-retinal fibrous tissue, which, along with the vitreous, can contract, resulting in traction retinal detachment.

Clinical Features

- Early stages: Asymptomatic.
- Following symptoms develop as the disease progresses:
  - Blurred vision
  - Floaters
  - Dark areas in vision
  - Impaired color vision
  - Sudden vision loss (with proliferative diabetic retinopathy or diabetic macular edema)

Diagnosis

- Fundoscopy: May show microaneurysms, retinal hemorrhages, exudates , cotton wool spots, venous changes, neovascularization, vitreous hemorrhage, and fibrosis **(Fig. 9.20)**.
- Color fundus photography
- Fluorescein angiography
- Optical coherence tomography.

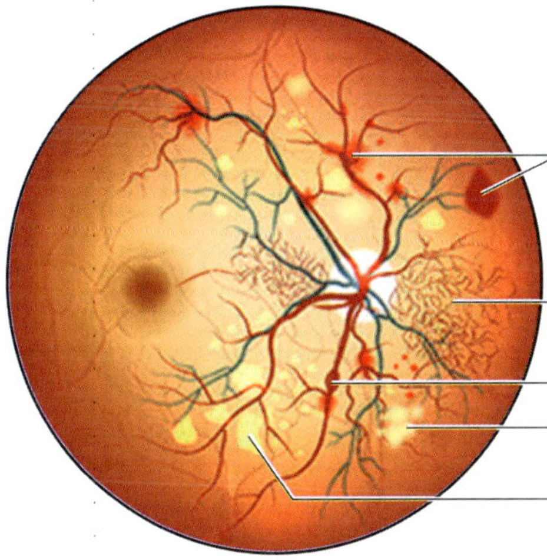

Figure 9.20: Diabetic retinopathy

Management

- Severe non-proliferative and proliferative retinopathy is treated with retinal laser photocoagulation. Photocoagulation is used to destroy areas of retinal ischemia which stimulate neovascularization, to seal leaking microaneurysms and reduce macular edema, and to gliose new vessels directly on the retinal surface.
- Clinically significant macular edema is treated with intraocular injection of anti-VEGF drugs (e.g. ranibizumab, bevacizumab, aflibercept) and/or with focal laser photocoagulation.
- Vitrectomy may be used in selected cases where visual loss is due to recurrent vitreous hemorrhage which has failed to clear, or retinal detachment resulting from retinitis proliferans.

Prevention

- Good control of blood sugar and blood pressure
- Regular screening for retinopathy at least once a year in all diabetic patients.

Q. Discuss the classification, pathology, clinical features, investigations and management of diabetic neuropathy.

Q. Autonomic neuropathy.

- Diabetic neuropathy is the most common complication of diabetes mellitus (DM), affecting as many as 50% of patients with type 1 and type 2 DM.
- It is asymptomatic in the majority, although it can cause disabling symptoms in a few patients. Its prevalence is higher with long duration of diabetes and poor control of blood sugar.

Classification

Symmetric polyneuropathy

- Most common form

Polyradiculopathies

- Lumbar polyradiculopathy (diabetic amyotrophy)
- Thoracic polyradiculopathy

Mononeuropathies
- Cranial mononeuropathy (e.g. CN III, VI, VII)
- Peripheral mononeuropathy (e.g. median, ulnar, peroneal nerves)

Mononeuropathy multiplex
Autonomic neuropathy

Pathology and Pathogenesis

- Diabetic neuropathy is a result of metabolic and microvascular injury to nerves.

Metabolic Factors

- Hyperglycemia-induced oxidative stress
- Polyol pathway activation (glucose → sorbitol → fructose) leading to osmotic injury
- Advanced glycation end-products (AGEs) damaging nerves
- Reduced nerve growth factor.

Vascular Factors

- Microangiopathy of vasa nervorum → ischemia of peripheral nerves.

Inflammatory and Autoimmune Factors

- Particularly relevant in diabetic amyotrophy and autonomic neuropathy.

Pathological Findings

- Axonal degeneration of both myelinated and unmyelinated fibers
- Thickening of Schwann cell basal lamina
- Patchy, segmental demyelination
- Thickened endoneural blood vessel walls and vascular occlusions.

Clinical Features

Symmetrical Polyneuropathy

- Distal symmetric sensorimotor polyneuropathy is the most common type of diabetic neuropathy. It is characterized by progressive loss of distal sensation, followed, in severe cases, by motor weakness.
- Symptoms include paresthesiae in the feet and, rarely, in the hands, pain in the lower limbs (dull, aching and/or lancinating, worse at night), burning sensations in the soles of the feet, cutaneous hyperesthesia and numbness in the feet.
- Examination shows loss of vibration sensation, altered proprioception distally and loss of tendon reflexes in the lower limbs. These features are due to large nerve fiber involvement. Impairment of pain, light touch and temperature is secondary to loss of small fibers.
- Muscle weakness and wasting develop only in advanced cases, but subclinical motor nerve dysfunction is common.
- All the above features start initially in the feet, but later as the disease advances, hands also get involved.

Polyradiculopathies

- *Lumbar polyradiculopathy (diabetic amyotrophy):* The most common type of diabetic polyradiculopathy is high lumbar radiculopathy involving the L2, L3, and L4 roots. Patients present with thigh pain followed by painful proximal weakness and wasting in one leg. Tendon reflexes may be absent on the affected side(s). This condition is thought to be due to acute infarction of the involved nerve roots. Although recovery usually occurs within 12 months, some deficits become permanent. Management is mainly supportive.
- *Thoracic polyradiculopathy:* This is less common than lumbar polyradiculopathy and affects the T4 through T12 roots. Patients present with abdominal pain, sometimes in a band-like pattern. Diagnosis is confirmed by EMG studies.

Mononeuropathies

- Mononeuropathies are usually severe and of rapid onset but eventually recover.
- Cranial mononeuropathy: Cranial nerves 3, 6 and 7 are commonly affected. Patients present with unilateral pain, ptosis, and diplopia, with sparing of pupillary function. Facial mononeuropathy (Bell's palsy) occurs more frequently in diabetic than in nondiabetics.
- Peripheral mononeuropathy: Median, femoral and sciatic nerves are commonly involved. These are usually compression palsies. Median nerve gets compressed at the wrist commonly leading to carpal tunnel syndrome. Lateral popliteal nerve compression occasionally causes foot drop. Ulnar mononeuropathy, either at the elbow or, less commonly, at the wrist can also occur.

Mononeuropathy Multiplex

- Multiple mononeuropathies in the same patient are known as mononeuropathy multiplex (or asymmetric polyneuropathy).

Autonomic Neuropathy

- It can affect many organ systems, including cardiovascular, gastrointestinal, genitourinary, pupillary, sudomotor and neuroendocrine systems.
- Either parasympathetic or sympathetic nerves may be predominantly affected in one or more visceral system.

Investigations

- Autonomic testing: Simple clinical tests such as heart rate variation during deep breathing, heart rate response to standing and blood pressure response to standing. Baroreflex sensitivity using power spectral analysis of heart rate.
- Nerve conduction studies (not routinely required).
- Assess glycemic control by FBS, PPBS and HbA1c.

Management

- Good control of diabetes
- Pain control: Neuropathic pain can be controlled by tricyclic antidepressants (amitriptyline), anticonvulsants (gabapentin, carbamazepine, phenytoin, pregabalin), topical capsaicin, opiates (tramadol, oxycodone) and duloxetine. Any one or more of these can be used.
- Autonomic neuropathy: Postural hypotension can be reduced by full length elastic stockings, increasing salt intake, fludrocortisone and α-adrenoceptor agonist (midodrine). Gastroparesis may respond to prokinetic agents such as metoclopramide and domperidone. Diarrhea responds to diphenoxylate, loperamide and broad-spectrum antibiotics. Constipation can be managed by stimulant laxatives (senna). Bladder dysfunction can be managed by intermittent self-catheterization. Erectile dysfunction (impotence) by phosphodiesterase-5 inhibitors (sildenafil, vardenafil, tadalafil).
- Foot care education to prevent ulcers and amputation.

Complications

- Foot ulcers, infections, gangrene
- Charcot neuroarthropathy
- Amputation
- Falls due to proprioceptive loss
- Silent myocardial infarction (due to autonomic neuropathy).

Q. Diabetic foot.

- Diabetic foot refers to infection, ulceration, or destruction of tissues of the foot associated with neuropathy and/or peripheral vascular disease in patients with diabetes mellitus.
- Foot complications are common in diabetics and if neglected can lead to amputation. Hence, foot care is very important in diabetics.

Etiology

- Both neuropathy and peripheral vascular disease play an important role in the causation of diabetic foot. Neuropathy promotes ulcer formation by decreasing pain sensation and perception of pressure. Peripheral vascular disease also contributes to ulcer formation and gangrene due to decreased blood supply.
- Infection occurs as a secondary phenomenon following disruption of the protective epidermis.

Investigations

Basic

- Blood glucose, HbA1c
- Complete blood count (CBC)—leukocytosis in infection
- ESR/CRP—elevated in infection or osteomyelitis
- Wound culture and sensitivity.

Vascular Assessment

- Ankle-Brachial Index (ABI): <0.9 suggests PVD
- Doppler ultrasound
- Angiography in selected cases.

Neuropathy Assessment

- Monofilament test (10 g), tuning fork, vibration, pinprick, temperature.

Imaging

- X-ray foot: Foreign body, gas, osteomyelitis
- MRI: For deep infection or early osteomyelitis.

Clinical Features

- *Due to neuropathy*—pain, paraesthesiae and numbness, neuropathic ulcer.
- *Due to ischemia*—rest pain, cluadication, ischemic ulcer, gangrene.
- *Due to infection*—cellulitis, abscess, osteomyelitis and sepsis.

Management

- Good control of blood sugar
- Removal of callus skin
- Treatment of infection with appropriate antibiotics
- Avoid weight-bearing on calluses and ulcers
- Treatment of peripheral vascular disease
- Amputation if there is extensive tissue necrosis, gangrene and/or bony destruction
- Specially manufactured and fitted orthotic footwear to prevent recurrence of ulceration and protect the feet of patients with Charcot neuroarthropathy.
- Use of foot wear made of microcellular rubber is helpful to prevent callus formation and ulcers.

Prevention

- Daily foot inspection
- Proper footwear
- Avoid walking barefoot
- Control of blood sugar, BP, and lipids
- Smoking cessation
- Regular podiatric care.

Q. What is gestational diabetes mellitus? Discuss the pathophysiology, risk factors, diagnostic criteria, and management of gestational diabetes.

- Gestational diabetes mellitus (GDM) is defined as diabetes with first onset or recognition during pregnancy.
- Most GDM cases begin during pregnancy, but some GDM cases may be actually previously undetected type 1 or type 2 diabetes.
- It usually resolves postpartum but may increase the risk of developing type 2 diabetes later in life.

Pathophysiology

- Pregnancy is characterized by insulin resistance particularly during the second half of pregnancy which may predispose some women to develop diabetes.
- Insulin resistance is due to placental secretion of diabetogenic hormones such as growth hormone, cortisol, placental lactogen, and progesterone, as well as increased maternal adipose tissue deposition, decreased exercise, and increased caloric intake.

- GDM develops when pancreas fails to compensate for increased insulin resistance.

Risk Factors for Gestational Diabetes

- Obesity
- Age greater than 25 years
- Ethnicity (South Asian, black, Hispanic, Native American)
- Family history of diabetes
- Previous GDM or impaired glucose tolerance
- Previous macrosomia
- Polyhydramnios
- Polycystic ovarian syndrome (PCOS).

Diagnosis of GDM

75-g OGTT

- Perform a 75-g OGTT, with plasma glucose measurement when patient is fasting and at 1 and 2 hours, at 24–28 weeks of gestation in women not previously diagnosed with diabetes.
- The OGTT should be performed in the morning after an overnight fast of at least 8 h.
- The diagnosis of GDM is made if any one of the following is met:
  - Fasting: ≥92 mg/dl
  - 1-hour glucose: ≥180 mg/dl
  - 2-hour glucose: ≥153 mg/dl.

Significance of GDM (effects on mother and fetus)

- Gestational diabetes is associated with an increased risk of later development of type 2 diabetes. Maternal morbidity is increased and there is a high chance of caesarean section. Pregnancy is also associated with an increased risk of ketoacidosis.
- Increased risk of perinatal mortality and morbidity for the baby. Maternal hyperglycemia stimulates fetal insulin production which stimulates fetal growth leading to macrosomia. Fetal macrosomia increases the risk of birth injury during delivery, and of subsequent neonatal hypoglycemia. There is also increased risk of polycythemia, hyperbilirubinemia and hypocalcemia in the fetus.

Management of GDM

Targets recommended for blood glucose control in gestational diabetes mellitus:

- Fasting glucose <95 mg/dl and
- One-hour postprandial glucose <140 mg/dl or
- Two-hour postprandial glucose <120 mg/dl.

Medical Nutrition Therapy (MNT)

- All women with GDM should receive nutritional counseling and nutrition therapy. Total calories should be distributed wisely throughout the day. Consumption of refined carbohydrates should be reduced. When nutritional therapy fails to maintain glucose at normal levels, insulin should be used.
- Moderate exercise like walking after meals improves glucose control.

Pharmacological Therapy

- Indicated if glycemic targets not met in 1–2 weeks with lifestyle therapy.
- All the oral antidiabetic agents are contraindicated during pregnancy except metformin and glibenclamide although insulin is preferred. Metformin is sometimes given for PCOS and can be continued.
- Insulin is the gold standard treatment for GDM; does not cross placenta. Only human insulin should be used during pregnancy. 3–4 injections of short acting insulin may be required to achieve good glucose control.
- Blood glucose should be monitored daily. Do not strive for normoglycemia at the expense of hypoglycemia.
- Insulin can be stopped after delivery when blood sugar tends to return to normal levels.

Postpartum Care

- OGTT at 6 weeks postpartum to assess for persistent diabetes.
- Annual screening for type 2 diabetes in future.

Q. Metabolic syndrome (insulin resistance syndrome; Syndrome X).

- The co-occurrence of metabolic risk factors (abdominal obesity, hyperglycemia, dyslipidemia, and hypertension) is termed "metabolic syndrome". Patients with metabolic syndrome are at risk of developing type 2 diabetes and cardiovascular disease.
- Abdominal obesity increases the risk of metabolic syndrome. Excess abdominal fat leads to excess free fatty acids in the portal vein, increasing fat accumulation in the liver. Fat also accumulates in muscle cells leading to insulin resistance and hyperinsulinemia. Glucose metabolism is impaired, and dyslipidemia and hypertension develop. Serum uric acid level is usually elevated (increasing the risk of gout).

Diagnostic Criteria

- Metabolic syndrome is diagnosed when any three of the following five criteria are present:

- Abdominal obesity, defined as a waist circumference in men >40 inches and in women >35 inches.
- Serum triglycerides ≥150 mg/dl or drug treatment for elevated triglycerides.
- Serum HDL cholesterol <40 mg/dl in men and <50 mg/dl in women or drug treatment for low HDL-C.
- Blood pressure ≥130/85 mm Hg or drug treatment for elevated blood pressure.
- Fasting blood sugar ≥100 mg/dl or drug treatment for elevated blood glucose.

Risk Factors

- Lifestyle-related:
  - Physical inactivity
  - High-calorie, high-fat diet
  - Smoking

- Genetic predisposition.
- Aging.
- Ethnicity (South Asians, Hispanics at higher risk).
- Low birth weight or intrauterine malnutrition.
- Polycystic ovary syndrome (PCOS).

Clinical Features

- Often asymptomatic
- May present with:
    - Central obesity (abdominal fat)
    - Signs of insulin resistance (e.g. acanthosis nigricans).
    - Hypertension
    - Features of T2DM or cardiovascular disease.

Clinical Implications

The risk of following conditions is increased in people with metabolic syndrome:

- Type 2 diabetes
- Cardiovascular diseases (MI, stroke, atherosclerosis)
- Nonalcoholic fatty liver disease (NAFLD)
- Polycystic ovarian disease
- Obstructiv+dney disease.

Investigations

- Fasting blood glucose
- Lipid profile
- Blood pressure monitoring
- Waist circumference measurement
- Oral glucose tolerance test (OGTT) (if needed)
- HbA1c.

Treatment

- Reduction of obesity is the main therapeutic goal. This can be achieved by regular exercise, low fat, and high fiber diet.
- Control of hypertension, dyslipidemia and hyperglycemia by appropriate drugs. Metformin is used to treat insulin resistance.
- Cessation of smoking.

Chapter 10

Diseases of Immune System, Connective Tissue and Joints

Q. What are rheumatic diseases?

- Rheumatic diseases are autoimmune and inflammatory diseases that primarily affect the joints, bones, muscles, tendons, ligaments, and sometimes internal organs. These are usually painful, chronic, and progressive diseases.
- These diseases are different from orthopedic problems which also affect musculoskeletal system.

Q. Describe the genetic basis and pathophysiology of autoimmune disease.

- Autoimmune diseases arise from an inappropriate immune response against the body's own tissues due to loss of self-tolerance. The result is chronic inflammation, tissue damage, and organ dysfunction.

Genetic Basis of Autoimmune Diseases

HLA (human leukocyte antigen) Associations

- Strongest genetic risk factor.
- HLA molecules (especially class II) present self-antigens to $CD4^+$ T cells.
- Certain HLA alleles predispose to specific autoimmune diseases, e.g. HLA-DR2, HLA-DR3 predispose to SLE and HLA-DR4 to rheumatoid arthritis.

Non-HLA Genetic Factors

- Many non-HLA genetic factors predispose to autoimmune diseases. Examples are PTPN22, CTLA-4, and STAT4. All these regulate the immune system.

Pathophysiology of Autoimmune Disease

Loss of Self-tolerance

- Normally there is deletion of autoreactive T and B cells during development. Failure to delete leads to escape of self-reactive lymphocytes into circulation.
- Failure in the following mechanisms responsible to prevent autoimmunity.
  - Anergy: Non-responsiveness to self-antigen.
  - Regulatory T cells (Tregs): Suppress immune responses.
  - Activation-induced cell death (AICD): Eliminates activated T cells.

Environmental Triggers

- Infections:
  - Molecular mimicry (e.g. rheumatic fever post-Streptococcus infection).
  - Bystander activation.
- UV radiation: Increases apoptosis and self-antigen exposure (e.g. in SLE).
- Drugs: Can alter self-antigens or promote autoantibody production (e.g. drug-induced lupus).
- Microbiota dysbiosis: Alters mucosal immunity.

Mechanisms of Autoimmune Tissue Injury

Type II Hypersensitivity (antibody-mediated cytotoxicity)

- Autoantibodies bind to cell surface antigens → cell lysis.
- *Examples*: Autoimmune hemolytic anemia, myasthenia gravis.

Type III Hypersensitivity (immune complex-mediated)

- Immune complexes deposit in tissues → inflammation.
- *Examples*: SLE (glomerulonephritis, vasculitis).

Type IV Hypersensitivity (T cell-mediated)

- Autoreactive T cells destroy tissues.
- *Examples*: Type 1 diabetes, multiple sclerosis.

Role of Cytokines and B Cells

- In a healthy immune system, there's a balance among T-helper subsets. In autoimmune diseases, there is upregulation of Th1 and Th17 immune responses, which are proinflammatory and tissue-damaging.
- Interferon-α (IFN-α): Drives SLE pathology.
- B cells: Autoantibody production, antigen presentation.

Q. What are the presenting complaints of rheumatic diseases (musculoskeletal diseases)?

Articular manifestations

- Joint pain
- Back pain
- Joint stiffness (subjective feeling of inability to move freely)
- Swelling of joints
- Deformity (Joint, bone)

Extra-articular/systemic complaints

- Fever
- Fatigue
- Skin rash
- Weight loss
- Eye involvement (uveitis, scleritis)
- Mouth ulcers

Q. What are the investigations done in rheumatic diseases?

Investigations in rheumatic diseases help in:

- Confirming the diagnosis.
- Assessing disease activity and organ involvement.
- Monitoring treatment response.

Blood Investigations

- C-reactive protein (CRP) and erythrocyte sedimentation rate (ESR): these are acute phase reactants and elevated in infections and inflammation.
- Autoantibodies: Rheumatoid factor (RF), antinuclear antibodies (ANA), antiphospholipid antibodies and anti-CCP (cyclic citrullinated peptide) antibodies. Anti-CCP has more specificity for diagnosing rheumatoid arthritis than RF.
- Biochemical tests (calcium, phosphorous, uric acid, alkaline phosphatase).

Imaging Studies

- Plain X-rays: It may show joint erosions in rheumatoid arthritis, joint space narrowing in osteoarthritis, sacroiliitis in ankylosing spondylitis, and calcifications in pseudogout.
- Ultrasonography: Useful in confirming soft tissue changes such as a hip joint effusion, popliteal cyst or tenosynovitis.
- CT and MRI: Useful to assess anatomically complex structures, such as the spine.
- Bone mineral density (BMD) measurements: Useful to diagnose and quantify osteoporosis. Dual energy X-ray absorptiometry (DEXA) is the current method of choice.
- Radionuclide bone scans (useful in detecting Paget's disease, and primary or secondary bone tumors).

Synovial Fluid Analysis

- Cell count, crystals, culture, Gram's stain.
- Helps in diagnosis of gout/pseudogout (crystals), septic arthritis (infection).

Urine Tests

- Proteinuria, hematuria due to renal involvement (e.g. lupus nephritis).

Biopsy

- Skin biopsy (SLE, vasculitis)
- Muscle biopsy (myositis)
- Renal biopsy (lupus nephritis)
- Temporal artery biopsy (giant cell arteritis).

Q. What is arthrocentesis? Enumerate the indications for arthrocentesis.

- Arthrocentesis is a procedure performed to collect synovial fluid from joint spaces by inserting a needle.

Indications

- Diagnosis of joint infection (septic arthritis)
- Diagnosis of crystal induced arthropathy (e.g. pseudogout)
- Administration of medications for acute or chronic arthritis
- Symptomatic relief in large joint effusion
- Evacuation of possible hemarthrosis in a traumatic effusion
- Identifying communication between the joint space and a laceration.

Contraindications

- Periarticular infection (chances of introducing the infection into the joints.
- Coagulopathy.

Q. Enumerate the causes of monoarthritis.

- Monoarthritis refers to inflammation of only one joint.

Causes

- Septic arthritis
- Crystal Induced arthritis (gout, pseudogout)
- Trauma
- Osteoarthritis
- Hemarthrosis
- Foreign body reaction (e.g. plant thorn)
- Avascular necrosis
- Subchondral collapse or fracture
- Monoarticular presentation of oligo-or polyarthritis (reactive arthritis, psoriatic arthritis, Rheumatoid arthritis, etc.)

Q. Enumerate the causes of oligoarthritis.

- Oligoarthritis refers to arthritis affecting 2–4 joints.

Causes

- Osteoarthritis
- Seronegative spondyloarthropathies (reactive arthritis, psoriatic arthritis, ankylosing spondylitis, IBD associated arthritis)
- Juvenile idiopathic arthritis
- Oligoarticular presentation of polyarthritis
- Infections (bacterial endocarditis, Neisseria, mycobacteria)

Q. Enumerate the causes of polyarthritis.

- Polyarthritis refers to arthritis involving 5 or more joints simultaneously.

Infections: Gonococcal arthritis, rheumatic fever tuberculous arthritis, syphilitic arthritis, bacterial endocarditis, Lyme's disease, viral arthritis.

Autoimmune/inflammatory diseases: Rheumatoid arthritis, ankylosing spondylitis, SLE, systemic vasculitis, systemic sclerosis, polymyositis/dermatomyositis, Still's disease, Behçet's syndrome, sarcoidosis.

Mechanical: Degenerative joint disease-osteoarthritis.

Malignancy: Paraneoplastic arthropathies.

Metabolic: Hypothyroidism, hyperparathyroidism, Cushing's disease, hemochromatosis, Wilson's disease, ochronosis, hyperlipoproteinemias.

Drug-induced: Hydralazine, procainamide (drug induced lupus).

Q. Enumerate the causes of bone pain.

- Bone pain refers to discomfort, aching, or tenderness originating specifically from bone tissue.
- It is distinct from joint, muscle, or nerve pain, and may arise from a variety of mechanical, metabolic, infectious, or neoplastic causes.

Causes of Bone Pain

- Malignancy (primary or secondary bone tumors)
- Hematological malignancies such as myeloma and leukemia
- Fracture
- Paget's disease
- Osteoporosis (microfractures, vertebral compression fractures cause pain)
- Osteomalacia
- Chronic infection (osteomyelitis)
- Osteonecrosis

Q. Discuss the etiology, clinical features, investigations and management of osteoarthritis.

- Osteoarthritis (OA, osteoarthrosis) is the most common form of arthritis.
- It is characterized by degeneration of articular cartilage, subchondral bone changes, and osteophyte formation. Inflammation is not a prominent feature of OA.

Epidemiology

- The prevalence of osteoarthritis increases with ageing. By 65 years of age, 80% of people have radiographic evidence of OA.
- It mainly affects weight bearing joints though certain small joints can also be involved. The knee and hip are most often involved.
- Knee OA is prevalent in all racial groups but hip, hand and generalized OA are only prevalent in Caucasians.
- OA is more common in females.

Etiology and Pathogenesis

- OA was previously thought to be a normal consequence of aging, thereby leading to the term degenerative joint disease. However, it is now realized that multiple factors play a role in the causation of OA.
- There are many risk factors for the development of OA which are as follows:

- Advanced age
- Female sex
- Obesity
- Occupation which involves repetitive loading of particular joints (e.g. shipyard workers)
- Sports activities
- Previous injury to joint
- Muscle weakness
- Proprioceptive deficits
- Genetic factors
- Acromegaly
- Calcium crystal deposition disease

- Many insults such as trauma, repetitive loading, metabolic, genetic or constitutional insults may damage a synovial joint and trigger the repair process.
- The repair process involves new bone formation and remodeling of joint shape. New bone formation occurs at the margins of the joint and are called osteophytes. This may result in anatomically altered but pain-free functioning joint ('compensated' OA). However, poor repair process may result in progressive symptoms and joint failure.
- Pathologically there is fissuring of the articular cartilage surface ('fibrillation'), development of deep vertical clefts, localized chondrocyte death and decrease in cartilage thickness. Decrease in the thickness of articular cartilage results in decrease in joint space. The bone immediately below the damaged articular cartilage develops cysts and there is increase in its trabecular thickness. The synovium also undergoes variable degrees of hyperplasia. These synovial changes may sometimes resemble those of rheumatoid arthritis.

Clinical Features

- The main symptoms of OA are pain and restriction of joint movement. Patient is usually above 45 years (often over 60 years).
- Pain is of insidious onset over months or years. Usually, one or few joints are affected and weight bearing joints are commonly involved (such as knee and hip). It is variable or intermittent over time ('good days, bad days'). It is worse on movement and weight-bearing, and relieved by rest. Morning stiffness is less (<30 minutes) compare to rheumatoid arthritis (>1 hour).
- Examination of the involved joint shows restricted movement (due to capsular thickening and blocking by osteophyte), coarse crepitus on movement (due to rough articular surfaces), bony swelling (osteophyte) around joint margins, joint deformity, and joint-line tenderness.
- Muscle wasting is present around the involved joint.

- Generalized OA involves multiple joints. It initially starts at interphalangeal joints (IPJs) of fingers affecting distal interphalangeal joints (DIP) more than proximal interphalangeal joints (PIP). Affected joints develop posterolateral swellings on each side of the extensor tendon which enlarge and harden to become Heberden's (DIP) and Bouchard's (PIP) nodes.

Investigations

- Blood counts, ESR and CRP are normal.
- Plain X-ray: This shows reduced joint space, marginal osteophytes and joint deformities **(Fig. 10.1)**.
- Synovial fluid analysis: Predominantly viscous with low turbidity; calcium pyrophosphate crystals may be seen.

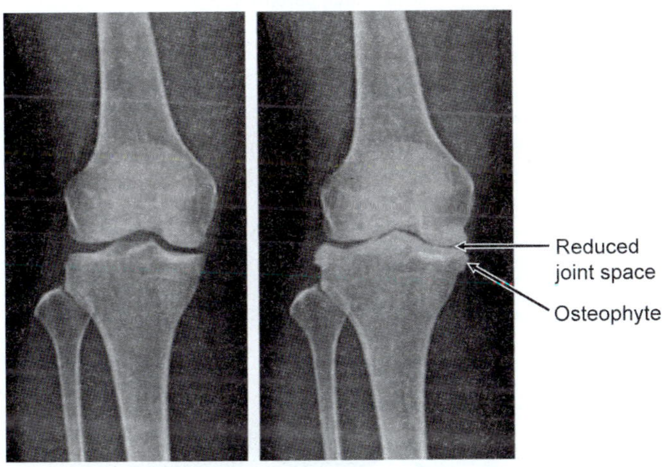

Figure 10.1: Normal knee (left) and osteoarthritis of knee (right)

Management

Nonpharmacologic Therapy

- Short periods of rest during acute pain.
- Reduction of risk factors: Weight loss if obese, pacing of activities, use of a walking stick for painful knee or hip OA, etc.
- Physiotherapy including muscle strengthening exercises.

Pharmacologic Therapy

- Analgesics: Paracetamol up to 4 g/day. Oral NSAIDs such as ibuprofen, diclofenac or aceclofenac, etc. can be used. Topical NSAIDs and capsaicin are also helpful in relieving the pain and inflammation.
- Steroids: Intra-articular injection of corticosteroid can be tried for severe pain.

Surgical Therapy

- Surgery is indicated if there is severe pain, progressive immobility and functional impairment in spite of conservative measures. Osteotomy (for mal-aligned joints), arthroscopic debridement, arthroplasty, joint replacement, etc. are options.

Q. Discuss the etiology, clinical features, investigations and management of rheumatoid arthritis.

Q. Systemic features of rheumatoid arthritis (or rheumatological diseases).

- Rheumatoid arthritis (RA) is a chronic autoimmune disease primarily involving joints. Its main feature is symmetric, peripheral polyarthritis.
- RA occurs all over the world. Highest prevalence is in Pima Indians of Arizona and lowest in black Africans and Chinese. It is more common in females.

Etiology

- The exact cause of RA is unknown. It is an autoimmune disease and is thought to result from the interaction between patients genotype and environment.
- RA might be a manifestation of the response to an infectious agent in a genetically susceptible host. A number of infectious agents have been suspected which include mycoplasma, Epstein-Barr virus (EBV), cytomegalovirus, parvovirus, and rubella virus.
- Evidence for genetic predisposition is suggested by higher incidence of RA in monozygotic twins than in dizygotic twins and increased frequency of disease in first-degree relatives of patients. The risk of developing rheumatoid arthritis has been associated with HLA-DR4 and HLA-DR1.
- Female gender and cigarette smoking are risk factors for the development of RA.
- Changes in the composition of intestinal bacteria have also been implicated in rheumatoid arthritis.

Pathogenesis/Pathology

- Autoimmunity is triggered by genetic and environmental factors (e.g. smoking, infection).
- Loss of self-tolerance → Activation of CD4+ T cells against self-antigens in synovium.
- The earliest change is swelling and congestion of the synovial membrane which becomes infiltrated with lymphocytes (CD4+ T cells), plasma cells and macrophages. These inflammatory cells release cytokines which stimulate the activation, proliferation and differentiation of B-cells into antibody-producing plasma cells. These plasma cells produce antibodies (rheumatoid factor, anti cyclic citrullinated peptide [anti-CCP]) which contribute to joint destruction.
- Inflammation of synovium leads to synovial hypertrophy and effusion of synovial fluid into the joint space leading to joint swelling. There is formation of inflammatory granulation tissue (pannus) which spreads over and under the articular cartilage, and damages it. Involved joint may develop fibrous or bony ankylosis **(Fig. 10.2)**.
- Muscles adjacent to inflamed joints atrophy and there may be focal infiltration with lymphocytes.
- Subcutaneous nodules consist of a central area of fibrinoid necrosis surrounded by radially arranged (palisade) mononuclear cells with strands of collagen.
- Rheumatoid vasculitis involves medium and small arteries and venules, with infiltration by lymphocytes.

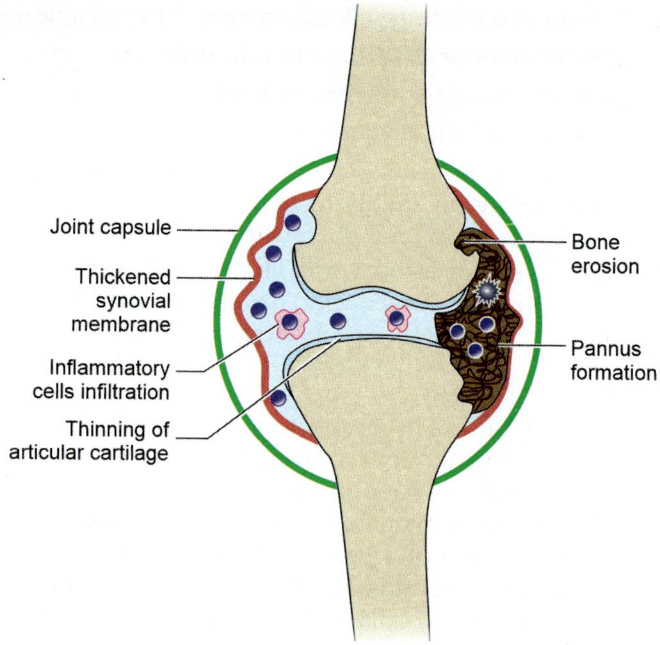

Figure 10.2: Pathology of RA

Clinical Features

Articular Features

- RA is more common in females. The peak age of onset is in the fourth decade in females and slightly later in males.
- The onset can be monoarticular, oligoarticular or polyarticular.
- The most common presentation is insidious onset of symmetric polyarthritis. The joints involved are wrist, metacarpophalangeal (MCP) joints, wrist, proximal interphalangeal (PIP) joints, elbow, shoulder, knee, ankle, and MTP joints. Wrists, and metacarpophalangeal joints of index and middle fingers are most commonly involved. The distal interphalangeal (DIP) joints of the fingers are usually spared. Symmetrical joint involvement is common in middle-aged women.
- Acute onset with asymmetrical polyarthritis is more often seen in elderly patients.
- Asymmetrical presentation becomes symmetrical as the disease progresses.
- In the palindromic-onset type, joints are affected and resolve completely within hours to days and recur after a period of time. This type may finally evolve into classical symmetrical polyarticular pattern.
- Predominant symptoms are stiffness, and swelling of involved joints.
- Morning stiffness is a common feature of RA and is defined as slowness or difficulty moving the joints when getting out of bed or after staying in one position too long. Stiffness usually lasts more than one hour.
- Deformities in long-stand RA **(Figs 10.3 to 10.5)**.
  - Swan neck deformity: Hyperextension of PIP, flexion of DIP
  - Boutonnière deformity: Flexion of PIP, hyperextension of DIP

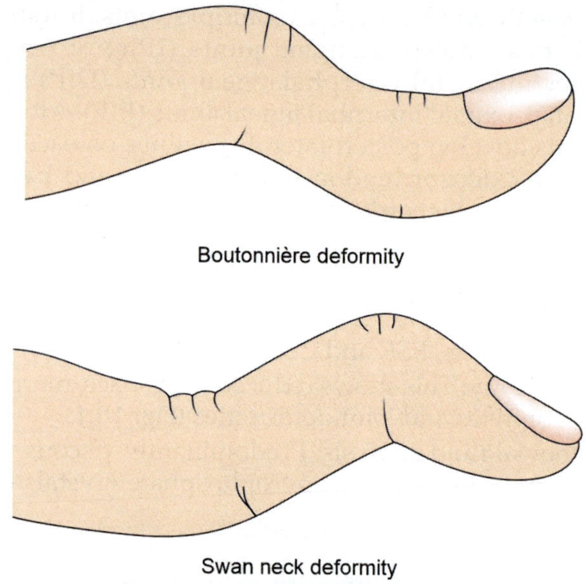

Figure 10.3: Deformities of fingers in RA

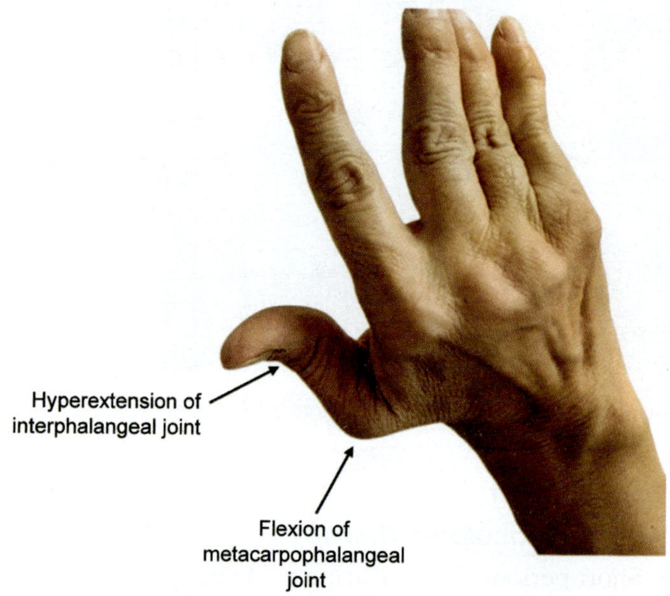

Figure 10.4: Z deformity of thumb

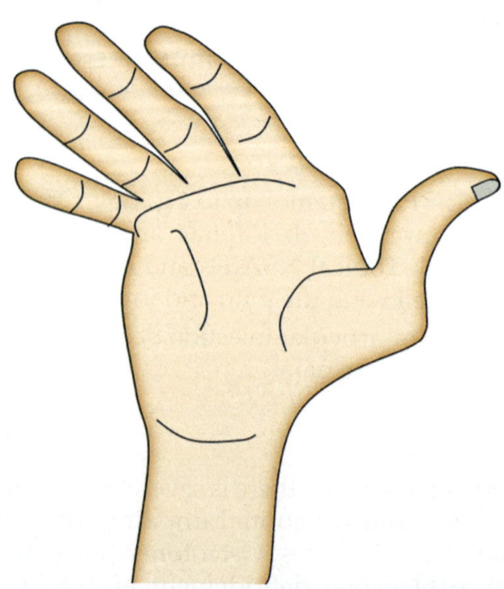

Figure 10.5: Ulnar deviation of fingers

- Z thumb: Flexion of MCP and hyperextension of IP joint
- Ulnar deviation of fingers
- Wrist subluxation
- Foot deformities: Hammer toes, hallux valgus.

Extra-articular Features (systemic features)

Constitutional symptoms

- Low grade fever, weight loss, loss of appetite, and fatigue.

Musculoskeletal

- Muscle wasting, bursitis, tenosynovitis and osteoporosis. Osteoporosis and muscle-wasting result from systemic inflammation.

Skin

- Rheumatoid nodules—are subcutaneous nodules seen in 25% of patients with RA. They are firm, round masses and vary in size. They are seen over the pressure points like the olecranon process, scapula, sacrum, Achilles tendon and the occiput. Visceral structures like heart, lungs and CNS may also be involved. Most skin nodules do not require any treatment. For painful nodules or those that interfere with joint motion or impinge upon nerves, local injection with a mixture of a steroid and local anesthetic may cause regression.
- Other skin manifestations are ulcers, vasculitis, gangrene and pyoderma gangrenosum.

Eye

- Episcleritis, scleritis.

Respiratory

- Pleural effusion is usually bilateral with low pleural fluid glucose.
- Interstitial lung disease.
- Caplan's syndrome—is a combination of rheumatoid arthritis and pneumoconiosis which manifests as multiple nodules in the lungs and interstitial lung disease. This is seen in coal miners.

Cardiac

- Pericarditis, myocarditis, and endocarditis
- Coronary vasculitis—can lead to myocardial infarction
- Aortitis/aortic regurgitation
- Conduction disturbances including complete heart block.

Hematological/reticuloendothelial

- Normocytic normochromic anemia
- Thrombocytosis
- Eosinophilia
- Splenomegaly (Felty's syndrome)

Neurological

- Compression neuropathies—are due to compression of peripheral nerves by hypertrophied synovium or joint subluxation, e.g. carpal and tarsal tunnel syndromes.
- Cervical cord compression—due to subluxation of atlantoaxial joint or at a subaxial level.
- Peripheral neuropathy
- Mononeuritis multiplex.

Others

- Systemic vasculitis (skin, CNS, lungs, etc.)
- Amyloidosis is a rare complication of chronic active disease and usually presents with nephrotic syndrome.

Diagnosis of Rheumatoid Arthritis

- Diagnosis should be suspected in any patient who presents with chronic symmetric polyarthritis. American College of Rheumatology (ACR) and the European League against Rheumatism (EULAR) criteria for the classification of rheumatoid arthritis is as follows (**Table 10.1**).

TABLE 10.1: Diagnostic criteria for rheumatoid arthritis

Feature	Score
Joint involvement	
• 1 large joint (shoulder, elbow, hip, knee, ankle)	0
• 2–10 large joints	1
• 1–3 small joints (MCP, PIP, thumb IP, MTP, wrists)	2
• 4–10 small joints	3
• >10 joints (at least 1 small joint)	5
Serology	
• Negative RF (rheumatoid factor) and negative anti-CCP (anti-citrullinated protein antibody)	0
• Low-positive RF or low-positive anti-CCP antibodies (3 times ULN)	2
• High-positive RF or high-positive anti-CCP antibodies (>3 times ULN)	3
Acute-phase reactants	
• Normal CRP and normal ESR	0
• Abnormal CRP or abnormal ESR	1
Duration of symptoms	
• <6 weeks	0
• ≥6 weeks	1

- A total score ≥6/10 is classified as definite RA.
- These criteria are meant for classification, not strict diagnosis, and should be applied only in patients with at least 1 joint with clinical synovitis (swelling), not explained by another disease.
- Ultimately RA is a clinical diagnosis. The above criteria has many caveats and hence should be used only as a guideline to help the diagnosis of RA.

Investigations

- Complete blood count: Anemia of chronic disease (normocytic, normochromic anemia).
- ESR and CRP are elevated.
- Rheumatoid factor is present in more than 80% of cases.
- Anticitrullinated peptide (anti-CCP) antibody: This is more specific (~95%) than rheumatoid factor for the diagnosis of RA.
- Antinuclear antibodies (ANA) may be positive but nonspecific.
- X-rays—of the hands, wrists and both feet show periarticular osteopenia and marginal erosions. Bone

erosions may not be seen initially up to 6 months. Deformities in advanced cases (e.g. ulnar deviation, subluxation).

- Ultrasound (musculoskeletal): Detects early synovitis and joint effusions. Power Doppler detects active inflammation.
- MRI: More sensitive than X-ray. Detects bone marrow edema, early erosions, synovitis.
- Synovial fluid analysis–Done in monoarthritis to rule out other causes like septic arthritis and gout. Usually shows a white cell count of 5000–20,000/mm^3, with predominant neutrophils. Synovial fluid glucose is usually normal, but may be low.

Management

- The goals of treatment are (1) relief of pain, (2) reduction of inflammation, (3) protection of articular structures, (4) maintenance of function, and (5) control of systemic involvement.

Pharmacologic Therapy

Analgesics (symptomatic relief only)

- Acetaminophen (paracetamol), and NSAIDs (diclofenac, ibuprofen, aceclofenac) have both analgesic and anti-inflammatory properties but do not alter disease outcomes. Opioid analgesics such as propoxyphene, tramadol, oxycodone, etc. are also useful to control pain. Topical analgesic preparations (e.g. capsaicin or diclofenac) can be combined along with oral agents.

Steroids

- Examples are prednisolone, triamcinolone, etc. these are used to suppress inflammation, and may be administered orally, intravenously, or by intra-articular injection. Prednisolone 7.5 mg/day or less is relatively safe and can be used for extended periods of time. Doses higher than 7.5 mg/day should be used for the shortest time possible. Steroids are especially useful during initial control of the disease and during flare ups.

Disease-modifying antirheumatic drugs (DMARDs)

- These are slow-acting anti-rheumatic drugs. They can reduce or prevent joint damage, preserve joint integrity and function, and maintain economic productivity. These include hydroxychloroquine, sulfasalazine, methotrexate, and leflunomide. Out of these, methotrexate and hydroxychloroquine are commonly used. Other less commonly used DMARDs are gold salts, D-penicillamine, azathioprine, and cyclosporine.
- Methotrexate is given once a week in a dose of 7.5–25 mg per week. Folic acid should be given along with methotrexate to prevent hematological side effect. Hydroxychloroquine is given at a dose of 200–400 mg daily. Sulfasalazine is given at a dose of 1 g twice daily.

Biologic agents

- These are biologic response modifiers and have immunosuppressive effect.
- These are anti-TNF (tumor necrosis factor) agents such as adalimumab, etanercept, and infliximab. Other biologic agents are tocilizumab (interleukin-6 inhibitor), abatacept (inhibits T-cell costimulation), and rituximab (anti-B cell).

Immunosuppressive agents

- Examples are azathioprine and cyclophosphamide. These are 3rd line agents and are rarely used. They have serious side effects. IV cyclophosphamide may be life saving in acute vasculitis causing organ damage.

Nonpharmacological Measures

- Patient education and counseling: Patient should be explained about the chronic nature of disease and the need for long-term therapy. The side effects of drugs should be explained and the need for follow up stressed.
- Rest: This helps during acute arthritis and during flare ups.
- Exercise: Lack of exercise can result in loss of joint mobility, contractures, and muscle atrophy. Patients should exercise regularly to prevent and reverse these problems.
- Physiotherapy: This involves application of heat or cold to relieve pain or stiffness, ultrasound to tenosynovitis, passive and active exercises to improve and maintain joint motion range.

Surgery

- Synovectomy of the wrist or finger tendon sheaths may be required for pain relief or to prevent tendon rupture when medical therapy fails.
- Osteotomy, arthrodesis or arthroplasties may be required in advanced disease when joint destruction and deformities take place.

Q. Felty syndrome.

- Felty syndrome refers to severe rheumatoid arthritis (RA) complicated by neutropenia and splenomegaly. Although the pathophysiology of Felty syndrome is not fully understood, evidence points to splenic sequestration and subsequent neutrophil destruction.

Clinical Features

- Felty syndrome is characterized by rheumatoid arthritis, neutropenia, and splenomegaly.
- More common in middle-aged to elderly women.
- Usually associated with severe, long-standing RA (>10 years).
- Both articular and extra-articular features of rheumatoid arthritis are more severe in Felty syndrome.
- Neutropenia (neutrophil count <2000/mm^3) predisposes to recurrent bacterial infections. Respiratory tract and skin infections due to bacteria are most common.
- Splenomegaly can be detected clinically in most patients and sometimes can be massive.

Investigations

- Low neutrophil count (<2000/mm^3) is required for the diagnosis of Felty syndrome.

- Peripheral blood smear to rule out any other hematological abnormality.
- Bone marrow shows myeloid hyperplasia with a relative excess of immature forms.
- Ultrasound abdomen may be required to demonstrate splenomegaly.
- Strongly seropositive for RF and anti-CCP antibodies.

Management

- Treatment is generally same as for rheumatoid arthritis.
- Granulocyte colony stimulating factor (G-CSF) may be required to rapidly reverse neutropenia in patients with life-threatening or refractory bacterial infection.
- Splenectomy is required for severe persistent neutropenia and severe thrombocytopenia due to hypersplenism.

Q. Rheumatoid factor (RF).

- Rheumatoid factor (RF) is an antibody directed against the Fc portion of IgG.
- RF is usually of IgM class, although IgG and IgA are also seen rarely.
- RF was first identified in patients with rheumatoid arthritis but also occurs in other conditions and in some normal adults.
- It has more sensitivity than specificity in the diagnosis of rheumatoid arthritis. Its principal use is as a prognostic marker; a high titer at presentation associates with a poorer prognosis.

Diseases Associated with RF Positivity

Autoimmune diseases
- Rheumatoid arthritis
- Sjögren's syndrome
- Mixed connective tissue disease
- SLE
- Polymyositis/dermatomyositis

Nonrheumatic disorders
- Chronic infections (subacute bacterial endocarditis, hepatitis B or C virus infection)
- Sarcoidosis
- Malignancy
- Primary biliary cirrhosis.

Healthy individuals
- RF can be positive in up to four percent of healthy individuals.

Prognostic Value in RA

High RF titers are associated with:
- More severe joint disease
- Extra-articular manifestations (e.g. rheumatoid nodules, vasculitis, Felty syndrome)
- Radiographic joint erosions
- Worse prognosis.

Limitations

- False-positives: In infections, liver disease, elderly
- False-negatives: ~20–30% of RA patients may be seronegative.
- Not useful alone; must be interpreted with clinical findings and other markers (e.g. anti-CCP, ESR, CRP).

Q. Anticyclic citruillinated peptide (anti-CCP) antibody.

- Anti-CCP antibody is an autoantibody directed against citrullinated proteins. Citrullinated peptide is found in the keratin and synovium. It is IgG class autoantibody.
- Anti-CCP antibodies are helpful in the diagnosis of rheumatoid arthritis. Anti CCP antibodies are more specific but less sensitive than rheumatoid factor in the diagnosis of RA. It has a sensitivity of around 60% and specificity of around 95% for RA. Testing for both rheumatoid factor and anti-CCP is more useful in the diagnosis of RA than either of the tests alone. Anti-CCP is especially useful in early diagnosis of RA when classic features are not present.
- High titers are associated with: More severe disease, early erosive changes on imaging, extra-articular manifestations, greater risk of joint destruction, and poorer long-term outcome.
- Anti-CCP antibody may also be positive in other conditions such as active tuberculosis, SLE, Sjögren's, polymyositis, dermatomyositis, and scleroderma. However, titers are less in these conditions than in RA.

Q. What is spondyloarthritis (seronegative spondyloarthropathies)? Discuss the pathology and general features of spondyloarthritis.

- The term, spondyloarthritis (formerly spondyloarthropathy), is used to refer to a group of inflammatory joint diseases sharing similar pathogenesis, distinct from rheumatoid arthritis. They usually involve both spine and peripheral joints (*spondylo* means spine and *arthro* means joints).
- They have overlapping articular and extra-articular features.
- They have strong association with HLA-B27.
- Rheumatoid factor (RF) and anti-CCP are negative. Hence, they are also known as seronegative spondyloarthropathies.
- They are:
  - Ankylosing spondylitis (AS)
  - Reactive arthritis (ReA) including Reiter's syndrome
  - Psoriatic arthritis
  - Enteropathic arthritis (associated with inflammatory bowel disease (IBD))
  - Undifferentiated spondyloarthritis
- *Mnemonic to Remember the Seronegative Spondyloarthropathies "PEAR"*
  - *P–Psoriatic arthritis*
  - *E–Enteropathic arthritis*
  - *A–Ankylosing spondylitis*
  - *R–Reactive arthritis*

Pathology

- Strong association with HLA-B27. HLA-B27 misfolds in the endoplasmic reticulum (ER), causing ER stress and unfolded protein response (UPR) → Leads to activation of T-cells and production of proinflammatory cytokines like TNF-α, IL-17, and IL-23.
- In addition to synovitis, there is prominent extra-synovial inflammation involving tendon insertion sites (enthesitis), joint capsule, periarticular periosteum, cartilage and subchondral bone.
- Inflammation at entheses leads to erosion followed by abnormal bone formation (ankylosis).
- In contrast to RA, bone formation (not erosion) is more prominent.
- The inflammation resolves leaving behind fibrosis which may calcify and ossify leading to joint fusion. In the spine, periarticular osteitis and periostitis may result in bony spurs that bridge adjacent vertebral bodies (syndesmophytes) or protrude at sites of ligament attachment (e.g. calcaneal or olecranon 'spurs').
- Large central cartilaginous joints (sacroiliac, intervertebral, symphysis pubis) are particularly involved.
- Microbial infections may trigger spondyloarthritis in genetically predisposed individuals (as happens in reactive arthritis after UTI). This is due to molecular mimicry, i.e. microbial antigens mimic self-antigens leading to autoimmunity.

Clinical Features Common to Seronegative Spondyloarthritis

- Asymmetrical inflammatory oligoarthritis (lower limb >upper limb)
- Involvement of spine (spondylitis) and sacroiliac joints
- Inflammation at tendon or ligament insertion sites (enthesitis)
- Strong association with HLA-B27 and tendency for familial aggregation
- Rheumatoid factor is usually negative

Extra-articular features

- Inflammation of mucosal surface: Conjunctivitis, buccal ulceration, urethritis, prostatitis, bowel ulceration
- Inflammation in the eyes—uveitis
- Pustular skin lesions, nail dystrophy
- Aortic root fibrosis (aortic incompetence, conduction defects)
- Erythema nodosum

Q. Discuss the etiology, clinical features, investigations and management of ankylosing spondylitis.

- Ankylosing spondylitis (AS) is a chronic, systemic inflammatory arthritis that primarily affects the axial skeleton, especially the sacroiliac joints and spine, leading to progressive spinal fusion (ankylosis).
- Ankylosis refers to a fibrous or bony bridging of joints. In the spine this includes bridging of one or more intervertebral discs.

Etiology

- Exact etiology is unknown.
- Genetic factors: Most patients are HLA-B27 positive (~90–95% of patients). Close relatives of patients with AS have increased risk of developing AS.
- Infections: Increased fecal carriage of *Klebsiella aerogenes* occurs in patients with ankylosing spondylitis.
- Immunologic mechanisms: There is overactivation of Th17 cells, increased cytokines, leading to inflammation of entheses and adjacent bone → aberrant new bone formation (syndesmophytes) and spinal ankylosis.

Clinical Features

- It characteristically affects young adults with a peak age of onset between 20 and 30 years.
- Males are more commonly affected (male: female ratio 3:1).

Articular Features

- Spine (mainly lumbosacral) and sacroiliac joints are commonly affected.
- Insidious onset of low back pain and stiffness. Pain and stiffness are worse in the morning and after inactivity and are relieved by movement. Lumbosacral area is usually the first and worst affected region, but rarely thoracic or cervical spine can get affected first.
- As the disease progresses, whole spine is affected. As the spine becomes progressively ankylosed, spinal rigidity and secondary osteoporosis predispose to spinal fracture, presenting as acute, severe, well-localized pain. Secondary spinal cord compression is a rare complication.
- Examination shows restricted spinal mobility in all directions, pain on sacroiliac compression, and diminished chest expansion. Increasing flexion of the neck, increased thoracic kyphosis and loss of normal lumbar lordosis may lead to a stooped posture **(Fig. 10.6)**.
- Peripheral arthritis is seen in 30% of patients. Hips, knees, ankles and shoulders are mainly involved. Peripheral arthritis may precede spinal involvement in 10% of cases.

Extra-articular Features

- Enthesitis–inflammation at tendon or ligament insertion sites (Achilles tendon, iliac crest and greater trochanter)
- Eye—anterior uveitis, conjunctivitis (20%)
- Prostatitis (80% men)
- CVS—aortic regurgitation, pericarditis, MVP
- RS—upper lobe fibrosis
- CNS—cervical myelopathy (secondary to atlantoaxial dislocation), cauda equina syndrome
- Kidneys—IgA nephropathy, secondary amyloidosis
- GIT—mucosal ulcers.

Investigations

- ↑ ESR and CRP
- Rheumatoid factor is negative or present in low titer
- HLA B_{27} is usually positive

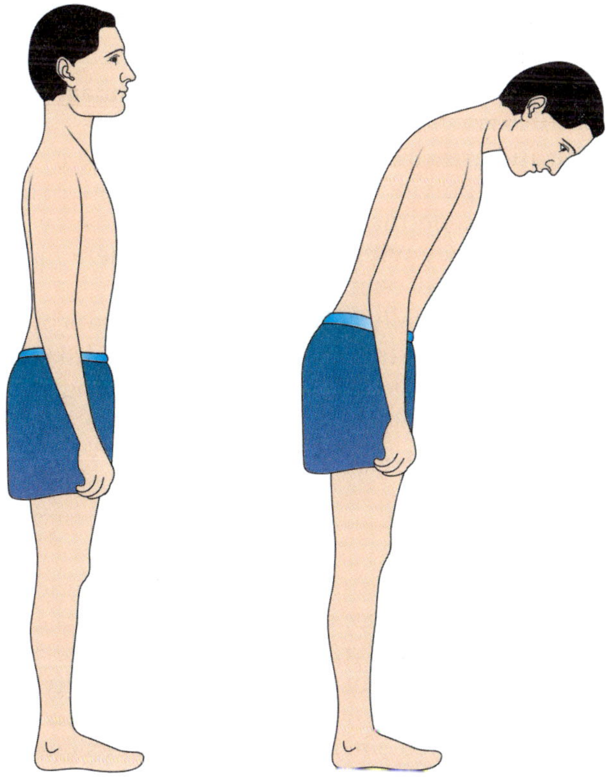

Figure 10.6: Normal posture (left) and stooped posture in AS (right)

- Radiographs: Sacroiliac joint is usually first involved. X-ray of sacroiliac joint may show irregularity and loss of cortical margins, widening of the joint space, sclerosis, narrowing and fusion. Lateral thoracolumbar spine X-ray may show anterior 'squaring' of vertebrae due to erosion and sclerosis of the anterior corners, bridging syndesmophytes, ossification of the anterior longitudinal ligament and facet joint fusion. All these changes produce the typical **'bamboo spine' (Fig. 10.7)**. Erosive changes may be seen in the symphysis pubis, the ischial tuberosities and peripheral joints. Osteoporosis and atlantoaxial dislocation can occur.
- MRI (Sacroiliac joints): Detects early sacroiliitis before X-ray changes. Bone marrow edema and active inflammation.

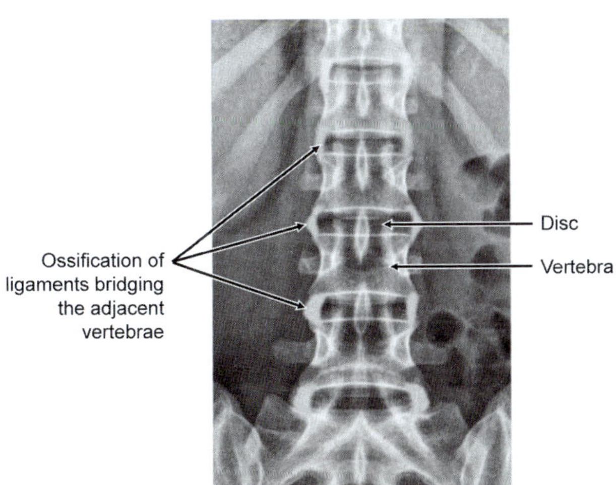

Figure 10.7: Bamboo spine in AS

Management

- The goals of treatment are to relieve pain and stiffness, maintain skeletal mobility and prevent deformity.

Nonpharmacological Measures

- Education of the patient about the disease
- Regular daily back extension exercises, including a morning 'warm-up' routine
- Avoid prolonged periods of inactivity
- Poor bed and chair posture must be avoided
- Smoking cessation.

Drug Therapy

- *NSAIDs* relieve the symptoms but do not alter the course of the disease.
- A long-acting NSAID at night is particularly helpful for marked morning stiffness.
- *Anti-rheumatic drugs*—sulfasalazine, methotrexate or azathioprine may control peripheral arthritis but have little effect on spine inflammation.
- *Anti-TNF agents*—etanercept, infliximab, and adalimumab have been shown to improve signs and symptoms of AS, including spinal mobility.
- *IL-17 inhibitors*—secukinumab, ixekizumab (especially in TNF-failure).
- *Steroids*—local corticosteroid injections are helpful in persistent plantar fasciitis and enthesitis. Oral steroids are useful in acute uveitis but should otherwise be avoided.

Surgery

- Severe hip, knee or shoulder restriction may require surgery. Total hip replacement (total hip arthroplasty), cervical fusion for atlantoaxial subluxation, and wedge osteotomy for severe flexion deformities of the spine are the surgical procedures that may be required.

Q. Discuss the etiology, clinical features, investigations, and management of reactive arthritis.

Q. Reiter syndrome.

- The term "reactive arthritis" refers to aseptic arthritis that is associated with a recent or coexisting extra-articular infection usually gastrointestinal or genitourinary infections.
- Reiter syndrome refers to the triad of reactive arthritis, urethritis, and conjunctivitis.

Etiology

- *Gastrointestinal infections*: Salmonella, shigella, Campylobacter and Yersinia.
- *Genitourinary infections:* Chlamydia (most common), *N. gonorrhea*.
- *Genetic predisposition:* Strong association with HLA-B27 (seen in ~60–80% cases).

Pathogenesis

- Bacterial antigens which mimic self antigens may persist in synovial fluid or tissue, even though the organism is no longer viable. This causes T-cell–mediated autoimmune attack on joint tissues in genetically predisposed individuals.

- Note that there are no viable bacteria in the joints, hence it is not an infection, it is only reactive inflammation to bacterial antigens.

Clinical Features

- Reactive arthritis commonly affects young men aged <40 years. However, it may occur at any age.
- Presentation is usually acute onset oligoarthritis predominantly affecting the large of the lower limbs (knees, ankles) 1–3 weeks following UTI or an attack of dysentery. Symptoms and signs of urethritis or conjunctivitis may be minimal or absent and there may be no clear history of prior dysentery.
- Extra-articular features are Achilles tendonitis, plantar fasciitis, circinate balanitis, keratoderma blennorrhagica, nail dystrophy and buccal ulcers. Circinate balanitis is superficial erosions in a circular pattern on the coronal margin of the glans penis. Keratoderma blennorrhagica are hyperkeratotic skin lesions with desquamating margins.
- Systemic features like fever, fatigue and weight loss can occur.

Investigations

- ESR and CRP are raised
- Normocytic, normochromic anemia
- Urine culture may grow *N. gonorrhea* or Chlamydia.
- Stool culture—may grow the causative organism but are usually negative by the time arthritis develops.
- Serologic testing—detection of antibodies against the organism may help confirm previous dysentery.
- Rheumatoid factor and ANA are negative.
- Radiographic features: Initially there are no changes. With chronic disease, periarticular osteopenia, joint space narrowing and marginal proliferative erosions may develop. Periostitis, especially of metatarsals, phalanges and pelvis, and large 'fluffy' calcaneal spurs may be seen. Asymmetrical or unilateral sacroileitis and syndesmophytes can occur.
- Synovial fluid analysis—shows features of inflammation such as low viscosity, turbid appearance and presence of giant macrophages (Reiter's cells).

Management

- NSAIDs—control the pain and inflammation of arthritis.
- Steroids—intra-articular or local corticosteroid injections are helpful in relieving the symptoms of arthritis or enthesitis. Systemic steroids are used for anterior uveitis.
- Antirheumatic drugs—sulfasalazine has been shown to be effective in reactive arthritis. Azathioprine or methotrexate may be required in severe progressive arthritis and intractable keratoderma blennorrhagica.
- Antibiotics—are used to treat acute infection. Chlamydial urethritis is treated with doxycycline.

Q. Discuss the clinical features, diagnosis, and management of psoriatic arthritis.

- Psoriatic arthritis (PsA) is a seronegative inflammatory arthritis associated with psoriasis.
- Psoriatic arthritis usually occurs in patients with current or previous skin psoriasis. In some patients it may precede the onset of psoriasis or may start simultaneously with psoriasis. Rarely there may be arthritis without skin lesions.
- The onset is usually between 25 and 40 years of age.
- The exact cause of psoriatic arthritis is unknown. However, genetic (HLA-B27), immunologic, and environmental factors all play a role in the causation of the disease.

Clinical Features

Articular Features

- Psoriatic arthritis usually presents as asymmetrical oligoarthritis. Both upper and lower limb joints can be affected. The distal interphalangeal (DIP) joints of fingers and toes are especially affected. Hand deformity often results from tenosynovitis and soft tissue contractures. Knees are affected often with very large effusions.

Extra-articular Features

- Enthesitis—affects Achilles tendon, plantar fascia and the pelvic bones.
- Tenosynovitis—affects the flexor tendons of the hands, the extensor carpi ulnaris, or other sites.
- Dactylitis (sausage digits): Dactylitis is uniform diffuse swelling of an entire finger or toe giving it a sausage-like appearance **(Fig. 10.8)**. It is due to inflammation of the soft tissues of the digits, synovium, and tendons. Dactylitis is a key diagnostic clue in PsA and other spondyloarthropathies.
- Skin lesions—plaques with silvery white scales.
- Nail changes—include pitting, onycholysis, nailbed hyperkeratosis, and splinter hemorrhages.
- Eyes—conjunctivitis and uveitis.

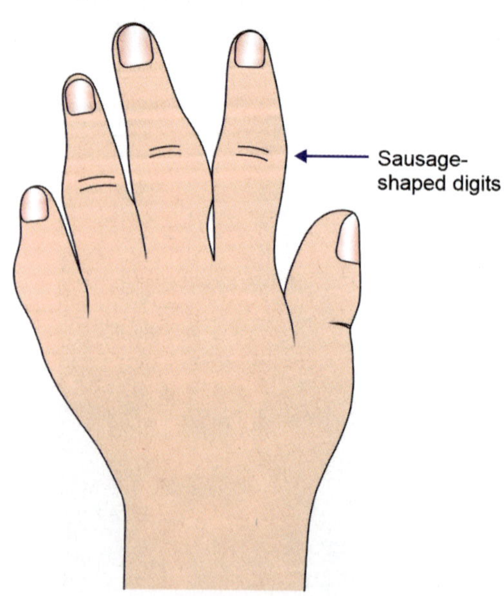

Figure 10.8: Dactylitis (sausage shaped digits)

Investigations

- ESR and CRP are elevated.
- Rheumatoid factor and ANA are usually negative.
- X-rays may be normal or show erosive changes with new bone formation in the distal joints.
- MRI is more sensitive than plain X-rays in detecting articular, periarticular, and soft-tissue inflammation.

Management

- *General measures:* Regular exercise and attention to posture should be prescribed as in those with spondylitis. Splints and prolonged rest are avoided because of the increased tendency to fibrous and bony ankylosis.
- *NSAIDs:* These are first choice and help in pain relief and control inflammation.
- *Second line drugs:* These are indicated for persistent arthritis. Examples are sulfasalazine methotrexate or azathioprine. Antimalarial agents such as hydroxychloroquine should be avoided because it can exacerbate psoriatic skin lesions.
- *Surgery:* It may be required for severe joint destruction causing immobility.

Q. Inflammatory bowel disease (IBD)-associated arthritis (enteropathic arthritis).

- IBD-associated arthritis refers to the arthropathies associated with Crohn's disease or ulcerative colitis.
- It is an acute inflammatory oligoarthritis mainly involving large lower limb joints (i.e. knees, ankles, hips) but upper limb joints such as wrists, elbows and small joints of the fingers and toes can also be involved. Sacroiliac and spinal joint involvement is rare.
- Onset of arthritis may coincide with exacerbations of inflammatory bowel disease.

Treatment

- NSAIDs
- Sulfasalazine
- Azathioprine and methotrexate in refractory cases.

Q. Enumerate the crystal induced arthropathies.

Q. Discuss the etiology, clinical features, investigations and management of gout.

- Crystal-induced arthropathies are joint diseases caused by the deposition of crystals in the joints or periarticular tissues, leading to inflammation.
- These are as follows:

- Gout: due to uric acid
- Pseudogout: due to calcium pyrophosphate
- Acute arthritis in dialysis patients: calcium oxalate

Gout

- Gout is a crystal-induced inflammatory arthritis caused by deposition of monosodium urate (MSU) crystals in joints and tissues due to hyperuricemia.

Etiology

- It occurs due to hyperuricemia (normal value less than 7 mg/dl). Causes of hyperuricemia are as follows:

Increased Intake
- Intake of purine-rich foods (e.g. liver, kidney, meat, mushrooms)
- Beer is particularly rich in guanosine, a purine nucleoside.

Increased production
- Hypoxanthine-guanine phosphoribosyltransferase (HGPRT) deficiency
- Phosphoribosylpyrophosphate (PRPP) synthetase overactivity
- Glucose-6-phosphatase deficiency (glycogen storage disease, type I)
- Increased nucleoprotein turnover in hematologic conditions: Lymphoma, leukemia, hemolytic anemia
- Increased rates of cellular proliferation and cell death: Psoriasis, cancer chemotherapy, radiation therapy, malignancies
- Obesity

Decreased renal excretion (most common cause of hyperuricemia)
- Inherited isolated renal tubular defect ('under-excretors')
- Renal failure
- Lead poisoning
- Diabetic ketoacidosis
- Lactic acidosis
- Hypothyroidism
- Drugs (thiazides, pyrazinamide, cyclosporine)

Epidemiology

- Gout is more common in males (male:female ratio >10:1). Prevalence increases with age and increasing serum uric acid concentration.

Clinical Features

Gout can present in the following ways:
1. Acute gouty arthritis
2. Chronic tophaceous gout.

Acute gout

The typical attack of acute gouty arthritis, includes the following clinical features:
- Usually involves single distal joint. Most commonly involved joint is base of the great toe (first metatarsophalangeal joint, known as podagra), or the knee. Other common sites (in order of decreasing frequency) are the ankle, midfoot, knee, small joints of hands, wrist and elbow. Spine and large proximal joints are rarely involved and never as the first site.
- Onset of arthritis is sudden and there is severe pain, redness, and swelling of the affected joints. Complete resolution occurs within a few days to several weeks.
- There may be periarticular swelling and erythema, accompanying fever, malaise and even confusion, especially if a large joint such as the knee is involved. As the attack subsides, pruritus and desquamation of overlying skin are common.
- Acute attacks may also manifest as bursitis, tenosynovitis or cellulitis.

Chronic tophaceous gout

- Tophaceous gout is characterized by collections of solid urate in connective tissues (which may be calcified).

- These collections produce irregular firm nodules ('tophi') at the usual sites for nodules around extensor surfaces of fingers, hands, forearm, elbows, Achilles tendons and sometimes the helix of the ear. They may be clinically visible or detected by imaging.
- Tophi are usually painless and nontender. Large tophi may ulcerate, discharging white gritty material.

Renal and urinary tract manifestations

- Uric acid stones may form and cause renal colic.
- Urate crystal deposition in the interstitium of the medulla and pyramids leads to chronic inflammation, fibrosis, glomerulosclerosis and secondary pyelonephritis.

Investigations

- Polarizing microscopy—definitive diagnosis requires identification of needle-shaped, negatively birefringent monosodium urate crystals in the aspirate from a joint, bursa or tophus.
- Histologic examination—birefringent urate crystals may be visible in biopsy specimens.
- Uric acid levels in the blood—are elevated (>7 mg/dl). However occasionally it can be normal (<7 mg/dl).
- 24-hour urinary uric acid excretion—can identify uric acid over-producers.
- Urea, creatinine should be measured to rule out renal dysfunction.
- Complete blood picture, ESR and peripheral blood smear should be done to rule out any myeloproliferative disorders.
- X-rays—can assess the degree of joint damage. In early disease they are usually normal, but in advanced disease, narrowing of joint space, sclerosis, cysts and osteophyte (changes of OA) may develop (rat bite erosions with overhanging edges). Calcified tophi may be visible on X-rays.

Management

Acute attack

- Oral NSAID (e.g. naproxen, diclofenac, indomethacin) can give effective pain relief and is the standard treatment.
- Oral colchicine is effective in acute attacks but can cause vomiting and diarrhea.
- Steroids, either oral or intra-articular can give rapid relief. Can be used if symptoms are very severe.
- Aspiration of the joint gives instant relief and, when combined with an intra-articular corticosteroid injection effectively aborts the attack.
- Note that allopurinol and uricosuric drugs should not be given during acute attack because they can worsen the attack.

Long-term management

- Lifestyle changes: Correct obesity and reduce alcohol consumption. Avoid high purine diet (seafood, red meat and offal). Stop diuretics if possible.
- Hypouricemic drugs: These drugs are started after the acute attack subsides. Indications are ≥2 attacks/year, tophaceous gout, chronic kidney disease, and uric acid stones.
- *Allopurinol* inhibits xanthine oxidase and reduces conversion of hypoxanthine and xanthine to uric acid. Dosage is 100–300 mg daily. The sharp reduction in tissue uric acid levels after allopurinol therapy can dissolve monosodium urate crystals and trigger acute attacks. This risk can be minimized by starting at low dose (100 mg). Since it can exacerbate acute attacks, it should be withheld till the acute attack subsides. *Febuxostat,* is a new drug and is a nonpurine selective inhibitor of xanthine oxidase. Febuxostat is given orally and is metabolized mainly in the liver. In contrast, allopurinol and its metabolites are excreted primarily by the kidney. Therefore, febuxostat can be used in patients with renal impairment with no dosage adjustment.
- The goal of treatment is to reduce serum uric acid level to lower half of normal range. In most cases allopurinol will need to be continued indefinitely.
- Uricosuric drugs such as probenecid or sulfinpyrazone also have equal efficacy to allopurinol but require more frequent dosing. Uricosurics are contraindicated in over-producers (they already have gross uricosuria), those with renal impairment (ineffective), and in patients with urolithiasis (increased stone formation).
- Pegloticase is a pegylated form of recombinant uricase an enzyme that converts urate to allantoin, which is more soluble. Pegloticase is used in patients with gout in whom other treatments have been unsuccessful in lowering the serum urate level.
- Asymptomatic hyperuricemia need not be treated unless the levels are very high (>10 mg/dl) or there is strong family history of gout or urolithiasis.

Q. Calcium pyrophosphate arthritis (pseudo gout; chondrocalcinosis).

- Pseudogout is a crystal-induced arthropathy caused by the deposition of calcium pyrophosphate dihydrate (CPPD) crystals in the joints.
- The term "pseudogout" is commonly used because the symptoms of the disorder are very similar to those caused by gout but not due to gout. Chondrocalcinosis refers to crystal deposition in hyaline and/or fibrocartilage without signs of arthritis.
- Pseudogout is most common in the elderly (>60 years). The knee (hyaline cartilage and menisci) is the most commonly affected site, followed by the wrist and pelvis.

Etiology

- The exact cause of crystal formation is not clear. The crystals first develop in the joint cartilage and eventually move to synovium and joint fluid where they cause inflammation. This causes pain and swelling.
- Frequent association with joint trauma (including surgery), hypomagnesemia, hyperparathyroidism, gout, hemochromatosis, and old age, suggests that calcium pyrophosphate crystal deposits are secondary to degenerative or metabolic changes in the affected tissues. Some cases are familial.

- Recent studies indicate that the ankyrin protein plays a major role in increased CPPD crystal formation.

Clinical Features

- Patients present with acute monoarthritis. Acute attack resembles acute gout and is characterized by severe pain, stiffness and swelling of affected joint. Knee is the commonest site, followed by wrist, shoulder, ankle and elbow. Some patients may develop chronic arthritis, early morning stiffness, and functional impairment. Acute attacks may be superimposed on chronic arthritis.
- Joint trauma, intercurrent illness or surgery may trigger an acute attack of pseudogout.
- Pseudogout should be differentiated from acute gouty arthritis and septic arthritis.

Investigations

- Demonstration of CPPD crystals in synovial fluid.
- X-rays may show chondrocalcinosis.
- Screening for metabolic or familial causes should be done in young patients.

Management

- Aspiration of joint effusion quickly reduces pain and may alone be sufficient.
- Intra-articular injection of corticosteroid
- Oral NSAIDs and colchicine.

Q. Approach to a case of joint pain.

Approach to a case of joint pain involves the following components:

- Duration of joint pain
- Is it articular (joint) pain or non-articular pain (e.g. ligaments, muscles)?
- Inflammatory *vs.* non-inflammatory
- Mono *vs.* oligo *vs.* polyarticular
- Pattern and distribution
- Determine pathophysiologic cause
- Investigations
- Management.

Duration of Joint Pain

Joint pain can be classified based on duration into acute, subacute, and chronic, which helps guide diagnosis and management.

- Acute: <6 weeks
- Subacute: 6–12 weeks
- Chronic: >12 weeks.

Acute Causes of Joint Pain (<6 weeks)

- These often present suddenly with redness, warmth, swelling, and severe pain.
- ***Infectious:*** Septic arthritis (bacterial/fungal), viral arthritis (parvovirus B19, chikungunya, Hepatitis B/C), reactive arthritis (post-enteric or urogenital infection).
- ***Crystal-induced:*** Gout (monosodium urate), pseudogout (calcium pyrophosphate deposition)
- ***Trauma-related:*** Ligament injuries, meniscal tear, hemarthrosis (e.g. hemophilia).

Subacute Causes of Joint Pain (6–12 weeks)

- ***Post-viral arthritis***: Self-limiting arthritis after viral infections (e.g. parvovirus, rubella).
- Early phase of inflammatory arthritis (RA, SLE, etc.).

Chronic Causes of Joint Pain (>12 weeks)

- Usually due to chronic inflammation, degeneration, or autoimmune processes.
- ***Chronic inflammatory arthritis***: Rheumatoid arthritis, psoriatic arthritis, ankylosing spondylitis, juvenile idiopathic arthritis, SLE.
- ***Degenerative disorders***: Osteoarthritis, avascular necrosis.
- ***Metabolic disorders***: Chronic tophaceous gout, hemochromatosis.
- ***Other autoimmune disorders***: Sjögren's syndrome, sarcoidosis.
- ***Chronic infections (rare):*** Tubercular arthritis, fungal arthritis.

Identify if Pain is Articular *vs.* Non-articular (Table 10.2)

TABLE 10.2: Differences between articular and non-articular pain

Feature	Articular (Joint)	Non-articular (Periarticular)
Pain location	Deep, diffuse	Localized (e.g. tendons, bursae)
Movement	Limited active and passive	Pain in active, not passive movement
Swelling	May be present	Typically absent
Crepitus/Instability	Common	Rare

Determine Inflammatory *vs.* Non-inflammatory Pathophysiology (Table 10.3)

TABLE 10.3: Differences between inflammatory and non-inflammatory arthritis

Inflammatory arthritis	Non-inflammatory/mechanical
Morning stiffness >30 minutes	<30 minutes
Soft tissue swelling (synovitis) present	Swelling due to bony enlargement
Warmth/erythema often present	Rare
Systemic symptoms such as fever, fatigue, rash often present	Absent
Symptoms worsen after a period of immobility	Symptoms aggravated by motion and weight bearing and relieved by rest
Typical joints involved: small joints (hands, wrists, ankles)	Weight-bearing joints (hip, knee)
ESR/CRP elevated	Normal
Examples: RA, SLE, gout, septic arthritis	OA, trauma, tendinitis

Assess Number of Joints Involved (Table 10.4)

TABLE 10.4: Number of joints involved and common causes

Involvement type	Definition	Common causes
Monoarthritis	1 joint	Gout, trauma, septic arthritis, OA
Oligoarthritis	2–4 joints	Psoriatic arthritis, reactive arthritis
Polyarthritis	≥5 joints	RA, SLE, viral arthritis

Determine Pattern and Distribution (Table 10.5)

TABLE 10.5: Pattern and distribution of joint pain and possible diagnosis

Feature	Clue toward diagnosis
Symmetric *vs* asymmetric	RA (symmetric), PsA/reactive (asymmetric)
Axial *vs* peripheral	Ankylosing spondylitis (axial), RA (peripheral)
Small *vs* large joints	RA (small joints), Osteoarthritis (weight-bearing joints)
Migratory pattern	Acute rheumatic fever, gonococcal arthritis
Additive pattern	RA
Intermittent	Gout, pseudogout, palindromic rheumatism

Identify Underlying Pathophysiologic Category (Table 10.6)

TABLE 10.6: Underlying pathology and common causes

Pathophysiology	Common causes	Diagnostic features
Inflammatory (autoimmune)	RA, SLE, PsA, AS	↑ ESR/CRP, autoantibodies, joint effusion
Crystal-induced	Gout, pseudogout	Crystals in synovial fluid (MSU/CPPD)
Infectious (septic)	Bacterial, viral, TB	Fever, high WBC, positive cultures
Degenerative (mechanical)	Osteoarthritis, trauma	Crepitus, bony hypertrophy, normal labs
Neuropathic	Charcot joint (diabetes, syphilis)	Painless swelling, deformity, X-ray destruction
Endocrine/ metabolic	Hemochromatosis, hyperparathyroidism	Systemic signs, specific biochemical markers
Neoplastic	Leukemia, bone tumors	Night pain, systemic signs, radiologic abnormalities
Referred pain	Hip pathology → knee pain. Spine → limb	No local joint findings

Order Targeted Investigations

Blood Tests

- CBC, ESR, CRP.
- Rheumatoid factor (RF), anti-CCP.
- ANA, anti-dsDNA.
- Uric acid.
- HLA-B27 (if suspecting spondyloarthritis).
- Blood cultures (if septic arthritis suspected).

Synovial Fluid Analysis (arthrocentesis) (Table 10.7)

TABLE 10.7: Synovial fluid analysis

Parameter	Inflammatory	Non-inflammatory	Septic
Appearance	Cloudy	Clear	Purulent
WBC count	>2,000–50,000/ mm^3	<2,000/mm^3	>50,000/mm^3
Crystals	+ (Gout or CPPD)	–	–
Gram's stain/ culture	Negative	Negative	Often positive

Imaging

- X-ray: Joint space, erosions, osteophytes
- MRI: Synovitis, early cartilage loss
- Ultrasound: Effusion, crystal deposits, synovial thickening.

Management Based on Pathophysiology (Table 10.8)

TABLE 10.8: Management based on pathophysiology

Pathophysiology	Management approach
Inflammatory	NSAIDs, steroids, DMARDs (e.g. MTX, biologics)
Crystal-induced	Colchicine, NSAIDs, allopurinol (gout), hydration
Septic arthritis	Emergency → IV antibiotics + joint drainage
Osteoarthritis	Weight reduction, physiotherapy, NSAIDs, surgery
Neuropathic	Offloading, treat underlying neuropathy
Endocrine/metabolic	Treat underlying disorder (e.g. phlebotomy in hemochromatosis)
Neoplastic	Oncology referral, biopsy if needed

Q. Differentiate between arthralgia and arthritis (Table 10.9).

TABLE 10.9: Differences between arthralgia and arthritis

Feature	Arthralgia	Arthritis
Definition	Joint pain without objective signs of inflammation	Joint pain with inflammation (swelling, redness, warmth)
Signs	No visible joint swelling or warmth	Swelling, erythema, warmth, effusion, tenderness

(Contd.)

TABLE 10.9: Differences between arthralgia and arthritis *(Contd.)*

Feature	Arthralgia	Arthritis
Mobility	Normal or slightly restricted	Often restricted due to pain/inflammation
Causes	Viral illness, systemic diseases, fibromyalgia	RA, SLE, gout, OA, septic arthritis
Investigations	Often normal labs/ imaging	Raised ESR/CRP; imaging may show erosions or joint space loss

Q. How do you differentiate between articular and periarticular pain (Table 10.10).

TABLE 10.10: Differences between articular and periarticular pain

Feature	Articular	Periarticular
Origin	From within the joint capsule	From structures around the joint (tendons, bursae, ligaments)
Pain location	Deep, diffuse, often poorly localized	Localized to a specific area (e.g. lateral shoulder)
Pain with movement	Pain with both active and passive movement	Pain with active only, not passive motion
Swelling	Present within joint (effusion)	Localized swelling (bursa, tendon sheath)
Examples	RA, OA, septic arthritis	Bursitis, tendinitis, tenosynovitis, enthesitis
Tests	Joint aspiration, imaging	MRI, local tenderness, USG

Q. Discuss the etiology, pathogenesis, clinical features, diagnosis, and management of systemic lupus erythematosus (SLE).

- Systemic lupus erythematosus (SLE) is a chronic autoimmune disease which affects multiple organ systems. It is the most common multisystem connective tissue disease.
- Immunologic abnormalities, especially the production of a number of antinuclear antibodies, are another prominent feature of the disease.
- The prevalence is 50–150 per lakh population. 90% of affected patients are females, with peak onset in the second and third decades. It is more common in urban than rural areas.

Etiology

- Exact etiology is unknown. Thought to be autoimmune.
- *Genetic factors:* There is a high concordance rate of SLE in monozygotic twins. It is more common in relatives of SLE patients. Risk of SLE is increased in those with HLA-B8, HLA-DR2, and HLA-DR3.
- *Hormonal factors:* Female sex and hormonal influence is a significant risk factor for SLE. Use of estrogen-containing contraceptive agents is associated with increased risk of developing SLE. Elevated levels of prolactin are seen in patients with SLE.
- *Immune abnormalities:* SLE is primarily a disease with abnormalities in immune regulation. Affected patients are not tolerant to their self-antigens, and consequently develop an autoimmune response. Phagocytosis and clearing of immune complexes and of apoptotic cells are defective in SLE.
- *Environmental factors:* Smoking, some viruses, ultraviolet rays and silica dust may increase the risk of developing SLE.
- *Drugs:* Hydralazine, procainamide, isoniazid, and others (drug-induced lupus).

Pathogenesis (Fig. 10.9)

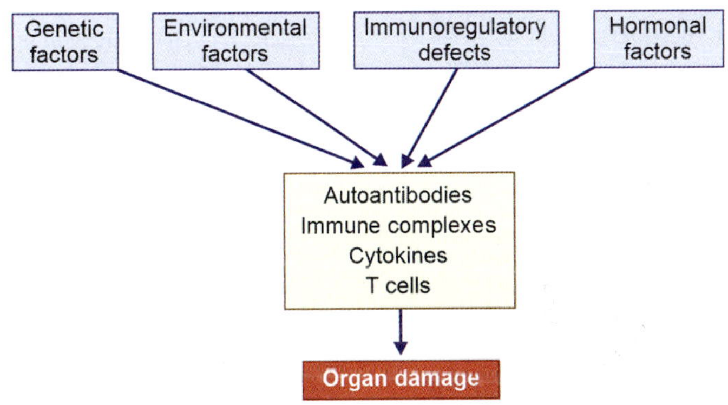

Figure 10.9: Pathogenesis of SLE

- SLE is characterized by loss of self-tolerance and formation of autoantibodies, especially against nuclear components. Many components of intracellular and intra-nuclear machinery act as autoantigens in SLE. In normal health these antigens are 'hidden' from the immune system and do not provoke an immune response.
- Interactions between susceptibility genes and environmental factors result in abnormal immune responses.
- This abnormal immune response results in the production of pathogenic autoantibodies and immune complexes that deposit in tissues, activate complement, cause inflammation, and over time lead to irreversible organ damage.

Clinical Features

- SLE affects almost all the organ systems.

Constitutional Symptoms

- Fatigue, fever, myalgia, weight loss and mild lymphadenopathy.

Raynaud's Phenomenon

- Cold or emotion-induced color changes of the digits of the hands and/or feet is a frequent problem.

Musculoskeletal Features

- Arthritis and arthralgias: Joint symptoms occur in over 90% of patients with SLE. The arthritis tends to be migratory and asymmetrical. Only a few joints are usually affected, especially those of the hands. Joint deformities are usually rare.

- Avascular necrosis
- Tenosynovitis.

Mucocutaneous Features

- The most common lesion is butterfly rash (erythema over the cheeks and nose, which appears after sun exposure (**Fig. 10.10**). It spares the nasolabial folds. The absence of papules and pustules helps distinguish SLE from rosacea.
- Discoid rashes are characterized by hyperkeratosis and follicular plugging with a tendency to scar.
- Vasculitic skin lesions may include mottled erythema on the palms and fingers, periungual erythema, nail-fold infarcts, urticaria, and palpable purpura.
- Other skin manifestations include livedo reticularis, photosensitivity, Raynaud's phenomenon, and alopecia (hair loss).
- Mucus membrane manifestations are painless oral and/or nasal ulcers.

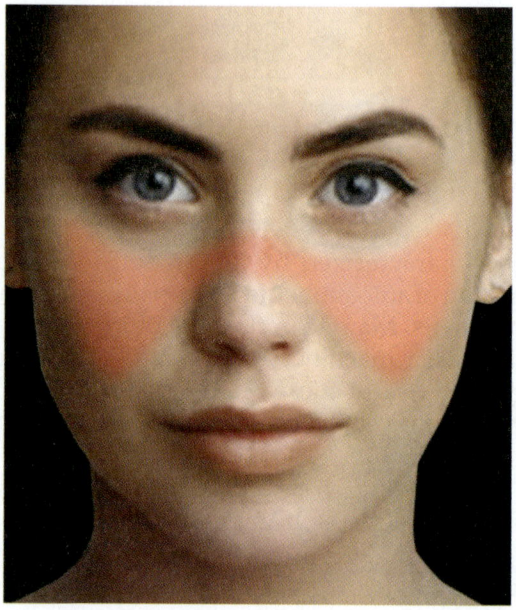

Figure 10.10: Butterfly rash of SLE

Renal Features

- Kidney is the most commonly involved visceral organ in SLE.
- Initially it may be asymptomatic. Hence, regular urine analysis for proteinuria, and serum creatinine measurements are important.
- Proliferative glomerulonephritis (lupus nephritis) characterized by hematuria, proteinuria and urinary casts.

Cardiovascular Features

- Pericarditis leading to chest pain and pericardial effusion.
- Myocarditis and sterile Libman-Sacks endocarditis. Libman-Sacks endocarditis is characterized by noninfectious vegetations, formed as a result of procoagulability in association with antiphospholipid antibodies.
- Increased risk of venous thromboembolism due to the presence of antiphospholipid antibodies.
- Coronary vasculitis causing angina is rarely reported.

Pulmonary Features

- Pleuritis and pleural effusion
- Pneumonitis
- Interstitial lung disease
- Pulmonary hypertension
- Alveolar hemorrhage
- Shrinking or vanishing lung syndrome
- Pulmonary embolism.

Neuropsychiatric Features

- Fatigue, headache, poor concentration
- Visual hallucinations
- Chorea (also associated with antiphospholipid antibody syndrome)
- Organic psychosis
- Transverse myelitis
- Lymphocytic meningitis
- Seizures.

Hematological Features

- Coombs' positive hemolytic anemia.
- Pancytopenia (anemia, leukopenia and thrombocytopenia) due to antibody-mediated destruction of peripheral blood cells
- Splenomegaly and lymphadenopathy.

Gastrointestinal Features

- Nonspecific abdominal pain
- SLE vasculitis can lead to pancreatitis, peritonitis, and colitis
- Mesenteric vasculitis
- Hepatosplenomegaly.

Ophthalmologic Features

- Keratoconjunctivitis sicca due to secondary Sjögren's syndrome.
- Rare features are cotton wool exudates due to retinal vasculitis, episcleritis or scleritis, and uveitis.

Diagnosis

Investigations

- Complete blood count and differential count: anemia or pancytopenia is seen.
- Serum creatinine, urine analysis with microscopy, and 24-hour urinary protein excretion to rule out renal involvement.
- ESR, CRP are elevated and complement levels (C3, and C4) are decreased.
- Autoantibody testing-antinuclear antibodies (ANA), antiphospholipid antibodies, antibodies to double

stranded DNA (anti-dsDNA) and anti-Smith (Sm) antibodies may be positive. Antinuclear antibody (ANA) test is the best diagnostic test for SLE. ANA is positive in significant titer (usually 1:160 or higher) in virtually all patients with SLE. However, ANA is not specific for SLE and it can be positive in Sjögren's syndrome, scleroderma, and rheumatoid arthritis. Anti-dsDNA and anti Sm antibodies—are highly specific for SLE. Other antibodies that can be positive in SLE are antibodies to single-stranded DNA and nucleoprotein (NP), antibodies to ribonucleoprotein (anti-RNP), antibodies to Ro (SS-A) and La (SS-B).

- Chest X-ray—to look for pneumonitis, interstitial lung disease, etc.
- CT or MRI brain in people who present with seizures
- Biopsy—of an involved organ (e.g. skin or kidney) is necessary in some cases.

Management

- Educate the patient to avoid sun and UV light exposure, and to use sun block preparations.
- NSAIDs are enough for mild joint pain.
- Hydroxychloroquine (200–400 mg daily) is indicated for all patients with SLE regardless of disease severity because it decreases disease flares and decreases mortality. It is especially useful in troublesome cutaneous and joint symptoms.
- Steroids—are required for mild to moderate disease activity (e.g. rashes, synovitis, pleuro-pericarditis). High dose steroids (oral prednisolone 40–60 mg daily or i.v. methylprednisolone 500 mg-1 g) in combination with pulse IV cyclophosphamide is required for life-threatening disease (i.e. renal, cerebral involvement, systemic vasculitis, diffuse alveolar hemorrhage). For maintenance therapy oral prednisone ≤7.5 mg once a day or its equivalent can be used along with hydroxychloroquine or azathioprine.
- Immunosuppressive drugs (azathioprine, methotrexate, ciclosporin, tacrolimus, mycophenolate mofetil)–these are useful either alone or in combination with steroids for severe but non-life-threatening manifestations or as step-down therapy after cyclophosphamide.
- Belimumab inhibits the production of antibodies by preventing the maturation of B cells into plasma cells. It is indicated for active, autoantibody-positive SLE which is not responding to standard therapy.
- Rituximab can be used in CNS lupus including transverse myelitis. It is also helpful in refractory cases of hemolytic anemia and thrombocytopenia.
- Anticoagulants—such as warfarin is required life-long for patients with the antiphospholipid antibody syndrome with thrombotic events.

Q. Autoantibodies in SLE.

- SLE is characterized by the production of a variety of autoantibodies, many directed against nuclear antigens. These autoantibodies play diagnostic, prognostic, and sometimes pathogenic roles (**Table 10.11**).

TABLE 10.11: Autoantibodies in SLE

Test	Description
Antinuclear antibody (ANA)	Antinuclear antibodies are autoantibodies that bind to contents of the cell nucleus. ANA is used as a screening test for diagnosing connective tissue diseases; ANA is positive in significant titer (usually 1:160 or higher) in virtually all patients with SLE. However, ANA is not specific for SLE and it can be positive in Sjögren's syndrome, scleroderma, and rheumatoid arthritis. There are many subtypes of ANA which are anti-dsDNA, anti-Sm, anti-SSA, anti-SSB, anti-ribosomal P, anti-RNP (ribonucleic protein), etc.
Anti-dsDNA (double-stranded DNA)	Has high specificity for the diagnosis of SLE; sensitivity only 70%. Anti-dsDNA levels correlate with disease activity in SLE; high levels indicate more active lupus.
Anti-Smith (anti-Sm)	Most specific antibody for SLE 99%), but only 30–40% sensitivity. They are associated with central nervous system involvement, kidney disease, lung fibrosis and pericarditis in SLE, but they are not associated with disease activity
Anti-SSA (Sjögren syndrome A) or Anti-SSB (Sjögren syndrome B)	Present in 15% of patients with SLE and other connective-tissue diseases such as Sjögren syndrome
Anti-ribosomal P protein antibodies	Uncommon antibodies that may correlate with risk for CNS disease, including increased risk of psychosis.
Anti-Ro (SSA) (ribonucleic protein)	Presence of this antibody indicates mixed connective-tissue disease with overlap SLE, scleroderma, and myositis
Anti-U1 RNP (Ribonucleoprotein)	Associated with mixed connective tissue disease (MCTD) (very high titers). Associated with Raynaud's phenomenon, arthritis, and mild renal disease.
Anticardiolipin	These are IgG/IgM antiphospholipid antibodies used to screen for antiphospholipid antibody syndrome (APLA) which can occur in SLE.
Lupus anticoagulant (LA)	LA is tested along with anticardiolipin antibody to diagnose APLA. It can be positive in SLE. Lupus anticoagulant is a misnomer, as it is actually a prothrombotic agent.
Direct Coombs' test	Positive test indicates presence of antibodies on RBCs
Antihistone	Drug-induced lupus ANA antibodies are often of this type (e.g. with procainamide or hydralazine. p-ANCA is positive in minocycline-induced drug-induced lupus)

Q. Raynaud's syndrome (Raynaud's phenomenon).

- Raynaud's syndrome is characterized by recurrent vasospasm of the fingers and toes on exposure to cold temperature or emotional stress. It is due to an exaggerated vascular response and was first described by Maurice Raynaud, a medical student.

Types

Primary Raynaud's Syndrome

- This is characterized by the occurrence of the vasospasm alone, without any underlying disorder.

Secondary Raynaud's Syndrome

- This is occurrence of the vasospasm which is associated with an underlying disorder, most commonly an autoimmune disease.

Etiology

Primary (idiopathic) (80–90% cases)

- Cause is unknown. Common in young women (age 15–30).

Secondary

- *Autoimmune diseases:* Progressive systemic sclerosis (scleroderma), SLE, mixed connective-tissue disease, dermatomyositis and polymyositis, rheumatoid arthritis, Sjögren's syndrome, vasculitis.
- *Occupational:* Vibration-induced (e.g. jackhammer use).
- *Arterial diseases:* Atherosclerosis, Buerger's disease.
- *Infectious diseases:* Hepatitis B and C, mycoplasma.
- *Neoplastic diseases:* Lymphoma, leukemia, myeloma, Waldenstrom macroglobulinemia, carcinoid syndrome, paraneoplastic disorders.
- *Environmental factors:* Vibration injury, vinyl chloride exposure, frostbite.
- *Endocrine disorders:* Acromegaly, myxedema, pheochromocytoma.
- *Hematologic diseases:* Paroxysmal nocturnal hemoglobinuria, polycythemia, cryoglobulinemia.
- *Drugs:* Beta blockers, oral contraceptives, ergot alkaloids, nicotine, cocaine, bromocriptine, sympathomimetics.

Pathophysiology

- Various abnormalities have been found in the vessels of patients with Raynaud's syndrome. These include endothelial dysfunction, deficiency of vasodilators such as nitric oxide, calcitonin gene-related peptide, and increase in vasoconstrictors such as endothelin-1, neuropeptide Y and thromboxane A2. Various neural abnormalities leading to an exaggerated vasospasm have also been documented.

Clinical Features

- Females are affected more commonly than males.
- Acral areas such as digits of the fingers are affected commonly, but toes, nose, and ears are affected occasionally.
- Affected areas show color changes usually in the order of white (pallor), blue (cyanosis), and red (hyperemia) **(Fig. 10.11)**. Pallor is due to vasospasm. Cyanosis is due to reduction of blood flow. Red color is due to compensatory increase in blood flow (hyperemia). These color changes are usually transient but may rarely lead to local ischemia and gangrene. Numbness and pain in the affected areas may be present.
- There may be signs and symptoms of an underlying disorder (such as connective tissue disease).

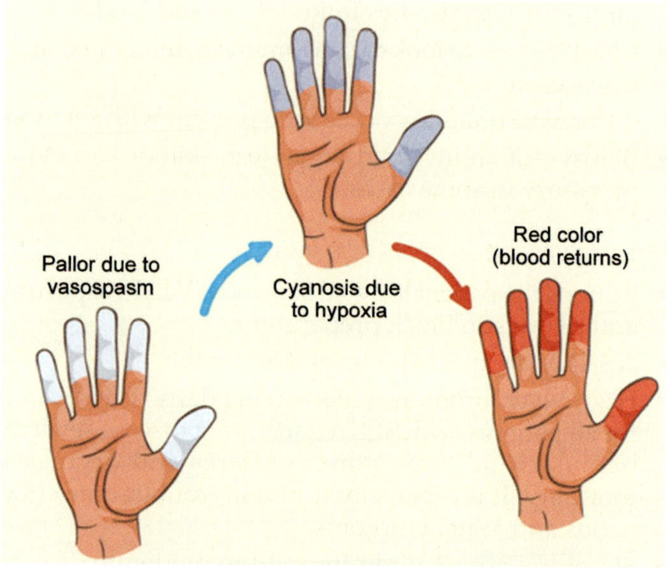

Figure 10.11: Raynaud's phenomenon

Investigations

- Routine blood tests
- Doppler flow studies (if digital ischemia is suspected)
- Antinuclear antibody (ANA) and rheumatoid factor—may be positive in autoimmune diseases
- *Hepatitis panel:* Positive for B or C infection in many patients with cryoglobulinemia
- Other tests as per the suspected underlying disease.

Treatment

- *General measures:* These include reassurance, application of warmth to affected areas, stopping of any offending drugs. Patient should avoid cold environment.
- Vasodilators such as calcium channel blockers are useful as they prevent vasospasm. Nifedipine is most commonly used. Other drugs such as nicardipine, amlodipine, or diltiazem can also be used. Transdermal nitroglycerin can be added in severe cases.
- Parenteral prostaglandins such as prostaglandin E1 (PGE1), prostacyclin (PGI2), and iloprost (a PGI2 analog) have been shown to be of benefit in severe attacks causing digital ischemia.
- Cervical sympathectomy is useful for patients with recurrent attacks. It is more useful in patients with primary Raynaud's syndrome. Localized microsurgical digital sympathectomy has been gaining support as an alternative to cervical sympathectomy.
- Any underlying disorder should be treated.

Q. Discuss the etiology, pathogenesis, clinical features, diagnosis, and treatment of systemic sclerosis (scleroderma, CREST syndrome).

- Systemic sclerosis (previously called 'scleroderma') is a multisystem connective tissue disorder affecting the skin, internal organs and vasculature.
- Thickened skin (scleroderma) is the hallmark of this disease.
- It is more common in females (4:1 female: male ratio) and the peak age of onset is in the fourth and fifth decades.
- It is subdivided into diffuse cutaneous systemic sclerosis (DCSS) and limited cutaneous systemic sclerosis (LCSS). LCSS may have features of 'CREST' syndrome (calcinosis, Raynaud's, esophageal involvement, sclerodactyly, telangiectasia).

Etiology

- The exact etiology is unknown. It is multifactorial.
- ***Environmental factors:*** Many environmental factors such as exposure to silica dust, vinyl chloride, epoxy resins and trichloroethylene have been suspected to play a role in the causation of the disease.
- ***Genetic predisposition***: HLA-DQB1, DRB1.
- ***Autoimmunity:*** Production of specific autoantibodies.
- ***Hormonal factors***: F >M (4:1).

Pathogenesis

Involves 3 main pathological processes:

- ***Vascular injury***: Endothelial dysfunction → Raynaud's phenomenon, pulmonary HTN.
- ***Autoimmune activation***: ↑ T cells, autoantibodies.
- ***Fibrosis***: Excessive collagen deposition due to fibroblast activation Fibrosis can happen in any organ leading to organ damage and functional impairment.
- Systemic sclerosis can overlap with other autoimmune rheumatic disorders.

Clinical Features

Skin features

- Edematous swelling and erythema of the skin may precede skin thickening.
- Thickening and hardening of the skin. The skin of fingers, hands and face is first affected. Skin becomes taut and shiny. Skin creases disappear. Thickening of facial skin results in mask-like-facies and microstomia (small mouth).
- Skin involvement restricted to sites distal to the elbow or knee (apart from the face) is classified as 'limited cutaneous disease' or CREST syndrome. Involvement proximal to the knee and elbow and on the trunk is classified as 'diffuse cutaneous disease'.

Vascular

- Raynaud's phenomenon (first sign in many)
- Telangiectasias
- Digital ischemia/gangrene.

Musculoskeletal features

- Arthralgia
- Morning stiffness
- Tenosynovitis
- Myositis

Gastrointestinal features

- Smooth muscle atrophy and fibrosis in the esophagus lead to esophageal reflux, dysphagia and odynophagia (painful dysphagia).
- Involvement of the stomach causes early satiety and occasionally outlet obstruction.
- Vascular ectasia in the stomach ("watermelon stomach") is frequent, and may cause recurrent gastrointestinal bleeding and anemia.
- Small and large bowel involvement may lead to malabsorption due to bacterial overgrowth, bloating, pain or constipation and pseudo-obstruction.

Pulmonary features

- Interstitial lung disease.
- Pulmonary hypertension leading to progressive dyspnea, right heart failure and angina.
- Increase in the incidence of lung cancer.

Cardiac features

- Right heart failure and angina due to pulmonary hypertension
- Pericarditis
- Myocardial fibrosis
- Arrhythmias.

Renal features

- Proteinuria
- Scleroderma renal crisis—this is a life-threatening renal disease and is more frequent in patients with DCSS. It is characterized by acute onset of renal failure and malignant hypertension.

Neurological features

- Cranial, entrapment, peripheral, and autonomic neuropathies.
- CNS involvement, including headache, seizures, stroke, vascular disease, radiculopathy, and myelopathy.

Genitourinary features

- Erectile dysfunction in men
- Decreased vaginal lubrication or constriction of the vaginal introitus in women leading to dyspareunia.

Diagnosis

- Systemic sclerosis is mainly a clinical diagnosis based on the presence of typical skin thickening and hardening (sclerosis) along with the presence of extra-cutaneous features and characteristic autoantibodies.
- ESR is elevated. Anemia may be present.
- Skin biopsy—is usually not essential but required if the diagnosis is in doubt. It is also helpful to differentiate from other causes of skin thickening.
- Autoantibodies—presence of many autoantibodies support the diagnosis of systemic sclerosis. These include anti-centromere, anti-topoisomerase-I (Scl-70), anti-RNA polymerase, or U3-RNP antibodies. ANA with a nucleolar staining pattern is frequently present.
- X-ray and CT scan chest if there is suspicion of ILD.

- Echocardiogram to rule out pulmonary hypertension and cardiac involvement.
- RFT and urine analysis to rule out renal damage.

Management

- Regular monitoring of BP, renal function tests and blood counts.
- Intravenous cyclophosphamide has been shown to slow the progression of the disease, but the drug has significant side effects.
- Corticosteroids and immunosuppressive agents are indicated in patients with myositis or interstitial lung disease.
- Raynaud's phenomenon—avoidance of cold exposure and use of vasodilators such as calcium channel blockers (nifedipine, amlodipine) or angiotensin II receptor blockers (e.g. valsartan) may be helpful. Sympathectomy may be tried in patients who do not respond to medical therapy.
- Esophageal dysmotility and acid reflux—this can be improved by proton pump inhibitors, and prokinetic agents such as itopride.
- Infection of ulcerated skin should be treated with prompt antibiotic therapy.
- For severe digital ischemia, intermittent infusions of epoprostenol may be helpful.

Q. Sarcoidosis.

Definition

- Sarcoidosis is a chronic, systemic disease of unknown etiology characterized by the presence of noncaseating granulomas in one or more organ systems.
- Although it is a systemic disease, lungs and lymphatic system are affected more commonly.
- The clinical picture can vary from asymptomatic to multi organ failure.

Epidemiology

- Sarcoidosis has worldwide distribution, but more common in northern Europe, North America, and Japan. It mainly affects whites. It is less common in Asian countries like China, Africa, India, and Russia.
- Most patients present between 20 and 40 years of age. Women are affected more often than men.
- It occurs more commonly in nonsmokers unlike other lung diseases which occur in smokers.

Etiology

- Exact cause of sarcoidosis is unknown. Available evidence implicates exaggerated cellular immune response as the etiological factor. Immunological response is triggered by some antigens. Genetic factors may also make a person more susceptible.
- A variety of exogenous agents, both infectious and non-infectious, have been hypothesized as possible causes of sarcoidosis. It has been suggested that an exogenous agent induces immunologic sensitization, by acting as a "hapten" that binds to peptides or alters major histocompatibility complex molecules. Some of the agents implicated are *Mycobacterium tuberculosis*, atypical mycobacteria, viruses, fungi, protozoa, pine pollen, etc. Beryllium can produce an identical illness in human beings. Recent workers have found evidence of mycobacterial DNA in sarcoid tissue.
- Recurrence of disease can occur in the transplanted lung of patients who receive a transplant for end-stage sarcoidosis. In addition, sarcoidosis has been reported to develop in the transplant recipient of tissue from a donor with sarcoidosis.

Pathogenesis

- The unknown antigen triggers a cell-mediated immune response. The first manifestation of sarcoidosis is an accumulation CD4+ T lymphocytes and mononuclear phagocytes in affected organs. This inflammatory process is followed by the formation of noncaseating granulomas, aggregation of macrophages, epithelioid cells, and multinucleated giant cells. Organ dysfunction results from the granulomas and accumulated inflammatory cells distorting the architecture of the affected tissue. Chronic inflammation in the organs may lead to fibrosis and permanent damage.
- Hypercalcemia may occur because vitamin D analogs are produced by activated macrophages. Nephrolithiasis and nephrocalcinosis may occur, sometimes leading to chronic kidney disease.

Clinical Manifestations

- Sarcoidosis is notable for its protean manifestations and variable course. Any organ can be affected, but the respiratory system is most commonly affected.
- *General symptoms*: Fever, malaise, weight loss, night sweats (resemble TB).
- *Respiratory system:* 90% of patients with sarcoidosis have pulmonary involvement on chest X-ray. Upper lobes tend to be more affected than the lower lobes. Pleura and airways can also be affected. Severe disease may lead to irreversible fibrosis and honeycombing. Patients usually present with respiratory symptoms, such as dyspnea and cough. Crepitations may be heard on auscultation of lungs. Extrapulmonary disease can occur without concomitant pulmonary involvement but rare.
- *Hematologic:* Lymphocytopenia, anemia of chronic disease, pancytopenia due to granulomatous infiltration of bone marrow, splenic sequestration causing thrombocytopenia, leukopenia.
- *CVS:* Involvement results in conduction defects, arrhythmias, and heart failure.
- *Nervous system:* Manifestations include facial nerve palsy (most common manifestation), seizures, meningitis, peripheral neuropathy, and psychiatric symptoms. Virtually any part of the nervous system can be involved.
- *GIT:* Hepatosplenomegaly is common. Parotid involvement leads to bilateral swelling. Pancreas also can be involved.

- *Skin:* Cutaneous manifestations include papules, plaques, nodules, erythema nodosum, infiltration of old scars, and lupus pernio.
- *Eye:* Involvement takes the form of anterior or posterior uveitis, conjunctival involvement, and papilledema. Heerfordt's syndrome or uveoparotid fever, is a form of sarcoidosis in which anterior uveitis is accompanied by parotid gland enlargement and often fever and facial palsy.
- *Musculo-skeletal system:* Effusion into joints, myalgia and arthralgia may occur.
- *Endocrine system:* Diabetes insipidus may result from hypothalamus lesions. Diabetes mellitus can occur due to pancreas involvement. Hypopituitarism and hypothyroidism have also been recorded.

Investigations

- *Elevation of angiotensin-converting enzyme (ACE) and calcium:* Hypercalcemia may be due to elevated levels of 1, 25-dihydroxyvitamin D produced by macrophages within the granulomas. Elevation in ACE is believed to be due to production of the enzyme by epithelioid cells and macrophages within the granulomas.
- *Histopathology (gold standard):* Noncaseating granulomas without central necrosis in the affected organs. Flexible bronchoscopy with transbronchial lung biopsy is particularly useful.
- *Kveim test:* It is done by intradermal injection of a validated antigen. Formation of a typical granuloma is highly specific and sensitive. Not done nowadays.
- Tuberculin test is usually negative in sarcoidosis.
- *Chest X-ray:* It shows hilar lymphadenopathy, and involvement of the pulmonary parenchyma. Interstitial, alveolar and nodular pattern opacities may also be seen.
- *High-resolution CT scan of chest:* It shows mediastinal lymphadenopathy and opacities better than chest X-ray
- *PET scan:* It is very helpful in assessing extent of disease. Whole-body imaging helps in mapping multi-organ involvement and clinically silent lesions.

Treatment

- All cases of sarcoidosis do not require treatment. Indications for treatment are: symptomatic disease, organ dysfunction (ocular, cardiac, CNS, severe pulmonary), and hypercalcemia. Intrathoracic lymph node involvement does not require treatment, but lung parenchymal involvement requires treatment.
- Corticosteroids are the drugs of choice to suppress inflammation. Prednisolone is started at a dose of 0.5–1 mg/kg/day, and continued for several weeks and then tapered to a lower dose which is continued for 6–12 months. The optimum duration of therapy is not known and needs to be individualized based on response. Premature discontinuation of therapy may lead to recurrence of disease. Alternative agents include methotrexate (7.5–15 mg per week), or other immunosuppressive or cytotoxic agents such as cyclophosphamide and azathioprine.
- Hydroxychloroquine has been used for serious and disfiguring cutaneous sarcoidosis. Dose is 250–750 mg/day for 6–9 months.
- Tumor necrosis factor (TNF) receptor antagonists such as etanercept and infliximab have shown benefit in some trials.
- In patients with severe, end-stage pulmonary disease, lung transplantation is an important option, but the disease may affect the transplanted lungs also.

Natural History and Prognosis

- Often self-limiting. 2/3rd recover without treatment.
- Patients with progressive disease can become disabled from significant organ system involvement, particularly respiratory failure from interstitial lung disease.

Q. What are idiopathic inflammatory myopathies?

Q. Discuss the etiology, classification, clinical features, diagnosis, and management of polymyositis-dermatomyositis.

- Idiopathic inflammatory myopathies are rare connective tissue disorders characterized by the presence of muscle inflammation (myositis) and weakness.
- These include polymyositis, dermatomyositis and inclusion body myositis.
- The term polymyositis is used when the condition spares the skin and the term dermatosmyositis is used when the condition involves the skin.
- They are more common in females (2:1 ratio).

Etiology

- The exact etiology is unknown.
- Genetic factors may play a role.
- Other connective tissue diseases such as SLE or vasculitis can cause myositis.
- They may be associated with malignancy.

Clinical Features

Polymyositis

- The onset is usually between 40 and 60 years of age and is insidious.
- The most common presentation is symmetrical proximal muscle weakness, usually affecting the lower limbs first. There is difficulty in getting from sitting position and climbing stairs. Muscle pain may be present. Respiratory or pharyngeal muscle involvement leads to dyspnea and aspiration.
- Systemic features such as fever, weight loss and fatigue may be present.
- Interstitial lung disease causes progressive dyspnea and dry cough.

Dermatomyositis

Muscle manifestations

- These are similar to polymyositis.

Skin manifestations

- Gottron's papules are scaly erythematous plaques or papules occurring over the extensor surfaces of interphalangeal joints.
- Heliotrope rash is a violaceous eruption on the upper eyelids, often accompanied by eyelid edema.
- Shawl sign and V sign: Shawl sign is an erythematous lesion occurring over the chest and shoulders (shawl distribution) or in a V–shaped distribution over the anterior neck and chest.
- Periungual nail-fold capillaries are often abnormal.
- Mechanic's hands: This is roughening and cracking of the skin of the tips and lateral aspects of the fingers resembling those of a manual laborer.
- Systemic features such as fever, weight loss and fatigue may be present.

Diagnosis

- These conditions should be suspected when there is proximal muscle weakness without neuropathy, and there is evidence of systemic disease.
- Creatine kinase (CK) is usually elevated.
- Electromyography (EMG) to confirm myopathy and exclude neuropathy.
- Muscle biopsy (gold standard for diagnosis) shows features of inflammation, necrosis, and regeneration.
- MRI is useful to visualize muscle inflammation and also identify areas of abnormal muscle for biopsy.

Management

- ***Steroids:*** Oral steroids (e.g. prednisolone 40–60 mg daily) are the mainstay of treatment. Intravenous steroids (methylprednisolone 1 g daily for 3 days) may be required for severe weakness or respiratory or pharyngeal weakness. Steroids should be tapered slowly to a maintenance dose of 5–7.5 mg per day.
- ***Immunosuppressive agents:*** These are required if there is inadequate response to steroids. Azathioprine and methotrexate are the first choice and ciclosporin, cyclophosphamide, tacrolimus and intravenous immunoglobulin are alternatives.
- ***General measures:*** Physiotherapy, avoidance of sunlight, prevention of opportunistic infections, etc.

Q. Marfan's syndrome.

- Marfan's syndrome is an autosomal dominant inherited disorder of connective tissue.

Pathogenesis

- It occurs due to mutation of fibrillin-1 gene (FBN1) on chromosome15q21. Fibrillin-1 is a glycoprotein essential for elastic fiber formation in connective tissue.
- Mutant fibrillin-1 leads to weak connective tissue. This leads to: aortic root dilation, lens dislocation, skeletal overgrowth and joint laxity.

Clinical Features

- It affects approximately 1 in 5000 population.

Skeletal Features

- Tall, thin body habitus
- Long limbs and fingers (arachnodactyly)
- Arm span >height
- Scoliosis
- Pectus deformities (pectus excavatum/carinatum)
- Joint hypermobility
- High-arched palate.

Cardiovascular

- Aortic root dilation, aneurysm, and dissection
- Aortic regurgitation
- Mitral valve prolapse (MVP).

Ocular

- Ectopia lentis (superotemporal lens dislocation)
- Myopia
- Retinal detachment (less common).

Skin

- Striae (stretch marks not due to obesity)
- Recurrent hernias.

Pulmonary

- Spontaneous pneumothorax
- Apical blebs
- Restrictive lung disease due to chest wall abnormalities.

Investigations

- Ophthalmologic examination–for lens subluxation
- Echocardiography to assess aortic root and valve
- Genetic study to confirm FBN1 mutation.

Management

- Beta-blocker therapy slows the rate of dilatation of the aortic root.
- Prolonged exertion should be avoided because of cardiac defects.
- Aortic root diameter of 5 cm or more requires aortic root replacement.

Q. Inclusion body myositis.

- This is the most common acquired myopathy in patients over the age of 50.
- Etiology is unknown, but involves both autoimmune and degenerative mechanisms (abnormal protein accumulation similar to neurodegenerative diseases).
- It affects men more often than women.
- Distal muscle weakness is more common than proximal weakness which is in in contrast to other myopathies where proximal muscle weakness is the rule. Other clinical features are similar to polymyositis.
- Investigation findings are similar to polymyositis and dermatomyositis. However, muscle biopsy shows characteristic rimmed vacuoles and filamentous inclusions in the nucleus and cytoplasm of muscle fibers (hence called inclusion body myositis).

- Treatment is with steroids and immunosuppressive agents. However, the response is poor.

Q. Discuss the clinical features, investigations and management of Sjögren's syndrome.

Q. Keratoconjuctivitis sicca.

- Sjögren's syndrome (SS) is an autoimmune disorder of unknown etiology characterized by lymphocytic infiltration of exocrine glands, leading to glandular fibrosis and exocrine failure. Salivary and lacrimal glands are commonly involved.
- Sjögren's syndrome can be classified into primary SS or secondary SS. Primary SS is not associated with other diseases. Secondary SS occurs as a complication of other rheumatic disorders such as rheumatoid arthritis, SLE, polymyositis or scleroderma.

Clinical Features

- Patients are generally old (mean age 50 years) and more than 90% are women.

Exocrine Gland Involvement

- Dry eyes (keratoconjunctivitis sicca) occur due to lacrimal gland involvement. It is the hallmark of Sjögren's syndrome, but can also occur due to other conditions such as vitamin-A deficiency, contact lens use, etc. The ocular symptoms of dry eyes are irritation, grittiness, and a foreign body sensation. Conjunctivitis and blepharitis are frequent but keratitis can also occur.
- Dry mouth (xerostomia) occurs due to salivary gland involvement. Salivary glands may be enlarged. Decreased salivary secretion leads to difficulty swallowing dry food without water. Oral dryness leads to increased risk of dental caries and periodontal disease.
- Vaginal dryness can lead to dyspareunia.
- Exocrine gland involvement in the skin may lead to xerosis.

Extraglandular Features

- Musculoskeletal system: arthralgia, myalgia, non-erosive arthritis
- Nervous system: Peripheral neuropathy
- Kidneys: Glomerulonephritis, renal tubular acidosis
- Heart: Pericarditis
- RS: Interstitial lung disease
- GIT: Dysphagia
- Lymphadenopathy
- Thyroid–hypothyroidism
- Vascular: Vasculitis, Raynaud's phenomenon
- Increased incidence of lymphoma
- Low-grade fever, fatigue.

Investigations

- Anemia, leukopenia, thrombocytopenia
- Elevated ESR
- Cryoglobulinemia.
- Autoantibodies: ANA and rheumatoid factor are usually positive. Other antibodies which can be present are anti-Ro/SS-A, anti-La/SS-B and gastric parietal cell antibodies.
- Schirmer test: It is done by placing absorbent paper strips in the lower lacrimal sac for 5 minutes. Less than 5 mm of wetting is abnormal.
- Biopsy: Diagnosis can be confirmed by finding lymphocytic infiltrate in the minor salivary glands on lip biopsy.

Management

- Artificial lubrication is the mainstay of symptomatic treatment. Artificial tears such as hypromellose drops can be used for the eyes. Occlusion of the lacrimal ducts can increase the tear content of the eyes.
- Artificial saliva and oral gels can be tried for xerostomia. Stimulation of saliva flow by sugar-free chewing gum or lozenges may be helpful. Oral hygiene is important to prevent caries and gum problems. Vaginal dryness is treated with lubricants such as K-Y jelly.
- Extraglandular manifestations can be treated by steroids and immunosuppressive drugs such as azathioprine. Immunosuppression has no effect on sicca symptoms.

Q. Define vasculitis. Discuss the classification, clinical features, investigations and management of vasculitis (systemic vasculitis).

- Vasculitis refers to inflammation of blood vessels. Vasculitis can affect any blood vessel; arteries, arterioles, veins, venules, or capillaries.
- Vasculitis may be primary or secondary. Primary vasculitis mainly affects blood vessels and has no known cause. Secondary vasculitis may be triggered by an infection, a drug, or a toxin or may occur as part of another inflammatory disorder or cancer.
- Vasculitis may lead to blockage of the involved blood vessels and this leads to ischemia of the tissues supplied by the vessel.

Etiology

- Primary (idiopathic)—autoimmune (e.g. ANCA-associated vasculitis).
- Secondary—due to:
  - Infections (e.g. hepatitis B/C, HIV)
  - Drugs (e.g. hydralazine, minocycline)
  - Malignancies
  - Connective tissue diseases (e.g. SLE, RA).

Classification

- Vasculitis has been classified based on the predominant size of blood vessels affected. However, there is often substantial overlap.

Large vessel vasculitis
- Giant cell arteritis
- Takayasu's arteritis

Medium vessel vasculitis
- Polyarteritis nodosa (PAN)
- Kawasaki disease

Small vessel vasculitis
- Microscopic polyangiitis
- Wegener's granulomatosis
- Churg-Strauss syndrome
- Henoch-Schönlein purpura (IgA vasculitis)
- Hypersensitivity vasculitis (due to drugs, etc.)
- Vasculitis secondary to connective tissue disorders (SLE, RA)
- Vasculitis secondary to viral infection (hepatitis B and C)

Clinical Features

- Clinical features are produced due to a combination of local tissue ischemia caused by vessel block and the systemic inflammation.
- Systemic vasculitis should be suspected in a patient with fever, weight loss, fatigue, multisystem involvement, rashes, raised inflammatory markers and abnormal urinalysis.

Systemic: Fever, night sweats, weight loss
Skin: Palpable purpura, pulp infarcts, ulceration, livedo reticularis
Musculoskeletal: Arthralgia, myalgia
Ear, nose and throat: Epistaxis, recurrent sinusitis, deafness
Ophthalmologic: Scleritis, uveitis, vision loss in giant cell arteritis (temporal arteritis)
Respiratory: Cough, hemoptysis, wheezing
Gastrointestinal: Mouth ulcers, bleeding, abdominal pain (due to mucosal inflammation or enteric ischemia)
Neurological: Mononeuritis multiplex, polyneuropathy, radiculopathy, stroke
Renal: Hematuria, proteinuria, rapidly progressive glomerulonephritis

Investigations

- ESR and CRP are elevated
- Routine biochemistry
- Autoantibodies (ANA, antineutrophil cytoplasmic antibodies (ANCA), RA factor, cryoglobulins)
- Complement levels (C3, C4): Low in cryoglobulinemia, lupus vasculitis
- Hepatitis-B and C serology
- HIV ELISA
- Urinalysis (may show proteinuria and hematuria)
- CT/MRI angiography: Large/medium vessel vasculitis.
- Biopsy: Biopsy from an involved site such as skin, nasal mucosa can show vessel wall inflammation.

Management

- Management depends on the nature and severity of the vasculitis.
- Hypersensitivity vasculitis may respond to withdrawal of the offending drug, antihistamines and a short course of steroids.
- Oral steroids plus cytotoxic (cyclophosphamide) drugs are required for severe systemic vasculitis with multi-organ involvement.
- Azathioprine and methotrexate can be used in less severe forms of vasculitis and as maintenance therapy after remission has been induced by cyclophosphamide.

Q. Giant cell arteritis (Temporal arteritis).

- Temporal arteritis (giant cell arteritis) is a systemic inflammatory vasculitis occurring commonly in older individuals.
- Giant cell arteritis (GCA) commonly affects the large and medium sized arteries, especially superficial temporal arteries and its branches—hence the term temporal arteritis. In addition, GCA also affects the ophthalmic, occipital, vertebral, and posterior ciliary arteries. It can cause permanent blindness by causing occlusion of the posterior ciliary or central retinal arteries.

Pathophysiology

- Basically, there is granulomatous inflammation of the vessel wall leading to edema of the vessel wall and occlusion. Biopsy shows inflammatory cell infiltration into all three layers of the vessel wall.

Clinical Features

- Age: >50 years (peak ~70–80 years).
- Sex: Female >Male (2:1).
- GCA may begin with constitutional symptoms such as fever, anorexia, fever, malaise, and myalgia.
- Headache, orbital or frontotemporal, dull and constant in nature, aggravated by cold temperatures.
- Jaw claudication noted as fatigue or discomfort of the jaw muscles during chewing. Jaw claudication is almost pathognomonic of temporal arteritis, and it is a result of ischemia of the maxillary artery supplying the masseter muscles.
- Ophthalmologic symptoms: Occur due to ischemic optic neuropathy. Unilateral visual blurring or vision loss, or occasionally diplopia. A partial field defect may progress to complete blindness over days. Fundus examination may show pale or swollen optic disc, retinal splinter hemorrhages or a pale retina, and cherry-red spot (i.e. central retinal artery infarction).
- Tenderness may be present on the scalp and over the temporal artery.

Investigations

- ESR is the best screening test and is usually markedly elevated (i.e. >50, often >100). A normal ESR does not rule out GCA.
- CRP is also elevated.
- Temporal artery biopsy is required for definitive diagnosis.

- Ultrasound of temporal artery has emerged as an alternative or complement to biopsy. "Halo sign" (hypoechoic wall thickening) may be seen.
- MRI/PET-CT: For large vessel involvement (aorta, subclavian, carotid).

Treatment

- No vision loss: Prednisolone 40–60 mg/day. Treatment with steroids should be initiated promptly on suspecting temporal arteritis. Otherwise, permanent visual loss can occur.
- Vision loss or high risk: Intravenous methylprednisolone (500–1000 mg every day for 3 days, followed by oral prednisone with a gradual taper.
- Steroid sparing agents are used for relapsing/refractory cases. These are cyclosporin, azathioprine, methotrexate.

Q. Takayasu arteritis (pulseless disease; occlusive thromboaortopathy; aortic arch syndrome).

- Takayasu arteritis is a large vessel vasculitis. It mainly affects aorta and its major branches especially the subclavian, carotid, and renal arteries.
- It leads to vessel wall thickening, stenosis, occlusion, or aneurysm formation.
- The etiology is unknown.
- It is more common in women (female: male ratio 8:1) between 25–30 years.
- Clinical features are claudication with systemic symptoms (fever, arthralgia and weight loss). There may be absent pulses and bruits.
- Investigations show high ESR and anemia. Angiography shows coarctation, occlusion and aneurysmal dilatation.
- Treatment is with steroids (oral prednisolone). Additional therapy with methotrexate or cyclophosphamide is usually required.

Q. Discuss the etiology, clinical features, diagnosis, and management of polyarteritis nodosa (PAN).

- PAN is a systemic necrotizing vasculitis which mainly affects medium-sized arteries.
- It affects all age groups, with a peak incidence in the fourth and fifth decades.
- It is more common in males (male: female ratio of 2:1).

Etiology

- Primary type is idiopathic which accounts for most cases.
- Secondary type is due to hepatitis B and C, HIV, hairy cell leukemia, drugs (e.g. minocycline, sulfonamides).

Pathology

- Inflammation of vessel wall leads to narrowing of the lumen and occlusion of the vessel. Inflammation also leads to weakening of vessel wall leading to aneurysmal dilatation at multiple points which gives rise to string of beads appearance in angiogram **(Fig. 10.12)**.

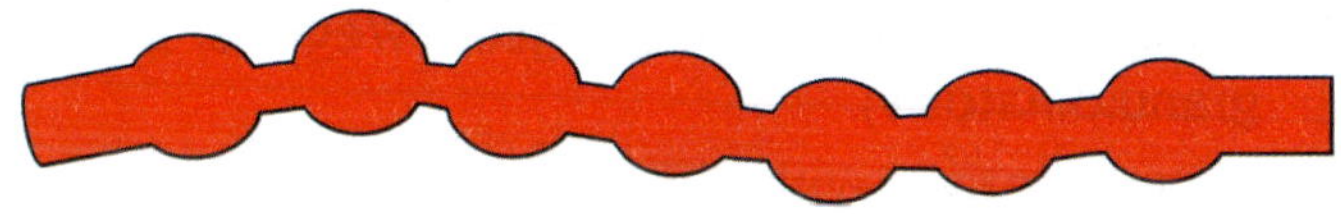

Figure 10.12: String of beads appearance

Clinical Features

- *Systemic symptoms:* Fever, weight loss, arthralgia and myalgia.
- *Skin lesions:* Palpable purpura, ulceration, livedo reticularis, infarction and gangrene of fingers or toes.
- *Nervous system:* Involvement of vasa nervosum (vessels supplying nerves) leads to neuropathy which commonly presents as mononeuritis multiplex. CNS involvement can present with headache, seizures and ischemic stroke.
- *Cardiac:* Involvement of coronary arteries can cause angina and heart failure.
- *Gastrointestinal:* Vasculitis of the liver or gallbladder causes right upper quadrant pain. Vasculitis of mesenteric arteries causes abdominal pain, bloody diarrhea, malabsorption, intestinal perforation, and acute abdomen.
- *Renal:* Hypertension, oliguria, uremia. Renal failure may occur due to multiple renal infarctions.
- *Genital:* Orchitis with testicular pain and tenderness can occur.

Diagnosis

- Raised ESR and anemia
- Angiography shows multiple aneurysms and smooth narrowing of medium sized arteries such as mesenteric, hepatic or renal arteries.
- Testing for hepatitis B and C
- Anti-neutrophil cytoplasmic antibodies (ANCA) are usually absent.
- Autoantibody testing to rule out other connective tissue diseases which can cause vasculitis. These are ANCA, rheumatoid factor, anticyclic citrullinated peptides (CCP), ANA, complement levels, anti-Smith, anti-Ro/SSA, anti-La/SSB, and anti-RNP), etc.
- Urinalysis may show proteinuria and hematuria. RBC casts are absent because there is no glomerular involvement.
- Angiography (renal, mesenteric, hepatic arteries): Microaneurysms, stenosis, occlusion, "beading" appearance.
- CT/MR angiography can also be used.
- Tissue biopsy (muscle or sural nerve) may show vessel wall inflammation.

Treatment

- Steroids and cyclophosphamide to control vessel wall inflammation.
- Treat the underlying cause such as hepatitis B or C infection.

Q. Granulomatosis with polyangiitis (Wegener's granulomatosis).

- Granulomatosis with polyangiitis (formerly known as Wegener's granulomatosis) is a type of small and medium-sized vasculitis characterized by necrotizing granulomatous vasculitis which predominantly affects respiratory tract and kidneys.

Etiology

- Autoimmune in origin
- Often associated with cytoplasmic ANCA (c-ANCA).

Pathogenesis

- Environmental or infectious trigger → activation of neutrophils
- ANCA antibodies (esp. PR3-ANCA) bind neutrophils → release of lytic enzymes → endothelial damage
- Leads to necrotizing granulomatous inflammation of vessels and surrounding tissue.

Clinical Features

- Most common presentation is with upper airway involvement which may produce epistaxis, nasal crusting and sinusitis, mucosal ulceration and deafness due to serous otitis media. Untreated nasal disease leads to destruction of bone and cartilage.
- Lower respiratory tract involvement may produce cough, dyspnea and hemoptysis.
- Renal involvement produces acute glomerulonephritis, hematuria, and proteinuria.
- Proptosis may be present due to inflammation of the retro-orbital tissue.

Investigations

- Chest X-ray: Migratory pulmonary infiltrates and nodules.
- C-ANCA (cytoplasmic antineutrophil cytoplasmic antibodies) is usually positive.
- Biopsy of the involved tissue: Lung biopsy may show characteristic necrotizing granulomatous vasculitis. Renal biopsy may show necrotizing crescentic glomerulonephritis without immunoglobulin deposition (pauci-immune).

Treatment

- Treatment is same as microscopic polyangiitis.

Q. Eosinophilic granulomatosis with polyangiitis (Churg-Strauss syndrome).

- Eosinophilic granulomatosis with polyangiitis (EGPA, formerly called Churg-Strauss syndrome) is a systemic small and medium vessel vasculitis, characterized by extravascular granulomas, eosinophilia, and tissue infiltration by eosinophils.

Etiology

- Exact cause is unknown. It is probably due to an allergic or autoimmune reaction to an environmental agent or drug.

Clinical Features

- The most common organ involved is lung, followed by skin. However, any organ can get affected.
- Clinical manifestations occur in several sequential phases:
  - Prodromal phase—is characterized by atopic disease, allergic rhinitis, and asthma.
  - Eosinophilic phase—is peripheral blood eosinophilia and eosinophilic infiltration of many organs, especially the lung and gastrointestinal tract.
  - Vasculitic phase—is life-threatening systemic vasculitis of the small and medium vessels. Vasculitis phase may be associated with systemic symptoms such as fever, weight loss, and fatigue.
- Skin manifestations include purpura or nodules.
- Pulmonary infiltrates and pleural or pericardial effusions due to serositis may be present.
- Abdominal symptoms may be present due to mesenteric vasculitis.

Investigations

- Elevated ESR and CRP
- Peripheral blood eosinophilia (>10%)
- Urine shows RBC casts and proteinuria
- Chest X-ray may show infiltrates and pleural or pericardial effusions
- P-ANCA is usually positive
- Biopsy of the affected tissue shows vasculitis with extravascular eosinophils.

Treatment

- Same as microscopic polyangiitis.

Q. Henoch-Schönlein purpura (HSP) or IgA vasculitis.

- HSP (now called IgA vasculitis) is a small vessel vasculitis which mainly occurs in children and young adults.
- HSP is self-limited in majority of cases.

Etiology

Often follows infections or immune triggers:

- Preceding upper respiratory tract infection (especially group A Streptococcus).
- Viral infections (e.g. Parvovirus B19)
- Drugs (e.g. antibiotics)
- Vaccinations
- Foods and insect bites (rare).

Pathogenesis

- Immune complex (IgA1)-mediated vasculitis
- Deposition of IgA immune complexes in small vessel walls → complement activation (especially alternate pathway) → inflammation
- Predominantly involves dermal capillaries, glomerular mesangium, and GI submucosal vessels.

Clinical Features

- Typically seen in children (age 3–15) but may affect adults.
- The classic tetrad of HSP includes—palpable purpura, arthritis/arthralgia, abdominal pain and renal disease. The onset usually follows an upper respiratory tract infection.
- Palpable purpura is due to vasculitis involving skin blood vessels and mainly found over the buttocks and lower legs.
- Abdominal symptoms include colicky pain and bleeding.
- Arthritis/arthralgia usually involves knee or ankle.
- Renal involvement produces hematuria, proteinuria and in some cases renal failure.

Investigations

- ESR and CRP are elevated.
- Serum IgA levels may be elevated.
- Abnormal renal function tests and proteinuria.
- Biopsy of the skin (purpuric spot) or kidney may show IgA deposition within and around blood vessel walls.

Treatment

- Steroids are effective for gastrointestinal and joint involvement.
- Renal involvement requires treatment with both pulse IV steroids and immunosuppressants (cyclophosphamide, azathioprine).
- Plasmapheresis may be effective in delaying the progression of kidney disease.

Q. Behçet disease.

- Behçet disease is a chronic, relapsing, autoimmune disease characterized by triple-symptom complex of recurrent oral aphthous ulcers, genital ulcers, and uveitis.

Etiology

- Exact cause is unknown.
- Immunologic (including autoimmune) and viral or bacterial triggers have been suggested, and HLA-B51 is associated with some cases.

Clinical Features

- Behçet disease involves multiple systems. The most common feature is the presence of recurrent mucocutaneous ulcers.
- *Oral ulcerations*: Most patients have recurrent oral aphthous ulcerations. The ulcers are painful and range in size from a few millimeters to two centimeters. These ulcers heal spontaneously but recur again and again.
- *Genital ulcers*: These are similar to oral ulcers and are painful. They commonly occur on the scrotum and vulva.
- *Skin lesions*: They include acneiform lesions, papulo-vesiculo-pustular eruptions, nodules, erythema nodosum, superficial thrombophlebitis, and pyoderma gangrenosum. Pathergy refers to an erythematous papular or pustular response to local skin injury. It is defined as a greater than 5 mm lesion that appears 24–48 hours after skin prick by a needle.
- *Ocular disease*: Uveitis is the main feature. It is bilateral and episodic. Other manifestations are retinal vasculitis, vascular occlusion, and optic neuritis. All these may lead to blindness if untreated.
- *Vascular disease*: Behçet's disease can involve blood vessels of all sizes. Most clinical manifestations of Behçet's disease are believed to be due to vasculitis.
- Other features are arthritis, meningoencephalitis, epididymitis, intestinal ulcerations, renal, cardiac and lung involvement.

Diagnosis

Criteria for the diagnosis of Behçet disease

Recurrent oral ulcers (≥3 episodes/year) plus any two of:

- Recurrent genital ulcers
- Eye lesions (anterior/posterior uveitis or retinal vasculitis)
- Skin lesions (erythema nodosum, papulopustular, acneiform)
- Positive Pathergy test

Treatment

- Oral ulcers are treated with topical steroid preparations. Thalidomide is very effective for resistant oral and genital ulceration but is teratogenic and neurotoxic.
- Colchicine is effective for erythema nodosum and arthralgia.
- Systemic disease requires oral steroids with other immunosuppressive drugs.

Q. Fibromyalgia (myofascial pain syndrome; fibrositis; fibromyositis).

- Fibromyalgia is a chronic pain disorder of unknown etiology. It is a very common cause of multiple regional musculoskeletal pain and disability.

Etiology/Risk Factors

- Exact etiology is unknown but is multifactorial.
- Current evidence suggests fibromyalgia may be a centrally mediated disorder of pain sensitivity with enhanced pain perception.
- Risk factors are genetic predisposition, psychosocial stresses, sleep disturbances, infections, and psychiatric comorbidities (e.g. depression, anxiety).
- It may be associated with other chronic pain disorders like: Irritable bowel syndrome (IBS), chronic fatigue syndrome, and temporomandibular joint (TMJ) disorders.

Pathophysiology

- Abnormal central pain processing: Hyperexcitability of neurons in the dorsal horn of the spinal cord.
- Decreased pain threshold.
- Increased substance P, decreased serotonin, norepinephrine, and dopamine in CSF.
- Dysregulation of HPA (hypothalamic-pituitary-adrenal) axis.

Clinical Features

- It is more common in females and increases with age.
- Widespread musculoskeletal pain (lasting >3 months). Pain does not respond to analgesics and NSAIDs. Reduced threshold to pain perception and tolerance are present.
- Fatigability is another major problem. Often severe, unrefreshing sleep.
- Tender points: Pain on pressure at specific sites (e.g. neck, shoulders, elbows, hips, knees).
- Cognitive symptoms: "Fibro fog"—memory/concentration difficulties.
- Examination of musculoskeletal and neurological system is normal. The main finding is hyperalgesia at tender sites.
- Other features are low mood, irritability, weepiness, swelling of hands and fingers, numbness and tingling of fingers, nonthrobbing bifrontal headache.

Investigations

- Mainly to exclude other causes
- CBC, ESR, CRP—typically normal
- TSH—to rule out hypothyroidism
- ANA, RF—to exclude autoimmune diseases
- Polysomnography (if sleep disorder suspected).

Differential Diagnosis

- Chronic fatigue syndrome (CFS) can cause similar generalized myalgias and fatigue and laboratory test results are typically normal.
- Polymyalgia rheumatica can cause generalized myalgias. However, it usually affects older adults, tends to affect proximal muscles selectively, and ESR is high.

Management

Nonpharmacological (mainstay of treatment)

- Patient education and reassurance
- Aerobic exercise (e.g. walking, swimming, cycling)
- Cognitive behavioral therapy (CBT)
- Sleep hygiene
- Yoga, tai chi, acupuncture, and meditation
- Physiotherapy.

Pharmacological

- Tricyclic antidepressants (e.g. *Amitriptyline*)
- SNRIs: *Duloxetine*, *Milnacipran*
- Anticonvulsants: *Pregabalin*, *Gabapentin*
- NSAIDs: Limited benefit, mostly for associated symptoms.

Q. Polymyalgia rheumatica (PMR).

- Polymyalgia rheumatica is a rheumatic condition associated with muscle pain and stiffness and, an increased ESR.
- It is not a true vasculitis but there is a close association with giant cell arteritis. Polymyalgia rheumatica occurs in about 50% of patients with giant cell arteritis.
- People over 50 years of age are mainly affected. Women are affected more often than men (3:1 ratio).

Etiology and Pathogenesis

- Exact cause unknown
- Suspected immune-mediated inflammatory process
- Genetic predisposition (e.g. HLA-DR4)
- Overlaps with giant cell arteritis, possibly representing different manifestations of the same disease spectrum.
- Triggered by environmental factors (e.g. infections).

Clinical Features

- Main features are subacute or chronic onset of muscle stiffness and pain in the shoulders, hip girdles, neck and torso in patients over the age of 50. There is marked early morning stiffness, often with night pain. No synovitis or joint swelling.
- Examination shows stiffness and restriction of active movements but passive movements are normal. There may be muscle tenderness but no muscle-wasting. If muscle wasting is there, then primary muscle or neurological disease should be suspected.
- Systemic features are weight loss, fatigue, and night sweats.

Investigations

- Elevated ESR and CRP
- Normochromic, normocytic anemia
- RF, anti-CCP, ANA: Negative (to rule out RA/SLE).

Management

- Treatment is with steroids (prednisolone). There is dramatic response within 72 hours. If there is no response by 72 hours or an incomplete response by 7 days, then other conditions should be suspected.
- Most patients need steroids for an average of 12–18 months. Immunosuppressants such as methotrexate or azathioprine can be considered if steroids cannot be withdrawn at 2 years.

Q. Antineutrophil cytoplasmic antibodies (ANCA).

- ANCA are autoantibodies directed against certain proteins in the cytoplasm of neutrophils and monocytes. They are mainly of the IgG type.
- There are two major types of ANCA: c-ANCA and p-ANCA. C-ANCA (cytoplasmic ANCA) refers to cytoplasmic staining pattern observed by immunofluorescence microscopy when serum antibodies bind to indicator neutrophils. P-ANCA (perinuclear ANCA) refers to perinuclear or nuclear staining pattern of the indicator neutrophils.

Significance

- ANCA are positive in systemic vasculitis syndromes, particularly Wegener's granulomatosis and microscopic polyangiitis, and in patients with necrotizing and crescentic glomerulonephritis.

- ANCA can also be positive in nonvasculitic rheumatic diseases such as rheumatoid arthritis, systemic lupus erythematosus (SLE), Sjögren's syndrome, etc. Hence, ANCA positivity alone is not diagnostic of vasculitis.
- The levels of ANCA do not correlate with disease activity.

Q. Antinuclear antibodies (ANA).

- ANA are autoantibodies directed against various nuclear antigens. They are a hallmark of systemic autoimmune diseases, especially systemic lupus erythematosus (SLE).

Conditions Associated with Positive ANA

Systemic autoimmune diseases
- Systemic lupus erythematosus (SLE)
- Scleroderma
- Mixed connective tissue disease
- Polymyositis/dermatomyositis
- Rheumatoid arthritis
- Sjögren's syndrome

Specific organ autoimmune disease
- Hashimoto's thyroiditis
- Graves' disease
- Autoimmune hepatitis
- Primary biliary cirrhosis
- Idiopathic pulmonary arterial hypertension

Infections
- Hepatitis C infection
- Subacute bacterial endocarditis
- Tuberculosis
- HIV infection

Significance

- ANA is a screening test for autoimmune connective tissue diseases.
- Very high concentrations of antibody (titer >1:640) should arouse suspicion of an autoimmune disorder even in a patient without any symptoms.
- ANA is also useful to monitor disease activity and to determine the specific type of disease.

Types of ANA

Certain types of antinuclear antibodies are somewhat specific to certain diseases. The main types of ANA are as follows:
- *Antibodies to double-stranded DNA (anti dsDNA)*: These are found in SLE and rheumatoid arthritis.
- *Antibodies to histone proteins*: These are found in SLE and drug-induced lupus.
- *Antibodies to chromatin*: These are especially prevalent in SLE patients with renal disease.

False-positive Tests

- The ANA test is said to be false positive when a person tests positive but does not have any other features of autoimmune disease. False-positive result occurs often in women and elderly people. Drugs such as hydralazine, isoniazid, and procainamide can cause false-positive results.

Q. Antiphospholipid syndrome (antiphospholipid antibody syndrome; APLA).

- The antiphospholipid syndrome (APS) also known as antiphospholipid antibody syndrome (APLA) is a multisystemic autoimmune disorder. It is characterized by the presence of antiphospholipid antibodies (APLA), arterial and venous thrombosis, and recurrent abortions.
- These antiphospholipid antibodies (APLA) include lupus anticoagulant ((also known as lupus antibody) and anticardiolipin (aCL) antibody. The antibodies in APLS have prothrombotic effect and also have action on vascular tone causing the clinical manifestations of APLS.

Etiology

- APLS can be primary without any underlying cause or it can be secondary to an underlying cause which are as follows.
- *Autoimmune diseases:* SLE, Sjögren syndrome, rheumatoid arthritis.
- *Infections:* syphilis, Hepatitis C infection, HIV infection
- *Drugs:* Procainamide, quinidine, propranolol, hydralazine, phenytoin, chlorpromazine.
- *Genetic predisposition:* Relatives of persons with known APS are more likely to have APS.
- *HLA associations:* individuals who carry certain HLA genes *DR7* and *DR4 have increased risk of developing APS.*

Clinical Features

- These patients may have a variety of clinical manifestations including venous and arterial thrombosis, recurrent fetal losses, neurologic events, and thrombocytopenia.
- *Thrombotic events:* Deep vein thrombosis and pulmonary embolism, ischemic stroke, peripheral and intra-abdominal vascular occlusion.
- *Obstetric complications:* Recurrent spontaneous abortions and fetal growth retardation, which probably are due to thrombosis of placental vessels.
- Catastrophic APS1 is the most severe form of APS with clinical evidence of multiple organ involvement developing over a short time with histopathological evidence of small vessel occlusions. It is a medical emergency with high mortality.

Diagnosis

- Diagnosis of antiphospholipid syndrome is based on a combination of clinical history and laboratory testing. APLS should be suspected if there is:
  - Occurrence of one or more otherwise unexplained thrombotic or thromboembolic events.
  - Recurrent abortions.
  - Unexplained thrombocytopenia or prolongation of a test of blood coagulation (e.g. PT or aPTT).
- Presence of lupus anticoagulant and anticardiolipin antibodies should be tested.

Treatment

Prophylactic Therapy to Prevent Thrombosis

- Long-term anticoagulation: Warfarin or any other oral anticoagulant.
- Low-dose aspirin or clopidogrel can be added in arterial disease.
- Lifelong treatment may be required for patients with recurrent thrombotic events.

Pregnant Women with APS

- Treatment of antiphospholipid syndrome during pregnancy reduces the risks of pregnancy loss, preeclampsia, placental insufficiency, preterm birth, and thrombosis. Women with antiphospholipid syndrome and no history of thrombosis should receive heparin and low-dose aspirin during pregnancy and for six to eight weeks postpartum. Patients who require heparin administration throughout pregnancy should receive calcium and vitamin D supplementation to help avoid heparin-induced osteoporosis.
- Some studies have shown that aspirin alone is as efficacious as heparin plus aspirin.

Q. Lupus anticoagulant.

- Lupus anticoagulant (LA) is a type of antiphospholipid antibody that interferes with phospholipid-dependent coagulation tests in vitro but paradoxically increases the risk of thrombosis *in vivo*. It is one of the diagnostic antibodies in antiphospholipid syndrome (APS).
- It is an IgG or IgM autoantibody.

Associated Conditions

- Antiphospholipid syndrome (APS)
- Systemic lupus erythematosus (SLE)
- Infections (e.g. HIV, hepatitis C)
- Malignancies
- Drug-induced (e.g. chlorpromazine, phenytoin, quinidine).

Clinical Significance

- Thrombosis: Arterial or venous (e.g. DVT, stroke, PE).
- Pregnancy morbidity: Recurrent fetal loss, preeclampsia, IUGR.
- Prolonged aPTT without bleeding tendency.
- May cause false-positive VDRL test (due to anticardiolipin activity).

Testing for Lupus Anticoagulant

- Presence of lupus anticoagulant should be suspected in cases of a markedly prolonged APTT without clinical bleeding. APTT fails to correct when the patient's plasma is mixed with normal plasma.
- The Russell viper venom (RVV) time is test of choice to detect the presence of lupus anticoagulant.

Treatment

- Asymptomatic patients do not require treatment unless high-risk.
- Anticoagulant therapy should be started for patients with thrombosis. Heparin therapy is difficult to monitor due to already prolonged APTT and hence, low-molecular-weight heparin is preferred.
- LA in pregnancy: Use low-dose aspirin + LMWH to prevent obstetric complications.

Q. Enumerate the causes of low backache.

Mechanical Problems

- Lumber strain
- Degenerative process of disks and facets
- Intervertebral disc prolapse
- Spinal stenosis
- Osteoporotic compression fracture
- Spondylolisthesis
- Traumatic fracture
- Congenital disease (severe kyphosis and scoliosis)
- Spondylolysis.

Nonmechanical Problems

- Neoplasia (multiple myeloma, metastatic carcinoma, lymphoma, leukemia, etc.)
- Infection (osteomyelitis, discitis, paraspinal abscess, shingles)
- Inflammatory arthritis (ankylosing spondylitis, psoriatic spondylitis)
- Paget's disease of bone.

Visceral Disease

- Disease of pelvic organs (prostatitis, endometriosis, pelvic inflammatory disease)
- Renal disease (nephrolithiasis, pyelonephritis, perinephric abscess)
- Aortic aneurysm
- Gastrointestinal disease (pancreatitis, cholecystitis, penetrating ulcer).

Chapter 11

Nutritional Disorders

Q. Nutritional assessment in adults.

- Nutritional assessment is the systematic evaluation of an individual's dietary intake, physical status, and biochemical data to determine nutritional status.

Components of Nutritional Assessment (A useful mnemonic is "ABCD")

- A–Anthropometry: Measurement of body size and composition.
- B–Biochemical tests: Lab tests to assess nutritional status.
- C–Clinical examination: Physical signs of malnutrition.
- D–Dietary assessment: Evaluation of food intake.

Anthropometric Measurements (Table 11.1)

TABLE 11.1: Anthropometric measurements

Parameter	Normal range
Body weight	Varies with height, sex, and age; compare with ideal body weight (IBW) for assessment
Height	For BMI calculation
Body mass index (BMI)	Weight (kg)/Height^2 (m^2) Normal 8.5–24.9
Mid-upper arm circumference (MUAC)	Assesses muscle mass. Normal 23.5–32 cm. <23.5 cm suggests undernutrition
Skinfold thickness (triceps, biceps)	Estimates subcutaneous fat stores. Normal: Males: 12–20 mm, Females: 16–25
Waist-hip ratio	Assesses central obesity. This is a better predictor of cardiovascular/metabolic risk than BMI alone. Normal: Males: <0.90, Females: <0.85
Weight loss (%)	Significant if >5% over 6 months

Biochemical Parameters (Table 11.2)

TABLE 11.2: Biochemical parameters

Test	Usefulness
Serum albumin	Chronic protein malnutrition (↓ in illness)
Prealbumin (transthyretin)	Short-term marker of protein status
Transferrin	Protein status, iron transport
Total lymphocyte count	Immunity status, protein-energy malnutrition
CRP (C-reactive protein)	Helps interpret nutritional markers (e.g. albumin)
Micronutrients	Iron, B_{12}, folate, vitamin D, zinc

Clinical Assessment

Looks for signs of malnutrition:

- Pallor
- Muscle wasting, loss of fat
- Skin changes: Dry, scaly, hyperpigmented
- Hair: Dry, thin, sparse
- Mouth: Cheilitis, glossitis
- Edema (protein deficiency)
- Functional decline (handgrip strength).

Dietary Assessment (Table 11.3)

TABLE 11.3: Dietary assessment

Method	Description
24-hour recall	Patient recalls all food in past 24 hours
Food frequency questionnaire	Frequency of various foods over time
Food diary (3–7 days)	Self-reported log of food intake
Calorie counts	Often done in hospital setting

Q. Body mass index (BMI).

- Body mass index (BMI) is a measure of weight adjusted for height, calculated as weight in kilograms divided by the square of height in meters (kg/m^2). Although BMI is often considered an indicator of body fatness, it is a surrogate measure of body fat because it measures excess weight rather than excess fat.

$$\text{BMI} = \frac{\text{Weight (kg)}}{\text{Height (m)}^2}$$

Uses of BMI

- BMI is a simple, inexpensive, and noninvasive surrogate measure of body fat which can be used bedside.
- BMI levels correlate with body fat and with future health risks. High BMI predicts future morbidity and death. Therefore, BMI is an appropriate measure for screening for obesity and its health risks.
- Use of BMI at the population level has resulted in an increased availability of published population data that allows public health professionals to make comparisons across time, regions, and population subgroups.

Limitations of BMI

- BMI is a surrogate measure of body fatness because it is a measure of excess weight rather than excess body fat.
- Factors such as age, sex, ethnicity, and muscle mass can influence the relationship between BMI and body fat.
- Cannot assess fat distribution (visceral *vs.* subcutaneous).
- BMI does not distinguish between excess fat, muscle, or bone mass. For example, older adults tend to have more body fat than younger adults for an equivalent BMI. Women have more body fat than men with the same BMI. Muscular individuals may have a high BMI because of increased muscle mass.

Interpretation of BMI

BMI	Interpretation
<18.5	Underweight
18.5–24.9	Normal
25–29.9	Overweight
30–34.9	Obese class I
35–39.9	Obese class II
>40	Obese class III (extreme obesity)

Alternatives to BMI

- Other measures of body fat, such as skinfold thicknesses, bioelectrical impedance, underwater weighing, and dual energy X-ray absorption, may be more accurate than BMI. But, most of these methods are cumbersome for routine clinical use.

Q. Describe the calorie requirements of normal person.

Calorie Requirement

- The average requirement for men is around 2500 kcal/day and for women, it is 2000 kcal. This requirement is not static and depends on many factors which are as follows:
  - Age
  - Gender
  - Height
  - Weight
  - Physical activity
  - Certain conditions like pregnancy or lactation.
- Simple formula to calculate calorie requirement for healthy adults:

Calorie Needs	Kcal/kg/day
Sedentary	25–30 kcal/kg
Moderately active	30–35 kcal/kg
Very active	35–40+ kcal/kg

Macronutrient Distribution for Healthy Adult

Carbohydrate

- At least 45–55% of total calories should be derived from carbohydrates.

Protein

- For adults, the recommended dietary allowance (RDA) for protein is about 0.6 g/kg desirable body mass per day. Current recommendations for a healthy diet call for at least 10–14% of calories from protein.

Fat

- Fats are a concentrated source of energy. For optimal health, fat intake should not be more than 30% of calories. Saturated fat and transfat should be limited to <10% of calories, and polyunsaturated fats to <10% of calories, with monounsaturated fats comprising the remainder of fat intake.

Water Intake

- The daily recommended water intake for men and women is 3.7 L/day and 2.7 L/day, respectively.

Other Nutrients

- Such as fiber, vitamins and minerals should be taken in the recommended quantity.

Q. Discuss the causes and consequences of protein-calorie malnutrition in the hospital.

Introduction

- Protein-calorie malnutrition (PCM)—also called Protein-energy malnutrition (PEM)—in hospitalized patients is a common but often under-recognized problem. It refers to inadequate intake or assimilation of protein and calories, resulting in tissue wasting and functional decline.
- Prevalence: Up to 30–60% of hospitalized patients have some degree of PCM.
- At-risk groups: Elderly, critically ill, surgical patients, cancer patients, and those with chronic diseases.

Causes of Protein-calorie Malnutrition in the Hospital

Inadequate nutritional intake

- Poor appetite/anorexia due to illness, medications (e.g. opioids, chemotherapy).
- Nil per oral (NPO) status for procedures or investigations.
- Dysphagia (e.g. stroke, neurological disorders)
- Altered mental status or coma
- Depression or delirium
- Unpalatable hospital food or dietary restrictions.

Increased Nutritional Requirements

- Sepsis and systemic infections
- Surgery and trauma
- Burns, wounds, pressure ulcers
- Fever, inflammation, or catabolic states
- Malignancy or chronic inflammatory diseases (e.g. IBD, TB).

Nutrient Losses

- Vomiting, diarrhea
- Fistulas or drainage tubes
- Renal replacement therapy (dialysis)
- GI bleeding or malabsorption (e.g. celiac disease, pancreatitis).

Malabsorption and Maldigestion

- Pancreatic insufficiency
- Short bowel syndrome
- Chronic liver disease
- Post-surgical states (e.g. gastric bypass).

Iatrogenic Factors

- Polypharmacy affecting appetite or GI function
- Prolonged use of IV fluids without nutritional value ("IV starvation")
- Over-restriction (e.g. diabetic or renal diets).

Consequences of Protein-calorie Malnutrition in the Hospital

- *Immunological consequences:* Impaired immune response, increased susceptibility to infections (e.g. pneumonia, wound infection, sepsis), delayed recovery from infections
- *Musculoskeletal and functional decline:* Loss of lean body mass and muscle wasting, weakness, fatigue
- *Impaired wound healing:* Delayed recovery after surgery or trauma
- *Hematologic effects:* Anemia (iron, B_{12}, folate deficiency), impaired oxygen delivery and reduced healing capacity
- *Gastrointestinal effects:* Mucosal atrophy, malabsorption, decreased digestive enzyme production
- *Metabolic and endocrine effects:* Electrolyte imbalances (e.g. hypokalemia, hypophosphatemia), hypoglycemia
- *Psychological and cognitive effects:* Depression, apathy, confusion
- *Increased morbidity and mortality:* Prolonged hospital stay, increased complications, increased mortality, especially in ICU or surgical patients.

Prevention and Management

Nutritional Assessment

- Within 24–48 hours of hospital admission.

Nutritional Support

- Oral nutrition: High-protein, high-calorie diets; oral nutritional supplements.
- Enteral feeding: Nasogastric, PEG tube if oral intake is inadequate.
- Parenteral nutrition: If GI tract is nonfunctional.
- Micronutrient supplementation: Vitamins and trace elements.

Q. Describe nutritional assessment and calorie requirement during illness.

- During illness, energy needs increase due to stress metabolism, tissue repair, fever, infection, and inflammation. Proper nutrition is needed to prevent and recover from illness. Malnutrition during illness deceases immunity; increases susceptibility to nosocomial infections; decreases wound healing and promotes organ failure.
- Caloric estimation helps guide nutritional support.
- Nutrition support refers to oral, enteral, or parenteral provision of calories, protein, electrolytes, vitamins, minerals, trace elements, and fluids.
- Carbohydrates are the preferred energy source during illness because fat mobilization is impaired.

Assessment of Nutritional Status during Illness

- Nutritional Assessment in sick especially critically ill patient is difficult. It can be done by anthropometric measurements, biochemical tools, clinical assessment, and dietary assessment as is done for a normal individual (remember ABCD).

Anthropometric Measurements

- It measures the current nutritional status.
- Body weight: 10% loss is considered significant, 20% loss is considered critical, and 30% loss is considered lethal.
- Other measurements include mid-arm circumference, skinfold thickness, head-circumference, head chest ratio, and BMI (body mass index). BMI is an independent predictor of mortality in seriously ill patients.

Biochemical Tests

- Measuring hemoglobin, albumin, transferrin, prealbumin, lymphocyte count. Decreased levels correlate with malnutrition.

Clinical Assessment

- It is the simplest and most practical method.
- Nutritional history, general physical examination, loss of subcutaneous fat (chest and triceps), and presence of edema and ascites are often found in malnutrition.

Dietary Assessment

- It can be assessed by 24 hours dietary recall, frequency of food intake, and actual observation of food intake.

Nutritional Requirements

Calorie Requirements

- Energy requirements depend on the severity of illness as follows;
- Normal requirements: 25–30 kcal/kg/day
- Mild stress (e.g. minor surgery): 30–35 kcal/kg/day
- Moderate stress (e.g. sepsis): 35–40 kcal/kg/day
- Severe stress (e.g. burns, trauma): 40–50 kcal/kg/day.

Fluid Requirements

- Baseline water requirement for adults is 30–35 ml/kg/hour. Addition must be made for fever (300–500 ml/24 hour) for 10°C above normal and for other losses.

Protein Requirement

- Normal adult: 0.8–1.0 g/kg/day
- Illness (moderate stress): 1.2–1.5 g/kg/day
- Severe catabolic illness (e.g. burns): up to 2.0 g/kg/day.

Carbohydrate Requirement

- 50–60% of total calories.

Fats

- 20–30% of total calories (monitor triglycerides).

Micronutrients Supplementation

- Micronutrient requirements increase during stress, infection, or inflammation
- Routine supplementation is recommended in critically ill, malnourished, or elderly patients
- Almost all the vitamins and minerals can be supplemented during illness. Fat-soluble vitamins (A, D, E, K) require caution due to toxicity risk.
- Specific illnesses requiring specific micronutrient supplements are as follows:
  - Anemia: Iron, vitamin B_{12}, and folic acid depending on the cause.
  - Sepsis/critical illness: Thiamine, vitamin C, selenium, zinc
  - Burns: High-dose vitamin C, A, zinc
  - Chronic kidney disease: Vitamin D, B-complex (excluding A, E–fat-soluble toxicity risk).
  - Gastrointestinal losses: Electrolytes, vitamin B_{12}, folate.

Route of Nutrition

- Nutritional Support can be given through one of the three routes oral, enteral, and parenteral.

Oral

- If the patient can eat then they should be encouraged to do so. It is the preferred route if the patient can tolerate oral feeds, but it is important to monitor whether he is taking adequate nutrition or not.

Enteral

- Indicated when oral intake has been inadequate for 1–3 days.
- Methods of enteral feeding include nasogastric tube (most common method), nasoduodenal tube, nasojejunal tube, percutaneous feeding gastrostomy and jejunostomy tube.
- Early enteral nutrition (within 24–48 hours after an acute illness) is indicated in severe trauma, major burns, ARDS, cancer surgery, and acute malnutrition.
- There are many commercially prepared feeds available or feeds can be prepared immediately before administration. There are disease specific formulae available: These are usually designed for liver diseases (contain low sodium and altered aminoacids contents to reduce encephalopathy), for renal disease (contain low phosphate and potassium), for respiratory disease (contain high fat to reduce CO_2 production).
- Contraindications include circulatory shock, intestinal ischemia, complete mechanical bowel obstruction or ileus, severe diarrhea, and pancreatitis.

Parenteral Nutrition

- Parenteral nutrition (PN) is the intravenous administration of nutrients—such as glucose, amino acids, lipids, vitamins, and minerals—when the gastrointestinal (GI) tract is non-functional or inaccessible.
- Parenteral nutrition can be given as separate components but is more commonly given as a sterile emulsion of water, protein, lipids, carbohydrates, electrolytes, vitamins and trace elements. It is given through peripheral or central venous line.

Indications for Parenteral Nutrition

- Short bowel syndrome (inadequate bowel length to absorb nutrients)
- Severe intestinal obstruction
- Paralytic ileus
- High-output fistula (>500 ml/day). Feeding worsens output
- Mesenteric ischemia/infarction
- Intractable vomiting/diarrhea
- Severe pancreatitis (acute phase)
- Severe mucositis (e.g. postchemotherapy)
- Postoperative patients (GI surgery).

Monitoring and Reassessment

- Regular weight monitoring
- Serum albumin/prealbumin (trends more useful than absolute values)
- Clinical signs of improvement or deterioration
- Adjust caloric goals based on recovery, complications, or organ failure.

Q. Discuss the classification, etiology, clinical features, investigations and management of malnutrition; protein energy malnutrition (PEM); under-nutrition.

- Malnutrition is a broad term that includes under-nutrition (deficiency) and over-nutrition (excess). The following discussion focuses on under-nutrition, particularly protein-energy malnutrition (PEM), a major public health problem, especially in developing countries.
- BMI less than <18.5 is called undernutrition.

Classification

Undernutrition

- Wasting (low weight-for-height)
- Stunting (low height-for-age)
- Underweight (low weight-for-age).

Micronutrient Deficiencies

- Iron, iodine, vitamin A, zinc, etc.

Etiology of Undernutrition and Weight Loss

- Famine
- Endocrine disorders (hyperthyroidism, pheochromocytoma, adrenal insufficiency)
- Uncontrolled diabetes mellitus
- GI disorders (malabsorption syndromes, chronic pancreatitis, IBD, parasitic infestation)
- Malignancy
- Infections (tuberculosis, HIV, subacute bacterial endocarditis)
- COPD
- Chronic renal failure
- Psychiatric disorders (depression, mania, anorexia nervosa, schizophrenia)
- Chronic alcoholism
- Drugs (opiates, amphetamines, digoxin, metformin, NSAIDs, anticancer drugs)
- Treatment of obesity
- Anorexic drugs amphetamines and derivatives
- Distance runners, models, ballet dancers, gymnasts
- Excessive physical activity (e.g. marathon runners)

Clinical Features

General Features of PEM

- Growth failure
- Muscle wasting
- Fat loss (especially in marasmus)
- Behavioral changes (apathy, irritability)
- Delayed milestones.

Kwashiorkor (protein deficiency)

- Edema (pitting, bilateral)
- Moon face
- Dermatosis (flaky paint skin)
- Hair changes (flag sign, sparse)
- Fatty liver
- Enlarged abdomen
- Apathy and irritability.

Marasmus (calorie and protein deficiency)

- Severe wasting (muscle and fat)
- "Old man" face
- No edema
- Ribs prominent
- Alert but irritable child
- Wrinkled skin, sunken eyes.

Clinical Features of Specific Nutrient Deficiency

(Table 11.4)

TABLE 11.4: Clinical features of specific nutrient deficiency

Nutrient	Features of deficiency
Vitamin A	Night blindness, xeropthalmia, ulceration and necrosis of the cornea (keratomalacia), perforation, endophthalmitis. Xerosis and hyperkeratinization of the skin
Vitamin D	Rickets, osteomalacia
Vitamin E	Areflexia, ataxia, ophthalmoplegia, hemolytic anemia
Vitamin K	Coagulation disorder
Thiamin (Vitamin B_1)	Beriberi, Wernicke-Korsakoff syndrome
Riboflavin (Vitamin B_2)	Cheilosis, angular stomatitis, glossitis
Niacin (vitamin B_3)	Pellagra (dementia, diarrhea, dermatitis)
Vitamin B_6 (Pyridoxine)	Peripheral neuropathy, anemia
Biotin	Dermatitis, alopecia, paranesthesia
Vitamin B_{12} (Cobalamin)	Anemia, peripheral neuropathy, subacute combined degeneration
Vitamin C (Ascorbic acid)	Scurvy
Folate	Anemia
Iron	Anemia, platynychia, koilonychia
Iodine	Goiter
Calcium	Tetany, pathologic fractures due to osteomalacia, muscular irritability
Zinc	Anorexia, weakness, tingling, impaired taste

Investigations

- Mild anemia, leukopenia and thrombocytopenia. ESR is normal unless there is infection
- Low blood glucose
- Plasma free fatty acids are increased and there is ketosis and a mild metabolic acidosis because of breakdown of fat for energy production
- Albumin may be low but concentration is often normal because of normal liver function
- Micronutrients are low: Iron, vitamin A, B_{12}, folate, zinc
- Insulin secretion is low, glucagon and cortisol secretion is high
- Urine has a fixed specific gravity and creatinine excretion becomes low.

- Tests of delayed skin hypersensitivity, e.g. to tuberculin, are falsely negative.
- ECG shows sinus bradycardia and low voltage.

Management

- People with mild malnutrition do not require any active treatment. Those with moderate malnutrition need extra feeding. Severe malnutrition needs hospital care.
- In severe malnutrition, initial efforts should be directed at correcting fluid and electrolyte abnormalities and infections. The second phase of treatment is directed at repletion of protein, carbohydrates, and micronutrients. In severe malnutrition, there is atrophy of the intestinal epithelium and of the exocrine pancreas, and the bile is dilute. Hence, refeeding should be initiated with small amounts of food which is easily digestible. Food should be palatable and similar to the usual staple meal-for example, a cereal with some sugar, milk powder and oil. Either the enteral or parenteral route can be used, although the former is better.
- About 1500–2000 kcal/day will prevent progressive undernutrition, but additional calories are required to regain weight. A weight gain of 5% body weight per month is satisfactory. Patients should be followed up closely.

Q. Causes of weight loss.

- Weight loss refers to a reduction in total body weight. It may be:
  - Intentional: Due to diet, exercise, or lifestyle changes.
  - Unintentional: Significant concern, often indicating underlying illness.
- Unintentional weight loss of >5% of body weight over 6–12 months is considered clinically significant.
- Mild weight loss (<5%) can result from temporary factors (e.g. acute illness, stress). >5 loss often indicates an underlying disease (e.g. malignancy, infection, depression, hyperthyroidism, etc.).

Causes of Weight Loss (Table 11.5)

TABLE 11.5: Causes of weight loss
Nutritional causes
• Starvation or fasting
• Malnutrition (e.g. poverty, poor intake)
• Eating disorders (anorexia nervosa, bulimia)
• Dysphagia (stroke, neurological diseases)
Gastrointestinal causes
• Malabsorption (celiac disease, chronic pancreatitis, inflammatory bowel disease)
• Worm infestation
• Peptic ulcer disease
• Post-surgical: Gastrectomy, bowel resection.
Endocrine causes
• Hyperthyroidism (↑ metabolism)
• Diabetes mellitus (uncontrolled)
• Adrenal insufficiency (Addison's disease)
• Pheochromocytoma
Infectious diseases
• Tuberculosis
• HIV/AIDS
• Chronic fungal or parasitic infections
• Endocarditis
Neoplastic causes (cancers)
• Any advanced malignancy
Psychiatric causes
• Depression and anxiety
• Dementia or Alzheimer's disease
• Schizophrenia
• Substance abuse (alcohol, cocaine, amphetamines)
• Anorexia nervosa or bulimia nervosa
Chronic organ diseases
• Chronic kidney disease
• Chronic liver disease (cirrhosis)
• Heart failure
• Chronic obstructive pulmonary disease (COPD)
Medication-related causes
• Chemotherapy or radiation therapy
• Antidepressants or antipsychotics
• Anti-TB drugs
• Digoxin, levodopa
• Amphetamines or laxative abuse
Social and environmental causes
• Poverty, neglect, or abuse
• Old age and isolation

(Contd.)

(Contd.)

Q. Define obesity.

Q. Discuss the etiology, clinical features, complications, investigations and management of obesity.

- Obesity is a chronic, multifactorial disease characterized by excessive accumulation of body fat.
- Obesity is one of the most common disorders in medical practice and among the most frustrating and difficult to manage.

Diagnosis of Obesity

- Accurate quantification of body fat requires sophisticated techniques but physical examination is usually sufficient to detect excess body fat.

Body Mass Index (BMI)

- Body mass index (BMI) closely correlates with excess adipose tissue and obesity can be graded based on BMI.
- BMI ≥30 kg/m² defines obesity (as per WHO). Indian criteria define BMI ≥25 kg/m² as obese, unlike the global WHO threshold of ≥30. Due to higher body fat percentage and central obesity in South Asians, lower BMI cut-offs are recommended for Indians.

Waist Circumference (WC)

- Abdominal obesity is a greater health hazard than generalized obesity. Visceral fat within the abdominal cavity is more hazardous to health than subcutaneous fat.

- Assesses abdominal (central) obesity, which is a key concern in Indians.
- Gender cutoff for central obesity: Men >90 cm, Women >80 cm.

Waist-to-hip Ratio (WHR)

- Also indicates central fat distribution.
- Gender High Risk WHR: Men >0.90, Women >0.85.

Etiology/Risk Factors

- Obesity is the result of an imbalance between daily energy intake and energy expenditure resulting in excessive weight gain. There are multiple factors which can cause obesity which are as follows.

Modifiable Risk Ractors

These are factors that can be changed or controlled.

- Sedentary lifestyle
- Dietary factors: Overeating, high fat diet
- Endocrine disorders: Hypothalamic disease, hypothyroidism, Cushing's syndrome, polycystic ovary syndrome, hypogonadism.
- Psychiatric disorders: Night eating syndrome, binge-eating.
- Drugs: Steroids, clozapine, amitriptyline, cyproheptadine, thiazolidinediones.

Nonmodifiable Risk Factors

These are inherent or genetic factors not easily influenced by lifestyle changes.

- Genetic factors: Mutations in leptin, leptin receptor, interaction of multiple genes with environmental triggers.
- Age: Basal metabolic rate (BMR) decreases with age.
- Sex: Females have higher body fat percentage than males. Hormonal changes (e.g. menopause) affect fat distribution.
- Ethnicity: South Asians, including Indians, have higher central fat at lower BMI, increasing risk of metabolic syndrome.
- Family history of obesity: Increases the likelihood of being obese due to shared genes and lifestyle.

Grading of Obesity

BMI	Classification
18.5–24.9	Normal
25–29.9	Overweight
30–34.9	Mild obesity
35–39.9	Moderate obesity
>40	Extreme obesity

Pathophysiology

- Association of genetics and obesity is already well established.
- Leptin is an adipocyte hormone which reduces food intake and body weight. Cellular leptin resistance is associated with obesity.
- Adipose tissue secretes adipokines and free fatty acids causing systemic inflammation which causes insulin resistance and increased triglyceride level which subsequently contributes to obesity. Adipocytes have prothrombotic activity which can increase the risk of strokes.
- Obesity can cause increased fatty acid deposition in the myocardium causing left ventricular dysfunction. It has also been shown to alter the renin-angiotensin system causing increasing salt retention and elevated blood pressure.
- Adiponectin has insulin-sensitizing and anti-inflammatory properties and its levels are low in those with visceral obesity.

Clinical Features

General Features

- Increased body weight
- Fat accumulation (central or generalized)
- Shortness of breath on exertion
- Fatigue, reduced exercise tolerance
- Excessive sweating.

Associated Signs

- Acanthosis nigricans (insulin resistance)
- Striae, hirsutism (esp. in PCOS)
- Joint pain (esp. knees, hips)
- Snoring/sleep apnea.

Complications of Obesity

- Hypertension
- Type 2 diabetes mellitus
- Hyperlipidemia
- Coronary artery disease
- Degenerative joint disease (osteoarthritis)
- Increased incidence of cancers (colon, rectum, and prostate in men; uterus, biliary tract, breast, and ovary in women)
- Thromboembolic disorders
- Digestive tract diseases (gallstones, reflux esophagitis)
- Nonalcoholic steatohepatitis (NASH)
- Obstructive sleep apnea
- Respiratory failure (Pickwickian syndrome)
- Psychosocial problems (low self esteem, depression)
- Varicose veins.

Clinical Assessment

History

- Age of onset, recent weight changes
- Family history of obesity
- Cigarette and alcohol use
- Complete nutrition history
- Physical activity
- Sleep patterns
- H/o any depression and eating disorders
- Use of any drugs and nutritional supplements.

Physical Examination

- Anthropometric measurements: BMI, waist circumference (>102 cm in men, >88 cm in women = high risk), Waist-hip ratio
- Degree and distribution of body fat, overall nutritional status, and signs of secondary causes of obesity
- Look for any complication of obesity such as hypertension, atherosclerosis, etc.

Investigations

- Blood sugar
- Lipid profile
- Urea, creatinine
- Electrolytes
- Liver function tests (for NAFLD)
- Thyroid function tests and other endocrine work up if necessary
- ECG to look for evidence of coronary artery disease
- Polysomnography (if sleep apnea suspected)
- Ultrasound abdomen (fatty liver, PCOS).

Treatment

- Obesity needs multiprong treatment strategies and may require lifelong treatment.

Dietary Therapy

- Calorie-restricted balanced diet (500–1000 kcal/day deficit)
- Emphasis on fruits, vegetables, whole grains, lean protein
- Avoid processed food, sugars, saturated fats.

Exercise

- ≥150 minutes/week moderate-intensity aerobic exercise.
- Increasing energy expenditure through physical activity helps in losing weight. Aerobic exercise is particularly useful for long-term weight maintenance. When compared with no treatment, exercise alone results in small amounts of weight loss. Exercise plus diet results in greater weight loss than diet alone. A greater intensity of exercise causes greater amount of weight loss. Up to 1 hour of moderate exercise per day is associated with long-term weight maintenance in individuals who have successfully lost weight.

Drug Therapy (BMI ≥30, or ≥27 with comorbidities)

- Drug therapy may be considered for those with a BMI greater than 30 or those with BMI >27 with comorbid conditions. Obesity drugs may be used as part of a comprehensive weight loss program.
- Orlistat: This drug inhibits lipase and blocks fat absorption from the GI tract. Orlistat can cause diarrhea, oily stools, and reduced absorption of fat-soluble vitamins. The recommended dose of orlistat is 120 mg three times daily with meals.
- Liraglutide/semaglutide (GLP-1 agonists)
- Naltrexone-bupropion combination
- Metformin (especially in PCOS or insulin resistance).

Liposuction

- Removal of fat by aspiration after injection of saline has been used to remove and contour subcutaneous fat. However, it does not improve insulin sensitivity or risk factors for coronary heart disease.

Surgery

- Bariatric surgery is a treatment option for patients with severe obesity (BMI over 40, or over 35 if obesity-related comorbidities are present). These are as follows:
  - *Gastric banding*: This is a purely restrictive procedure that compartmentalizes the upper stomach by placing a tight, adjustable prosthetic band around the entrance to the stomach **(Fig. 11.1)**. Gastric banding results in less dramatic weight loss than RYGB and fewer short-term complications. Frequent follow-up is required to adjust the gastric band.
  - *Roux-en-Y gastric bypass (RYGB)*: Here a small proximal gastric pouch is created and connected to the rest of the gastrointestinal tract via a tight stoma and a Roux-en-Y small bowel arrangement **(Fig. 11.2)**. RYGB results in substantial amounts of weight loss. Complications include peritonitis due to anastomotic leak, abdominal wall hernias, staple line disruption, gallstones, neuropathy, marginal ulcers, stomal stenosis, wound infections, thromboembolic disease, gastrointestinal symptoms, and nutritional deficiencies.
  - *Vertical-banded gastroplasty*: This is a restrictive procedure in which the upper part of the stomach is partitioned by a vertical staple line with a tight outlet wrapped by a prosthetic mesh or band **(Fig. 11.3)**. It is often referred to as a stomach stapling operation. The small proximal pouch gets filled quickly by food and prevents consumption of a large meal.

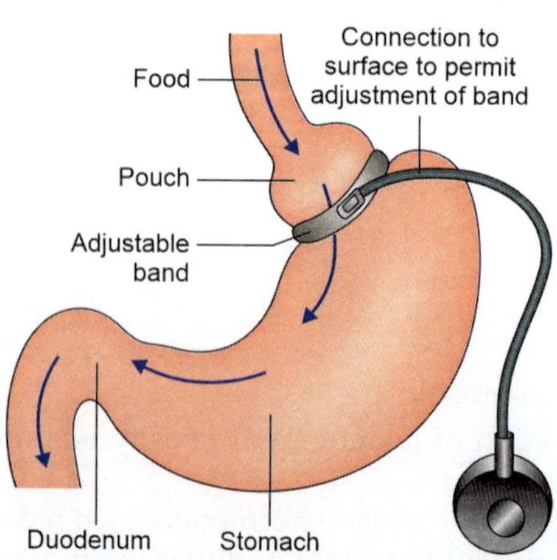

Fig. 11.1: Gastric banding

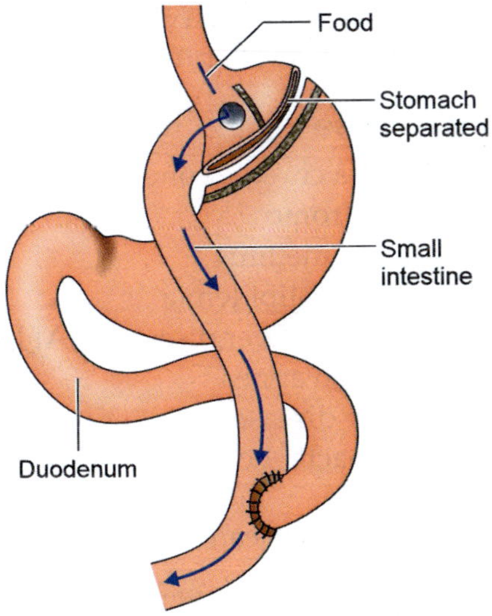

Fig. 11.2: Roux-en-Y gastric bypass

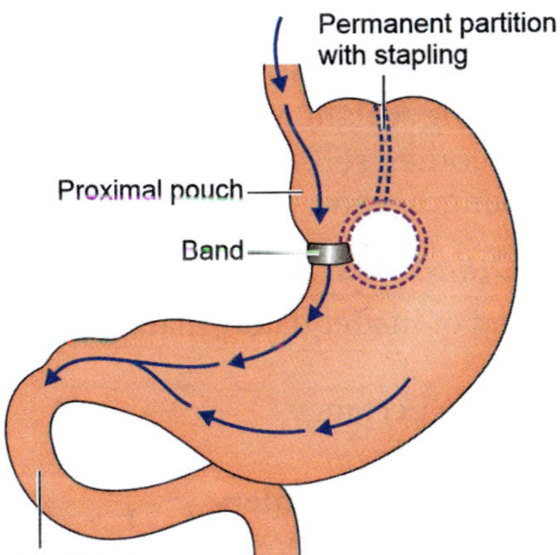

Fig. 11.3: Vertical-banded gastroplasty

Treatment of Underlying or Associated Conditions

- Hypothyroidism
- PCOS
- Depression
- Diabetes, hypertension.

Q. Describe the monogenic forms of obesity.

- Monogenic obesity refers to rare, single-gene mutations that cause severe early-onset obesity, often with associated endocrine or developmental features. These are inherited in a Mendelian pattern, typically autosomal recessive.
- These are rare (<5% of obesity cases) but important in pediatric severe obesity.

Pathophysiology

- Monogenic obesity primarily affects the hypothalamic leptin-melanocortin pathway, which regulates appetite and energy homeostasis.

Key Hormones and Pathways Involved

- Leptin (LEP) → produced by adipose tissue, signals satiety to hypothalamus.
- Leptin receptor (LEPR) → receives leptin signals.
- Pro-opiomelanocortin (POMC) → precursor for α-MSH, stimulates MC4R.
- Melanocortin 4 receptor (MC4R) → suppresses appetite.
- Mutations in any of these genes can cause hyperphagia and severe obesity.

Features Suggestive of Monogenic Obesity

- Early-onset obesity (<5 years)
- Severe obesity with BMI >3 standard deviations above mean
- Hyperphagia (constant hunger and food-seeking behavior)
- Family history of consanguinity or similarly affected siblings.
- May include endocrine abnormalities (e.g. hypogonadism, adrenal insufficiency).
- Some have dysmorphic features or developmental delays.

Diagnosis

- Clinical suspicion based on early-onset, severe obesity.
- Genetic testing: Next-generation sequencing (NGS), targeted gene panels.
- Hormonal assays: Low or undetectable leptin in LEP mutation; ACTH for POMC/PCSK1.

Q. Discuss the impact of environmental factors including eating habits, food, work, environment and physical activity on the incidence of obesity.

- Obesity is not solely a result of genetics or individual choices—it is strongly influenced by multiple environmental factors including eating habits, food choices, work environment, etc. The modern environment promotes obesity by making high-calorie food easily accessible and physical activity less necessary.

Eating Habits, Food Choices and their Impact on Obesity

- High-calorie diets. Increased intake of processed, calorie-rich, nutrient-poor foods leads to energy surplus.
- Frequent snacking and portion sizes: Large portion sizes, sugary drinks, fast food consumption promote passive overeating.
- Low fiber and high sugar/fat intake: Increases calorie intake, delays satiety and promotes fat storage.
- Eating out and food delivery culture: Increases exposure to high-fat, high-sodium, oversized meals.
- Emotional or binge eating: Triggered by stress or anxiety, contributes to irregular and excessive caloric intake.
- Skipping meals (especially breakfast): Disrupts metabolism and often leads to compensatory overeating later in the day.

Work and Occupational Environment

- Sedentary jobs (desk work): Reduces daily energy expenditure significantly and promotes weight gain.

- Long working hours: Limits time and motivation for physical activity or healthy meal preparation.
- Workplace stress: Triggers emotional eating, cortisol-related fat deposition (especially abdominal).
- Shift work/night shifts: Disrupts circadian rhythm, metabolism, and hormone regulation of hunger and satiety.

Built Environment and Urbanization

- Lack of open spaces/playgrounds: Reduces access to physical activity, especially for children.
- Vehicle dependent transport systems: Reduces opportunities for walking or cycling.
- Unsafe neighbourhoods: Discourages outdoor physical activity.
- High urban density and pollution: Limits physical activity and may contribute to metabolic stress.

Physical Inactivity

- Low participation in structured exercise: Reduces energy expenditure.
- High screen time (TV, mobile, computers): Sedentary behavior leads to energy imbalance.
- Lack of awareness about active lifestyle: Prevents self-regulation of weight and health habits.

Q. Describe the natural history of obesity.

- The natural history of obesity refers to its onset, progression, and long-term outcomes in the absence of effective intervention. Obesity typically develops gradually and progresses to cause multiple chronic diseases over time.

Phases in the Natural History of Obesity

Predisposing Phase (preobesity)

- Starts early in life: Intrauterine malnutrition or over-nutrition, high birth weight, formula feeding, early introduction of high-calorie foods.
- Genetic susceptibility: Family history of obesity.
- Environmental exposure: Sedentary behaviour, high-calorie diets.
- Early indicators: Rapid infant weight gain, childhood overweight.

Initiation Phase

- Gradual positive energy balance (caloric intake > expenditure)
- Weight gain begins, initially reversible with lifestyle changes
- Increased fat cell size (hypertrophy).

Progression Phase

- Sustained overnutrition leads to:
  - Further fat accumulation
  - Increase in number of fat cells (hyperplasia), especially in childhood and adolescence
  - Onset of insulin resistance, chronic low-grade inflammation.
- Fat accumulates centrally (visceral fat), which is metabolically active and harmful.

Complication Phase

- Obesity becomes a chronic condition, often with:
  - Metabolic syndrome
  - Type 2 diabetes mellitus
  - Hypertension, dyslipidemia
  - Nonalcoholic fatty liver disease (NAFLD)
  - Obstructive sleep apnea
  - Cardiovascular disease
- Psychosocial impacts: Low self-esteem, depression, social stigma.
- Increased risk of certain cancers (breast, endometrial, colon).

Chronic/Recurrent Phase

- Body develops leptin resistance and altered metabolic set-point, making weight loss harder.
- Basal metabolic rate (BMR) decreases after weight loss, promoting weight regain (yo-yo effect).
- Obesity becomes self-sustaining and resistant to lifestyle changes alone.

Long-term Outcomes

If left untreated or inadequately managed, obesity leads to:

- Reduced life expectancy
- Poor quality of life
- Increased healthcare burden
- Multi-organ complications and premature death.

Q. Describe the measures to prevent obesity and promote a healthy lifestyle.

- Obesity is a preventable disease. Effective prevention and lifestyle promotion require a multi-level approach, involving individuals, families, healthcare workers, and public health systems.

Patient and Public Education

Healthy Eating Habits

- Include fruits, vegetables, whole grains, lean proteins, and healthy fats.
- Avoid overeating and learn to recognize satiety cues.
- Reduce processed/junk foods, sugary drinks, and fried snacks.
- Maintain regular meal timings. A avoid skipping meals and late-night eating.
- Maintain good hydration by drinking 8–10 glasses of water daily; limit sweetened beverages.
- Mindful eating. Avoid eating while distracted by screens; eat slowly and intentionally.

Physical Activity

- Aerobic activity: At least 150–300 minutes/week of moderate-intensity (e.g. brisk walking, cycling).
- Strength training: At least 2 days/week to maintain muscle mass.

- Reduce sedentary behavior: Take breaks from sitting, walk during phone calls, limit screen time.
- Encourage family activities: Promote active play for children and family exercise routines.

Role of Healthcare Workers (HCWs)

- Screening and early detection: Use BMI, waist circumference, and lifestyle assessment tools.
- Educate patients: Offer simple, culturally appropriate nutrition and exercise advice.
- Develop individualized care plans: Tailored to patient age, gender, health status, and motivation.
- Encourage family involvement: Obesity prevention is more effective with family support.
- Involve dietitians, physiotherapists, psychologists, or bariatric specialists if needed.

Public Health and Community Level Interventions

- School-based programs: Include physical education, healthy lunch policies, and nutrition literacy.
- Workplace wellness: Walking breaks, and healthy canteens.
- Urban planning: Create safe parks, cycle paths, and walkable neighborhoods.
- Mass media campaigns: Spread awareness about healthy living and dangers of obesity.
- Regulate food marketing: Especially to children; front-of-pack labeling; taxes on sugary drinks.
- Train frontline workers: ASHAs, Anganwadi workers, nurses in basic obesity prevention counseling.

Q. Vitamin A (retinol) deficiency.

- Vit-A is a fat-soluble vitamin essential for vision, epithelial integrity, immune function, reproduction, and growth.
- Vitamin A was the first fat-soluble vitamin to be discovered.
- The recommended daily intake of vitamin A is 800–1000 µg.

Sources

- Vitamin A is obtained from diet in two forms: Preformed vitamin A (retinol and retinyl ester) and provitamin A (beta-carotenoid).
- Preformed vitamin-A is derived from animal sources such as meat, dairy products, and fish.
- Provitamin A (beta-carotene) is derived from fruits and vegetables.

Causes of Vitamin A Deficiency

- *Reduced intake*: It is endemic in areas such as southern and eastern Asia, where rice, devoid of β-carotene, is the staple food.
- *Interference with absorption:* Celiac disease, cystic fibrosis, pancreatic insufficiency, duodenal bypass, chronic diarrhea, bile duct obstruction, giardiasis, and cirrhosis.
- *Impaired storage:* Liver disorders (vitamin A is stored in hepatic stellate cells).

Clinical Features of Vitamin A Deficiency

Ocular Manifestations (most specific)

- Vitamin A deficiency is an important cause of blindness globally especially in Asia.
- Night blindness—is the earliest sign due to an impairment of the dark adaptation process.
- Xerophthalmia—is caused by inadequate function of the lacrimal glands and is characterized by Bitot's spots, corneal xerosis and keratomalacia.
- Bitot's spots—are glistening white plaques of desquamated thickened conjunctival epithelium, usually triangular in shape and firmly adherent to the conjunctiva.
- Keratomalacia—corneal dryness leading to softening and ulceration.
- Corneal scarring—can cause irreversible blindness.

Systemic Manifestations

- Growth retardation: In children due to impaired cell differentiation
- Skin changes: Dry, rough, scaly skin (follicular hyperkeratosis)
- Poor wound healing
- Impairment of humoral and cell mediated immunity via direct and indirect effects on the phagocytes and T cells.

Complications

- Irreversible blindness
- Severe infections and increased mortality in children
- Stunted growth and development
- Increased maternal morbidity.

Investigations

- Serum retinol level is low. A value of <20 µg/dl indicates deficiency.
- A serum RBP (retinol binding protein) is less expensive than a serum retinol study. Level is low in vitamin A deficiency.
- Conjunctival impression cytology: Detects keratinization of epithelial cells.

Treatment

- For treatment of xerophthalmia, vitamin A is given in three doses. The first dose (2 lakh U) is given immediately on diagnosis, the second on the following day, and the third dose at least two weeks later. If there is vomiting or severe diarrhea, vitamin A is given by intramuscular injection.
- In countries where vitamin A deficiency is endemic, pregnant women should be advised to eat dark green leafy vegetables and yellow fruits. A single prophylactic oral dose (2 lakh U) is given to pre-school children. Repeated oral administration of these doses to children every 4–6 months is used in some endemic areas.

Prevention

- **Dietary improvement:** Promote consumption of vitamin A-rich foods (liver, dairy, eggs, green leafy vegetables, orange/yellow fruits and vegetables).
- **Fortification:** Of staples like oil, milk, or sugar.
- **Periodic supplementation programs:** WHO recommends vitamin A doses every 6 months for children in high-risk areas.
- **Health education and breastfeeding promotion.**

Q. Hypervitaminosis A; vitamin A toxicity.

- Hypervitaminosis A refers to toxic effects resulting from excessive intake of vitamin A (preformed retinol). Provitamin A carotenoids (e.g. beta-carotene) found in plants are not toxic, even in high doses.

Etiology/Causes

- Excessive supplementation.
- High intake of liver (e.g. polar bear liver, which is extremely rich in vitamin A).
- Long-term use of vitamin A-containing medications (e.g. isotretinoin, acitretin).
- Errors in fortification or dosing.

Clinical Features

- Acute toxicity occurs in adults if >>300,000 IU of vitamin A is ingested over a short period. Symptoms include nausea, vomiting, increased intracranial pressure, skin desquamation, vertigo, and blurry vision (pseudotumor cerebri). In very high doses, drowsiness, malaise, and recurrent vomiting can follow the above symptoms. In infants under 6 months of age, even 20,000 IU may produce toxic effects.
- Chronic vitamin A toxicity may occur with intake of >25,000 IU/day for several months. Signs and symptoms include low-grade fever, headache, fatigue, anorexia, intestinal disturbances, hepatosplenomegaly, anemia, nocturia, joint and bone pain, and skin changes such as yellowing, dryness, alopecia, and photosensitivity.
- Vitamin A is highly teratogenic if taken during pregnancy. Hence pregnant women should not take vitamin A supplements unless there is deficiency.

Investigations

- Serum vitamin A levels: Elevated in toxicity.
- Liver function tests (LFTs): May be deranged.
- Imaging (X-rays): In chronic toxicity—hyperostosis of long bones.
- Intracranial pressure measurement: In cases of pseudotumor cerebri.

Management

- Immediate withdrawal of vitamin A sources
- Supportive care: Manage nausea, headache, intracranial hypertension, liver monitoring
- Hospitalization in severe acute toxicity
- Avoid retinoids during pregnancy—counsel regarding teratogenic risk.

Q. Beriberi.

Q. Vitamin B_1 (thiamine) deficiency.

Q. Wernicke-Korsakoff syndrome.

- Thiamine (vitamin B_1) is a water-soluble vitamin essential for carbohydrate metabolism and neural function.
- Deficiency causes impaired glucose metabolism, leading to neuronal and cardiovascular dysfunction.
- Thiamine is found in larger quantities in yeast, legumes, pork, rice, and cereals.

Activity

- Thiamine is required for carbohydrate metabolism. Thiamine pyrophosphate (TPP) is an essential co-enzyme in the conversion of pyruvate to acetyl CoA. This is the bridge between glycolysis and the tricarboxylic acid (Krebs) cycle.
- TPP is also the co-enzyme for transketolase of the pentose phosphate pathway.
- Thiamine is also important for nerve impulse conduction.

Causes of Thiamine Deficiency

- Inadequate intake: Malnutrition, polished rice diet (common in Asia), fad diets.
- Increased demand: Pregnancy, lactation, hyperthyroidism, fever.
- Excess losses: Diarrhea, dialysis, chronic alcoholism.
- Malabsorption: Chronic diarrhea, GI surgery.
- Alcoholism: Reduces thiamine absorption and liver storage.

Clinical Features

- In thiamine deficiency, cells cannot metabolize glucose aerobically leading to accumulation of pyruvic and lactic acids, which produce vasodilatation and increased cardiac output. There is also less ATP generation.
- *Infantile beriberi* is seen in exclusively breastfed infants of thiamin-deficient mothers, and is invariably fatal.
- *Dry beriberi* mainly affects peripheral nervous system. Onset of peripheral neuropathy is gradual and is characterized by peripheral neuropathy with wrist and/or foot drop. It is due to axonal degeneration in peripheral nerves.
- *Wet beriberi* mainly affects heart and causes congestive cardiac failure with pulmonary and peripheral edema.
- *Wernicke's encephalopathy* affects central nervous system. Onset is acute. Wernicke's encephalopathy is characterized by the classic triad of confusion, ataxia, and ophthalmoplegia. Nystagmus is often present. It is reversible with treatment.
- *Korsakoff's psychosis* follows untreated or chronic Wernicke's encephalopathy. It is characterized by severe memory loss (both anterograde and retrograde amnesia). There is confabulation, disorientation, and apathy. Confabulation is a memory disturbance where false memories are created to fill in gaps in memory

without the intention to deceive. The person believes these memories are true. Korsakoff's psychosis is irreversible in most patients.
- Both Wernicke's encephalopathy and Korsakoff's psychosis are almost exclusively seen in alcoholics with thiamine deficiency.

Treatment

- Thiamine is given at a dose of 100 mg for 7–14 days IV or IM. Then an oral dose of 100 mg per day is given until full recovery is achieved. Give thiamine before giving glucose, because glucose first can worsen symptoms by increasing thiamine demand.
- Korsakoff' psychosis is irreversible and does not respond to thiamin treatment.
- Treat underlying cause (e.g. alcoholism).
- Nutritional rehabilitation.

Q. Niacin deficiency (pellagra).

- Niacin (vitamin B_3) is a water soluble vitamin which exists as nicotinic acid and nicotinamide.
- Niacin is an essential component of the coenzymes nicotinamide adenine dinucleotide (NAD) and nicotinamide adenine dinucleotide phosphate (NADP), which are involved in many oxidation-reduction reactions.
- Pellagra is a clinical syndrome caused by deficiency, characterized by the "3 Ds": dermatitis, diarrhea, and dementia. If untreated, it may lead to death (the 4th D).

Sources of Niacin

- The major food sources of niacin are protein foods, cereals, vegetables, and dairy products.
- It is also synthesized by the body in small amounts from tryptophan.

Causes of Niacin Deficiency

Nutritional Deficiency

- Maize-based diets (low niacin and tryptophan).
- Poverty, famine.

Malabsorption

- Chronic diarrhea
- Inflammatory bowel disease
- Chronic pancreatitis.

Increased Requirements

- Pregnancy, lactation
- Hyperthyroidism, infections
- Pellagra is now uncommon except in parts of Africa, alcoholics and in patients with anorexia nervosa, or malabsorption.

Impaired Tryptophan Metabolism

- Pellagra can occur in Hartnup's disease which is characterized by impaired absorption of several amino acids, including tryptophan.
- It may also be seen in carcinoid syndrome, where tryptophan is utilized for the production of serotonin rather than the synthesis of niacin.
- Vitamin B_6 deficiency (needed for conversion of tryptophan to niacin).

Alcoholism

- Poor intake, absorption, and hepatic processing.

Deficiency (pellagra)

- Pellagra (meaning "raw skin") is characterized by three Ds: dermatitis, diarrhea, and dementia.
- *Dermatitis*—appears as erythema resembling severe sunburn, symmetrically over the areas of the body exposed to sunlight, particularly the dorsum of hands and feet, and neck are involved (Casal's necklace). Skin lesions are dark, dry, and scaling.
- *Diarrhea*—is often associated with glossitis, stomatitis and dysphagia, reflecting the presence of inflammation throughout the gastrointestinal tract.
- *Dementia*—begins with lethargy, insomnia and irritability, and progresses to confusion, memory loss, hallucinations, and psychosis.
- *Death*—in severe untreated cases.

Treatment

- Nicotinamide is given in a dose of 100 mg 8-hourly by mouth or by the parenteral route for 5 days.
- Intake of diet rich in niacin such as meats, milk, peanuts, green leafy vegetables, whole or enriched grains, and brewers' dry yeast.

Q. Vitamin B_{12} deficiency.

- Vitamin B_{12} deficiency causes megaloblastic anemia, and neurological degeneration.
- Vitamin B_{12} is required for the integrity of myelin. In severe deficiency there is demyelination. It may be clinically manifest as peripheral neuropathy or spinal cord degeneration affecting both posterior and lateral columns (subacute combined degeneration of the spinal cord). In addition, there may be cerebral manifestations (resembling dementia) or optic atrophy.
- Treatment is with parenteral hydroxocobalamin.
- Vitamin B_{12} is discussed in detail in hematology chapter.

Q. Vitamin C (ascorbic acid) deficiency; scurvy.

- Scurvy is a clinical syndrome resulting from a deficiency of vitamin C (ascorbic acid), characterized by impaired collagen synthesis, leading to bleeding, poor wound healing, and connective tissue weakness.
- Vitamin C is an essential vitamin for human beings. Vitamin C plays a role in collagen, carnitine, hormone, and amino acid formation. It is essential for wound healing and facilitates recovery from burns. Vitamin C is also an antioxidant, supports immune function, and facilitates the absorption of iron.
- It takes part in the hydroxylation of proline and lysine to hydroxyproline and hydroxylysine which is present in collagen.

- Daily requirement: Adults 75–90 mg/day. Higher in pregnancy, lactation, infections, and smokers.

Sources

- Citrus fruits (oranges, lemons)
- Guava, amla
- Tomatoes, strawberries
- Green leafy vegetables, peppers
- It is easily destroyed by heat. Hence many traditional cooking methods reduce or eliminate it.

Causes of Deficiency

- Lack of dietary fruit and vegetables >2 months
- Infants fed exclusively on boiled milk (low in vitamin C)
- Severely malnourished individuals
- Malabsorption syndromes
- Drug and alcohol abusers
- Extreme poverty
- Smoking (increases requirement)

Clinical Features

- Severe deficiency causes scurvy.
- Defective formation of collagen impairs wound healing, causes capillary hemorrhage and reduced platelet adhesiveness (normal platelets are rich in ascorbate).
- Symptoms develop after weeks to months of vitamin C depletion. Lassitude, weakness, irritability, weight loss, and vague myalgias and arthralgias may develop early.
- Gums become swollen, purple, spongy, friable and bleed easily. Eventually, teeth become loose and avulsed.
- Hemorrhagic manifestations—include perifollicular hemorrhages, petechiae and purpura, splinter hemorrhages, hemarthroses, and subperiosteal hemorrhages. Intracerebral hemorrhage can cause death.
- Anemia
- Impaired wound healing.

Diagnosis

- Diagnosis is based on clinical features. Serum ascorbic acid levels of <0.2 mg/dl indicates vitamin C deficiency, but this test is not routinely done.

Treatment

- Scurvy is treated with 300–1000 mg of ascorbic acid orally per day.
- Eating raw fruits and vegetables especially citrus fruits.

Q. Fluorosis.

- Fluorosis is a condition caused by excessive fluoride intake, primarily affecting bones and teeth.

Causes

- High fluoride content in drinking water (>1.5 ppm)
- Fluoride-rich groundwater (common in India: Andhra Pradesh, Rajasthan, Karnataka, etc.).
- Industrial exposure (e.g. aluminum smelting)
- Excessive use of fluoridated dental products (in children).
- Certain foods (e.g. tea leaves, rock salt) with high fluoride levels.

Clinical Features

- Fluorosis causes hypomineralization of the dental enamel. The earliest signs are chalky-white patches on the surface of the enamel. These patches become stained yellow or brown, producing a characteristic mottled appearance. Severe toxicity weakens the enamel, pitting its surface and teeth become brittle and easily breakable.
- Other features are sclerosis of the bones, especially of spine, pelvis and limbs. Ligament and tendon calcification also can occur.

Management

- Fluorosis is primarily a cosmetic concern, but it can make the teeth more susceptible to wear and breakage.
- Fluorosis can be prevented by avoiding excess fluoride consumption (e.g. avoiding swallowing of fluoridated toothpaste or mouth rinses).

Q. Vitamin D deficiency.

- Vitamin D is a fat-soluble vitamin. There are two chemical forms of vitamin D; ergocalciferol (vitamin D_2) and cholecalciferol (vitamin D_3).
- A minimum intake of 200 IU of vitamin D per day is recommended for adults. For pregnant and lactating women, a minimum of 400 IU per day is recommended.

Sources of Vitamin D

- Ergocalciferol (vitamin D_2) is present in plant foods. Cholecalciferol (vitamin D_3) is synthesized in the skin on exposure to sunlight from 7-dehydrocholesterol and also present in animal sources.
- Natural dietary sources of vitamin D include egg yolk, liver, fatty fish, butter and milk.

Actions

- Vitamin D is hydroxylated in the liver to 25-hydroxyvitamin D (calcidiol), which is the major circulating form of vitamin D and is the best index of vitamin D levels. Calcidiol is hydroxylated in the kidney to 1, 25-dihydroxyvitamin D (calcitriol), which is the most active form.
- Vitamin D has a variety of actions on calcium, phosphate, and bone metabolism.
- It increases serum calcium and phosphate concentration by increasing intestinal calcium and phosphate absorption, increasing renal calcium reabsorption, and enhancing PTH-mediated bone resorption.
- Vitamin D deficiency is present when serum levels of 25-hydroxyvitamin D is less than 20 ng/ml.
- Vitamin D deficiency produces defective mineralization of bone, leading to rickets in children and osteomalacia in adults.

Causes of Vitamin D Deficiency

- Deficient intake
- Malabsorption
- Increased requirements (Pregnancy, lactation, rapid growth)
- Inadequate sunlight exposure
- Loss of vitamin D binding protein (nephrotic syndrome)
- Defective 25-hydroxylation (e.g. cirrhosis of liver)
- Defective 1-alpha 25-hydroxylation (e.g. renal failure)
- Vitamin D-resistance
- Drugs that interfere with absorption: phenytoin, rifampin, glucocorticoids, orlistat

Clinical Features of Vitamin D Deficiency

- Vitamin D deficiency causes rickets in children and osteomalacia in adults. For details, *see* the following pages:

Investigations

- 25-hydroxyvitamin D level will be low. A level of less than 20 ng/ml indicates vitamin D deficiency.
- Serum calcium ↓ or normal.
- Serum parathyroid hormone level will be elevated. But PTH measurement is not routinely required.

Treatment of Vitamin D Deficiency

- Mild to moderate deficiency: Initial treatment with 60,000 units of vitamin D_2 or D_3 orally once per week for 6–8 weeks, and then 800–1000 IU of vitamin D_3 daily thereafter. Vitamin D_3 is better than vitamin D_2 for vitamin D supplementation. Loading dose is not recommended in pregnant women.
- Severe deficiency or malabsorption: Higher oral doses or intramuscular vitamin D.
- All patients should maintain a daily calcium intake of at least 1000 mg per day.

Prevention

- Adequate sun exposure (15–30 min/day)
- Fortification of foods (milk, cereals)
- Supplementation in:
  - Pregnant/lactating women
  - Infants exclusively breastfed
  - Elderly or housebound individuals

Q. Osteomalacia.

- Osteomalacia is a disorder of impaired bone mineralization in adults, due to deficiency or resistance to vitamin D. It is the adult counterpart of rickets in children.
- Osteomalacia is characterized by defective bone mineralization, bone pain, muscle weakness, increased bone fragility and fractures.
- Osteomalacia has to be differentiated from osteoporosis. Osteoporosis refers to decreased bone mass due to imbalance between bone formation and bone resorption. In osteoporosis, the bones are porous and brittle, whereas in osteomalacia the bones are soft. Osteopenia is a condition in which bone mineral density is lower than normal, but not severe enough to call it as osteoporosis. Osteopenia is a precursor to osteoporosis.

Etiology

Vitamin D deficiency—causes

- Deficient intake
- Malabsorption
- Inadequate sunlight exposure
- Loss of vitamin D binding protein (nephrotic syndrome)
- Defective 25-hydroxylation (e.g. cirrhosis of liver)
- Defective 1-alpha 25-hydroxylation (e.g. renal failure)
- Vitamin D-resistance
- Drugs: Phenytoin, rifampicin, glucocorticoids.

Clinical Features

- It can be asymptomatic and present radiologically as osteopenia.
- Diffuse bone pain (especially hips, ribs, lower back)
- Proximal muscle weakness (difficulty climbing stairs, getting up, waddling gait)
- Tenderness over bones.
- Fractures may occur with little or no trauma.
- Bone deformities can occur in severe osteomalacia of long duration.

Investigations

- *Radiologic findings*
  - Reduced bone density with thinning of the cortex. Bowing of long bones.
  - Changes in vertebral bodies—loss of radiologic distinctness of the vertebral body trabeculae, concavity of the vertebral bodies, the codfish vertebrae. The vertebral disks appear large and biconvex. There may be spinal compression fractures.
  - Looser's zones—these are pseudo-fractures, fissures, or narrow radiolucent lines, and are characteristic radiologic finding in osteomalacia **(Fig. 11.4)**. They

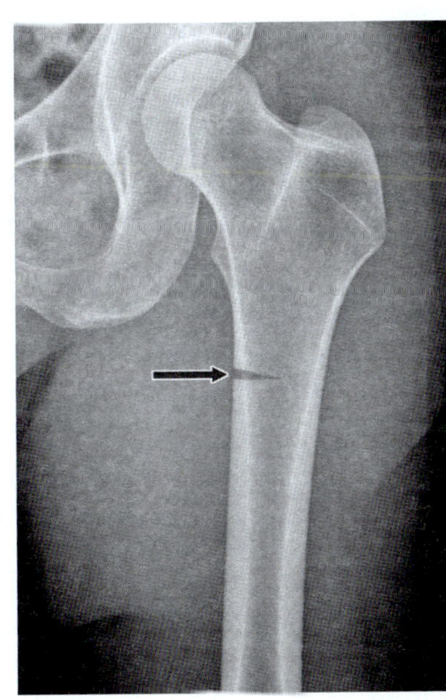

Figure 11.4: Looser's zone (arrow)

are usually found at the femoral neck, femoral shaft, and the pubic and ischial rami. The term "Milkman syndrome" refers to the combination of multiple, bilateral and symmetric pseudofractures in a patient with osteomalacia.

- Low vitamin D level
- Hypocalcemia or hypophosphatemia
- High alkaline phosphatase (ALP) level
- Parathyroid hormone (PTH): ↑ (secondary hyperparathyroidism)
- Low bone mineral density (BMD)
- Iliac crest bone biopsy is the gold standard for establishing the diagnosis but should be done only when the diagnosis is in doubt. It shows increased unmineralized osteoid.

Treatment

- Vitamin D supplementation: Cholecalciferol: 60,000 IU weekly × 6–8 weeks. Maintenance dose is 800–1000 IU/day.
- Calcium supplementation: 1–1.5 g/day.
- Underlying cause should be treated.

Q. Rickets.

- Rickets is a disorder of growing bones in children, caused by defective mineralization of the osteoid matrix, primarily due to vitamin D deficiency.
- Hypocalcemic rickets is due to calcium deficiency.
- Hypophosphatemic rickets is due to phosphate deficiency.

Etiology

- Same as osteomalacia.

Pathophysiology

- ↓ Vitamin D → ↓ intestinal absorption of calcium and phosphate.
- Hypocalcemia → ↑ parathyroid hormone (secondary hyperparathyroidism).
- Bone resorption increases → defective mineralization of osteoid → soft, deformed bones.

Clinical Manifestations

- Rickets manifests initially at sites of rapid bone growth such as distal forearm, knee, and costochondral junctions (**Fig. 11.5**).

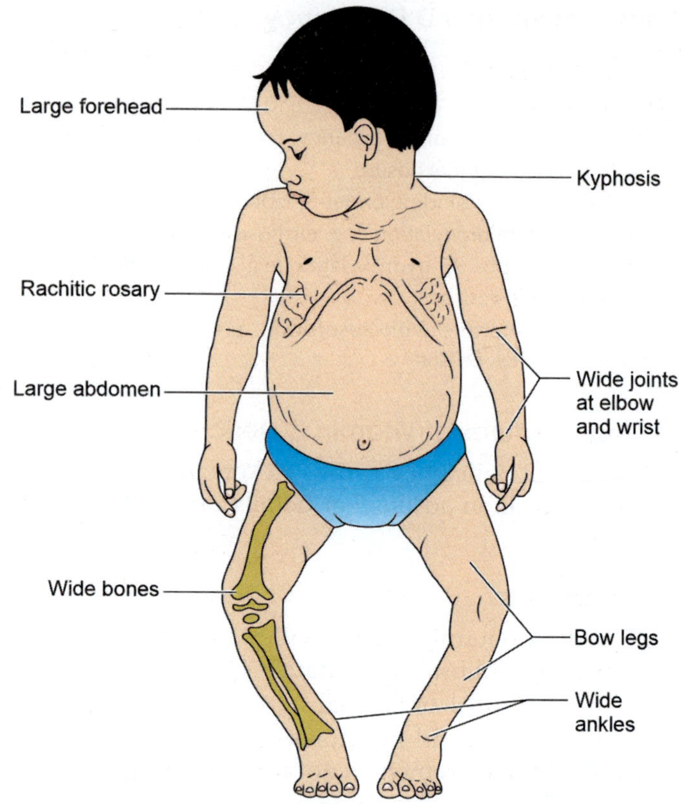

Figure 11.5: Clinical features of rickets

Skeletal Findings

- Delay in the closure of the fontanelles
- Parietal and frontal bossing
- Craniotabes (soft skull bones)
- Enlargement of the costochondral junction visible as beading along the anterolateral aspects of the chest (the "rachitic rosary").
- Development of Harrison sulcus caused by the muscular pull of the diaphragmatic attachments to the lower ribs
- Enlargement of the wrist and bowing of the distal radius and ulna
- Progressive lateral bowing of the femur and tibia.

Extraskeletal Findings

- Decreased muscle tone, seizures, increased sweating and hypoplasia of the dental enamel are seen in hypocalcemic rickets.
- Abscesses of the teeth occur in hypophosphatemic rickets.

Laboratory Findings

- Alkaline phosphatase is markedly increased
- Low serum calcium and phosphorus
- Parathyroid hormone level is elevated in hypocalcemic rickets and normal in hypophosphatemic rickets.
- Serum concentration of 25-hydroxyvitamin D is low in vitamin D deficiency.
- Measurement of serum creatinine to exclude renal insufficiency as the primary etiology.
- Measurement of liver enzymes to exclude liver disease as the etiology of elevated alkaline phosphatase activity.

Radiographic Findings

- Widening of the epiphyseal plate and loss of definition of the zone of provisional calcification at the epiphyseal/metaphyseal interface.
- Disorganization of the growth plate with cupping, splaying, formation of cortical spurs, and stippling.
- Delayed appearance of epiphyseal bone centers.
- The shafts of the long bones are osteopenic, with thin cortex. Trabecular pattern is reduced and becomes coarse. Bone deformities are usually present and in severe rickets, pathological fractures and Looser zones may be noted.

Treatment

- Vitamin D supplementation: 60,000 IU orally once weekly × 6 weeks, then maintenance dose (400–600 IU/day).
- Calcium supplementation: 500–1000 mg/day.
- Adequate sunlight exposure.
- Treatment of hypophosphatemic rickets is with phosphate supplements, combined with vitamin D to promote intestinal calcium and phosphate absorption.

Q. Discuss the etiology, clinical features, investigations and management of osteoporosis.

- Osteoporosis is characterized by a decrease in bone mass and density with normal mineralization. In osteomalacia, the ratio of bone mineral to bone matrix is low. Osteoporosis means "porous bone." The rate of bone formation is often normal, whereas the rate of bone resorption is increased.
- WHO definition (based on DEXA scan): T-score ≤–2.5 at lumbar spine, femoral neck, or total hip.
- Osteoporosis is associated with increased risk of fractures especially the spine and hip. It is a leading cause of morbidity and mortality in elderly people.

Etiology

Primary osteoporosis

- Most common cause and most cases occur in postmenopausal women and elderly people.

Secondary osteoporosis

- Cancer (e.g. multiple myeloma, lymphoma, leukemia).
- COPD (chronic obstructive pulmonary disease) due to the disorder and its treatment with glucocorticoids, tobacco use, and decreased physical activity.
- Chronic kidney disease
- Drugs (e.g. glucocorticoids, phenytoin, heparin, alcohol, proton pump inhibitors)
- Endocrine disease (e.g. Cushing's disease, hyperparathyroidism, hyperthyroidism, hypogonadism, hyperprolactinemia, diabetes mellitus).
- Hypervitaminosis A
- Hypophosphatemia
- Vitamin D deficiency
- Immobilization
- Liver disease
- Malabsorption syndromes
- Prolonged weightlessness (as occurs in space flight).

Clinical Features

- Osteoporosis = "Silent thief of bone"–often asymptomatic until fracture.
- Backache or spontaneous fracture or collapse of vertebra.

Investigations

- X-rays show osteopenia.
- Serum calcium and phosphate to rule out hypocalcemia.
- ALP may be slightly elevated, following a fracture.
- Parathyroid hormone level to screen for primary hyperparathyroidism.
- Serum vitamin D level
- Thyroid function tests
- Serum testosterone in men (hypogonadism)
- Serum and urine protein electrophoresis to rule out multiple myeloma
- 24-hour urinary free cortisol if features of Cushing's syndrome are present
- Bone mineral density test using dual energy X-ray absorptiometry (DEXA).

Treatment

General Measures

- Good diet containing adequate protein, calories, calcium, and vitamin D
- Physical activity increases bone density.
- Subjects who already have osteoporosis should take precautions to avoid falls (e.g. adequate lighting, handrails on stairs, handholds in bathrooms).
- Bed-ridden patients should be given active or passive exercises.
- Alcohol and smoking should be avoided.
- If on steroids, dose should be reduced or discontinued if possible.

Specific Measures

- Treatment is indicated for all patients with osteoporosis and for those who have had fragility fractures. Prophylactic treatment should also be considered for patients with advanced osteoporosis.
- *Vitamin D and calcium supplementation*: Oral vitamin D is given in doses of 800–1000 IU daily and calcium supplementation in a dose of 1000–1200 mg/day including dietary consumption.
- *Bisphosphonates*: They are the first line therapy to treat osteoporosis. They inhibit osteoclast-induced bone resorption and reduce the incidence of both vertebral and nonvertebral fractures. Both oral and parenteral bisphosphonates are available. Examples are alendronate, risedronate, zoledronic acid and pamidronate. Osteonecrosis of the jaw has been associated with use of bisphosphonates; however, this condition is rare in patients taking oral bisphosphonates.
- *Hormone replacement therapy*: Reserved for symptomatic postmenopausal women. However, it is associated increased risk of thromboembolism, endometrial cancer and breast cancer.
- *Selective estrogen receptor modulators*: Raloxifene, 60 mg/day orally, can be used by postmenopausal women instead of estrogen for the prevention of osteoporosis. Unlike estrogen, raloxifene does not cause endometrial hyperplasia, uterine bleeding, or cancer. The risk of breast cancer is also reduced. However, since raloxifene is a potential teratogen, it is contraindicated in premenopausal women. It also increases the risk of thromboembolism.
- *Teriparatide*: This is an analog of PTH. It stimulates production of new bone matrix that must be mineralized. Patients should take sufficient vitamin D and calcium

along with this drug. When given to patients with osteoporosis daily subcutaneously for 2 years, teriparatide dramatically improves bone density. Hypercalcemia is a risk with this medicine. Following a course of teriparitide, a course of bisphosphonates should be considered to retain the improved bone density.

- *Denosumab* is a monoclonal antibody and reduces bone resorption by osteoclasts.
- *Teriparatide and denosumab* are used in patients who cannot tolerate other forms of therapies.

Q. Hypervitamiosis D.

- Hypervitaminosis D is a condition resulting from excessive intake of vitamin D leading to toxicity, most notably hypercalcemia.
- The upper limit of vitamin D intake is 2000 IU daily. Chronic intake >10,000 IU/day over months can lead to toxicity.
- Toxic serum level: 25(OH)D >150 ng/ml.

Causes

- Vitamin D intoxication may occur in fad dieters who consume "mega doses" of supplements or in patients on vitamin D replacement therapy.
- Empirical administration of very high doses of intramuscular vitamin D injections at frequent intervals is one of the most common causes of hypervitaminosis D.
- Primary hyperparathyroidism, MEN I and II syndrome
- Malignancies such as Hodgkin's lymphoma and non-Hodgkin's lymphoma (increase vitamin D activation).
- Granulomatous diseases like sarcoidosis and tuberculosis (macrophages produce excess calcitriol).

Pathophysiology

- Excess vitamin D → Increased calcium absorption from the gut → Hypercalcemia → Calcification of soft tissues, kidney damage, and altered CNS function.

Clinical Features

- Vitamin D excess results in hypercalcemia which is responsible for widespread systemic effects.
- *Gastrointestinal:* Nausea, vomiting, constipation, anorexia.
- *Renal:* Hypercalciuria, polyuria, polydipsia, dehydration, nephrocalcinosis, renal stones, acute kidney injury.
- *Neurological:* Confusion, lethargy, stupor.
- *Cardiac:* Hypertension, arrhythmias.
- *Others:* Bone pain, muscle weakness, ectopic calcification (e.g. in lungs, blood vessels).

Investigations

- Serum 25-hydroxyvitamin D level is >100 ng/ml. serum calcium and urine calcium level is high.

Treatment

- Stop vitamin D intake immediately
- Restriction of dietary calcium intake
- Hydration with IV normal saline to promote calcium excretion.
- Glucocorticoids—reduce intestinal calcium absorption and vitamin D activity.
- Bisphosphonates or calcitonin—inhibit bone resorption and reduce calcium.
- Dialysis—in cases of life-threatening hypercalcemia or renal failure.

Q. Vitamin K deficiency.

- The name "K" comes from the German/word *koagulations* vitamin (clotting vitamin).

Importance of Vitamin K

- Vitamin K plays an important role in coagulation by acting as a cofactor for the posttranslational carboxylation of coagulation factors II, VII, IX, and X. Without carboxylation, coagulation reactions occur slowly and hemostasis is impaired.
- Vitamin K also plays a role in bone health by promoting carboxylation of osteocalcin, a bone matrix protein.
- Vitanub K is a fat-soluble vitamin. Pancreatic and biliary function need to be intact for proper vitamin K absorption. Dietary vitamin K is protein-bound and requires pancreatic enzymes in the small intestine for liberation. Bile salts then solubilize vitamin K into luminal micelles for absorption.
- Daily Requirement (RDA): Men: ~120 µg/day, Women: ~90 µg/day.

Types and Sources of Vitamin-K

- *Vitamin K_1 (Phylloquinone):* Found in green leafy vegetables (e.g. spinach, kale, broccoli).
- *Vitamin K_2 (Menaquinones):* Produced by gut bacteria and found in fermented foods, dairy, and meat.

Causes of Vitamin K Deficiency

- Deficiency develops because of inadequate diet, use of broad-spectrum antibiotics, liver and pancreatic disorders. A patient not taking orally and is put-on broad-spectrum antibiotics can develop vitamin K deficiency in as little as 1 week.

Clinical Features

- There are no specific clinical features. Bleeding can occur at any site. Vitamin K deficiency is common in the newborn and can manifest as hemorrhagic disease of the newborn. Hence, parenteral vitamin K is given routinely to newborns.

Laboratory Findings

- In mild vitamin K deficiency, only the PT is prolonged.
- In severe vitamin K deficiency both PT and aPTT are prolonged, but PT is more prolonged than aPTT.
- Clotting factor assay: Reduced levels of II, VII, IX, X.

Treatment

- Vitamin K should be replaced parenterally either subcutaneously or intravenously. A single dose of 15 mg will completely correct laboratory abnormalities in 12–24 hours.

Chapter 12

Psychiatric Disorders

Q. Give the classification of psychiatric disorders.

- Psychiatric disorders are mental disorders characterized by disturbances in emotion, cognition, motivation, and socialization.
- They can impair daily life, relationships, and occupational or academic performance.
- All psychiatric disorders currently lack well-defined neuropathology and *bona fide* biologic markers. Therefore, diagnosis continues to be made solely from clinical features.
- Psychiatric disorders are classified based on symptomatology, etiology, and clinical course. The two most widely accepted classification systems are:
  - ICD-11: International Classification of Diseases, 11th Revision (by WHO)
  - DSM-5-TR: Diagnostic and Statistical Manual of Mental Disorders, 5th Edition Text Revision.

Classification of Psychiatric Disorders (based on ICD-11 and DSM-5-TR)

- Neurodevelopmental disorders
- Schizophrenia and other psychotic disorders
- Mood (Affective) disorders
- Anxiety disorders
- Obsessive-compulsive and related disorders
- Trauma- and stressor-related disorders
- Somatic symptom and related disorders
- Dissociative disorders
- Feeding and eating disorders
- Elimination disorders (enuresis, encopresis)
- Sleep-wake disorders
- Sexual dysfunctions
- Gender dysphoria
- Disruptive, impulse-control, and conduct disorders
- Substance-related and addictive disorders
- Neurocognitive disorders
- Personality disorders
- Paraphilic disorders
- Other mental disorders

Q. Differences between neurotic *vs* psychotic disorders.

Q. Differences between organic *vs* functional disorders.

Neurotic *vs* Psychotic Disorders (Table 12.1)

TABLE 12.1: Neurotic vs psychotic disorders

Feature	Neurotic disorders	Psychotic disorders
Definition	Disorders characterized by distressing symptoms but intact reality testing	Severe mental disorders with loss of contact with reality
Reality testing	Preserved	Impaired (delusions, hallucinations)
Insight	Usually present	Often absent
Examples	• Generalized anxiety disorder • Phobias • OCD • Depression (mild to moderate)	• Schizophrenia • Bipolar disorder (mania) • Severe depression with psychosis
Behavior	Usually socially appropriate	May be disorganized or inappropriate

Organic *vs* Functional (nonorganic) Disorders (Table 12.2)

TABLE 12.2: Organic *vs* functional (nonorganic) psychiatric disorders

Feature	Organic psychiatric disorders	Functional (nonorganic) psychiatric disorders
Definition	Mental disorders due to identifiable physical/biological cause, especially brain pathology	Mental disorders with no demonstrable structural or biochemical brain lesion
Cause	Secondary to medical or neurological illness	Primary psychiatric in origin
Investigations	Abnormal findings on MRI, EEG, blood tests	Usually normal
Examples	• Delirium • Dementia • Alcohol-related brain damage • Brain tumors	• Schizophrenia • Depression • Anxiety disorders • OCD

Q. Psychosis.

- Psychosis is a clinical syndrome characterized by a loss of contact with reality, manifesting as disturbances in thinking, perception, emotion, and behavior.
- It is a hallmark of several mental illnesses, notably schizophrenia and other psychotic disorders.

Clinical Features

- *Hallucinations*: These are false sensory perceptions occurring in any of the five sensory modalities. Auditory hallucinations are the most common, followed by visual, tactile, olfactory, and gustatory.
- *Delusions*: False beliefs that are firmly held despite obvious evidence to the contrary, and not typical of the patient's culture, faith, or family, are classified as delusions. Examples are persecutory, grandiose, religious, somatic, and other delusions.
- *Disorganized thinking*: Disruption of the logical process of thought may manifest as nonsensical speech, or bizarre behavior. Disorganized thinking may prevent the patient from giving a coherent history or meaningful consent to treatment.
- *Disorganized or abnormal motor behavior*: Ranges from agitation to catatonia. Agitation is an acute state of anxiety, heightened emotional arousal, and increased motor activity. Acts or threats of violence may occur in patients with persecutory delusions, thought disorganization, and poor impulse control.
- *Negative symptoms*: Diminished emotional expression, anhedonia, avolition, alogia.
  - Anhedonia is the inability to experience pleasure from activities that are normally found enjoyable, such as hobbies, social interactions, or sexual activity.
  - Avolition is marked decrease in the motivation to initiate and sustain purposeful activities.
  - Alogia is reduction in the quantity or quality of speech output.

Disorders Associated with Psychotic Features

Primary Psychiatric Illnesses

- Schizophrenia
- Bipolar disorder (mania with psychosis)
- Severe major depressive disorder (with psychotic features).

Secondary (organic) Causes

- Neurological (e.g. epilepsy, brain tumors, dementia)
- Substance use (e.g. alcohol, LSD, cannabis, amphetamines)
- Medical illnesses (e.g. (CNS infections, seizures, endocrine problems, hypoxia, hypercarbia, hypoglycemia, fluid or electrolyte abnormalities, hepatic and renal disorders).

Diagnosis

- Based on clinical history and mental status examination.
- Exclude medical and substance-related causes (labs, imaging)
- Use tools like DSM-5-TR criteria.

Treatment

- Antipsychotic drugs are the mainstay of treatment. Examples of antipsychotic drugs are risperidone, olanzapine, quetiapine, clozapine, etc.
- Psychosocial interventions (cognitive behavioral therapy, family therapy, rehabilitation).
- Treat any underlying cause if present.

Q. Discuss the etiology, clinical features and management of schizophrenia.

Q. Enumerate the positive symptoms (first rank symptoms) of schizophrenia.

- Schizophrenia is a chronic, severe psychiatric disorder characterized by a distortion of thinking, perception, emotions, language, sense of self, and behavior.
- It typically presents with psychotic symptoms, including hallucinations, delusions, disorganized speech/behavior, and cognitive impairment.
- It is one of the most disabling and economically catastrophic disorder, because of lifelong course, debilitating symptoms, and lack of social acceptability.

Etiology

- *Genetic factors*: Schizophrenia can be transmitted genetically. There is 50% concordance rate between monozygotic twins and 10% concurrence rate for first-degree relatives.
- *Environmental factors*: Advanced paternal age, first and second trimester insults to fetal development, including viral infection, starvation, and toxic exposure, perinatal insults such as anoxia and birth trauma are associated with an increased risk of schizophrenia. Urban upbringing, and exposure to psychoactive drugs in adolescence and young adulthood has also been linked to development of schizophrenia.
- *Psychological stresses*: Adverse life events and highly emotional family environment may precipitate episodes of schizophrenia. Early childhood trauma and neglect has been linked to schizophrenia.
- *Neurochemical dysregulation*: ↑ Dopamine activity in mesolimbic pathway (midbrain to limbic system) → positive symptoms. ↓ Dopamine in mesocortical pathway (midbrain to cortex) → negative symptoms. Abnormal glutamate and GABA also implicated.
- *Structural abnormalities of the brain*: Schizophrenic brains are smaller than normal brains, with enlarged ventricles. Abnormalities in prefrontal cortex and hippocampus.
- Schizophrenia can be associated with temporal lobe epilepsy, Huntington's chorea, cerebral tumors and demyelinating diseases. This is known as symptomatic schizophrenia.

Clinical Features

Positive Symptoms (first-rank symptoms)

- These are excess or distortion of normal functions. Positive symptoms are synonymous with psychosis. "Positive" refers to the active quality of these symptoms and are of the 'first rank' in importance when making the diagnosis of schizophrenia. These can be remembered by the mnemonic ABCD.
  - *A = Auditory hallucinations:* these are commonly of voices heard outside the head that talk to the person or talk about the person. Sometimes the voices repeat the person's thoughts. Hallucinations of other sensory modalities also occur.
  - *B = Broadcasting, insertion/withdrawal of thoughts:* Disturbances of the normal private boundary of thinking manifests as belief that their thoughts are being broadcast to others and others thoughts are being 'inserted' into their mind.
  - *C = Control of feelings, impulses or acts by others.*
  - *D = Delusions (false fixed beliefs).*

Negative Symptoms (loss of normal functions)

- *Flattened (blunted) affect*: This is loss of capacity to express feelings, resulting in a blank appearance, monotonous voice, and absence of meaningful gestures.
- *Apathy and loss of drive (avolition)*: Lack of motivation) o involve in constructive activity, social interaction, and recreation, etc.
- *Social withdrawal*: It includes a loss of interest in interactions with family, friends, colleagues, neighbors, and others.
- *Poverty of speech (alogia)*: Decreased speech and terse replies to questions, creating the impression of inner emptiness. The speech may be circumstantial (i.e. the patient takes a long time and uses many words in answering a question) or tangential (i.e. the patient speaks at length but never actually answers the question).
- *Poor self-care.*

Cognitive Symptoms

- Poor attention, memory, executive functioning.
- Difficulty with planning, abstract thinking.

Other Symptoms

- *Catatonia*: This refers to adoption of awkward postures for prolonged periods.

Diagnostic Criteria

- *Diagnostic and Statistical Manual of Mental Disorders, Fifth Edition*, (*DSM-5*) criteria for the diagnosis of schizophrenia are as follows:

- Diagnosis requires two or more symptoms (at least one positive symptom) for ≥1 month with signs of disturbance for ≥6 months:
  - Delusions
  - Hallucinations
  - Disorganized speech
  - Grossly disorganized or catatonic behavior
  - Negative symptoms
- Symptoms must cause social or occupational dysfunction and not be attributable to other conditions or substances.

Management

Antipsychotic Agents

- Antipsychotics (also called neuroleptics) may be divided into conventional (typical, or first-generation) drugs such as chlorpromazine and haloperidol, and newer (atypical, or second-generation) drugs such as clozapine, olanzapine, quetiapine and risperidone.
- These drugs work by blocking D_2 dopamine receptors in the brain. Newer drugs also block 5HT2 receptors and are less likely to produce extrapyramidal side-effects, but clozapine can cause agranulocytosis and requires regular monitoring of WBC count.
- They take 2–3 weeks to be maximally effective. After symptoms are controlled, treatment is continued for 1–2 years to prevent relapse. In patients with multiple psychotic episodes, treatment may be required for many years.

Psychological Treatment

- General support for the patient and his or her family and family education.
- Cognitive behavioral therapy may help patients to cope with their symptoms and also to adhere to treatment with antipsychotic drugs.

Social Treatment

- After symptoms of schizophrenia have been controlled by drugs, social and occupational rehabilitation is required to obtain employment and to re-establish a social network.

Q. Define anxiety. Discuss briefly the clinical features and management of anxiety disorders.

Q. Generalized anxiety disorder.

- **Anxiety** is a distressing, unpleasant emotional state of nervousness and uneasiness. Anxiety can be anticipatory before a threat, persist after a threat has passed, or occur without an identifiable threat.
- It differs from **fear**, which is a response to a real or perceived external threat, whereas anxiety is often internal and anticipatory.
- Anxiety is one of the most common psychiatric disorders in the general population.

Types of Anxiety Disorders

- Generalized anxiety disorder (GAD)
- Panic disorder
- Phobias (e.g. social phobia, specific phobia)
- Agoraphobia
- Separation anxiety disorder
- Selective mutism.

Clinical Features

- Initial manifestations appear at the age of 20–35 years, and it is more common in women.
- Symptoms include excessive anxiety and worry about a number of events or activities, irritability, difficulty in concentrating, and insomnia for at least 6 months.
- Somatic manifestations include increased heart rate, palpitations; Shortness of breath, rapid breathing; chest pain or pressure; choking sensation; dizziness; sweating; dyspepsia; trembling; tingling or numbness in arms and legs; faintness; and dry mouth.
- *Generalized anxiety disorder:* The key feature of this disorder is persistent and excessive worry about various domains, including work and school performance. This is the most common clinically significant anxiety disorder.
- *Separation anxiety*: Pathological anxiety atypical for his/her age due to separation from attachment figures.
- *Specific phobia:* Individuals with specific phobias are fearful or anxious about specific objects or situations which they avoid or endure with intense fear or anxiety.
- *Social anxiety:* This disorder is characterized by marked or intense fear or anxiety of social situations in which one could be the subject of scrutiny.
- *Panic disorder:* Panic attacks are abrupt surges of intense fear or extreme discomfort that reach a peak within minutes, accompanied by physical and cognitive symptoms such as palpitations, sweating, shortness of breath, fear of going crazy, or fear of dying.
- *Selective mutism:* This is a childhood anxiety disorder characterized by a consistent failure to speak in specific social situations (e.g. at school or with unfamiliar people) despite speaking in other settings (e.g. at home).
- *Anxiety disorder due to medical conditions:* Medical conditions such as hyperthyroidism, hypoglycemia, and pheochromocytoma can cause anxiety disorder.

Treatment

- Antidepressants such as escitalopram and venlafaxine are effective in anxiety disorder. Other useful drugs are benzodiazepines and buspirone.
- Psychotherapy (cognitive-behavioral therapy), relaxation and biofeedback may be of some help.

Q. Generalized anxiety disorder (GAD).

Definition

- GAD is characterized by excessive, uncontrollable worry and anxiety about various aspects of life (e.g. work, health, finances) lasting ≥6 months, with associated symptoms.

Diagnostic Criteria (DSM-5)

- Excessive anxiety and worry, occurring more days than not for at least 6 months
- Difficult to control the worry
- Associated with ≥3 of the following:
    - Restlessness or feeling keyed up
    - Being easily fatigued
    - Difficulty concentrating
    - Irritability
    - Muscle tension
    - Sleep disturbance
- Causes significant distress or impairment.

Management of GAD

Pharmacotherapy

- SSRIs, or SNRIs are the preferred initial drugs of choice. Duration of therapy is at least 1 year.
- Selective serotonin reuptake inhibitors (SSRIs): Paroxetine, Escitalopram, Sertraline.
- Serotonin-norepinephrine reuptake inhibitors (SNRIs): Venlafaxine, Duloxetine.
- Buspirone: Nonsedating, nonaddictive.
- Benzodiazepines: Short-term use only for severe cases.

Psychotherapy

- Cognitive behavioural therapy (CBT) is the treatment of choice.
- Relaxation and mindfulness-based stress reduction.

Supportive Measures

- Lifestyle changes
- Patient education
- Family involvement
- Stress reduction techniques.

Q. Phobic disorder.

- A phobia is an abnormal or excessive fear of an object or situation, which leads to avoidance of it.
- *Social phobia*: It is marked and persistent fear of social or performance situations such as attending social functions, dating, participation in small groups, etc. They often live alone and work at solitary jobs.
- *Agoraphobia*: Agoraphobia refers to a fear of any place where escape may be difficult, including large open spaces or crowds, as well as various means of travel.
- *Claustrophobia*: This is opposite of agoraphobia, i.e. fear of closed spaces, e.g. fear of MRI when head goes into the MRI machine.
- *Specific phobia*: There are several other types of specific phobias, some of which are acrophobia (fear of heights), aviophobia (fear of flying), trypanophobia (fear of injections), zoophobia (fear of animals, usually spiders, snakes, or mice), etc.

Etiology

- Genetic predisposition
- Traumatic experience (e.g. being bitten by a dog leading to animal phobia)
- Learned behavior (via classical conditioning)
- Personality traits (e.g. shy, inhibited children more prone to social phobia).

Clinical Features

- Sudden anxiety or panic on exposure to the phobic object or situation
- Anticipatory anxiety
- Avoidance behavior
- Physical symptoms: Palpitations, sweating, trembling, chest discomfort, dizziness
- Affects daily functioning or quality of life.

Treatment

- Exposure therapy: patients are encouraged to seek out, confront, and remain in contact with what they fear until their anxiety is gradually relieved through a process called habituation.
- SSRIs: Example—paroxetine, sertraline—effective for social anxiety and agoraphobia.
- Benzodiazepines (lorazepam) or beta-blockers (propranolol) are helpful to prevent phobia if taken before getting exposed to the object of fear.
- Relaxation techniques: Deep breathing, progressive muscle relaxation, mindfulness.

Q. Panic attack and panic disorder.

- *Panic attack* is the sudden onset of a brief period of intense discomfort, anxiety, or fear accompanied by somatic symptoms. Can occur in healthy individuals or in other mental disorders (e.g. depression, phobia).
- *Panic disorder* is occurrence of repeated unprovoked panic attacks accompanied by fears about future attacks or changes in behavior to avoid situations that might predispose to attacks.
- Somatic symptoms include chest pain, palpitations, dizziness, nausea and carpopedal spasm. These symptoms are in part due to involuntary overbreathing (hyperventilation). Patients often fear they are suffering from a serious illness such as a heart attack or stroke, and may seek emergency medical care.
- Panic attacks may occur in any anxiety disorder (such as phobias). For example, a person with a phobia of snakes may panic at seeing a snake.

Etiology (Causes)

Biological Factors

- Genetic predisposition
- Dysregulation of neurotransmitters (e.g. serotonin, norepinephrine)
- Abnormal activity in brain areas such as the amygdala.

Psychological Factors

- Cognitive distortions
- Learned responses to stress.

Environmental Factors

- Stressful life events
- Substance use (e.g. caffeine, stimulants).

Treatment

- SSRIs (e.g. fluoxetine, sertraline, paroxetine) are the first line agents to treat panic disorder. Other options are SNRIs (e.g. venlafaxine), benzodiazepines (short-term use only, e.g. clonazepam, alprazolam), and beta-blockers (for controlling physical symptoms like palpitations).
- Psychotherapy in the form of exposure therapy and cognitive-behavioral therapy are used along with drugs.
- Lifestyle and supportive measures: Avoid caffeine, alcohol, and stimulants. Stress management techniques (e.g. breathing exercises, mindfulness).

Q. Obsessive-compulsive disorder (OCD).

- Obsessions are persistent intrusive thoughts. Compulsions are repetitive behaviors or mental acts performed in response to the obsessions.
- In the obsessive-compulsive disorder, an irrational idea or impulse persistently intrudes into the mind, leading to repetitive actions (such as washing the hands many times). These actions are recognized by the individual as absurd, but anxiety is alleviated only by ritualistic performance of the action. Under extreme stress, these patients may exhibit paranoid and delusional behaviors, which can mimic schizophrenia.
- These patients are usually predictable, orderly, and intelligent. Highest prevalence is in the young, divorced, separated, and unemployed. Males and females are equally affected.
- There is a high correlation between OCD and depression; two-thirds of OCD patients will develop major depression during their lifetime.

Etiology

Biological

- Dysfunction in serotonin neurotransmission.
- Abnormal activity in corticostriatothalamocortical circuits.
- Genetic predisposition.

Psychological

- Maladaptive beliefs (e.g. inflated sense of responsibility).
- Behavioral reinforcement (relief after compulsion reinforces the behavior)

Environmental

- Stressful life events.
- Childhood abuse or infections.

Treatment

- Exposure and ritual prevention therapy is often effective; it involves gradually exposing patients to situations or people that trigger obsessions and rituals while requiring them not to perform their rituals.
- Antidepressants such as SSRIs (Selective serotonin reuptake inhibitors) and clomipramine are also effective in OCD.

Q. Posttraumatic stress disorder (PTSD).

- PTSD is recurring, intrusive recollections of an overwhelming traumatic event (e.g. rape, severe burns, accident, military combat). Recollections last >1 month and begin within 6 months of the event.
- Women are more affected than men.

Etiology and Pathophysiology

- Direct exposure to actual or threatened death, serious injury, or sexual violence
- Witnessing it in person
- Learning that it occurred to a close family member or friend
- Repeated exposure to traumatic details (e.g. first responders)
- It is hypothesized that in PTSD there is excessive release of norepinephrine from the locus coeruleus in response to stress and increased noradrenergic activity at projection sites in the hippocampus and amygdala. These changes facilitate the encoding of fear-based memories.
- Risk factors for the development of PTSD include a past psychiatric history and personality characteristics of high neuroticism and extroversion. Twin studies show a substantial genetic influence.

Clinical Features

- PTSD usually starts after a few days or months after the traumatic event. Generally, events likely to evoke PTSD are those that invoke feelings of fear, helplessness, or horror.
- Typical symptoms are recurrent intrusive memories (flashbacks) of the traumatic event, as well as sleep disturbance, nightmares (usually of the traumatic event) from which the patient awakes in a state of anxiety, symptoms of autonomic arousal, and emotional blunting. Patients often actively avoid stimuli that precipitate recollections of the trauma.
- These patients are at risk of developing other disorders related to anxiety, mood, and substance abuse.

Treatment

- Psychotherapy: It involves exposure therapy. Here the person is exposed to situations which he avoids because they may trigger recollections of the trauma. Repeated exposure in fantasy to the traumatic experience itself usually lessens distress after some initial increase in discomfort.
- Selective serotonin reuptake inhibitors (SSRI) such as sertraline are also effective in PTSD. Prazosin is effective for nightmares and sleep disturbances.
- Most patients recover within 2 years.

Q. What are mood disorders (affective disorders)? Discuss the etiology, clinical features diagnosis, and management of depression.

- Mood disorders are emotional disturbances consisting of prolonged periods of excessive sadness, excessive joyousness (mania), or both. They include depression, bipolar disorder (combining episodes of both mania and depression) and dysthymia.

Depression

- Depression is characterized by persistent low mood and loss of interests/pleasure. Prolonged depression is called dysthymia.
- Depression may be mild, moderate or severe, and episodic, recurrent or chronic. It can be both a complication of a medical condition or can be a cause of medical condition.

Etiology

Biological factors

- Genetic predisposition
- Decreased levels of serotonin and norepinephrine in the brain
- Abnormal hypothalamo-pituitary-adrenal axis (HPA) regulation, which results in elevated cortisol levels that do not suppress with dexamethasone.
- Medical conditions causing/predisposing depression: hypothyroidism, severe anemia, hyperparathyroidism, Cushing's disease, Addison's disease, tuberculosis, HIV, dementia, post-traumatic brain injury syndromes, malignancy, SLE, etc.

Social and environmental factors

- Stressful life events (e.g. job loss, bereavement), lack of social support, poverty, isolation.

Psychological factors

- Negative thinking patterns, poor coping strategies, early childhood trauma or loss.

Drugs

- Alcohol, beta blockers, withdrawal from cocaine and amphetamines.

Diagnosis

- For diagnosis, at least 5 of the following must be present for at least 2-week period, and one of them must be depressed mood or loss of interest or pleasure:

- Depressed mood most of the day
- Markedly diminished interest or pleasure in most activities (anhedonia)
- Appetite/weight change (Significant gain or loss)
- Sleep disturbances (insomnia or hypersomnia)
- Psychomotor agitation or retardation observed by others (not self-reported)
- Fatigue
- Feelings of worthlessness or excessive guilt
- Diminished ability to think or concentrate or indecisiveness
- Recurrent thoughts of death or suicide, a suicide attempt, or a specific plan for committing suicide.

Investigations

- Diagnosis is mainly based on clinical criteria. However, investigations are useful to exclude physical conditions that can cause depression.
- Tests include CBC, TSH levels, and routine electrolyte, vitamin B_{12} and folate levels.
- Testing for illicit drug use if suspected.

Management

Antidepressants

- *Selective serotonin re-uptake inhibitors (SSRIs):* These are the first-line agents as they have less anticholinergic effects, are less cardiotoxic, and cause less sedation. Examples are citalopram, escitalopram, fluoxetine, sertraline and paroxetine.
- *Serotonin-norepinephrine reuptake inhibitors (SNRIs):* These are venlafaxine, and duloxetine.
- *Tricyclic antidepressants (TCAs):* They inhibit the re-uptake of noradrenaline and 5-HT at synaptic clefts. Their main side effects are anticholinergic effects, postural hypotension and cardiotoxicity. Examples are imipramine and amitriptyline.
- *Monoamine oxidase inhibitors (MAOIs):* These drugs inhibit the metabolism of noradrenaline (norepinephrine) and 5-HT. They are rarely used now because of side effects like hypertensive crisis when given along with tyramine containing foods. Examples are phenelzine and selegiline. Moclobemide is a selective inhibitor of monoamine oxidase subtype A, which is less likely to cause hypertensive crisis.
- *Melatonergic antidepressant:* Agomelatine is a melatonergic (MT1/MT2) agonist and a 5-HT-2c receptor antagonist. It is used for major depressive episodes. It has fewer adverse effects than most antidepressants and does not cause daytime sedation.
- *Others:* e.g. mirtazepine.
- Almost all the antidepressants are equally effective, but newer agents have fewer side effects. Improvement may take 2–4 weeks.

Psychological treatments

- Both cognitive behavioral therapy and interpersonal therapy are as effective as antidepressants for mild to moderate depression.

Electroconvulsive therapy (ECT)

- May be required for severe depression complicated by psychosis, catatonia, treatment resistance or suicidal risk

Q. Red flag signs of depression requiring referral to a specialist (psychiatrist).

- Referral to a mental health specialist is urgent or necessary when the patient exhibits any of the following red flag signs:

- Suicidal risk (suicidal ideation or plan, previous suicide attempts, self-harming behavior, expressed hopelessness or worthlessness)
- Psychotic symptoms (delusions, hallucinations, severe thought disorganization)
- Severe functional impairment
- Treatment-resistant depression
- Rapid deterioration (agitation or aggression, risk of harm to self or others)
- Manic or hypomanic features (suggesting bipolar disorder)
- Comorbid substance abuse
- Comorbid psychiatric conditions
- Depression in special populations (children, pregnant or postpartum women)

Q. Bipolar disorder (manic depression).

Q. Discuss the clinical features and management of mania.

- Bipolar disorders are characterized by episodes of mania and depression, which may alternate, although many patients have a predominance of one or the other.

Etiology

- Genetic factors: Bipolar disorder is strongly heritable.
- There is also evidence of dysregulation of serotonin and norepinephrine.
- Stressful life events and physical illness may trigger the episodes.
- Drugs (e.g. cocaine, amphetamines), alcohol, and certain antidepressants (e.g. tricyclics, MAOIs) may play a role in triggering episodes.

Clinical Features

Manic Episodes

- Abnormally and persistently elevated mood lasting for at least one week and 3 or more (4 if mood is irritable only) of the following symptoms are present:
  - Inflated self esteem or grandiosity.
  - Decreased need for sleep
  - More talkative than usual
  - Racing thoughts or flight of ideas
  - Distractibility (easily drawn to irrelevant stimuli)
  - Increase in goal-directed activity
  - Excessive involvement in pleasurable activities such as spending money or sexual indiscretion.

Depressive Episodes

- Depression is characterized by features described under depression.

Investigations

- Investigations are done to rule out hyperthyroidism and stimulant drug abuse which can mimic bipolar disorder.

Management

- Drugs for bipolar disorder include mood stabilizers and 2nd generation antipsychotics.
- Mood stabilizers include lithium, sodium valproate, and lamotrigine. Second-generation antipsychotics include aripiprazole, olanzapine, quetiapine, risperidone, and ziprasidone.
- Antidepressants (e.g. SSRIs) are sometimes added for severe depression, but they are not recommended as sole therapy for depressive episodes.
- Electroconvulsive therapy (ECT) is sometimes used for depression refractory to treatment and is also effective for mania.

Q. Attention-deficit hyperactivity disorder (ADHD).

- ADHD is a neurodevelopmental disorder characterized by a persistent pattern of inattention and/or hyperactivity-impulsivity that interferes with functioning or development.

- It typically begins in childhood, often before age 12, and can persist into adolescence and adulthood.

Pathogenesis

- The pathogenesis of attention deficit hyperactivity disorder (ADHD) in adults is not known. The most noticeable deficits in the area of attention are, in general, related to frontal-subcortical dysfunction and deal with executive function.
- It is likely that a network of interrelated brain areas is involved in the attentional-executive impairments of individuals with ADHD.

Clinical Features

Inattention

- Difficulty sustaining attention in tasks/play
- Easily distracted
- Does not seem to listen
- Fails to finish schoolwork or chores
- Disorganized work habits
- Avoids or dislikes tasks requiring sustained effort
- Often forgetful in daily activities.

Hyperactivity

- Fidgets or squirms in seat
- Leaves seat in situations when remaining seated is expected
- Runs about or climbs excessively
- Talks excessively
- Difficulty engaging in leisure activities quietly.

Impulsivity

- Blurts out answers
- Difficulty waiting for turn
- Interrupts or intrudes on others
- Impulsivity in adults often results in more serious consequences than during childhood and may include premature termination of relationships or quitting jobs without having any alternative. Impulsivity can contribute to the driving errors, traffic tickets, and speeding.

Emotional Dysregulation

- Mood lability, irritability, anger outbursts, low frustration tolerance, and motivational deficits are commonly seen in adults with ADHD.
- These mood symptoms are commonly referred to as emotional dysregulation, which is the inability to manage uncomfortable emotions when necessary.

Diagnostic Criteria (DSM-5)

- Symptoms must be present before age 12
- Occur in two or more settings (e.g. school, home)
- Clear evidence of impairment in social, academic, or occupational functioning
- Symptoms are not better explained by another disorder (e.g. anxiety, mood disorders).

Etiology

- *Genetic factors*: Strong hereditary component
- *Neurobiological*: Dopamine/noradrenaline dysregulation, delayed cortical maturation
- *Environmental risk factors*: Prenatal exposure to alcohol/tobacco, low birth weight, psychosocial adversity.

Management

Nonpharmacological Interventions

- Behavioral therapy: Positive reinforcement, structured routines
- Parent management training
- Classroom interventions (e.g. seating arrangements, cueing, breaks)
- Psychoeducation for child and parents.

Pharmacological Treatment

- **Stimulants:** *Methylphenidate, amphetamines*. Stimulants are preferred over nonstimulant medication because they have a clinical effect almost immediately after starting.
- **Nonstimulants:** *Atomoxetine* (a selective norepinephrine reuptake inhibitor), *guanfacine* and *clonidine* (α_2-agonists).

Prognosis

- 60–70% may continue to have symptoms into adolescence/adulthood.
- Early diagnosis and comprehensive treatment improve academic, social, and emotional outcomes.

Q. Autism spectrum disorder (ASD)

- Autism spectrum disorder (ASD) is a neurodevelopmental disorder characterized by persistent deficits in social communication and social interaction and restricted, repetitive patterns of behavior, interests, and activities.
- These symptoms appear in early childhood and cause clinically significant impairments in social, academic, or occupational functioning.

Etiology

- Genetic: Strong heritability; multiple genes involved.
- Neurobiological: Abnormalities in brain structure and connectivity.
- Environmental: Advanced parental age, prenatal exposure to infections or toxins (not vaccines).

Clinical Features

Deficits in Social Communication and Interaction

- Deficits in social-emotional reciprocity, e.g. abnormal social approach, reduced sharing of emotions, failure to initiate/respond to social interaction
- Deficits in nonverbal communicative behaviors, e.g. poor eye contact, lack of facial expressions, difficulty understanding gestures.

- Deficits in developing, maintaining, and understanding relationships, e.g. difficulty adjusting behavior in social contexts, lack of interest in peers.

Restricted and Repetitive Behaviors

- Stereotyped or repetitive motor movements, speech, or use of objects (e.g. hand flapping, rocking behaviors, echolalia).
- Resistance to change, insistence on following the same routines, extreme distress at small changes.
- Re-enacting or repeating scenes or scripts that have been heard (e.g. from videos or cartoons).
- Highly restricted, fixated interests (e.g. strong attachment to unusual objects, narrow topics).
- Lack of or unusual reaction to sensory stimuli (e.g. noise, texture, smells).

Associated Features

- There may be intellectual disability, language impairment, anxiety, ADHD, and seizure.

Diagnosis

- Symptoms must be present in early developmental period.
- Must cause clinically significant impairment.
- No better explained by intellectual disability or global developmental delay.

Management

Nonpharmacological Interventions

- Early intensive behavioral intervention
- Speech and language therapy
- Occupational therapy for sensory integration and motor skills
- Social skills training
- Structured educational support (special education).

Pharmacological Treatment

Used for associated symptoms, not core ASD symptoms:

- Irritability, aggression: *Risperidone, aripiprazole*
- Hyperactivity, impulsivity: *Methylphenidate, atomoxetine*
- Anxiety or mood symptoms: *SSRIs* (e.g. fluoxetine) — used cautiously.

Prognosis

- Varies widely; early diagnosis and intensive intervention improve outcomes.
- Some individuals achieve independence; others may require lifelong support.
- Language development and IQ are key predictors of long-term outcome.

Q. Describe common psychosexual disorders.

- Psychosexual disorders (also called sexual dysfunctions or sexual disorders) involve problems with sexual desire, arousal, orgasm, or pain that cause significant distress or interpersonal difficulties. These conditions can be influenced by psychological, physiological, or relational factors.
- They are broadly classified into five categories:
  - Sexual desire disorders
  - Sexual arousal disorders
  - Orgasmic disorders
  - Sexual pain disorders
  - Paraphilic disorders (formerly paraphilias)

Etiology

- Psychological: Anxiety, depression, trauma, negative sexual experiences.
- Biological: Hormonal imbalances, chronic illnesses, neurological conditions.
- Social/relational: Poor communication, relationship conflict, cultural/religious beliefs.
- Medications/substances: Antidepressants (SSRIs), alcohol, antihypertensives.

Sexual Desire Disorders

Hypoactive Sexual Desire Disorder

- Persistently low or absent sexual desire/fantasies
- Common in both males and females, especially post-menopausal women
- Causes: Depression, relationship issues, hormonal changes, medications.

Sexual Aversion Disorder

- Active avoidance of sexual contact due to fear, anxiety, or disgust. Often linked to past sexual trauma or phobias.

Sexual Arousal Disorders

Female Sexual Interest/Arousal Disorder

- Reduced interest in sex and lack of genital or nongenital arousal. No lubrication, minimal sexual excitement.

Male Erectile Disorder (erectile dysfunction)

- Persistent difficulty in achieving or maintaining an erection. Often due to anxiety, cardiovascular disease, diabetes, substance use.

Orgasmic Disorders

Female Orgasmic Disorder

- Delay in, infrequency of, or absence of orgasm after sexual stimulation.
- Often related to anxiety, guilt, inadequate sexual knowledge.

Male Orgasmic Disorder (delayed ejaculation)

- Delay or absence of orgasm despite adequate stimulation.

Premature Ejaculation

- Ejaculation that occurs within one minute of penetration or before the person desires it. Common in younger men; often anxiety-related.

Sexual Pain Disorders

Genitopelvic Pain/Penetration Disorder

- Pain, fear, or difficulty during vaginal intercourse or penetration. It includes:
  - Dyspareunia: Pain during intercourse.
  - Vaginismus: Involuntary muscle contractions preventing penetration.

Paraphilic Disorders (formerly paraphilias)

- These involve intense sexual urges or behaviors involving unusual objects, activities, or situations, which cause distress or harm. Paraphilic behaviors become disorders when they cause distress or involve non-consenting individuals. Examples are as follows:
  - Exhibitionistic disorder: Urge to expose genitals to strangers.
  - Fetishistic disorder: Sexual fixation on non-living objects (e.g. shoes, leather).
  - Frotteuristic disorder: Urge to touch or rub against a non-consenting person.
  - Pedophilic disorder: Sexual focus on prepubescent children.
  - Sexual masochism/sadism disorder: Sexual arousal from being hurt or causing pain.
  - Voyeuristic disorder: Urge to observe unsuspecting individuals naked or in sexual activity.

Management

Psychotherapy

- Cognitive behavioral therapy (CBT)
- Sex therapy
- Couple/marital therapy.

Medical Treatment

- Hormonal therapy (e.g. testosterone)
- Medications (e.g. sildenafil for erectile dysfunction, SSRIs for premature ejaculation).

Education and Counseling

- Sex education
- Addressing myths, fears, and misconceptions.

Q. Medicolegal, societal, ethical, and humanitarian principles in dealing with the LGBTQA+ community.

- The LGBTQA+ community (table) is a diverse group of individuals whose sexual orientations, gender identities, and expressions differ from the societal norms traditionally associated with heterosexuality and cisgender identities.
- Healthcare providers must uphold medicolegal, ethical, societal, and humanitarian responsibilities while working with the LGBTQA+ community. This includes respecting identity, ensuring non-discriminatory practices, providing inclusive care, and advocating for social justice.

LGBTQA+ Stands for (Table 12.3)

TABLE 12.3: Meaning of LGBTQA+

Letter	Meaning
L	**Lesbian:** A woman who is romantically or sexually attracted to other women.
G	**Gay:** A person (often a man) who is attracted to people of the same gender.
B	**Bisexual:** A person attracted to more than one gender.
T	**Transgender:** A person whose gender identity differs from the sex assigned at birth.
Q	**Queer or questioning:** *Queer* is an umbrella term for nonheterosexual identities; *Questioning* refers to those still exploring their gender or sexuality.
A	**Asexual or Ally:** *Asexual* refers to people who experience little or no sexual attraction; *Ally* refers to supportive non-LGBTQ individuals.
+	Represents **inclusion of other identities** not specifically listed, such as intersex, pansexual, non-binary, genderfluid, and others.

Medicolegal Principles

- *Legal recognition of gender and sexual diversity*: In many countries (including India), gender identity and sexual orientation are protected by law.
- *Right to confidentiality and informed consent:* LGBTQA+ individuals have the legal right to confidentiality about their gender identity, sexual orientation, and medical history. Information about them should not be disclosed without their consent. Informed consent must be obtained for all procedures, especially in gender-affirming care.
- *Right to nondiscrimination*: Discrimination in healthcare settings based on sexual orientation or gender identity is prohibited by law. Legal mechanisms exist for redressal in case of violation of rights.

Ethical Principles

- *Autonomy:* Respect for the individual's right to self-identify, choose their gender, and make decisions regarding their body and medical care. Healthcare providers must support informed decision-making and gender-affirming care without coercion.
- *Beneficence and nonmaleficence*: Provide care that benefits the individual without causing harm. Avoid unnecessary psychiatric labeling or conversion therapies, which are unethical and harmful.
- *Justice:* Ensure equal access to healthcare, education, and employment opportunities. Advocate for social equity and challenge structural barriers.
- *Respect and dignity*: Use correct pronouns, preferred names, and provide culturally competent care. Create a nonjudgmental, inclusive environment in clinical settings.

Societal Principles

- *Inclusion and acceptance:* Promote awareness and acceptance of LGBTQA+ individuals in schools,

workplaces, and communities. Address stigma, myths, and misinformation through education and advocacy.
- *Antistigma campaigns*: Encourage public health initiatives that address mental health, substance use, and HIV/STI prevention in the LGBTQA+ community.
- *Support systems*: Facilitate peer support groups, community-based resources, and mental health counseling tailored to LGBTQA+ needs.
- *Educational reforms*: These include gender and sexuality education in medical and public health curricula. Train healthcare professionals in LGBTQA+ cultural competence.

Humanitarian Principles

- *Right to health*: The LGBTQA+ community has the fundamental human right to health, including physical, mental, reproductive, and sexual health.
- *Right to life with dignity*: Support the right to live free from fear, violence, and discrimination. Address mental health vulnerabilities (e.g. higher rates of depression, suicide, and substance abuse) compassionately.
- *Protection in crisis and vulnerability*: Ensure that LGBTQA+ individuals are protected in emergencies, refugee camps, shelters, and during pandemics or disasters. Advocate for antiviolence laws and protective shelters.

Q. Anorexia nervosa.

Definition

- Anorexia nervosa is an eating disorder characterized by restriction of energy intake relative to requirements, leading to a significantly low body weight.
- Patients have intense fear of gaining weight and distorted body image so that they regard themselves as fat even when grossly underweight.

Clinical Features

- It is common in women.
- *Restricting type*: Weight loss achieved through dieting, fasting, or excessive exercise.
- *Binge eating/purging type*: Regular episodes of binge eating or purging (vomiting, laxatives, diuretics).
- Associated anxiety and depressive symptoms are common. Downy hair (lanugo) may develop on the back, forearms and cheeks. Extreme starvation may affect multiple organ systems, especially heart and skeletal system. Amenorrhea is also common.

Etiology

- Exact etiology is unknown, but a combination of psychological, biological, family, genetic, environmental, and social factors play a role.
- Social pressure on women to be thin also plays a role.

Investigations

- Rule out other causes of weight loss such as malabsorption syndromes (e.g. due to inflammatory bowel disease or celiac disease), new-onset type 1 diabetes, adrenal insufficiency, and cancer. Amphetamine abuse may cause similar symptoms.

Management

- All other causes of weight loss should be ruled out (e.g. malabsorption, cancer, etc.).
- The goals of treatment are: To ensure patient's physical well-being, to maintain normal body weight, and to correct the psychological disturbances.
- Patients can be treated on outpatient basis. Admission is required if there is severe weight loss or if there is a risk of death from medical complications or from suicide.
- Cognitive behavioral therapy helps the patient manage the anxiety related to eating and poor body image by developing more adaptive thoughts and coping strategies. Family therapy encourages family members to refeed patients at home with the support of a family therapist.
- Psychotropic drugs are helpful if there is associated depression.

Q. Bulimia nervosa.

- Bulimia nervosa is an eating disorder characterized by episodes of binge eating, followed by compensatory behavior of the purging type (self-induced vomiting, laxative abuse, diuretic abuse) or nonpurging type (excessive exercise, fasting, or strict diets).
- Note that bulimia nervosa (normal weight) is different from binge-eating/purging type of anorexia nervosa (significantly underweight).
- Binge eating disorder is also different from bulimia nervosa. Binge eating disorder is characterized by recurrent episodes of consuming large amounts of food without any compensatory behavior.

Clinical Features

- It is more common in women and the etiology is same as anorexia nervosa.
- Patients typically describe binge-purge behavior. Binges involve rapid consumption of large amounts of high calorie foods. Binge eating episodes can occur several times a day and triggered by psychological stress. Binge eating is followed by compensatory behaviors: self-induced vomiting, use of laxatives or diuretics, excessive exercise, and/or fasting.
- There is dissatisfaction with body shape and weight but weight is maintained within normal limits (note that in anorexia nervosa there is significant weight loss).
- Physical signs of repeated self-induced vomiting include pitted teeth (from gastric acid), calluses on knuckles and parotid gland enlargement.

Management

- Cognitive behavioral therapy (gold standard).
- Drugs: Antidepressants like fluoxetine, amitriptyline have been shown to reduce binge eating. Other helpful drugs are topiramate and ondansetron.

Q. Somatic symptom disorders.

- Somatic symptom disorders (earlier called somatoform disorders) are a group of psychiatric conditions characterized by the presence of physical (somatic) symptoms that are distressing or disruptive, but cannot be fully explained by a medical condition.
- Somatic symptom disorders include the following **(Table 12.4)**:

TABLE 12.4: Somatic symptom disorders	
Somatic symptom disorder	One or more distressing physical symptoms, e.g. pain, fatigue
Illness anxiety disorder (formerly hypochondriasis)	Preoccupation with having or acquiring a serious illness
Conversion disorder	Neurological symptoms (e.g. paralysis, blindness, seizures) without neurological disease
Psychological factors affecting other medical conditions	A psychological factor (e.g. anxiety) worsens a real medical illness (e.g. asthma, diabetes)
Factitious disorder	Intentional production or feigning of physical or psychological symptoms Motivation is to assume the sick role (not for external gain)

Etiology

- Exact cause is unknown.
- Contributory factors include depression or anxiety, erroneous interpretation of somatic symptoms as evidence of disease, and preoccupation with physical illness.
- Family history or previous history of a particular condition may provoke concerns about illness.

Clinical Features

- Physical complaints usually begin before age 30. Most patients have multiple somatic symptoms such as pain, headache, etc. The somatic symptoms are not explained by a medical condition and are also not part of depressive or anxiety disorder. Physical symptoms may involve one or more organ systems and are not intentional. Symptoms persist for a long time. The symptoms themselves or excessive worry about them is distressing or disrupts daily life. Some patients become overtly depressed.
- When physical complaints accompany another medical disorder, patients over-respond to the implications of the medical disorder; for example, patients who have had an MI may constantly worry about having another MI or think themselves as unfit. Such patients are very anxious about their health problems and are difficult to reassure.
- Whatever the manifestations, the essence of somatic symptom disorder is the patient's excessive or maladaptive thoughts, feelings, or behaviors in response to the symptoms.

Treatment

- Cognitive-behavioral therapy.
- Insight-oriented therapy or stress management
- Treatment of concurrent mental disorders (e.g. depression).
- Selective serotonin reuptake inhibitors (SSRIs) and serotonin-norepinephrine reuptake inhibitors (SNRIs) have shown benefit.

Q. Conversion disorder (hysteria; dissociative disorder).

- Conversion disorder (also known as functional neurological symptom disorder) consists of neurologic symptoms or deficits that develop unconsciously and nonvolitionally without a definable organic cause.
- "Conversion" is characterized by conversion of psychic conflict into physical symptoms. The coping mechanisms used in this condition are repression (a barring from consciousness) and isolation (a splitting of the affect from the idea).

Etiology (causes)

- *Psychological stress/conflict:* Emotional trauma (e.g. abuse, war, loss), internal conflict or repressed emotions.
- *Personality factors*: Histrionic or dependent traits. Low stress tolerance.
- *Social/environmental factors*: Secondary gain (e.g. attention, relief from responsibilities).
- *Neurobiological factors*: Abnormalities in brain circuits related to emotion and movement (e.g. limbic system dysfunction).
- *Preexisting psychiatric illness*: Depression, anxiety, PTSD.

Clinical Features

- It is more common in young and uneducated women from lower socioeconomic class.
- Symptoms often develop abruptly, and onset can often be linked to a stressful event. Patients may present with impaired coordination or balance, weakness, paralysis of an arm or a leg, loss of sensation in a body part, seizures, unresponsiveness, blindness, double vision, deafness, aphonia, difficulty—swallowing, sensation of a lump in the throat, or urinary retention. The manifestations are not in the conscious control of the patient.
- There is apparent unconcern (La belle indifference) even in the face of gross physical disability.
- Clues pointing toward conversion disorder are: history of similar episode in the past, presence of a serious precipitating emotional event, presence of associated depression, etc. temporal correlation between the precipitating event and the symptom, and a temporary "solving of the problem" by the conversion.
- A complete physical and neurological examination is important to rule out physical causes.

Treatment

- Reassurance
- Explanation of the cause of symptoms. It is helpful to explain the physiological mechanism for the symptom that emphasizes the link with psychological factors such as stress.
- Advice on how to cope with stress and relaxation techniques.
- Antidepressant drugs are helpful even if the patient is not depressed.
- Cognitive behavioral therapy and other psychological treatments are helpful.

Q. Factitious disorder imposed on self (Munchausen syndrome).

- Factitious disorder imposed on self is a psychiatric disorder in which patients deliberately produce or falsify symptoms and/or signs of illness for the purpose of assuming the sick role. It is also known as Munchausen syndrome named after German Baron Freiherr von Munchausen, who told fanciful tales only to entertain others.
- Patients with factitious disorders differ from malingerers because, there are no obvious external incentives (e.g. economic gain) for their behavior. It is unclear what they gain beyond medical attention for their suffering.

Clinical Features

- Approximately two-thirds of patients with Munchausen syndrome are males. They are usually older with a solitary lifestyle.
- They present frequently with dramatic symptoms. Examination may show previous multiple surgical scars. They often present at night when junior doctors and residents are on duty. The history can be convincing enough to persuade doctors to undertake investigations or initiate treatment, including exploratory surgery.

Management

- Management is by gentle but firm confrontation with clear evidence of the fabrication of illness, together with an offer of psychological support. Any underlying psychological disorders (anxiety, depression) should be treated.

Q. Substance abuse.

- Substance abuse (also known as substance use disorder), refers to excess or harmful use of psychoactive substances—including alcohol and illicit drugs. It involves compulsive use, loss of control, and continued use despite adverse consequences.
- Substance dependence (addiction) refers to substance use associated with psychological dependence (craving), physiologic dependence (withdrawal symptoms on stopping the drug) and tolerance.
- Substance abuse and dependence are major problems world-wide. They affect all races, and all socioeconomic strata. They are more common in men than in women although the gap is narrowing.

Etiology

- Cultural pressures, particularly within a peer group
- Easy availability of a drug
- Medical over-prescribing
- Psychiatric problems such as depression.

Commonly Abused Psychoactive Substances

- Alcohol
- Nicotine (smoking and smokeless tobacco)
- Cannabis (*bhang*, *ganja*, *charas*)
- Opioids (heroin, codeine, tramadol, opium)
- Sedatives and hypnotics (benzodiazepines)
- Inhalants (used more in adolescents)
- Stimulants (less common: cocaine, amphetamines).

Diagnosis

- History
- Physical examination—needle marks in IV drug users; evidence of localized or systemic infections; staining of teeth, respiratory problems in inhalation drug abuse
- Drug screening of samples of urine or blood.

Management

- Psychological counseling
- Harm minimization—for example, advice to use clean needles.
- Substitute prescribing (example methadone in opiate dependence).
- Identifying and treating problems associated with the drug misuse.
- Treatment of complications of drug misuse.

Q. Alcohol use disorder (alcohol abuse and alcohol dependence).

Q. Complications of chronic alcohol abuse.

Definitions

Alcohol use Disorder

- Alcohol use disorder is defined as a problematic pattern of alcohol use leading to clinically significant psychosocial, behavioral, or physiologic impairment.
- It includes alcohol abuse and alcohol dependence, which are now outdated terms and merged into single term 'alcohol use disorder'.
- It is categorized by severity (mild, moderate, severe) based on the number of diagnostic criteria met.

Diagnostic Criteria for Alcohol Use Disorder

At least **2 of the following within 12 months:**

1. Drinking more or longer than intended
2. Persistent desire or unsuccessful efforts to cut down
3. Much time spent obtaining, using, or recovering from alcohol
4. Craving
5. Failure to fulfill major obligations
6. Continued use despite social/interpersonal problems
7. Giving up important activities
8. Use in physically hazardous situations

9. Continued use despite physical/psychological harm
10. Tolerance (need more to get same effect)
11. Withdrawal symptoms when not drinking

- **Mild:** 2–3 symptoms
- **Moderate:** 4–5
- **Severe:** 6 or more

Risk Factors for Alcohol Use Disorder

- Availability of alcohol and social patterns of use
- Genetic factors
- As a measure to relieve anxiety or depression
- Many who abuse alcohol have certain personality traits: feelings of isolation, loneliness, shyness, depression, dependency, hostile and self-destructive impulsivity, and sexual immaturity.
- Social problems: Broken home, disturbed relationship with their family.

Complications of Alcohol Misuse

Acute intoxication: Emotional and behavioral disturbance, hypoglycemia, aspiration, respiratory depression and even death

Nervous system: Peripheral neuropathy, cerebellar degeneration, cerebral hemorrhage, Wernicke's encephalopathy, dementia

Liver: Alcoholic liver disease (hepatitis, fatty liver and cirrhosis), liver cancer

GIT: Esophagitis, gastritis, pancreatitis, esophageal cancer, Mallory-Weiss syndrome

RS: Pulmonary TB, pneumonia

CVS: Cardiomyopathy, hypertension, arrhythmias

Hematologic:

- Anemia (macrocytic from B_{12}/folate deficiency)
- Thrombocytopenia
- Leukopenia

Musculoskeletal: Myopathy, fractures

Endocrine and metabolic: Pseudo-Cushing's syndrome, hypoglycemia, gout.

Reproductive: Hypogonadism, fetal alcohol syndrome, infertility.

Psychiatric problems: Depression, anxiety, alcohol withdrawal, alcoholic hallucinosis, alcoholic 'blackouts'.

Social and legal complications:

- Domestic violence
- Job loss
- Legal issues
- Marital problems

Management

- Advice about the harmful effects of alcohol and safe levels of consumption.
- Supportive psychotherapy
- Pharmacotherapy: Naltrexone, disulfiram, and acamprosate are helpful to treat alcohol dependence.
- Naltrexone (opiate antagonist) can be started while the patient is still drinking. It lessens the pleasurable effects of alcohol. It also reduces craving for alcohol.
- Disulfiram should be used by abstinent patients to maintain abstinence.
- Acamprosate should be used once abstinence is achieved. It reduces craving and helps maintenance of abstinence.

Q. Alcohol withdrawal syndrome (delirium tremens).

- Alcohol withdrawal syndrome (AWS) is a set of symptoms that occur when a heavy or prolonged alcohol user suddenly stops or significantly reduces alcohol intake.
- Alcohol is a CNS depressant, hence, withdrawal symptoms are caused by unmasking of compensatory over-activity of certain parts of the nervous system, including sympathetic autonomic outflow.
- The most severe form of withdrawal is delirium tremens—a life-threatening medical emergency characterized by confusion, hallucinations, tremors, and autonomic instability.

Pathophysiology

- Chronic alcohol use enhances GABAergic activity. Alcohol withdrawal causes a functional decrease in the inhibitory neurotransmitter GABA. This leads to increased activity of excitatory neurotransmitters such as norepinephrine, glutamate, and dopamine.
- Alcohol also acts as an NMDA receptor antagonist. Withdrawal leads to increased activity of these excitatory neuroreceptors, resulting in tremors, agitation, hallucinations, seizures, tachycardia, hyperthermia, and hypertension.

Clinical Features

- Symptoms usually occur within eight hours of stopping alcohol, reach a peak on the 2nd or 3rd day, and diminish by the 4th or 5th day.
- Symptoms include anxiety, tremor, insomnia, decreased cognition, irritability, headache, diaphoresis, palpitations, and in severe cases delirium tremens.
- Delirium tremens (DTs) is the most severe form of alcohol withdrawal manifested by altered mental status (global confusion) and sympathetic hyperactivity, which can progress to cardiovascular collapse. It is characterized by mental confusion, visual hallucinations (often of snakes, bugs, etc.), agitation, tremor, tachycardia,hypertension, diaphoresis, dehydration, and seizures.

Investigations

- Rule out hepatic encephalopathy, gastrointestinal bleeding, cardiac arrhythmia, infection, and glucose or electrolyte imbalance by appropriate tests.
- CT or MRI of brain may be required to rule out intracranial pathology.

Complications

- Delirium tremens (DTs)—medical emergency
- Seizures
- Wernicke's encephalopathy (due to thiamine deficiency)
- Cardiac arrhythmias due to electrolyte imbalance.

Treatment

- Benzodiazepines (drug of choice)—diazepam or chlordiazepoxide are commonly used, but other agents can also be used. Benzodiazepines exert their effect via stimulation of gamma-aminobutyric acid (GABA) receptors, causing a decrease in neuronal activity and relative sedation. They alleviate most symptoms of withdrawal. The average patient requires 25–50 mg of chlordiazepoxide or 10 mg of diazepam given PO every 4–6 hours on the first day and then tapered off over a period of 3–5 days. Oral therapy is enough in most cases, but parenteral therapy may be required in severe cases associated with delirium tremens and seizures.
- Thiamine supplementation should be given to all patients.
- Supportive therapy: ICU care, IV fluids, nutritional support.

Q. Nicotine abuse.

- Nicotine abuse refers to the compulsive use of tobacco products, despite harmful health consequences. It is commonly seen in the form of smoking cigarettes, chewing tobacco, snuff, or vaping. The key substance responsible for dependence is nicotine, an alkaloid with powerful psychoactive and addictive properties.

Epidemiology

- Tobacco is the leading preventable cause of death worldwide.
- In India, over 267 million people use tobacco in some form.
- Common in adolescents, young adults, and low socio-economic groups
- Forms in India include: cigarettes, bidis, gutka, khaini, zarda, etc.

Pathophysiology

- Nicotine activates nicotinic acetylcholine receptors in the brain, releasing dopamine, producing pleasure and reinforcing use.
- Chronic use leads to tolerance, dependence, and withdrawal symptoms.

Clinical Features

Acute Effects

- Increased alertness and attention
- Appetite suppression
- Mild euphoria
- Increased heart rate and blood pressure.

Chronic Effects

- Persistent cough, wheezing
- Dyspnea (shortness of breath)
- Bad breath, stained teeth
- Physical dependence (cravings, tolerance)
- Behavioral compulsion to smoke or chew.

Withdrawal Symptoms

- Irritability, anxiety, depression
- Insomnia
- Increased appetite and weight gain
- Difficulty concentrating
- Intense cravings.

Complications of Chronic Nicotine Use

Respiratory

- Chronic bronchitis
- Chronic obstructive pulmonary disease (COPD)
- Lung cancer.

Cardiovascular

- Coronary artery disease
- Hypertension
- Stroke.

Gastrointestinal

- Peptic ulcers
- Oral and esophageal cancers (especially with smokeless tobacco).

Reproductive

- Reduced fertility
- Complications in pregnancy (low-birth weight, miscarriage).

Diagnosis

- Clinical history and physical examination.
- Use of Fagerstrom test for nicotine dependence. This is a standardized questionnaire used to assess the intensity of physical addiction to nicotine.
- Carbon monoxide monitoring (in smokers)
- Cotinine (nicotine metabolite) levels in blood/urine.

Management

Behavioral Interventions

- Counseling (individual or group)
- Cognitive-behavioral therapy (CBT)
- Motivational interviewing
- Quitlines and mobile health interventions.

Pharmacotherapy

- Nicotine replacement therapy (NRT): Patches, gums, lozenges, inhalers
- Nonnicotine medications: Bupropion—has anti-depressant with anticraving effects. Varenicline (Chantix)—partial nicotinic receptor agonist.

Prevention and Public Health Measures

- School and community education programs
- Legislation: Bans on tobacco ads, public smoking
- Graphic warnings on packaging
- Increased taxes on tobacco products.

Q. Complications of smoking.

Q. Management of smoking cessation.

- Smoking refers to the inhalation of smoke from burning tobacco, most commonly through cigarettes, but also bidis, cigars, pipes, or hookah. It is a leading cause of preventable morbidity and mortality worldwide.
- Cigarette smoke contains more than 4,000 substances. The main active ingredient is nicotine. Other important substances include carbon monoxide, tar, aromatic hydrocarbons, benzopyrine, nitrosamine, vinyl chloride, trace metals, phenol, cresol and catechol. Most of these are carcinogens.
- Passive smoking (secondhand smoke) refers to involuntary exposure of nonsmokers to tobacco smoke from the smoking of others. Passive smoking is a mixture of side stream smoke given off by the burning cigarette and of mainstream smoke that is exhaled by the smoker. Side stream smoke, generated under the lower temperature conditions in the smoldering cigarette, has higher concentrations of many of the toxic compounds than the mainstream smoke. Passive smoking is also associated with all the complications of active smoking.

Complications of Chronic Smoking

CVS
- Increased risk of angina and MI
- Hypertension
- Aortic aneurysm
- Peripheral vascular disease

RS
- Increased incidence of respiratory tract infections
- COPD
- Laryngeal cancer
- Lung cancer

GIT
- Periodontitis
- Discoloration of teeth, reduced taste and smell
- Acid peptic disease
- Increased risk of cancers of oral cavity, esophagus, stomach, colon and pancreas

Nervous system
- Irritability
- Increased risk of stroke

Genitourinary system
- Impotence
- Infertility
- IUGR
- Increased risk of spontaneous abortion, fetal death and sudden infant death
- Cancer of urinary bladder

Blood
- Polycythemia

Management of Smoking

- Same as management of nicotine abuse (*see* previous topic).

Q. Cannabis abuse.

- Cannabis (marijuana, weed, *ganja*, *charas*, *bhang*) is a psychoactive substance derived from the *Cannabis sativa* or *Cannabis indica* plant. It is one of the most commonly used illicit drugs worldwide, especially among adolescents and young adults.
- Main psychoactive component: Δ^9-tetrahydrocannabinol (THC)—responsible for most of the psychoactive effects.

Modes of Use

- Smoking (joints, pipes, chillums, bongs)
- Edibles (cookies, brownies)
- Vaping
- Bhang (in India, especially during festivals).

Clinical Presentation

- Euphoria, relaxation
- Red eyes, increased appetite
- Altered perception (time slows down)
- Impaired coordination, reaction time
- With chronic use: Amotivation, memory impairment, psychosis.

Withdrawal (mild)

- Irritability, sleep disturbances, anxiety.

Management

- Supportive psychotherapy
- Cognitive behavioral therapy (CBT)
- Treatment of comorbid psychiatric symptoms (e.g. anxiety, psychosis).

Q. Opioid abuse (e.g. heroin, opium, prescription painkillers).

- Opioids are a class of drugs that include natural, semi-synthetic, and synthetic compounds that bind to opioid receptors in the brain and body to produce pain relief and euphoria.

Types of Opioids

- *Natural:* Opium, morphine, codeine
- *Semi-synthetic*: Heroin, oxycodone, hydrocodone
- *Synthetic:* Fentanyl, methadone, tramadol, pethidine.

Clinical Presentation

- Euphoria, drowsiness ("nodding off")
- Pinpoint pupils
- Respiratory depression (can be fatal)
- Bradycardia, hypotension, constipation, itching
- With chronic use: Dependence, needle marks (IV users), infections.

Withdrawal

- Runny nose, lacrimation, yawning
- Body aches, diarrhea, goosebumps ("cold turkey")

Management

- Detoxification: Clonidine (for autonomic symptoms), antidiarrheals, NSAIDs, antiemetics
- Maintenance therapy (opioid substitution treatment): Methadone or buprenorphine
- Relapse prevention: Naltrexone is opioid antagonist; prevents relapse after detoxification
- Psychosocial therapy, group support.

Q. Sedative-hypnotic abuse (e.g. benzodiazepines).

- Sedative-hypnotic abuse refers to the nonmedical use, overuse, or dependence on central nervous system (CNS) depressants, especially:
  - Benzodiazepines (e.g. diazepam, alprazolam, lorazepam).
  - Barbiturates (e.g. phenobarbital).
  - Z-drugs (e.g. zolpidem, zaleplon).
- They enhance GABA-A receptor activity, increasing inhibitory neurotransmission, leading to—sedation, muscle relaxation, anxiolysis, and anticonvulsant effects.

Clinical Presentation

- Sedation, slurred speech, euphoria
- Dizziness, unsteady gait
- Memory impairment
- Chronic use → dependence
- Severe overdose: Respiratory depression, hypotension, coma, death (especially with alcohol/opioids)
- *Withdrawal (can be dangerous):* Anxiety, tremors, seizures, delirium.

Management

- Tapering the dose gradually
- Switching to long-acting agents (e.g. diazepam)
- Psychological support.

Q. Inhalant abuse.

- Inhalant abuse refers to the intentional inhalation of volatile substances (vapors, gases, or aerosols) to achieve a psychoactive or mind-altering effect. These substances are not intended for human consumption and are often legal household products.
- Inhalants are CNS depressants, enhancing GABA activity or directly affecting neuronal membranes.

Common Inhalants

- *Volatile solvents*: Glue, paint thinners, nail polish remover, correction fluid
- *Aerosols*: Spray paints, deodorants, hair sprays, air fresheners
- *Gases*: Butane, propane, nitrous oxide ("laughing gas"), whipped cream chargers
- *Nitrites* (often used sexually): Amyl nitrite ("poppers"), butyl nitrite.

Clinical Presentation

- Dizziness, euphoria, hallucinations
- Slurred speech, loss of coordination
- Sudden sniffing death (cardiac arrest)
- Chronic use → brain, liver, kidney damage.

Management

- Supportive care
- Family therapy and counseling
- Monitoring for complications.

Q. What are the sleep disorders?

Q. Discuss the causes and management of insomnia.

- Sleep disorders are conditions that disrupt the normal pattern, quality, timing, or amount of sleep. They can significantly affect physical health, emotional well-being, and daytime functioning.
- Sleep consists of two phases: (1) REM (rapid eye movement) sleep, also called dream sleep, and (2) NREM (non-REM) sleep. NREM sleep is divided into stages 1, 2, 3, and 4 which can be recognized by different EEG patterns. Stages 3 and 4 are "delta" or deep sleep. Dreaming occurs mostly in REM sleep.
- Sleep is a cyclic phenomenon, with REM and NREM sleep alternating throughout the night. Stage 3 and 4 sleep decreases as the age advances.

Sleep disorders can be divided into 2 broad categories:

- Parasomnias: These are unusual experiences or behaviors that occur during sleep; they are sleep terror, sleepwalking and nightmare disorder.
- Dyssomnias: These are characterized by abnormalities in the amount, quality, or timing of sleep; they are insomnia and hypersomnia, narcolepsy, and circadian rhythm sleep disorder.

Insomnia

- Insomnia is characterized by an inadequate quantity or quality of sleep.
- Affected patients complain of difficulty initiating or maintaining sleep, resulting in nonrestorative sleep and impairment of daytime functioning.

Causes

Transient insomnia

- Change of sleeping environment
- Jet lag
- Changes in work shift
- Physical discomfort (excessive noise, unpleasant room temperature)
- Stressful life events (e.g. loss of a loved one, divorce, loss of employment, preparing to take an examination)
- Acute medical or surgical illnesses
- Stimulant medications (theophylline, quinolones, caffeine)

Chronic insomnia

- Depression
- Mania
- Abuse of alcohol
- Heavy smoking

- Neurological disorders (fatal familial insomnia, Alzheimer's disease, Parkinson's disease, cerebral hemispheric and brain stem strokes, brain tumors)
- Chronic medical disorders (COPD, CCF, AIDS)
- Primary sleep disorders (restless legs syndrome, sleep apnea).

Evaluation

History

- Duration of symptoms and h/o any events (e.g. work change, new drug, new medical disorder) that coincided with onset
- Determine the quality and quantity of sleep by asking: Time of going to bed, latency of sleep (time from bedtime to falling asleep), number and time of awakenings, final morning awakening and arising times, frequency and duration of naps
- Ask about bedtime events (e.g. food or alcohol consumption, physical or mental activity)
- H/o of snoring, interrupted breathing patterns, and other nocturnal respiratory disturbances suggest sleep apnea syndromes
- H/o depression, anxiety, mania, and hypomania suggest mental sleep disorders
- Ask about any medical disorders that can interfere with sleep, including COPD, asthma, heart failure, hyperthyroidism, gastroesophageal reflux, neurologic disorders (particularly movement and degenerative disorders), and painful disorders (e.g. rheumatoid arthritis).
- Ask about any drug intake that could interfere with sleep (e.g. SSRIs, phenytoin, amphetamines, aminophyline).

Physical examination

- Look for any upper respiratory tract abnormalities that can cause obstructive sleep apnea and snoring.
- Look for evidence of diseases that could interfere with sleep.

Investigations

- Appropriate tests to rule out any medical disorder that can cause insomnia.

Management

- *Good sleep hygiene*—go to bed only when sleepy, get up early, discontinue caffeine and nicotine, daily exercise, avoid alcohol, and practice relaxation techniques.
- *Pharmacologic measures*—hypnotic medications such as lorazepam (0.5 mg at night), zolpidem (5–10 mg at bedtime), and zaleplon (5–10 mg at bedtime). In general, medications should be used for short courses of 1–2 weeks. Melatonin (a hormone secreted by pineal gland) is effective for delayed sleep onset. Suvorexant is a new treatment for insomnia that acts by blocking brain orexin receptors, thereby blocking orexin-induced wakefulness signals and enabling sleep initiation. Tasimelteon, a melatonin receptor agonist, can increase nighttime sleep duration and decrease daytime sleep duration.
- *Treatment of underlying cause*—such as COPD, CCF, etc.

Q. Narcolepsy.

- Narcolepsy is characterized by chronic excessive daytime sleepiness, often with sudden loss of muscle tone (cataplexy).

Etiology

- In narcolepsy there is dysregulation of the timing and control of REM sleep. Therefore, REM sleep intrudes into wakefulness and into the transition from wakefulness to sleep.
- Genetic factors: Narcolepsy is strongly associated with specific HLA haplotypes, and children of patients with narcolepsy have increased risk.
- Deficiency of neuropeptide hypocretin-1 is found in CSF of narcoleptic animals and human patients.

Clinical Features

- The disease typically begins in the teens and early twenties, affects both sexes equally, and usually levels off in severity at about 30 years of age.
- Narcolepsy is characterized by the following features:
  - Daytime sleepiness—sudden and brief attacks of sleep during any type of activity.
  - Cataplexy—sudden loss of muscle tone which may cause the person to slump to the floor or unable to move.
  - Sleep paralysis—is a complete inability to move for one or two minutes immediately after awakening.
  - Hypnagogic hallucinations—visual or auditory, occur just as the patient is falling asleep or upon awakening.
- Diagnosis can be confirmed by polysomnography and multiple sleep latency testing.

Treatment

- Modafinil, a nonamphetamine wakefulness promoting agent has become a first line agent because of less abuse potential.
- CNS stimulant drugs such as methylphenidate or amphetamine derivatives are used instead of or with modafinil if patients do not respond to modafinil.
- Tricyclic antidepressants (clomipramine) and SSRIs may be useful for cataplexy, sleep paralysis, and hypnagogic and hypnopompic hallucinations.

Q. Sleepwalking (somnambulism).

- Sleepwalking also known as somnambulism involves getting up and walking around or performing a complex motor activity while in a state of sleep.
- It generally occurs in deep non rapid eye movement (NREM) (stages 3 and 4) sleep.

Causes

- Somnambulism may be precipitated by a variety of conditions such as insufficient sleep resulting from an irregular sleep schedule, staying up late, giving up a daily nap or waking early in the morning.
- In elderly, it may be a feature of dementia.

- Drugs (phenothiazines, chloral hydrate, lithium), marijuana, alcohol and medical conditions (e.g. complex partial seizures) can also cause sleep walking.
- It may be familial.

Clinical Features

- It affects mostly children aged 6–12 years. Patients with this disorder carry out automatic motor activities during sleep that range from simple to complex. There is no memory of the event. Individuals may walk, urinate inappropriately, eat, or exit from the house while remaining only partially aware. Attempt to awaken them may rarely lead to agitation or even violence.

Treatment

- Reassurance is the mainstay of treatment. Patients and parents should be told that sleepwalking is benign and eventually disappears.
- Auditory, tactile, and visual stimuli should be avoided early in the sleep cycle as these may induce sleepwalking.
- Parents should be instructed to lock windows and doors, remove obstacles and sharp objects from the room to avoid injuries.
- Low-dose clonazepam is the drug of choice if the episodes are very frequent. Tricyclic antidepressants and trazodone are also beneficial.

Q. Describe intellectual disability disorder (mental retardation).

- Intellectual disability disorder (previously called mental retardation) is a neurodevelopmental disorder characterized by:
  - Deficits in intellectual functioning
  - Deficits in adaptive functioning
  - With onset during the developmental period (before age 18).
- These deficits result in impairments in academic, social, and practical domains.

Core Diagnostic Criteria

- Intellectual functioning deficit: Impairment in reasoning, problem-solving, planning, abstract thinking, judgment, learning from experience. Measured by IQ testing (IQ <70).
- Adaptive functioning deficit: Difficulty in coping with everyday life demands in:
  - Conceptual (e.g. academic skills)
  - Social (e.g. communication, social judgment)
  - Practical (e.g. self-care, money handling)
- Onset during developmental period: Symptoms must appear in childhood or adolescence.

Classification Based on Severity

See **Table 12.5**.

TABLE 12.5: Classification of intellectual disability disorder

Severity	Approximate IQ range	Adaptive functioning
Mild	50–69	Can achieve basic education, may live independently with support
Moderate	35–49	Can learn self-care and simple communication; supervised living
Severe	20–34	Limited language and self-care; needs close supervision
Profound	<20	Dependent in all areas of functioning; may have physical disabilities

Etiology

- **Prenatal factors:** Genetic syndromes (e.g. Down syndrome, Fragile X), infections (e.g. rubella, CMV), maternal substance abuse (e.g. fetal alcohol syndrome).
- **Perinatal factors:** Birth asphyxia, prematurity, low birth weight.
- **Postnatal factors:** Infections (e.g. meningitis, encephalitis), head trauma, malnutrition, environmental deprivation.

Clinical Features

- Developmental delays in speech, motor, or cognitive milestones
- Poor academic performance
- Problems with self-care, social interaction, and decision-making
- May have associated conditions like ADHD, autism spectrum disorder, seizures.

Diagnosis

- Clinical history and developmental assessment
- IQ testing
- Adaptive behavior scales
- Genetic and neurological investigations if needed.

Management

Educational and Behavioral Interventions

- Special education programs
- Occupational and speech therapy
- Social skills training
- Behavioral modification techniques

Medical

- Treat associated conditions (e.g. epilepsy, behavioral issues)
- Genetic counseling if hereditary cause

Family Support

- Counseling and training
- Legal support for guardianship, disability rights, and benefits

Prognosis

- Depends on severity and cause.

- Many with mild Intellectual disability disorder can lead semi-independent lives.
- Early intervention significantly improves outcomes.

Q. Electroconvulsive therapy.

- Electroconvulsive therapy (ECT) is a medical treatment in which a controlled electrical stimulus is applied to the brain under general anesthesia to induce a brief seizure for therapeutic benefit.
- ECT causes a generalized central nervous system seizure (peripheral convulsion is not necessary) by means of electric current. Electrical current insufficient to cause a seizure produces no therapeutic benefit.
- The mechanism of action is not known, but it is thought to involve major neurotransmitter responses at the cell membrane.
- Modified ECT is the standard and safest form of ECT used today. Modified ECT is performed under general anesthesia and muscle relaxation to ensure comfort and reduce the risk of injury.

Procedure

- ECT is done under general anesthesia. A short-acting anesthetic (e.g. propofol) along with muscle relaxant (e.g. succinylcholine) is used.
- An electric current (70–120V) is applied to head to induce seizure (20–60 seconds).
- Patient is monitored until recovery after the procedure.
- Usually 6–12 sessions, 2–3 times per week are given.

Indications for ECT

- Major depression refractory to antidepressants, with psychotic features or suicidal risk
- Bipolar mood disorder
- Schizophrenia
- Organic delusional disorder
- Obsessive-compulsive disorder
- Catatonia.

Contraindications

- Recent myocardial infarction
- Unstable or severe cardiovascular disease
- Increased intracranial pressure
- Space-occupying intracranial lesion
- Recent cerebral hemorrhage or stroke
- Venous thrombosis
- Bleeding or otherwise unstable vascular aneurysm.
- Severe pulmonary condition.

Side Effects

- Memory disturbance
- Headache
- Aspiration of gastric contents.

Common Misconceptions about ECT (Table 12.6)

TABLE 12.6: Misconceptions about ECT

Misconception	Reality
ECT is painful.	Not true–Modified ECT is done under general anesthesia and muscle relaxants.
ECT causes brain damage.	No scientific evidence supports brain damage from ECT. Memory loss may occur but is usually temporary.
Only for dangerous or insane people.	ECT is used for severe depression, catatonia, mania, and treatment-resistant psychiatric illnesses, not just violent behavior.
ECT is outdated.	Modern modified ECT is safe, effective, and widely recommended in psychiatry.
ECT is the last resort.	It may be the first-line treatment in emergencies (e.g. suicidal depression, catatonia).

Chapter 13

Fluid and Electrolyte Disorders

Q. Write briefly about the normal distribution of water and electrolytes in the body.

Normal Distribution of Water in the Body

- In a typical adult male, the total body water (TBW) is approximately 60% of the body weight (i.e. 40 liters in a 70 kg male). Out of this, two-thirds (25 liters) is intracellular fluid (ICF), and one-third (15 liters) is extracellular fluid (ECF). ECF is further divided into interstitial fluid (12 liters) and plasma (3 liters) **(Fig. 13.1)**.
- The main difference between the plasma and interstitial fluid is the presence of high concentration of protein in the plasma.

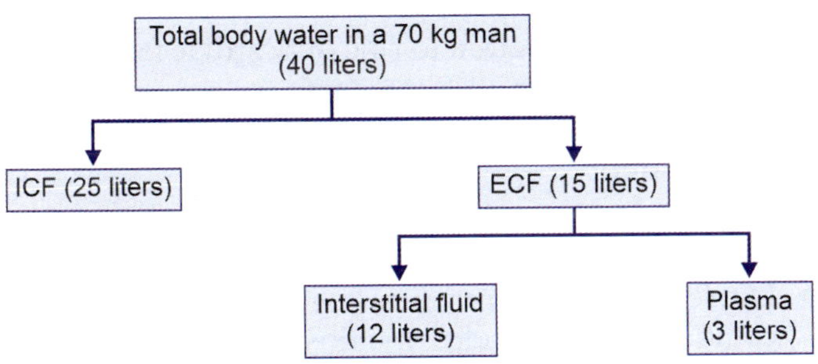

Figure 13.1: Distribution of fluid in the body

Normal Distribution of Electrolytes in the Body

- The major electrolytes in the body are sodium (Na), potassium (K), chloride (Cl) and bicarbonate (HCO_3). Other important electrolytes are calcium, phosphorus and magnesium.
- Most of the sodium, chloride and bicarbonate are present in the ECF. Most of the potassium and phosphates are present in ICF. The major force maintaining the differences in the distribution of Na and K is sodium-potassium pump which is present in all cell membranes. This difference is important for many cell processes, including the excitability of conducting tissues such as nerve and muscle. High concentration of protein in the plasma favors fluid retention within the capillaries, thus maintaining an adequate circulating plasma volume.

Electrolytes	Normal plasma values
Na^+	135–145 mEq/L
K^+	3.5–5 mEq/L
Cl^-	98–107 mEq/L
HCO_3^-	22–28 mEq/L
Mg	1.6–3 mg/dl
Serum osmolality	285–295 mosm/kg water
Blood pH	7.36–7.44

Q. Fluid volume depletion (dehydration).

- Volume depletion occurs when fluid is lost from the extracellular fluid at a rate exceeding net intake.
- The terms hypovolemia and dehydration are often used interchangeably, but they have different meanings in clinical medicine.
- Hypovolemia is loss of intravascular fluid (blood plasma volume). Dehydration is loss of total body water, primarily from intracellular space. Note that one can lead to the other.

Etiology

- ***Gastrointestinal losses***: Vomiting, diarrhea, bleeding, and external drainage.
- ***Renal losses***: Diuretics, osmotic diuresis, salt wasting nephropathies, hypoaldosteronism.
- ***Skin or respiratory losses***: Insensible losses, sweating, and burns.
- ***Third-space sequestration***: Intestinal obstruction, crush injury, major bone fracture, peritonitis, and acute pancreatitis.

Clinical Features

- Symptoms are easy fatigability, thirst, muscle cramps, postural dizziness, and decreased urine output.
- Examination reveals tachycardia, reduced or absent tears, reduced skin turgor, dry mucous membranes, altered mental status, hypotension and shock.

Laboratory Abnormalities

- Serum sodium concentration may be high when more water is lost and may be low in combined salt and water loss.
- Blood urea and creatinine may be elevated.
- Urine sodium concentration is less than 25 mEq/L in extrarenal causes of volume depletion, because of sodium retention by the kidneys whereas in renal causes of volume depletion it is more than this.
- Urine osmolality often exceeds 450 mosmol/kg in volume depletion except in osmotic diuresis, administration of diuretics, and diabetes insipidus.
- Hematocrit may be high except when there is blood loss.

Treatment

- Mild to moderate cases can be corrected by oral supplementation of fluids in the form of oral rehydration salt.
- Severe volume depletion requires intravenous hydration using ringer lactate or normal saline.

Q. Generalized edema.

- Edema is defined as a palpable swelling produced by expansion of the interstitial fluid volume.
- Edema becomes clinically apparent when the interstitial volume has increased by 2.5–3 L, an amount that is almost equal to the plasma volume.
- When edema affects the entire body, it is called generalized edema. Extreme, life-threatening generalized edema is called anasarca.

Causes

- Heart failure
- Renal failure
- Cirrhosis of liver
- Hypoalbuminemia (nephrotic syndrome, protein-losing enteropathy, malnutrition)
- Hypothyroidism
- Pregnancy and premenstrual edema
- Refeeding edema
- Inflammation or sepsis
- Allergic reactions, including certain forms of angioedema
- Drugs: Minoxidil, diazoxide, thiazolidinediones, calcium channel blockers, NSAIDs, fludrocortisone, estrogens.

Pathophysiology

- For generalized edema to occur, two factors must be present:
  1. An alteration in capillary hemodynamics that favors the movement of fluid from the vascular space into the interstitium. Such movement requires a change in one or more components of Starling's law: increased capillary hydrostatic pressure, decreased capillary oncotic pressure, and increased capillary permeability.
  2. Retention of sodium and water by the kidneys. The retention of sodium and water can either be a primary event, as in renal failure, or a secondary event due to reduction in cardiac output (e.g. heart failure) or systemic vascular resistance (e.g. cirrhosis).

Clinical Manifestations

- Peripheral edema manifests as pitting on pressure in dependent areas, i.e. lower limbs in ambulatory patients and sacrum in patients at bed rest. Non-pitting edema is seen in lymphatic obstruction or thyroid disease. Patients with the nephrotic syndrome may also have prominent periorbital edema due to the low tissue pressure in this area.
- Abdominal distension due to ascites. In cirrhosis, ascites is seen first followed by peripheral edema. In cardiac failure, peripheral edema is seen first followed by ascites.
- Dyspnea, orthopnea and bilateral basal lung crepitations due to pulmonary edema. Pleural effusion may be present.
- JVP is raised.
- There may be signs of underlying disease.

Investigations

- Hematocrit may be low due to hemodilution.
- Hyponatremia may be present (dilutional hyponatremia) except in cases of primary renal sodium retention.
- Thyroid function tests
- Serum albumin and liver function tests
- Renal function tests
- Urine analysis to look for proteinuria
- ECG, echocardiogram to rule out cardiac failure
- Abdominal ultrasound (ascites).

Management

- Treat underlying cause
- Salt and fluid restriction
- Diuretics: Loop diuretics (e.g. furosemide). May combine with thiazides or aldosterone antagonists.
- Albumin infusion (in selected cases like nephrotic syndrome or hypoalbuminemia).

Q. Discuss the etiology, clinical features, investigations and management of hyponatremia.

- Hyponatremia is defined as a serum sodium concentration <135 mEq/L. Normal serum sodium level is between approximately 135 and 145 mEq/liter.
- It is the most common electrolyte disorder encountered in clinical practice.
- Hyponatremia is classified into 3 types based on the volume status: Euvolemic, hypovolemic, and hypervolemic.
  - *Euvolemic hyponatremia*: Total body water (TBW) is increased slightly, enough to dilute the serum sodium, but not enough to cause edema. Total body sodium remains normal, but serum level is low because of dilution. Since there is no clinically obvious edema, it is called euvolemic hyponatremia.

- *Hypovolemic hyponatremia*: Both TBW and sodium decrease, but sodium decreases to a greater extent. The extracellular fluid (ECF) volume is decreased.
- *Hypervolemic hyponatremia*: Both TBW and total body sodium increase, but TBW increases to a greater extent (leading to hyponatremia). The ECF is increased markedly with the presence of edema.

Causes of Hyponatremia

Euvolemic hyponatremia

- SIADH (syndrome of inappropriate antidiuretic hormone secretion)
- Adrenal insufficiency
- Hypothyroidism
- Stress
- Drugs (SSRIs, antipsychotics, barbiturates, carbamazepine, NSAIDs).

Hypovolemic hyponatremia

- Integumentary loss: Sweating, burns
- Gastrointestinal loss: Vomiting, diarrhea
- Renal loss: Diuretics, osmotic diuresis, salt-wasting nephropathy, mineralocorticoid deficiency
- Third space loss: Pancreatitis, intestinal obstruction, peritonitis
- Cerebral salt wasting syndrome

Hypervolemic hyponatremia

- Congestive heart failure
- Nephrotic syndrome
- Renal failure
- Cirrhosis
- Iatrogenic

Other Causes of Hyponatremia

- ***Redistributive hyponatremia:*** Here water shifts from the intracellular to the extracellular compartment, causing dilutional hyponatremia. The TBW and total body sodium are unchanged. It occurs with hyperglycemia or administration of mannitol. It causes hypertonic (hyperosmolar) hyponatremia.
- ***Pseudohyponatremia:*** Occurs as a result of decrease in aqueous portion of plasma due to excessive proteins or lipids. The TBW and total body sodium are unchanged. This condition is seen with hypertriglyceridemia and multiple myeloma.

Pathophysiology of Hyponatremia

- Most causes of hyponatremia are associated with low serum osmolality. In general, hypotonic hyponatremia is due either to a primary water gain (and secondary Na^+ loss) or a primary Na^+ loss (and secondary water gain).
- Isotonic (or slightly hypotonic) hyponatremia may complicate transurethral resection of the prostate because large volumes of iso-osmotic (mannitol) or hypo-osmotic (sorbitol or glycine) bladder irrigation solution can be absorbed and result in a dilutional hyponatremia.
- Hypertonic hyponatremia is usually due to hyperglycemia or, occasionally, intravenous administration of mannitol. Glucose is an effective osmole and draws water from muscle cells, resulting in hyponatremia. Plasma Na^+ concentration falls by 1.4 mmol/L for every 100 mg/dL rise in the plasma glucose concentration.
- Diuretic-induced hyponatremia is almost always due to thiazide diuretics, because loop diuretics decrease the tonicity of the medullary interstitium and impairs maximal urinary concentrating capacity. This limits the ability of ADH to promote water retention.

Effects of Hyponatremia on Brain

- The fall in serum osmolality due to hyponatremia creates an osmolar gradient that favors water movement into the cells, leading to brain edema.
- Hyponatremia-induced cerebral edema occurs primarily with rapidly (over one to three days) developing hyponatremia. In slowly developing hyponatremia, there is time for adaptation of neuronal cells and hence, this can be clinically asymptomatic.

Clinical Manifestations

- Acute hyponatremia (<48 hours) is more symptomatic than chronic hyponatremia (>48 hours).
- Mild hyponatremia (plasma sodium level >120 mEq/L) is usually asymptomatic. Nausea and malaise are the earliest findings seen with mild hyponatremia.
- Headache, lethargy, obtundation, seizures, coma, and respiratory arrest may be seen at sodium level below 115 mEq/L.
- Chronic hyponatremia may be asymptomatic or associated with nonspecific features such as fatigue, nausea, dizziness, gait disturbances, forgetfulness, confusion, lethargy, and muscle cramps.

Approach to a Case of Hyponatremia

(Fig. 13.2)

Elicit Appropriate Clinical History and Perform Clinical Examination

- Ask about symptoms and their duration.
- Enquire about drug intake (especially diuretics, antiepileptics).
- Elicit diet history.
- Enquire about history of volume loss, i.e. diarrhea, vomiting, etc.
- Determine volume status, i.e. look for dehydration, edema, and ascites. Hypervolemia is suggested by the presence of peripheral edema, raised JVP, ascites and pleural effusion. Hypovolemia (dehydration) is suggested by orthostatic hypotension, tachycardia, dry mucus membranes, and decreased skin turgor.
- Look for signs of hypothyroidism or adrenal insufficiency.
- Look for any signs of CNS or lung disease.

Determine Serum Osmolality

- Either by lab estimation or calculation using the formula, serum osmolality (in mosm/kg) = $(2 \times Na)$ + (glucose/18) + (BUN/2.8).

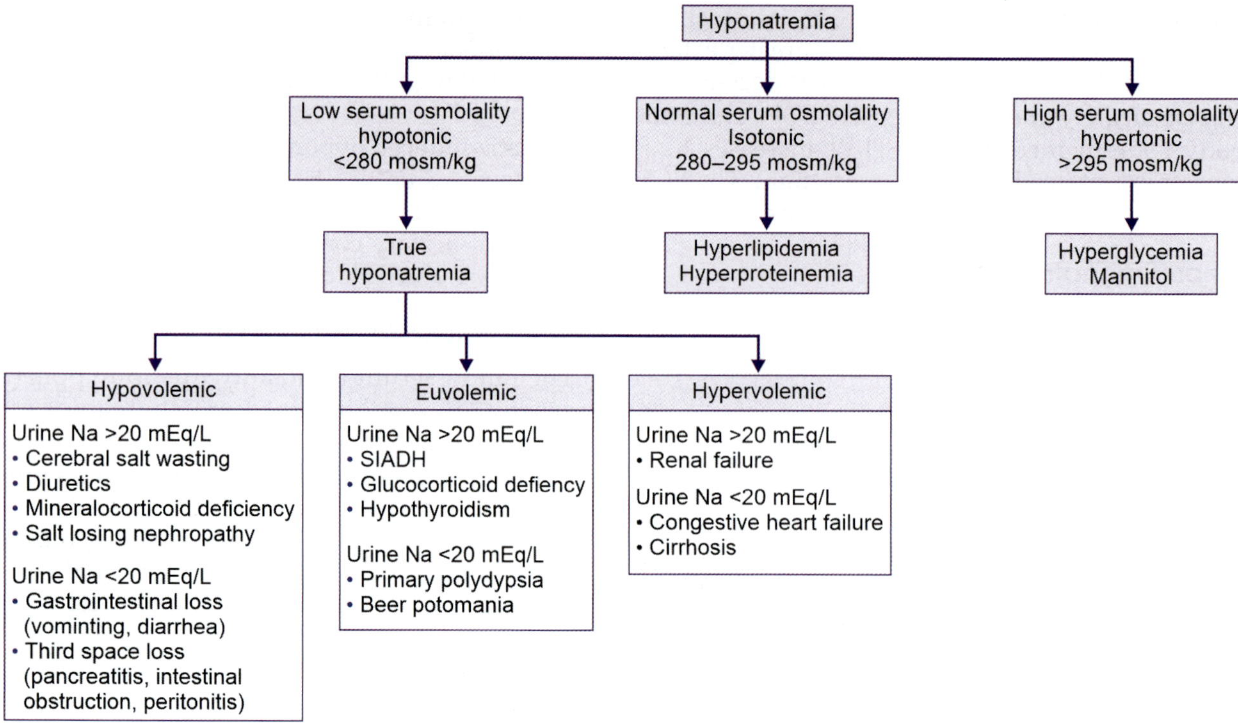

Figure 13.2: Approach to a case of hyponatremia

- True hyponatremia is associated with low serum osmolality.

Determine Volume Status

- To further narrow down the causes of true hyponatremia, determine the volume status of the patient by clinical examination. Based on the volume status, true hyponatremia can be divided into hypovolemic, euvolemic, and hypervolemic hyponatremia.

Determine Urinary Sodium Excretion

- Based on urinary sodium excretion (>20 or <20) causes of hyponatremia can be further narrowed down.

Investigations

- Serum sodium level is less than 135 mEq/L
- Serum osmolality
- Urine sodium and urine osmolality is inappropriately increased in SIADH.
- Appropriate tests to rule out cardiac, renal, or liver disease.
- Thyroid function tests and cortisol levels.

Management

- Treatment of hyponatremia depends on the degree and rapidity of development of hyponatremia.
- Mild hyponatremia (Na >120) may not require any treatment.
- Rapid development of hyponatremia (over hours to days) has high morbidity due to cerebral edema, and may be associated with altered sensorium or seizures. It is generally safe to correct this relatively rapidly using hypertonic saline infusions (1.6% or 3% saline).
- On the other hand, rapid correction of hyponatremia which has developed slowly (over weeks to months) can be hazardous to the brain. In these situations, an abrupt increase in extracellular osmolality can lead to neuronal dehydration and detachment from their myelin sheaths (central pontine myelinolysis–CPM)). CPM presents as quadriparesis, dysarthria, dysphagia and altered sensorium and is generally fatal. Hence, in chronic hyponatremia, correction should be slow and not exceed 10 mEq/L/day.
- Underlying cause of hyponatremia should be corrected always. For hypovolemic patients, this will require intravenous saline infusion. SIADH requires fluid restriction and treatment with conivaptan or tolvaptan which are ADH receptor antagonists and are useful in SIADH. Hypervolemic patients (due to CCF) are treated with a combination of diuretics and fluid restriction.

Q. Syndrome of inappropriate antidiuretic hormone secretion (SIADH).

- SIADH is a condition where excess antidiuretic hormone (ADH) is released inappropriately (not due to actual need for water retention), leading to water retention, dilutional hyponatremia, and low serum osmolality.
- Hypovolemia and hyperosmolality are physiological stimulations for ADH secretion, so the diagnosis of SIADH is made only if these are absent.
- Normal regulation of ADH release occurs from both CNS and chest via baroreceptors and neural input. Hence, disorders affecting CNS and lungs commonly produce SIADH.

Causes

CNS disorders: Head trauma, stroke, subarachnoid hemorrhage, brain tumor, encephalitis, meningitis.
Lung diseases: Tuberculosis, pneumonia, bronchiectasis, neoplasms.
Malignancies: Bronchogenic carcinoma, malignant lymphoma, leukemia.
Drugs: Carbamazepine, phenytoin, haloperidol, fluoxetine, cyclophosphamide.
Others: Postoperative state, sustained pain, stress, nausea, AIDS, idiopathic.

Pathophysiology

- ADH (vasopressin) is normally secreted in response to hypovolemia or hyperosmolality.
- In SIADH, ADH is secreted independently of osmolality or volume status.
- This causes water retention, dilution of serum sodium → hyponatremia, concentrated urine (high urine osmolality).
- There is no peripheral edema because sodium is not retained.

Clinical Features of SIADH

- These are same as those given under hyponatremia. Clinical features of underlying disease may also be present.

Diagnosis of SIADH

- Hyponatremia
- Low plasma osmolality <270 mmol/kg
- High urine osmolality >100 mosml/kg. Normally urine should be maximally dilute in the presence of low serum osmolality, but is typically >100 in SIADH, i.e. inappropriately concentrated due to ADH action.
- Urine sodium concentration >30 mEq/L
- Normal renal function tests, uric acid
- Exclusion of other causes of hyponatremia
- Appropriate clinical context.

Treatment

- Severe symptomatic hyponatremia should be corrected using hypertonic saline.
- Fluid restriction to 800–1000 ml/day (most important treatment).
- Treatment of the cause of SIADH (e.g. withdrawal of a drug causing SIADH).
- Demeclocycline (600–900 mg/day) may enhance water excretion, by interfering with collecting duct responsiveness to ADH (rarely used now).
- Oral urea therapy (30–45 g/day) induces osmotic diuresis.
- ADH receptor antagonists are the new drugs available to treat SIADH. These are conivaptan and tolvaptan. They promote the excretion of free water (aquaretics). Tolvaptan is hepatotoxic and should not be given to patients with liver disease.

Q. Hypernatremia.

- Serum sodium level of >145 mEq/L is called hypernatremia.
- Hypernatremia is either due to excess water loss from the body or due to excess sodium intake. Most of the cases are due to excess free water loss from the body.
- An intact thirst mechanism usually prevents hypernatremia. Hence, whatever may be the underlying cause, hypernatremia occurs only if adequate water intake is not possible, as with unconscious patients.

Causes

Loss of free water (most common cause)

- Excessive diuretic therapy due to relatively more water loss than sodium loss.
- Primary water loss due to diarrhea, excessive sweating, fever, burns.
- Diabetes insipidus (central or nephrogenic).
- Impaired thirst mechanism or no access to water, e.g. debilitated and elderly patients, infants, unconscious or paralyzed patients.

Sodium Gain

- Excess sodium intake (IV or oral salt administration)
- Hyperaldosteronism (rare).

Clinical Features

- Thirst, lethargy, weakness, restlessness are seen with mild to moderate hypernatremia (Na^+ <160 mEq/L).
- Confusion, irritability, muscle twitching, seizures and coma are seen with severe hypernatremia (Na^+ >160 mEq/L).
- Signs of dehydration may be present in infants and elderly due to primary water loss (dry mucous membranes, sunken eyes, poor skin turgor, and hypotension).

Investigations

- Serum sodium: >145 mEq/L.
- Serum osmolality: >295 mosm/kg.
- Urine osmolality: High in extrarenal losses of free water (diarrhea), low in diabetes insipidus.
- ADH level: For suspected diabetes insipidus (low).
- Water deprivation test: Differentiates between central and nephrogenic DI.

Treatment

- Correction of underlying cause
- Fluids without sodium, such as 5% dextrose should be administered to correct hypernatremia. Fluids should be administered over a 48-hour period, aiming for a decrease in serum sodium by no more than 10–12 mEq/L per day.

Q. Discuss briefly about the normal handling of potassium by the body.

- Potassium is a major intracellular cation (about 98% of total body K^+ is inside cells).

- Since, most of the body's potassium is intracellular, massive destruction of cells (e.g. hemolysis, rhabdomyolysis) can release large amount of potassium into the circulation.
- Potassium is abundant in meat, fruits (especially bananas), and coconut water. The usual dietary intake of potassium is between 80 and 160 mEq per day. Serum concentration is between 3.5–5 mEq/L.
- An excess potassium load is handled by: Uptake into cells, renal excretion and extra-renal losses (e.g. gastrointestinal).
- Uptake of potassium into cells is governed by the activity of the Na/K ATPase in the cell membrane and by hydrogen ion concentration. Uptake is stimulated by insulin, beta-adrenergic stimulation and alkalosis. Uptake is decreased by alpha adrenergic stimulation and acidosis (K^+ exchanged for H^+ across cell membrane).
- Kidneys are responsible for the excretion of 90% of the potassium taken in diet. Renal excretion of potassium is increased by aldosterone, which stimulates K^+ and K^+ secretion in exchange for Na^+ in the collecting duct. Because H^+ and K^+ are interchangeable in the exchange mechanism, acidosis decreases and alkalosis increases the secretion of K^+. Aldosterone secretion is stimulated by hyperkalemia and inhibited by hypokalemia. Many drugs affect K^+ homeostasis by affecting aldosterone release (e.g. heparin, NSAID, ACE inhibitors) or by directly affecting renal potassium handling (e.g. diuretics). In the presence of decreased potassium intake, reduction of renal excretion of potassium may take 1–2 weeks. During this time hypokalemia may develop.
- About 10% of daily potassium intake is excreted in the gastrointestinal tract. Excessive vomiting, diarrhea, and colorectal villous adenomas can lead to hypokalemia.

Q. Enumerate the causes of hypokalemia. Discuss briefly the clinical features, ECG manifestations, approach and management of hypokalemia.

- Hypokalemia is defined as plasma K^+ concentration of < 3.5 mEq/L.

Etiology

Reduced intake

- Diet containing less K^+, starvation, potassium free IV fluids.

Urinary loss

- Diuretics (loop, thiazide)
- Hyperaldosteronism (Conn's syndrome)
- Cushing's syndrome
- Salt-wasting nephropathies including Bartter's or Gitelman's syndrome
- Renal tubular acidosis
- Metabolic acidosis
- Hypomagnesemia
- Amphotericin B, certain antibiotics

Gastrointestinal loss

- Vomiting
- Diarrhea
- Aspiration of gastric contents (direct loss of K^+ plus loss of acid from stomach creates alkalosis which shifts K^+ into cells)
- Laxative abuse
- Villous adenoma

Increased entry into cells

- Alkalosis, increased availability of insulin, beta-2 agonists, hypokalemic periodic paralysis.

Clinical Features

- Muscular weakness and paralysis. Respiratory muscle weakness can lead to respiratory failure and death. Gastrointestinal muscle weakness leads to paralytic ileus.
- Cardiac arrhythmias—include ectopic beats, sinus bradycardia, paroxysmal atrial or junctional tachycardia, atrioventricular block, and ventricular tachycardia or fibrillation.
- Renal—polyuria, polydipsia, nephrogenic DI. This happens because hypokalemia reduces the responsiveness of collecting duct cells to ADH, and also impairs the concentrating ability of loop of Henle and distal tubule.
- Muscle cramps leading to rhabdomyolysis and myoglobinuria.

Investigations

- Serum electrolytes, calcium and magnesium
- Urine potassium excretion—is increased in hypokalemia due to renal loss and decreased in extrarenal loss.
- Plasma renin activity and aldosterone levels will identify patients with primary hyperaldosteronism.
- ECG changes—depression of ST segment, flattening or inversion of T wave, and presence of U waves at the end of the T wave. U waves are often seen in leads V4 to V6. Ventricular arrhythmias (ectopics, VT) are seen in severe cases.

Approach to Hypokalemia

See **Fig. 13.3**.

Management

- Treatment of the underlying cause.
- Potassium replacement: This can be done by oral (as syrup) or IV potassium chloride supplementation.
- For mild hypokalemia (K^+ 3.0–3.5 mEq/L), about 20–80 mEq per day of oral potassium chloride is given in 3–4 divided doses.
- In moderate to severe hypokalemia (K^+ <3.0 mEq/L), give IV potassium chloride (KCl) cautiously: Typical: 10–20 mEq/hr (max 40 mEq/hour in ICU with ECG monitoring). Use central line if concentration >40 mEq/L. Never give IV potassium as a rapid bolus.
- Potassium sparing diuretics–such as spironolactone or amiloride can be used along with other measures to correct hypokalemia.

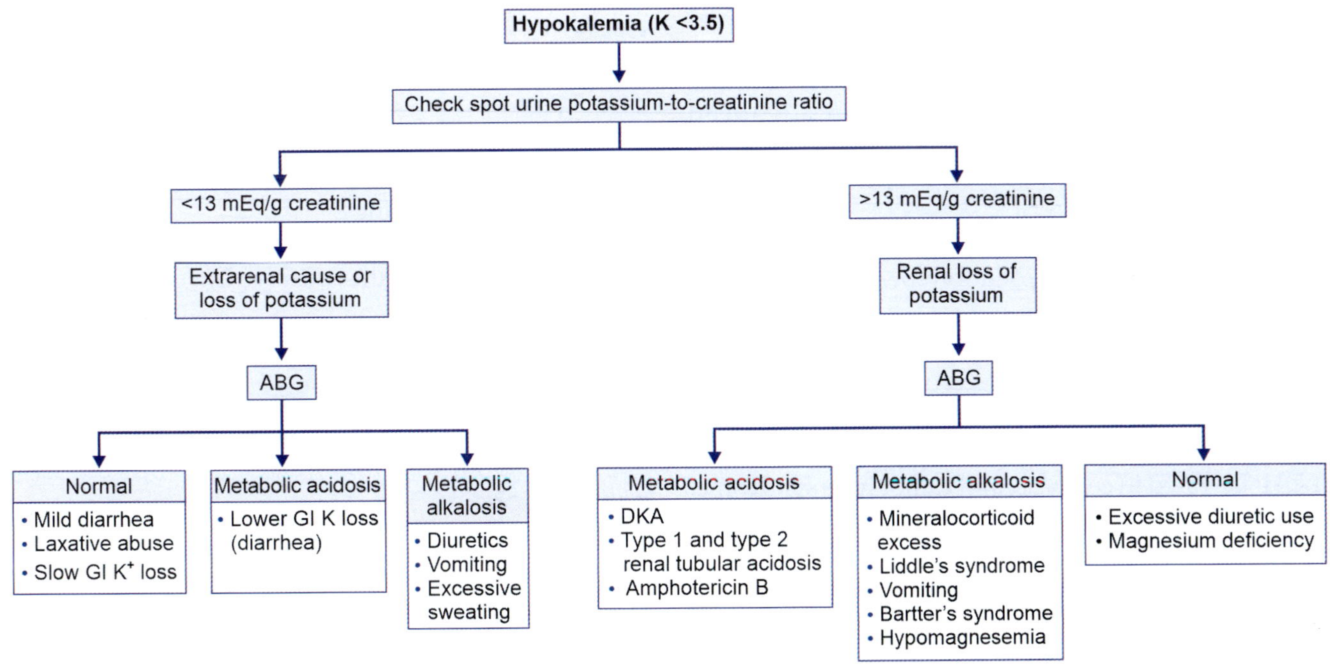

Figure 13.3: Approach to a case of hypokalemia

- Magnesium replacement (if low): IV magnesium sulfate helps stabilize membrane and retain potassium.

Q. Enumerate the causes of hyperkalemia. Discuss briefly the clinical features, ECG manifestations and management of hyperkalemia.

- Hyperkalemia is defined as a plasma K^+ concentration of >5 mEq/L.
  - Mild: 5.1–5.9 mEq/L
  - Moderate: 6.0–6.4 mEq/L
  - Severe: ≥6.5 mEq/L. Can be life-threatening due to cardiac arrhythmias.

Causes

Excess intake

- K^+ rich foods, intravenous fluid containing K^+

Impaired excretion

- Acute or chronic kidney disease
- Addison disease (due to hypoaldosteronism)
- Drugs (K^+ sparing diuretics, ACE inhibitors, ARBs, NSAIDs)

Release of intracellular K^+

- Hemolysis, rhabdomyolysis, crush injury, burns, tumorlysis syndrome.

Shift of K^+ out of cell

- Metabolic acidosis
- Insulin deficiency (e.g. DKA)
- Hyperkalemic periodic paralysis
- Drugs: Succinylcholine, digitalis

Pseudohyperkalemia

- Hemolyzed blood sample
- Repeated fist clenching during phlebotomy, with release of K^+ from forearm muscles
- Specimen drawn from arm with K^+ infusion.

Clinical Features of Hyperkalemia

- Symptoms generally do not occur until the plasma potassium concentration exceeds 7 mEq/L, unless the rise in potassium concentration has been very rapid.
- Hyperkalemia interferes with normal neuromuscular function and causes muscle weakness and, rarely, flaccid paralysis. This happens repeatedly in hyperkalemic periodic paralysis.
- Paralytic ileus and abdominal distention may occur.
- Hyperkalemia causes depolarization, leading to decreased cardiac excitability, hypotension, and bradycardia. Ventricular fibrillation and cardiac arrest are terminal events.
- *ECG changes* **(Fig. 13.4)**: Tall peaked T waves with shortened QT interval are the first changes seen on the ECG. This is followed by progressive lengthening of the PR interval and QRS duration. The P wave may

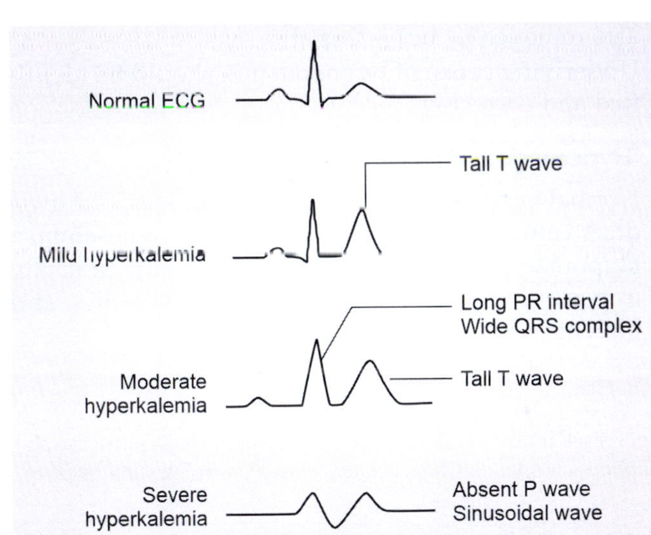

Figure 13.4: ECG changes in hyperkalemia

disappear, and QRS widens giving rise to "sine wave" pattern. A variety of other conduction disturbances, including right bundle branch block, left bundle branch block, bifascicular block, and advanced atrioventricular block may also be seen.

Investigations

- Repeat serum potassium and confirm hyperkalemia, especially in suspected pseudohyperkalemia.
- ECG
- Renal function tests
- Endocrine tests (serum aldosterone, cortisol, renin)
- ABG
- CK-NAC: Elevated in rhabdomyolysis
- LDH: Elevated in cell lysis, and tumor lysis syndrome.

Treatment

- Discontinue exogenous K^+ intake by eliminating K^+ rich foods such as fruits, coconut water, etc.
- Calcium gluconate decreases membrane excitability and prevents cardiac arrhythmias. The usual dose is 10 ml of a 10% solution intravenously over 2–3 min.
- Insulin plus dextrose infusion shifts K^+ into the cells and temporarily lowers the plasma K^+ concentration. 50 ml of 50% dextrose plus 10 units of regular insulin is given every 6th–8th hourly.
- Sodium bicarbonate increases blood pH and results in a shift of K^+ into cells. 1–2 ampoules can be given intravenously.
- B_2 adrenergic agonists such as salbutamol promote cellular uptake of K^+. They can be given parenterally or in nebulized form every 4th–6th hourly.
- K^+ excretion can be enhanced by diuretics (frusemide, thiazides) and cation-exchange resin. Sodium polystyrene sulfonate (e.g. K-BIND) is a cation-exchange resin that binds to K^+ in the gastrointestinal tract which is then excreted in the stools.
- Hemodialysis is the most rapid way of removing the K^+ from the body. It is indicated in patients with renal failure and those with severe hyperkalemia unresponsive to other measures. Peritoneal dialysis also removes K^+ but is less effective.
- Underlying cause of hyperkalemia should be identified and corrected.

Q. Hypomagnesemia.

- Normal magnesium level in the plasma is 1.7–2.4 mg/dl. A value <1.7 mg/dl is called hypomagnesemia.
- Hypomagnesemia is often overlooked but clinically important, especially in critically ill, alcoholics, and patients with electrolyte disturbances.

Causes

Decreased intake or absorption: Malnutrition, alcoholism, malabsorption, chronic diarrhea, laxative abuse, gastrointestinal suction, total parenteral nutrition.

Increased renal loss: Diuretics, hyperaldosteronism, hyperparathyroidism, hyperthyroidism, hypercalcemia, tubulointerstitial diseases.

Others: Diabetes mellitus, post parathyroidectomy (hungry bone syndrome), respiratory alkalosis, pregnancy.

Clinical Features

- *General symptoms:* Anorexia, nausea, vomiting, lethargy, and personality change.
- *Neuromuscular:* Weakness, tremors, fasciculations, muscle cramps, seizures, positive Chvostek/Trousseau signs.
- *Cardiac:* Palpitations, arrhythmias (e.g. torsades de pointes).
- *Electrolyte effects:* Can cause or worsen hypokalemia and hypocalcemia.

Investigations

- Serum magnesium: To confirm diagnosis.
- Urinary excretion of magnesium–more than 10–30 mg/day indicates renal magnesium loss.
- Hypocalcemia and hypokalemia may be present.
- ECG shows prolonged QT interval, ST depression, wide QRS, flat T waves, and sometimes torsades de pointes (polymorphic ventricular tachycardia).

Treatment

- In mild, asymptomatic cases, oral magnesium gluconate (500–1000 mg two to three times daily is given for 3–4 days.
- In symptomatic cases, IV infusion of 1–2 g of magnesium sulfate, followed by an infusion of 6 g magnesium sulfate in at least 1 L of fluids over 24 hours, repeated for up to 7 days to replete magnesium stores. Magnesium sulfate may also be given intramuscularly.

Q. Hypermagnesemia.

- Hypermagnesemia is a serum Mg concentration >2.5 mg/dl.
- It is a rare but potentially life-threatening condition, often seen in patients with renal failure or excessive magnesium containing drugs, such as antacids or purgatives. Other causes are administration of magnesium sulfate intravenously (as a treatment for eclampsia and aluminum phosphide poisoning).
- Symptoms and signs include hyporeflexia, hypotension, respiratory depression, and cardiac arrest.
- Treatment of severe Mg toxicity consists of intravenous calcium gluconate. IV furosemide can increase Mg excretion when renal function is adequate. Hemodialysis may be considered in severe hypermagnesemia.

Q. Discuss the normal physiology of acid base balance.

OR

Q. Discuss how the body maintains normal pH.

- The concentration of hydrogen ions in both extracellular and intracellular compartments is tightly controlled. The pH of ECF including blood is maintained between 7.36–7.44 (average 7.40).

Maintenance of pH within this range is important; otherwise, all the metabolic functions of the body get affected leading ultimately to death.

- A decrease in extracellular fluid pH is called acidosis which is equivalent to raising the hydrogen ion concentration. An increase in extracellular fluid pH is called alkalosis which is equivalent to lowering the hydrogen ion concentration.
- Acidosis is two types; metabolic acidosis and respiratory acidosis. Metabolic acidosis is associated with a low pH and low bicarbonate concentration. Respiratory acidosis is associated with a low pH and high PCO_2.
- Alkalosis is also of two types; metabolic alkalosis and respiratory alkalosis. Metabolic alkalosis is associated with a high pH and high bicarbonate concentration. Respiratory alkalosis is associated with a high pH and low PCO_2.
- Body maintains the pH within normal limits by a variety of physiological mechanisms.

Maintenance of Normal pH by the Body

The body uses three main systems to tightly regulate acid–base balance. These are:

1. Buffer systems (immediate response)
2. Respiratory regulation (minutes)
3. Renal regulation (slow–hours to days)

Buffer Systems (immediate response)

Bicarbonate buffer system

- Most important buffer in ECF. It immediately corrects the swing in pH. Any acid load in the form of H^+ ions combine with bicarbonate to form carbonic acid, which, then dissociates to form CO_2 and water. CO_2 thus produced is excreted by the lungs.

$$CO_2 + H_2O \rightleftharpoons H_2CO_3 \rightleftharpoons H^+ + HCO_3^-$$

- Bone contains large amount of bicarbonate which can buffer acid load.

Protein buffers (e.g. albumin, hemoglobin)

- Important in both ICF and plasma.
- Hemoglobin buffers H^+ in RBCs.

Phosphate buffer system

- Active mainly in intracellular fluid and renal tubules.
- $H_2PO_4^- \rightleftharpoons H^+ + HPO_4^{2-}$.
- Dihydrogen phosphate ($H_2PO_4^-$): Weak acid → can donate H_2.
- Monohydrogen phosphate (HPO_4^{2-}): Weak base → can accept H_2.

Respiratory Regulation (minutes)

- Respiratory compensation for acid-base disturbances can occur quickly, by controlling the level of CO_2 in blood.
- In acid accumulation, ventilation is increased, thus washing out CO_2 which is equivalent to carbonic acid thus increasing the pH. Conversely, alkalosis leads to inhibition of ventilation and accumulation of CO_2 leading to decrease in pH.

Renal Regulation (slow–hours to days)

- Kidneys provide third line of defense against acid base disturbances. When acid accumulates, kidneys increase urinary excretion of acid, and conserve bicarbonate.

Q. Discuss the causes, clinical features, investigations and management of metabolic acidosis.

- Metabolic acidosis is defined as a disorder associated with a low pH and low bicarbonate concentration.
- It can be produced by three major mechanisms:
  - Increased acid production (e.g. ketoacidosis and lactic acidosis).
  - Loss of bicarbonate (e.g. diarrhea or type 2 renal tubular acidosis).
  - Decreased renal acid excretion (e.g. renal failure or type 1 renal tubular acidosis).
- The pH fall is compensated by hyperventilation, resulting in a reduced PCO_2. Kidneys try to compensate by increasing the excretion of acid load and conserving bicarbonate. Respiratory compensation is immediate, but renal compensation takes many days.
- Based on the nature of accumulating acid, two types of metabolic acidosis can be defined; high anion gap acidosis and normal anion gap acidosis.
- In high anion gap acidosis, an accumulating acid is accompanied by its corresponding anion, which adds to the unmeasured anion gap, while the chloride concentration remains normal. Examples are ketoacidosis and lactic acidosis.
- In normal anion gap acidosis, a mineral acid (HCl) accumulates, or there is a primary loss of bicarbonate buffer from the ECF. Here, there is no addition of new acidic anion to the plasma. Hence, the anion gap $(Na^+ + K^+) - (Cl^- + HCO_3^-)$, remains normal (15 mmol/L) since the plasma chloride increases to replace the depleted bicarbonate levels. Normal anion gap is due to anions such as phosphate, sulphate and multiple negative charges on plasma protein molecules. Examples of normal anion gap metabolic acidosis are diarrhea and type-2 renal tubular acidosis.

Causes

High anion gap metabolic acidosis (HAGMA)

Mnemonic: MUDPILES

- M–Methanol
- U–Uremia
- D–Diabetic ketoacidosis (DKA)
- P–Propylene glycol
- I–Isoniazid/Iron Toxicity → lactic acidosis
- L–Lactic acidosis (shock, sepsis, hypoxia)
- E–Ethylene glycol (antifreeze)
- S–Salicylates (Mixed disorder, also respiratory alkalosis)

Normal anion gap (hyperchloremic) metabolic acidosis

- Diarrhea
- Ureterosigmoidostomy (absorption of urinary acids from bowel)
- Renal tubular acidosis
- Acetazolamide (carbonic anhydrase inhibition)
- Addison's disease (aldosterone deficiency → H^+ retention)

Clinical Features

- *RS:* Kussmaul breathing—deep sighing respiration
- *Cardiac:* Hypotension, arrhythmias (severe acidosis)
- *GIT:* Abdominal pain and vomiting
- *Neurological:* Irritability, lethargy, seizures and coma
- *Others:* Features of underlying cause (e.g. dehydration in DKA, sepsis signs).

Investigations

- Arterial blood gas analysis–pH, PCO_2, and the bicarbonate concentration can be known by this. Low serum bicarbonate and low pH confirms the diagnosis of metabolic acidosis. PCO_2 is decreased due to respiratory compensation.
- Renal function tests
- LFT
- Serum electrolytes such as sodium, potassium, and chloride to calculate anion gap
- Blood sugar and urinary ketones (to rule out diabetic ketoacidosis)
- Serum lactic acid levels → elevated in lactic acidosis
- Serum levels of methanol, ethanol, paracetamol, salicylates and ethylene glycol if indicated.

Management

- Identify and correct the underlying cause.
- Use of sodium bicarbonate infusion is indicated when the underlying disorder cannot be readily corrected or when the acidosis is severe (pH <7).
- Sodium bicarbonate and potassium supplements are needed to achieve normal plasma bicarbonate and potassium levels in proximal and distal renal tubular acidosis.

Q. Anion gap.

- The anion gap is the difference in the measured cations (positively charged ions) and the measured anions (negatively charged ions) in serum, plasma, or urine.
- Normally, plasma is electrically neutral: total cations = total anions.
- Measured cations: Na^+ ($\pm K^+$)
- Measured anions: Cl^- and HCO_3^-
- Unmeasured anions: proteins (albumin), phosphate, sulfate, lactate, organic acids. Anion gap reflects these unmeasured anions.

$$\text{Anion gap} = Na^+ - (Cl^- + HCO_3^-)$$

- Normal value for the serum anion gap is 8–12 mEq/L. Anion gap can be high, normal or low.
- Anion gap is useful in knowing the cause of metabolic acidosis, because the causes of high and normal anion gap acidosis are different.

Causes of High Anion Gap Acidosis

- *See* under metabolic acidosis.

Causes of Normal Anion Gap Acidosis

- *See* under metabolic acidosis.

Low Anion Gap

- Decrease in unmeasured anions (albumin, dilution).
- Increase in unmeasured cations (multiple myeloma, hypercalcemia, hypermagnesemia, lithium, polymixin B).

Q. Metabolic alkalosis.

- Metabolic alkalosis is characterized by an increase in plasma pH and bicarbonate concentration. There is a compensatory rise in PCO_2 due to hypoventilation.

Causes

- GI loss of hydrogen ion, e.g. vomiting or aspiration of gastric contents
- Renal loss of hydrogen, e.g. primary and secondary hyperaldosteronism, diuretic use, Bartter syndrome, Gitelman syndrome
- Intracellular shift of hydrogen, due to hypokalemia
- Alkali administration.

Clinical Features

- *Neuromuscular:* Muscle cramps, weakness, tetany (carpopedal spasm) due to increased neuromuscular irritability as the plasma ionized calcium falls. Confusion, lethargy, seizures (in severe alkalosis).
- *CVS:* Alkalosis lowers threshold for anginal symptoms and arrhythmias.
- *Respiratory:* Hypoventilation (compensatory to retain CO_2).
- Manifestations of underlying cause.

Investigations

- ABG: Confirm metabolic alkalosis (↑ pH, ↑ HCO_3^-).
- Serum electrolytes ↓ K^+, ↓ Cl^-, ↑ HCO_3^-.

Management

- Treat the underlying cause
- Replacement of potassium in hypokalemia induced alkalosis.

Q. Respiratory acidosis.

- Respiratory acidosis occurs when there is accumulation of CO_2 due to reduced alveolar ventilation. Renal retention of bicarbonate partially compensates for acidosis; hence, there is rise in plasma bicarbonate concentration.
- Respiratory acidosis can be acute or chronic.

Causes

- Conditions that impair CNS respiratory drive: Encephalitis, brainstem disease, drugs (opioids, benzodiazepines, barbiturates).
- Respiratory muscle weakness, e.g. myasthenia gravis, Guillain-Barré-syndrome, muscular dystrophy, cervical cord lesions.
- Lung diseases: COPD, acute exacerbation of asthma, interstitial lung disease, pneumothorax.

- Chest wall disorders: Severe kyphoscoliosis, flail chest.
- Obesity-hypoventilation syndrome, obstructive sleep apnea (OSA).

Clinical Features

- CNS: Headache, confusion, drowsiness, seizures, coma, due to CO_2 accumulation.
- CVS: Tachycardia, bounding pulse, hypertension, arrhythmias (in severe cases).
- Features of underlying disease.

Investigations

- ABG: Confirms respiratory acidosis (↑ $PaCO_2$, ↓ pH).
- Serum electrolytes: Mild ↑ HCO_3^- in chronic cases.
- Chest X-ray/CT: To identify lung pathology (COPD, pneumonia).
- Pulmonary function tests: Assess chronic lung disease (obstructive or restrictive).
- Toxicology screen: Suspected drug overdose (benzodiazepines, barbiturates).
- Neurological evaluation: To rule out neuromuscular diseases.

Management

- Correct the underlying cause.
- Ventilatory support if required.
- Bicarbonate is almost always contraindicated, because HCO_3^- can be converted to PCO_2 in serum.

Q. Respiratory alkalosis.

- Respiratory alkalosis develops when there is reduction of PCO_2 due to hyperventilation resulting in increase in plasma pH. If hyperventilation is prolonged, renal compensation occurs so that acid secretion is reduced and bicarbonate excretion is increased.
- Causes of hyperventilation include anxiety states, over-vigorous assisted ventilation, pregnancy, pulmonary embolism, chronic liver disease, and salicylate poisoning.
- Clinical features include those of underlying cause. Reduction in ionized calcium due to alkalosis produces agitation, perioral and digital tingling, carpopedal spasm, Trousseau's sign and Chvostek sign. Seizures may develop in severe cases.
- Management involves correction of the underlying cause. In acute hyperventilation due to anxiety, rebreathing into a paper bag will increase the PCO_2. Sedation may be needed if anxiety and hyperventilation persists.

Chapter 14

Oncology

Q. What is cancer? Describe the epidemiology and common cancers encountered in clinical practice?

- Cancer refers to unregulated cell growth with tissue invasion/metastasis. Unregulated cell growth without invasion is called *benign neoplasms*, or new growths. Cancer is a synonym for *malignant neoplasm*.
- Cancers of epithelial tissues are called *carcinomas*; cancers of nonepithelial (mesenchymal) tissues are called *sarcomas;* Cancers arising from hematopoietic or lymphoid cells are called *leukemias* or *lymphomas*.

Epidemiology of Cancer

- Cancers are among the leading causes of morbidity and mortality worldwide and the incidence of cancer is increasing every year.
- More than 60% of the world's new cancer cases occur in Africa, Asia, and Central and South America. 70% of the world's cancer deaths also occur in these regions.
- Tobacco is the most important identified cause of cancer followed by dietary practices, inadequate physical activity, alcohol consumption, infections due to viruses and sexual behavior.
- In general cancer incidence is more in old age compared to younger age group.
- In general cancer is more common in men than women except breast, thyroid, and gallbladder cancers. In females, breast cancer is the leading site of cancer especially in urban areas followed by cancer cervix (in rural areas).
- Lung cancer is the most common cancer in males. The highest rates are among men in eastern Europe, North America, and the rest of Europe, whereas the lowest rates are observed in Africa, excluding South Africa Lung cancer is more strongly associated with cigarette smoking than any other cancer.
- Cancers that are strongly related to infectious etiologies, for example, stomach, liver, and uterine cervix are, in general, decreasing globally. Cancers that were common only in wealthy countries are now increasing in middle- and low-income countries also (these are cancers of the lung, breast, prostate, and colon/rectum).
- Deaths due to cancers are more in developing countries because of late diagnosis and inadequate treatment.

Common Cancers Encountered in Clinical Practice

Men	Women
Lung cancer	Breast cancer
Oral cancer	Cervical cancer
Esophageal cancer	Ovarian cancer
Stomach cancer	Colorectal cancer
Colorectal cancer	Oral cancer

Q. Discuss briefly the risk factors/etiology of cancer.

- The etiology of cancer is multifactorial, involving genetic mutations and environmental exposures. Risk factors can be divided into modifiable and nonmodifiable factors.

Nonmodifiable Risk Factors (cannot be changed)

Aging

- Age is most significant factor for cancer development. Two-third of all cancers occur above the age of 65 years. This is due to alteration of host cells, longer exposure to carcinogens, and decreased immunity.

Gender

- Some cancers have gender preference (e.g. prostate cancer in males, breast cancer in females).

Genetic factors

- This is the most important cause of cancer development. Most tumors exhibit chromosomal abnormalities such as deletions, inversions, translocations, or duplications. This leads to activation of proto-oncogenes to oncogenes or deletion of tumor suppressor genes—or both. Both these changes cause abnormal cellular proliferation and cancer formation.

Family History

- First-degree relatives with cancer may increase individual risk.

Ethnicity/Race

- Certain ethnic groups have higher risk for specific cancers (e.g. Indians are prone to develop oral, breast, and cervix cancer. People of China and Japan have high risk of stomach cancer. African Americans have very high incidence and mortality from prostate cancer.

Personal History of Cancer

- Prior cancer or radiation therapy increases risk of secondary cancers.

Modifiable Risk Factors (can be controlled or avoided)

Infections

- ***Viruses:*** The role of viruses in carcinogenesis is well known. Epstein-Barr virus (EBV) is associated with Burkitt's lymphoma and nasopharyngeal cancer. Hepatitis B and C virus can lead to hepatocellular carcinoma. Helicobacter pylori infection is associated with non-Hodgkin's lymphoma and stomach carcinoma. Human T-lymphotrophic virus type I (HTLV-I) is associated with adult acute T-cell leukemia. Kaposi's sarcoma is seen in HIV infection. Human papilloma viruses (HPV) can cause cervical cancer in women.
- ***H. pylori:*** Risk factor for stomach cancer.

Radiation Exposure

- ***Ionizing radiation:*** Natural sources (cosmic rays, soil) or man-made ionizing radiation (diagnostic, therapeutic, atomic bomb explosion) can lead to skin cancer and leukemia.
- ***UV (ultraviolet) radiation:*** UV rays from the sun, particularly (UV-B spectrum 240–230 nm) can cause skin cancer or melanoma.

Tobacco

- Smoking and chewing tobacco has been identified as a major cause of lung and oral cancer. Cancers of esophagus, stomach, bladder, kidney, liver and larynx are also related to tobacco carcinogens which are primarily polycyclic hydrocarbons and cyclic N-nitrosamine.

Occupational Hazards

- Chimney sweepers had a high incidence of scrotal cancer which was attributed to soot. Bladder cancer has been noted in aniline dye workers. Asbestos exposure is associated with mesothelioma and lung cancer.

Environmental Pollution

- Air pollution caused by industries and exhaust from vehicles contains polycyclic hydrocarbons; these hydrocarbons cause lung cancer.
- Asbestos → mesothelioma.

Drugs and Toxins

- Cancer chemotherapeutic drugs can cause leukemia. Aflatoxin increases the chance of hepatocellular carcinoma.
- Hormone replacement therapy (HRT) increases breast/endometrial cancer risk.

Diet and Alcohol

- Meat and fat increase the risk of colon cancer. Salt intake and salted fish in diet increase the risk of stomach cancer and nasopharyngeal cancer, respectively.
- Alcohol increases oral, liver, breast, esophageal, and colorectal cancer risk.

Obesity

- Risk factor for breast, endometrial, colorectal, kidney, and pancreas cancers.

Q. Discuss briefly about the genetic factors in the causation of cancer.

Q. Genetic basis of transformation of a normal cell into a malignant cell.

Q. Proto-oncogene, oncogene and tumor suppression genes.

- Cancer is fundamentally a genetic disease caused by mutations that lead to uncontrolled cell growth, evasion of apoptosis, and metastasis. These mutations may be inherited (germline) or acquired (somatic). Most tumors exhibit genetic abnormalities such as deletions, inversions, translocations, or duplications.
- Most genetic abnormalities lead to activation of proto-oncogenes to oncogenes or deletion of tumor suppressor genes—or both. Both these changes cause abnormal cellular proliferation and cancer formation.

Proto-oncogenes and Oncogenes

- Oncogenes were initially discovered in the genome of retroviruses capable of causing cancers in chickens, mice, and rats. Proto-oncogenes in the normal state stimulate the normal growth of cells. Activated proto-oncogenes are called oncogenes and are responsible for the development of cancers. Activation of proto-oncogenes to oncogenes can occur due to point mutation, DNA amplification, chromosomal rearrangement and viral infections.
- *Point mutation*—is a common mechanism of oncogene activation. Point mutations occur due to ionizing radiation, ultraviolet rays, and carcinogens.
- *DNA amplification*—DNA sequence amplification is another mechanism of proto-oncogene activation and leads to overexpression of the gene product. Numerous genes have been reported to be amplified in cancer. Because the region amplified often extends to hundreds of thousands of base pairs, more than one oncogene may be amplified in some cancers. Demonstration of amplification of a cellular gene is often a predictor of poor prognosis. For example, *ERBB2/HER2* and *NMYC* are often amplified in aggressive breast cancers and neuroblastoma, respectively.
- *Chromosomal Rearrangement*—in Burkitt's lymphoma, the c-*myc* oncogene is activated by translocation of genetic material from chromosome 8 to chromosome 14. CML is caused by reciprocal translocation of the

long arms of chromosomes 9 and 22, resulting in the generation of a fusion protein (BCR-ABL) with tyrosine kinase activity. Amplification of the HER-2/*neu* oncogene in breast cancer has been associated with more aggressive tumors.

- *Viruses*: Viral DNA may integrate within a proto-oncogene and may activate it. Viral DNA may also contain proto-oncogene which may be transferred to the host after infection. Viruses may also activate growth-promoting pathways and inhibit tumor-suppressor products in the infected cells.

Tumor Suppressor Genes

- These genes normally suppress cell growth or promote apoptosis. Mutation or inactivation leads to uncontrolled cell division.
- For example, the *p53* gene triggers programmed cell death (apoptosis). Mutations in the *p53* gene lead to abnormal cell proliferation and cancer formation. *RB* gene is a tumor suppressor gene, and its inactivation leads to development of retinoblastoma. Many soft tissue sarcomas are produced due to inactivation of tumor suppressor genes.

Q. Cancer screening.

- Cancer screening is the process of detecting cancer or precancerous conditions at an early, asymptomatic stage using various tests, examinations, or procedures.
- Early detection of cancer offers a chance of cure, improves treatment outcomes, and reduces mortality. When patients are diagnosed with a cancer on the basis of symptoms, the cancer may have already spread in a significant proportion, so that curative treatment (usually surgical) is not possible. Early detection of cancer in an asymptomatic population can identify people with cancer which may be curable.

Requirements of a Screening Program

- Acceptable to the population
- Capable of detecting high percentage of early cancers
- Low false-positive rate (reducing unnecessary interventions)
- Cost effective
- Early treatment should be more effective than late treatment.
- Availability of an effective intervention.

Cancers with Potential for Screening (Table 14.1)

TABLE 14.1: Cancers with potential for screening

Malignancy	Method of screening	Population to be screened
• Breast cancer	Mammography, breast self examination	Females 40 and above, every year
• Cervical cancer	Cervical smear cytology (pap smear) HPV DNA testing	Females: 18–65, every 1–3 years
• Prostate cancer	Serum prostate-specific antigen (PSA) level	Males of 50 years of age and above, every year
• Colorectal cancer	Fecal occult blood test Colonoscopy	50 years of age and above Fecal occult blood test every year Colonoscopy every 5–10 years
• Oral cancer	Oral visual examination by trained health workers	Adults >30 years, especially tobacco users, every 3 years
• Lung cancer	Low-dose CT (LDCT) for high-risk smokers	Age 55–80 years with heavy smoking history. Every year

Limitations and Challenges

- False-positives/negatives
- Overdiagnosis and overtreatment
- Low awareness and poor participation
- Limited infrastructure in rural areas.

Q. Tumor markers.

- Tumor markers are substances (usually proteins) produced either by cancer cells or by the body in response to cancer. They can be found in blood, urine, tissues, or other body fluids.

Examples of Tumor Markers

- **Carcinoembryonic antigen (CEA):** Cancers of gastrointestinal tract, lung, breast
- **CA-19:** Colon and pancreas
- **CA-125:** Ovarian cancer
- **Alpha-fetoprotein (AFP):** Hepatocellular carcinoma and malignant teratoma
- **Lactate dehydrogenase (LDH):** Most cancers, reflecting tumor burden or necrosis
- **Prostate-specific antigen (PSA):** Prostate cancer
- **β_2 –Microglobulin:** Elevated in multiple myeloma
- **Human chorionic gonadotropin (hCG):** Germ cell tumors of testes and ovaries, choriocarcinoma
- **Calcitonin:** Medullary carcinoma thyroid
- **Thyroglobulin:** Postoperative marker for thyroid cancer (but not for medullary cancer)
- **Chromogranin-A:** Neuroendocrine tumor.

Uses of Tumor Markers

- To detect the presence of cancer
- Levels may reflect the extent (stage) of the cancer
- To follow response to therapy
- To screen for recurrence of cancer.

Limitations

- Lack of specificity (elevated in benign conditions too)
- Not useful for early detection in all cancers

- False positives and negatives possible
- Should not be used alone for diagnosis.

Q. Enumerate oncologic emergencies.

Due to local effect: Spinal cord compression, superior vena cava syndrome, malignant effusions.

Systemic effects: Tumor lysis syndrome, hypercalcemia, opportunistic infections, hyperuricemia, SIADH.

Hematologic: Hypercoagulability, thrombocytopenia, febrile neutropenia, DIC.

Q. Tumor lysis syndrome.

- Tumor lysis syndrome is a life-threatening oncologic emergency caused by the massive and rapid destruction of cancer cells, leading to the release of intracellular contents into the bloodstream.
- It typically occurs after chemotherapy, but can also happen spontaneously, especially in highly proliferative tumors.
- It is commonly seen in lymphomas, leukemias and multiple myeloma.

Pathophysiology (Fig. 14.1)

- Lysis of large number of tumor cells releases intracellular potassium and phosphate causing hyperkalemia and hyperphosphatemia. Sudden destruction of tumor cells also leads to hyperuricemia. Uric acid crystals may get deposited in renal tubules leading to renal failure.
- Hypocalcemia is a consequence of acute hyperphosphatemia with subsequent precipitation of calcium phosphate in soft tissues.
- Acute renal failure and the liberation of large amounts of endogenous intracellular acids from cellular catabolism result in metabolic acidosis.

Clinical Features

- Dysuria, oliguria, hematuria may be present due to uric acid deposition in kidneys and consequent AKI. Uremia due to AKI may produce fatigue, weakness, nausea, vomiting and anorexia.
- Hyperkalemia may produce muscle weakness and cardiac arrhythmias.
- Hypocalcemia may produce muscle camps, tetany, and seizures.

Investigations

- Serum uric acid, phosphate and potassium are elevated. Serum calcium decreased (hypocalcemia).
- Urea and creatinine are elevated due to renal failure.
- ABG shows metabolic acidosis.
- ECG
- Other routine investigations.

Treatment

- Hydration: Volume depletion is a major risk factor for tumor lysis syndrome and must be corrected vigorously. Intravenous fluids along with loop diuretics are given to maintain high urine output so that uric acid crystals are easily washed out in the urine thus preventing uric acid nephropathy.
- Hyperuricemia is treated with *allopurinol and rasburicase*. Allopurinol blocks conversion of hypoxanthine and xanthine to uric acid. Rasburicase is a recombinant urate oxidase which converts uric acid into an inactive and soluble metabolite (allantoin) which is easily excreted by the kidneys. *Febuxostat* is a new xanthine oxidase inhibitor which is long acting and does not require dose modification in renal failure. Febuxostat can be used instead of allopurinol.

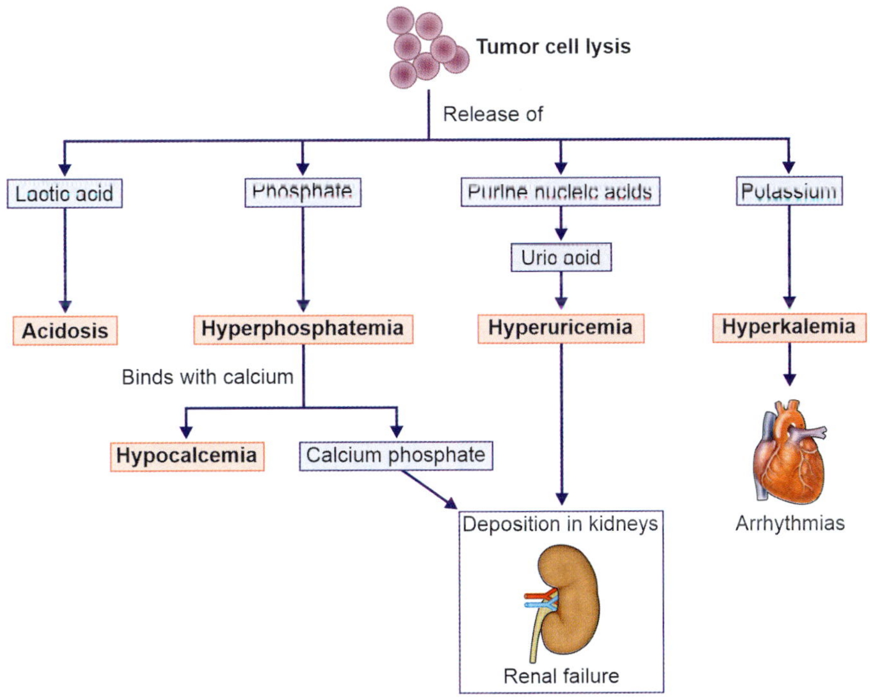

Figure 14.1: Pathogenesis of tumor lysis syndrome

- Hyperkalemia is treated with antihyperkalemia measures such as beta-2 agonists, insulin plus dextrose infusions and potassium binding resins.
- Hypocalcemia is treated with intravenous infusion of calcium gluconate.
- Hyperphosphatemia is managed with oral phosphate binders and insulin plus dextrose solution used for the control of hyperkalemia.
- Urinary alkalinization will convert uric acid to more soluble urate salt, thus preventing deposition of uric acid crystals in the renal tubules and consequent renal failure. Sodium bicarbonate is given intravenously for this purpose.
- Hemodialysis should be considered in severe cases.

Q. Spinal cord compression due to tumor.

- Spinal cord compression is a neurological emergency caused by extrinsic, intradural, or intramedullary compression of the spinal cord by a tumor.
- Early recognition is critical to prevent permanent paralysis.

Clinical Features

- Thoracic spine is most commonly affected.
- Back pain at the level of the spinal cord lesion.
- Progressive weakness and sensory loss below the level of compression.
- Radiculopathy due to nerve root compression.
- Bowel and bladder dysfunction.

Investigations

- Plain X-rays may show bony destruction.
- MRI is essential to demonstrate tumor detail and spinal cord compression.
- Biopsy of the lesion may be required to confirm the diagnosis of malignancy.

Treatment

- Immediate diagnosis and treatment is essential to prevent permanent neurological deficits.
- Inj dexamethasone 10 mg is given IV stat followed by 4 mg mg IV 6-hourly.
- Urgent radiotherapy
- Surgery is indicated if neurologic deficits worsen despite nonsurgical treatment, a biopsy is needed, spine is unstable or tumor recurs after radiation therapy.

Q. Paraneoplastic syndromes.

- Paraneoplastic syndromes are disorders due to the remote effects of malignancy that cannot be attributed either to direct invasion or metastatic lesions.
- They may affect up to 15% of patients with cancer. The most common cancer associated with paraneoplastic syndromes is small cell cancer of the lung.
- These syndromes may be the first sign of a malignancy and provide an early clue to the presence of certain types of cancer. Treatment of the cancer leads to resolution of the syndrome, and, conversely, recurrence of the cancer may be heralded by the return of the syndromes.

Mechanism of Paraneoplastic Syndromes

- Paraneoplastic syndromes result from the production and release of physiologically active substances by the tumor. Tumors may produce hormones, hormone precursors, a variety of enzymes, or cytokines. Paraneoplastic syndromes associated with ectopic hormone production are the best-characterized entities. Examples are hypercalcemia due to production of parathyroid hormone (PTH) or PTH-related peptide by squamous cell carcinoma of lung and SIADH (syndrome of inappropriate secretion of antidiuretic hormone) due to ADH secretion by small cell carcinoma.
- Antibodies produced against tumor cells may cross react and destroy normal tissues producing paraneoplastic manifestations. Many neurologic paraneoplastic syndromes have been found to be caused by the production of antineuronal antibodies.
- In some cases the pathophysiology of paraneoplastic syndromes is unknown.

Manifestations of Paraneoplastic Syndromes

Systemic
- Anorexia
- Cachexia
- Weight loss
- Fever
- Suppressed immunity

Endocrine
- Cushing's syndrome
- SIADH
- Hypercalcemia
- Hypoglycemia
- Carcinoid syndrome

Neuromuscular
- Peripheral neuropathy (most common neurologic paraneoplastic syndrome)
- Subacute cerebellar degeneration
- Eaton-Lambert syndrome
- Stiff man syndrome

Hematologic
- Erythrocytosis
- Pure red cell aplasia
- Eosinophilia
- Thrombocytosis
- Coagulopathy

Rheumatologic
- Arthropathies
- Hypertrophic osteoarthropathy
- Dermatomyositis/polymyositis

Cutaneous
- Itching
- Dermatomyositis
- Acanthosis nigricans
- Sweet's syndrome

Others
- Amyloidosis
- Hypertrophic pulmonary osteoarthropathy

Management

- Treatment of underlying cancer leads to resolution of paraneoplastic syndromes. Life threatening paraneoplastic emergencies such as hypercalcemia should be treated appropriately.
- Immunosuppression (steroids), intravenous immunoglobulins, or plasma exchange can be used in patients with autoantibodies causing paraneoplastic manifestations.

Q. Targeted therapy in the treatment of cancer.

- Conventional cancer therapy (radiotherapy and chemotherapy) does not adequately discriminate between rapidly dividing normal cells and cancer cells. Hence normal dividing cells also get killed leading to many side effects such as bone marrow suppression, alopecia, mucositis, etc.
- Targeted therapy uses specific molecular targets present exclusively on cancer cells (and not on normal cells) thus avoiding the side effects of conventional chemotherapy. These targets may be receptors or enzymes in the tumor cells. To be effective, molecular targets should have a role in cancer cell division and growth.
- Targeted therapy is often used with chemotherapy and radiotherapy for additive or synergistic effect.

Examples of Targeted Therapies

- Hormone therapies
- Signal transduction inhibitors
- Gene expression modulators
- Apoptosis inducers
- Angiogenesis inhibitors
- Immunotherapies.

Hormone Therapies

- Hormone therapies block a certain hormone required by the tumor to grow. Hormone therapies are used in the treatment of breast and prostate cancer.

Signal Transduction Inhibitors

- Block the activities of molecules that stimulate cell division.
- Examples are imatinib, a tyrosine kinase inhibitor used in the treatment of CML. Gefitinib and erlotinib inhibit tyrosine kinase in the epidermal growth factor receptors (EGFR). They have been tried in advanced non small cell lung cancer.

Gene Expression Modulators

- Oncogene expression can be inhibited by triplex forming oligonucleotides, as well as peptide nucleic acids. Research is going on this.

Apoptosis Inducers

- They induce the cancer cells to undergo apoptosis (spontaneous cell death). Examples include *proteosome inhibitors*, such as bortezomib and carfilzomib. Proteosome-ubiquitin pathway is an essential intracellular system that degrades many labile proteins regulating cell cycle, apoptosis, and transcription. These drugs are used in refractory multiple myeloma.

Angiogenesis Inhibitors

- They block the growth of blood vessels supplying the tumor. Lack of blood supply interferes with tumor growth. Many of these drugs work by blocking *vascular endothelial growth factor* (VEGF) proteins or the VEGF receptors.
- Examples of angiogenesis inhibitors include bevacizumab and ramucirumab.

Immunotherapies

- They trigger the immune system to destroy cancer cells.
- Examples are monoclonal antibodies that recognize specific molecules on the surface of cancer cells. Binding of the monoclonal antibody to the target molecule results in the immune destruction of cells that express that target molecule. *Rituximab* is a monoclonal antibody against the B lymphocyte antigen CD20. It is used in the treatment of resistant or relapsed lymphomas.
- *Trastuzumab* is a recombinant monoclonal antibody directed against the HER-2/*neu* gene product (a cells surface receptor) and is effective in the treatment of HER-2/*neu* expressing breast cancer.
- Monoclonal antibodies can also be used to deliver toxic molecules to cancer cells specifically (immunotoxin therapy). Once the antibody has bound to its target cell, the toxic molecule that is linked to the antibody—such as a radioactive substance or a toxin is taken up by the cell, ultimately killing that cell. Immunotoxin therapy is used in Hodgkin's lymphoma since the Reed-Sternberg cells express a large number of antigens that occur in only a small fraction of normal cells.

Q. Enumerate the various modes of treatment of cancer.

- Cancer treatment is often multimodal, meaning that more than one type of therapy may be used to treat cancer, Various modes of cancer treatment are as follows.

Surgery

- Surgery refers to physical removal of the tumor. Surgery has a pivotal role in the management of cancer.
- It can be either curative or palliative. Surgery can be curative for most solid tumors if detected early. Palliative surgeries relieve the symptoms without curing the cancer. Examples of palliative surgeries are debulking the tumor to relieve pressure symptoms, colostomy in colon cancer, and fixation of pathological fractures.

Chemotherapy

- Chemotherapy makes use of various cytotoxic drugs with different modes of action. Examples are melphalan, methotrexate, cyclophosphamide, etc.

Radiotherapy

- Radiotherapy makes use of ionizing radiation to kill or shrink cancer cells.

Hormonal Treatments

- Makes use of hormones/hormone modifiers for the treatment of cancer.
- Examples: Reducing estrogen levels can reduce the proliferation of breast cancer cells and increase their loss through apoptosis. Antiandrogen therapy can help in prostate cancer.

Targeted Therapies

- These therapies target a particular pathway in cancer cells with minimal or no effect on normal cells. This creates the potential to target cancer cells more selectively, with reduced toxicity to normal tissues.
- Example is imatinib which inhibits the *BCR-ABL* gene product tyrosine kinase that is responsible for chronic myeloid leukemia.
- Rituximab is a monoclonal antibody against the B-cell antigen CD20. It increases response rates and survival in non-Hodgkin's lymphoma.

Immunotherapy

- These therapies stimulate or enhances the body's immune system to recognize and destroy cancer cells.
- Example: Immune checkpoint inhibitors like Nivolumab, Pembrolizumab.

Q. Write briefly about cancer chemotherapy.

Q. Classification of anticancer drugs.

Q. Complications of cancer chemotherapy.

- Cancer chemotherapy refers to the use of cytotoxic drugs to treat malignancies by destroying rapidly dividing cancer cells. It may be used alone or in combination with surgery and radiotherapy.
- Nitrogen mustard was the first anticancer drug to be found, followed by discovery of other agents. Anticancer drugs (cytotoxic agents) have a broader range of intracellular effects than radiotherapy.

Classification of Anticancer Drugs

- Cancer chemotherapeutic drugs can be classified by their mode of action.

Alkylating agents
- Mechanism: Cross-link DNA, inhibiting replication
- Examples: Melphalan, carmustine, chlorambucil, cyclophosphamide, cisplatin, busulphan, ifosfamide

Antitumor antibiotics
- Mechanism: Intercalate DNA, inhibit topoisomerase.
- Examples: Bleomycin, mitomycin, etoposide, doxorubicin and daunorubicin, mitoxantrone

Antimetabolites
- Mechanism: Inhibit DNA/RNA synthesis by mimicking normal substrates
- Examples: Methotrexate, 5-fluorouracil, cytarabine (cytidine)

Natural products
- Mechanism: interfere with microtubule function.
- Examples: Vincristine, vinblastine, docetaxel, paclitaxel

Hormones/hormone modifiers
- Mechanism: act against the natural hormones and thus inhibit the growth of tumors which depend on these hormones.
- Examples: Steroids, antiandrogens (flutamide), antiestrogens (tamoxifene), aromatase inhibitors (letrozole)

Targeted therapy
- Mechnaism: Specifically target molecular pathways involved in cancer cell growth.
- Examples: Monoclonal antibodies (rituximab, trastuzumab), tyrosine kinase inhibitors (imatinib).

Immunotherapy
- Mechnaism: Stimulates or enhances the body's immune system to recognize and destroy cancer cells.
- Examples: Immune checkpoint inhibitors like Nivolumab, Pembrolizumab.

Objectives of Chemotherapy

- *Curative:* To eliminate cancer entirely (e.g. some leukemias, lymphomas).
- *Palliative:* To relieve symptoms and prolong life in advanced cancers.
- *Neoadjuvant:* Before surgery/radiotherapy to shrink tumors.
- *Adjuvant:* After surgery to eliminate residual disease.

Combination Chemotherapy

- It overcomes drug resistance and limits the side effects of different drugs.
- Combinations usually include drugs from different classes, each of which may be independently active and the combination of which should not have additive toxic effects.
- Each tumor has specific regimens that are used at various stages of the disease.

Administration

- Drugs are conventionally given by intravenous injection every 3–4 weeks, allowing enough time for the patient to recover from short-term toxic effects such as bone marrow suppression.
- Between four and eight such cycles of treatment are usually given in total.

Complications of Cancer Chemotherapy

- Most cytotoxics have a narrow therapeutic index. They cannot specifically target malignant cells. They have various effects on normal cells (especially rapidly dividing cells) which is responsible for their side effects.

Skin

- ***Alopecia***—hair loss due to damage to hair follicles. Psychological support and the use of wigs can be encouraged.
- ***Tissue necrosis***—is common if extravasation of the drug occurs during intravenous administration.

GIT

- ***Nausea and vomiting***: This is the most common side effect of chemotherapy. This can be prevented and treated by various antiemetic drugs such as ondansetron, domperidone, prochlorperazine, etc.
- ***Diarrhea***: This is common with fluorouracil infusions. It responds to antimotility agents such as "high-dose" loperamide.
- ***Mucositis***: Irritation and inflammation of the mucous membranes may affect oral, anal mucosa, and also rest of the gastrointestinal tract. Mucositis is due to damage to the proliferating cells at the base of the mucosal squamous epithelia or in the intestinal crypts.

Hematological

- ***Bone marrow suppression***: Almost all the agents cause bone marrow suppression which manifests as cytopenias. Marrow is susceptible because of high number of rapidly dividing cells. Leukopenia leads to various infections, thrombocytopenia leads to bleeding manifestations, and anemia leads to easy fatigability.

Reproductive

- ***Gonadal dysfunction***: Cessation of ovulation and azoospermia occurs with most chemotherapeutic agents leading to infertility. Sperm banking before treatment may be considered to support patients likely to be sterilized by treatment.

Secondary Malignancies

- Development of secondary malignancies especially leukemias can happen with alkylating agents.

Organ Toxicity

- Cardiotoxicity (doxorubicin)
- Nephrotoxicity (cisplatin)
- Neurotoxicity (vincristine, peripheral neuropathy)
- Hemorrhagic cystitis (cyclophosphamide).

Other Side Effects

- Tumor lysis syndrome.

Q. Write briefly about radiotherapy of cancer.

- Radiotherapy means the treatment of cancer with ionizing radiation. It can be curative or palliative. For localized cancers it may be curative. Source of ionizing radiation can be from the decay of a radioactive isotope (gamma rays) or produced by linear accelerators (X rays).

Mechanism of Action

- Radiation is a physical form of treatment that damages any tissue in its path. Radiation causes breaks in DNA and generates free radicals from cell water that may damage cell membranes, proteins and organelles. Its selectivity for cancer cells is due to defects in a cancer cell's ability to repair sublethal DNA and other damage.
- Radiation damage is dependent on oxygen; hypoxic cells are more resistant.

Modes of Delivery of Radiation

- Total required dose of radiation is given in 20–30 fractions given daily, 5 days a week over 4–6 weeks. This allows normal cells to recover from radiation damage, but recovery is less in cancer cells. Radiation can be delivered by three methods:
  - *External beam radiotherapy (teletherapy):* Radiation is delivered from a machine outside the body, directed precisely at the tumor.
  - *Brachytherapy (internal radiotherapy):* It involves placing a source of radiation into or adjacent to the tumor. This allows the delivery of a very high localized dose of radiation. It is used in the management of localized cancers of the head and neck and cancer of the cervix and endometrium.
  - *Systemic radiotherapy:* Radioactive substances (e.g. radioactive iodine) are taken orally or intravenously to target specific cancers. Examples, intravenous injection of iodine-131 is used to treat thyroid cancer and Strontium 89 is used to treat bone metastases.

Uses

- Curative: To completely eliminate the tumor
- Adjuvant: After surgery to kill remaining microscopic disease
- Palliative: To relieve symptoms like pain or bleeding in advanced cancers.

Indications for Palliative Radiotherapy

- Radiotherapy can be extremely useful for the alleviation of symptoms which are as follows:
  - Bone pain
  - Hemoptysis
  - Spinal cord compression
  - Superior vena caval obstruction
  - Brain metastases.

Side Effects of Radiotherapy

Acute

- Mucositis
- Skin erythema (ulceration in severe cases)
- Bone marrow toxicity.

Late

- Hypothyroidism, cataracts and retinal damage after radiation to head and neck area.
- Brachial plexopathy, chronic constrictive pericarditis, and lung fibrosis after radiation to thoracic area.
- Shrinkage and fibrosis of the bladder after treatment for bladder cancer.
- Risk of secondary cancer induction.

Q. Relation between infection and cancers.

- Many infectious agents including bacteria and viruses can cause cancers by various mechanisms. Viruses are the most common infectious agents causing cancers.

- ***Mechanisms of virus causing cancer:*** Viral DNA may integrate within a proto-oncogene and may activate it. Viral DNA may also contain proto-oncogene which may be transferred to the host after infection. Viruses may also activate growth-promoting pathways and inhibit tumor-suppressor products in the infected cells.

Viruses Associated with Human Cancers

- *Epstein-Barr virus (EBV):* Burkitt's lymphoma, Hodgkin lymphoma, nasopharyngeal carcinoma
- *Hepatitis B virus (HBV):* Hepatocellular carcinoma
- *Hepatitis C virus (HCV):* Hepatocellular carcinoma
- *Human papillomavirus:* Ca cervix, genital tumors, oropharyngeal cancer
- *Human immunodeficiency virus*: AIDS-related malignancies
- *Human T-cell lymphotropic virus 1 (HTLV1):* Adult T-cell leukemia
- *Kaposi sarcoma herpesvirus/human herpesvirus*: Kaposi sarcoma
- *Markel cell virus*: Markel cell carcinoma

Other Infectious Agents Causing Cancers

- *Helicobacter pylori*: Gastric cancer
- *Chlamydia trachomatis*: Ca cervix
- *Streptococcus bovis*: Colorectal cancer
- Liver flukes: Cholangiocarcinoma
- *Schistosomes*: Bladder cancer.

Q. Breast cancer.

- Breast cancer is the most common cancer diagnosed in women.
- Breast cancer always evolves silently. Most of the patients discover their disease during their routine screening. Others may present with an accidentally discovered breast lump, change of breast shape or size, or nipple discharge.
- The survival rate improves with early diagnosis.

Etiology

Risk factors for breast cancer are as follows:

- Age: Incidence of breast cancer increases with advancing age. The median age of women at the time of breast cancer diagnosis is 61 years.
- Family history of breast cancer and genetic risk factors: First-degree relatives of patients with breast cancer have a 2–3-fold risk of developing the disease. A 5–10% of all breast cancer cases are due to genetic factors. BRCA1 and BRCA2 are the 2 most important genes responsible for increased breast cancer susceptibility.
- Reproductive risk factors: Reproductive milestones that increase a woman's lifetime estrogen exposure are thought to increase the breast cancer risk. These include the onset of menarche before 12 years of age, late childbirth (after age 30 years), nulliparity, and menopause after age 55 years.
- Exogenous hormone use: Therapeutic or supplemental estrogen and progesterone increase the risk of breast cancer.
- Other risk factors: Obesity, alcohol use, radiation exposure.

Pathology

- Breast cancer arises from the cells of the breast, most commonly from the ducts (ductal carcinoma) or lobules (lobular carcinoma).
- Breast cancer develops due to DNA damage and genetic mutations that can be influenced by exposure to estrogen. Sometimes there will be an inheritance of DNA defects or procancerous genes like BRCA1 and BRCA2. Thus the family history of ovarian or breast cancer increases the risk for breast cancer development. In a normal individual, the immune system attacks cells with abnormal DNA or abnormal growth. This fails in those with breast cancer disease leading to tumor growth and spread. Breast cancer can be invasive or non-invasive according to its relation to the basement membrane. The tumor tends to spread lymphatically and hematologically, leading to distant metastasis and poor prognosis.

Clinical Features

- Most early breast cancers are asymptomatic and are discovered during screening mammography.
- With increasing size, the patient may discover cancer as a painless lump that is felt accidentally, mostly during combing or showering. Breast pain is rare.
- Nipple retraction, discharge (may be bloody)
- Skin changes (peau d'orange appearance)
- Axillary lymphadenopathy
- Advanced cases: Weight loss, bone pain, liver or lung metastases.

Investigations

- Mammography is the most commonly used modality for the diagnosis of breast cancer. Most of the asymptomatic cases are diagnosed during screening mammography. Breast cancer is seen as calcification, dense lump, with or without architecture distortion in mammography. Mammography is not sensitive in young women because dense breasts and for them breast ultrasonography is more useful.
- Ultrasonography of breast: More useful in young women. It is useful in assessing the consistency and size of breast lumps. It is also useful for guided needle biopsy.
- MRI: It is indicated if there are occult lesions, or suspicion of multifocal or bilateral malignancy, and in the assessment of response to neoadjuvant chemotherapy, or when planning for breast conservation surgery and screening in the high-risk patient.
- Biopsy: Tissue biopsy is an important step in the evaluation of a breast cancer patient. There are different ways to take a tissue specimen, and include fine-needle aspiration cytology (FNAC), core biopsy (Trucut), and incisional or excisional biopsy.
- PET/CT scans to assess spread.

Treatment/Management

Surgery

- Mainstay for localized disease. Breast-conserving surgery is removal of the tumor with a margin of normal tissue. Mastectomy is removal of entire breast. Axillary lymph node dissection is done if nodes are positive for metastases.

Radiotherapy

- Used after breast conserving surgery to reduce local recurrence.
- Post-mastectomy: In high-risk patients (large tumor, node-positive).
- Delivered as external beam radiotherapy.

Chemotherapy

- Used in node-positive or high-grade tumors, large tumors (≥2 cm), before surgery (neoadjuvant) to shrink tumor, after surgery (adjuvant) to reduce recurrence.
- Common drugs used are anthracyclines (doxorubicin), taxanes (paclitaxel, docetaxel), cyclophosphamide, 5-fluorouracil.

Hormonal (endocrine) Therapy

- Used for estrogen and/or progesterone receptor positive tumors.
- Examples are tamoxifen (selective estrogen receptor modulator) and anastrozole (aromatase inhibitor).

Targeted Therapy

- Trastuzumab (a monoclonal antibody) used in HER2-positive tumors. May be combined with chemotherapy.

Staging

- Breast cancer staging is done by clinical examination and imaging studies (PET/CT scans) before treatment, and after surgery pathological findings can be used to determine the stage.
- Breast cancer is classified with the TNM classification system, which uses primary tumor size (T), the regional lymph nodes status (N), and if there is any distant metastasis (M).

Prognosis

- Prognosis for early breast cancer is (stage 0 and stage I) excellent. When there are distant metastases, prognosis is poor.
- Death in breast cancer is most commonly caused by distant metastasis, especially to the lungs, liver, brain, or bones, and the complications arising from them, such as organ failure or sepsis.

Q. Mammography.

- Mammography is a X-ray imaging technique used to detect and evaluate abnormalities in the breast, especially early-stage breast cancer.
- Mammography is currently the gold standard screening tool for breast cancer and has been shown to decrease breast cancer mortality and reduce treatment morbidity.
- Patients with equivocal or suggestive mammographic screening results require further imaging with a diagnostic mammogram, ultrasound, breast MRI, biopsy, or combination thereof.

Technique

- Mammography utilizes X-rays to image the breast. The breast is compressed between two plates. Low-dose X-rays are taken from different angles. Compression helps spread tissue for better imaging and lowers radiation dose.
- Mammography can be used to evaluate the breast based on the differential attenuation characteristics of the tissues. Fat attenuates fewer X-rays than fibroglandular tissue and stromal elements and appears gray on mammography. Dense mineral deposits such as skin calcifications or calcifications within a neoplastic lesion appear bright white. Superimposition poses a challenge in mammography, as tissue structures that overlie or overlap one another may obscure a small mass. Hence, screening mammograms are performed in at least two standard views, which include the craniocaudal view (CC) and the mediolateral oblique (MLO). By comparing these two different viewpoints, structures that are superimposed upon one another in one view may be separated in the other. In cases of uncertainty, additional diagnostic views may be obtained.

Indications for Mammography

- Annual mammography is recommended for all women from the age of 40 onwards.
- High risk patients should undergo mammogram starting at an earlier age. Such high-risk patients include patients with atypical ductal hyperplasia or lobular neoplasia on a prior breast biopsy, women with specific gene mutations, including BRCA 1 and 2, those with a strong family history of breast cancer, and patients who have received radiation therapy of the chest between 10 to 30 years of age.
- It is recommended that women undergo a risk assessment by age 30 to determine the appropriate screening timeline.

BI-RADS System—Grading of Mammogram Findings

- The BI-RADS (breast imaging reporting and data system) is a standardized system for interpreting and reporting breast imaging results (including mammograms). It guides clinical decisions on whether to observe, biopsy, or treat.

BI-RADS Categories and their Meaning

See **Table 14.2.**

TABLE 14.2: BIRADS categories for mammogram

BI-RADS	Category name/Interpretation	Recommendation
0	Incomplete. Need additional imaging or comparison with prior studies	Additional views or ultrasound
1	Negative. No abnormal findings	Routine screening (usually yearly)
2	Clearly benign findings (e.g. simple cyst, fibroadenoma)	Routine screening
3	Probably benign. <2% chance of cancer; features suggest nonmalignancy	Short-term follow-up (e.g. 6 months)
4	Suspicious; not classic for cancer, but biopsy is advised abnormality	Biopsy recommended
5	Highly suggestive of malignancy	Appropriate action (usually biopsy and surgery)
6	Known malignancy. Biopsy-proven cancer before treatment	Ensure appropriate treatment is ongoing

Q. Differences between curative and palliative care of cancers.

- Curative and palliative care have long been associated with life or death, but palliative care today is focused on relieving pain and stress. In fact, both curative care and palliative care can be used simultaneously to enhance a patient's life. Both types of care are used concurrently with surgery, radiation therapy and chemotherapy.

Differences between Curative and Palliative Care of Cancers (Table 14.3)

TABLE 14.3: Differences between curative and palliative care of cancers

Feature	Curative care	Palliative care
Goal	To completely eliminate the cancer and achieve a cure	To relieve symptoms, improve quality of life, not necessarily to cure
Applicable stage	Early or localized cancer	Advanced, metastatic, or terminal stages
Treatment intensity	Often aggressive (surgery, chemo, radiotherapy)	Focused on comfort and symptom control
Examples of treatment	Tumor resection, curative chemotherapy, radiation	Pain management, antiemetics, palliative radiation
Duration of treatment	Often time-limited, aimed at cure	Long-term or continuous, based on patient needs
Outcome goal	Cancer-free survival, long-term remission	Comfort, dignity, emotional and psychosocial support
Team involvement	Oncologists, surgeons, radiotherapists	Multidisciplinary: palliative care doctors, nurses, counselors
Patient prognosis	Potential for long-term survival	Focused on end-of-life care or improving remaining life

Q. Discuss the mechanisms of pain and its implications in patient with cancer.

Q. Assessment of severity of pain in cancer patients using pain scale.

- Pain is an unpleasant sensory and emotional experience associated with actual or potential tissue damage.
- It is the most fearful and the most distressful symptom in cancer patients. 75% of advanced cancer patients experience pain.
- Inadequate pain control leads to profound alteration in nearly all aspect of wellness (activity, mood, rest, nutrition, etc.). Optimal pain control increases quality of life in all aspects.

Mechanisms of Cancer Pain

- Due to tumor infiltration/metastases: Metastatic bone pain, retroperitoneal lymphadenopathy pain, liver capsule pain, headache, cranial neuralgias
- Nerve compression or infiltration
- Spinal cord compression
- Thalamic tumor (causes thalamic pain)
- Treatment related-surgical incision pain, phantom limb pain, peripheral neuropathy, radiation fibrosis of brachial plexus, lumbosacral plexus, radiation myelopathy.

Pain Assessment

- *Detailed history of pain should be asked:* Type and quality of pain, onset, duration, course, intensity (i.e. pain experienced at rest; with movement; interference with activities); location, radiation of pain; aggravating and relieving factors, prior pain therapies; family and other support.
- Diagnose the etiology and pathophysiology (somatic, visceral, or neuropathic) of the pain.
- Assessment of pain severity. There are many ways of assessing pain. Two methods are given below:
  - *Verbal descriptor scale:* Uses words like: "no pain", "mild", "moderate", "severe", "very severe", "worst possible pain". Disadvantage is, there is limited selection of pain descriptors.
  - *Verbal numeric rating scale:* Patient rates pain from 0 (no pain) to 10 (worst possible pain). Easy to use and widely applicable.
  - *Visual analog scale:* A 10 cm line, one end labeled "no pain", the other "worst pain imaginable" **(Fig. 14.2)**. Patient marks a point on the line corresponding to their pain level. Advantages are simplicity, reproducibility, easy comprehensibility, and sensitivity to small changes in pain.
  - *Wong-Baker faces pain rating scale:* Especially useful for children or elderly with cognitive impairment. Patient selects a face image that best represents their pain **(Fig. 14.3)**.

Management

Treatment of underlying pathology (cancer): By surgery, radiation therapy, chemotherapy, etc.

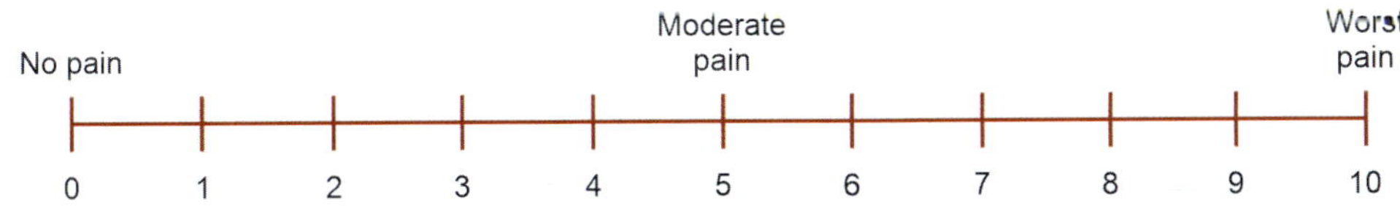

Figure 14.2: Visual analog scale

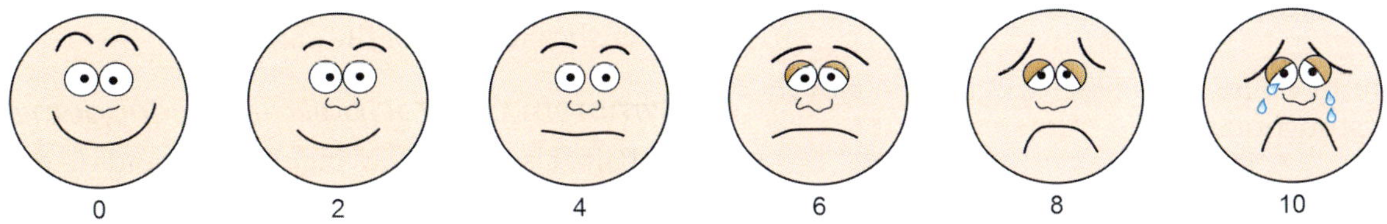

Figure 14.3: Wong-Baker faces pain rating scale

Analgesics:
- Non-opioid analgesics: Paracetamol, NSAIDs.
- Opioid analgesics: Morphine, methadone, codeine, tramadol.

Nondrug methods: Massage, heat pads, psychological-relaxation, cognitive behavioral therapy.

Interruption of pain pathways: Local anesthesia, neurolysis (by using alcohol, phenol, cryotherapy, thermo-coagulation), neurosurgery (e.g. cervical cordotomy).

Modification of way of life and environment: Avoid precipitating activity, immobilization of painful part (e.g. cervical collar, slings), walking aid.

Q. Describe the indications, use, side effects of narcotics in pain alleviation in patients with cancer.

- Opioids (narcotics) are the mainstay of moderate to severe cancer pain management, especially in advanced or terminal stages. They act on opioid receptors in the brain and spinal cord to modulate pain perception.

Indications for use of Narcotics in Cancer Pain

- Moderate to severe pain not responsive to nonopioids (e.g. NSAIDs, paracetamol).
- Chronic cancer-related pain, e.g. due to bone metastasis or tumor compression.
- Breakthrough pain episodes in patients already on regular analgesics.
- Postoperative pain following cancer surgery.
- Pain due to chemotherapy or radiation-induced tissue injury.
- Neuropathic cancer pain not controlled by other medicines.
- Palliative and end-of-life care: To relieve suffering and improve comfort.

Commonly used Narcotics in Cancer Pain

Drug	Remarks
Morphine	Gold standard; dose titratable
Fentanyl	Good for opioid-tolerant patients
Oxycodone	Useful in renal dysfunction
Hydromorphone	Potent; used in opioid rotation
Methadone	Long-acting; also NMDA antagonist
Buprenorphine	Partial agonist; good safety margin
Tramadol	Weak opioid; useful for mild-moderate pain
Tapentadol	Similar to tramadol

Use of Narcotics in Cancer Pain: WHO Analgesic Ladder

WHO Three-step Ladder for Cancer Pain Relief

- Step 1: Mild pain → Non-opioid (e.g. paracetamol, NSAIDs).
- Step 2: Moderate pain → Weak opioids (e.g. codeine, tramadol) ± nonopioids.
- Step 3: Severe pain → Strong opioids (e.g. morphine) ± non-opioids ± adjuvants.
- Adjuvants: Antidepressants (e.g. amitriptyline), anticonvulsants (e.g. gabapentin), corticosteroids.

Key Principles in Use

- Start with low dose and titrate upward
- Use oral route when possible.
- Provide regular dosing with rescue doses for breakthrough pain.
- Assess pain regularly and adjust
- Prevent and manage side effects (e.g. give laxatives with opioids).

Side Effects of Narcotics

Common Side Effects

- Constipation—most persistent; prophylactic laxatives required
- Nausea and vomiting
- Drowsiness and sedation
- Dry mouth
- Urinary retention
- Sweating
- Pruritus (itching).

Less Common/Serious Side Effects

- Respiratory depression—especially in opioid-naive patients or overdose
- Tolerance—requiring higher doses over time
- Physical dependence—expected with long-term use; tapering needed
- Opioid-induced hyperalgesia—paradoxical increase in pain
- Delirium or hallucinations—especially in elderly or renal dysfunction.

Q. Describe the common issues encountered in patients at the end of life and principles of management of end-of-life care.

Common Issues Encountered in Patients at the End of Life

- Patients nearing the end of life, especially due to cancer or chronic illness, often face complex physical, psychological, social, and spiritual challenges. These include:

Physical Symptoms

- Pain (most common and feared symptom)
- Dyspnea (breathlessness due to lung metastasis, effusion, or heart failure)
- Fatigue and weakness
- Nausea and vomiting (due to drugs, GI obstruction)
- Anorexia and cachexia
- Constipation (from opioids, immobility)
- Delirium or agitation (due to metabolic imbalances, infections, drugs)
- Incontinence or retention of urine due to spinal cord or nerve damage.

Psychological Issues

- Depression and anxiety
- Fear of death, abandonment, or being a burden
- Grief and anticipatory loss
- Delirium or terminal restlessness.

Social Issues

- Family distress and caregiver fatigue
- Financial burdens
- Unresolved interpersonal conflicts.

Spiritual and Existential Issues

- Loss of meaning or purpose
- Desire for forgiveness or closure
- Fear of afterlife or nonexistence
- Spiritual distress: "why me?" or belief of punishment.

Principles of Management of End-of-life Care

- End-of-life care is patient-centered, holistic, and compassionate, aiming to improve quality—not quantity—of life.
- Strives to help patients and families address physical, psychological, social, spiritual and practical issues, and their associated expectations, needs, hopes and fears
- Prepares the patient and others for managing self-determined life closure and the dying process
- Aims to relieve patient suffering and improve the quality of living and dying
- Learn/understand/implement the patient/family's wishes for end of life care.

Symptom Control (palliative management)

- Pain: Use analgesics including opioids (e.g. morphine) as needed
- Dyspnea: Oxygen (if hypoxic)
- Anxiety: Use anxiolytics (e.g. lorazepam)
- Nausea/vomiting: Antiemetics (ondansetron, haloperidol)
- Delirium: Haloperidol, midazolam; calm environment
- Secretions: Anticholinergics (glycopyrrolate, scopolamine)
- Fatigue: Gentle reassurance, low-dose corticosteroids sometimes used.

Communication

- Clear, honest communication about prognosis and goals of care.
- Use of advance care planning, including:
  - Do not resuscitate (DNR) orders
  - Living wills or advanced directives
  - Naming a healthcare proxy

Psychosocial and Emotional Support

- Counseling and reassurance for patient and family
- Support groups and bereavement services
- Social work involvement for financial/legal assistance.

Spiritual Care

- Facilitate access to spiritual leaders or chaplains
- Support patient's personal beliefs and rituals
- Explore meaning and help in finding peace or closure.

Care Setting and Team Approach

- Can be delivered at home, hospice, or hospital depending on patient preference.
- Multidisciplinary team approach: Physicians, nurses, psychologists, social workers, chaplains.
- Involve the family in patient care: The family can be the primary caregiver for the patient if preferred. During final moments family can visit frequently, allow home-cooked meals, which may be preferred by patient and gives the family a chance to participate in care. The family can perform simple care activities such as feeding the patient, washing the face, combing hair. Teach and demonstrate to family feeding techniques, bathing, mouth care, and hygiene measures.

Ethical and Legal Aspects

- Respect for patient autonomy

- Informed decision-making about life-sustaining treatments.
- Withholding or withdrawing futile treatments when appropriate.

Q. Ethical and the medico legal issues involved in end-of-life care.

- End-of-life (EOL) care involves complex ethical and legal challenges, particularly in balancing patient autonomy, medical responsibility, and societal norms. The goal is to ensure compassionate care while respecting the patient's rights and legal framework.

Ethical Issues in End-of-life Care

Autonomy

- The patient has the right to make informed decisions about their care, including the right to refuse or discontinue treatment.
- Includes advance directives and informed consent.

Beneficence

- The healthcare team must act in the best interest of the patient to relieve suffering and provide comfort.

Nonmaleficence

- "Do no harm." Avoid unnecessary or futile interventions that may prolong suffering or dying.

Justice

- Fair allocation of limited healthcare resources (e.g. ICU beds, ventilators), especially in terminally ill patients.

Truth-telling and Transparency

- Open, honest communication about diagnosis, prognosis, and realistic outcomes is ethically essential.

Dignity

- Respecting the patient's values, beliefs, and preferences at the end of life is a moral obligation.

Medicolegal Issues in End-of-life Care

Informed Consent

- Legally required before initiating or withholding any treatment.
- Patients (or their legal surrogates) must understand the risks, benefits, and alternatives.

Advance Directives/Living Will

- A legal document where a person specifies their preferences for medical treatment if they become incapacitated. May include:
  - Do not resuscitate (DNR) orders: Legally binding instruction to avoid CPR or advanced life support in case of cardiac arrest. Requires written consent and documentation.
  - Withholding life-support
  - Designating a healthcare proxy.

Withholding vs Withdrawing life Support

- Both are legally permissible if aligned with the patient's wishes or best interest.
- Withdrawing (e.g. stopping ventilator) is ethically and legally equivalent to withholding (e.g. not initiating).

Palliative Sedation

- Use of sedatives to relieve intractable suffering in terminal cases.
- Legal and ethical if the intent is relief of suffering, not hastening death.

Euthanasia and Physician-assisted Dying

- Not legal in India
- Active euthanasia (administering a lethal dose) is illegal
- Passive euthanasia (withholding or withdrawing life-sustaining treatment) was legalized in india by the supreme court judgment in 2018 under specific conditions.

Professional Negligence

- Failure to provide appropriate palliative care or ignoring patient's EOL preferences can result in legal liability.

Chapter 15

Genetic Disorders

Q. What is genetics? Define the terms 'gene' and 'chromosome'.

- The word genetics comes from ancient Greek word '*genetikos*' meaning "genitive" and from '*genesis*' meaning "origin". Genetics deals with the molecular structure and function of genes, and gene behavior in context of a cell or organism, patterns of inheritance from parent to offspring, and gene distribution, variation and change in populations.
- A gene is a specific sequence of DNA that contains the instructions to make a particular protein or RNA molecule. It is the basic unit of heredity and determines specific traits in an organism.
- Chromosomes: A chromosome is a thread-like structure made of DNA and proteins (mainly histones) that carries genes. Humans have 46 chromosomes (23 pairs) in each somatic cell, with one set inherited from each parent.

Q. Mutation.

- Mutation is defined as a permanent change in the DNA sequence of a gene or chromosome. Mutations may be lethal or of no functional consequence. Mutations can occur in the germline (sperm or oocytes) which can be transmitted to progeny or in somatic tissue after conception. Some somatic mutations are associated with neoplasia because they confer a growth advantage to cells.
- Acquired mutations in somatic cells are fairly common, but most mutations are rectified by repair mechanisms. Causes of increased mutation rate include: ionizing and non-ionizing radiation, chemical mutagens. Loss of DNA repair enzymes increases mutation rate and susceptibility to cancer. Example is xeroderma pigmentosum (XP).

Types of Mutations

Gene Point Mutations

Affect single or few nucleotides:

- **Substitution** (e.g. A replaced by G)
- **Insertion** (addition of nucleotides)
- **Deletion** (removal of nucleotides)
- **Frameshift mutation**—caused by insertions or deletions not in multiples of 3, altering the reading frame.

Chromosomal Mutations

Affect the structure or number of chromosomes:

- **Deletion:** Loss of a chromosome segment
- **Duplication:** Repetition of a chromosome segment
- **Inversion:** Reversal of a chromosome segment
- **Translocation:** Transfer of a segment to a non-homologous chromosome
- **Aneuploidy:** Abnormal number of chromosomes (e.g. trisomy 21 in Down syndrome)

Q. Human genome project.

- Human genome project (HGP) was an international scientific research initiative aimed at mapping and sequencing the entire human genome, that is, all the DNA present in human cells.
- This project began in 1990 and was completed in 2003. It has produced a reference database of sequence of human genome which is used worldwide in biomedical sciences. It is available to anyone on the internet.
- It has been found that only 1.5% of the total length of human genome encodes proteins and rest of the genome is junk DNA.

Applications of the Human Genome Project

- Improved diagnosis of genetic disorders
- Personalized medicine and targeted drug therapy
- Better understanding of human evolution and genetic variation
- Foundation for studying complex diseases like cancer, diabetes, and Alzheimer's
- Development of gene therapy.

Q. Prenatal diagnosis.

- Prenatal diagnosis refers to medical procedures used to detect genetic, chromosomal, or structural abnormalities in a fetus before birth.

- If any abnormality is found genetic counseling and termination of pregnancy may be offered to parents.

Techniques Used in Prenatal Diagnosis

- Ultrasound
- Fetal blood sampling
- Chorionic villus biopsy
- Amniocentesis
- Analysis of maternal serum
- Fetal MRI.

Indications for Prenatal Diagnosis

- Advanced maternal age (>35 years)
- Family history of genetic disorders
- Previous child with genetic or congenital anomaly
- Abnormal results from screening tests (e.g. triple test, ultrasound)
- Exposure to teratogens (e.g. drugs, infections).

Q. Prevention of genetic diseases.

- Prevention of genetic diseases involves strategies at different levels to avoid the occurrence, recurrence, or severity of inherited disorders.

Primary Prevention (prevention before disease occurs)

- Genetic counseling: Educating at-risk couples about the risk of passing on genetic disorders.
- Carrier screening: For diseases like thalassemia, sickle cell anemia, cystic fibrosis.
- Consanguinity avoidance: Discouraging marriage among close relatives in high-risk populations.
- Folic acid supplementation: To prevent neural tube defects.
- Avoidance of teratogens: e.g. alcohol, certain drugs, radiation.

Secondary Prevention (early detection)

- Prenatal diagnosis and screening.
- Newborn screening (e.g. for congenital hypothyroidism, phenylketonuria).
- Preimplantation genetic diagnosis: In IVF, embryos are tested for genetic disorders before implantation.

Tertiary Prevention (limiting complications)

- Early treatment and rehabilitation.
- Enzyme replacement therapies (e.g. for Gaucher disease).
- Genetic-based therapies (e.g. gene therapy in clinical trials).

Q. Genetic counseling.

- Genetic counseling is a process of communication and education that helps individuals or families understand the medical, psychological, and familial implications of genetic conditions.
- It involves assessing the risk of a hereditary disorder, discussing available testing options, and providing support for decision-making.
- Genetic counseling can be provided by a medical geneticist, a specialist nurse counselor or obstetrician or pediatrician. The key requirement for genetic counseling is the provision of adequate time in a quiet place free of disturbance.
- Strict patient confidentiality should be observed at all times and information from medical records obtained only with prior consent.

Aims of Genetic Counseling

- To help individuals understand the nature and inheritance of genetic disorders.
- To assess the risk of recurrence in future pregnancies.
- To explain diagnostic tests, their results, and implications.
- To support individuals in making informed reproductive choices.
- To help families cope with psychological and social issues.

Indications for Genetic Counseling

- A known or suspected hereditary disease in the patient or a family member.
- Maternal age of 35 years or older during a pregnancy.
- Consanguineous marriage.
- Teratogen exposure during pregnancy.
- Ethnic background associated with an increased prevalence of a heritable disorder.
- Presence of birth defects, chromosomal abnormality, or mental retardation in a parent, a child, or the child of a family member.
- Identification of one or more significant abnormalities during an antenatal ultrasound.
- Abnormal results on first or second trimester screening (e.g. Down syndrome, neural tube defects, trisomy 18).

Q. Proteome.

Q. Proteomics.

- The word proteome is blend of the words "protein" and "genome" and refers to all the proteins produced by an organism just like genome refers to all the genes.
- Proteomics refers to study of protein expression in tissues, serum, and other biologic samples. Human body may contain more than 2 million proteins each having different functions. Compared to the study of DNA or RNA expression patterns, proteomics may provide a more accurate understanding of human diseases.
- Proteomics research will enhance our understanding of tumor biology, particularly the aberrant cellular signaling that characterizes malignant disease.
- Understanding the structure and function of each protein and the complexities of protein-protein interactions will be critical for developing the most effective diagnostic techniques.

- Proteomics will facilitate identification of potential novel biomarkers.
- Proteomics will play an important role in developing new drugs. For example, if a certain protein is implicated in a disease, its 3D structure provides the information to design drugs to interfere with the action of the protein.

Q. Epigenetics.

- The term epigenetics (*epi* = over; above genetics) refers to changes in phenotype (appearance) or gene expression caused by mechanisms other than changes in the underlying DNA sequence.
- There are many nongenetic factors which cause the organism's genes to behave (or "express themselves") differently.
- The molecular basis of epigenetics involves modification, inhibition and activation of certain genes, but not the basic structure of DNA. Additionally, the chromatin proteins associated with DNA may be activated or silenced.

Q. Classify genetic disorders with examples.

- Genetic disorders can be broadly divided into following categories;
  - *Monogenic (Mendelian) disorders*: These are due to single gene defect.
  - *Polygenic (multifactorial)*: These are due to interaction of multiple genetic factors and environment.
  - *Chromosomal disorders*: These are due to abnormal number or structure of chromosomes.
  - *Mitochondrial disorders*: These are caused by mutations in mitochondrial DNA and are maternally inherited.

Monogenic (Mendelian) Disorders

- Genetic disorders caused by a single gene abnormality are easiest to analyze and the most well understood **(Fig. 15.1)**. If expression of a trait requires only one copy of a gene (one allele), that trait is called dominant. If expression of a trait requires 2 copies of a gene (2 alleles), that trait is called recessive.
- However, X-linked disorders can be expressed in males even if the trait is recessive, because males have only one X- chromosome and hence, there is no paired allele to offset the effects of abnormal allele on the X chromosome.

Autosomal Dominant Disorders

- Autosomal dominant disorders **(Fig. 15.2)** occur when there is mutation in even one allele of a gene. The affected person who has one normal and one abnormal allele is called heterozygous. If both alleles are affected then the person is said to be homozygous.
- Males and females are equally affected.
- Often associated with structural proteins or receptors rather than enzymes.
- There is a 50% risk that the child of an affected parent will be affected.
- Every generation typically has affected individuals. No skipping of generations.
- Both sexes transmit and receive the disorder.
- Father-to-son transmission is possible (unlike X-linked disorders).
- Some persons who carry an abnormal gene may not have signs of the disease. This is due to reduced penetrance of the disease. Penetrance is all or none: either the person has the disease or does not.

Autosomal Recessive Disorders

- Autosomal recessive disorders **(Fig. 15.3)** are conditions that result from the presence of mutations in both alleles (homozygous) of a gene on an autosome. Those who have one normal and one abnormal allele (heterozygous) are carriers and do not suffer from the disease.
- Males and females are affected equally.

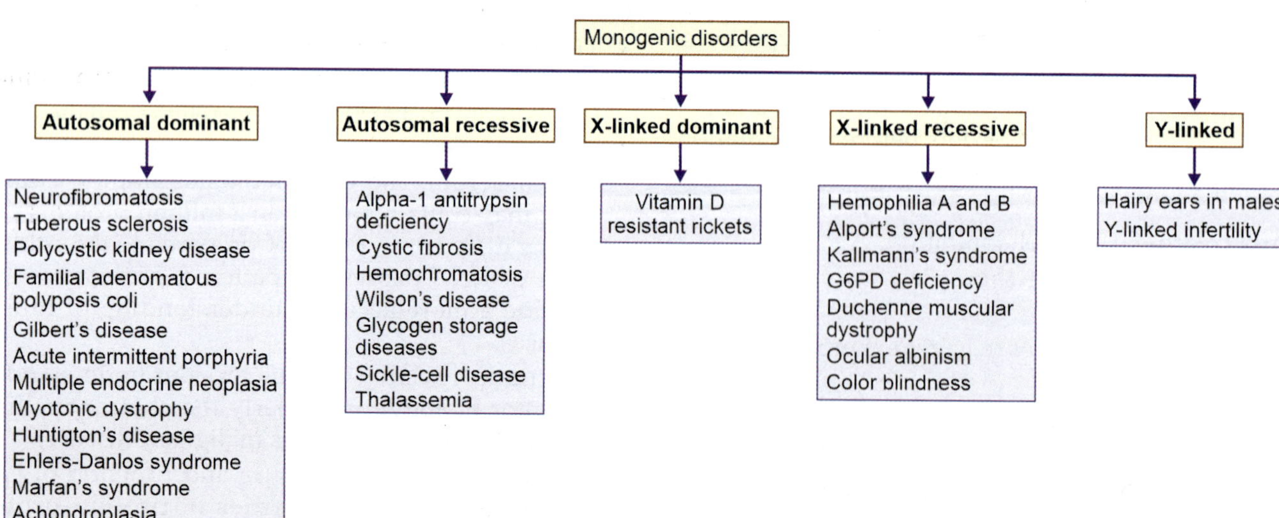

Figure 15.1: Monogenic disorders

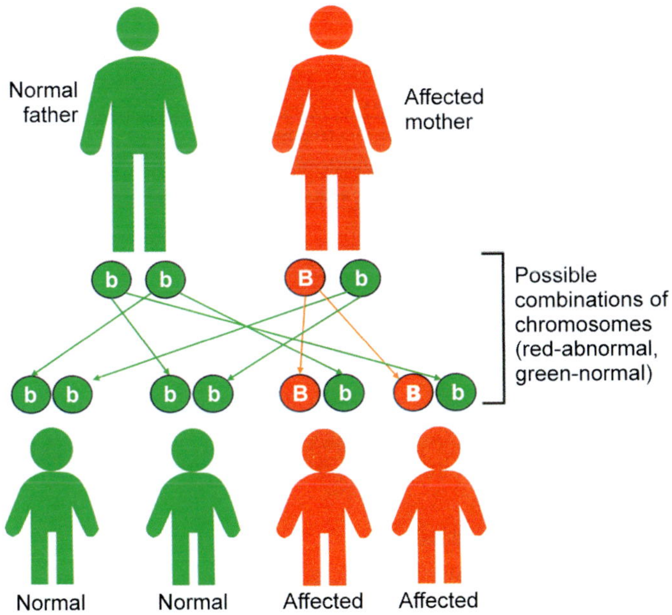

Figure 15.2: Autosomal dominant disorder

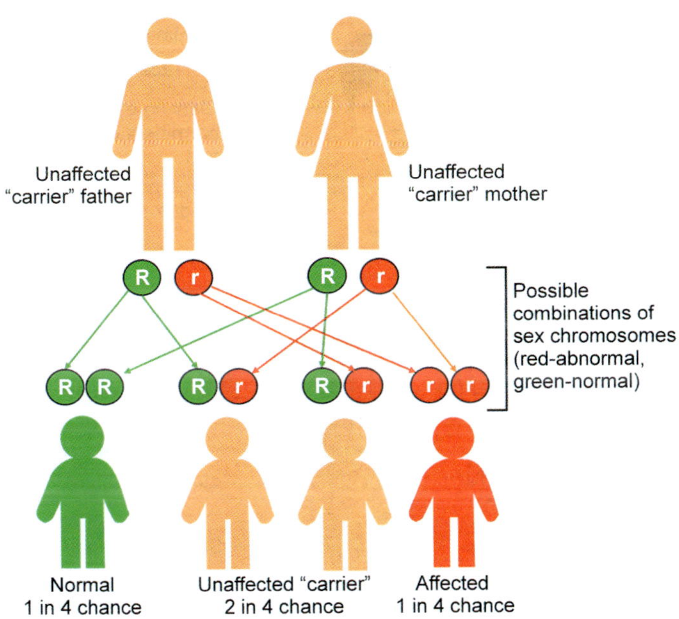

Figure 15.3: Autosomal recessive disorder

- Each offspring of two carriers has a 25% chance of being affected, a 50% chance of being a carrier, and a 25% chance of inheriting neither mutant allele. Thus, two-thirds of all clinically unaffected offspring are carriers.
- Both parents are typically carriers (heterozygous, unaffected). However, if one of the parent is affected with an autosomal recessive disease because both alleles are abnormal, then all the children will be carriers because each child will inherit one normal allele from the unaffected parent and one abnormal allele from the affected parent.
- Often skips generations.
- More common in consanguineous marriages.
- Usually involve enzyme deficiencies.

X-linked Dominant Diseases

- Mutant gene is present on X-chromosome.
- Disease will manifest even if single X-chromosome has abnormal gene, hence no carriers.
- Affected father cannot transfer the disease to son as the son's X chromosome is from mother. But affected father can transfer the disease to all daughters as the daughters get an abnormal X from the father.
- If mother is affected and father is normal, 50% chance of male child getting affected and 50% chance of female child getting affected.
- In general males are more severely affected than females.

X-linked Recessive Diseases

- Mutant gene is present X-chromosome
- Affected father cannot transfer the disease to son as the son's X chromosome is from mother. Females are carriers and can transfer the gene to sons and daughters
- It manifests only in males as they have only one X chromosome. It does not manifest in females because they have two X chromosomes one of which is normal. However, rarely females can also be affected, if they have only one X-chromosome (Turner's syndrome) or one X-chromosome is inactivated (Lyonization).

Y-linked Disorders

- Only males are affected
- Affected father transfers the disorder to all his sons but not to daughters.

Polygenic (multifactorial) Disorders

- Polygenic or multifactorial disorders are caused by the combined effect of multiple genes (polygenic inheritance) along with environmental factors. They do not follow Mendelian inheritance patterns.
- Each gene has a small effect individually but together contribute to the disease. Environmental factors like lifestyle, diet, stress, infections, etc. influence disease expression. Disease occurs when a certain number of risk genes + environmental triggers cross a threshold.
- Risk is higher in close relatives but not predictable with a fixed ratio.
- *Examples*:
    - Type 2 diabetes mellitus
    - Hypertension
    - Coronary artery disease (CAD)
    - Asthma
    - Epilepsy
    - Schizophrenia
    - Depression
    - Cleft lip and palate.

Chromosomal Disorders

- Chromosomal abnormalities are genetic disorders caused by changes in the number or structure of chromosomes. These changes can affect autosomes or sex chromosomes, leading to developmental delays, congenital anomalies, or infertility.

- Chromosomal disorders are very common and may affect more than half of all conceptions. However, most affected offspring spontaneously miscarry.
- Both autosomal and sex-linked abnormalities can be of following two broad types:
  - Numerical abnormalities
  - Structural abnormalities.

Numerical Abnormalities (Aneuploidy)

- Caused by nondisjunction (failure of chromosomes to separate during meiosis).
- Results in trisomy (one extra chromosome) or monosomy (one missing chromosome).
- Autosomal aneuplodies: Down syndrome (trisomy-21; 47,XX/XY,+21), Patau's syndrome (trisomy-13; 47XY, +13), Edward's syndrome (trisomy-18; 47XY, +18).
- Sex chromosome aneuploidies: Turner's syndrome (45,X), Klinefelter's syndrome (47,XXY).

Structural Abnormalities

- In structural abnormality, there is an alteration in the structure of one or more chromosomes due to translocations, deletions, duplications or inversions. Example is translocation between 9 and 22 chromosomes resulting in Philadelphia (Ph) chromosome causing CML.

Q. Down syndrome (mongolism).

- Down syndrome is a genetic disorder caused by the presence of an extra (third) copy of chromosome 21—hence also known as trisomy 21. This extra-chromosome 21 is almost always maternally derived.
- It is the most common chromosome abnormality among live born infants.
- Incidence—one in 1000 live births. Incidence increases with increasing maternal age.

Clinical Features

- Down syndrome affects multiple systems and causes both structural and functional defects **(Fig. 15.4)**.

General
- Short stature
- Obesity
- Single palmar crease (simian crease, in 50% of cases)
- Increased risk of sleep apnea

Head and neck
- Brachycephalic small skull
- Short neck
- Low set ears
- Hearing loss
- Short flat nose

Eyes
- Upslanting palpebral fissures with epicanthic fold at inner canthus (Mongolian eyes).
- Brushfield spots on the iris (small, white or gray spots on the periphery of the iris).
- Refractory errors
- Congenital cataract, glaucoma

Developmental and cognitive
- Intellectual disability (mild to moderate)
- Delayed developmental milestones
- Speech and language delay, mental retardation
- Autistic behavior

GIT
- Duodenal atresia
- Intestinal defects

CVS
- Congenital heart disease (especially VSD and atrioventricular canal defects)
- Increased risk of mitral valve prolapse and aortic regurgitation

Hematology
- Increased risk of leukemia
- Thrombocytopenia

Endocrine
- Diabetes mellitus
- Hypothyroidism

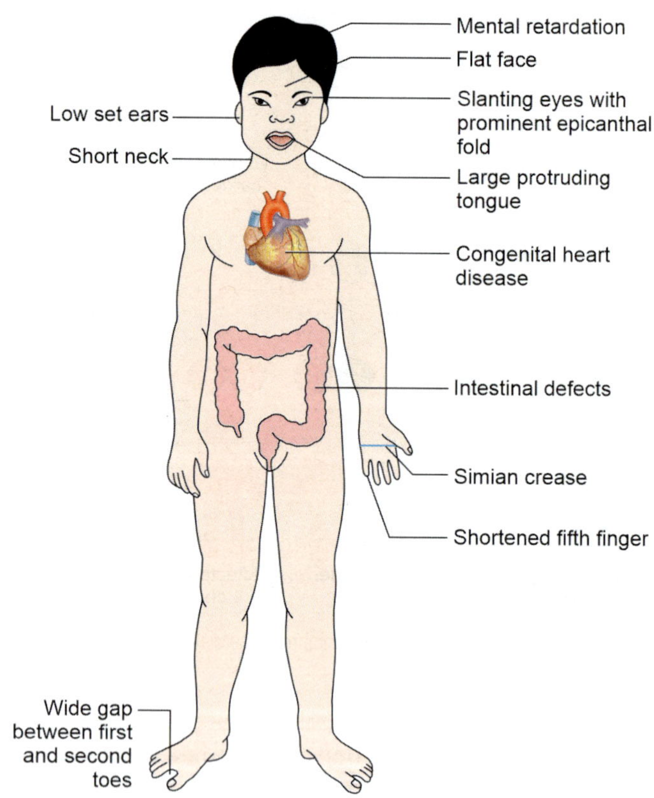

Figure 15.4: Down syndrome

Investigations

- Prenatal diagnosis: First trimester – nuchal translucency, serum β-hCG and PAPP-A (pregnancy-associated plasma protein A). In Down syndrome (trisomy 21), PAPP-A levels are decreased and β-hCG levels are increased. Second trimester – Quad screen (AFP, hCG, Estriol, Inhibin A). Prenatal chorionic villus sampling and/or amniocentesis with karyotype analysis. Free fetal DNA analysis of maternal blood sample.

- Karyotype analysis of the child will show trisomy-21.
- IQ testing.
- Echocardiogram to identify congenital heart disease.
- Ultrasound abdomen to identify duodenal atresia.
- Thyroid function tests to identify hypothyroidism.
- Hearing evaluation to identify deafness.
- Ophthalmology evaluation.
- Growth monitoring—height, weight, and head circumference plotted at each health visit using a Down syndrome growth chart.
- Other routine blood tests.

Treatment

- There is no treatment for the underlying disorder.
- If prenatal diagnosis suggests Down syndrome, genetic counseling and medical termination of pregnancy may be offered.
- Surgical treatment for duodenal atresia and congenital heart disease.
- Hypothyroidism is treated with thyroid hormone replacement.
- Other problems are treated as per standard guidelines.
- Provide social and educational support.
- No medical treatment has been proven to affect the intellectual capacity.

Q. Klinefelter's syndrome.

- Klinefelter's syndrome is a genetic condition that affects males, caused by the presence of one or more extra X chromosomes.
- The most common genotype is 47 XXY. Other genotypes are 48 XXXY and 46 XY/46 XXY mosaicism.
- Incidence – 1 in 1000 live male births.

Pathophysiology

- The 47,XXY karyotype of Klinefelter's syndrome spontaneously arises when paired X chromosomes fail to separate (nondisjunction during meiosis, during oogenesis or spermatogenesis).
- The X chromosome carries genes that play roles in testis function, brain development, and growth. Extra X chromosome results in many physical and mental abnormalities. Phenotypic abnormalities are directly related to the number of supernumerary X chromosomes. Higher the number of supernumery X chromosome, more severe are the manifestations.
- Klinefelter's syndrome is a form of primary testicular failure, with low serum testosterone levels, and elevated gonadotropin levels due to lack of feedback inhibition of the pituitary gland. Low testosterone level causes poor development of male genitalia and male secondary sexual characters.

Clinical Features (Fig. 15.5)

- Patients are actually males who develop some feminine features due to extra X chromosome.
- Affected males are normal in appearance before puberty.

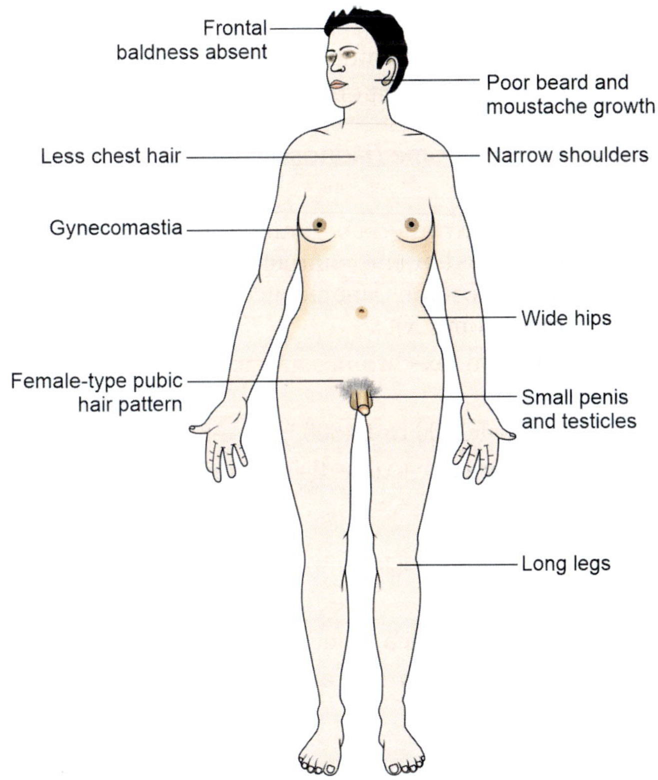

Figure 15.5: Klinefelter's syndrome

- After puberty, they develop disproportionately long legs and arms, and failure of growth of external genitalia. Penis and testes remain small.
- Testosterone deficiency causes sparse or absent facial, axillary, and pubic hair; decreased muscle mass and strength; gynecomastia; small testes and penis; diminished libido; decreased physical endurance; and osteoporosis.
- Infertility due to azoospermia.
- Increased incidence of mental retardation and behavioral abnormalities.

Differential Diagnosis

- Klinefelter's syndrome has to be differentiated from other causes of male hypogonadism such as Kallmann syndrome, Noonan syndrome, Prader Willi syndrome, cryptorchidism, panhypopituitarism, and other diseases causing testicular failure.

Investigations

- Low serum testosterone and elevated FSH and LH after puberty.
- Karyotyping—confirms 47,XXY or other variants. Diagnosis can also be made prenatally based on cytogenetic studies of fetus.

Treatment

- Testosterone should be given after puberty. It promotes normal growth of body and development of secondary sexual characteristics but will not restore fertility.
- Fertility treatment, e.g. assisted reproductive techniques.

- Speech and language therapy, educational support.
- Psychological counseling, if needed.
- Surgical management of gynecomastia, if severe.

Q. Turner's syndrome (Monosomy X; Gonadal Dysgenesis).

- Turner's syndrome is a genetic disorder affecting females, caused by the complete or partial absence of one X chromosome. The most common karyotype is 45,X (monosomy X).
- Most common sex-chromosome abnormality in female conceptions.
- Incidence—1:2000 to 1:4000 in live-born females.
- Most cases are due to nondisjunction, resulting in 45,X karyotype.

Clinical Features (Fig. 15.6)

- Short stature
- Primary amenorrhea, infertility
- Poorly developed breast and other secondary sexual characters
- Webbed neck
- Broad shield like chest
- Renal anomalies (horseshoe kidney)
- Coarctation of aorta
- Cubitus valgus
- High arched palate
- Short 4th metacarpal or metatarsal
- Peripheral lymphedema
- Increased incidence of mental retardation
- Increased risk of malignancy.

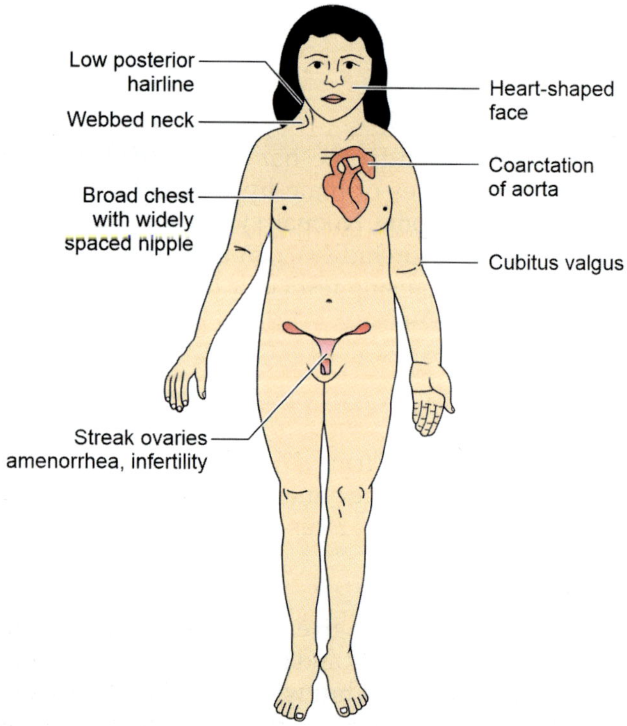

Figure 15.6: Turner's syndrome

Investigations

- Karyotyping: Confirms 45,X.
- Hormonal profile: ↓ estrogen, ↑ FSH and LH (hypergonadotropic hypogonadism).
- Ultrasound/MRI: Evaluate uterus and ovaries.
- Prenatal diagnosis: Increased nuchal translucency on ultrasound, cystic hygroma, hydrops fetalis. Amniocentesis or chorionic villus sampling.

Treatment

- Prenatal diagnosis and offering of genetic counseling and termination of pregnancy.
- Surgical correction of cardiovascular anomalies.
- Growth hormone therapy to improve final adult height (start in early childhood).
- Estrogen therapy to induce and maintain sexual development and cyclic uterine bleeding.

Q. Gene therapy.

- Gene therapy is a technique that involves the introduction, removal, or alteration of genetic material (DNA or RNA) within a patient's cells to treat or prevent disease.
- Gene therapy is one of the most powerful concepts in modern medicine and has the potential to address a host of diseases for which there are currently no cures. However, gene therapy is still in the stage of clinical trials and not yet come into clinical practice.

Types of Gene Therapy

Somatic Cell Gene Therapy

- Targets nonreproductive cells
- Not passed on to offspring
- Used to treat genetic disorders, cancer, etc.
- Ethically accepted.

Germline Gene Therapy

- Targets sperm or egg cells.
- Changes are heritable (passed to next generations) that could result in new or altered traits in the population. It is banned globally as unethical.

Procedure of Gene Therapy

- Gene transfer involves three elements: (1) a vector, (2) a gene to be delivered, and (3) a target cell to which the gene is delivered. The series of steps in which the donated gene enters the cell and begins expression is referred to as *transduction*.
- Since genes (DNA or RNA) cannot be directly transferred into a cell, it is done by using a vector, or gene delivery vehicle.
- Gene delivery can be done by using viruses, liposomes or plasmids to carry the therapeutic gene to target cells.
- Viral vehicles are most popular way of delivering the genes to target cells. They are prepared by deleting some or all of the viral genome and replacing it with the therapeutic gene of interest. Many viruses such

as retroviruses, lentiviruses, adenovirus, adeno-associated virus (AAV), herpes simplex virus, and sarcoma virus have been found to be useful as vectors. Recombinant AAV (adeno-associated virus) has especially emerged as attractive gene delivery vehicle. Engineered from a small replication-defective DNA virus, they are devoid of viral coding genes and do not cause any illness in experimental animals.

- Gene therapy can be *in vivo*, in which the vector is directly injected into the patient or, *ex vivo* in which target cells are removed from the patient and returned to the patient after gene transfer in the laboratory.

Diseases with Potential for Gene Therapy

Genetic Disorders

- Here the missing or defective gene is replaced. Examples are hemophilia A, sickle cell disease, Duchenne muscular dystrophy, X-linked severe combined immunodeficiency disease (SCID), Wiskott-Aldrich syndrome and cystic fibrosis.

Cancer

Many strategies are used in cancer gene therapy which are as follows:

- Intratumoral injection of an adenoviral vector expressing the thymidine kinase (TK) gene. Cells which take up and express the TK gene are killed after the administration of gancyclovir, which is phosphorylated to a toxic nucleoside by TK.
- Use of adenoviral-mediated expression of the tumor suppressor gene p53.
- Use of oncolytic viruses that selectively replicate in tumor cells and destroy them but not in normal cells.
- Promotion of recognition of tumor cells by the immune system by transduction of tumor cells with immune-enhancing genes.
- Inhibition of tumor angiogenesis by enhancing the expression of angiogenesis inhibitors such as angiostatin and endostatin.
- Protection of normal cells from the toxicities of chemotherapy by transduction of cells with genes encoding resistance to chemotherapeutic agents.

Cardiovascular Disease

- Strategies include induction of angiogenesis in limbs (in limb ischemia) or cardiac muscle (in angina/myocardial ischemia). The major transgene used has been VEGF (vascular endothelial growth factor), because of its specificity for endothelial cells. The design of most of the trials involved direct IM (or myocardial) injection of either a plasmid or an adenoviral vector expressing the transgene.

Neurodegenerative Disorders

- In Parkinson's disease, AAV vectors expressing enzymes required for enhanced synthesis of dopamine have been introduced into affected areas of the brain (striatum, subthalamic nucleus) by stereotactic neurosurgery.
- In Alzheimer's disease, autologous fibroblasts are transduced with a retroviral vector expressing nerve growth factor, and then reimplanted into the basal forebrain.

Problems with Gene Therapy

- Immune response against viral vectors making them ineffective.
- Short term expression of the gene by cells or limited transduction of cells by vectors.
- Potential for producing disease by recombining with other viruses or getting activated by host genes.
- Risk of insertional mutagenesis (may cause cancer).
- Activation of proto-oncogenes leading to secondary cancers such as leukemia.

Q. Human leukocyte antigen (HLA) system.

- Human leukocyte antigen (HLA) system is a group of genes located on chromosome 6 that code for cell-surface proteins responsible for the regulation of the immune system in humans. These proteins are part of the major histocompatibility complex (MHC) in humans.
- MHC antigens are integral to the normal functioning of the immune response. Essential role of HLA antigens lies in the control of self-recognition and thus defence against microorganisms and surveillance.

Classification of HLA

Class I HLA Molecules

- HLA-A, HLA-B, HLA-C.
- Found on all nucleated cells.
- Present endogenous (intracellular) antigens (e.g. viral peptides) to CD8+ cytotoxic T cells.
- Important for transplantation.

Class II HLA Molecules

- HLA-DR, HLA-DQ, HLA-DP.
- Expressed on antigen-presenting cells (APCs) such as macrophages, dendritic cells, and B cells.
- Present exogenous (extracellular) antigens to CD4+ helper T cells.

Class III HLA Molecules

- Include genes encoding complement proteins (C2, C4, factor B) and some cytokines (e.g. TNF-α).
- Not directly involved in antigen presentation.

HLA Typing Methods

- Serology used to be the 'gold' standard. Now being superseded by molecular techniques.
- Cellular methods rarely used now. Originally used for class II typing.
- Molecular methods are now becoming the method of choice.

Functions of HLA System

- Antigen presentation: HLA molecules bind antigenic peptides and display them to T lymphocytes for immune recognition.

- Immune response regulation: Helps in distinguishing self from non-self.
- Transplant compatibility: HLA matching is crucial for organ and bone marrow transplantation to reduce the risk of rejection.
- Disease association: Certain HLA alleles are associated with increased susceptibility to specific autoimmune diseases.

Q. Immune deficiency disorders.

- Immune deficiency disorders are conditions in which the immune system's ability to fight infectious diseases and cancer is compromised or entirely absent.
- They may be congenital (primary) or acquired (secondary).

Classification of Immunodeficiency Disorders

Primary (Congenital)

- Result from some genetic or congenital defect. Manifestations are seen in infants and young children.
- *Types*:
  - B-cell (Humoral) deficiencies, e.g. X-linked agammaglobulinemia, selective IgA deficiency (most common humoral deficiency).
  - T-cell (Cellular) deficiencies, e.g. DiGeorge syndrome.
  - Combined B and T cell deficiencies, e.g. severe combined immunodeficiency (SCID), Wiskott-Aldrich syndrome (WAS).
  - Phagocytic cell defects, e.g. Chediak-Higashi syndrome.
  - Complement deficiencies, e.g. C3 deficiency.

Acquired

- Develop as a direct consequence of some other recognized cause.
- Examples:
  - HIV/AIDS
  - Malnutrition
  - Chemotherapy or radiation
  - Immunosuppressive therapy (e.g. after organ transplantation)
  - Chronic diseases—diabetes, chronic kidney disease, malignancy
  - Protein-losing conditions—nephrotic syndrome, intestinal lymphangiectasia
  - For example, HIV infection, chemotherapy.

Clinical Features

- Recurrent infections (especially respiratory, gastrointestinal, skin)
- Poor response to antibiotics
- Growth retardation in children
- Autoimmune manifestations
- Unusual or opportunistic infections
- Multiple family members affected
- Patients may appear normal or there may be growth retardation due to recurrent infections.
- Gingivitis, dental erosions, signs of sinusitis.
- Cervical lymph nodes, adenoid and tonsillar tissue are typically very small or absent in X-linked agammaglobulinemia, X-linked hyper-IgM syndrome, and severe combined immunodeficiency (SCID).
- Ataxia, telangiectasia and neurodeficits are seen in ataxia telangiectasia.
- Eczema and petechiae (Wiskott-Aldrich syndrome).
- Oculocutaneous albinism (Chediak-Higashi).
- Dermatomyositis-like rash (X-linked agammaglobulinemia).
- Generalized molluscum, extensive warts, candidiasis (T-Cell defects).

Diagnosis

- Complete blood count with differential.
- Serum immunoglobulin levels (IgG, IgA, IgM).
- T-cell, B-cell, and NK cell counts (flow cytometry).
- Nitroblue tetrazolium test or DHR for phagocyte function.
- Complement levels (CH50, C3, C4).
- Genetic testing (for primary disorders).

Management

- Infections: Prompt and aggressive treatment.
- Immunoglobulin replacement therapy (IVIG – intravenous immunoglobulin or subcutaneous immunoglobulin—SCIG).
- Prophylactic antibiotics.
- Hematopoietic stem cell transplantation (HSCT)—especially in SCID.
- Gene therapy—under development for some primary immunodeficiency diseases.
- Avoid live vaccines in many immunodeficient patients.

Q. Antioxidants.

- Antioxidants are substances that prevent or slow damage to cells caused by free radicals.
- Free radicles are unstable molecules produced during normal cellular metabolism or due to environmental exposures (e.g. radiation, pollution, smoking).
- Oxygen is an element indispensable for life. When cells use oxygen to generate energy, free radicals are created as a consequence of ATP production by the mitochondria. These by-products are generally reactive oxygen species (ROS) as well as reactive nitrogen species (RNS). These species can be either harmful or helpful to the body. ROS and RNS are generated from either endogenous or exogenous sources. Some internal sources of these species are: mitochondria, xanthine oxidase, Fenton reaction, phagocytes, inflammation, ischemia, etc. Many external sources of free radicals and oxidants include: pollutants, cigarette smoke, radiation, medication, etc
- At low or moderate levels, free radicals and oxidants exert beneficial effects on cellular responses and immune function. At high concentrations they generate oxidative stress, a deleterious process that

can damage cell structures, including lipids, proteins, and DNA

- Oxidative stress plays a major part in the development of chronic and degenerative ailments such as cancer, autoimmune disorders, rheumatoid arthritis, cataract, aging, cardiovascular and neurodegenerative diseases, etc.
- The body has several mechanisms to counteract oxidative stress by producing antioxidants, either naturally generated in situ (endogenous antioxidants), or externally supplied through foods (exogenous antioxidants). The roles of antioxidants are to neutralize the excess of free radicals, to protect the cells against their toxic effects and to contribute to disease prevention.

Types of Antioxidants

Endogenous (naturally produced in the body)

Enzymatic antioxidants

- Superoxide dismutase (SOD)
- Catalase
- Glutathione peroxidase

Non-enzymatic

- Glutathione
- Uric acid
- Coenzyme Q10
- Melatonin

Exogenous (obtained from diet)

- Vitamin E (tocopherol)
- Vitamin C (ascorbic acid)
- Vitamin A (beta-carotene)
- Selenium, Zinc
- Flavonoids (in fruits/vegetables)
- Polyphenols (in tea, coffee, grapes)

Uric Acid

- Uric acid is by-far the highest concentration antioxidant in human blood. Uric acid (UA) is produced from xanthine by the enzyme xanthine oxidase, and is an intermediate product of purine metabolism. Studies of high-altitude acclimatization show that urate mitigates the oxidative stress caused by high-altitude hypoxia. Serum UA levels are inversely associated with the incidence of multiple sclerosis in humans. Moreover, the administration of UA is therapeutic in experimental animal model of multiple sclerosis.

Vitamin A

- Vitamin A supplementation as been shown to reduce the incidences of leukoplakia, lung cancer, fewer episodes of respiratory tract infections in children. Vitamin A levels were found to be lower in patients with measles, Alzheimer's disease, etc.

Ascorbic Acid (Vitamin C)

- Ascorbic acid is redox catalyst which can reduce, and thereby neutralize reactive oxygen species such as hydrogen peroxide. There are many studies showing the beneficial effects of vitamin C in conditions such as infertility, mood disorders, longevity, cataract formation, blood pressure, etc.

Vitamin E

- Vitamin E is the collective name for a set of eight related tocopherols and tocotrienols, which are fat-soluble vitamins with antioxidant properties. Of these, alpha-tocopherol is the most important. alpha-tocopherol protects membranes from oxidation by reacting with lipid radicals produced in the lipid peroxidation chain reaction. Many studies have documented the benefits of Vitamin E supplementation in reducing the symptoms of intermittent claudication, rheumatoid arthritis, and parkinsonism. It has also been shown to reduce the incidence of cataract formation and enhances immune response.

Glutathione

- Glutathione is a cysteine-containing peptide and is synthesized in the body. Glutathione has antioxidant properties since the thiol group in its cysteine moiety is a reducing agent and can be reversibly oxidized and reduced.
- In cells, glutathione is maintained in the reduced form by the enzyme glutathione reductase.
- Due to its high concentration and its central role in maintaining the cell's redox state, glutathione is one of the most important cellular antioxidants.

Melatonin

- Melatonin is a powerful antioxidant. Melatonin easily crosses cell membranes and the blood-brain barrier. Melatonin, once oxidized, cannot be reduced to its former state because it forms several stable end-products upon reacting with free radicals. Therefore, it has been referred to as a terminal (or suicidal) antioxidant.

Should We Routinely Prescribe/Take Antioxidants?

- Antioxidants are being studied as treatments for stroke and neurodegenerative diseases
- Antioxidants are widely used in dietary supplements and have been investigated for the prevention of diseases such as cancer, coronary heart disease and even altitude sickness.
- Although initial studies suggested that antioxidant supplements might promote health, later large clinical trials with a limited number of antioxidants detect no benefit and even suggested that excess supplementation may be harmful.
- An advisory statement published by the American Heart Association says that there is no good reason for people to take antioxidant supplements. This conclusion was reached by the AHA's nutrition committee after an extensive review of the medical literature.

Chapter 16

Diseases of the Skin

Q. Enumerate and define the terms used to describe skin lesions.

- **Primary skin lesions:** Primary lesions are those that occur de novo on a normal skin (**Table 16.1**).
- **Secondary skin lesions:** These occur on pre-existing primary lesions and modify them or follow as a consequence of the primary lesions (**Table 16.2**).

TABLE 16.1: Primary skin lesions

Term	Description	Examples
Macule	A small flat area of altered color <1 cm in diameter	Tinea versicolor, measles
Patch	Flat area of altered color >1 cm in diameter. This differs from a macule only in size.	Vitiligo
Papule	Solid lesions raised above the surface of the skin, generally <1 cm in size. Larger papules are called nodules	Acne, warts
Plaque	A large (>1 cm), flat-topped, raised lesion.	Psoriasis
Vesicle	A small, fluid-filled lesion, <1 cm in diameter, raised above the surface of skin. Fluid is often visible, and the lesions are translucent	Herpes simplex, chickenpox
Pustule	Similar to vesicle but filled with pus.	Folliculitis
Bulla	A fluid-filled, raised, often translucent lesion >1 cm in diameter.	Impetigo, pemphigus, pemphigoid, toxic epidermal necrolysis
Wheal	A raised, erythematous, edematous lesion , usually due to short-lived vasodilatation and vasopermeability.	Urticaria
Nodule	Firm, deeper lesion >1 cm	Lipoma
Telangiectasia	Dilated superficial blood vessels visible on the skin surface	Rosacea
Petechiae, purpura and ecchymosis	Petechiae are small pinhead-sized (1–3 mm) hemorrhages in the dermis and are not palpable. Purpura are similar to petechiae, but larger (3–10 mm) and may be palpable. Ecchymosis ('bruise') is bleeding into deeper structures and is more than 1 cm.	Thrombocytopenia

TABLE 16.2: Secondary skin lesions

Term	Description
Lichenification	Thickened, leathery skin due to chronic scratching or rubbing
Scale	Excessive accumulation of stratum corneum
Crust	Dried exudate of body fluids that may be yellow (serous crust) or red (hemorrhagic crust)
Erosion	Loss of epidermis without an associated loss of dermis
Ulcer	Loss of epidermis and at least a portion of the underlying dermis
Fissure	Linear crack in the skin (e.g. athlete's foot)
Excoriation	Linear, angular erosions caused by scratching
Atrophy	Thinning of skin due to diminution of the epidermis, dermis or subcutaneous fat
Scar	Replacement of normal structure by fibrous tissue

Q. Discuss the etiology, clinical features, diagnosis and management of scabies.

Q. Norwegian or crusted scabies.

- Scabies is due to infestation of the skin by the mite *Sarcoptes scabiei* mite resulting in an intensely pruritic eruption.
- Crowded conditions increase the prevalence of scabies in the population.

Transmission

- It spreads from person to person by direct contact.
- It also spreads by wearing or handling contaminated clothing, or by sleeping in an unchanged bed recently occupied by an infested individual.

Etiologic Agent

- *Sarcoptes scabiei*, is a whitish-brown eight-legged mite which looks like a turtle **(Fig. 16.1)**. Its small size (0.4 × 0.3 mm) and burrowing habits prevent it from being observed by patients.
- The female mite burrows into the epidermis, lays eggs and dies in place after one to two months. Larvae hatch, leave the burrow for the surface, copulate, and continue the cycle.

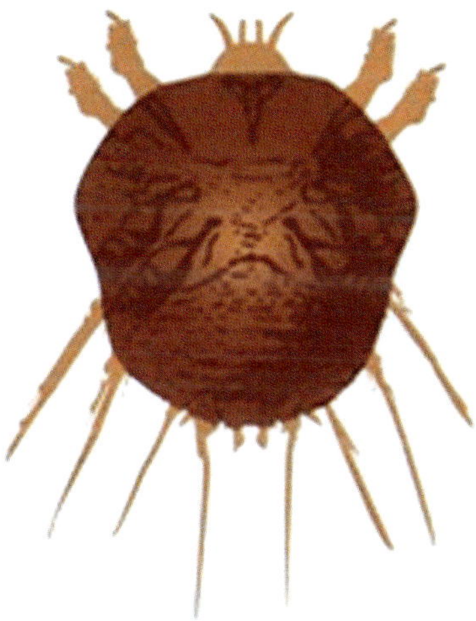

Figure 16.1: *Sarcoptes scabiei*

Clinical Features

- The prominent clinical feature is itching. It is worse at night. Itching is due to delayed type-IV hypersensitivity reaction to the mite, mite feces, and mite eggs.
- Small, erythematous papules, often excoriated may be seen. Miniature wheals, vesicles, pustules, and rarely bullae may also be present **(Fig. 16.2)**.

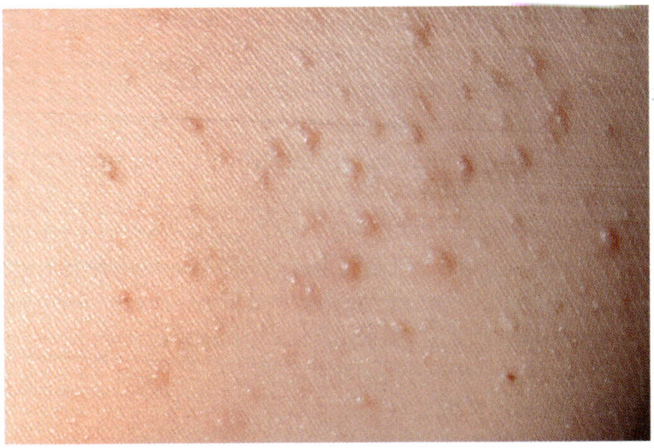

Figure 16.2: Papular lesions in scabies

- The pathognomonic sign of scabies is burrow. It appears as a thin, grayish, reddish, or brownish line 2–15 mm long. Burrows may be absent or obscured by excoriation or secondary infection.
- The distribution of scabies usually involves web spaces of fingers, flexor aspects of the wrists, axillae, waist, genitalia, knees, buttocks and adjacent thighs. Head is spared except in very young children. In young children involvement of the palms, soles and head is common.
- Secondary infection with Staphylococcus or Streptococcus can occur.

Crusted or Norwegian Scabies

- Norwegian scabies (so called because it was first described in Norwegian patients with leprosy) occurs in AIDS, leprosy, lymphoma, and other conditions where cellular immunity is compromised. Normally, cellular immunity prevents multiplication of scabies mites and when it is reduced, there can be unrestricted multiplication of mites. It may also be seen in patients with Down syndrome.
- Norwegian scabies begins as erythematous patches which quickly develop a prominent scale. Any area may be affected, but the scalp, hands, and feet are prominently involved. If untreated, it spreads extensively and may involve the entire body. Scales and crusts appear. The lesions are malodorous. Crusts and scales contain hundreds of thousands of mites. Nails may be discolored and dystrophic. Itching may be minimal or absent.

Diagnosis

- Diagnosis can be made from history and the distribution of lesions.
- Other members of the family are also affected.
- Presence of burrows.
- Diagnosis is confirmed by finding the mite or eggs on microscopic examination of scrapings from burrows or papules.

Treatment

Eradication of Mites

- Topical agents—permethrin cream (5%) is commonly used and is safe even in infants. Permethrin is applied to the entire body including head in infants and washed after 8 hours. A repeat application is required after 1 week. Other topical agents are benzyl benzoate, crotamiton, lindane, malathion, and sulfur in petrolatum.
- Ivermectin: This is an oral anthelmintic. A single dose of ivermectin 200 μg/kg with a repeat dose two

weeks later is as effective as permethrin cream. This is very easy to administer and compliance is very good compared to topical agents. However, it is not recommended in pregnant or lactating women and safety has not been established in children with less than 15 kg weight.

- For Norwegian scabies, two doses of ivermectin two weeks apart should be given along with topical permethrin at the same time. Permethrin should be continued weekly until all scales and crusts are gone.

Control of Itching

- Antihistamines, such as diphenhydramine or cetirizine can be used. Severe itching can be controlled by topical or oral steroids.

Secondary Infection

- This is treated with appropriate systemic antibiotics.

Control of Transmission

- All family members should be treated at the same time to avoid reinfestation.
- Clothing and linen should be bagged for several days, machine washed, and then dried in a hot dryer to kill mites.
- Patients with Norwegian scabies should be isolated and treated.

Q. Describe the pathogenesis, diagnostic features and management of pediculosis.

- Pediculosis refers to infestation by lice, which are obligate ectoparasites. It can affect both adults and children, with *Pediculus humanus capitis* (head louse), *Pediculus humanus corporis* (body louse), and *Phthirus pubis* (pubic or crab louse) being the primary types affecting humans.

Pathogenesis of Pediculosis

Transmission

- Head lice: Direct head-to-head contact; rarely via combs, caps.
- Body lice: Through infested clothing, poor hygiene.
- Pubic lice: Sexually transmitted or via close personal contact.

Infestation Mechanism

- The female louse lays eggs (nits) on hair shafts or clothing fibers.
- Nits hatch in 7–10 days, and lice mature in 9–15 days.
- Lice feed on blood several times a day by piercing the skin and injecting saliva, which causes hypersensitivity reactions.

Immune Response

- Lice saliva contains anticoagulants and vasodilators, provoking a types I and IV hypersensitivity reaction, leading to itching, erythema, and secondary bacterial infection due to scratching.

Clinical Features

General Symptoms (all types)

- Intense pruritus (itching)
- Excoriations, erythematous papules
- Secondary infection: impetigo, lymphadenopathy.

Pediculosis Capitis (head lice)

- Common in children aged 3–11 years
- Occipital, temporal, and postauricular regions are commonly affected.
- Nits seen on hair shafts, especially behind the ears and nape.
- Lice may be visible on combing wet hair.

Pediculosis Corporis (body lice)

- Seen in homeless or unhygienic individuals.
- Lice and nits found in seams of clothing, not on the body.
- Lesions: Excoriations on trunk, especially waist, axillae, and shoulders.

Pediculosis Pubis (crab lice)

- Found in pubic region, but may involve eyelashes (pediculosis ciliaris), chest, or axilla.
- Symptoms: Itching, bluish macules (maculae ceruleae) from louse bites
- Lice are short, broad, and crab-shaped.

Diagnosis

- Wood's lamp: Nits fluoresce pale blue.
- Wet combing: Most effective for detecting head lice.
- Microscopy: Confirms presence of lice/nits.

Management

General Principles

- Kill live lice and eradicate nits
- Treat close contacts
- Improve hygiene and launder clothing and bedding
- Treat secondary bacterial infection if present.

Topical Pediculicides (Table 16.3)

TABLE 16.3: Topical pediculicides

Drug	Application
Permethrin 1% lotion	First-line for head lice. Apply to scalp/hair for 10 minutes; repeat after 7–10 days
Malathion 0.5% lotion	Apply for 8–12 hours. Not safe for infants
Benzyl alcohol 5% lotion	Suffocates lice. Safe in children >6 months
Ivermectin 0.5% lotion	Single application; kills lice and nits
Lindane 1% lotion	Neurotoxic; use only if other treatments fail. Avoid in children and pregnant women

Oral Therapy

- Oral ivermectin (200 μg/kg) repeated after 7–10 days. Used in resistant or widespread infestations.

Nonpharmacological Measures

- Wet combing every 3–4 days for 2 weeks.
- Hot laundering (≥60°C) of clothing, bedding.
- Items that cannot be washed can be sealed in plastic bags for 2 weeks.

Q. What are the common dermatophytoses? How do you diagnose and treat them?

- Dermatophytoses, also known as ringworm or tinea, are superficial fungal skin infections caused by dermatophytes.
- Dermatophytes are keratinophilic fungi and infect skin, hair, and nails.
- Dermatophytes belong to three genera: Microsporum, Trichophyton, and Epidermophyton.
- These infections differ from candidiasis in that they are rarely if ever invasive.

Types

Depending on the site of infection, dermatophytoses are classified as follows:

- *Tinea corporis*: Involvement of the body (trunk and limbs). Waist is a common site especially in obese women. Lesions are erythematous, annular and scaly, with a well-defined edge and often central clearing. They may be single or multiple and are usually asymmetrical.
- *Tinea capitis:* Involvement of the scalp and associated hair. There may be alopecia of the area involved. A soft, boggy mass with loose, easily detachable hairs may be seen (kerion). Tinea capitis is common in children.
- *Tinea barbae:* Involvement of the beard and moustache area. It presents with perifollicular pustules, erythema, crusting, seropurulent discharge and local loss of hairs.
- *Tinea facici:* Face involvement, excluding the beard area.
- *Tinea cruris*: Involvement of the groins. Features are similar to those of tinea corporis.
- *Tinea pedis* (athlete's foot)–involvement of the foot, usually interdigital spaces. It usually presents with fissuring, scaling or maceration in the interdigital areas or as scaly areas all over the soles.
- *Tinea manuum:* Infection of the hands.
- *Tinea unguium (onychomycosis):* Involvement of nails. It presents as white discolored nails and chalky crumbling nails. There may be subungual hyperkeratosis and partial separation of nail plate. Risk factors for onychomycosis are diabetes mellitus, nail trauma, occlusive foot wear, and immunosuppression.

Clinical Features

- Distribution and morphology of lesions is as described above. Lesions are scaly, have slightly raised border with central clearing **(Fig. 16.3)**.

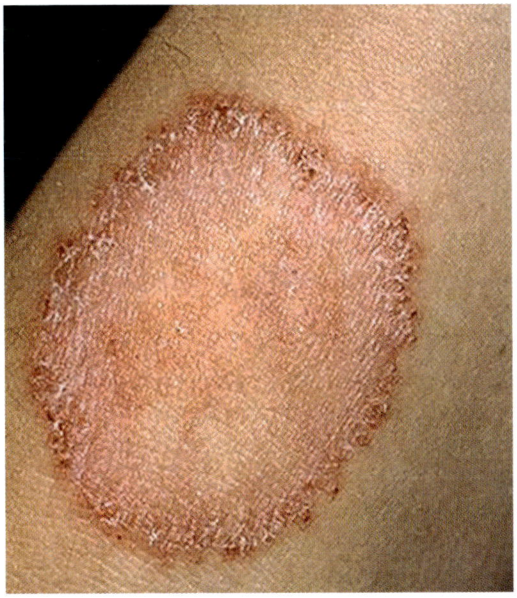

Figure 16.3: Tinea infection (ring worm)

- Patients complain of itching in the lesions which is often worse at night.
- Secondary bacterial infection of the skin lesion may occur producing pustules.

Diagnosis

- Based on history and clinical findings.
- Potassium hydroxide (KOH-10%) mount of skin scrapings-fungi are seen as long, branched and septate hyphae.
- Skin or nail biopsy.
- Culture: on Sabouraud's medium.
- Wood's lamp examination: Lesions of *Tinea versicolor* and certain types of *Tinea capitis* fluoresce when examined under Wood's lamp, emitting ultraviolet rays.

Treatment

- Topical preparations of clotrimazole, miconazole, terbinafine or ketoconazole can be applied twice daily for 4 weeks. Topical therapy is not effective for nail infections.
- For tinea capitis and barbae, ketoconazole shampoo can be used as additional therapy.
- For severe and unresponsive lesions, oral antifungal agents can be used. These are griseofulvin, ketoconazole, fluconazole, itraconazole and terbinafine. Duration of therapy is 4–8 weeks. For tinea unguam, duration of therapy is 3 months.

Q. Tinea versicolor (pityriasis versicolor).

- *Tinea versicolor*, also called pityriasis versicolor, is a superficial fungal infection of the stratum corneum caused by *Malassezia species* (lipophilic yeasts, especially *Malassezia furfur*). It leads to hypo-or hyperpigmented scaly macules on the upper trunk and shoulders.

Etiology

- Malassezia is part of normal skin flora but becomes pathogenic under certain conditions:
  - Hot and humid climate
  - Excessive sweating
  - Oily skin
  - Immunosuppression
  - Hormonal changes (e.g. adolescence)

Clinical Features

- Lesions are discrete hypopigmented or hyperpigmented or erythematous oval macules with fine scaling **(Fig. 16.4)**. Versicolor refers to the variety of colors of lesions.
- Lesions are most common on the upper trunk and extremities, and less common on the face. Seborrhoeic areas are the sites of predilection as sebum facilitates proliferation of the fungi. Lesions may coalesce to form large patches.
- Most patients are asymptomatic, but some may complain of mild itching. It is mildly contagious, and other family members may be affected.

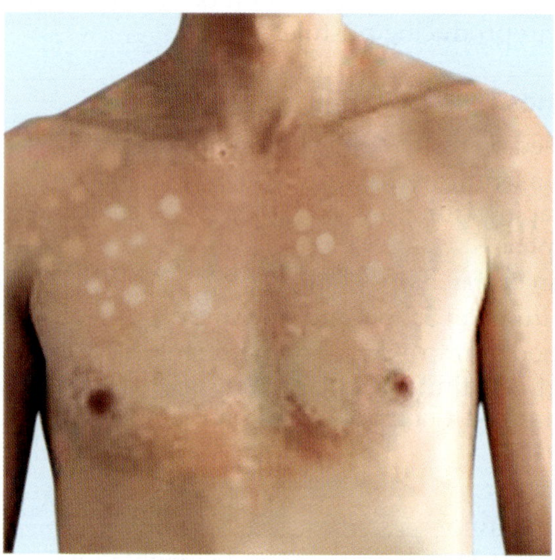

Figure 16.4: *Tinea versicolor*

Diagnosis

- Diagnosis can be confirmed by examination of scrapings from lesions with 10% potassium hydroxide (KOH). Both hyphae and budding cells are seen in a pattern described as "spaghetti and meatballs" **(Fig. 16.5)**.
- A Wood light examination reveals yellowish-green fluorescence.

Treatment

- Topical antifungals like clotrimazole, miconazole, terbinafine or ketoconazole are effective.
- Selenium sulfide shampoo applied thrice weekly 10–30 minutes before bath for about 15 applications or ketoconazole 2% shampoo once daily for three days is also effective.

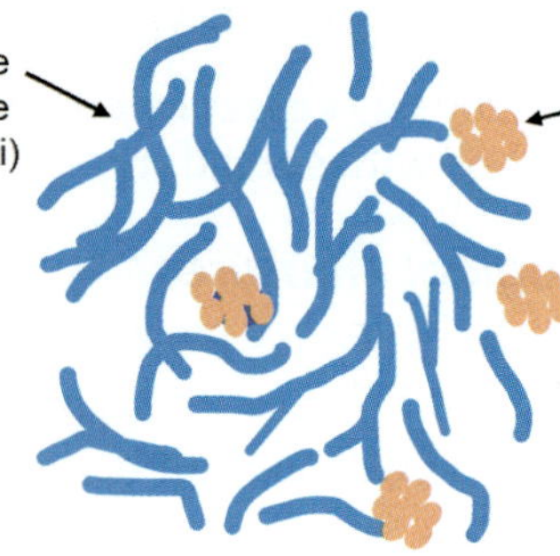

Figure 16.5: Spaghetti and meat-ball appearance

- Oral therapy is more convenient for patients with extensive disease. Two convenient regimens are a single 400-mg dose of ketoconazole or fluconazole 150 mg/week for 2–4 week.

Q. Enumerate various types of dermatitis (eczema). Discuss the clinical features and management of dermatitis.

- Dermatitis (also called eczema) is a broad term for inflammation of the skin characterized by itching, redness, and varying degrees of swelling, blistering, oozing, and scaling.

General Features of Dermatitis

- Redness and swelling
- Itching
- Papules, vesicles and, rarely, large blisters
- Oozing and crusting
- Fissures and scratch marks
- Pigmentation changes (hypo- and hyper)
- Scaling
- Lichenification, secondary to rubbing and scratching.

Types of Dermatitis and Clinical Features

- **Atopic dermatitis:** Chronic, relapsing eczema often associated with a personal/family history of atopy (asthma, allergic rhinitis).
- **Contact dermatitis**
  - *Irritant contact dermatitis*: Due to direct toxic effect of chemicals. Dermatitis is due to direct damage caused by non-immune mechanisms as opposed to allergic contact dermatitis. Examples of irritants are cleansers, soaps, detergents, organic solvents, alkalies, and vegetables like chillies.
  - *Allergic contact dermatitis*: This occurs due to delayed hypersensitivity reaction mediated by T-lymphocytes against certain chemicals (allergens) on coming in contact with the skin. Most contact allergens are haptens (incomplete allergens) which become complete allergens after combining with epidermal proteins. Examples are hair dye, shampoos, cement, etc.
- **Seborrheic dermatitis:** This is a chronic dermatitis characterized by greasy scales overlying erythematous patches or plaques. It mainly involves areas rich in sebaceous glands such as scalp, retroauricular and

nasolabial folds, eyelids, trunks and axillae. It is probable due to overgrowth of *Malassezia furfur*.

- **Nummular (discoid) eczema:** This is characterized by pruritic circular or oval lesions with closely set papulovesicles on an erythematous base. It is seen most often on the limbs of elderly males.
- **Dyshidrotic eczema (Pompholyx):** Vesicular eczema on palms and soles.
- **Stasis dermatitis:** Seen in lower legs due to venous insufficiency.
- **Lichen simplex chronicus:** Thickened skin due to chronic scratching.
- **Asteatotic eczema:** Dry, cracked skin in elderly, especially in winter.
- **Photoallergic/phototoxic dermatitis:** Caused by sun exposure + drugs or chemicals.
- **Juvenile plantar dermatitis:** Seen in children; localized to soles.

Investigation of Dermatitis

- Patch tests—useful in suspected cases of allergic contact dermatitis.
- IgE levels—are useful in atopic dermatitis.
- Bacterial and viral swabs for microscopy and culture in suspected secondary infection.
- Skin biopsy—Rarely needed, in atypical or resistant cases.

General Management of Dermatitis

- Explanation and reassurance.
- Avoidance of contact with triggers (allergens, irritants, sweating, rough fabrics).
- Avoidance of dryness by regular use of emollients.
- Topical corticosteroids: Mainstay (low to high potency based on area/severity).
- Antihistamines: For itching (give at night due to sedating effect).
- Seborrhoeic eczema is treated with antipityrosporal agents such as ketoconazole shampoo and creams, supplemented with weak corticosteroids.
- Systemic therapy–Required in severe/refractory cases. Agents used are oral steroids (short-term), immunosuppressants (e.g. cyclosporine, methotrexate), and biologics (e.g. dupilumab for atopic dermatitis).

Q. Contact Dermatitis.

- Contact dermatitis is an inflammatory skin reaction caused by direct contact with an external substance. It can be either irritant or allergic in nature.

Etiology

- Irritant contact dermatitis (ICD) accounts for 80% of all cases of contact dermatitis. It is caused by substances which directly cause irritation and inflammation of the skin. Immune system is not involved here. Common substances include:
  - Chemicals (e.g. acids, alkalis, solvents, metal salts)
  - Soaps (e.g. abrasives, detergents)
  - Plants (e.g. parthenium, peppers)
  - Body fluids (e.g. urine, saliva)
- Allergic contact dermatitis (ACD) is a type IV cell-mediated hypersensitivity reaction to allergens. Requires prior sensitization. Some of the substances triggering ACD are ragweed pollen, hair dye, cosmetics, poison ivy, latex rubber, etc.

Clinical Features (Table 16.4)

TABLE 16.4: Clinical features of dermatitis

Feature	Irritant CD	Allergic CD
Onset	Immediate to few hours	24–72 hours after exposure
Lesion distribution	Confined to contact area	May spread beyond contact site
Symptoms	Burning, stinging	Itching (pruritus) prominent
Skin findings	Erythema, scaling, fissures	Papules, vesicles, oozing, crusting

- In both the cases, skin changes often occur at the site of contact with allergen, but later may spread due to scratching. Hands are commonly involved due to handling of allergens.
- Chronic exposure leads to lichenification and fissuring.

Diagnosis

- Clinical history and examination.
- Sometimes patch testing. Here, standard contact allergens are applied to the upper back using adhesive-mounted patches containing minute amounts of allergens.

Treatment

- Identify and avoid the offending agent.
- Protective clothing/gloves.
- Symptomatic treatment: Dressings for excoriation and ulceration, antihistamines for itching.
- Topical corticosteroids: Mainstay for both types (mild to potent depending on severity).
- Oral corticosteroids: For severe or widespread reactions.
- Antihistamines: For itching.

Q. Discuss the etiology, clinical features and management of psoriasis.

- Psoriasis is a chronic immune-mediated inflammatory disease of the skin, characterized by well-defined erythematous plaques with silvery scale.
- It is more common in European community and less common in African and Asian communities.
- It affects men and women equally. Although psoriasis can begin at any age, there seem to be two peaks in onset: one between ages 20 and 30 and another between 50 and 60.

Etiology

- Psoriasis is considered to be an autoimmune disease with a genetic basis. It has a strong genetic predilection

in the form of polygenic autosomal dominant inheritance with variable penetrance. Certain genes and HLA antigens (Cw6, B13, B17) are implicated in psoriasis.
- Precipitating and aggravating factors include hormonal changes of puberty and pregnancy, infections, physical trauma (including sunlight), obesity, smoking, alcohol consumption and mental stress.
- Drugs like beta-blockers, antimalarials, NSAIDs, lithium, etc. are known to cause psoriasiform drug reactions and also to precipitate the disease.
- Patients with HIV and AIDS can have severe and resistant disease at a young age.

Pathology

- There are two main abnormalities noted in psoriatic plaques:
  - Inflammatory cell infiltrate in the skin.
  - Hyperproliferation of keratinocytes with a grossly increased mitotic index.

Clinical Features

- Psoriasis is characterized by well demarcated plaques, which may vary from few millimeters to several centimeters in diameter. The lesions are red, with a silvery-white scale **(Fig. 16.6)**.
- Extensor aspects such as elbows, knees and lower back are commonly affected. Other sites of predilection include scalp, nails, flexures and palms.
- Nails may show pitting, onycholysis (separation of the nail from the nail bed), and subungual hyperkeratosis.
- Some patients may have seronegative arthritis (psoriatic arthropathy) involving spine and/or peripheral joints.
- Auspitz sign: Pinpoint bleeding when scales are scraped off.
- Koebner phenomenon: Lesions appear at sites of trauma.

Investigations

- Diagnosis is made clinically.
- Rarely skin biopsy or scraping may be required to rule out other disorders.
- X-rays and MRI may be needed if there is arthritis.

Management

General Measures

- Explanation and reassurance.
- Avoid triggers (trauma, infections, offending drugs).
- Moisturizers/emollients for scaling.
- Lifestyle changes (stop smoking, reduce alcohol).

Topical Therapy

- *Topical therapies*: They are the first-line treatment for mild-to-moderate psoriasis and are also used as adjuncts in more severe cases.
- *Topical corticosteroids*: These are the most commonly used agents. They have anti-inflammatory, immunosuppressive, and anti-proliferative action. Main side effects are local skin atrophy. Psoriasis tends to return when steroids are stopped. Examples are hydrocortisone, betamethasone, and clobetasol.
- *Vitamin-D analogs (calcipotriene, calcitriol)*: These agents have cytostatic and cytotoxic effects on proliferating keratinocytes. They also suppresses the underlying inflammation. They reduce the thickness and scaling of the psoriatic plaque, but do not clear the plaque. They are applied once or twice daily. Often combined with steroids to reduce irritation and increase efficacy.
- *Topical retinoids (e.g. Tazarotene)*: Normalizes keratinocyte differentiation and has anti-inflammatory effects. Often causes irritation—usually combined with a corticosteroid.

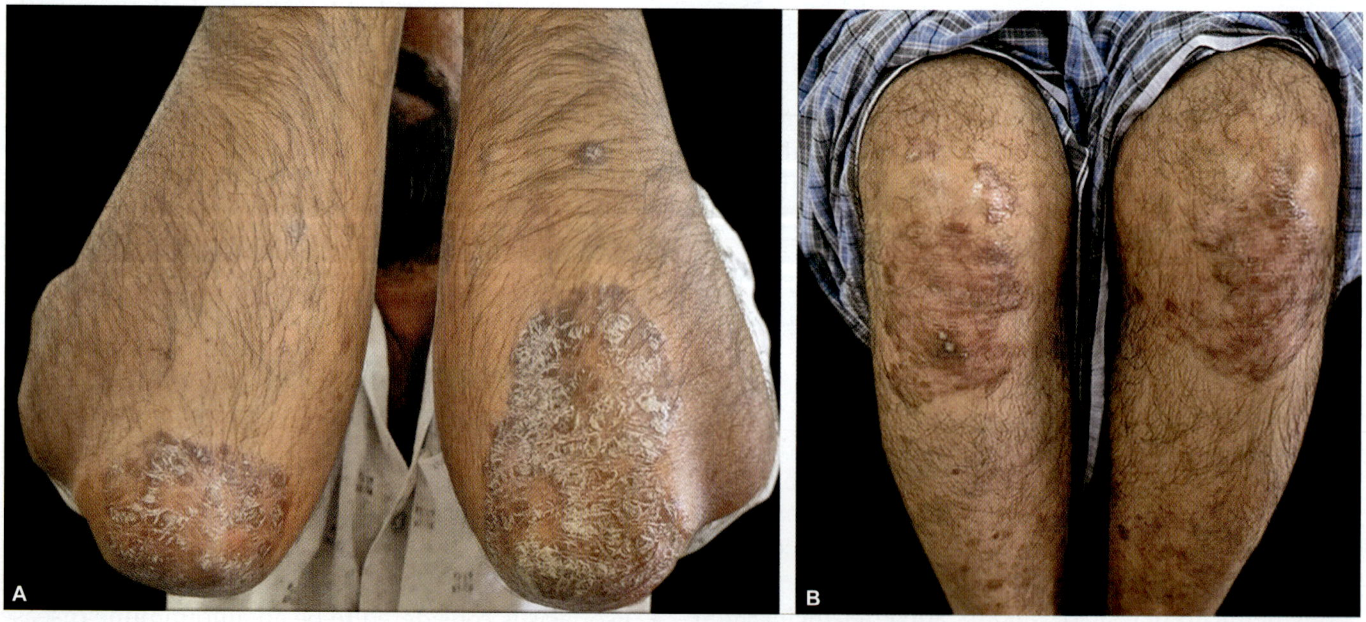

Figure 16.6: Psoriasis on the elbows (A) and knees (B)

- *Calcineurin inhibitors* (e.g. tacrolimus, pimecrolimus): Useful in sensitive areas (face, intertriginous zones). Off-label use in psoriasis.
- *Coal tar:* Coal tar has antimitotic effects and is effective in the treatment of psoriasis. Less commonly used now due to messiness, odor, and staining.
- *Anthralin (dithranol)*: It has antiproliferative effect. Applied for short-contact therapy. Can cause skin irritation and stains skin/clothing.
- *Salicylic acid*: It is keratolytic. Helps remove scales and improves penetration of other agents. Often used in combination (especially with steroids or coal tar).

PUVA Therapy

- Psoralen along with ultraviolet A (PUVA) is very effective for treatment of psoriasis. Psoralens are natural photosensitizers found in plants. Psoralen is given orally and is distributed all over the body. It gets activated only in those sites that are exposed to UVA. Psoralen intercalates into DNA and upon UVA exposure, forms cross-links, which inhibit DNA synthesis and cell proliferation. It is given 2–5 times a week and clearance occurs in the majority within 8 weeks. Main concern is increased risk of skin cancers. NBUVB (narrowband UVB light) is equally effective without the side effects of psoralen like gastrointestinal upset, cataract formation, and carcinogenic effect. It can safely be given to children, pregnant and lactating females and even elderly.

Systemic Therapy

- Systemic therapy is used for moderate to severe psoriasis, particularly when topical treatments and phototherapy are insufficient.
- Indications:
  - Extensive disease (>10% BSA)
  - Psoriatic arthritis
  - Nail or scalp psoriasis
  - Failure of topical/phototherapy
  - Significant impact on quality of life
- *Methotrexate* is highly effective for psoriasis and is the drug of choice. It can be given as long as the disease remains active. It acts by suppressing the immune system.
- *Oral retinoids* such as acitretin, etretinate are also effective in some patients with psoriasis. Retinoids are teratogens, hence pregnancy should be avoided for at least 2 years following their use.
- *Cyclosporine* can be used to induce a clinical response but its use should be intermittent.
- Biological agents such as infliximab, etanercept, efaluzimab have varying degrees of activity against psoriasis. They are expensive and may be considered when other treatment agents have failed.

Distinguishing Psoriasis from Other Lesions

See **Table 16.5.**

Q. Grattage test (scraping test)

- The Grattage test is a clinical test used in dermatology to help diagnose psoriasis by demonstrating characteristic scaling and pinpoint bleeding.

Procedure

A psoriatic plaque is gently scraped with a glass slide or blunt scalpel. There are 3 steps:

- Step A: Gently scrape lesion with a glass slide. This accentuates the silvery scales (Grattage test positive). Scrape off all the scales.
- Step B: Continue to scrape the lesion. A glistening white adherent membrane (Burkley's membrane) appears. Indicates end of epidermal layers.

TABLE 16.5: Distinguishing psoriasis from other lesions

Feature	Psoriasis	Eczema (dermatitis)	Tinea (fungal infection)	Lichen planus	Seborrheic dermatitis
Lesion appearance	Well-defined, erythematous plaques with silvery white scales	Poorly defined, red, itchy, oozy patches	Annular, scaly ring like lesion with central clearing	Violaceous, flat-topped papules with white streaks (Wickham striae)	Greasy, yellowish scales over red patches
Common sites	Extensor surfaces (elbows, knees), scalp, lower back	Flexural areas (elbows, knees, neck)	Groin, feet, body folds	Wrists, ankles, mucosa	Scalp, eyebrows, nasolabial folds
Scaling	Thick, dry, silvery-white scaling	Thin, flaky scaling	Peripheral scaling, central clearing	Fine white lines on surface	Greasy, yellowish scaling
Itching	Mild to moderate	Prominent itching	Moderate to severe	Mild-to-moderate	Mild itching
Auspitz sign	Positive (pinpoint bleeding on scale removal)	Negative	Negative	Negative	Negative
Koebner's phenomenon	Present	Can be present	Can be present	Present	Rare
Nail involvement	Pitting, onycholysis, subungual hyperkeratosis	Rare	Rare	Rare	—

- Step C: On removing the membrane, pinpoint bleeding spots appear due to capillary exposure in dermal papillae-positive Auspitz sign.

Clinical Relevance

- Positive Grattage test indicates psoriasis vulgaris. It is particularly useful in early or doubtful lesions.
- Negative in eczema, fungal infections, lichen planus.

Q. Pityriasis rosea.

- Pityriasis rosea is a self-limited, inflammatory disease characterized by diffuse, scaling papules or plaques.
- The cause may be viral infection (human herpesviruses 6, 7 and 8). Drugs may cause a similar eruption.

Clinical Features

- Affects mainly children and young adults. It affects women more often.
- Characterized by sudden appearance of oval, papulosquamous, pink or salmon colored lesions on the trunk and proximal limbs. The eruption usually begins with a **"herald" or "mother" patch**, a single oval pink or salmon-colored lesion on the chest, neck, or back. It is 2–5 cm in diameter with cigarette paper-like scales at the edges.
- A few days or weeks later oval lesions similar to the herald patch, but smaller, appear on the trunk and proximal areas of the limbs. The long axes of these oval lesions tend to be arranged along the cleavage lines of the skin. This arrangement of lesions on the back parallel to ribs gives rise to **"Christmas tree pattern"**.
- Mild-to-moderate pruritus may be present.
- The rash subsides within 6–8 weeks without significant consequences.
- Differential diagnosis includes secondary syphilis, psoriasis, lichen planus and drug reactions.

Treatment

- Generally, requires no treatment.
- Topical or oral steroids and antihistamines may be required to relieve itching.
- Ultraviolet light B (UVB) is helpful to reduce post-inflammatory hypopigmentation.
- Erythromycin has shown benefit in some trials. Benefit is probably due to its anti-inflammatory and immune modulating effects.

Q. What is pemphigus? Write briefly about pemphigus vulgaris.

Q. Nikolsky's sign.

- Pemphigus is a group of rare, chronic, autoimmune blistering disease affecting skin and mucus membranes (Greek pemphix = bubble).
- There are four major types of pemphigus:
  - Pemphigus vulgaris
  - Pemphigus foliaceus
  - Paraneoplastic pemphigus
  - Pemphigus vegetans.

Etiology

- It is an autoimmune disease characterized by the presence of IgG antibodies directed against desmoglein an adhesion molecule on the surface of keratinocytes. Blister formation occurs in the epidermis due to loss of cohesion between epidermal cells, a process known as acantholysis.

Clinical Features

Pemphigus Vulgaris

- Most common and severe form of pemphigus ("vulgar" means "common").
- Blisters are flaccid, nonpruritic, and easily break down, leaving behind erosions. Any area of the skin can be affected.
- Mucus membrane of oral cavity is commonly involved. Blisters are often found in areas subjected to friction such as cheek mucosa, tongue, palate and lower lip. Pharynx and larynx may be affected leading to pain on eating, and hoarseness of voice.
- Level of blister is suprabasal (intraepidermal).
- Nikolsky's sign is positive.

Pemphigus Foliaceous

- Milder form.
- Blisters are more superficial than pemphigus vulgaris, which easily rupture. Hence, erosions, rather than blisters, are the presenting feature.
- Lesions first appear on the face and scalp and later on the chest and back.
- There may be associated scaling, and crusting.
- Unlike pemphigus vulgaris, mucous membrane is not affected.
- Nikolsky's sign is positive.

Para-neoplastic Pemphigus

- Associated with malignancies, such as non-Hodgkin's lymphoma, CLL, and thymoma. Both skin and mucus membrane are affected.

Diagnosis

- The characteristic sign is Nikolsky's sign. It is elicited by applying lateral pressure to normal-looking skin at the periphery of active lesions, causing a shearing away of the epidermis leading to formation of new blisters.
- Tzanck smear—shows acantholytic cells.
- Biopsy of skin lesions—shows intraepithelial acantholysis without disruption of the basement membrane.
- Direct immunofluorescence shows deposits of IgG between epidermal cells.
- ELISA—detects circulating antibodies to desmogleins.

Differential Diagnosis

- In case of predominant mucous membrane lesions, herpes simplex, aphthous ulcers, lichen planus, and erythema multiforme have to be ruled out. In case of widespread erosions, pyoderma, impetigo, bullous pemphigoid, and bullous drug eruptions should be ruled out.

Treatment

- Without treatment pemphigus has high morbidity and mortality.
- High-dose systemic corticosteroids (e.g. prednisone 1 mg/kg/day) are the mainstay of therapy. Mild pemphigus may be treated with local steroids.
- Azathioprine and cyclosphosphamide are used as additional immunosuppressive agents. They reduce steroid requirement, decrease steroid side-effects and improve remission rate.
- Rituximab, alone or in combination with intravenous immunoglobulin (IVIG), is the treatment of choice in severe pemphigus refractory to above therapies.
- Silver sulphadiazine may be used to prevent secondary infection.

Q. Bullous pemphigoid or pemphigoid.

- Bullous pemphigoid is a subepidermal blistering disease usually seen in the elderly (>60 years of age). It is less aggressive than pemphigus vulgaris and usually not life-threatening.

Etiology

- It is an autoimmune disease characterized by linear deposits of IgG at the epidermal basement membrane. The antibodies are directed against hemidesmosomes which attach epithelial cells to the basement membrane). Hence there is a split between the epidermis and dermis. (Note that in pemphigus the split is within the epidermis).
- Drug-induced bullous pemphigoid develops due to penicillamine, furosemide, captopril, and antibiotics such as penicillin and nalidixic acid.
- It can be associated with systemic malignancies.

Clinical Features

- Usually affects people of >60 years of age.
- Blisters are large and tense, arising on a normal or erythematous skin. They occur anywhere on the body but common in flexural areas, groin, and axillae.
- Mucous membranes are not involved.
- Blisters are associated with marked itching. They may contain hemorrhagic fluid.
- Nikolsky's sign is negative.
- Blisters heal without scarring.
- Some patients go into spontaneous remission.

Diagnosis

- Skin biopsy: Subepidermal bulla with eosinophilic infiltrate. Direct immunofluorescence shows linear deposits of IgG and complement at the epidermal basement membrane.

Treatment

- Systemic steroids (e.g. prednisolone, 1 mg/kg per day).
- Azathioprine or cyclophosphamide can be used as additional immunosuppressive and steroid sparing agents.

Q. Discuss the causes, clinical features, investigations and management of Stevens-Johnson syndrome.

OR

Q. Toxic epidermal necrolysis.

- Stevens-Johnson syndrome (SJS) and toxic epidermal necrolysis (TEN) are severe mucocutaneous reactions, most commonly drug-induced, characterized by extensive epidermal necrosis and detachment.
- SJS and TEN are similar except for the amount of area involved. Involvement of <10% of body surface area is called SJS and >30% of body surface area is called TEN; involvement of 10–30% of body surface area is considered SJS/TEN overlap.

Causes

Drugs (most common cause)

- *Antigout agents:* Allopurinol
- *Antibiotics:* Sulfonamides (cotrimoxazole, sulfasalazine), penicillins, cephalosporins, fluoroquinolones.
- *Antipsychotics and antiepileptics:* Carbamazepine, phenytoin, valproate, lamotrigine, and phenobarbital.
- *NSAIDs:* Ibuprofen, piroxicam.

Infections

- *Mycoplasma pneumoniae*
- Herpes simplex virus

Rare

- Vaccinations, systemic diseases, chemical exposure, herbal medicines, and foods.

Clinical Features

- Prodrome of malaise and fever, followed by the onset of erythematous or purpuric macules and plaques.
- Lesions are symmetrically distributed, and start first on the face and thorax before spreading to other areas.
- Skin lesions progress to epidermal necrosis and sloughing.
- Target lesions may be present.
- Mucosal membranes (ocular, oral, and genital) are involved in most patients. Oral and esophageal involvement causes difficulty and pain while swallowing. Genitourinary involvement causes dysuria and difficulty to void. Bronchial epithelium may also slough, causing cough, dyspnea, pneumonia, pulmonary edema, and hypoxemia.
- Glomerulonephritis and hepatitis may develop.

Investigations

- Anemia and neutropenia may be present.
- AST and ALT may be elevated.
- Skin biopsy (gold standard): Full-thickness epidermal necrosis.

Differential Diagnosis

- Erythema multiforme.
- Viral exanthems.
- Drug rashes.
- Toxic shock syndrome.

- Exfoliative erythroderma (usually spares mucous membranes).
- Paraneoplastic pemphigus.

Management

- Treatment of underlying cause (e.g. withdrawal of causative agent).
- Maintenance of fluid and electrolyte balance.
- Antihistamines and local steroids are enough for mild cases.
- Silver-impregnated nanocrystalline gauze for topical wound care.
- Systemic corticosteroids are indicated in severe cases. Prednisolone, 1–3 mg/kg daily or an equivalent amount of other steroids can be used.
- IV immunoglobulin (1 gram/kg daily for three consecutive days) is also useful in severe cases of SJS and TEN.
- Sepsis is the major cause of death. Systemic antibiotics should be given at the first sign of wound infection.

Q. Erythroderma (exfoliative dermatitis).

- Erythroderma (also called exfoliative dermatitis) is a life-threatening dermatologic emergency characterized by generalized erythema and scaling involving >90% of the body surface area. It is a manifestation of various underlying skin or systemic diseases.

Causes of Erythroderma

- *Preexisting skin diseases:* Psoriasis, atopic dermatitis, seborrheic dermatitis, contact dermatitis.
- *Drug reactions:* Antiepileptics (phenytoin), antibiotics (penicillins, sulfa drugs), allopurinol.
- *Malignancies:* Cutaneous T-cell lymphoma (Sezary syndrome), leukemia.
- *Idiopathic:* ~25% cases.

Clinical Features

- Widespread erythema and scaling (>90% of BSA).
- Skin thickening and exfoliation.
- Intense pruritus, burning sensation.
- Facial edema, periorbital swelling.
- Alopecia, nail changes (ridging, shedding).
- Chills, fever, and malaise.
- Lymphadenopathy.

Investigations

- *CBC:* Eosinophilia, anemia.
- *LFTs, RFTs, electrolytes*: For systemic involvement.
- *Skin biopsy*: Helps identify underlying disease.
- *Blood cultures*: If febrile (rule out sepsis).
- *HIV test*: In immunocompromised.
- *Lymph node biopsy*: If lymphadenopathy.

Complications

- Fluid and electrolyte imbalance (due to transepidermal loss).
- Hypothermia (due to loss of temperature through skin).
- High-output cardiac failure due to widespread cutaneous vasodilatation.
- Protein loss → hypoalbuminemia due to skin exfoliation.
- Secondary bacterial infections.
- Sepsis.
- Nutritional deficiencies.

Management

- Erythroderma (exfoliative dermatitis) is a dermatological emergency that requires prompt hospitalization, supportive care, and targeted treatment based on the underlying cause.
- All cases of erythroderma should be considered for urgent referral or admission, preferably to a dermatology or intensive care unit.
- Airway, breathing, circulation: Stabilize ABCs, ensure oxygenation if needed.
- Temperature regulation: Keep patient warm (avoid hypothermia), cover with blankets.
- Fluid and electrolyte management: IV fluids if dehydration; monitor input/output.
- Nutritional support: High-protein diet; consider enteral nutrition.
- Infection control: Monitor for signs of sepsis, obtain cultures, start empirical antibiotics if indicated.
- Emollients and wet wraps: Liberal application of emollients (e.g. petroleum jelly) to prevent water loss.
- Symptomatic relief: Antihistamines for pruritus, paracetamol for fever.
- Systemic steroids (if inflammatory).
- Treatment of underlying cause (withdrawal of offending drug, psoriasis, lymphoma, drug rash, etc.).

Q. Fixed drug eruption (FDE).

- Fixed drug eruption is a distinctive type of cutaneous drug reaction characterized by recurring skin or mucosal lesions at the same site each time the offending drug is taken.

Etiology and Pathogenesis

- Type IV hypersensitivity reaction (cell-mediated).
- Caused by CD8+ T-cell activation at specific skin sites sensitized by previous drug exposure.
- Upon re-exposure, inflammatory mediators cause localized skin damage.

Common Offending Drugs

- *Antibiotics:* Sulfonamides, tetracyclines, fluoroquinolones.
- *NSAIDs:* Ibuprofen, naproxen, aspirin.
- *Antimalarials:* Quinine.
- *Anticonvulsants:* Barbiturates, phenytoin, carbamazepine.
- *Others:* Pseudoephedrine, food dyes.

Clinical Features

- Single or multiple well-demarcated erythematous patches or plaques.
- Initially red and swollen → evolve into dusky or violaceous patches.
- Central blistering may occur.
- Lesions typically appear ½–8 hours after drug intake.
- Heal with residual hyperpigmentation.
- Recur at same site(s) with repeated exposure.
- Common sites:
  - Lips, genitalia, hands, face, trunk.
  - Mucosal involvement (oral or genital) is common.

Diagnosis

- Clinical diagnosis based on history of recurrence at same site.
- Drug provocation test (oral rechallenge)—gold standard but rarely needed.
- Skin biopsy (if required): shows basal cell degeneration, necrotic keratinocytes, pigment incontinence.

Management

- Discontinue the offending drug: This is the most important step. Educate patient to avoid the culprit drug and cross-reacting agents.
- Topical corticosteroids (e.g. mometasone, clobetasol).
- Oral antihistamines for itching/burning.
- Topical anesthetics, antiseptic mouthwash for oral lesions.
- Short-course oral corticosteroids: Severe/bullous cases (rarely needed).
- Document the culprit drug in medical records.
- Provide drug allergy card to patient.

Q. Erythema multiforme.

- Erythema multiforme (EM) is an acute, immune-mediated hypersensitivity reaction affecting the skin and mucous membranes. It is characterized by the sudden appearance of target-like (iris) lesions, most commonly on the extremities.
- Earlier, erythema multiforme major was being equated with Stevens-Johnson syndrome. But now most authorities think that these two entities are different.

Etiology

- Majority of cases are caused by herpes simplex virus (HSV) infection (HSV-1 more so than HSV-2).
- Some cases are caused by drugs (sulfonamides, NSAIDs, and anticonvulsants), vaccines, other viral diseases (especially hepatitis C), and SLE.

Clinical Features

- Classic manifestation is target lesion, consisting of three concentric zones of color change; a central dark spot, surrounded by a pale area, and then a red outer ring (**Fig. 16.7**). Such classic lesions are found in herpes simplex infection. They are most often found on the hands and feet. Wheals, vesicles, and bullae can also be seen.

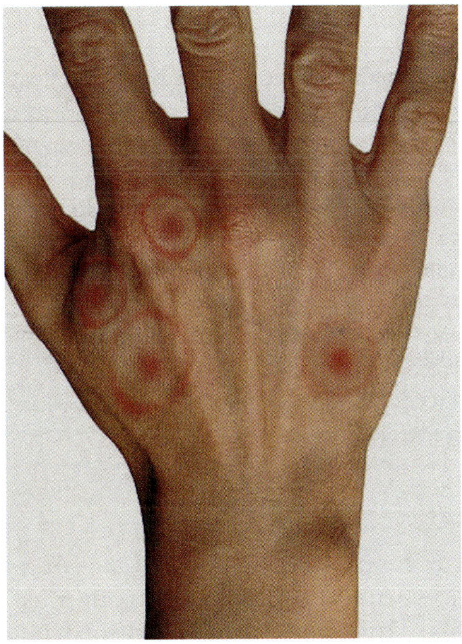

Figure 16.7: Erythema multiforme

Differential Diagnosis

- Stevens-Johnson syndrome (more mucosal involvement and skin detachment)
- Urticaria
- Drug eruptions
- Paraneoplastic pemphigus.

Treatment

- Withdrawal of offending agent
- Antihistamines (e.g. cetirizine) for itching
- Treatment of infection
- Topical steroids for mild cases
- Systemic steroids in severe cases.

Q. Define urticaria. Describe the etiology, pathogenesis, clinical features, investigations and management of urticaria.

- Urticaria, commonly known as hives, is a vascular reaction of the skin characterized by transient, pruritic wheals (raised, erythematous lesions with central pallor).
- It is a common dermatological condition affecting 15–20% of the population at least once in their lifetime.
- Urticaria may occur alone or in association with angioedema, which involves deeper dermal or subcutaneous tissue swelling.
- The wheals are typically short-lived, resolving within 24 hours without residual pigmentation or scaling.

Classification (based on duration)

- **Acute urticaria:** Duration <6 weeks
- **Chronic urticaria:** Duration >6 weeks.

Causes

- **Allergic (IgE-mediated):** Foods, drugs, insect bites, latex.
- **Nonallergic (Non-IgE-mediated):** Direct mast cell activation (e.g. opioids, radiocontrast media). Complement-mediated (e.g. hereditary angioedema).
- **Physical urticaria:** Dermatographism, cold, heat, pressure, cholinergic (heat/exercise-induced), solar urticaria.
- **Autoimmune urticaria:** Autoantibodies against IgE receptor and IgE antibody.
- **Infectious:** Viral (especially in children), bacterial (e.g. *Helicobacter pylori*), parasitic.
- **Drug-induced:** NSAIDs, antibiotics, ACE inhibitors.
- **Idiopathic:** No identifiable cause.

Pathogenesis

- Urticaria results from the release of vasoactive substances, mainly histamine, from mast cells and basophils. This leads to vasodilation and increased vascular permeability, producing erythema and edema.
- Triggering factor (allergens, insect bite, etc.) → Degranulation of mast cells → Release of histamine, leukotrienes, prostaglandins.
- Histamine effects:
  - Vasodilation → Erythema.
  - Increased vascular permeability → Edema (wheals/angioedema).
  - Nerve stimulation → Pruritus and burning.

Clinical Features

- The clinical presentation of urticaria is characterized by the sudden appearance of wheals—raised, erythematous swellings with well-defined borders and central pallor.
- These lesions are intensely pruritic and vary in size and shape, often coalescing into larger plaques.
- They typically appear on the trunk, limbs, or face but can occur anywhere on the body. One hallmark feature is their transient nature—each individual wheal usually resolves within 24 hours without leaving behind any residual pigmentation or scarring.
- The itching associated with urticaria can be severe and may worsen at night, interfering with sleep and quality of life.
- urticaria may be accompanied by angioedema, which is a deeper dermal and subcutaneous tissue swelling, often affecting the lips, eyelids, tongue, or genitalia.
- urticaria may present episodically or recur chronically, depending on the underlying cause.

Investigations

- Investigations are usually not required for acute urticaria. However, required in chronic/recurrent cases to find out any underlying cause:
  - CBC, ESR, CRP
  - Thyroid function tests (hyperthyroidism can present with chronic urticaria)
  - ANA, anti-thyroid antibodies
  - Autologous serum skin test (ASST)
  - Skin prick test (for allergens)
  - Complement levels (C4, C1 esterase inhibitor for angioedema).

Differential Diagnosis

- Urticarial vasculitis (lesions last >24 hours, painful, may leave pigmentation)
- Mastocytosis
- Erythema multiforme
- Drug reactions.

Management

General Measures

- Identify and avoid triggering factors
- Cool compresses, loose clothing
- Reassurance and education.

Pharmacological Treatment

- **First-line treatment:** Antihistamines (most commonly used drugs). Examples are cetirizine, loratadine, fexofenadine. H_2 blockers such as ranitidine, famotidine can be used in addition to H_1 antihistamines. They block type-2 histamine receptors which may provide additional action along with H_1 antihistamines.
- **Second-line therapies:** Montelukast, especially useful in NSAID-induced urticaria. Short-course corticosteroids for severe flares.
- **Third-line/advanced therapies:** Omalizumab (anti-IgE monoclonal antibody) for refractory chronic spontaneous urticaria. Cyclosporine for autoimmune or treatment-resistant cases.

Q. Define angioedema. Describe the etiology, pathogenesis, clinical features, investigations and management of angioedema.

- Angioedema is a localized, transient swelling of the deeper layers of the skin and mucous membranes, resulting from increased vascular permeability.
- It may occur alone or in association with urticaria. Unlike the superficial wheals of urticaria, angioedema involves the deeper dermis and subcutaneous or submucosal tissues and can be potentially life-threatening if it involves the upper airway.

Etiopathogenesis

- Angioedema results from increased vascular permeability, leading to fluid leakage and tissue swelling.
- May be histamine-mediated (allergic, idiopathic) or bradykinin-mediated (hereditary/acquired, ACE inhibitor-induced).
- Bradykinin-mediated forms do not respond to antihistamines or steroids.

Causes

- These are same as those of urticaria.

Clinical Features

- Swelling of deeper dermis/subcutaneous tissues. The overlying skin usually appears normal or slightly erythematous but not urticarial.
- Common sites: Eyelids, lips, tongue, genitalia, hands, feet
- Can be painful, usually not itchy.
- Involvement of airway or GI tract may cause respiratory distress or abdominal pain.
- Lesions last longer (up to 72 hours).

Differential Diagnosis

- Cellulitis (typically unilateral, painful, with systemic signs)
- Contact dermatitis
- Facial trauma
- Orbital cellulitis (if periorbital involvement).

Management

Histaminergic (allergic) Angioedema

- First-line: Non-sedating H_1-antihistamines (e.g. cetirizine).
- Systemic corticosteroids: For moderate-to-severe reactions.
- Epinephrine (IM): If associated with anaphylaxis or airway compromise.

Bradykinin-mediated Angioedema

- Not responsive to antihistamines or steroids.
- Hereditary angioedema (HAE):
  - C1-INH concentrate (plasma-derived or recombinant)
  - Icatibant (bradykinin receptor antagonist)
  - Ecallantide (kallikrein inhibitor).
- Long-term prophylaxis:
  - Attenuated androgens (e.g. danazol)
  - Antifibrinolytics (e.g. tranexamic acid)
  - Lanadelumab (monoclonal antibody against plasma kallikrein).

ACE Inhibitor-induced Angioedema

- Discontinue ACE inhibitor immediately
- Supportive management, airway protection
- Icatibant may be effective in severe cases.

Q. Discuss the etiopathogenesis, clinical features and management of acne vulgaris.

- *Acne vulgaris* is a chronic skin condition involving blockage and/or inflammation of pilosebaceous units (hair follicles and their accompanying sebaceous gland).
- Acne is seen in most teenagers. Peak severity is in the late teenage years but acne may persist into the third decade and beyond, particularly in females.

Etiopathogenesis

- Acne occurs through the interplay of 4 major factors: increased sebum production, follicular plugging with sebum and keratinocytes, colonization of follicles by *Propionibacterium acnes*, and release of multiple inflammatory mediators.
- Increased sebum production—with the onset of puberty, sebaceous glands enlarge and sebum production increases. There is a clear relation between severity of acne and sebum production. In the complete absence of sebum, acne does not occur. Androgens are mainly responsible for increased sebum production.
- Follicular plugging with sebum and keratinocytes: blockage of pilosebaceous duct due to retention of keratinous material and sebum leads to formation of small cysts, called *comedones*.
- Colonization and activity of bacteria (*Propionibacterium acnes*) within the comedones releases free fatty acids from sebum, causes inflammation within the cyst and rupture.
- Rupture of the cyst releases oily and keratinous debris leading to an inflammatory foreign-body reaction in the skin.

Risk Factors for Acne

Hormonal Factors

- Androgen excess (puberty, PCOS, congenital adrenal hyperplasia)
- Menstrual irregularities
- Pregnancy or postpartum hormonal shifts.

Genetic Predisposition

- Family history of acne increases risk. Often more severe and earlier onset.

Increased Sebum Production

- Stimulated by androgens
- Oily skin types more prone to acne.

Follicular Hyperkeratinization

- Leads to comedone formation due to blocked pores.

Bacterial Colonization

- Especially *Cutibacterium acnes* (formerly *Propionibacterium acnes*).
- Triggers inflammation within follicles.

Diet

- High glycemic index foods (sugary, refined carbs)
- Dairy products (especially skim milk)
- Whey protein supplements.

Mechanical and External Factors

- Friction or pressure (e.g. helmets, backpacks—acne mechanica)
- Cosmetic products (comedogenic cosmetics)
- Occlusive clothing or humid environments.

Stress

- Can worsen acne via hormonal and inflammatory pathways.

Medications (drug-induced acne)

- Corticosteroids (topical/systemic)
- Testosterone and anabolic steroids
- Lithium
- Isoniazid
- Phenytoin.

Clinical Features

- The clinical hallmark of acne vulgaris is the comedone, which may be closed (whitehead) or open (blackhead).
- Closed comedones appear as 1–2 mm white papules. Open comedones have a large follicular orifice and are filled with oxidized, darkened, oily debris.
- Inflammatory papules, nodules and cysts occur and healing may lead to scarring.
- Lesions are maximum on the face, but may also occur on shoulders, upper chest and back.

Clinical Grading of Acne

- Clinical grading of acne vulgaris helps determine the severity and guides treatment. It is commonly graded as mild, moderate, or severe, based on the number and type of lesions, distribution, and presence of scarring.

Mild Acne (Grade I)

- Lesions: Mostly comedones (open and closed)
- Few papules or pustules
- No nodules or scarring
- Location: Typically limited to face.

Moderate Acne (Grade II)

- Increased number of papules and pustules
- Comedones still present
- No nodules or cysts
- Mild inflammation
- May involve face, upper trunk.

Moderately Severe Acne (Grade III)

- Numerous inflammatory lesions (papules, pustules)
- Occasional nodules
- Risk of post-inflammatory hyperpigmentation or scarring
- Involves face, chest, and/or back.

Severe Acne (Grade IV/Nodulocystic Acne)

- Multiple nodules, cysts, abscesses
- Severe inflammation
- Extensive scarring
- May be painful
- Involves large body areas.

Management

- Treatment of acne vulgaris is directed toward elimination of comedones by normalization of follicular keratinization, decreasing sebum production, decreasing the population of *P. acnes*, and decreasing inflammation.

General Measures

- Gentle cleansing
- Avoid picking/squeezing lesions
- Avoid oily cosmetics and comedogenic skincare products.

Local Measures

- Enough for mild-to-moderate acne.
- Topical keratolytic agents-retinoic acid, benzoyl peroxide, or salicylic acid. They alter the pattern of epidermal desquamation and prevent the formation of comedones.
- Topical antibacterial agents-azelaic acid, topical erythromycin, or clindamycin. They inhibit *Proprionobacterium acnes*.
- Incision and drainage of cysts
- Intraleisonal injection of triamcinolone acetonide reduces inflammation and hastens the resolution of cysts.
- Dermabrasion and excision of scars to improve skin appearance.

Systemic Measures

- Useful in severe acne with prominent inflammatory component.
- Antibiotics–tetracycline (250–500 mg bid), or doxycycline (100 mg bid). These antibiotics have anti-inflammatory effect in addition to their antibacterial effect. Oral antibiotics should be given for at least 6 months. Other antibiotics such as amoxicillin, erythromycin, and trimethoprim/sulfamethoxazole are sometimes used.
- Oral isotretinoin is useful in severe acne unresponsive to other therapies. It is the only acne medication that combats all four factors in acne pathogenesis. It is given over a course of several months as monotherapy. It has significant adverse effects including teratogenicity.

Q. Miliaria (heat rash).

- Miliaria, commonly known as heat rash or prickly heat, is an acute inflammatory skin condition caused by blockage of the sweat ducts, leading to sweat retention and leakage into the epidermis or dermis.
- Blockage of seat ducts can be due to cutaneous debris or bacteria such as *Staphylococcus epidermidis* with its formation of biofilms.
- It occurs in hot and humid weather.

Clinical Features

- Lesions are small, superficial, red, thin-walled, discrete but closely aggregated vesicles, papules, pustules or vesicopustules. Itching and burning is usually present.
- Miliaria occurs most commonly on the covered areas of skin such as trunk and intertriginous areas. In hospitalized patients, it occurs commonly on the back.

Treatment

- Patient should keep cool and wear loose and light clothing.
- Local application of triamcinolone acetonide, or a mid-potency corticosteroid in a lotion or cream base.
- Antibiotics for secondary infections (clindamycin).
- Anticholinergic drugs may be helpful in severe cases (glycopyrrolate, 1 mg twice daily). They help by decreasing sweating.

Q. How do you identify herpes simplex virus (HSV) infection of skin and mucous membrane?

Q. Differentiate herpes simplex virus (HSV) infection from other lesions.

- Herpes simplex virus (HSV) is a DNA virus from the Herpesviridae family that causes vesicular infections of the skin, mucous membranes, and sometimes the nervous system. There are two types of herpes simplex.
- Herpes simplex virus type 1 (HSV-1): Mainly affects oral/facial area (herpes labialis).
- Herpes simplex virus type 2 (HSV-2): Mainly genital involvement.
- Causes recurrent, grouped vesicular eruptions on erythematous base.

Clinical Features of Herpes Labialis (cold sores)

- Herpes labialis typically affects the lips, perioral area, nose, and chin.
- It is often preceded by a prodrome of tingling, burning, or itching sensations at the site of the impending outbreak.
- The characteristic lesion consists of grouped vesicles on a red, erythematous base, which may eventually rupture, forming shallow ulcers that then crust over and heal within 7–10 days.
- Recurrences are common, especially triggered by factors such as fever, sunlight, and emotional stress.
- Systemic symptoms, such as mild fever and malaise, may accompany primary infections, but are usually absent in recurrent episodes.

Clinical Features of Genital Herpes

- Multiple painful vesicles/ulcers on genitalia, perianal area, or inner thighs.
- May have: Fever, malaise, lymphadenopathy, dysuria, vaginal/urethral discharge, and tender inguinal lymphadenopathy.
- Lesions crust over and heal in 2–4 weeks.

Differentiation of Herpes Simplex from Other Lesions

See **Table 16.6.**

TABLE 16.6: Differentiation of herpes simplex from other lesions

Condition	Features	How it is different from HSV?
Impetigo	Honey-colored crusts, especially in children	No grouped vesicles; usually bacterial; no prodrome
Aphthous ulcer	Painful shallow ulcers inside oral mucosa (not lips)	No vesicles; occurs on mucosal surfaces (e.g. buccal mucosa)
Hand-foot-mouth disease	Vesicles in mouth, palms, soles (Coxsackievirus)	Distribution includes extremities and oral mucosa, especially in children
Herpes zoster	Unilateral dermatomal vesicles with pain (shingles)	Follows dermatome, not typically perioral; usually in older adults
Contact dermatitis	Itchy, red rash with vesicles or blisters in contact area	No grouped vesicles or prodrome; related to irritant/allergen
Pemphigus vulgaris	Flaccid bullae and oral erosions	Widespread, not grouped; positive Nikolsky's sign
Angular cheilitis	Cracks and redness at mouth angles	No vesicles; associated with saliva pooling, candidiasis, or deficiency

Q. How do you differentiate between herpes zoster from varicella and also from other skin lesions.

Differences between Herpes Zoster and Varicella (Chicken pox)

See **Table 16.7.**

TABLE 16.7: Herpes zoster *vs* varicella

Feature	Varicella (chickenpox)	Herpes zoster (shingles)
Age group	Common in children, rarely in adults	Mainly in adults/ elderly
Onset	Generalized rash	Localized, dermatomal
Lesion type	Vesicles in multiple stages	Grouped vesicles in same stage
Distribution	Centripetal (trunk >limbs)	Unilateral, along dermatome
Prodrome	Fever, malaise	Pain, burning, tingling in dermatome
Recurrence	Rare	Can recur, especially in immunosuppressed
Complication	Secondary infection	Postherpetic neuralgia, vision loss

Differentiation from Other Skin Lesions

See **Table 16.8.**

TABLE 16.8: Differentiation of herpes zoster and varicella from other lesions

Condition	Key features
Herpes zoster	Unilateral, dermatomal grouped vesicles, painful, postherpetic neuralgia
Varicella	Generalized polymorphic lesions, centripetal spread, occurs in children, more on trunk, itchy
Herpes simplex	Grouped vesicles on lips/genitals, recurrent
Impetigo	Honey-colored crusts, mainly in children. No vesicles on red base; more superficial and bacterial in origin
Hand-foot-mouth disease	Vesicles on palms, soles, and mouth; often in children. No dermatomal pattern
Contact dermatitis	Vesicular lesions in contact area, with itching. Usually bilateral and related to allergen/irritant exposure
Eczema herpeticum	Diffuse vesicular eruption, associated with eczema, not dermatomal

Q. Molluscum contagiosum.

- Molluscum contagiosum is a common viral skin infection caused by a poxvirus (Molluscum contagiosum virus, MCV). It presents as umbilicated, skin-colored papules, and is often self-limiting.

Etiology

- Caused by molluscum contagiosum virus (MCV), a double-stranded DNA virus of the Poxviridae family.

Transmission

- Direct skin-to-skin contact (including sexual contact).
- Fomites (e.g. towels, toys, gym equipment).
- Autoinoculation (scratching spreads lesions).
- More common in children, immunocompromised (e.g. HIV), and atopic dermatitis patients.

Clinical Features

- Asymptomatic, but may cause itching or irritation.
- Lesions are small (2–5 mm), firm, skin-colored to pearly white papules with characteristic central umbilication **(Fig. 16.8)**. Can become inflamed or red before resolving.

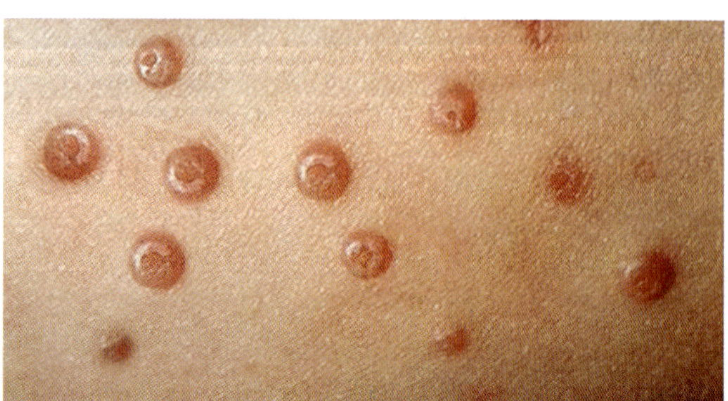

Figure 16.8: Molluscum contagiosum

- Common sites: Children → face, trunk, limbs. Adults → genitalia, lower abdomen, inner thighs (STD-related). Immunocompromised → face, neck, widespread or atypical lesions.

Diagnosis

- Clinical based on characteristic umbilicated lesions.
- Dermoscopy: It shows central pore with polylobulated white-to-yellow papules.
- Histopathology: Molluscum bodies (Henderson-Patterson bodies). These are large eosinophilic cytoplasmic inclusions in keratinocytes.
- PCR: Rarely needed. Detects viral DNA.

Management

- Often self-limiting (resolves in 6–12 months), so treatment may not be needed in children with few lesions.
- Treatment indicated in adults (especially genital lesions), extensive or cosmetically concerning lesions, and immunocompromised patients.

Local Treatment

- Cryotherapy (liquid nitrogen)
- Curettage
- Needle extraction (express core)
- Laser therapy (CO_2 laser)
- Topical treatments: Potassium hydroxide 5–10% solution, tretinoin 0.05% cream, cantharidin, and imiquimod (immune modulator).

Systemic Therapy

- Cidofovir (topical or IV) in HIV/AIDS with extensive disease.

Q. Lichen planus.

- Lichen planus (LP) is a chronic, inflammatory, autoimmune disease affecting the skin, mucous membranes, nails, and hair.

Etiology

Lichen planus is primarily considered an immune-mediated disorder, although its exact cause remains unknown. Following are the proposed etiological factors:

- ***Autoimmunity:*** The immune system, particularly CD8+ T cells, targets basal epidermal cells, possibly due to altered antigen expression. Associated with other autoimmune diseases such as alopecia areata, vitiligo, and ulcerative colitis.
- ***Genetic predisposition:*** Family history may be present, suggesting a possible genetic component.
- ***Infections:*** Hepatitis C virus (HCV) infection is significantly associated, especially with oral lichen planus. Rarely associated with other viruses like EBV and HPV.
- ***Drugs (lichenoid drug eruption):*** Certain medications can cause a lichen planus-like eruption (lichenoid

reaction), including: antihypertensives (e.g. ACE inhibitors, beta-blockers), antimalarials, NSAIDs, thiazide diuretics, gold salts, penicillamine.

- ***Dental materials:*** Dental amalgams and other materials may trigger oral lichenoid reactions, especially in lesions adjacent to fillings.
- ***Stress and psychological factors:*** Emotional stress is often reported as a precipitating or exacerbating factor.
- ***Allergens and contact sensitizers:*** Contact with certain dyes or fragrances may induce a lichenoid eruption.

Clinical Features

- Lichen planus typically affects adults between 30 and 60 years of age.
- Presents with characteristic skin lesions that are purple, polygonal, flat-topped, and intensely pruritic papules or plaques. These lesions most commonly appear on the flexor surfaces of the wrists and forearms, ankles, lower back, and genital region. A hallmark of lichen planus is the presence of **Wickham striae**, which are fine, white, lacy lines seen on the surface of the papules, especially noticeable in mucosal lesions **(Fig. 16.9)**.
- Oral involvement is common and manifests as white, reticular patches on the buccal mucosa, which can be asymptomatic or cause painful erosions.
- The disease may also involve the nails, leading to longitudinal ridging, thinning.
- Scalp involvement, known as lichen planopilaris, may result in scarring alopecia.
- The **Koebner phenomenon**, where lesions develop at sites of skin trauma, is often observed.

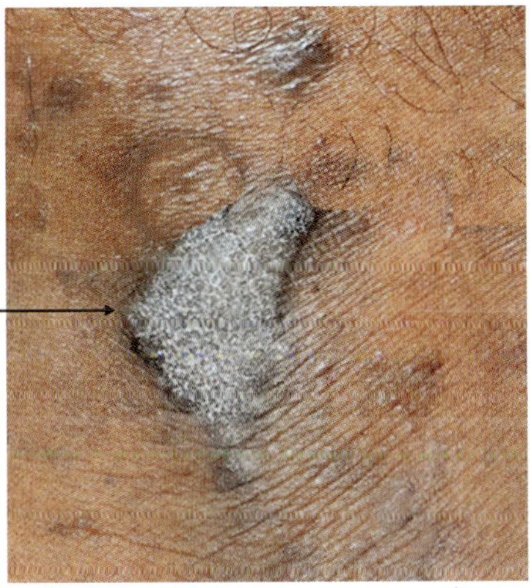

Figure 16.9: Lichen planus

Diagnosis

- Clinical examination.
- Dermoscopy: Wickham striae, violaceous hue.
- Biopsy: To confirm diagnosis (especially in atypical or treatment-resistant cases). It reveals hyperkeratosis, a dense band-like lymphocytic infiltrate along the dermoepidermal junction, and saw-toothing of the rete ridges due to basal cell degeneration.
- DIF (Direct immunofluorescence): Fibrin and IgM in a shaggy band at the basement membrane zone.
- Investigations for triggers: Hepatitis C serology (especially for oral LP), Drug history (ACE inhibitors, thiazides, NSAIDs may trigger LP).

Management of Lichen Planus

General Measures

- Identify and eliminate any triggering factor (e.g. drugs, dental amalgam).
- Reassure the patient: lesions often resolve in 1–2 years but may recur.

Topical Therapy

- Potent corticosteroids (e.g. clobetasol propionate) applied to lesions.
- For oral LP: Topical corticosteroids (e.g. triamcinolone in orabase).
- Adjuncts: Emollients, antihistamines (for pruritus).

Systemic Therapy (for widespread, severe, or resistant disease)

- Systemic corticosteroids: Prednisolone 0.5–1 mg/kg/day, tapering dose.
- Retinoids: Acitretin for cutaneous LP.
- Immunosuppressants: Methotrexate, azathioprine, or cyclosporine in severe/recalcitrant cases
- Phototherapy: NB-UVB or PUVA for widespread disease.

Q. Warts.

- Warts are mucocutaneous manifestation of human papillomavirus (HPV) infection.
- Viral warts are extremely common and most people suffer from one or more at some point during their life. HPV spreads by direct or sexual contact.

Clinical Features

- Common warts (verruca vulgaris) have smooth surface initially, but as they enlarge, their surface becomes irregular and hyperkeratotic, producing the typical warty appearance. They are most common on the hands but may also be seen on the face, genitalia, arm and leg. They are usually multiple.
- Plane warts (verruca plana) are smooth, flat-top papules seen most commonly on the face and backs of hands.
- Plantar warts (verruca plantaris) have a rough surface, surrounded by a horny collar. Plantar warts may be painful and disabling.
- Other types of wart are mosaic warts (mosaic-like plaques of tightly packed individual warts), facial warts (often filiform), and genital warts, which may be papillomatous and protuberant.

Treatment

- Wait and watch–spontaneous regression occurs in two-thirds of warts within two years. However, it is better to treat to avoid the risk of spread.

- Warts can be destroyed by local application of liquid nitrogen, salicylic acid, CO_2 laser, bichloroacetic acid, or cantharidin. Surgical excision and electrocautery are other options.
- Bleomycin injection into warts has a high cure rate for plantar and common warts.
- Podophyllum resin and the immunomodulator imiquimod are useful in anogenital warts.

Q. Erythema Nodosum.

- Erythema nodosum (EN) is a specific form of panniculitis (inflammation of subcutaneous fat) characterized by tender, red or violet, palpable, subcutaneous nodules.
- Most likely represents a delayed hypersensitivity reaction to antigens associated with the various infectious agents, drugs, and other diseases.

Causes

Infections
- Streptococcal pharyngitis (most common)
- Tuberculosis
- Yersinia, Salmonella, Campylobacter
- Viral infections (EBV, CMV, hepatitis B/C)

Drugs
- Sulfonamides
- Oral contraceptive pills
- Penicillin

Systemic diseases
- Sarcoidosis
- Inflammatory bowel disease (Crohn's disease, ulcerative colitis)
- Behçet's disease

Others
- Pregnancy
- Idiopathic (in up to 50% cases)

Clinical Features

- EN primarily affects people in their 20s and 30s but can occur at any age; women are more often affected.
- The lesions are deep nodules, 1–10 cm in diameter, red or violet in color and tender.
- They are most often located on the anterior surfaces of the legs below the knees (shin) but may rarely occur on the arms, trunk, and face.
- Fever, malaise, and arthralgia usually accompany the lesions.
- Lesions last about 6 weeks and heal without scarring
- Recurrence may occur.

Diagnosis

- Diagnosis is mainly based on clinical features.
- WBC, ESR and CRP are elevated.
- Appropriate tests to identify the underlying cause (chest X-ray, montoux test, ANA, ASO titre, etc.).
- Biopsy may be required in atypical cases.

Treatment

- Usually self-limited.
- Underlying cause should be identified and treated.
- Pain, arthralgia and fever can be treated by NSAIDs.
- Potassium iodide solution, 5–15 drops orally three times daily, results in prompt involution in many cases. Exact mechanism of action of potassium iodide is unknown.
- Oral corticosteroids in severe, extensive disease unless contraindicated by associated infection.

Q. Vitiligo.

- Vitiligo is skin depigmentation due to loss of melanocytes in the skin, mucosa, and hair.

Etiology

- In vitiligo there are focal areas of melanocyte loss which is considered to be due to cell-mediated autoimmune attack. Some patients have antibodies to melanin. It may be associated with other autoimmune diseases such as diabetes, Addison's disease and pernicious anemia.
- Genetic factors may play a role; 20–30% of patients may have a family history of vitiligo.
- Extrinsic factors also may play a role. Trauma, certain chemicals and sunburn may precipitate the appearance of vitiligo.

Clinical Features

- Lesions may start at any age, but generally in early adolescence or adult life.
- Segmental vitiligo is restricted to one part of the body.
- Generalized vitiligo is characterized by many widespread macules, often symmetrical and frequently involves the hands, wrists, knees and neck as well as the area around the body orifices.
- The patches of depigmentation are sharply demarcated **(Fig. 16.10)**.
- Sensation in the depigmented patches is normal unlike leprosy.
- Course is static or slowly progressive. Some patients may experience spontaneous repigmentation.

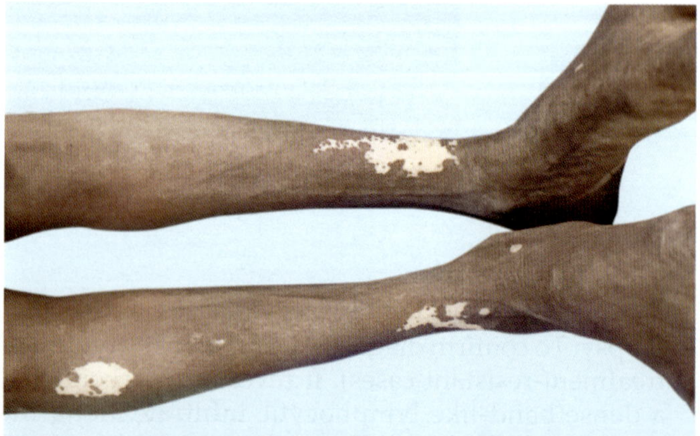

Figure 16.10: Vitiligo (well demarcated milky white lesions)

Differential Diagnosis

- Postinflammatory hypopigmentation
- Piebaldism (a rare autosomal dominant disorder; depigmented patches surrounded by hyperpigmented areas)
- Morphea (localized scleroderma)
- Leprosy (lesions are usually hypoesthetic)
- Lichen sclerosus
- Pityriasis alba
- Chemical leukoderma
- Leukoderma due to melanoma.

Management

- Corticosteroids: Topical corticosteroids are the first choice for patients with limited disease. Topical preparations of fluticasone propionate or mometasone, once a day for 4–6 months has to be applied. Oral corticosteroids may be helpful in progressive disease.
- Calcineurin inhibitors: Topical calcineurin inhibitors (e.g. tacrolimus) are also effective.
- Ultraviolet light: Topical or oral psoralens plus ultraviolet A radiation (PUVA), or ultraviolet B (UVB) radiation (phototherapy) is used in patients with extensive vitiligo. A total of 75–150 treatments (e.g. three times/week for 6–12 months) may be necessary.
- Surgery: Split-skin grafts and blister roof grafts can be used to cover vitiligo patches.
- Depigmentation therapy: If there is extensive vitiligo with only small areas of normal skin, these normal skin areas can be depigmented (by using hydroquinone) to make the skin look uniform.
- Patients should be advised to avoid excessive sun exposure and to use sunscreens to reduce the risk of skin cancer in the long run.
- Camouflage cosmetics may also be helpful to mask the patches.

Q. Differentiation of vitiligo from other causes of hypopigmented lesions.

- Many conditions can mimic hypopigmented patches of vitiligo. Differentiating vitiligo from these is crucial for accurate diagnosis and treatment.

Vitiligo

- Cause: Autoimmune destruction of melanocytes.
- Age group: Most cases begin in early adolescence or adult life (peak onset between 10 and 30 years of age).
- Lesion: Well-defined, depigmented (milky white) macules/patches.
- Onset: Gradual
- Distribution: Symmetrical; often on face, hands, genitalia, and over bony prominences.
- Wood's lamp: Enhances contrast—lesions appear bright white.
- Sensation: Normal
- Scaling: Absent
- Course: Progressive.

Pityriasis Alba

- Exact cause: Unknown
- Age group: Children and adolescents
- Lesion: Hypopigmented, ill-defined patches, mainly on face
- Wood's lamp: Minimal enhancement
- Sensation: Normal
- Scaling: Fine scaling often present
- Course: Self-limited, resolves with moisturizers.

Tinea Versicolor (pityriasis versicolor)

- Cause: Malassezia infection
- Lesion: Hypo/hyperpigmented macules with fine scaling, often confluent
- Distribution: Trunk, neck, upper arms
- Wood's lamp: Yellow-green fluorescence
- Sensation: Mild itch sometimes
- Scaling: Prominent (scraping reveals scaling-"scratch sign")
- Diagnosis: KOH mount shows "spaghetti and meatballs" appearance.

Post-inflammatory Hypopigmentation

- Cause: Follows trauma, dermatitis, or infection.
- Lesion: Hypopigmented patch in area of prior inflammation.
- Wood's lamp: No sharp contrast.
- Scaling: Absent.
- Course: Gradual repigmentation over time.

Leprosy (hypopigmented macule of tuberculoid leprosy)

- Cause: *Mycobacterium leprae*
- Lesion: Hypopigmented patch with ill-defined margin
- Sensation: Loss of sensation is hallmark
- Nerve involvement: Thickened peripheral nerves nearby
- Wood's lamp: No enhancement
- Diagnosis: Skin smear, biopsy.

Idiopathic Guttate Hypomelanosis

- Age group: Elderly
- Lesion: Multiple small, round/oval, hypopigmented macules
- Location: Forearms, shins
- Wood's lamp: No enhancement
- Sensation: Normal
- Course: Stable, not progressive.

Albinism

- Cause: Genetic defect in melanin synthesis
- Lesion: Generalized depigmentation since birth
- Eyes: Nystagmus, photophobia, reduced visual acuity
- Hair and skin: White or very light
- Wood's lamp: Whole skin appears depigmented.

Summary of Key Differentiating Points

See **Table 16.9.**

Q. Melanocytic nevi (moles).

- Melanocytic naevi (moles) are localized benign proliferations of melanocytes that appear as well-circumscribed pigmented macules, papules, or nodules on the skin or mucosa. Moles are a usual feature of most human beings. They are used as identification marks.
- They probably occur due to abnormalities of the normal migratory pattern of the melanocytes during development.

Clinical Features

Congenital Nevi

- These are present at birth or appear shortly after.

Acquired Nevi

- These appear in early childhood, at adolescence, and during pregnancy or oestrogen therapy. They can be divided into 3 types based on the location of clumps of melanocytes.
- *Junctional nevi*: These are present in the dermal-epidermal junction. They are common on the acral surfaces but may occur anywhere. They appear as flat, pigmented macules.
- *Compound nevi*: These are present in the dermo-epidermal junction as well as dermis. They are often raised, and may be papillomatous.
- *Dermal nevi*: These are present in the dermis only. They are typically flesh colored.

Significance of Moles

- Most moles are benign and do not cause any problems. Rarely there may be malignant transformation. Malignant change is most likely in large congenital melanocytic nevi.

Danger Signs Indicating Malignant Transformation of Moles

- Itching
- Increase in size
- Change in color
- Change in shape
- Bleeding
- Irregular margin or surface
- Inflammation
- Ulceration

Management

- Most nevi do not require any treatment.
- Excision may be considered if malignancy is suspected or when they repeatedly become inflamed or traumatized or for cosmetic reasons.

Q. Alopecia (baldness).

- Alopecia refers to hair loss from the scalp or other parts of the body. It can be scarring or nonscarring, localized or diffuse, and has various causes.
- It is a sign rather than a diagnosis.
- The hair cycle consists of three phases: The growth phase, which is called anagen, the resting phase, which is called catagen, and the shedding phase, which is the telogen phase. Different hairs will be at different phase at any given time.
- Anagen is long growing phase which lasts 2–6 years. Catagen is a brief transitional phase where the hair follicle shrinks in size. Telogen is a short resting phase lasting 1–4 months. At the end of the resting phase, the hair falls out (exogen) and new hair starts growing in the follicle, beginning the cycle again.
- Alopecia can be broadly classified into scarring and nonscarring types. It can be localized or diffuse.
- Scarring alopecia refers to hair loss associated with fibrosis that replaces and often permanently destroys the hair follicle.
- Nonscarring alopecia refers to hair loss without permanent destruction of the hair follicle.

Causes of Alopecia

Scarring alopecia

- Herpes zoster
- Chemical or physical trauma
- Discoid lupus erythematosus
- Scleroderma
- Severe folliculitis

TABLE 16.9: Differentiation of hypopigmented skin lesions

Condition	Scaling	Sensation	Wood's lamp	Distribution	Key feature
Vitiligo	Absent	Normal	Bright white	Symmetrical, exposed areas	Depigmented patches, autoimmune
Pityriasis alba	Fine	Normal	Minimal	Face (children)	Ill-defined patches, dry skin
Tinea versicolor	Present	Normal/mild itch	Yellow-green	Trunk, neck	Fungal, KOH positive
Leprosy (TT)	Absent	↓ Sensation	No	Extremities, face	Sensory loss, thickened nerves
Post-inflammatory	Absent	Normal	No	Site of prior lesion	History of trauma/inflammation
Guttate hypomelanosis	Absent	Normal	No	Shins, arms	Elderly, tiny discrete macules
Albinism	General	Normal	Generalized	Entire body	From birth, ocular signs

- Lichen planopilaris
- Dissecting cellulitis
- Tumors
- Radiotherapy
- Idiopathic

Nonscarring alopecia

- Androgenetic alopecia (most common cause)
- Tinea capitis
- Alopecia areata
- Traumatic (trichotillomania, traction)
- Syphilis
- Telogen effluvium
- Hypo and hyperthyroidism
- Hypopituitarism
- Diabetes mellitus
- HIV
- Nutritional deficiency (e.g. iron)
- Liver disease
- Postpartum
- Drugs (anticancer drugs, antithyroid drugs, oral contraceptives, allopurinol, gentamicin, and levodopa).

Clinical Features

- Note the onset and duration of hair loss, whether hair shedding is increased, and whether hair loss is localized or diffuse. Hair loss can be local or diffuse depending on the cause. Both scalp and body hair loss is seen in alopecia universalis. Loss of up to 100 hairs per day is normal. More than this is significant.
- H/o recent exposures to noxious agents (e.g. drugs, toxins, radiation) and stressors (e.g. surgery, chronic illness, fever, psychologic stressors) suggests toxic or stress induced hair loss.
- H/o weight gain, fatigue and cold intolerance suggests hypothyroidism. H/o virilization in women (hirsutism, deepening of the voice, and increased libido) suggests adrenal disorder or polycystic ovary syndrome. H/o gynecologic/obstetric complaints in women may suggest hormonal problems.
- A family history of hair loss should be recorded.
- Alopecia areata appears as sharply demarcated bald patches, with pathognomonic 'exclamation mark' hairs (broken-off hairs 3–4 mm long, which taper off towards the scalp). The hair usually regrows in small bald patches, but may be incomplete in larger patches.
- Androgenetic alopecia or male-pattern baldness is physiological in men over 20 years old. Hair loss usually occurs in an M-shaped pattern (bitemporal recession and then crown involvement) in the frontal hair line. It also occurs in females, usually after menopause, but hair loss is often diffuse.
- Hair loss associated with pruritus, erythema, and scaling is seen in chronic cutaneous lupus and tinea capitis.
- Asymmetric, bizarre, irregular hair loss pattern is seen in trichotillomania.

Investigations

- Serum testosterone, DHEA
- Iron, total iron binding capacity
- Urea, creatinine, electrolytes, LFT
- Thyroid function tests
- ANA
- HIV, VDRL and TPHA
- Fungal stain in localized hair loss with scaling
- Scalp biopsy, with direct immunofluorescence, if lichen planus or discoid lupus erythematosus is suspected.

Management

- Support and reassurance
- Treatment of underlying cause
- Alopecia areata sometimes responds to topical or intralesional corticosteroids such as triamcinolone.
- Systemic finasteride or topical 2% minoxidil solution are useful in severe androgenetic alopecia. In females, anti-androgen therapy such as cyproterone acetate can be used.
- Scalp reduction surgery and autologous hair transplantation are also options in irreversible alopecia.
- Wig may be useful for irreversible extensive alopecia.

Q. Pyoderma.

- Pyoderma refers to bacterial skin infections characterized by pus formation. It is a common dermatological condition and may be primary (arising on healthy skin) or secondary (occurring over previously diseased skin).

Classification of Pyoderma

- **Primary pyoderma:** Direct bacterial infection of healthy skin
  - *Impetigo (nonbullous and bullous)*
  - *Ecthyma*
  - *Folliculitis*
  - *Furuncle*
  - *Carbuncle*
  - *Cellulitis*
  - *Erysipelus*
- **Secondary pyoderma:** Infection over preexisting skin conditions
  - *Infected scabies*
  - *Infected eczema*
  - *Infected wounds or ulcers*

Causative Organisms

- *Staphylococcus aureus* (most common)
- *Streptococcus pyogenes*
- Others (less common): Pseudomonas, Proteus, Klebsiella.

Clinical Features

- Localized erythema, swelling, pain, warmth
- Pustules, vesicles, crusts, ulcers
- Possible regional lymphadenopathy
- May be mild to severe, with or without systemic symptoms like fever.

Common Types (Table 16.10)

TABLE 16.10: Clinical features of common types of skin infections	
Type	**Features**
Impetigo	Superficial infection; honey-colored crusts, mostly in children
Ecthyma	Deeper form of impetigo; ulcerative lesion with thick crust
Folliculitis	Infection of hair follicles; pustules centered on follicles
Furuncle	Boil; deeper infection of follicle and surrounding tissue
Carbuncle	Multiple interconnected furuncles; common in diabetics
Cellulitis	Spreading infection of dermis/subcutis; red, warm, tender skin
Erysipelas	Acute, superficial cellulitis with well-demarcated borders; often facial
Necrotizing fasciitis	Rapidly spreading deep soft tissue infection. Skin discoloration, bullae, necrosis, crepitus. Systemic toxicity and shock.
Staphylococcal scalded skin syndrome (SSSS)	Caused by *Staphylococcus aureus* (exfoliative toxin). There is widespread erythema followed by exfoliation. Flaccid bullae and skin peeling, especially in infants and young children. Nikolsky's sign positive (skin sloughs off with gentle pressure).

Diagnosis

- Clinical examination
- Gram stain and bacterial culture of pus
- Blood tests if systemic involvement is suspected.

Management

- Local care: Gentle cleansing, antiseptics (e.g. povidone-iodine)
- Topical antibiotics: Mupirocin, fusidic acid for localized lesions
- Systemic antibiotics:
  - Cloxacillin, cephalexin, or amoxicillin-clavulanate
  - For MRSA: Clindamycin, doxycycline, or TMP-SMX
- Treat underlying conditions in secondary pyoderma.
- Prevent recurrence by hygiene measures, treating carriers, etc.

Q. Discuss briefly the common skin malignancies.

Basal Cell Carcinoma (BCC) (rodent ulcer)

- This is the most common skin cancer. It arises from the basal layer of epidermis and its appendages.
- Both environmental and genetic factors contribute to the development of BCC. Chronic exposure to ultraviolet (UV) radiation in sunlight is the most important risk factor. Other risk factors are chronic arsenic exposure, therapeutic radiation, immunosuppression, and the basal cell nevus syndrome.
- It is common in Europeans and at least 3 times more common than squamous cell carcinoma.
- It is more common in men than in women probably due to more exposure to sun.
- Incidence increases with age.

Clinical Features

- Most BCCs occur on the face.
- Most common type is noduloulcerative form. The earliest lesion is a small papule, with fine telangiectatic vessels on the surface, which slowly enlarges. Central necrosis may occur, leaving an ulcer surrounded by a rolled pearly edge.
- The tumor invades locally but rarely metastasizes.
- The superficial (multifocal) variant is seen most often on the trunk; it appears as a slowly enlarging pink or brown scaly plaque.

Management

- Since metastasis is extremely rare, most BCCs can be treated by local destruction.
- Treatment options include surgery, cryotherapy, radiotherapy, photodynamic therapy or the topical immunostimulant imiquimod. Surgery is usually the first choice, as it allows histological assessment of the tumor and examination of tumor margins.

Squamous Cell Carcinoma (SCC)

- SCC is the second most common skin cancer after BCC.
- Risk factors for SCC are similar to BCC. Additional risk factors are chronic cutaneous ulcer, genetic disorders such as dystrophic epidermolysis bullosa and xeroderma pigmentosum, human papilloma virus infection, and smoking.

Clinical Features

- SCC arises most commonly in areas frequently exposed to the sun, such as the head and neck (most common site), dorsum of the hands and forearms, and legs.
- Varying clinical presentations include nodules, plaques, infiltrating tumors and ulcers.
- Histological grade varies from well-differentiated to anaplastic. SCCs of the lip behave more aggressively and show a greater frequency of metastasis.

Management

- Surgical excision is the preferred option because of the definite risk of metastasis.
- Other options are cryotherapy, electrosurgery (i.e. curettage and electrodesiccation), topical treatment (5-fluorouracil, or imiquimod) and radiotherapy.

Malignant Melanoma

- Incidence of malignant melanoma has increased in recent decades. There is no effective treatment for metastatic melanoma and hence, the main focus is on primary prevention and early detection.

- Malignant melanoma has very poor prognosis with a case fatality rate of approximately 20–25%.
- The main risk factors for melanoma are ultraviolet rays exposure, pale skin, melanocytic naevi, immunosuppression, and family history of melanoma. About 30–50% of melanomas develop in a preexisting melanocytic naevus. Development of any danger sign in a nevus should raise the suspicion of malignant transformation.

Clinical Features

- *Superficial spreading*: This is characterized by superficial and radially expanding, pigmented macule or plaque. Its margin is usually irregular.
- *Lentigo maligna*: This is the *in situ* phase of superficial spreading melanoma. It occurs most often on the exposed skin of the elderly. Lentigo maligna may have been present for many years before invasive melanoma develops from it.
- *Nodular*: Appears as a pigmented nodule.
- *Acral lentiginous*: It occurs on the palms and soles.
- In amelanotic melanomas, pigmentation is minimal or absent.
- Subungual melanomas present as painless, expanding areas of pigmentation under a nail.
- *Clinical stages of malignant melanoma*
  - Stage I: Primary lesion only
  - Stage II: Involvement of regional lymph nodes
  - Stage III: Distant metastases (nodal or visceral)

Management

- Surgical excision is the treatment choice. Palpable local nodes in stage II patients should be removed by block dissection.
- Chemotherapy is rarely curative but can be palliative in stage III disease or earlier.
- Alpha-interferon may reduce recurrences in patients with high-risk melanomas.

Q. Skin manifestations of internal disease (Table 16.11).

- Many systemic diseases manifest as skin diseases which can serve as a clue to systemic disease. The type of lesion typically relates to a specific disease or type of disease.

TABLE 16.11: Skin manifestations of internal disease

- **Erythema nodosum:** TB, leprosy, syphilis, sarcoidosis, inflammatory bowel disease, SLE
- **Acanthosis nigricans:** Internal malignancy, insulin resistance
- **Pyoderma gangrenosum:** Inflammatory bowel disease
- **Hyperpigmentation:** Hemochromatosis, Addison disease, ectopic ACTH syndrome, vitamin B_{12} deficiency, pellagra
- **Hypopigmentation:** Oculocutaneous albinism, Chediak-Higashi syndrome, phenylketonuria, systemic sclerosis (scleroderma), leprosy, tuberous sclerosis
- **Xanthomas and xanthelasma:** Elevated serum triglycerides
- **Acanthosis nigricans, necrobiosis lipoidica, and scleraderma:** diabetes mellitus
- **Thick and dry skin:** Hypothyroidism
- **Striae and skin fragility:** Cushing disease
- **Skin ulcers:** Vasculitis, sickle cell anemia, cryoglobulinemia, diabetes mellitus
- **Vesicles/bullae:** Paraneoplastic pemphigus, porphyrias
- **Purpura:** Thrombocytopenia, clotting factor defects, Ehlers-Danlos syndrome, scurvy, DIC, APLA, thrombotic thrombocytopenic purpura, cholesterol and fat emboli, systemic vasculitis, acute meningococcemia
- **Alopecia:** SLE, secondary syphilis, hypothyroidism, hyperthyroidism, deficiencies of protein, biotin, zinc, and iron
- **Urticaria:** Urticarial vasculitis, hepatitis B or C infection, serum sickness
- **Acneiform Eruptions:** Cushing's disease, congenital adrenal hyperplasia, polycystic ovary syndrome
- **Telangiectasias:** Carcinoid syndrome, ataxia-telangiectasia, hereditary hemorrhagic telangiectasia
- **Spider angioma:** Cirrhosis
- **Pruritus:** Occult cancer, often lymphoma.

Chapter 17

Poisoning, Venomous Bites and Environmental Diseases

Q. Discuss the general management/initial stabilization of a patient who has ingested a poison/drug overdose.

- A poison is any substance that can cause a disturbance of structure or function of the body when absorbed in relatively small amounts by a living organism.
- Poisoning may be accidental, intentional (suicidal) or homicidal. Accidental ingestion of poison is common in children. Over-dosage of 'recreational' drugs is frequent in young adults. Intentional (suicidal) poisoning is seen in adults of all ages. Homicidal poisoning (with the intention of murdering) is less common.
- Commonly ingested poisons are organophosphorus and organochloride insecticides, vegetable poisons (oleander), aluminum phosphide, methyl and ethyl alcohol, hypnotics and sedatives. Insecticide and vegetable poisoning is common in rural areas because of easy availability. Sedative overdosage is mainly encountered in urban areas.

General Management of a Case of Poisoning

Management of poisoning involves the following steps:

- Resuscitation and initial stabilization
- Diagnosis of type of poison
- Prevention of further absorption of poison
- Administration of antidote
- Increasing the clearance of absorbed poison
- Prevention of recurrence of poisoning.

Resuscitation and Initial Stabilization

- Airway, breathing and circulation (A, B and C) should be attended to first, even before obtaining a history.

Airway

- Airway may be compromised by aspiration of pharyngeal secretions or vomitus, by laryngeal edema in corrosive poisoning and anaphylaxis, or stridor in strychnine poisoning. Airway can be opened by positioning, suction, or insertion of a nasal or oropharyngeal airway. Endotracheal intubation is required if the patient is deeply comatose without any gag or cough reflex. Emergency tracheostomy is required if there is laryngeal obstruction.

Breathing

- Once the airway is opened by the above procedures, assess the patient for the rate and depth of breathing. Pulse oximetry can be useful to assess the adequacy of breathing, but is not reliable in methemoglobinemia or carbon monoxide poisoning. An urgent ABG (arterial blood gas analysis) provides important information about blood pH, PaO_2 and PCO_2. If breathing is inadequate, it should be assisted by bag-mask device or mechanical ventilation. Supplemental oxygen should be given.

Circulation

- Next, assess the patient for adequacy of circulation by measuring pulse rate and BP. Tissue perfusion can be assessed by urinary output, skin signs, and arterial blood pH. If BP is low, a large-bore IV line should be inserted and infusion of fluids (DNS or NS) started. Bradycardia can occur in sedative and OP compound ingestion and should be corrected by atropine injection intravenously. If BP does not pick up even after infusion of fluids, inotropes such as dopamine or noradrenaline infusion should be started. Patient should be put on continuous electrocardiographic monitoring.
- Before any fluid is given, blood should be drawn for complete blood count, glucose, electrolytes, serum creatinine and liver tests, and toxicologic screening.

Diagnosis of Type of Poison

- The diagnosis and treatment of poisons must proceed rapidly without waiting for the results of toxicologic screening.
- Type of poison, quantity and time of ingestion can be obtained by history, physical examination and laboratory tests. Relatives and bystanders may be able to give useful information. They should be asked to get the container of the suspected poison or drug.

Odor or appearance of the stomach contents may help in identification of the poison. A toxicological analysis of blood can be performed if the poison cannot be identified by the above means.

Identification of Poison based on Clinical Features (Table 17.1)

TABLE 17.1: Identification of poison based on clinical features

Clinical feature	Possible poison/drug
Coma	Narcotics, benzodiazepines, barbiturates, alcohol, methanol, organophosphorus
Pupil size	*Constricted*—opioid, phenothiazines, organophosphorus *Dilated*—alcohol, anticholinergics, dhatura, botulism, carbon monoxide
Respiratory rate	*Decreased*—opioids, benzodiazepines *Increased*–salicylates, methanol, ethylene glycol
Blood pressure	*Hypotension*—TCAs, antihypertensives *Hypertension*—cocaine, amphetamines, sympathomimetics
Heart rate	*Bradycardia*—organophosphorus, digoxin, betablockers, opioids. *Tachycardia*—coccaine, theophylline, anticholinergics
Body temperature	*Increased*—dhatura, atropine, SSRIs *Decreased*—sedatives, opioids
Jaundice	Phosphorus, isoniazid, rifampicin, carbon tetrachloride, paracetamol
Cyanosis	Methemoglobinemia—aniline dyes, sulfonamides, nitrates
Cherry-colored skin and mucous membranes	Carbon monoxide
Bullous rash	Barbiturates
Dystonias, muscle spasms	Phenothiazines, metoclopramide, strychnine
Burns and ulcers in the lips and mouth	Corrosive poison

Prevention of Absorption of Poison

Emesis

- Vomiting can remove unabsorbed poison from the stomach when performed within 3–4 hours of ingestion. Patient must be fully conscious and have stable breathing and circulation. Emesis is contraindicated in corrosive and hydrocarbon (like kerosene) ingestion. Kerosene can cause fatal chemical pneumonitis if aspirated during vomiting.
- Emesis can be induced by drinking 200–400 ml of a fully saturated sodium chloride solution, subcutaneous apomorphine, or syrup of ipecac (10–30 ml). Apomorphine and syrup of ipecac act by stimulation of vomiting centre.
- Emesis is less commonly used now, because of the risk of aspiration.

Gastric Lavage

- It is performed by passing a wide-bore nasogastric tube. Patient should be in lateral decubitus position with the head 15–20° lower than the feet (Trendelenburg position).
- Stomach contents are emptied, and then lavage is performed by introducing 200–300 ml fluid into the somach at a time. The fluid is allowed to drain out by gravity. Lavage is performed till the draining fluid is clear. Upto 3–5 liters of water may be required. Warm normal saline or tap water is used as lavage fluid to prevent hypothermia. Food particles may block the tube and prevent adequate emptying of the stomach. Intact tablets are incompletely recovered by gastric lavage.

Activated Charcoal

- Activated charcoal is fine charcoal powder which is heated with steam, air, or carbon dioxide to add more surface area.
- It has an extensive network of interconnecting pores that bind (adsorb) and trap chemicals, thereby preventing their absorption and toxicity.
- It is usually given after gastric lavage. The dose is 1 g/kg body weight (maximum 50–60 g) as a single dose. Multiple doses can be used in cases of poisons which undergo enterohepatic circulation. Side effects of charcoal include nausea, vomiting, and diarrhea or constipation.

Whole Bowel Irrigation

- Whole bowel irrigation (WBI) refers to the administration of large volumes of a balanced electrolyte solution with polyethylene glycol, via a nasogastric tube, to decontaminate the GI tract without causing fluid or electrolyte shifts. 1–1.5 liters of solution per hour is given until the rectal effluent is clear, which usually takes 4–6 hours.
- WBI is particularly useful in ingestion of enteric-coated pills, sustained-release preparations, illicit drug packets, and large ingestions of substances poorly bound by charcoal, such as iron, lithium and lead.

Administration of Antidote

- Antidotes counteract the effects of poisons by neutralizing them or by antagonizing their physiologic effects. Antidotes are available only for few poisons.

Commonly used Antidotes (Table 17.2)

TABLE 17.2: Commonly used antidotes

Poison/drug	Antidote
Organophosphates	Atropine, pralidoxime (PAM)
Paracetamol	N-acetylcysteine
Cyanide	Hydroxocobalamin or sodium thiosulfate + Sodium nitrite

(Contd.)

TABLE 17.2: Commonly used antidotes *(Contd.)*

Poison/drug	Antidote
Methanol	Fomepizole, ethanol
Amanita phalloides	Benzyl penicillin
Calcium-channel blockers	Calcium chloride
Methotrexate	Folinic acid
Anticholinergics	Physostigmine
Beta-blockers	Glucagon
Benzodiazepines	Flumazenil
Warfarin like compounds	Vitamin K
Lead, arsenic, mercury	Dimercaprol (BAL), D-penicillamine
Iron overdose	Deferrioxamine
Opioids	Naloxone
Digitalis	Digoxin immune Fab (Digibind)

Increasing the Clearance of Absorbed Poison

Alkaline Diuresis

- Alkalinization of urine enhances excretion of acidic drugs by increasing the ionic form of the drug in urine, thereby preventing its reabsorption by tubules.
- It is effective in poisoning due to salicylates, barbiturates, sulfonamides, barium, bromides, and calcium, etc.

Hemodialysis and Hemoperfusion

- Dialysis is based on the property of drugs and toxins to diffuse down a concentration gradient across a semipermeable membrane. Hemodialysis is useful in poisoning of methanol, ethylene glycol, isopropanol, salicylates, theophylline, and lithium.
- Hemoperfusion refers to the circulation of blood through an extracorporeal circuit containing an adsorbent such as activated charcoal or polystyrene resin. It is useful in poisoning due to amanita mushroom, amitriptyline, barbiturates, digitalis, methotrexate, paraquat, phenytoin and theophylline.

Prevention of Recurrence of Poisoning

- Some patients may make another suicidal attempt by consuming poison. Hence, all patients should be referred for psychiatric evaluation.

Q. Describe various types of toxidromes and possible poisons.

- A toxidrome (short for toxic syndrome) is a set of characteristic signs and symptoms that consistently occur together and are associated with a specific class of toxins or poisons.
- Recognizing these patterns is critical for early diagnosis and management, especially when the exact poison/drug is unknown.

Major Toxidromes

See **Table 17.3.**

TABLE 17.3: Major toxidromes

Toxidrome	Key features	Common agents
Cholinergic	DUMBBELSS symptoms	OPs, carbamates
Anti-cholinergic	• "Mad as a hatter, hot as a hare, dry as a bone, red as a beet, blind as a bat" • Delirium, hallucinations, agitation • Hyperthermia, dry flushed skin • Mydriasis (dilated pupils) • Urinary retention, decreased bowel sounds • Tachycardia	Antihistamines, dhatura, tricyclic antidepressants, atropine
Opioid	• Miosis (pinpoint pupils) • Respiratory depression • CNS depression (coma, low GCS) • Bradycardia, hypotension	Morphine, heroin, fentanyl
Sympatho-mimetic	• Agitation, anxiety • Mydriasis, tachycardia • Hypertension, hyperthermia • Diaphoresis (important difference from anticholinergic!) • Tremor, seizures (in severe cases)	Cocaine, amphetamines
Sedative-hypnotic	• CNS depression, slurred speech, ataxia • Normal pupils • Respiratory depression (in severe cases) • Bradycardia, hypotension	Benzodiazepines, barbiturates
Serotonin syndrome	• Hyperreflexia, clonus (esp. lower limbs) • Agitation, confusion • Fever, sweating, tremor • Diarrhea	SSRIs, MAOIs, MDMA
Neuroleptic malignant syndrome (NMS)	• Hyperthermia • "Lead pipe" rigidity • Delirium, autonomic instability • Elevated CPK	Antipsychotics
Hallucinogenic	• Visual/auditory hallucinations • Mydriasis • Anxiety, paranoia, panic • Tachycardia, hypertension • Phencyclidine (PCP): Aggression, vertical nystagmus	LSD, psilocybin, PCP

Q. Discuss the clinical features, diagnosis and management of organophosphorus or carbamate poisoning.

Q. Intermediate syndrome.

- Organophosphate (OP) and carbamate compounds are widely used as insecticides. Poisoning with these substances is common in agricultural areas and can occur accidentally or intentionally (suicidal).
- OP compounds are widely used as pesticides in agriculture. OP nerve agents are used in chemical warfare.
- Carbamates were synthesized after OP compounds. The use of OP compounds has declined after the introduction of carbamates.

Organophosphorus Compounds

Agricultural/household insecticides

- Malathion
- Parathion
- Chlorpyrifos
- Diazinon
- Phorate
- Dimethoate
- Methyl parathion
- Fenthion
- Monocrotophos
- Quinalphos

Chemical warfare agents (nerve agents)

- Sarin, tabun, soman

Carbamates

- Carbaryl, aldicarb and propoxur

Mechanism of Toxicity

- OP compounds are well absorbed through the skin, lungs, and gastrointestinal tract. Both OP compounds and carbamates inactivate the enzyme acetylcholinesterase (AChE) by phosphorylation leading to the accumulation of acetylcholine (ACh) at muscarinic, nicotinic, and central nervous system (CNS) receptors, resulting in cholinergic overstimu lation.
- Organophospates bind irreversibly with acetylcholinesterase receptors. This ACh esterase receptor and OP compound undergoes a conformational change, known as "aging," which renders the enzyme irreversibly resistant to reactivation by oximes.
- Unlike OP compounds, carbamates are transient reversible acetylcholinesterase inhibitors, which spontaneously hydrolyze from acetylcholinesterase site within 48 hours. Hence, carbamate toxicity tends to be of shorter duration than that caused by equivalent doses of organophosphates. However, the mortality rates are similar to OP compounds.
- Recovery follows the reappearance of active AChE following synthesis or spontaneous hydrolysis of phosphorylated AChE.

Clinical Features

Clinical features can be divided into following 3 phases:

- Acute cholinergic phase
- Intermediate syndrome (IMS)
- Organophosphate-induced delayed neuropathy (OPIDN).

Acute Cholinergic Phase

- This is due to acetylcholine excess at the synapses. Symptoms usually start within one hour of exposure.
- Features of cholinergic excess can be divided into muscarinic, nicotinic and CNS manifestations.

Muscarinic manifestations ("DUMBBELSS" Mnemonic)

- Diarrhea
- Urination
- Miosis
- Bronchorrhea, bronchospasm, bradycardia
- Emesis
- Lacrimation
- Salivation
- Sweating

Nicotinic manifestations

- Fasciculations.
- Muscle weakness and paralysis due to depolarizing block at neuromuscular junctions similar to succinylcholine.

CNS manifestations

- Anxiety, restlessness, unconsciousness, convulsions, respiratory depression.

Intermediate Syndrome (IMS)

- Intermediate syndrome (IMS) is a distinct clinical phase of organophosphate (OP) poisoning that occurs after the acute cholinergic crisis and before the onset of delayed neuropathy. It typically begins 1–4 days hours after exposure.
- The exact cause is unknown, but there are several postulations regarding the mechanism of intermediate syndrome: Persistence of nicotinic effects due to lack of early use of oximes; release of organophosphates from the adipose tissue acting on the nicotinic receptors; and neuromuscular junction dysfunction.
- Clinical manifestations of IMS are mainly neurological and are as follows:
  - Muscle weakness (symmetrical): Neck flexors, proximal limb muscles (especially lower limbs), respiratory muscles → can lead to respiratory failure.
  - Cranial nerve involvement: Facial weakness, dysphonia, dysarthria, dysphagia
  - Absent deep tendon reflexes
  - No muscarinic or nicotinic signs of cholinergic crisis at this point.

- Consciousness is preserved (unless hypoxia occurs).
- Paralysis may continue for 2–18 days. Recovery from IMS is complete with adequate ventilatory care unless OPIDN develops.

Organophosphate-induced Delayed Neuropathy (OPIDN)

- Organophosphate-induced delayed neuropathy (OPIDN) is a rare, distal, symmetric sensorimotor polyneuropathy, predominantly affecting the lower limbs due to certain lipophilic OP compounds. Agents like triorthocresyl phosphate (TOCP), malathion and chlorpyrifos are frequently associated with OPIDN. Carbamates are only rarely associated with OPIDN.
- OPIDN is caused by inhibition of neuropathy target esterase (NTE)—an enzyme critical for maintaining the integrity of long axons. Axonal degeneration occurs mainly in long motor neurons (especially in the lower limbs), and in spinal cord tracts (in severe cases).
- It usually occurs 7–21 days after exposure to OP compounds.
- Affected patients present with transient, painful "stocking-glove" paresthesias followed by a symmetrical motor polyneuropathy characterized by flaccid weakness of the lower limbs, which ascends to involve the upper limbs. Sensory loss is often mild. Recovery from OPIDN is usually incomplete. In severe cases, pyramidal tract signs (spasticity, Babinski) amy be seen.

Diagnosis

- History and examination findings
- Cholinesterase activity:
  - Plasma (pseudocholinesterase)–↓ within hours
  - RBC AChE–more specific, reflects neural inhibition
- Atropine challenge test—may support diagnosis
- Toxicology screening (rarely helpful acutely).

Management

Initial Stabilization

- Airway: Suction secretions; intubate if necessary.
- Breathing: Oxygen; ventilator support if required.
- Circulation: IV fluids if hypotensive.

Decontamination

- Further exposure is prevented by removing the contaminated clothing and washing skin thoroughly.
- Gastric lavage
- Activated charcoal
- Patient is admitted to ICU and vital parameters are continuously monitored.

Antidotes

- Atropine antagonizes the muscarinic effects of acetylcholine by blocking muscarinic receptors. Atropine does not reverse nicotinic effects such as muscle fasciculation. Initially 2–5 mg is given IV. If no effect is noted, the dose is doubled every 5–10 minutes until the muscarinic signs and symptoms are reversed. Atropine infusion is usually required for several days after the exposure. Signs of adequate atropinization are tachycardia, dilatation of pupils, and dryness of mucous membranes. Excess atropine causes agitation, confusion, urinary retention, ileus, and hyperthermia.
- Oximes such as pralidoxime (PAM) and obidoxime are cholinesterase reactivating agents and are effective in treating both muscarinic and nicotinic effects of OP compound. Dose of PAM is 2 g IV infusion over 30 minutes. Oximes are not needed for carbamate poisoning because carbamate–AChE binding is reversible and short-lived and hence the enzyme recovers spontaneously within a few hours.
- Intermediate syndrome is treated by ventilator support.
- There is no specific therapy for OPIDN. Regular physiotherapy may reduce deformities and muscle-wasting.

Q. Discuss the clinical features and management of sedative-hypnotic (benzodiazepines, barbiturates) overdose.

- Sedative-hypnotics are a class of CNS depressants commonly used to treat anxiety, insomnia, and seizures. The two most important groups in this class are:
  - Benzodiazepines (BZDs), e.g. diazepam, lorazepam, alprazolam
  - Barbiturates, e.g. phenobarbital, pentobarbital.
- Overdose of these agents can cause life-threatening CNS and respiratory depression, especially in combination with alcohol or opioids.

Mechanism of Action

- All the sedative-hypnotics are general CNS depressants. Most stimulate the activity of GABA, an inhibitory neurotransmitter in the CNS.

Clinical Features of Acute Intoxication

- Clinical features are mainly due to CNS depression and include the following:
  - Slurred speech
  - Incoordination and unsteady gait
  - Impaired attention or memory
  - Impaired consciousness ranging from stupor to coma
  - Nystagmus and decreased reflexes
  - Severe overdose may lead to respiratory depression.
- Psychiatric manifestations include inappropriate behavior, labile mood, and impaired judgment and social functioning
- Bradycardia and hypotension
- Bullous skin lesions may be seen in barbiturate poisoning in addition to above features. Additionally respiratory and CNS depression are common and more severe with barbiturate poisoning. Mortality also is high with barbiturates.

Investigations

- Complete blood count (CBC)
- Arterial blood gas (ABG)
- Blood glucose, electrolytes
- ECG
- Toxicology screen.

Management

General Measures

- Patient is admitted to ICU and vital parameters are continuously monitored
- Oxygen
- Gastric lavage is not advised in pure benzodiazepine overdose. However, it is required in mixed and other sedative hypnotic drug poisoning.
- Activated charcoal. Repeated doses are necessary in barbiturate poisoning.
- IV fluids
- Endotracheal intubation and ventilator support if required.

Specific Measures

- *Benzodiazepines*: Flumazenil is a benzodiazepine antagonist which can be used in acute benzodiazepine intoxication. The starting dose of flumazenil is 0.2 mg intravenously (IV) over 30 seconds. Further doses of 0.5 mg may be given every 60 seconds up to a total of 5 mg. It can provoke withdrawal seizures in patients with benzodiazepine dependence.
- *Barbiturates*: There is no specific antidote for barbiturates. Alkaline diuresis and hemodialysis are helpful in enhancing barbirurate removal.

Q. Aluminum and zinc phosphide poisoning.

- Aluminum phosphide (ALP) and zinc phosphide (ZnP) are highly toxic pesticides commonly used to protect grains from pests and rats. Ingestion of these agents can cause rapid, fatal systemic toxicity due to the release of phosphine gas (PH_3) in the stomach upon contact with water or acid.
- Aluminum phosphide is a solid fumigant pesticide available in tablet form (sometimes referred to as rice tablets). Zinc phosphide usually comes as a black powder.
- The following description applies to both aluminum and zinc phosphide.

Mechanism of Toxicity

- After ingestion, both aluminum and zinc phosphide reacts with water or acid in the stomach to release phosphine gas which has local as well as systemic toxicity.
- Local effects are severe burning retrosternal pain and vomiting. Systemic toxicity occurs after absorption from GI tract.
- Mechanism of systemic toxicity include cellular hypoxia due to the effect on mitochondria, inhibition of cytochrome C oxidase and formation of highly reactive hydroxyl radicals. This leads to multi-organ dysfunction.

Clinical Features

- Hypotension, cardiac failure due to myocarditis, acute kidney failure, liver cell necrosis, acute lung injury, gastrointestinal symptoms (nausea, vomiting, and diarrhea), and metabolic acidosis.
- Hypo or hypermagnesemia can occur.

Investigations

- ABG: Metabolic acidosis, hypoxia
- ECG: ST-T changes, conduction blocks, arrhythmias
- Chest X-ray: Pulmonary edema
- Electrolytes: Hypomagnesemia, hypokalemia
- Cardiac markers: Troponin, CK-MB (for myocarditis)
- LFT/RFT: Organ dysfunction
- Serum phosphine levels: Rarely available, mostly clinical diagnosis.

Management

- Gastric lavage with $KMnO_4$ (1:10000) or with magnesium sulfate ($MgSO_4$) to oxidize the unabsorbed poison. Gastric lavage with coconut oil has also been found to be helpful.
- Activated charcoal orally or through nasogastric tube to adsorb phosphine from the gastro intestinal tract.
- Antacids or H_2 blockers to reduce burning pain in the stomach and to reduce the absorption of phosphine.
- Magnesium sulfate ($MgSO_4$) is very effective in counteracting the toxic effects of aluminum phosphide. Magnesium has antihypoxic, antiarrhythmic, and antioxidant properties, hence is effective in reducing the morbidity and mortality of aluminum phosphide poisoning. Dose is 1 g IV stat, followed by 1 g every 8th hourly for 5–7 days.
- Sodium bicarbonate infusion can be given to correct metabolic acidosis.
- Mortality is high and most patients die despite optimal supportive care. Death usually from refractory shock or arrhythmia.

Q. Paracetamol (acetaminophen) poisoning.

- Paracetamol poisoning is common because of its wide availability as an over-the-counter drug.
- Maximum recommended daily dose is 4 g in adults.
- Toxicity is likely to occur at doses greater than 150 mg/kg per day (>7.5–10 g). Almost all patients who ingest >350 mg/kg develop severe liver toxicity.

Mechanism of Toxicity

- Paracetamol is metabolized by conjugation in the liver to nontoxic compounds. In acute overdose, metabolism by conjugation becomes saturated, and excess paracetamol is oxidatively metabolized by the CYP enzymes to the hepatotoxic metabolite, N-acetyl-p–benzoquinone imine (NAPQI) which causes hepatic injury.

Clinical Features

- Initial complaints are nausea, vomiting, diaphoresis, pallor, lethargy, and malaise.
- Liver damage usually develops 1–3 days after ingestion. Jaundice, hepatic encephalopathy, hyperammonemia, bleeding diathesis and marked elevation of liver enzymes (AST and ALT >1000 IU/L) develop.
- Rarely, renal failure and acute pancreatitis may occur.
- Confirmation of diagnosis and severity of poisoning can be assessed by measurement of serum paracetamol levels.

Investigations

- Serum paracetamol level (ideally between 4–24 hours post-ingestion)
- Liver function tests (AST, ALT, bilirubin)
- Prothrombin time (PT/INR)–to assess coagulation status
- Renal function—urea, creatinine
- ABG—for metabolic acidosis
- Glucose—hypoglycemia may occur
- Serum electrolytes.

Management

- Gastric lavage
- Activated charcoal
- The antidote is N-acetylcysteine (NAC), which is most effective if given within 10 hours of the overdose. NAC works through multiple routes. It prevents binding of NAPQI to hepatic macromolecules, acts as a substitute for glutathione, is a precursor for sulfate, and reduces NAPQI back to acetaminophen. It can be given either intravenously or orally.
  - IV NAC regimen (most common): 150 mg/kg over 1 hour → 50 mg/kg over 4 hours → 100 mg/kg over 16 hours (total 21 hours).
  - Oral NAC: 140 mg/kg loading dose, then 70 mg/kg every 4 hours × 17 doses (total 72 hours).
- Methionine 12 g orally 4th-hourly, to a total of four doses, is an alternative if NAC is not available. It acts as a glutathione precursor, helping replenish hepatic glutathione stores.
- Liver transplantation should be considered in patients who develop acute liver failure.

Q. Salicylate (aspirin) poisoning.

- Salicylate poisoning (commonly due to aspirin overdose) is a medical emergency. Aspirin is widely used as antiplatelet agent in patients with cardiovascular and cerebrovascular disease. Other salicylates, such as salicylic acid (a topical keratolytic agent and wart remover) and methyl salicylate (oil of Wintergreen), can also cause intoxication when ingested.
- Ingestion of greater than 150, 250 and 500 mg aspirin/kg body weight produces mild, moderate and severe poisoning respectively.

Mechanism of Toxicity

- Aspirin (acetylsalicylic acid) is rapidly converted to salicylic acid in the body.
- Salicylate directly stimulates medullary respiratory center and causes hyperventilation and respiratory alkalosis. As it is metabolized, it causes an uncoupling of oxidative phosphorylation in the mitochondria. This leads to anaerobic metabolism and increase in lactic acid levels resulting in metabolic acidosis. Hyperventilation worsens in an attempt to compensate for the metabolic acidosis. Eventually, the patient fatigues and is no longer able to compensate via hyperventilation, and metabolic acidosis prevails. This results in hemodynamic instability and end-organ damage.
- Other effects: Altered mental status, platelet dysfunction, and fluid and electrolyte imbalance.

Clinical Features

- Nausea and vomiting due to irritation of the gastric mucosa and stimulation of the chemoreceptor trigger zone.
- Tinnitus and deafness
- Hyperventilation due to direct stimulation of the respiratory center. Kussmaul's breathing (deep, rapid respirations) occurs due to metabolic acidosis.
- Petechiae and subconjunctival hemorrhages can occur due to reduced platelet aggregation.
- Renal failure and CNS effects such as agitation, confusion, coma and fits can occur in severe poisoning. Rarely, pulmonary and cerebral edema can occur.
- Death can occur as a consequence of CNS depression and cardiovascular collapse.
- Key points to remember: Tinnitus + hyperventilation + acidosis = Think of salicylate poisoning.

Investigations

- Plasma salicylate concentration helps in assessing the severity of poisoning
- Serum lactate level
- Serum electrolytes, including calcium and magnesium
- ABG
- LFTs
- CBC
- Coagulation studies
- ECG to evaluate for arrhythmias
- Consider a CT head if the patient has altered mental status.

Management

- Multiple doses of activated charcoal
- Intravenous fluid should be administered. 5% dextrose with 3 amps of sodium bicarbonate helps in correcting both dehydration and metabolic acidosis.
- Urinary alkalization enhances the clearance of salicylate. Give IV sodium bicarbonate to target urine pH to 7.5–8.

- Hemodialysis is very effective at removing salicylate and should be considered if there is cerebral or pulmonary edema, renal failure or serum salicylate concentration is >100 mg/dl.

Q. Cyanide poisoning.

- Cyanide is among the most rapidly lethal poisons known to man. It causes death within minutes to hours of exposure.
- Cyanide exists in gaseous (hydrogen cyanide), liquid, and solid (potassium cyanide) forms. Depending on its form, cyanide may cause toxicity through inhalation, ingestion, dermal absorption, or parenteral administration. Smoke inhalation, suicidal ingestion, and industrial exposures are the most frequent sources of cyanide poisoning. Inhalation of hydrocyanic acid or ingestion of inorganic cyanide salts or cyanide releasing substances such as cyanamide result in poisoning. Infusion of sodium nitroprusside used in hypertensive emergencies can also cause cyanide toxicity. Amigdal from bitter almonds also releases cyanide on digestion.

Mechanism of Toxicity

- Cyanide is a mitochondrial toxin. Cyanide binds to cytochrome C oxidase (complex IV) in the mitochondrial electron transport chain.
- This inhibits oxidative phosphorylation, blocking aerobic ATP production.
- Cells switch to anaerobic metabolism, causing lactic acidosis, hypoxia, and death—despite normal oxygen levels in the blood ("histotoxic hypoxia").
- Lethal dose: 50–60 mg of hydrogen cyanide (HCN) can be fatal within minutes. Inhalation or ingestion routes are especially dangerous.

Clinical Features

- There may be characteristic smell of bitter almonds.
- After inhaling cyanide, there is headache, anxiety, nausea, and a metallic taste. There may be eye and mucous membrane irritation, bronchorrhea, cough, and dyspnea.
- Ingestion of cyanide salts results in gastric irritation, causing vomiting and abdominal pain.
- Multi-organ failure: Renal failure, hepatic necrosis, pulmonary edema, rhabdomyolysis
- Hypotension, bradycardia, and arrhythmias
- Skin appears flushed and cherry-red due to non-utilization of oxygen by cells.
- Convulsions, coma and death occur within few hours.
- Cyanide poisoning should be differentiated from carbon monoxide poisoning which can present with similar features.
- Metabolic (lactic) acidosis
- Respiratory failure and death
- Classic triad (in severe cases): Altered mental status, severe lactic acidosis, bright red venous blood.

Investigations

Arterial and Venous Blood Gases

- Arterial oxygen tension is normal and venous oxygen tension is abnormally high due to nonutilization of oxygen by cells, resulting in a decreased arteriovenous oxygen difference (<10%). A high-anion-gap metabolic acidosis is seen due to lactic acidosis as a result of anaerobic metabolism.

Blood Lactate Level

- Elevated due to anaerobic metabolism. It is a sensitive marker for cyanide toxicity.

RBC or Plasma Cyanide Concentration

- The preferred test is red blood cell cyanide concentration. This test can be used for confirmation of cyanide poisoning, but results may not be available early to start treatment.

Methemoglobin Level

- Presence of methemoglobin in the blood is reassuring because it indicates that there is no free cyanide available for binding, because methemoglobin vigorously binds cyanide to form cyanomethemoglobin.
- Methemoglobin level can also be used a guide for the use of methemoglobin-inducing antidotes, such as sodium nitrite. Elevated level of methemoglobin (>10%) indicate that further nitrite therapy is not indicated.

Investigations

- Routines tests: Complete blood count, electrolytes, urinalysis, LFT, RFT.
- Carboxyhemoglobin level (if in a fire).
- ABG usually shows high anion gap metabolic acidosis. Venous PO_2 level is high.
- Serum lactate level is elevated.
- Plasma cyanide concentration level.
- Chest X-ray and ECG

Treatment

General Measures

- 100% oxygen via non-rebreather mask or intubation if needed
- Gastric lavage
- Activated charcoal
- IV sodium bicarbonate for severe metabolic acidosis.

Specific Antidotes

- Hydroxocobalamin, a precursor of vitamin B_{12}, contains a cobalt moiety which binds to cyanide, forming cyanocobalamin. This molecule is stable, with few side effects, and is easily excreted in the urine. Hydroxocobalamin is considered the first choice therapy for cyanide poisoning. It is given intravenously.

- Sodium thiosulfate: Acts as a sulfur donor, enhancing conversion of cyanide → thiocyanate (less toxic, excreted in urine). It is often given along with hydroxocobalamin or sodium nitrite.
- Sodium nitrite (alternative): Sodium nitrite is given intravenously. It induces methemoglobinemia, which binds to cyanide to form less toxic cyanomethemoglobin. Not preferred in hypoxic patients (e.g. fire victims) since it reduces oxygen delivery.
- Use of hyperbaric oxygen remains controversial.

Q. Methanol (methyl alcohol) poisoning.

- Methanol (wood alcohol) is used as a denaturant and is a component of varnishes, paint removers, windshield washers, copy-machine fluid, antifreeze solutions, and industrial solvents.
- Ingestion of methyl alcohol usually occurs with ingestion of cheap illicit liquor (*hooch*). The toxic dose is 30 ml of a 40% solution.

Mechanism of Toxicity

- Methanol itself is not very toxic except CNS depression.
- Toxicity is mainly due to its metabolites such as formaldehyde and formic acid which are produced by alcohol dehydrogenase in the liver.

Clinical Features

- Initial manifestations are due to methanol itself and include inebriation, gastritis, abdominal pain, nausea and vomiting. High dose causes obtundation, convulsions and coma.
- Late manifestations are due to formic acid and include retinal injury, metabolic acidosis, seizures, coma and death. Ocular toxicity manifests as diminished vision, flashing spots, dilated or fixed pupils, hyperemia of the optic disc, retinal edema and blindness.
- Classic triad of severe poisoning: Visual symptoms ("snowfield vision", blurred vision, blindness), high anion gap metabolic acidosis, and CNS depression (confusion, coma, seizures).

Investigations

- Serum methanol levels.
- Arterial blood gas (ABG) shows high anion gap metabolic acidosis.
- Renal function tests and liver function tests.
- CT scan of the brain shows bilateral putamen necrosis.

Management

General Measures

- Correction of acidosis by sodium bicarbonate infusion.
- Gastric lavage is useful if performed within 1 hour of ingestion. Activated charcoal is not useful.
- Control of seizures
- IV fluids.

Specific Measures

- *Fomepizole (preferred antidote):* Blocks alcohol dehydrogenase and prevents the formation of toxic metabolites.
- *Ethanol (alternative antidote):* If fomepizole is not available, ethanol is given to saturate alcohol dehydrogenase in the liver and prevent the formation of the toxic metabolites of methanol. Ethanol is given IV. Maintain serum level of 100–150 mg/dl.
- *Folic or folinic acid (adjunctive therapy):* Enhances conversion of formic acid to CO_2 and water.
- IV sodium bicarbonate to correct metabolic acidosis.
- Hemodialysis should be done if there is severe metabolic acidosis, or evidence of end-organ damage (e.g. visual changes, renal failure).

Q. Describe the clinical features, prognosis and management of and ethylene glycol poisoning.

- Ethylene glycol is a toxic alcohol commonly found in—antifreeze (de-icing solutions), brake fluids, and solvents
- It is odorless, colorless, sweet-tasting, and often ingested accidentally or intentionally.

Toxic Dose

- As little as 1 ml/kg can be fatal.
- Lethal dose ≈ 100 ml (in adults) if untreated.

Pathophysiology

- The toxicity of ethylene glycol is not due to itself but due to its metabolites.
- It is metabolized in the liver by alcohol dehydrogenase (ADH) into:
  - Glycolaldehyde
  - Glycolic acid
  - Glyoxylic acid
  - Oxalic acid → binds calcium → calcium oxalate crystals
- These metabolites lead to:
  - Metabolic acidosis (due to glycolic acid)
  - Renal failure (due to oxalate crystals in renal tubules)
  - Hypocalcemia (due to calcium oxalate formation).

Clinical Features

- Symptoms appear in three stages, within 6–72 hours.

Stage 1: Neurological phase (30 min–12 hours)

- CNS depression (like ethanol intoxication)
- Slurred speech, ataxia, confusion
- Seizures, coma in severe cases.

Stage 2: Cardiopulmonary phase (12–24 hours)

- Tachycardia, hypertension or hypotension
- Pulmonary edema, tachypnea
- Congestive heart failure.

Stage 3: Renal phase (24–72 hours)

- Flank pain
- Oliguria or anuria
- Acute tubular necrosis → acute renal failure
- Hypocalcemia—tetany, QT prolongation, seizures.

Investigations

- Arterial blood gas (ABG): High anion gap metabolic acidosis
- Serum osmolality: Increased
- Serum calcium: ↓ (due to oxalate binding)
- Urinalysis:
  - Calcium oxalate crystals (envelope or needle-shaped)
  - Fluorescence under UV light (if fluorescein is added to antifreeze)
- Serum ethylene glycol level (if available)
- Urea, creatinine—to assess renal function
- ECG: QT prolongation if hypocalcemic.

Management

Initial Stabilization

- ABCs (airway, breathing, circulation)
- IV fluids
- Correct hypoglycemia, electrolyte imbalances
- Seizure control, if needed.

Specific Antidotes

- Fomepizole (1st line): Inhibits alcohol dehydrogenase.
- Ethanol (if fomepizole unavailable): Competes with ethylene glycol for ADH. Requires ICU-level monitoring.

Adjunct Therapies

- Sodium bicarbonate—for metabolic acidosis.
- Thiamine (100 mg IV) and pyridoxine (50 mg IV)—Promote conversion of toxic metabolites to less harmful ones.

Hemodialysis

- Indicated if there is severe acidosis (pH <7.3), renal failure, ethylene glycol level >50 mg/dl, electrolyte disturbances unresponsive to treatment, and pulmonary edema or worsening symptoms.

Prognosis

- Good prognosis with early diagnosis and antidote use
- Poor outcomes if:
  - Treatment is delayed >12–24 hours
  - Severe renal failure, coma
  - Multiple organ failure
- Mortality rate is high without antidote or dialysis.

Q. Opioid/morphine poisoning.

- Opioids include heroin, morphine, methadone, codeine, pethidine, dihydrocodeine and dextropropoxyphene. Heroin (diacetylmorphine, diamorphine) is an artificial alkaloid derived from morphine, is the most dangerous drug of addiction.
- Opioids are commonly used as drugs of abuse. They give a rapid, intensely pleasurable experience, often accompanied by heightened sexual arousal. Physical dependence occurs within a few weeks of regular use.
- Overdose may occur due to therapeutic use, recreational use, intended self-harm, attempt to hide drugs from law enforcement agencies ("body stuffing"), swallowing packaged drugs in order to transport them across borders ("body packing"), and unintentional pediatric exposures.

Mechanism of Toxicity

- Opioids bind to μ (mu), κ (kappa), and δ (delta) receptors, mainly in the CNS and GI tract.
- Activation of μ-receptors leads to:
  - CNS depression
  - Respiratory depression
  - Miosis (pinpoint pupils)
  - Reduced gastrointestinal motility.

Investigations

- ABG: To assess respiratory acidosis/hypoxia
- Toxicology screen: Urine drug screen (detects morphine, heroin)
- ECG: Rule out cardiac arrhythmias or QT prolongation
- Chest X-ray: Evaluate for aspiration or pulmonary edema.

Clinical Features of Overdose

- The classic triad of opioid intoxication include:
  - CNS depression (drowsiness → coma).
  - Respiratory depression (slow, shallow or absent breathing).
  - Pinpoint pupils (miosis)—may dilate terminally due to hypoxia.
- There may be signs of intravenous drug abuse (e.g. needle track marks).
- Other features: Hypotension, bradycardia, hypothermia, cyanosis, decreased bowel sounds, pulmonary edema (especially with heroin), seizures (rare; more common with tramadol or meperidine).

Management

General Measures

- Maintenance of airway
- Supplementary high-flow oxygen
- Endotracheal intubation and ventilatory support if required.
- Gastric lavage and activated charcoal are usually not indicated because of risk of aspiration.

Specific Measures

- Naloxone is a specific opioid antagonist which reverses the features of opioid toxicity. It is given as IV bolus (0.8–2 mg) and repeated every 2 minutes until the level of consciousness and respiratory rate increase and the pupils dilate. This is followed by intravenous infusion of naloxone.
- May precipitate acute withdrawal in opioid-dependent individuals. Withdrawal symptoms can be managed by substitution with oral methadone.

Q. Enumerate the common plant poisons.

Common plant poisons are as follows:

- Poison hemlock
- Strychnos nux vomica
- Cannabis sativa
- Belladonna
- Datura
- Oleander
- Castor beans
- Abrus precatorius
- Argemone Mexicana
- Poisonous mushrooms.

Q. Oleander poisoning (cerbera thevetia; cerbera odollam; yellow oleander).

- This is an ornamental plant that is grown for its yellow bell-shaped flowers in the gardens of India.
- It contains highly toxic cardiac glycosides which are responsible for various heart blocks, brady-arrhythmias and tachy-arrhythmias.
- All parts of the plant contain toxin, but seeds have maximum amount.
- The roots and seeds are used as abortifacients, for suicidal and homicidal purposes and also as cattle poisons.

Clinical Features

- GI symptoms—dryness of the throat, vomiting, diarrhea.
- CNS effects—dizziness, dilated pupils, muscular weakness, tetanic convulsions.
- Cardiac effects—bradycardia, irregular pulse, heart blocks, cardiogenic shock.
- Death may occur from circulatory failure.

Diagnosis

- Clinical suspicion based on history and symptoms.
- ECG findings—sinus bradycardia, AV block, junctional rhythm, ventricular ectopics, bidirectional VT.
- Serum electrolytes—look for hyperkalemia.

Management

- Gastric lavage.
- Repeated doses of activated charcoal.
- Correction of acidosis, fluid and electrolyte disturbances.
- Atropine and pacing for bradycardia and heart blocks.
- Digoxin specific Fab antibodies can be used in severe poisoning.

Q. Datura poisoning.

- *Datura stramonium* (also known as thorn apple, angel's trumpet, Devil's trumpet, Devil's weed, etc.) is a common weed along roadsides, in cornfields and pastures and in waste areas. Its toxic components are tropane alkaloids (atropine, hyoscyamine, and scopolamine) which have potent anticholinergic action. It has been used voluntarily by teenagers for its hallucinogenic effect. Scopolamine, a muscarinic antagonist is thought to be mainly responsible for the toxic anticholinergic effects.
- The seeds and fruits are the most poisonous parts of the plant. 10–12 seeds or more can be fatal.
- Medicolegal Iiportance: Criminal use common (e.g. stupefying travelers). Suicidal or accidental ingestion (especially in children).

Clinical Features

- Datura produces anticholinergic syndrome.
- Skin: Flushed, hot, dry skin.
- Eyes: Dilated pupils, photophobia, blurred vision.
- Mouth: Dry mouth, thirst.
- CNS: Agitation, restlessness, confusion, hallucinations, delirium, seizures, coma.
- Initial symptoms are dry mouth and throat, burning pain in the stomach and difficulty in swallowing and talking.
- Heart: Tachycardia.
- GIT: Decreased bowel sounds.
- Genitourinary: Urinary retention.
- Death can occur from respiratory failure.
- Classically the effects of datura are described as "hot as a hare" (rise in skin temperature), "blind as a bat" (diplopia, loss of accommodation), "dry as a bone" (dryness of mouth, skin), "red as a beet" (cutaneous flushing) and "mad as a hatter" (delirium).

Management

- Gastric lavage.
- Activated charcoal.
- Cooling measures, if hyperthermic.
- Bladder catheterization if urinary retention occurs.
- Delirium is treated with sedatives.
- Cholinergic agents such as neostigmine, physostigmine or methacholine may be given to counteract anticholinergic effects of datura.

Q. Lead poisoning (plumbism).

- Lead poisoning, also known as plumbism, is a toxic condition resulting from the accumulation of lead in the body. It can affect multiple organ systems, particularly the hematopoietic, nervous, renal, and gastrointestinal systems. Both acute and chronic exposures may occur, but chronic low-level exposure is more common, especially in children.
- Lead exposure can occur in numerous work settings, such as manufacturing or use of batteries, solder, ammunitions, paint, car radiators, cable and wires, some cosmetics, ceramic ware with lead glazes, tin cans and lead pipes used in plumbing. Earlier lead was being added to gasoline and petrol to increase the octane level, but this practice has been discontinued and only unleaded fuel is available now. Lead is also found in some traditional Hispanic and Ayurvedic medicines. Lead-containing bullets lodged in the body can result in chronic lead toxicity.

Pathophysiology

- Lead is absorbed from the lungs or gastrointestinal tract. In adults, absorption of lead via the respiratory tract is the most significant route of entry. GI absorption can also be significant if working and/or eating in a lead-contaminated environment. GI absorption is the predominant route in children.
- Once absorbed, lead is distributed to the blood, soft tissues, and skeleton. In blood, 99% of lead is bound to the erythrocytes.
- Lead is a toxic metal that affects many organ systems and functions in humans. It inhibits sulfhydryl-dependent enzymes such as gamma-aminolevulinic acid dehydratase (ALA-D) and ferrochelatase which are important for heme synthesis. Causes microcytic hypochromic anemia with basophilic stippling of RBCs.
- Competes with calcium, accumulates in bone, and crosses the blood-brain barrier causing neurotoxicity.
- It also interferes with mitochondrial respiration and various nerve functions. Lead can also affect DNA and RNA. Lead has effects on cell membranes, interfering with various energy and transport systems.

Clinical Features

Acute Lead Poisoning

- Colicky abdominal pain, constipation, joint pains, muscle aches, headache, anorexia, decreased libido, difficulty concentrating and deficits in short-term memory, anemia, and nephropathy.
- Coma and convulsions may occur in severe poisoning.

Chronic Lead Poisoning

- ***Neurological:*** In children → developmental delay, behavioral issues, learning disabilities, encephalopathy. In adults → peripheral neuropathy (wrist drop, foot drop).
- ***Gastrointestinal:*** Abdominal pain, constipation, anorexia
- ***Hematologic:*** Anemia (microcytic), basophilic stippling.
- ***Renal:*** Interstitial nephritis.
- ***Reproductive:*** Infertility, miscarriage.
- ***Others:*** Lead lines on gums (Burton's line). Blue-black line at gingivodental junction. Lead lines in metaphyses on X-ray in children.

Diagnosis

- Blood lead levels: Whole blood lead levels above ≥5 µg/dl are diagnostic of lead poisoning. Level >10 µg/dl for extended period of time is associated with impaired neurobehavioral development in children. Level of >50 µg/dl may be associated with headache, irritability, subclinical neuropathy, colicky abdominal pain, etc. Level greater than 70 µg/dl is often associated with severe poisoning and acute encephalopathy.
- Peripheral blood smear: Microcytic hypochromic anemia with basophilic stippling.
- Elevated free erythrocyte protoporphyrin level is often inaccurate and is not used now.
- Urinary ALA (aminolevulinic acid) is increased.
- X-ray fluorescence is a new technology that can be used to make rapid, noninvasive measurements of lead in bone.

Treatment

- Maintain airway and treat coma and convulsions in severe poisoning.
- Avoid further exposure: If a large lead-containing object (e.g. fishing weight) has been ingested, it should be removed by repeated cathartics, whole bowel irrigation, endoscopy, or even surgical removal to prevent subacute lead poisoning. Workers with a single lead level greater than 60 µg/dl must be removed from the site of exposure.
- Chelation therapy: Patients with severe intoxication (encephalopathy or levels greater than 70 µg/dl) should receive dimercaprol (BAL). Calcium disodium EDTA can be used in addition to dimercaprol. An oral chelator, succimer (DMSA-dimercaptosuccinic acid) is available for use in children. Penicillamine is an alternative chelator (less commonly used now).

Prevention

- Ban on lead-based paints and gasoline
- Monitoring occupational exposure
- Public health surveillance in children (especially in high-risk areas).

Q. Arsenic poisoning.

- Arsenic is a metalloid element found in both organic and inorganic forms. The inorganic trivalent arsenic compounds (As^{3+}) are the most toxic. It is tasteless, odorless, and well absorbed after ingestion or inhalation.

Sources of Exposure

- Contaminated drinking water (especially in West Bengal, Bangladesh, Bihar)
- Occupational: Smelting, glass manufacturing, pesticide/insecticide factories
- Traditional medicines: Unregulated ayurvedic or homeopathic preparations
- Food: Rice, seafood (mostly organic arsenic, less toxic)
- Intentional poisoning: Homicide or suicide.

Mechanism of Toxicity

- Arsenic binds to sulfhydryl groups in enzymes → inhibits pyruvate dehydrogenase and other mitochondrial enzymes. This leads to disrupted energy system of the cell resulting in cell death.
- In exposed individuals, high concentrations of arsenic are present in bone, hair and nails.
- The primary target organs for arsenic toxicity are the gastrointestinal tract, skin, bone marrow, kidneys, and nervous system.

Clinical Features

Acute Poisoning

- Classic acute toxicity presents with gastroenteritis followed by hypotension.
- This can occur after ingestion or inhalation of arsenic dusts or fumes.
- Symptoms may develop within minutes or hours.
- Initially GI symptoms are seen and include nausea, vomiting, abdominal pain, and diarrhea. There may be a garlic odor of the breath and stool.
- These are followed by dehydration, hypotension, irregular pulse and cardiac instability.
- Acute encephalopathy may develop and lead to delirium, coma, and seizures.
- Renal injury can lead to proteinuria, hematuria, and acute tubular necrosis.
- In severe cases, shock, ARDS, and death may occur.
- If patients survive the initial illness, hepatitis, pancytopenia, and sensorimotor peripheral neuropathy may develop.

Chronic Poisoning

- Chronic arsenic exposure from drinking water has been reported in many parts of the world.
- Manifestations are peripheral neuropathy, skin eruptions, hepatotoxicity, bone marrow depression, and increased risk of cancers.
- Mee's lines (transverse white lines on finger nails) may be seen in some.

Investigations

- Urinary arsenic levels (preferred for recent exposure).
- Hair and nail analysis: For chronic exposure.
- Blood arsenic: Less useful due to rapid clearance from blood within hours. Only helpful in massive acute poisoning if taken very early. Not reliable for chronic poisoning.
- ECG, renal and liver function tests.
- Nerve conduction studies: For neuropathy.

Management

- Elimination of further exposure.
- Gastric lavage and activated charcoal in cases of ingestion.
- Chelation is indicated in patients with symptomatic arsenic poisoning. Dimercaprol (British anti-Lewisite, or BAL) and succimer (DMSA) are used as chelating agents.

Q. Enumerate the common corrosives. Describe their toxicology, clinical features, prognosis and approach to therapy.

- Corrosives are substances that cause tissue injury via chemical reaction. Common corrosive agents are as follows:

Common Corrosives

Acids
- Hydrochloric acid (toilet cleaner)
- Sulphuric acid (battery acid)
- Nitric acid
- Oxalic acid (bleaching agent, laundry cleaner)
- Carbolic acid (phenol)

Alkalis
- Sodium hydroxide (caustic soda)—drain cleaner
- Potassium hydroxide—soap industry
- Ammonia—cleaning agent
- Calcium hydroxide (lime)

Others
- Bleach (sodium hypochlorite)
- Hydrogen peroxide—antiseptic
- Formalin (formaldehyde solution)—used in laboratories
- Glacial acetic acid—used in pickling, labs

Toxicology

Corrosives cause coagulative necrosis (acids) or liquefactive necrosis (alkalis) of mucosal and deeper tissues, leading to:
- Protein denaturation.
- Cell membrane damage.
- Vascular thrombosis → tissue ischemia.
- Possible perforation of gastrointestinal tract.
- Systemic toxicity (especially with phenol, oxalic acid, or formalin).

Clinical Features

Local (immediately after ingestion or contact)

- Severe burning pain in mouth, throat, chest, abdomen.
- Drooling, dysphagia, odynophagia.
- Hoarseness, stridor, dyspnea if airway involved.
- Oral ulcers, white patches, burns on lips/tongue.
- Hematemesis, abdominal rigidity → suggests perforation.

Systemic Features

- Shock (due to fluid loss or perforation)
- Metabolic acidosis (especially with oxalic acid/ formalin)
- Renal failure (oxalic acid, phenol)
- Seizures, CNS depression (formalin, phenol).

Complications

- Oesophageal or gastric perforation
- Mediastinitis, peritonitis
- Strictures, especially of oesophagus (weeks later)
- Tracheoesophageal fistula
- Chronic dysphagia, malnutrition
- Increased risk of carcinoma esophagus (long-term).

Prognosis

- Depends on quantity, concentration, and time of exposure.

- Poor prognosis if:
  - There is shock or acidosis
  - Perforation is present
  - Delayed presentation (>24 hours)
- Children and suicidal adults are at higher risk for complications.

Investigations

- CBC, electrolytes, ABG.
- Chest and abdominal X-ray → look for perforation.
- Upper GI endoscopy within 12–24 hours to assess burn severity (NOT if perforation suspected).

Management

- Airway: Secure if stridor or airway edema
- Breathing, Circulation: IV fluids, O_2, manage shock
- Keep NPO (nil by mouth) strictly
- Avoid inducing vomiting or gastric lavage (risk of perforation). Also avoid giving activated charcoal as it is ineffective and obscures endoscopy.
- Proton pump inhibitors (PPIs) IV
- Antibiotics (if infection suspected or perforation)
- Nutritional support—parenteral or via feeding tube
- Surgical Intervention: For perforation, peritonitis, necrosis. Later strictures may need dilatation or surgical reconstruction.

Q. Classify poisonous snakes. Discuss the clinical manifestations, diagnosis and management of snake bites.

- Snake bite is a common life-threatening condition worldwide, especially in tropical countries. Farmers, hunters and rice-pickers are at particular risk of snake bite.
- More than 5 million poisonous snake bites occur annually worldwide, with >125,000 deaths. Regions with the highest incidence of venomous snakebites and snakebite deaths include Southeast and South Asia (e.g. India, Pakistan, Sri Lanka, and Bangladesh), sub-Saharan Africa, and Latin America. Nearly 40% of bites by venomous snakes do not produce signs of envenomation. The peak seasonal incidence is usually during the monsoon. Most of the bites occur in the evening, after sunset, when snakes come out for feeding. Nearly 75% of snake bites occur in outdoor and in rural settings. Males are bitten twice as often as females. Most frequent site of bite are lower limbs.

Major Families of Poisonous Snakes

Family	Main toxic effect
Elapidae: Cobras, kraits, mambas, coral snakes	Neurotoxic
Viperidae: Vipers and pit vipers	Severe local reaction, coagulation defects, renal failure
Hydrophidae: Sea snakes	Myotoxic
Colubridae: Boomslang	Mostly nonpoisonous. Some are mildly poisonous (e.g. boomslang)

Composition of Snake Venoms

Snake venoms are complex mixtures of enzymes, polypeptides, glycoproteins, and metal ions. Most snake venoms have multisystem effects. Major components are as follows:

- Hemorrhagins—cause vascular leakage and bleeding
- Procoagulants—activate clotting factors and cause consumptive coagulopathy
- Proteolytic enzymes—cause local tissue necrosis, coagulation defects, and organ damage
- Cardiotoxins—myocarditis, reduce cardiac output
- Neurotoxins—act at peripheral neuromuscular junctions and inhibit nerve impulses
- Myotoxins—local tissue necrosis, rhabdomyolysis.

Differentiating Venomous from Non-venomous Snakes

See **Table 17.4.**

Clinical Features of Venomous Snake Bite

- Snake bite victims usually develop anxiety and fear. This may lead to hyperventilation which causes paresthesia, and carpopedal spasm. Some may develop syncope, vasovagal shock and may even collapse. Clinical presentation of snakebite varies depending on the type of snake bitten, age of the patient, the area bitten, and the amount of poison injected.

Local Manifestations

- It manifests as pain, tenderness, paresthesia at local site followed by swelling of bitten limb. Entire limb with adjacent trunk can get involved. Severe local reaction leads to local tissue necrosis and bullae formation. Local bleeding and ecchymotic patches may develop due to hemostatic defects. Severe limb pain, absence of arterial pulse and cold limb suggest compartment syndrome (due to rise in the pressure of facial compartments which block the arteries) and may lead to ischemia and gangrene of the limb. Other complications like secondary infections, tetanus and gas gangrene may also develop.

Neurotoxicity

- Neurotoxic features are prominently seen with elapidae bites (cobra, krait, coral snakes). Features start within 6 hours but may be delayed.
- Paralysis first appears as bilateral ptosis followed sequentially by bilateral ophthalmoplegia, paralysis of muscles of palate, jaw, tongue, larynx, neck and muscles of deglutition. Pupillary reflexes are preserved till late stages. Diaphragm paralysis causes respiratory failure. Patients may become drowsy which may progress to coma. Neurotoxic effects are completely reversible, either spontaneously over several days or weeks, or immediately with antisnake venom and anticholinesterases (neostigmine).

Cardiotoxicity

- Features include tachycardia, hypotension, and ECG changes. Myocarditis can lead to congestive cardiac failure. Myocardial infarction and sudden cardiac arrest may occur.

TABLE 17.4: Differentiating venomous from nonvenomous snakes

Character	Venomous	Nonvenomous
Teeth	In upper jaw two fangs are present which are modified teeth 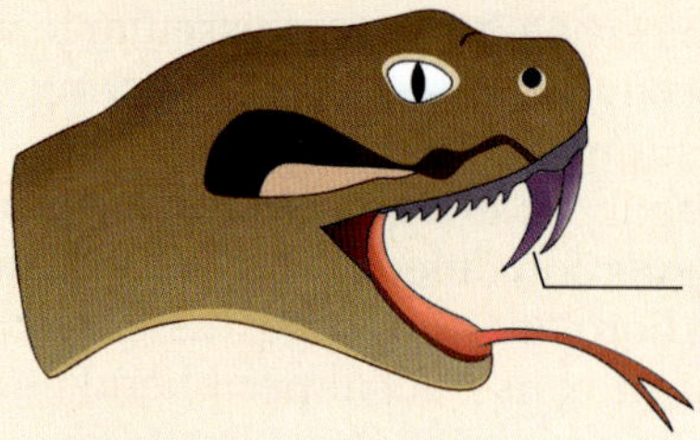 	All the teeth in the upper jaw are uniform and no fangs present 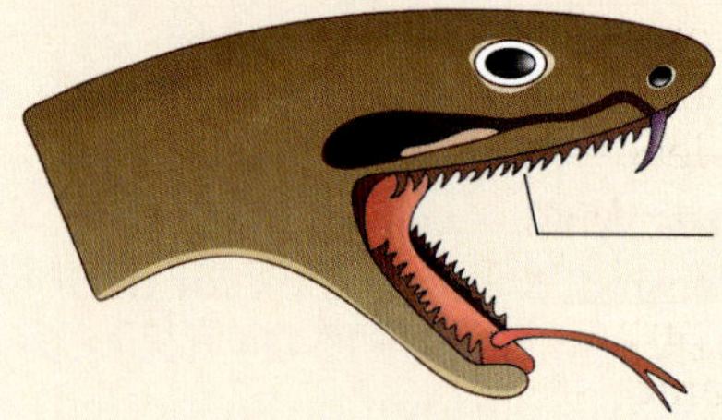
Snake bite mark	1 or 2 puncture on the skin by fangs 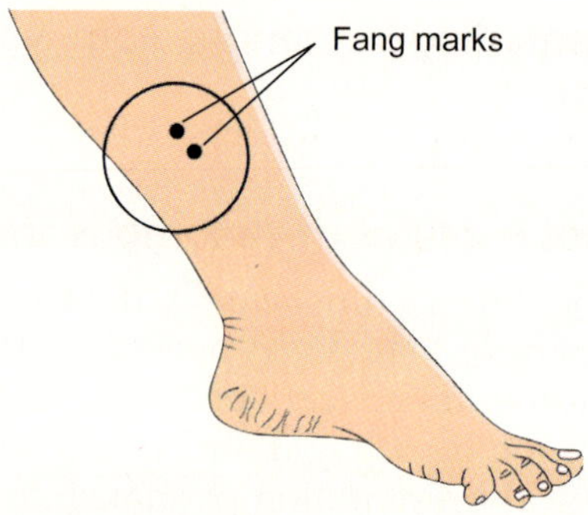 	Many punctures made by maxillary teeth but no fang marks 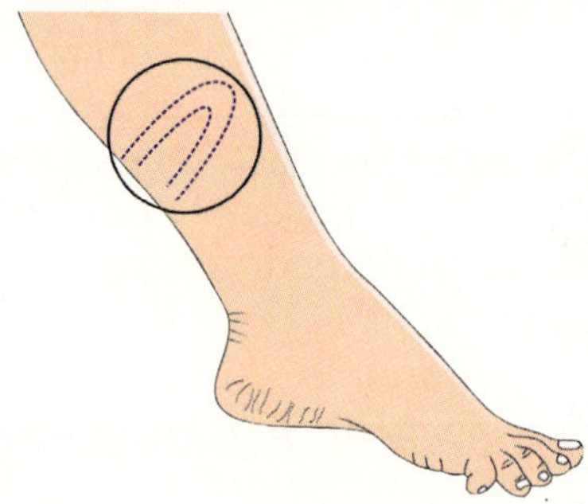
Pupil shape	Vertical slit like 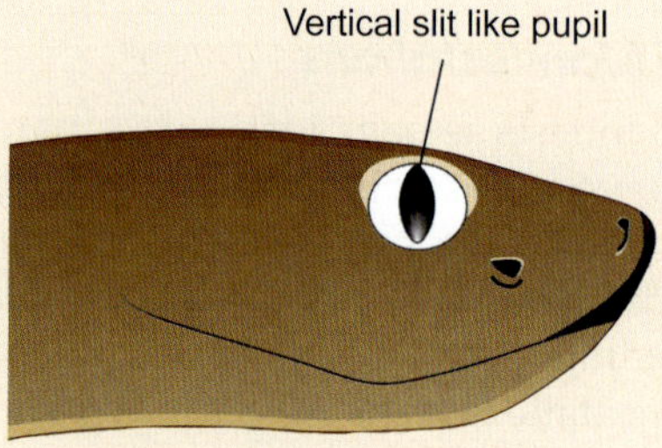 	Round 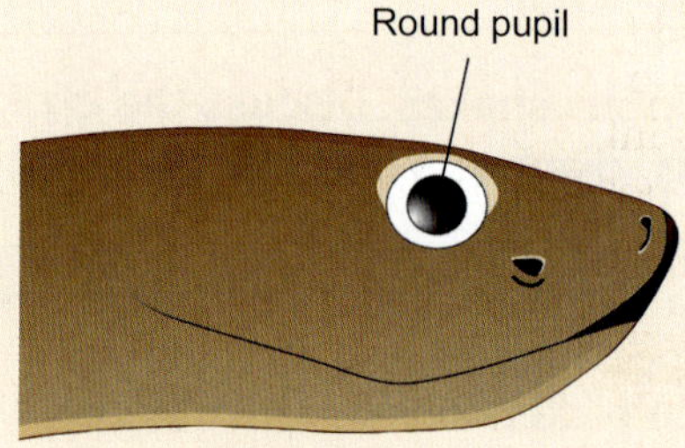
Head	Triangular and broad 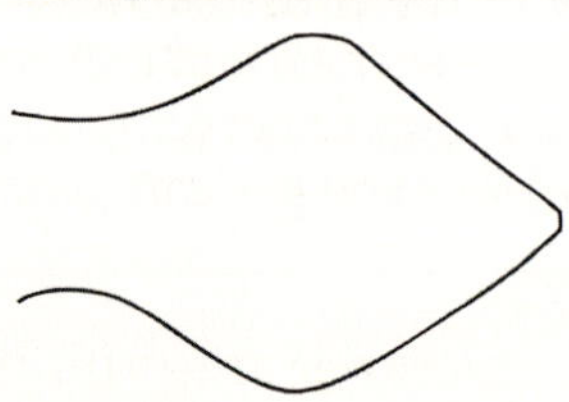	Elongated and oval 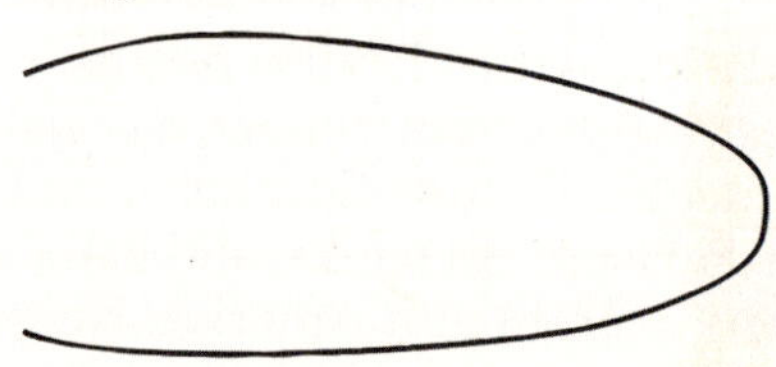
Tail	Often abruptly tapering	Tapers gradually
Belly scales	Large and cover the belly region completely 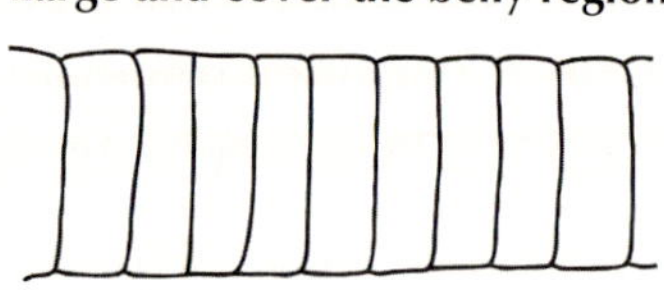	Small or large but not cover the belly region completely 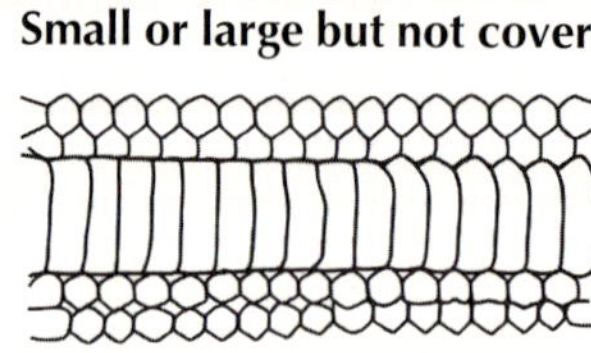
Heat sensing pits	Present in some (e.g. vipers, pit vipers)	Absent
Head scales	Small, irregular scales on top of head	Often have large, symmetrical head scales
Dorsal scales	Smaller (hexagonal in krait)	Large, not in hexagonal shape
Anal scale	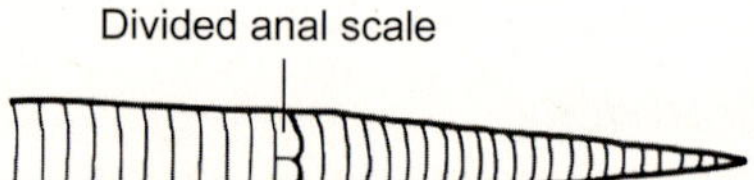 	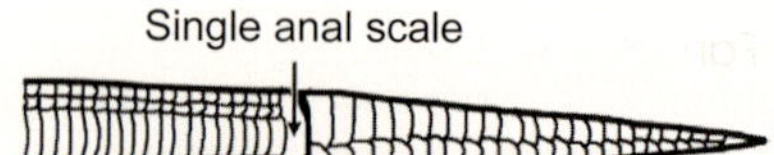
Color of snake	Bright color	Not bright (but some nonvenomous snakes such as python, sand boa, etc. are also brightly colored)

Hemostatic Abnormalities

- These are due hemorrhagins and consumption coagulopathy (DIC). Manifestations include bleeding from wound site, gums, nose and venipuncture site. Ecchymoses and bruising are common in the bitten limb. Hemoptysis, hematemesis, hematuria, and intracranial hemorrhage can also occur. Severe bleeding may lead to hypotension and shock. DIC with multiorgan dysfunction including ARDS can occur. Infarction of the anterior pituitary may occur causing acute pituitary adrenal insufficiency or, in survivors, chronic panhypopituitarism.

Nephrotoxicity

- Acute kidney injury commonly occurs in viper bites.

Myotoxicity

- Manifestations are generalized muscle pain, stiffness and myoglobinuria. Rhabdomyolysis is a prominent feature of sea snake bites.

Snake Bite without Envenomation (dry bites)

- This can happen when a person is bitten by a non-poisonous snake, or when a poisonous snake fails to inject poison. If a poisonous snake has bitten a prey prior to biting a person, then the poison would have been injected into the prey and hence, there will not be poison injection into the person **(Fig. 17.1)**. Similarly, when the snake bites into bony areas such as shin, or heel, there is little venom deposited because of the absence of adequate tissue space to accommodate the poison.

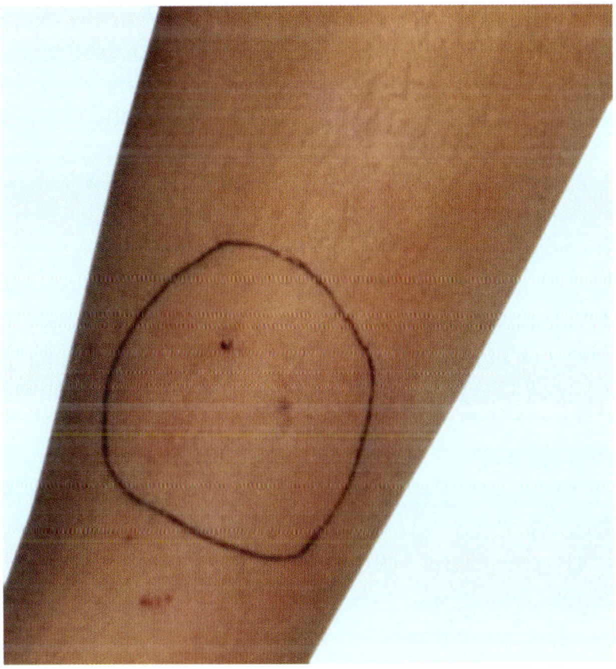

Figure 17.1: Fang marks in venomous snake bite

Investigations

- Snake venom detection kits are available in some countries. The venom is detected from a dry swab of the bite site using monoclonal antibody techniques.
- 20-minute whole blood-clotting test: 2–3 ml of venous blood is kept undisturbed in a bottle for at least 20 minutes. Absent coagulation indicates hemostatic defect from systemic envenomation.
- PT and aPTT may be elevated.
- Full blood count: Anemia may be present due to bleeding. Total WBC is elevated.
- Urea and creatinine may be elevated due to AKI.
- Electrolytes: Hyperkalemia may be present due to renal failure, hemolysis and rhabdomyolysis.
- Liver function tests may be altered.
- Creatine kinase may be high due to rhabdomyolysis.
- Troponins may be elevated due to myocardial damage.
- Blood grouping, typing and cross-matching as both venom and ASV can interfere with cross-matching.
- Urine examination may show RBCs, RBC casts, protein and myoglobin.
- ECG may show arrhythmias or changes due to electrolyte abnormalities.

Management of Snake Bite

Field Management

- Apply a splint to the bitten limb to immobilize it. Immobilization reduces the spread of poison.
- Application of pressure bandage: It limits the spread of poison, but concentrates the poison locally leading to greater local tissue damage and increased risk of amputation and loss of function, particularly with necrotic venoms such as viper venom. Pressure bandage can be used in Elapid bites which are primarily neurotoxic without much local effect. Pressure bandage is applied by wrapping the entire limb with a bandage (e.g. crepe or elastic). The wrap pressure must reach 40–70 mm Hg to be effective.
- Application of tourniquet is not recommended as most of the time it is not applied properly.
- Incision, cauterization and sucking out of venom are not recommended as they are not effective in removing poison and lead to more bleeding and local tissue damage.
- Transport the victim to a hospital as early as possible.
- The best first aid advice, as coined by Dr. Ian Simpson of the WHO's snakebite treatment group, is to "do it 'RIGHT'": **R**eassure the victim, **I**mmobilize the extremity, **G**et to the **H**ospital, and inform the physician of **T**elltale symptoms and signs.

Hospital Management

- Blood pressure, heart rate, respiration, coagulation, renal, and neurological status must be monitored.
- Administration of anti-snake venom (ASV)–this is the most important step. ASV should be given as soon as possible. ASV is most effective if given within 4 hours of bite, but can be given upto 24 hours or longer. Beneficial effects are reported even upto 7–10 days.
- ASV may be monovalent (effective against a particular snake species) or polyvalent (effective against several species).

Indications for antivenom

Evidence of systemic envenomation

- Neurotoxicity
- Coagulopathy
- Rhabdomyolysis
- Persistent hypotension
- Renal failure

Evidence of severe local envenomation

- Local tissue destruction
- Swelling
- Pain

Dosage of ASV

- Local reaction only at the site of bite—5 vials
- Local reaction with severe cellulitis: 5–15 vials
- Severe reactions with systemic envenomation: 15–30 vials.
- The recommended initial dose is 8–10 vials of polyvalent ASV diluted in 500 ml NS given as IV infusion over 1 hour. Can be repeated every 6 hours if no improvement. Maximum up to 20 vials initially; but more can be given in severe cases.
- Test dose is not recommended anymore for ASV. Monitor for anaphylaxis: wheeze, rash, hypotension. Treat with adrenaline 0.5 mg IM, antihistamines, corticosteroids if there is any allergic reaction to ASV.
- The newest available antivenom in the United States (CroFab) is an ovine, Fab fragment antivenom which is effective against all North American pit vipers. It requires less dosing and carries very low risk of allergic reactions.

Supportive measures

- IV fluids for hypotension and shock.
- Inj tetanus toxoid 0.5cc IM if not given in the last 5 years.
- Antibiotics: Gram-negative and anaerobic organisms should be covered. Augmentin plus metronidazole may be used intravenously. Antibiotics are not required routinely. They are required if there is significant local tissue damage with risk of infection.
- Fresh blood or FFP transfusion if bleeding manifestations occur.
- If neuromuscular paralysis is present. Neostigmine 1 mg IV stat plus atropine 1 mg IV should be given. It is repeated every half hourly and then taperd to hourly, 2nd hourly, and 4th hourly. It is most useful when there is respiratory muscle weakness pending ventilatory support and ASV administration.
- Artificial ventilation for respiratory paralysis.
- Surgical debridement for local necrosis and skin grafting.

Q. Scorpion stings.

- Scorpion stings are a common medical emergency in tropical and subtropical regions, including India. While many scorpion stings cause only local symptoms, some species (notably Mesobuthus tamulus in India) can cause severe systemic toxicity, especially in children.
- More than 80 species of scorpions are seen in India. Most important are black scorpions and red scorpions. Red scorpion is the most dangerous type. Stings occur most commonly at night, on the extremities.
- Scorpion venoms contain neurotoxins which stimulate synaptic sodium and potassium channels with release of catecholamines and acetylcholine.

Pathophysiology

- Scorpion venom is a neurotoxin that affects voltage-gated ion channels (mainly Na^+ and K^+).
- It causes massive release of catecholamines (adrenaline, noradrenaline) → "autonomic storm".
- In severe cases, myocarditis, pulmonary edema, and cardiogenic shock can occur.

Clinical Features

Local Features

- Most scorpion bites produce only local features.
- Severe local pain radiating throughout the affected dermatome.
- Swelling.

Systemic Features

- Red scorpion bites can cause severe systemic envenomation.
- Symptoms are due to cholinergic and adrenergic stimulation.
- Cholinergic symptoms include vomiting, increased gastrointestinal motility, profuse sweating, hypersalivation, pupillary constriction, bronchoconstriction, increased secretion of lacrimal, bronchial and pancreatic acinar glands, bradycardia, hypotension and priapism.
- Adrenergic features are hypertension, tachycardia, heart failure and pulmonary edema. Intracranial hemorrhage and convulsions may occur due to severe hypertension.
- In later stages, hypotension and shock may develop.
- ECG may show features of myocarditis or ischemia.
- Urinary excretion of vanillyl mandelic acid (VMA) is increased and cardiac enzymes are elevated.

Investigations

- ECG may show tachycardia, ST-T changes, arrhythmias.
- CXR may show pulmonary edema.
- Echocardiography (if myocarditis suspected).
- Serum electrolytes, cardiac enzymes.

Treatment

- Reassurance, rest, elevation of affected limb.
- Ice packs for pain relief.
- Severe local pain is treated by injection of local anaesthetic (0.1% lignocaine). Systemic analgesics (NSAIDs and opiates) may be needed.

- Hypertension and pulmonary edema are treated by selective alpha-1 adrenergic blockers such as prazosin. Prazosin reduces sympathetic overactivity and improves cardiac function.
- Dobutamine or milrinone for cardiogenic shock.
- Avoid beta blockers (may worsen condition).
- Hypotension may require fluid resuscitation.

Q. Bee Sting.

- Bee stings are common and typically cause mild local reactions, but in some individuals, especially those with allergies, they can lead to life-threatening anaphylaxis.

Toxin and Pathophysiology

- Bee venom contains:
  - Melittin (causes pain, inflammation)
  - Phospholipase A2 (cell membrane damage)
  - Hyaluronidase (spreads venom)
  - Histamine and kinins (vasodilation, allergic response).
- Venom causes:
  - Local inflammation
  - In allergic individuals: IgE-mediated hypersensitivity → anaphylaxis
  - Multiple stings: direct toxic effects (rhabdomyolysis, hemolysis, renal failure).

Clinical Features

Local Reaction

- Pain, redness, swelling, itching at sting site. Usually resolves in a few hours
- Extensive swelling involving the entire limb may develop over 24–48 hours, which lasts up to a week.

Systemic Allergic Reaction (anaphylaxis)

- Occurs within minutes
- Urticaria, angioedema
- Bronchospasm, wheezing, dyspnea
- Hypotension, shock
- Nausea, vomiting, abdominal pain
- May lead to collapse or death if untreated.

Toxic Reaction (multiple stings)

- Hemolysis
- Rhabdomyolysis
- Acute kidney injury
- Liver dysfunction
- Myocarditis.

Investigations (in severe/systemic cases)

- CBC, renal function, liver enzymes, electrolytes
- CPK (for rhabdomyolysis)
- Urinalysis (myoglobinuria)
- ECG, chest X-ray if cardiopulmonary involvement.

Management

Local Reaction

- Remove stinger (scrape, do not pinch)
- Wash area with soap and water
- Cold compress
- Oral antihistamines (e.g. cetirizine)
- Analgesics (e.g. paracetamol).

Anaphylaxis (medical emergency)

- IM Adrenaline (epinephrine): 0.5 mg in adults, 0.01 mg/kg in children, repeat every 5–15 min as needed.
- Oxygen, IV fluids
- Antihistamines, e.g. chlorpheniramine
- Steroids, e.g. hydrocortisone or methylprednisolone
- Beta-agonist nebulisation for bronchospasm (e.g. salbutamol).

Toxic Reaction

- Supportive care.
- IV fluids, renal protection.
- Dialysis if needed.

Q. Enumerate the causes of hyperthermia (hyperpyrexia).

- Hyperthermia is a condition in which the body's core temperature rises above the normal range (usually >38.5–39°C), not due to fever, but because of failed heat regulation mechanisms.

- Environmental exposure (heat stroke, working or exercising in hot, humid conditions)
- Cerebral and pontine hemorrhage
- Tetanus
- Thyroid storm
- Pheochromocytoma
- Malignant hyperthermia
- Neuroleptic malignant syndrome
- Catatonia
- Status epilepticus
- Alcohol, sedative-hypnotic withdrawal
- Drug overdose (sympathomimetics, anticholinergics)
- Dystonic reactions
- Serotonin syndrome

Q. Enumerate various heat related illnesses and the predisposing factors.

- Heat-related illnesses occur due to prolonged exposure to high environmental temperature, often worsened by humidity, exertion, and dehydration. They range from mild to life-threatening conditions. Various heat related illnesses are:
  - Heat edema: Mild swelling of hands, feet, ankles due to vasodilation and salt imbalance.
  - Heat syncope
  - Heat cramps
  - Heat exhaustion
  - Heat stroke (heat injury).

Predisposing Factors for Heat Related Illnesses

- High temperature
- High humidity
- Dehydration
- Elderly persons and infants
- Heavy exercise, particularly in the sun
- Heavy clothing
- Decreased sweating
- Associated Infection
- Obesity
- Alcohol withdrawal
- Mental illness
- Hyperthyroidism
- Drugs (anticholinergics, phenothiazines)

Q. Heat syncope

- This is sudden fainting due to cutaneous vasodilation in a hot weather leading to cerebral hypoperfusion. Often occurs after standing or exertion in heat. Skin is cool and moist, and there is weak pulse and hypotension.
- They are often seen in athletes, outdoor workers, soldiers, and laborers. Treatment consists of rest and recumbency in a cool place and fluid and electrolyte rehydration by mouth (or intravenously if necessary).

Q. Heat cramps

- Heat cramps are painful, involuntary muscle spasms that occur during or after vigorous physical activity in hot environments, typically due to loss of sodium and water through sweating.
- Blood shows hemoconcentration and reduced sodium and chloride concentration.
- Treatment involves moving the person to a cool environment and giving oral saline solution (4 tsp of salt per gallon of water) to replace both salt and water. For severe cramps 0.5–1 liter of normal saline is administered intravenously.
- It can be prevented by liberal salt intake.

Q. Heat exhaustion.

- Heat exhaustion is a moderate-to-severe heat-related illness caused by prolonged exposure to high temperatures, leading to fluid and electrolyte loss, dehydration, and inadequate cardiovascular response.
- If untreated, it can progress to heat stroke, a life-threatening emergency.

Pathophysiology

- In hot environments, the body tries to cool down via sweating and vasodilation.
- Prolonged sweating leads to fluid and salt loss, reducing plasma volume.
- This impairs cardiac output and tissue perfusion, causing hypovolemia and circulatory collapse.
- Core body temperature is usually <40°C, unlike heat stroke.
- Thermoregulation and CNS function are not impaired.

Clinical Features

- Temperature is elevated but <40°C
- Weakness, fatigue, malaise
- Features of dehydration such as dryness of tongue and mouth, excessive thirst, tachycardia, hypotension, oliguria and weakness.
- Nausea, vomiting, abdominal cramps
- Tachypnea may lead to tetany
- Irritability and incoordination may be present. Death may occur due to hypovolemic shock.

Investigations

- Elevation of the blood urea, sodium and hematocrit due to water depletion.
- Sodium level may be low in salt depletion type heat exhaustion due to water replacement without salt.

Treatment

- Removal of the patient from the heat
- Active cooling using cool sponging
- Fluid and salt replacement using oral rehydration mixtures containing both salt and water or intravenous isotonic saline. Hypertonic (3%) saline may be needed for severe hyponatremia.

Q. Heat stroke.

Heat stroke is a life-threatening medical emergency characterized by:

- Core body temperature ≥40°C (104°F)
- Central nervous system dysfunction (e.g. confusion, seizures, coma)
- Caused by failure of thermoregulatory mechanisms during prolonged exposure to high environmental temperature or exertion.

Pathophysiology

- Excessive heat production or impaired heat dissipation leads to hyperthermia.
- This results in:
  - Direct cellular injury.
  - Protein denaturation.
  - Endothelial damage, causing DIC and rhabdomyolysis.
  - Multiorgan dysfunction (MODS), including liver, kidneys, brain.

Clinical Features

There are two types of heat stroke; exertional and non-exertional (classic):

- Exertional heat stroke occurs in healthy individuals who engage in heavy exercise during high ambient temperature and humidity. Typical patients are athletes and military recruits in basic training.
- Nonexertional (classic) heat stroke occurs in individuals with an underlying disorder such as mental illness, hyperthyroidism, obesity, extremes of age, and use of drugs.

- Clinical features are due to shock, renal and liver damage, involvement of CNS and DIC.
- Rectal temperature is 40°C or more.
- Initial manifestations are faintness, dizziness, vertigo, nausea, and abdominal pain.
- CNS manifestations are altered sensorium, seizures and coma.
- Skin is flushed, hot and dry.
- Jaundice and petechiae may be present.
- Tachypnea, and bibasal lung crepitations may be present due to ARDS.
- Excessive bleeding may occur due to DIC.
- Death may occur due to ARDS, DIC, myocardial infarction and acute adrenal insufficiency.

Laboratory Features

- Investigations show hemoconcentration, leukocytosis, elevated urea and creatinine, proteinuria, coagulopathy and DIC, elevated liver enzymes, respiratory alkalosis and metabolic acidosis. Myoglobinuria may be present due to rhabdomyolysis.
- ECG may show non-specific ST depression and T wave inversion.

Treatment

- 100% oxygen
- Endotracheal intubation and ventilatory support if required.
- Reduction of body temperature
  - Augmentation of evaporative cooling is the treatment of choice because it is effective, noninvasive, and easily performed. The naked patient is sprayed with cool water and air is circulated with large fans.
  - Other cooling methods are immersing the patient in an ice-water tub (most rapid method of cooling), covering with water cooled sheets, keeping ice bags over of the body, intravenous or intraperitoneal administration of cool fluid, and gastric lavage or enema with ice-water.
- Hydrocortisone or dexamethasone injection IV 8 hourly helps to correct shock, cerebral edema and adrenal insufficiency.
- Renal failure may require hemodialysis.

Q. Neuroleptic malignant syndrome (NMS).

- Neuroleptic malignant syndrome (NMS) is a life-threatening medical emergency associated with the use of neuroleptic agents such as phenothiazines, butyrophenones and thioxanthines.
- It usually develops during the first two weeks of neuroleptic therapy. It is not a dose-dependent phenomenon, but is an idiosyncratic reaction.

Pathophysiology

- Caused by central dopamine receptor blockade, particularly in the hypothalamus, nigrostriatal pathways, and spinal cord.
- This leads to:
  - Thermoregulatory failure
  - Excessive muscle contraction
  - Autonomic dysfunction
  - Potential rhabdomyolysis and multi-organ failure.

Clinical Features

- NMS is characterized by mental status change, muscular rigidity, hyperthermia, and dysautonomia. The diagnosis should be suspected if any two of these four features appear in the setting of neuroleptic use.
- Mental status changes are delirium with confusion which may evolve to stupor and coma.
- Muscular rigidity is generalized. It can be lead pipe or cogwheel type rigidity. Other motor abnormalities include tremors, dystonia, opisthotonus, trismus, chorea, and other dyskinesias.
- Autonomic instability manifests as tachycardia, labile or high blood pressure, tachypnea, arrhythmias, and increased sweating.

Differential Diagnosis

- Malignant hyperthermia: Almost clinically indistinguishable from NMS, but the history of exposure to depolarizing muscle relaxants such as succinylcholine can help differentiate it from NMS.
- Serotonin syndrome: It has similar presentation to NMS but serotonin syndrome has prominent gastrointestinal manifestations. H/o use of SSRI is another important clue.
- Malignant catatonia: This has increased positive symptoms as compared to NMS and a behavioral prodrome of automatisms, agitation, or psychosis.
- Heat stroke.
- CNS infections (encephalitis, meningitis).

Laboratory Features

- Leukocytosis
- Elevated creatine kinase (CK) and hyperkalemia due to rhabdomyolysis
- Elevated liver enzymes
- Myoglobinuria and acute renal failure.

Treatment

- Admit to ICU
- Withhold neuroleptics
- Supportive measures
- Temperature should be lowered by external and internal cooling methods.
- **Dantrolene** (muscle relaxant) and **bromocriptine** (dopamine agonist; reverses dopamine blockade) may be considered in severe cases.

Q. Define hypothermia. Discuss the causes, clinical features and management of hypothermia.

- Hypothermia is defined as core body temperature below 35°C. Either rectal or esophageal temperature should be measured, as oral temperature is inaccurate.

Predisposing Factors for Hypothermia

- Elderly persons and infants
- Alcoholics
- Cold weather
- Immersion in cold water
- Mental retardation
- Malnutrition
- Stroke
- Cardiovascular disease.
- Hypothyroidism
- Hypopituitarism
- Addison's disease
- Transfusion of large amounts of refrigerated blood.
- Drugs: sedatives, phenothiazines

Clinical Features

- Core body temperature is below 35°C.
- Early manifestations are weakness, drowsiness, lethargy, irritability, confusion, shivering, and impaired coordination.
- Below 30°C there is cessation of all cerebral activity. Pulse and respiration become slow.
- Below 27°C, patient becomes unconscious, and deeply comatose at 25°C. Pulse and BP may be unobtainable, leading clinicians to believe that the patient is dead.
- Skin may appear blue or puffy.
- Other features are pulmonary edema, sluggish reflexes and generalized rigidity.
- Metabolic acidosis, pneumonia, pancreatitis, ventricular fibrillation, hypoglycemia or hyperglycemia, coagulopathy, and renal failure may occur.
- Death is usually due to cardiac asystole or ventricular fibrillation.

Investigations

- Hemoconcentration
- Hyperkalamia
- Arterial blood gas (ABG) analysis may show low PaO_2 and metabolic acidosis.
- ECG may show characteristic J waves of Osborn (positive deflection in the terminal portion of the QRS complex) and prolongation of the PR, QRS, and QT intervals.
- SGOT and CK may be elevated due to muscle damage.
- Thyroid function tests.
- Serum amylase may be elevated due to pancreatitis.
- If the cause of hypothermia is not obvious, additional tests may be done to identify any predisposing condition.

Management

- Goals of treatment are to rewarm the patient in a controlled manner and to treat the associated abnormalities.
- Any underlying condition should be treated promptly (e.g. hypothyroidism).
- Patient should be put in a warm room, and given additional thermal insulation (blankets and/or space film blanket). They should be given warm drinks. Core temperature will rise slowly over a few hours as a result of normal metabolic heat production.
- In severe hypothermia (core temperature <32°C), active external or internal rewarming methods are used to raise the core body temperature.
- Active external rewarming methods include heated blankets, forced hot air, radiant heat, and warm baths.
- Active internal rewarming methods include extracorporeal blood rewarming (method of choice), peritoneal or hemodialysis using warm dialysate fluid, administration of warm IV fluids, administration of heated, humidified air warmed to 42°C through a face mask or endotracheal tube, and gastric lavage with warm fluid.

Q. Discuss briefly the various cold related illnesses.

- Cold-related illnesses are medical conditions resulting from exposure to low environmental temperatures, and include both systemic hypothermia (discussed previously) and localized cold injuries.
- Various cold related illnesses are:
  - Hypothermia (discussed previously).
  - Localized cold injuries: Frostbite (freezing cold injury), trench or immersion foot (nonfreezing cold injury), and chilblains.

Frostbite (freezing cold injury)

- Frostbite is freezing injury of skin and underlying tissues due to exposure to sub-zero temperatures. It usually affects the exposed parts of the body such as fingers, toes, ears and face. It usually occurs in mountaineers, soldiers, those who work in the cold, the homeless, and individuals stranded outdoors in the winter.
- Tissue destruction occurs due to formation of ice crystals and subsequent inflammatory process.
- Predisposing factors are same as those listed under hypothermia.

Clinical Features

- Frostbitten tissue is initially pale and doughy to the touch and insensitive to pain. Once frozen, the tissue is hard.
- Other features are edema, hemorrhages, blisters and blebs.
- Local gangrene may occur.

Treatment

- Rewarming: This is done by immersing the affected area in a waterbath heated to 40–42°C. Higher temperatures may result in burns. Rubbing and direct heat should be avoided as they may exacerbate tissue injury. Thawing is usually complete in 15–30 minutes. Rewarming of frostbitten tissue is painful, hence, analgesics, generally opioids, should be administered.

- Tetanus prophylaxis, protection of the injured tissue and avoidance of infection.
- Because frostbite is associated with vascular thrombosis of the affected tissue, intravenous heparin along with thrombolytics (tPA) may improve outcome and prevent future amputation.
- Surgery may be required to remove dead tissue, but should be delayed, as surprisingly good recovery may occur over an extended period.

Nonfreezing Cold Injury

Trench or Immersion Foot

- This is soft tissue injury from prolonged exposure to cold and wet conditions above freezing temperatures (usually less than 10°C). Foot is commonly affected. Trench foot got its name during the first world war when many British and American soldiers developed the condition after spending long periods of time in the cold, wet trenches on the front line.
- Initial symptoms are cold and numbness, but there is no freezing of the tissue. Later manifestations are edema, blistering, swelling, redness, ecchymoses, hemorrhage, necrosis, peripheral nerve injury, or gangrene and secondary complications such as lymphangitis, cellulitis, and thrombophlebitis.
- Treatment involves gradual rewarming and recovery is usually complete. Tetanus prophylaxis is required.

Chilblains (pernio)

- Chilblains, also called perniosis, are an inflammatory skin condition related to an abnormal vascular response to the cold without actual freezing of the tissues. Pernio is most common in young women, but both sexes and all age groups may be affected.
- It typically presents as tender, pruritic red or bluish lesions located symmetrically on the dorsal aspect of the fingers, toes, ears and nose. Lesions usually resolve spontaneously.
- Treatment involves slow and passive rewarming of the affected part. Prazosin or nifedipine are useful for treatment and prevention of recurrence.

Q. Drowning.

- Drowning is defined as a process of experiencing respiratory impairment from submersion/immersion in a liquid medium. Drowning can lead to death, morbidity, or no morbidity. Terms like wet drowning, dry drowning and near-drowning are no longer accepted although they are still in use. Dry drowning refers to death due to intense laryngospasm without water entering the lungs.
- Fatal drowning: Death due to submersion.
- Nonfatal drowning: Survival after submersion (with or without complications).
- Drowning is a common cause of accidental death throughout the world and is particularly common in young children.
- Drowning is more common in males and during summer months.

Conditions that Increase Risk of Drowning/ Submersion Injury

- Suicide
- Use of alcohol or other sedative drugs
- Extreme fatigue
- Hyperventilation
- Sudden acute illness (e.g. hypoglycemia, seizure, arrhythmia, myocardial infarction)
- Muscle cramps while swimming
- Acute brain or spinal cord injury
- Venomous stings, bites, or injury in the water.

Pathogenesis

- Inhalation of water into the lungs leads to diffuse pulmonary edema, ARDS, ventilation-perfusion mismatching and intrapulmonary shunting, leading to hypoxemia. Hypoxemia causes diffuse organ dysfunction. CNS and heart are the two major organs which suffer hypoxic damage leading to death.
- Fresh water is hypotonic, and if absorbed into circulation in large amounts, may lead to hemolysis. Sea water is hypertonic and draws plasma into the alveoli leading to alveolar edema.
- Both salt water and fresh water wash out surfactant, leading to alveolar collapse and ventilation perfusion mismatching.
- Prolonged immersion in cold water may lead to hypothermia.
- Survival is possible after immersion for periods of up to 30 minutes in very cold water particularly in children.

Clinical Features

- Patients are often unconscious with absent breathing and may be in shock. Patients usually have anxiety, dyspnea, cough, wheezing, trismus, cyanosis, chest pain, arrhythmia, hypotension, vomiting, and diarrhea. A pink froth from the mouth and nose indicates pulmonary edema.
- *RS*—breathlessness, crepitations, and wheezing due to pulmonary edema and ARDS. Hemoptysis may occur due to alveolar damage.
- *Nervous system*—patients are in altered sensorium or unconscious due to cerebral hypoxia. Neuronal damage may lead to cerebral edema and raised ICT.
- *CVS*—hypothermia and hypoxemia can lead to arrhythmias. Sinus bradycardia and atrial fibrillation are common. Ventricular fibrillation or asystole may rarely occur.
- *Renal*—renal failure due to acute tubular necrosis may occur due to hypoxia, shock, hemoglobinuria, or myoglobinuria.

Laboratory Features

- Chest X-ray may show pulmonary edema or ARDS
- ABG shows hypoxemia
- ECG may show arrhythmias
- Metabolic acidosis may be present.

- Hypernatremia may occur due to absorption of swallowed seawater.

Management

- Cardiopulmonary resuscitation if pulse and respiration absent. Basic life support (BLS) protocol to be followed.
- Administration of oxygen.
- Airway should be cleared of foreign bodies. There is no need to try to drain the lungs of water since most inhaled water would have been absorbed.
- Intubation and ventilator support may be required for those unable to maintain oxygen saturation even after oxygen supplementation. Continuous positive airways pressure (CPAP) is useful in improving arterial oxygenation for spontaneously breathing patients.
- Cardiovascular support: Central venous pressure must be monitored to determine the intravascular volume status. Fluid overload and pulmonary edema should be treated with diuretics. Inotropic agents such as dopamine or noradrenaline should be used for persistent hypotension in spite of adequate intravascular volume.
- Prophylactic antibiotics are required only if drowning took place in contaminated water.

Q. Hanging.

- Hanging is a form of strangulation that involves suspension by the neck. Hanging can be complete or incomplete. In complete hanging, feet do not touch the ground and the entire weight of the victim is suspended at the neck. In incomplete hanging (partial hanging), some part of the body is touching the ground and the weight of the victim is not fully supported by the neck. Hanging may be suicidal, homicidal, accidental, or judicial.

Pathophysiology

- The following mechanisms are responsible for morbidity and mortality seen in cases of hanging.
- Fracture of the upper cervical spine (fracture of C_2 in the classic hangman fracture), and transection of the spinal cord. This is especially seen in judicial hanging where the body is dropped from a height. Partial injury to the spinal cord can also occur.
- Venous and arterial (carotids) obstruction, leading to cerebral edema, hypoxia, and unconsciousness, which in turn produces loss of muscle tone and airway obstruction.
- Vagal collapse, caused by pressure to the carotid sinuses and increased parasympathetic tone.

Clinical Features in Survivors (near hanging)

- Cough, stridor, muffled voice, respiratory distress and hypoxia may be present
- Altered mental status
- Abrasions, lacerations, contusions, edema and ligature mark may be observed on the neck.
- Subconjunctival hemorrhage and petechial spots may be seen in the head and neck area (Tardieu spots).
- Tenderness over the larynx may be present and indicates laryngeal fracture

Investigations

- Routine tests
- ABG analysis
- X-ray of cervical spine, anteroposterior and lateral view It may show fracture of cervical spine. X-ray should be taken after stabilizing the neck with hard collar.
- Chest X-ray
- CT or MRI of cervical spine provides details of spine and spinal cord injury.

Management

Prehospital Care

- C-spine stabilization and airway assessment are of paramount importance.
- Avoid endotracheal intubation in the field unless the airway is acutely compromised in view of possible C-spine fracture. Intubation is indicated if respiratory failure or airway obstruction is present.

In the Hospital

- Take care of airway and breathing. Endotracheal intubation and ventilator support is given for respiratory failure after ruling out C-spine injury. Cricothyroidotomy is performed if endotracheal intubation fails.
- Monitor the patient for cardiac arrhythmias.
- Mannitol is used to treat cerebral edema.
- Phenytoin is given IV to prevent hanging-induced seizures.
- Methylprednisolone 30 mg/kg IV bolus followed by infusion at a dose of 5.4 mg/kg/hour for next 23 hours is given if there is spinal cord injury, because it has been shown to prevent secondary cord damage due to edema and inflammation and improve final functional outcome.

Q. Electric shock/lightening injury.

- Electric shock is injury or death caused by the passage of electric current through the body.
- Lightning injury is a type of natural high-voltage electrical injury caused by a discharge of atmospheric electricity (lightning strike).
- Electric current is two types; alternating and direct current. Alternating current is more dangerous than direct current as the former can cause tetanic spasms which hook the victim to the source of current.
- Electrical injuries are almost always accidental and generally preventable.

Mechanism of Injury

- Injuries due to electricity occur by three mechanisms: (1) Direct effect of electrical current on body tissues; (2) Conversion of electrical energy to thermal energy, resulting in deep and superficial burns; (3) Blunt mechanical injury from lightning strike, muscle contraction, or as a complication of a fall after electrocution.

- The major determinant of injury is the amount of current flowing through the body. In addition, the type and extent of injury also depend on the voltage, resistance, type of current (AC or DC), the current pathway, and duration of contact. Voltage as low as 50 volts can be dangerous. The higher the voltage, the more the danger of cardiopulmonary arrest.
- Injuries can be generally divided into high voltage (>1000 volts) and low voltage (<1000 volts) injuries. Voltage in high-tension power lines is greater than 100,000 volts, while domestic voltage is 110–220 volts. Lightning strikes have a voltage of >10 million volts.
- Tissues with higher resistance have a tendency to heat up and coagulate, rather than transmit electric current. Skin, bone, and fat have high resistances, while nerves and blood vessels have lower resistances.
- DC current tends to cause a single muscle spasm that throws the victim from the source. This results in a shorter duration of exposure, but a higher likelihood of associated trauma. In contrast, AC repetitively stimulates muscle contraction. Often, the site of exposure is at the hand and, because the flexors of the arm are stronger than the extensors, the victim may actually grasp the source, prolonging the duration of contact and perpetuating tissue injury.

Clinical Features

- If the current passes through the heart or brainstem, death may be immediate due to ventricular fibrillation, asystole, or apnea.
- CVS: Cardiopulmonary arrest can be caused by low-voltage electric injury but is more common with high-voltage electric injury. Various cardiac arrhythmias can occur immediately or later and patients should undergo continuous ECG monitoring for at least 48 hours after electric injury. Vascular injury can result from a compartment syndrome or the electrical coagulation of small blood vessels.
- *Skin and internal organ burns*: Superficial, partial thickness, and full thickness thermal burns can occur following electrical injury. Burns occur due to exposure to electrical arc, clothes catching fire and the heating effect of electricity. Deep burns in the internal organs can occur along the path of current flow. Seemingly minor surface burns may coexist with massive muscle coagulation and necrosis as well as internal organ injury.
- *Nervous system*: Damage to both the central and peripheral nervous systems can occur after electrical injury. Manifestations include loss of consciousness, weakness or paralysis, respiratory depression, autonomic dysfunction, and memory disturbances. Current traversing peripheral nerves can cause acute or delayed neuropathy.
- *Renal*: Myoglobinuria due to rhabdomyolysis may lead to renal failure. Hypovolemia due to extravascular extravasation of fluid can also lead to prerenal azotemia and acute tubular necrosis.
- *GIT*: Direct liver injury, focal pancreatic and gall-bladder necrosis, and intestinal perforation have been reported, but are rare. Intestinal perforation may lead to infection, sepsis, and death.
- *Musculoskeletal*: Rhabdomyolysis is common after electrical injuries. It may lead to hyperkalemia, myoglobinuria and renal failure. Damaged muscles may swell and lead to compartment syndrome which may require fasciotomy. Since, bone has the highest resistance to electricity, it generates large amount of heat, resulting in periosteal burns, destruction of bone matrix, and osteonecrosis. In addition, bones can fracture from falls, blast injuries, or repetitive tetanic muscle contractions.
- *Eye*: Cataracts, hyphema, and vitreous hemorrhage may occur.
- *Ears*: Ruptured eardrums, sensorineural hearing loss, tinnitus, vertigo, and injury to the facial nerve may occur especially after lightening strike.

Investigations

- Cardiac monitoring and ECG
- Complete blood count
- Electrolytes
- Renal function tests, LFT
- Serum CK, and CK-MB
- Urinalysis, urine myoglobin.

Treatment

- Immediate removal of the patient from the electrical source. The rescuer must be protected. Turn off the power, sever the wire with a dry wooden-handled axe, or separate the victim using nonconductive objects such as dry clothing.
- Cardiopulmonary resuscitation
- All patients must undergo ECG monitoring in an ICU for 48 hours.
- IV fluids are required if there are extensive burns and wounds. If there is myoglobinuria, urine output should be maintained at more than 100 ml/hour to minimize intratubular cast formation and renal failure.
- Burns are treated in a similar manner to other thermal burns. Patients may require transfer to a burn unit, fasciotomy, escharotomy, and extensive skin reconstruction.
- Deep tissue damage due to high-voltage injury calls for surgical exploration for assessment of muscle function, and debridement of necrotic tissues to reduce the risk of infection and hyperkalemia. Extensive damage to muscles, nerves, tendons and vessels may call for amputation at a suitable level.
- If there is any evidence of injury to the abdominal organs, exploratory laparotomy may be required.
- Ophthalmologic examination is required to detect development of cataracts, particularly following

lightning injury. Cataracts generally develop several days after injury.

- Physical therapy to maintain functional status.
- Psychiatric consultation for any behavioral disturbances or posttraumatic stress disorder.

Q. High altitude illness.

Q. Acute mountain sickness.

- High altitude illness (HAI) refers to a group of clinical syndromes that occur when individuals ascend to high elevations too rapidly, typically above 2,500 meters (8,200 feet).
- Exposure to high altitude occurs during air travel and mountaineering. The barometric pressure falls as altitude increases. As a result, the higher one climbs, the lower the barometric pressure and the partial pressure of ambient oxygen. For example, on the summit of Mount Everest, barometric pressure is 253 mm Hg and the ambient oxygen tension is only 53 mm Hg. Reduction in oxygen tension results in a fall in arterial oxygen saturation. Acclimatization to hypoxemia at high altitude involves a shift in this dissociation curve (dependent on 2,3-DPG), erythropoiesis, polycythemia, and hyperventilation due to hypoxia. These changes take a few days to occur.
- Ascent to altitudes up to 2500 meters or travel in a pressurized aircraft cabin is harmless to healthy people. Above 2500 meters high-altitude illnesses may occur in healthy people, and above 3500 meters. They become common.
- Illnesses occurring at high altitude include the following.
  - Acute mountain sickness
  - High altitude periodic breathing of sleep
  - High altitude pulmonary edema
  - High altitude cerebral edema
  - High altitude retinal hemorrhage.
- In addition to the above, sudden ascent to altitudes above 6000 meters may result in decompression illness with the same clinical features as seen in divers. Rapid ascent to altitudes above 7000 meters may result in loss of consciousness.

Acute Mountain Sickness (AMS)

Cause

- Cerebral hypoxia → vasodilation → mild cerebral edema → headache and symptoms.
- Sleep disturbances due to periodic breathing.

Clinical Features

- Symptoms occur within 6–12 hours of an ascent.
- Symptoms include headache, fatigue, anorexia, nausea and vomiting, difficulty sleeping and dizziness. Ataxia and peripheral edema may also occur.

Treatment

- Most effective treatment is descent to a lower altitude.
- For mild cases, rest and simple analgesia are enough.
- For severe cases, acetazolamide, a carbonic anhydrase inhibitor can be used. It induces metabolic acidosis and stimulates ventilation leading to CO_2 wash out, which causes cerebral vasoconstriction and decreases intracranial pressure. Corticosteroids, diuretics and mannitol are also useful to decrease raised intracranial pressure.
- Acetazolamide may also be used as prophylaxis if a rapid ascent is planned.

Q. Low altitude illness/decompression sickness (Caisson's disease).

- Decompression sickness occurs when rapid pressure reduction (e.g. during ascent from a dive, exit from a caisson or hyperbaric chamber, or ascent to altitude) causes gas previously dissolved in blood or tissues to form bubbles and cause organ dysfunction.
- Decompression sickness is commonly seen among scuba divers.

Pathophysiology

- Ambient pressure under water increases by 1 atmosphere for every 10 meters of seawater depth. As the diver descends and breathes air under increased pressure, the tissues become loaded with increased quantities of nitrogen. As the diver ascends to the surface, there is liberation of free nitrogen gas from the tissues in the form of bubbles. The liberated gas bubbles can cause organ dysfunction by blocking blood vessels, rupturing or compressing tissue, or activating clotting and inflammatory cascades.

Clinical Features

- Symptoms usually occur during or within 4 hours of a dive.
- *General*—tender lymph nodes, edema, headache, nausea, vomiting, fatigue, general malaise.
- *Musculoskeletal*—osteonecrosis, pain in joints due to gas bubble formation.
- *Nervous system*—confusion, visual disturbances, weakness, paralysis, dizziness, paresthesias, aphasia, and coma.
- *RS*—gas embolism may lead to chest pain, cough, hemoptysis, dyspnea.
- *Skin*—itching, erythematous rash.
- *Audiovestibular*—ear and sinus barotrauma may lead to deafness, vertigo, tinnitus, nystagmus.

Management

- Patient is kept in horizontal position.
- Continuous administration of 100% oxygen or hyperbaric oxygen if available. This increases the washout of excess inert gas (nitrogen) and reduces tissue hypoxia due to gas embolism.
- Recompression, in a recompression chamber facility as soon as possible.
- IV fluids to correct the intravascular fluid loss from endothelial bubble injury and the dehydration associated with immersion.

- NSAIDs may be given for pain, but narcotics should be avoided.

Q. Bioterrorism.

- Bioterrorism is terrorism by intentional release or dissemination of biological (bacteria, viruses, or toxins) to cause illness or death in people, animals, or plants for political, religious, or ideological purposes.
- These agents may be in a naturally-occurring or in a human-modified form.
- Biological agents can be spread through the air, water, food or objects. Terrorists may use biological agents because they can be extremely difficult to detect and do not cause illness for several hours to several days.
- Bioterrorism is an attractive weapon because biological agents are relatively easy and inexpensive to obtain or produce, can be easily disseminated, and can cause widespread fear and panic beyond the actual physical damage they can cause. However, bioterrorism has some important limitations; it is difficult to employ a bioweapon in a way that only the enemy is affected and not friendly forces.

History of Bioterrorism

- Bioterrorism dates as far back as ancient Roman civilization, where feces was thrown into faces of enemies. In 14th century bubonic plague was used to infiltrate enemy cities. Over time, biological warfare became more complex. Countries began to develop weapons which were much more effective, and much less likely to cause infection to the wrong party.
- Recently anthrax became a weapon of choice because it is easily transferred, has a high mortality rate, and could be easily obtained. In 1993, a religious group Aum Shinrikyo released Anthrax in Tokyo. The attack was a total failure, infecting not a single person. In 2001 anthrax attacks, several cases of anthrax broke out in the United States. Letters laced with infectious anthrax were delivered to news media offices and the U.S Congress. The letters killed 5. Tests on the anthrax strand used in the attack pointed to a domestic source, possibly from the biological weapons program.

Agents Used in Bioterrorism

- Anthrax, smallpox, botulinum toxin, bubonic plague, brucellosis, glanders, *Vibrio cholerae*, viral hemorrhagic fever and tularemia.

Prevention and Preparedness

- Government agencies which would be called on to respond to a bioterrorism incident would include law enforcement, hazardous materials/decontamination units and emergency medical units.
- Medical profession must maintain a high index of suspicion especially when there are unusual clinical presentations or the clustering of cases of a rare disease.
- Many countries are creating specially trained forces to deal with bioterrorism.
- Laboratories are working on advanced detection systems to provide early warning, identify contaminated areas and populations at risk, and to facilitate prompt treatment. Forensic technologies are working on identifying biological agents, their geographical origins and/or their initial son.
- Some of the detection methods are: Tiny electronic chips that would contain living nerve cells to warn of the presence of bacterial toxins (identification of broad range toxins), fiber-optic tubes lined with antibodies coupled to light-emitting molecules (identification of specific pathogens, such as anthrax, botulinum, ricin), ultraviolet avalanche photodiodes detect anthrax and other bioterrorism agents in the air.
- In the United States, a Strategic National Stockpile (SNS) has been created by the CDC to provide rapid access to quantities of pharmaceuticals, antidotes, vaccines, and other medical supplies that may be of value in the event of biologic or chemical terrorism.

Management of Bioterrorism

- *Surveillance*: If an attack can be detected early, potential victims can be protected with prophylactic medicines or vaccines, and new cases can receive proper medical treatment. Enhanced surveillance should include ERs, primary care physicians, laboratories, pharmacists, and emergency response systems.
- *Public health response*: State and local health departments should work along with law enforcement agencies.
- *Confirmation/diagnostic testing*: Confirmation of the etiologic agent is important for planning preventive and treatment plans.
- *Decontamination*: It involves removal of clothing and personal effects, placing all items in plastic bags, and shower using copious quantities of soap and water. These items should be disposed appropriately or kept as evidence in a criminal trial or returned to the owner if the threat is unsubstantiated. Regular soap and water were as effective as antimicrobial soap and 2% chlorhexidine gluconate after contact with *B. anthracis*. For incidents involving possibly contaminated letters, the environment in direct contact with the letter or its contents should be decontaminated with a 0.5% hypochlorite solution.
- *Prophylaxis*: Chemoprophylaxis should be given to all exposed persons if appropriate. Vaccines are useful in control of a smallpox epidemic and prevention of a global pandemic. Postexposure prophylaxis against anthrax (along with antibiotics), protection of laboratory and health care providers working with these agents are also additional preventive measures.
- *Infection control*: This is done by isolation of infected patients, etc. Patients infected with smallpox require aerosol and contact precautions, while those with pneumonic plague require droplet precautions.
- *Specific treatment*: This involves specific antimicrobial drugs, antitoxins, antidotes and vaccines. If the agent is unknown, symptomatic treatment and treatment of

coexisting injuries should follow standard guidelines. If the etiologic agent is known, then specific treatment should be instituted against that agent.

- *Psychological support*: Panic among public should be allayed by assurance and educating the public about disease course and outcome.

Q. Describe the medico legal aspects of suspected suicidal or homicidal poisoning.

- The medicolegal aspects of suspected suicidal or homicidal poisoning are crucial because such cases often involve intent, criminal liability, and mandatory legal obligations for medical practitioners.
- Following are the medicolegal aspects of suspected suicidal or homicidal poisoning.

Mandatory Reporting to Authorities

- Under Section 39 CrPC (Code of Criminal Procedure) and various state laws:
    - Any suspected case of suicidal, homicidal, or criminal poisoning must be immediately reported to the nearest police station
    - This is a legal duty of the attending physician or hospital.

Medicolegal Case (MLC) Registration

- All cases of poisoning with suspicious intent should be registered as an MLC at the time of admission.
- Details must be recorded:
    - Patient identity
    - Alleged history
    - Circumstances (e.g. found unconscious, substance found nearby).

Proper Documentation

- Detailed medical records must be maintained:
    - Time of admission
    - Symptoms, vital signs
    - Clinical findings and treatment given
    - Statement of the patient (if conscious) about the incident
    - Names of people accompanying the patient
- Document all interventions clearly (antidotes, lavage, etc.)

Dying Declaration (if applicable)

- If patient is conscious and death is anticipated, a dying declaration may be recorded under:
    - Section 32 of the Indian Evidence Act
    - Preferably recorded by a Magistrate
    - If not possible, can be recorded by the doctor in presence of witnesses.

Preservation of Evidence

- Preserve samples for forensic toxicology:
    - Stomach contents
    - Blood and urine
    - Vomitus
    - Suspected poison container
- Seal and label with proper identification and hand over to the police with acknowledgment.

Involvement of Police and Magistrate

- Police must be informed for:
    - Site inspection (if patient was found unconscious at home, workplace, etc.)
    - Seizure of poison containers or evidence
- In case of death:
    - Postmortem examination is compulsory.
    - Inquest by police (Section 174 CrPC) or executive magistrate.

Postmortem Examination

- Conducted in all suspected suicidal or homicidal poisonings.
- Helps establish:
    - Cause of death
    - Nature and type of poison
    - Whether death was accidental, suicidal, or homicidal

Ethical and Legal Responsibilities of the Doctor

- Provide emergency care without delay, even if it is a medicolegal case (Article 21, Right to Life).
- Maintain confidentiality, except when disclosure is legally mandated (e.g. police report).
- Avoid any alteration or destruction of evidence.
- If the patient is a minor or mentally unstable, extra care should be taken in documentation and consent.

Q. Enumerate the indications for psychiatric consultation and describe the precautions to be taken in a patient with suspected suicidal ideation/gesture.

Indications for Psychiatric Consultation in Suspected Poisoning

- Suicidal attempt or ideation: Any case of deliberate self-poisoning (e.g. overdose, ingestion of corrosives, pesticides). Persistent thoughts of self-harm or suicide.
- Recurrent self-harm: History of multiple past suicide attempts.
- Psychiatric illness: Severe depression or mood disorders or schizophrenia
- Substance use disorders: Poisoning with alcohol, opioids, benzodiazepines, or other drugs of abuse.
- Altered behavior or delirium: Hallucinations, paranoia, agitation, or disorientation post-poisoning.
- Family conflict/domestic violence: Poisoning resulting from emotional stress, interpersonal conflict, or abuse.

Precautions in a Patient with Suspected Suicidal Ideation or Gesture

- Ensure immediate medical stabilization
- Never leave the patient unattended: Keep under constant supervision, especially during acute care and

observation. Use trained staff or attendants to monitor behavior.

- Safe environment: Remove all dangerous objects (belts, sharp tools, ropes, medication, glass items). Use restraints only if the patient is severely agitated or at risk of harming self or others (with ethical/legal documentation).
- Psychiatric evaluation before discharge: Do not discharge the patient without a psychiatric assessment. Evaluate for risk of repeat attempt, presence of mental illness, and the need for admission or therapy
- Family involvement and counseling: Inform and involve the family or caregivers. Educate about suicide warning signs, importance of emotional support and restriction of access to poisons or medications at home
- Medico-legal formalities: Report to police as a medicolegal case. Document patient's and caregiver's statements, time, and condition.
- Follow-up and referral: Arrange follow-up psychiatric care. May refer to de-addiction centres, social workers, or crisis helplines.

Q. Describe the functions and role of a poison center.

- A poison center (or poison control center) is a specialized medical facility that provides expert advice, guidance, and support in cases of actual or suspected poisoning—whether chemical, drug-related, environmental, or venomous.
- In India, examples include: National Poisons Information Centre (NPIC), AIIMS, New Delhi, State-level poison information centers and toxicology units in tertiary hospitals.

Functions and Roles of a Poison Center

Clinical Support and Emergency Advice

- Provides 24 × 7 expert guidance to healthcare professionals and the public during poisoning emergencies.
- Advises on:
  - Identification of the toxic agent.
  - Risk assessment (based on dose, timing, symptoms).
  - Treatment protocols, antidotes, decontamination.
  - Monitoring and follow-up advice.

Telephone Helpline Services

- Immediate telephone consultation with trained toxicologists or pharmacologists
- Toll-free numbers in some countries; available to both public and healthcare providers.

Database and Toxicology Information

- Maintains databases on:
  - Toxic substances (drugs, chemicals, plants, venom, etc.).
  - Antidotes
  - Management protocols and risk stratification tools
- Uses international databases like TOXBASE, Poisindex, INTOX, or local registries.

Identification of Poisons

- Helps identify poisons from patient history, packaging, chemical names, or clinical signs.
- May assist in toxicological testing through affiliated labs.

Public Health Surveillance and Reporting

- Monitors and reports poison trends (accidental, occupational, suicidal, or environmental).
- Assists in outbreak detection (e.g. methanol poisoning, pesticide mass exposure).
- Alerts authorities and helps develop public health interventions.

Education and Training

- Trains: Medical professionals, paramedics, pharmacists.
- Raises community awareness about poison prevention.
- Conducts workshops and CME programs on clinical toxicology.

Antidote Information and Logistics

- Provides details about availability, dosing, and administration of antidotes.
- Some poison centres coordinate antidote stocking and emergency distribution.

Research and Policy Support

- Participates in toxicovigilance (long-term tracking of poisoning trends).
- Supports policy-making in occupational health, pesticide regulation, and public safety laws.

In a case of suspected poisoning, a poison centre can help with (Table 17.5)

TABLE 17.5: Functions of poison centre in a case of suspected poisoning

Need	How the poison centre assists
Unknown substance ingestion	Identification and likely toxic effects
Risk stratification	Based on dose, time since ingestion, and patient status
Decision for decontamination	Whether to do gastric lavage, activated charcoal, etc.
Antidote guidance	Type, dose, availability
Monitoring and discharge criteria	What labs to monitor, when to admit/discharge
Poisoning clusters or epidemics	Detection, coordination with public health

Chapter 18

Emergency Medicine and Critical Care

Q. Shock.

- Shock is defined as a life-threatening clinical syndrome characterized by inadequate tissue perfusion, leading to cellular hypoxia, organ dysfunction, and if untreated, death.

Classification and Causes

- *Hypovolemic shock:* It occurs as a consequence of inadequate circulating volume. Examples: hemorrhage, dehydration, vomiting, diarrhea.
- *Obstructive shock:* This is caused by extracardiac obstruction of blood flow. Examples: Cardiac tamponade, pulmonary embolism, tension pneumothorax.
- *Cardiogenic shock:* This is caused by primary pump failure. Examples: Myocardial infarction, myocarditis, cardiomyopathy.
- *Distributive shock:* This is due to widespread vasodilatation leading to hypotension and maldistribution of blood flow and volume. Examples: Septic shock, anaphylactic shock and neurogenic shock.
- *Endocrine shock:* This results from hormonal pathology. Examples: Acute adrenal insufficiency, myxedema coma.

Pathophysiology

- The fundamental defect in shock is reduced perfusion of tissues. Reduced perfusion leads to tissue hypoxia leading to anaerobic metabolism with increased production of CO_2 and accumulation of lactic acid. Cellular function declines, and if shock persists, irreversible cell damage and death occur.
- During shock, both the inflammatory and clotting cascades may be triggered in areas of hypoperfusion. There is widespread endothelial dysfunction with increased capillary permeability leading to leakage of fluid and plasma proteins into the interstitial space. In the GI tract, increased permeability may allow the enteric bacteria to enter into the bloodstream, potentially leading to sepsis or metastatic infection. Inflammatory cascade also releases vasodilator substances such as nitric oxide (NO) leading to vasodilatation and hypotension. BP may be normal in the early stages of shock (although hypotension eventually occurs if shock is not reversed).
- In septic shock, blood flow to microvessels including capillaries is reduced due to fibrin deposition even though large-vessel blood flow is preserved.
- Compensatory measures occur to counteract tissue hypoxia and hypotension. Cells extract more oxygen from the blood and there is sympathetic stimulation due to hypotension leading to tachycardia and peripheral vasoconstriction. There is selective vasoconstriction (splanchnic circulation, skin) shunting blood to vital organs such as heart and brain.
- Ultimately, because of all these changes, multiple organ dysfunction syndrome (MODS) which is defined as the progressive dysfunction of ≥2 organs sets in leading to death **(Fig. 18.1)**.

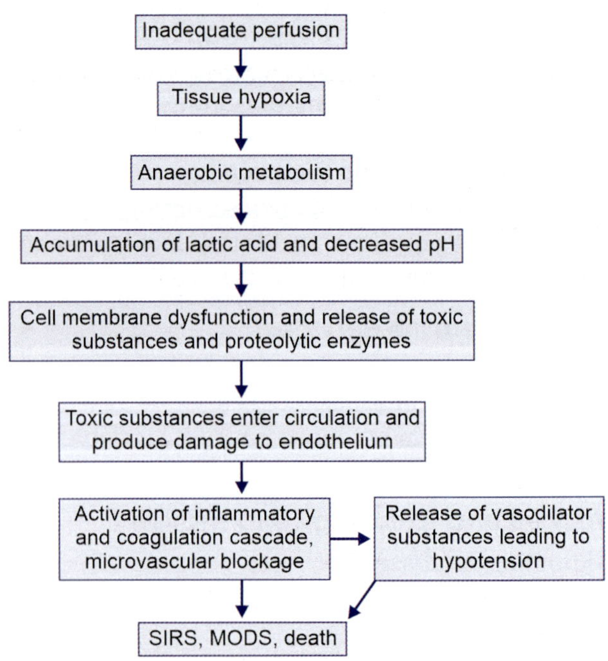

Figure 18.1: Pathophysiology of shock

Clinical Features

- Lethargy, confusion, and somnolence are common.
- The hands and feet are pale, cool, and clammy.

- Cyanosis may be present.
- Capillary filling time is prolonged.
- Peripheral pulses are weak, tachypnea and tachycardia may be present.
- BP is low (<90 mm Hg systolic) or not recordable. However, it may be normal in early stages of shock.
- In septic shock, skin may be warm, or fever may be present. Some patients with anaphylactic shock have urticaria or wheezing.
- Chest pain and dyspnea may be present in cardiogenic shock due to myocardial infarction.
- Evidence of multi-organ dysfunction (MODS) such as decreased urine output (kidney involvement), jaundice (liver involvement), dyspnea (ARDS), etc. may be present.

Investigations

- Complete blood count
- LFT, RFT
- Serum electrolytes
- PT, aPTT
- Serum cortisol (if suspecting adrenal insufficiency)
- ABG
- ECG, echocardiogram
- Monitoring of central venous pressure (CVP)
- Chest X-ray, ultrasound abdomen to identify any chest (pneumonia, ARDS) or abdominal pathology.

Treatment

- Admit the patient in ICU and monitor vital parameters.
- Supplemental oxygen by face mask.
- Intubation and mechanical ventilation if shock is severe or if ventilation is inadequate.
- Intravenous fluids: initially 1 liter of 0.9% saline is infused over 15 minutes. Further fluid therapy is based on the underlying condition and may require monitoring of CVP.
- If BP remains low even after giving fluid challenge, intravenous infusion of noradrenaline or dopamine is started. Dobutamine is preferred in cardiogenic shock.
- Cardiogenic shock is treated by percutaneous coronary interventions, intra-aortic balloon pump, etc.
- Parenteral antibiotics (meropenem or piperacillin-tazobactum) are started if there is suspicion of septic shock.
- Intravenous steroids (hydrocortisone or dexamethasone) are given for adrenal insufficiency.

Q. Define systemic inflammatory response syndrome (SIRS) and MODS (multiple organ dysfunction syndrome). Discuss the etiology, pathogenesis and management of SIRS.

- SIRS is a nonspecific, generalized inflammatory response to a variety of severe clinical insults, both infectious and noninfectious. SIRS is defined by the presence of ≥2 of the following conditions:
  - Fever (oral temperature >38°C) or hypothermia (<36°C).
  - Tachypnea (>20 breaths/min) or arterial carbon dioxide tension ($PaCO_2$) of less than 32 mm Hg.
  - Tachycardia (>90 beats/min).
  - Leukocytosis (>12,000/µl), or leukopenia (<4,000/µl), or >10% bands in peripheral blood.
- The etiology of SIRS may be infectious or noninfectious. SIRS that has a proven or suspected microbial etiology is referred to as 'sepsis'.
- MODS is severe form of SIRS where there is damage to 2 or more organs. It reflects the end stage of systemic inflammation such as that seen in severe sepsis or SIRS.

Causes of SIRS

- Infections (e.g. pneumonia, UTI, cellulitis, meningitis)
- Burns
- Trauma
- Drug reaction
- Electrical injuries
- Myocardial infarction
- Pancreatitis
- Seizure
- Extensive surgical procedures
- Transfusion reactions

Pathogenesis

- Basically microorganisms themselves and their products or the noninfectious insult cause activation of inflammatory cells such as macrophages, monocytes, neutrophils, etc. in the host. Activated inflammatory cells release immune mediators called cytokines such as IL-1, IL-6,IL-8 and TNF-alpha. Other cytokines that have a supposed role in sepsis are IL-10, interferon gamma, IL-12, macrophage migration inhibition factor (MIF), granulocyte colony-stimulating factor (G-CSF), and granulocyte macrophage colony-stimulating factor (GM-CSF).
- The release of all these cytokines lead to a systemic inflammatory response syndrome (SIRS) in the host characterized by diffuse endothelial damage, increased vascular permeability, vasodilation, and activation of coagulation cascade.
- Endothelial damage leads to increased capillary permeability leading to intravascular fluid loss and hypotension. Arterial vasodilation is another important cause of hypotension. Cause of vasodilation is multifactorial, but the primary factors are activation of ATP-sensitive potassium channels in vascular smooth muscle and activation of NO synthase. Initially counter-regulatory mechanisms like sympathetic over activity maintain BP but when these mechanisms fail, BP falls and septic shock develops.
- A combination of direct affection (as in infection), hypotension and DIC lead to multiple organ dysfunction as evidenced by bleeding (affection of blood), jaundice (affection of liver), decreased urine output (affection of kidney), altered mental status

(affection of CNS), ARDS (affection of lungs). 1 in 2 persons with multiorgan dysfunction and DIC die.

Clinical Features

- Fever or hypothermia
- Tachycardia
- Tachypnea or hyperventilation
- Hypotension (late finding)
- Confusion or altered mental status
- Signs of organ dysfunction (e.g. oliguria, hypoxemia).

Management of SIRS

- *Treat the underlying cause*: Such as infection, pancreatitis, burns, etc.
- *Supportive care:* Oxygen supplementation or mechanical ventilation, IV fluids, vasopressors if hypotension persists after fluid resuscitation.
- *Nutritional support*
- *Monitoring of vital signs, organ function, urine output.*
- *Prophylaxis against DVT and stress ulcers.*

Q. Define bacteremia, sepsis, severe sepsis and septic shock.

Q. Discuss the etiopathogenesis of sepsis. How do you investigate and manage a case of sepsis.

Definition

- *Bacteremia* means the presence of bacteria in the blood.
- *Sepsis* means SIRS that has a proven or suspected microbial etiology.
- *Septic shock* is sepsis with hypotension (arterial blood pressure <90 mm Hg systolic, or reduction of more than 40 mm Hg from baseline) in the absence of other causes of hypotension. Hypotension is not corrected by fluid resuscitation.

Etiology

- Sepsis may be due to any microorganisms like bacteria, virus, fungus, protozoa or rickettsiae. But majority of sepsis cases are due to gram-negative and Gram-positive bacteria.

Pathogenesis

- Is same as that described under SIRS.

Clinical Features

History

- Fever or hypothermia
- Tachypnea
- Decreased urine output
- Nausea, vomiting, diarrhea
- Disorientation and confusion.

Examination

General examination

- Patient may be confused and disoriented.
- Presence of tachycardia, tachypnea and hypotension.
- Temperature high or rarely low (oral temperature >38°C or <36°C, respectively) (low temperature may be seen in neonates, elderly patients, uremic patients, alcoholic patients and immunocompromised patients.
- Pallor and jaundice may be present.
- Peripheries may be cold and cyanosed.
- Cellulitis, pustules, bullae/hemorrhagic lesions may be there. These findings may be the cause or effect of sepsis.
- Petechiae or purpura may be seen in meningococcal infection and Rocky Mountain spotted fever.

RS

- Features of pneumonia and or ARDS may be there.

CVS

- Features of myocardial dysfunction may be present due to myocarditis such as S3, S4, dilated heart, etc.

Abdomen

- Paralytic ileus, hepatomegaly, splenomegaly.

CNS

- Encephalopathy, especially in elderly patients or those with prior neurologic impairment.

Investigations

- Complete blood count (CBC): Shows leukocytosis (WBC count >12,000/µl) or leukopenia (WBC count <4000) or normal WBC count with>10% immature forms. Thrombocytopenia (platelet count, <100,000/µl) may be present and may indicate direct effect of infections such as dengue or may indicate DIC.
- Blood cultures: Send at least two blood cultures from different sites preferably before administration of antibiotics. Culture of other specimens as clinically indicated. For example, urine culture in suspected urosepsis or CSF culture in suspected meningitis.
- Markers of inflammation: Elevation of C-reactive protein (CRP) and procalcitonin.
- RFT: Elevation of urea and creatinine.
- LFT: Elevation of bilirubin, AST, ALT and ALP.
- Coagulation abnormalities: INR >1.5 or aPTT >60 seconds.
- Arterial blood gases (ABG): They shows hypoxemia and usually metabolic acidosis.
- Serum lactate: It is elevated due to hypotension, tissue hypoxia and anaerobic metabolism.
- Procalcitonin: Elevated serum procalcitonin level is seen in sepsis. This test can be used to differentiate sepsis from SIRS.
- Chest X-ray: It may show presence of pneumonia, empyema (which may be cause of sepsis) or ARDS due to sepsis.
- Echocardiogram: It can rule out infective endocarditis as a cause of sepsis and may also show myocardial dysfunction in the form of poor ejection fraction.
- Imaging studies: Ultrasound or CT scan may be used to identify the source of sepsis in case of localized infections (example, intra-abdominal abscess).
- Other investigations as required to identify the infecting organism such as tests for malaria, WIDAL

test, HIV and HBsAg serology, dengue serology, tests for leptospirosis, scrub typhus, etc.

Management of Sepsis and Septic Shock

- The goals are to identify the causative organism, eradicate the focus of infection and pathogens from the bloodstream, and correct organ dysfunction.
- Prompt and aggressive treatment is often successful but once septic shock supervenes the mortality is high.

Antibiotics

- Initially a broad-spectrum antibiotic is chosen based on the suspected organism and the site of infection. Reasonable initial choice of antibiotics include carbapenems (imipenem, meropenem), or cefoperazone with sulbactam, or piperacillin-tazobactam. Antibiotics can be changed later, once the infecting organism is identified and culture sensitivity reports are available.
- Antibiotics should be administered intravenously.

Supportive Measures

- Intravenous fluids should be administered.
- If the BP is low in spite of giving adequate IV fluids BP should be maintained by giving infusions of noradrenaline or dopamine either alone or in combination. Noradrenaline is the drug of choice in septic shock to maintain BP.
- Respiratory function should be carefully monitored for the development of ARDS and timely intubation and mechanical ventilation instituted where necessary.
- Renal function, hepatic function, and disturbances in coagulation should be assessed and if abnormal managed accordingly. Renal failure may require hemodialysis.
- Deep vein thrombosis (DVT) prophylaxis is required. Use unfractionated heparin (UFH) or low molecular weight heparin (LMWH) unless contraindicated. If heparin is contraindicated, mechanical prophylactic device, such as compression stockings or an intermittent compression device can be used.

Corticosteroids

- Steroids are indicated in septic shock when hypotension responds poorly to fluid resuscitation and vasopressors (noradrenaline). Steroids should not be used in sepsis if hypotension is not present unless the patient's endocrine or corticosteroid history warrants it. Choice of steroid is hydrocortisone (50 mg 6th hourly).

Surgery

- Has a role when there is a well-defined abscess or a foreign body. Wherever there is an abscess it should be drained. Antibiotics alone may be inadequate without draining the abscess.
- Surgery also has a role when the tissues are necrosed and gangrenous and act as a source of infection and sepsis. Such necrosed and gangrenous foci should be removed.

Q. Acute respiratory distress syndrome (ARDS).

Q. Acute lung injury (ALI).

- ARDS is a severe, acute, inflammatory lung injury characterized by:
  - Increased pulmonary vascular permeability
  - Loss of aerated lung tissue
  - Noncardiogenic pulmonary edema
  - Severe hypoxemia
- ARDS is the severe end of the spectrum of acute lung injury (ALI).

Berlin Definition of ARDS

- ARDS definition **(Table 18.1)** was further refined in 2011 by a panel of experts who met at Berlin and is termed the Berlin definition of ARDS. In the Berlin definition, there is no use of the term acute lung injury (ALI). ALI corresponds to mild ARDS.

TABLE 18.1: ARDS definition

Timing	Within 1 week of a known clinical insult or new or worsening respiratory symptoms
Chest imaging (X-ray or CT scan)	Bilateral opacities—not fully explained by effusions, lobar/lung collapse, or nodules
Origin of pulmonary edema	Respiratory failure not fully explained by cardiac failure or fluid overload
Oxygenation (PaO_2/FiO_2)	Mild ARDS: PaO_2/FIO_2 200–≤300 mm Hg Moderate ARDS: PaO_2/FIO_2 100–≤200 mm Hg Severe ARDS: PaO_2/FIO_2 ≤100 mm Hg

Causes of ARDS

- ARDS is caused by diffuse lung injury due to many medical and surgical disorders **(Table 18.2)**.

TABLE 18.2: Causes of ARDS

Direct lung injury	Indirect lung injury
Pneumonia	Anaphylaxis (drugs, wasp, bee sting)
Aspiration of gastric contents	Drug overdose (heroin, barbiturates)
	Pancreatitis
Lung contusion	Cardiopulmonary bypass
Smoke inhalation	Sepsis
Amniotic fluid embolism	Shock
Fat embolism	Severe trauma
Near-drowning	Multiple bone fractures
Diffuse alveolar hemorrhage	Multiple blood transfusions
	Burns

Pathogenesis

- Inflammatory cells collect in the lungs because of direct or indirect lung injury listed above. Cytokines are released from inflammatory cells which cause damage to capillary endothelial cells and alveolar epithelial cells. Damage to these cells causes increased vascular permeability and decreased production of surfactant which result in interstitial and alveolar pulmonary edema, alveolar collapse, and hypoxemia.

- Three overlapping stages can be recognized in the evolution of ARDS; exudative, proliferative, and fibrotic stages.
- The exudative phase (1–7 days) is characterized by alveolar edema, neutrophil-rich leukocytic infiltration and hyaline membrane formation.
- Proliferative phase (7–21 days) occurs within 7 days and is characterized by interstitial inflammation and early fibrotic changes.
- Fibrotic phase (after day 21): Interstitial fibrosis and long-term lung damage (may or may not occur).

Clinical Features

- ARDS is marked by the rapid onset of dyspnea that usually occurs 12–48 hours after the initiating event.
- Physical examination reveals labored breathing, tachypnea, intercostal retractions, and diffuse crepitations.
- Many patients with ARDS have multiple organ failure.
- Signs of underlying disease (e.g. sepsis, trauma).

Investigations

- *Chest X-ray* shows diffuse or patchy bilateral infiltrates which become confluent with sparing of costophrenic angles. Air bronchograms may be seen. Heart size is normal, and pleural effusions are nil or minimal.
- *ABG* analysis shows marked hypoxemia that is refractory to supplemental oxygen.
- *Bronchoscopy and lung biopsy* can be considered in patients in whom the cause of ARDS is not clear.
- *BNP/echcardiography*: To rule out cardiogenic pulmonary edema.
- Blood cultures, inflammatory markers.

Treatment

- Treatment of ARDS must include identification and treatment of the underlying precipitating condition (e.g. sepsis, aspiration, trauma).
- Treatment of hypoxemia usually requires tracheal intubation and positive-pressure mechanical ventilation. The lowest levels of PEEP (used to recruit atelectatic alveoli) and supplemental oxygen required to maintain the SaO_2 above 90% should be used. Prone positioning may improve oxygenation by recruiting atelectatic alveoli. A variety of mechanical ventilation strategies like using volume-cycled ventilation with small tidal volumes (6 ml/kg of ideal body weight) have shown benefit in trials.
- Fluid administration should be restricted and enough to maintain pulmonary capillary wedge pressure at the lowest level compatible with adequate cardiac output. Crystalloid solutions should be used when intravascular volume expansion is necessary. Diuretics should be used to reduce intravascular volume if pulmonary capillary wedge pressure is elevated.
- Systemic corticosteroids have been studied extensively with variable and inconsistent results. Though steroids cannot be recommended routinely for all patients, studies have shown benefit in late-phase ARDS.
- Supportive care should be provided to minimize venous thromboembolism, gastrointestinal bleeding, and central venous catheter infections. Adequate nutrition should be provided for a good outcome.
- ECMO (extracorporeal membrane oxygenation) can be considered in patients who do not maintain oxygen saturation even on ventilatory support.

Course and Prognosis

- Mortality rate associated with ARDS is 30–40%. Median survival is about 2 weeks.
- Most survivors of ARDS are left with some pulmonary symptoms (cough, dyspnea, sputum production), which tend to improve over time.

Q. Respiratory failure.

- Respiratory failure is a condition in which the respiratory system fails in one or both of its gas exchange functions, i.e. oxygenation and/or elimination of carbon dioxide. Arterial blood gas criteria for respiratory failure are a PaO_2 under 60 mm Hg or a PCO_2 over 50 mm Hg.
- Respiratory failure can arise from an abnormality in any of the components of the respiratory system, including the airways, alveoli, central nervous system (CNS), peripheral nervous system, respiratory muscles, and chest wall.
- Respiratory failure can be classified as follows
  - *Hypoxemic respiratory failure (type 1)*: Hypoxemia present, PCO_2 normal or low. It is caused by processes that impair oxygen transfer in the lung. e.g. acute asthma, pulmonary edema, pulmonary embolism, pneumonia, ARDS.
  - *Hypercapnic respiratory failure (type 2):* Hypoxemia usually present, PCO_2 high. It is caused by inadequate ventilation leading to retention of CO_2, and hypoxemia, e.g. COPD, myasthenia gravis, brainstem stroke.
  - *Mixed respiratory failure:* Here, there is a combination of type I and type II respiratory failure (acute-on-chronic respiratory failure).
- Respiratory failure may be further classified as either acute or chronic. Acute respiratory failure develops over minutes to hours (e.g. pneumothorax, pulmonary edema). Chronic respiratory failure develops over several days or longer. (e.g. COPD).
- Respiratory failure is a serious condition associated with poor prognosis. Incidence and mortality from respiratory failure increase with age and in the presence of other comorbid conditions.
- Prognosis has improved now because of advances in mechanical ventilation and airway management. Even patients with irreversible chronic respiratory failure can now have a reasonably good quality of life with domiciliary ventilator support systems. Lung transplantation is another option for patients with chronic respiratory failure.

Causes of Respiratory Failure

Lung disorders
- Asthma
- COPD
- Bronchiolitis
- Obstruction of airways due to mass or foreign body
- Pulmonary edema
- Pneumonia
- Interstitial lung diseases
- Diffuse alveolar hemorrhage syndromes
- Aspiration
- Lung contusion
- Pulmonary embolism
- Pulmonary AV malformations

Muscular disorders
- Botulism
- Neuromuscular blocking agents
- Electrolyte disturbances: hypokalemia, hyperkalemia

Nervous system disorders
- Brainstem disorders
- CNS infections
- Guillain-Barré syndrome
- Myasthenia gravis
- Poliomyelitis
- Spinal cord injury

Chest wall, diaphragm, and pleural disorders
- Rib fracture
- Pneumothorax
- Pleural effusion
- Phrenic nerve injury or dysfunction
- Massive ascites

Drugs
- Sedative overdose
- Anesthetics

Clinical Features

- Symptoms and signs of acute respiratory failure are those of the underlying disease plus those of hypoxemia and/or hypercapnia.

Due to Hypoxemia

- Dyspnea, cyanosis, restlessness, confusion, anxiety, delirium, tachypnea, hypertension, cardiac arrhythmias, and tremor.

Due to Hypercarbia

- Dyspnea, headache, peripheral flushing, bounding pulses, hypertension, tachycardia, tachypnea, altered sensorium, papilledema, and flapping tremors (asterixis).

Investigations

- *Pulse oximetry* is a noninvasive method to determine arterial oxygen saturation.
- *Arterial blood gas (ABG)* analysis can accurately assess blood oxygen and carbon dioxide content.
- *Routine blood tests:* Complete blood count, renal function tests, liver functions tests, serum electrolytes. Abnormalities in electrolytes such as potassium and magnesium can cause or aggravate respiratory failure.
- *Chest X-ray* can show any lung pathology such as pneumonia, ARDS, etc.
- *Pulmonary function tests* if feasible.
- *Thyroid function tests* should be done to rule out hypothyroidism as the cause of respiratory failure.
- *CT thorax*, if indicated.
- *Cardiac evaluation* with ECG, ECHO and troponins are important to rule out cardiac problem as a cause of respiratory failure.

Treatment

- Treatment of respiratory failure consists of (i) treatment of underlying disease (ii) respiratory support and (iii) general supportive care.
- ***Treatment of underlying disease***: Treating pulmonary edema, COPD, myasthenia gravis, etc. which have caused respiratory failure.
- ***Respiratory support:*** Providing supplemental oxygen through mask or nasal cannula helps correcting hypoxemia. High concentrations of oxygen are needed for patients with ARDS, pneumonia, and other parenchymal lung diseases. Low flow oxygen should be used in COPD because their respiratory drive may be due to hypoxia. Noninvasive ventilation (NIV) such as BiPAP (bilevel positive airway pressure) and CPAP (continuous positive airway pressure) are helpful especially in COPD. Mechanical ventilator support is required if the patient is not responding to oxygen supplementation. It may be provided via face mask (noninvasive) or through tracheal intubation. Extracorporeal membrane oxygenation (ECMO) is a treatment that uses a pump to circulate blood through an artificial lung and back into the bloodstream. ECMO is indicated in severe respiratory failure not responding to even mechanical ventilation.
- ***General supportive care:*** This includes providing adequate hydration and nutrition, preventing stress ulcers in the stomach by using sucralfate syrup, preventing bedsores, and preventing deep vein thrombosis by using subcutaneous heparin or low molecular weight heparin.

Q. Discuss the causes, clinical features and management of hypoxia.

- Hypoxia is defined as lack of oxygen in tissues. Hypoxemia is decreased oxygen concentration of blood. Hypoxia is usually preceded by hypoxemia.

Causes of Hypoxia

- Hypoxia secondary to high altitude
- Anemic hypoxia
- Carbon monoxide intoxication
- Respiratory hypoxia (due to advanced respiratory disease)
- Hypoxia secondary to right-to-left shunting (tetralogy of Fallot, transposition of the great arteries, and Eisenmenger's syndrome).

- Stagnant hypoxia (heart failure, shock)
- Histotoxic hypoxia (cyanide poisoning).

Clinical Features

- Cyanosis, dyspnea, tachycardia.
- *CNS effects:* Impaired judgment, motor incoordination, fatigue, drowsiness, apathy, inattentiveness, delayed reaction time, and reduced work capacity.
- *CVS:* Pulmonary vasoconstriction, increase in pulmonary vascular resistance and right ventricular afterload. Increase in cardiac output due to generalized vasodilation.
- *Metabolic effects:* Anaerobic metabolism leading to lactic acid production and metabolic acidosis.
- *Blood:* Chronic hypoxia causes secondary polycythemia.

Investigations

- *Pulse oxymetry:* It may show decreased oxygen saturation.
- *ABG (arterial blood gases):* It shows decreased PaO_2 except in histotoxic hypoxia.
- *Chest X-ray:* To rule out any underlying lung disease.
- *Blood tests:* To rule out anemia.
- *ECG and echocardiogram* to rule out cardiac disorders.

Treatment

- *Oxygen supplementation:* This will correct hypoxia in all cases except in left to right shunts and ventilation perfusion mismatching. Oxygen can be given by nasal cannulae, face mask or through endotracheal intubation.
- Treatment of the underlying cause.

Q. Oxygen therapy.

- Oxygen therapy is the administration of oxygen at concentrations greater than ambient air (21%) to treat or prevent hypoxemia and tissue hypoxia.
- Oxygen is the vital gas. It should be treated like any other drug; it should be prescribed in writing, with the required flow rate and the method of delivery clearly specified. When administered correctly it is lifesaving.

Indications for Oxygen Therapy

- Cardiac and respiratory arrest
- Acute and chronic respiratory failure
- Asthma and COPD exacerbation
- ARDS, pneumonia, pulmonary edema
- Hypotension (systolic blood pressure <80 mm Hg)
- Cardiac conditions: Myocardial infarction, heart failure.
- Poisonings: CO poisoning, cyanide poisoning.

Recognizing Hypoxia

- Tissue hypoxia occurs within 4 minutes of stoppage of oxygen supply.
- Successful treatment of tissue hypoxia requires early recognition.
- Clinical features are often nonspecific and include altered mental state, dyspnea, cyanosis, tachypnea, arrhythmias, and coma.
- Arterial oxygen saturation (SPO_2) and PaO_2 are easily measured and are the main indicators for starting oxygen therapy. However, PaO_2 and SPO_2 can be normal when tissue hypoxia is caused by low output cardiac states, anemia, and failure of tissue to use oxygen.

How to give Oxygen?

Oxygen Masks

- The mask and valve design allows delivery of an inspired oxygen of 24–90%.
- There are two basic types of oxygen masks. High flow mask and low flow mask. High flow masks contain venturi valves, which use the principle of jet mixing (Bernoulli effect). When oxygen passes through a narrow orifice it produces a high velocity stream that draws a constant proportion of room air through the base of the venturi valve. Air entrainment depends on the velocity of the jet (the size of orifice and oxygen flow rate) and the size of the valve ports. It can be accurately controlled to give inspired oxygen levels of 24–60%.

Nasal Prongs

- Are simple and convenient to use. The FiO_2 depends on the flow rate of oxygen (1–6 liters/min). Nasal prongs prevent rebreathing, are comfortable for long periods, and allow talking and eating.

High-flow Nasal Oxygen Therapy

- High-flow nasal oxygen (HFNO) administration is a relatively new technique that is used in the intensive care unit (ICU), and increasingly in the operating theatres. HFNO has become popular in the ICU for management of patients with acute hypoxemic respiratory failure when attempting to avoid intubation or to help after extubation. HFNO has become a valuable tool in the management of COVID-19 patients with hypoxia. HFNO provides humidified, titrated oxygen therapy matching or even exceeding the patients' inspiratory demand. In addition, HFNO has been proposed to limit oxygen desaturation by prolonging apneic oxygenation during intubation both in ICUs and operating theatres.

Noninvasive Ventilation

- Supplemental oxygen may be provided through tight fitting nasal or full face masks during nasal intermittent positive pressure ventilation and continuous positive airways pressure.

Invasive Ventilation

- Patient is intubated and endotracheal tube is connected to an oxygen source or a ventilator. Inspired O_2 (FiO_2) can be varied by adjusting ventilator settings.

Monitoring Oxygen Therapy

- ABG measurements: ABG analysis provides accurate information on the pH, PaO_2, and $PacO_2$, but invasive.

- Pulse oximetry: Noninvasive, and provides continuous monitoring of the state of oxygenation.

Complications of Oxygen Therapy

- *Fire:* Oxygen promotes combustion. Facial burns and deaths of patients who smoke when using oxygen are well documented.
- **CO_2 retention** in COPD patients by decreasing hypoxic respiratory drive.
- *Oxygen toxicity:* 100% oxygen is both irritant and toxic, if inhaled for more than a few hours. Premature infants develop retrolental fibroplasia and blindness if exposed to excessive concentrations. High concentrations of oxygen (>60%) may damage the alveolar membrane when inhaled for more than 48 hours. Progression to the acute respiratory distress syndrome with high protein alveolar edema and pulmonary radiographic infiltrates is associated with high mortality.
- *Paul-Bert effect:* Breathing hyperbaric oxygen (for example, when diving) can cause severe cerebral vasoconstriction and epileptic fits.

Q. Mechanical ventilation.

- Mechanical ventilation is a life-support technique to mechanically assist or replace spontaneous breathing by using a ventilator.
- Mechanical ventilation can be noninvasive or invasive. In noninvasive method, tracheal intubation is not done and ventilation is provided through a tight fitting face mask, e.g. NPPV (noninvasive positive pressure ventilation). In invasive ventilation endotracheal intubation or tracheostomy is done and patient is ventilated through these.

Indications

- Bradypnea or apnea with respiratory arrest
- Severe hypercapnia not reversed by appropriate specific therapy
- ARDS
- Severe pneumonia
- COPD with respiratory failure
- Acute severe asthma
- Circulatory failure
- Pulmonary edema
- Coma
- Status epilepticus
- Respiratory muscle paralysis (e.g. Guillain-Barré, poliomyelitis, myasthenia gravis)
- Head injury—to reduce intracranial pressure by hyperventilation
- Brainstem disorders affecting respiratory center

Modes of Mechanical Ventilation

- Ventilator modes determine how breaths are delivered—either by the machine, by the patient, or both. Modes are chosen based on the patient's condition, ability to breathe spontaneously, and therapeutic goals (oxygenation vs ventilation).
- **Controlled mandatory ventilation (CMV):** This is a mode of mechanical ventilation in which the ventilator delivers a preset tidal volume or pressure at a fixed rate, regardless of any patient effort. Breaths are fully machine-triggered, controlled, and cycled. Patient cannot trigger spontaneous breaths. Patient effort is ignored if present, not sensed or used.
- **Assist-control ventilation (AC or A/C):** This allows breaths to be triggered either by the patient or by time. However, once a breath is triggered, the ventilator fully controls it—either by volume or pressure—and delivers a full mechanical breath. This mode provides full ventilatory support and is commonly used in ARDS or severe respiratory failure.
- **Synchronized intermittent mandatory ventilation (SIMV):** This mode delivers mandatory breaths that are either time- or patient-triggered and controlled by the ventilator. Between these breaths, the patient can breathe spontaneously. The cycle may be volume- or pressure-controlled. This mode is useful as a weaning strategy, as it allows partial patient participation in breathing.
- **Pressure support ventilation (PSV)** is entirely patient-triggered. The ventilator assists each spontaneous breath with a preset level of pressure but does not initiate breaths. This mode is commonly used during weaning or in conditions such as neuromuscular weakness.
- **Pressure-controlled ventilation (PCV)** can be triggered either by the patient or by the ventilator (time-based). The ventilator controls the pressure, and the breath is cycled based on time. It is often used in ARDS to avoid the risk of barotrauma due to high pressures.
- **Volume-controlled ventilation (VCV)** delivers breaths that are triggered either by time or the patient, but the ventilator controls the tidal volume. The breath ends when the preset volume is delivered. This mode ensures precise control of tidal volume, which is useful in many controlled ventilation scenarios.
- **Continuous positive airway pressure (CPAP)** is used in patients who are breathing spontaneously. Both triggering and control are done by the patient, and there is no mechanical cycling. It provides continuous positive airway pressure throughout the respiratory cycle and is used primarily in obstructive sleep apnea or mild respiratory distress.
- **Bi-level positive airway pressure (BiPAP)** is also a noninvasive mode where the patient initiates and controls the breath. It delivers two levels of pressure—higher during inspiration (IPAP) and lower during expiration (EPAP). This helps both oxygenation and ventilation and is commonly used in COPD patients or those with hypercapnic respiratory failure.

Weaning from Mechanical Ventilation

- Weaning is slowly taking off the ventilator support. It is done over a period of hours to days. Mechanical ventilation cannot be stopped suddenly as the patient is adapted to ventilator and may not be able to breathe.

- Weaning should be considered when the underlying cause of respiratory failure has resolved.

Complications of Mechanical Ventilation

- Migration of the tip of the endotracheal tube into a main bronchus can cause atelectasis of the contralateral lung and over distention of the intubated lung.
- Barotrauma can occur in patients ventilated with high tidal volumes and high pressures. There is rupture of alveoli and small airways due to high pressures. It is manifested by subcutaneous emphysema, pneumomediastinum, pneumothorax, or systemic gas embolism.
- Acute respiratory alkalosis can occur due to hyperventilation.
- Hypotension can occur in patients put on excessive PEEP, because excess intrathoracic pressure prevents venous return to heart and hypotension.
- Tracheal stenosis can occur if endotracheal tube is kept for long time.
- Ventilator-associated pneumonia is another serious complication.

Chapter 19

Role of Physician in the Community, Medicolegal and Ethical Issues in Health Care

Q. Enumerate and describe professional qualities of a Physician.

- A physician's role goes beyond medical knowledge and technical skills. To deliver holistic, ethical, and patient-centered care, a physician must embody certain professional qualities that foster trust, accountability, and excellence in clinical practice.

Professional Qualities Expected in a Doctor

Medical Knowledge and Clinical Competence

- A physician must have a strong foundation in medical sciences and the ability to apply this knowledge in diagnosing and managing illnesses accurately and efficiently. Clinical competence includes decision-making skills and procedural proficiency.

Compassion and Empathy

- A good physician treats patients not just as cases but as human beings with emotions and fears. Compassion helps provide emotional support, while empathy enables the doctor to understand the patient's perspective, leading to better care.

Ethical Integrity

- Physicians must uphold high ethical standards by practicing honesty, fairness, and justice. They should prioritize the patient's best interest, avoid conflicts of interest, and follow medical ethics including autonomy, beneficence, non-maleficence, and justice. Quality that ensures patient's rights, autonomy, modesty and privacy is respected at all times.

Confidentiality

- Respecting patient privacy and maintaining confidentiality of health information is a core legal and ethical duty of a physician. Breaches can damage trust and lead to legal consequences.

Professionalism and Accountability

- Being punctual, respectful, and responsible in one's duties is vital. Physicians must be accountable for their actions, admit errors when they occur, and strive to correct them.

Lifelong Learning

- Medicine is a continuously evolving field. Physicians must stay updated with new research, guidelines, and technologies through continuing medical education (CME) and professional development.

Teamwork and Collaboration

- Modern healthcare is delivered by multidisciplinary teams. A physician should work respectfully with nurses, technicians, pharmacists, and other professionals to provide coordinated and safe care.

Cultural Sensitivity and Respect

- Physicians should be aware of and sensitive to patients' cultural, religious, and personal beliefs. This ensures respectful and individualized care, especially in diverse societies.

Leadership and Advocacy

- Physicians often serve as leaders in healthcare settings and advocates for patients' rights, access to care, and public health. Leadership includes managing resources wisely and mentoring others.

Communication Skills and Bedside Manners

- Communication plays an important role between doctor and patients, colleagues or public.
- Effective verbal and nonverbal communication is crucial for understanding patient concerns, explaining conditions and treatments, and counseling families. It also reduces misunderstandings and improves compliance and outcomes.

Q. Describe and discuss the role of a physician in healthcare system.

- The GMR envisages the following roles that a doctor must perform in order to achieve the goal of the UG medical education program.

- ***Clinician***: Who understands and provides preventive, promotive, curative, palliative and holistic care with compassion.
- ***Leader and member of the healthcare team and system***: With capabilities to collect analyze, synthesize and communicate health data appropriately.
- ***Communicator***: With patients, families, colleagues and community.
- ***Lifelong learner***: Committed to continuous improvement of skills and knowledge.
- ***Professional***: Who is committed to excellence, is ethical, responsive and accountable to patients, community and profession.

Q. Describe the commitment to lifelong learning as an important part of physician growth.

- Medical science is an ever-changing field of practice with advances in medicine, expanded evidence sources, new treatment options, and changing governmental regulations and models of care. Most doctors are aware of the aphorism that learning should continue from the cradle to the grave.
- Lifelong learning offers individuals the opportunity to keep their knowledge current, learn new skills, and pursue a wide variety of interests through intellectual growth and expansion. We must continuously read and evaluate the literature, discuss it with colleagues, and formulate opinions that impact our practice.
- Lifelong learning is not an option in healthcare, it is required by healthcare workers to remain relevant and continue providing safe, effective patient care. The lifelong learning movement in healthcare provides benefit and welfare for everyone in society.
- Opportunities for lifelong learning can take place in the following ways:
  - E-learning
  - Attending CME and conferences
  - Reading journals and latest textbooks
  - Discussion with colleagues.

Q. Describe and discuss the role of nonmaleficence as a guiding principle in patient care.

- Nonmaleficence is one of the four fundamental principles of medical ethics, alongside beneficence, autonomy, and justice. Nonmaleficence means doing no harm. There is an obligation not to inflict harm on others either by omission or commission of an act. The guiding principle of *primum non nocere*, "First, do no harm," is found in the Hippocratic Oath. Actions or practices of a healthcare provider are "right" as long as they are in the interest of the patient and avoid negative consequences.
- Harm by an act of omission means that some action could have been done to avoid harm but was not done. Example of an act of omission would be failing to give adrenaline injection in case a case of anaphylactic shock. An act of commission is something actually done that resulted in harm. An example of an act of commission would be delivering a medication in the wrong dose or to the wrong patient.

Q. Describe the role of autonomy and shared responsibility as a guiding principle in patient care.

Autonomy in Patient Care

- Autonomy refers to the patient's right to make informed decisions about their own healthcare, free from coercion or undue influence.
- Respect for autonomy requires that patients be told the truth about their condition and be informed about the risks and benefits of treatment in order for them to make informed decisions. Under the law, they are permitted to refuse treatment even if the best and most reliable information indicates that treatment would be beneficial, unless their action may have a negative impact on the well-being of another individual. These conflicts set the stage for ethical dilemmas. Nowadays, patients are well informed and able to make decisions about their own care. Doctor should give all the options of diagnostic methods, treatment options, etc. and help make the patient make a decision.
- Autonomy, however, does not negate responsibility. Health care is a partnership between the provider and patient. Each owes the other a position of partner and respect in health care decision-making. Physician needs to guide the patient to make correct decisions which are beneficial and not harmful.
- The principle of autonomy does not extend to persons who lack the capacity (competence) to act autonomously; examples include infants and children and incompetence due to developmental, mental or physical disorder.

Examples

- Respecting a patient's refusal to take chemotherapy after understanding its risks and prognosis.
- Respecting a patient's choice to seek alternative or complementary therapies.

Shared Responsibility in Patient Care

- Shared responsibility refers to the collaborative partnership between healthcare professionals and patients in planning and implementing care.

Role in Patient Care

- **Collaborative decision-making:** Both parties contribute to decisions, ensuring care is medically sound and aligned with patient preferences.
- **Mutual accountability:** Healthcare providers guide and educate, while patients engage actively in their care, such as adhering to treatment and lifestyle changes.
- **Improved outcomes:** Fosters better compliance, satisfaction, and clinical outcomes by ensuring both medical expertise and patient values are integrated.

Examples

- A diabetic patient and physician codeveloping a realistic lifestyle modification plan.
- A mental health treatment plan adjusted based on the patient's input and daily experiences.

Q. Describe the role of beneficence of a guiding principle in patient care.

- The principle of beneficence is the moral obligation of healthcare providers to act for the benefit of the patient.
- Beneficence means actively doing good for the patient. Unlike nonmaleficence (which focuses on avoiding harm), beneficence emphasizes positive action—providing care that benefits the patient in a meaningful way. This principle states that health care providers must do all they can to benefit the patient in each situation. To ensure beneficence, medical practitioners must develop and maintain a high level of skill and knowledge, make sure that they are trained in the most current and best medical practices, and must consider their patients' individual circumstances.
- The principle calls for not just avoiding harm, but also to benefit patients and to promote their welfare. While physicians' beneficence conforms to moral rules, and is altruistic, it is also true that in many instances it can be considered a payback for the debt to society for education (often subsidized by governments), ranks and privileges, and to the patients themselves (learning and research).

Examples in Clinical Practice

- Administering lifesaving treatment during an emergency.
- Counseling a diabetic patient on diet and exercise to prevent complications.
- Providing vaccination to prevent serious illnesses.
- Rehabilitative care after a stroke to improve function and quality of life.
- Coordinating multidisciplinary care for complex chronic illnesses.

Balancing Beneficence with Other Principles

- **With autonomy:** A patient may refuse a treatment that the doctor believes is beneficial. In such cases, beneficence must be balanced with respect for autonomy.
- **With nonmaleficence:** Sometimes, beneficial actions may carry risks; clinicians must weigh benefits against potential harm.

Q. Describe the role of justice as a guiding principle in patient care.

- Justice is a fundamental ethical principle in health care that emphasizes fairness, equity, and impartiality in the distribution of medical resources, treatment, and care. It ensures that all patients are treated equally and with dignity, regardless of their background, socioeconomic status, age, gender, or other factors.
- In actual practice, a number of different factors may influence the application of this principle of justice especially when there are limited resources. When there are scarce resources, equality of distribution cannot be implemented and patients have to be prioritized. An example is younger patients get priority over old patients for kidney transplantation.

Role in Patient Care

Fair Access to Care

- All patients should have equal access to healthcare services, medications, and procedures. Healthcare systems must strive to reduce disparities in care delivery.

Equitable Allocation of Resources

- In times of resource scarcity (e.g. ICU beds, organ transplants, vaccines), decisions must be based on ethical and clinical criteria, not personal or social biases.

Nondiscrimination

- Justice mandates that treatment decisions are not influenced by race, religion, gender, social class, disability, or financial status.

Prioritizing Based on Need

- Patients with the greatest need or likelihood of benefit may be given priority in certain cases, such as emergency care or public health interventions.

Q. Discuss the medicolegal, sociocultural, economic and ethical issues as it pertains to rights, equity and justice in access to health care.

- Access to health care is a fundamental human right. However, it is influenced by multiple factors including medicolegal, sociocultural, economic, and ethical considerations. Ensuring equity and justice in healthcare access means that care is provided fairly and without discrimination, and that those with greater health needs receive appropriate services regardless of socioeconomic or demographic status.

Medicolegal Issues

- Legal right to health care: Many constitutions and international declarations (e.g. WHO, universal declaration of human rights) recognize health as a basic right. In practice, legal protections vary; some countries guarantee universal healthcare, while others do not.
- Discrimination and equal protection: Laws must protect individuals from denial of care based on race, gender, caste, religion, disability, or HIV status.
- Legal frameworks must ensure equal treatment and redress in case of violations.
- Above issues can be addressed by strong legal structures to protect vulnerable groups and enforce fair distribution of care. Laws must ensure that no one is unjustly denied treatment.

Sociocultural Issues

- Cultural beliefs and practices: Some communities avoid modern medical care due to traditional or religious beliefs.
- Language barriers and gender norms may restrict women or minorities from accessing care.
- Stigma and marginalization: Social stigma associated with diseases like HIV/AIDS, mental illness, or leprosy can discourage people from seeking help.
- Health literacy: Lack of awareness and education about health services can limit access, particularly in rural or tribal populations.
- Above sociocultural issues can be addressed by culturally sensitive care, community health education, and inclusion of local beliefs in healthcare planning.

Economic Issues

- Affordability and out-of-pocket costs: In many countries, high medical expenses prevent poor people from accessing care. Lack of insurance coverage further widens inequality.
- Urban–rural divide: Healthcare infrastructure and personnel are concentrated in urban areas, leaving rural populations underserved.
- Resource allocation: Limited resources may be inequitably distributed based on political influence or income levels.
- To address the above economic issues, publicly funded health insurance, subsidized care for the poor, and rural health missions are essential to bridge economic barriers and promote fairness in access.

Ethical Issues

- *Justice and fairness*: The ethical principle of justice demands that healthcare be distributed based on need, not wealth or social status. Equal access is essential to maintain public trust and moral integrity in medicine.
- *Right to health vs. Market forces*: Ethical tensions arise between treating healthcare as a right versus as a commodity.
- *Vulnerability and prioritization*: Ethical frameworks may support prioritizing care for the most vulnerable, e.g. the elderly, chronically ill, or disabled, to achieve equitable outcomes.
- To address the above ethical issues, healthcare systems must prioritize the common good while respecting individual rights. Equity in access is not just a policy goal but a moral duty.

Q. Discuss the medicolegal, socioeconomic and ethical issues as it pertains to organ donation.

- Organ donation is a vital, lifesaving intervention, but it also raises several complex medicolegal, socioeconomic, and ethical issues that must be carefully navigated to ensure safety, fairness, and respect for human dignity.

Medicolegal Issues

Consent Laws

- Informed consent is essential for both living and deceased donors.
- Legal systems may follow either:
  - Opt-in system: Donation occurs only with prior consent (e.g. India, USA).
  - Opt-out system (presumed consent): Everyone is considered a donor unless they explicitly refuse (e.g. Spain).

Definition of Death

- Organ retrieval must occur only after brain death or cardiac death is legally and medically confirmed.
- Standardized and legally recognized criteria must be used to avoid premature declaration.

Transplantation Laws and Regulations

- In India, the Transplantation of Human Organs and Tissues Act (THOTA), 1994 governs organ donation and prohibits organ trade.
- Establishes authorization committees to scrutinize unrelated living donations and prevent exploitation.

Prevention of Organ Trafficking

- Illegal organ trade is a serious medicolegal issue.
- Laws mandate stringent documentation and monitoring to ensure ethical procurement and prevent coercion.

Ethical Issues

- The following ethical criteria should be addressed in cases of living donor transplantation.
- The removal of the tissue or organ does not impair the health or functional integrity of the donor.
- The benefits expected to be given to the recipient bear an acceptable proportion to the harm likely to the donor.
- The donation should be altruistic and is given without any coercion or any other form of external pressure.
- The donor must be fully informed of the nature of the procedure and the possible even if rare complications. This entails the need for follow-up of the donor's health in the future.
- The views of close relatives such as the spouse or adult children are taken into account.
- There must be no element of commercialization or exploitation in the donation.

Socioeconomic Issues

- Organ transplantation is expensive, often excluding poor patients. Wealthier individuals may receive preferential access to organs or better post-transplant care.
- Poor and marginalized populations may be pressured to donate organs for financial compensation.

- "Transplant tourism" involves wealthier recipients traveling to developing countries to obtain organs unethically.
- Myths, fear, and religious misconceptions can reduce donation rates.

Q. Discuss the medicolegal, sociocultural and ethical issues as it pertains to confidentiality in patient care.

- All information about one's patient is confidential. It includes any information about the patient's identity, condition, diagnosis, investigations' results, treatment, and/or prognosis (whether chances of cure, disability, or death).
- Patients put their trust on doctors and other healthcare professionals during the course of treatment and share lot of information regarding their health and personal matters. It is important that information shared during this time is not shared with anyone who is not directly involved in the care of that patient. This unnecessary sharing of information may lead to problems for the patient. For example, if the patient is positive for HIV and his friends to come to know it, then the patient may face social stigma.
- A breach of confidentiality is a disclosure of private information to a third party not involved with the patient's care, without patient consent or court order. Disclosure can be oral or written, by telephone or fax, or electronically, for example, via e-mail or health information networks. Accessing the medical records of patient's without legitimate reason is also considered a breach of confidentiality.
- *Tips for maintaining confidentiality:* Discuss patient related matters with the authorized persons only. Avoid discussing about patient in nonprivate areas (e.g. elevator, hallway or cafeteria). Limit the accessibility to the medical records. Do not discuss the patient's medical information with unauthorized family members. Do not disclose patient's information without his/her consent except in established exceptions.

Q. Patient rights in health care.

- Right to Information: Physicians or their qualified assistants are required to provide adequate information about the illness, its diagnosis, proposed investigation and possible complications to the patient.
- Right to records and reports.
- Right to emergency medical care. Patient has the right to prompt emergency care by doctors without compromise on quality or safety and without having to pay full or an advanced fee to the hospital.
- Right to informed consent: The doctor primarily in charge of a patient has to explain the risks, consequences and procedure of the investigation or surgery in simple language before providing the protocol consent form to the patient or to the responsible caretaker.
- Right to confidentiality, human dignity and privacy: Unless it is an exceptional case where sharing this information is "in the interest of protecting other or due to public health considerations."
- Right to nondiscrimination.
- Right to safety and quality care according to standards.
- Right to choose alternative treatment options if available.
- Right to a second opinion.
- Right to transparency in rates, and care according to prescribed rates wherever relevant.
- Right to choose the source for obtaining medicines or tests.
- Right to proper referral and transfer, which is free from perverse commercial influences.
- Right to protection for patients involved in clinical trials.
- Right to protection of participants involved in biomedical and health research.
- Right to be discharged.
- Right to receive the body of a deceased person from the hospital.
- Right to patient education.

Q. Discuss the medicolegal, sociocultural and ethical issues as it pertains to decision making in health care including advanced directives and surrogate decision making

- Decision-making in health care is a complex process, particularly in situations where patients are unable to make decisions for themselves. It involves medicolegal, sociocultural, and ethical considerations that influence how and by whom decisions are made. This is especially relevant in cases involving advanced directives and surrogate decision-making.

Medicolegal Issues

- ***Advanced directives:*** These are legal documents in which a competent person outlines their preferences for future medical care in the event they become incapacitated. These include living wills (specific treatment preferences) and durable power of attorney for healthcare (appoints a proxy or surrogate).
- ***Legal validity and enforcement:*** Advanced directives must comply with jurisdictional laws to be considered valid. Health care providers are legally obligated to honor them unless they are ambiguous or unavailable at the time of care.
- ***Surrogate decision-makers:*** When no directive exists, the law provides a hierarchy for choosing a surrogate (e.g. spouse, adult children, legal guardian). Surrogates must act in accordance with the patient's known wishes or best interests.
- ***Do not resuscitate (DNR) orders:*** Legally binding decisions must be documented clearly. Improper application may result in legal liability.

Sociocultural Issues

- Family and community roles: In some cultures, family-centered decision-making is preferred over individual autonomy. Elders or male heads of family may be expected to make medical decisions, even when the patient is competent.
- Beliefs about death and dying: Some cultural or religious groups oppose advanced directives or withdrawal of life support due to beliefs about fate, divine will, or sanctity of life.
- Respect for cultural diversity requires sensitive, inclusive discussions with patients and families to honor their values while ensuring ethical care.

Ethical Issues

- *Autonomy:* Central to ethical decision-making. Advanced directives uphold patient autonomy when they can no longer express their wishes. Surrogate decisions should reflect the patient's prior preferences, not the surrogate's opinions.
- *Beneficence and nonmaleficence:* Decisions must aim to do good and avoid harm.

Q. Advance directives in health care.

- Some patients may have made plans with medical and/or legal professionals to determine their future preferences of medical care in case they are unable to communicate those preferences in the future. These are called advanced directives. Some of the common advance directives are Do Not Resuscitate (DNR) or Do Not Intubate (DNI) orders. These decisions may or may not have been made in discussion with and including input from their family.
- Patients with these advanced directives should have no difficulties fulfilling their preferred medical decisions; however, there are situations where this may present a problem. Sometimes, these advanced directives are not readily available, or the doctor may not know if a patient has a directive, especially if the patient is unable to give this information. In these cases, it is prudent to provide appropriate medical care whenever there is doubt regarding a patient's medical directive. Another potential issue is when family members of a patient with an advanced directive are not aware of a patient's wishes, or perhaps do not agree with them, and may attempt to intervene in the medical decision making. All health care providers need to keep the patient and the patient's wishes as their primary focus, and the medical decision should be guided by the information that is readily available. In the setting of an impaired elderly patient, healthcare professionals should see whether the patient has legally appointed anybody as the patient's medical decision-maker, such as medical power of attorney who can make decisions on behalf of patient.
- If the patient does not have such a legally appointed individual, medical professionals should determine if a living will or other documented medical directive is available. If no directive or medical power of attorney exists, and the patient is unable to communicate their directive, discussion with family members is appropriate and expected for decision making. This shared decision making will avoid conflict between the medical team and the family members of the patient. Remember that a patient with any advanced directive always retains the right to change their mind and accept further care.

Q. Discuss the medicolegal, sociocultural and ethical issues as it pertains to decision making in emergency care including situations where patients do not have the capability or capacity to give consent.

- Decision-making in emergency care often involves urgent situations where rapid intervention is required, but the patient may be unconscious, disoriented, or otherwise incapable of providing informed consent. These circumstances raise significant medicolegal, sociocultural, and ethical issues that healthcare providers must navigate carefully.

Medicolegal Issues

- *Implied consent in emergencies:* When a patient lacks decision-making capacity and immediate treatment is required to prevent serious harm or death, the law assumes "implied consent." This legal doctrine permits physicians to proceed without formal consent in life-threatening situations.
- *Assessment of capacity:* Patients must be assessed for capacity to consent, which includes the ability to understand, appreciate, and communicate decisions. Lack of capacity must be clearly documented.
- *Surrogate decision-makers*: If time permits and a surrogate (legal guardian, family member) is available, their consent should be obtained. In some jurisdictions, specific legal hierarchies exist for selecting a decision-maker.
- *Legal risk of delay:* Delaying emergency treatment to obtain consent or surrogate authorization can result in legal liability if harm occurs due to inaction.
- *DNR and advance directives*: Legally valid Do Not Resuscitate (DNR) orders or advance directives must be respected, even in emergencies. However, in their absence or ambiguity, resuscitative efforts are usually initiated.

Sociocultural Issues

- *Cultural beliefs and emergency care:* Some cultures may view invasive procedures, blood transfusions, or specific medications as unacceptable, even in emergencies. Families may resist emergency interventions due to religious or traditional beliefs.
- *Family-centered decision-making:* In collectivist societies, families play a central role in decisions, even if the patient is conscious. In emergencies, conflict may arise between medical urgency and cultural expectations of consultation with family or elders.

- *Language and communication barriers:* Language differences can impede rapid informed consent or understanding of the situation. Miscommunication may lead to mistrust or refusal of emergency care.
- *Stigma and social norms*: In some communities, emergency care for injuries like sexual assault or suicide attempts may be stigmatized, affecting willingness to seek or accept care.

Ethical Issues

- *Autonomy vs beneficence:* Ethical tension arises when respecting a patient's autonomy (e.g. refusal of treatment) may lead to serious harm. In emergencies, beneficence—acting in the patient's best interest—often takes precedence if autonomy cannot be confirmed.
- *Justice and fairness:* Resources must be allocated fairly, especially during mass casualty events or in resource-limited settings. No patient should be discriminated against due to race, gender, socioeconomic status, or mental health condition.
- *Nonmaleficence:* Efforts must be made to minimize harm even during urgent interventions. Invasive procedures without confirmed consent should only be performed when absolutely necessary.
- *Respect for known wishes:* If the patient has previously expressed wishes (verbally or in writing), efforts should be made to honor those preferences. Ignoring known DNR orders or prior refusal of blood products (e.g. Jehovah's witnesses) raises ethical concerns.

Q. Discuss the medicolegal, sociocultural and ethical issues as it pertains to research on human subjects.

- Research involving human subjects is essential for medical advancement, but it carries significant medicolegal, sociocultural, and ethical responsibilities. To protect the dignity, rights, and welfare of participants, strict standards must govern the planning, conduct, and reporting of research.

Medicolegal Issues

- *Informed consent:* Legally, all participants must provide voluntary, informed consent before participating. Consent should include information about the purpose, procedures, risks, benefits, and right to withdraw at any time without penalty.
- *Regulatory oversight:* Research must be approved by an Ethics Committee or Institutional Review Board (IRB), which ensures compliance with national and international laws (e.g. ICMR guidelines in India, the Declaration of Helsinki, and good clinical practice guidelines).
- *Vulnerable populations:* Special legal protections are required for groups such as children, prisoners, pregnant women, mentally ill individuals, and economically disadvantaged people. Research involving these groups must have a strong scientific justification and extra safeguards.
- *Privacy and confidentiality:* Participants' personal and health information must be protected under data protection laws (e.g. GDPR, HIPAA). Unauthorized disclosure can lead to legal action.
- *Compensation and injury:* Laws often require that participants be compensated for any research-related injury or adverse effects. Clinical trial rules in India mandate insurance or compensation for injury or death related to participation.

Sociocultural Issues

- *Cultural sensitivity and respect:* Research must be respectful of local customs, traditions, and beliefs. For instance, drawing blood samples or discussing reproductive health may be culturally sensitive in some communities.
- *Language and literacy*: Consent forms must be in a language understandable to participants, with accommodations for illiterate individuals. Miscommunication may lead to misunderstanding of the risks or purpose.
- *Community engagement*: Especially in field-based or epidemiological studies, researchers must build trust with communities through open communication and involvement in planning. Community leaders may be consulted, but individual consent must still be obtained.
- *Power imbalances*: Poor, illiterate, or marginalized individuals may feel pressured to participate, especially if offered incentives. Researchers must ensure that participation is truly voluntary and not exploitative.

Ethical Issues

- *Autonomy:* Participants must be free to make an informed and voluntary decision without coercion.
- Deceptive practices or withholding information undermines autonomy and is unethical.
- *Beneficence and nonmaleficence:* Research should aim to benefit participants or society while minimizing potential risks or harm. High risk research must be justified by potential high benefit.
- *Justice*: Fair selection of participants is essential. Exploiting low-income groups for research while the benefits go to wealthier populations violates ethical standards.
- *Transparency and honesty*: Full disclosure about the nature of research, potential conflicts of interest, and funding sources is required. Results (positive or negative) should be published to avoid research bias.
- *Ethical review and oversight*: Independent review ensures ethical soundness, risk-benefit balance, and participant safety. Continuing ethical oversight is essential during the course of the study.

Q. Discuss physician's role and responsibility to society and the community that she/ he serves.

- 'Some heroes do not wear caps, we call them doctors'. This saying summarises what the society expects from a doctor and what the doctor owes to society. The absolute first and the last event of a human are both certified by doctors, in maternity hospitals and morgue.

- It is the professional responsibility of physicians to use the medical knowledge, scientific expertise, and ethical training to work for better public health. A physician is not only a healer of individuals but also a servant of society. The role of a doctor extends beyond the confines of hospitals and clinics to encompass a deep social, ethical, and professional responsibility to the community.
- The doctor is expected to play following roles in the society.
- ***Medical expert at a societal level:*** Physicians acts as consultants by advising as per their expertise to identify healthcare problems in the society and solutions. Physicians should strive to save lives, extend lifespan, improve quality of life, and prevent epidemics.
- ***Organizer/administrator at the community level:*** physicians should also take the responsibility as administrator to supervise and implement health related policies. Physicians must have insights into management tasks at departmental and organizations level. It is also expected to have this knowledge in regional, national and international level
- ***Teacher/communicator at the community level:*** Physicians must educate the community to on how to prevent diseases and improve health.
- ***Researcher*:** Research is one of the ways to contribute to medical field and also to society. This can be improved or new diagnostic technique, new treatment, or development of vaccines which benefit society.

Q. Discuss the medicolegal, sociocultural, professional and ethical issues in physician-industry relationships.

- Physician–industry relationships—especially those involving pharmaceutical companies, medical device manufacturers, and biotechnology firms—can offer many benefits such as access to the latest innovations, education, and research funding. However, these relationships also raise ethical dilemmas, legal risks, sociocultural sensitivities, and professional challenges. Hence, such interactions must be managed carefully to preserve patient trust, professional autonomy, and public confidence in the medical profession.

Medicolegal Issues

- ***Conflict of interest*:** Physicians who accept gifts, honoraria, or sponsorships from industry may be legally vulnerable if their decisions are influenced. Under Indian laws and Medical Council regulations (such as MCI/NMC Ethics Regulations), accepting bribes, incentives, or kickbacks is considered professional misconduct.
- ***Disclosure obligations:*** There is a legal requirement in many jurisdictions (and in ethical guidelines) for physicians to disclose industry affiliations in publications, presentations, and prescriptions.
- ***Product liability:*** If a physician promotes or uses an industry product irresponsibly (e.g. off-label or experimental use without consent), legal liability for adverse outcomes may follow.
- ***Regulatory violations:*** Participation in unethical drug trials or data manipulation for industry sponsors may violate clinical trial regulations, including those under the ICMR, CDSCO, and DCGI in India.

Ethical Issues

- ***Patient welfare vs. commercial influence:*** Physicians must prioritize patient best interests over company profits. Accepting favors may compromise clinical judgment.
- ***Transparency:*** Full disclosure of industry ties to patients and institutions is ethically mandatory.
- ***Prescribing ethics*:** Writing prescriptions based on promotional bias rather than evidence violates non-maleficence and autonomy.
- ***Research integrity*:** Industry-funded research should be free from data suppression, ghostwriting, or selective reporting.

Professional Issues

- ***Professionalism and trust*:** Unethical relationships can damage the professional image of medicine and erode public trust.
- ***Independence:*** Physicians should maintain intellectual and clinical independence and avoid becoming agents of corporate marketing.
- ***Continuing medical education (CME):*** Industry-sponsored CMEs should be unbiased, scientifically accurate, and free of marketing agendas.
- ***Institutional codes*:** Medical institutions and associations often develop guidelines or codes of conduct for managing physician–industry relationships.

Sociocultural Issues

- ***Public perception*:** In cultures like India, physicians are viewed with reverence. Any appearance of financial conflict or bias can severely damage this image.
- ***Pharmaceutical marketing in LMICs*:** In low- and middle-income countries, aggressive industry marketing may exploit weaker regulatory oversight, and physicians may unknowingly promote irrational drug use.
- ***Inequity:*** Industry influence may cause doctors to favor expensive branded products, increasing the economic burden on poor patients.
- ***Cultural norms:*** Accepting gifts may be culturally normal in some regions but ethically problematic in professional healthcare settings.

Q. Discuss the medicolegal, sociocultural professional and ethical issues pertaining to medical negligence.

- Negligence is the breach of a legal duty to care. It means carelessness in a matter in which the law mandates carefulness. A breach of this duty gives a patient the right to initiate action against negligence.

- Medical malpractice occurs when a healthcare provider deviates from the recognized "standard of care" in the treatment of a patient. The "standard of care" is defined as what a reasonably prudent medical provider would or would not have done under the same or similar circumstances. In essence, it boils down to whether the provider was negligent.
- After Consumer Protection Act has come into force, many patients have filed legal cases against doctors, have established that the doctors were negligent in their medical service, and have claimed and received compensation.
- In medical negligence cases it is the duty of the patient or his/her relatives to establish that: 1. There was a duty which the medical practitioner owed to the patient; 2. There was a breach of duty; 3. The breach resulted in injury to the patient; 4. The injury resulted in causing damages.
- A doctor is not guilty of negligence if he has acted in accordance with practice accepted as proper by reasonable body of medical man skilled in that particular art.
- *Contract Act:* No legal duty to treat the patient except contract. Advice and consultation through TV and news Paper-not contract. No assurance of success of treatment. Discretionary power to choose mode of treatment.

Contributory Negligence

- These are negligence from patient side which lead to failure of treatment. These are failure to take care about himself, choosing wrongful doctor which is apparent, failure to furnish necessary information, refusal to submit for further test, and failure to follow doctor instructions.
- Contributory negligence is not absolute defense. Contributory negligence is applicable to conscious patient. In case of unconscious patient, duty is on doctor or guardian. Contributory negligence of guardian is attributed to patient.

Defences for Doctor

- Most of the time potential civil actions against health care providers are for the following reasons: (1) lack of informed consent, and (2) violation of the standard of care. To avoid this doctor should obtain informed consent as per the prescribed guidelines and keep his knowledge updated in the field of his practice. The standard of care emerges from a variety of sources, including professional publications, interactions of professional leaders, presentations and exchanges at professional meetings, and among networks of colleagues.
- Defense of consent: Obtaining informed consent goes a long way in protecting the doctor against legal cases. Inherent risks involved in the treatment, inevitable accident in the course of operation, unexpected response which requires higher care than prescribed by law are all defenses against the patient who files case against doctor. In emergency situation, doctor need not have necessary qualification and specialization.

Remember

- Things can go wrong when you do not follow ethics.
- Too many doctors increases confusion and litigations.
- We cannot hide our negligence for long.
- Tender, loving care reduces many conflicts.

Q. Discuss the medicolegal, sociocultural, professional, and ethical issues pertaining to malpractice.

- Medical malpractice and medical negligence are related to each other though there is difference between the two. The main difference between the two is intent. In medical negligence a mistake from the medical professional causes a patient unintended harm. Medical malpractice, on the other hand, is when a medical professional knowingly did not follow the proper standard of care. It does not mean that there was malicious intent to cause harm, but the harm could have been avoided if the medical professional had taken alternative measures. In malpractice, the healthcare provider knew something that could either help or harm the patient and consciously chose the option that harmed them. While all medical malpractice is negligence, not every instance of negligence is malpractice.

Types of Malpractice

- Errors in diagnosis, surgical mistakes, improper medication, failure to obtain informed consent, or ignoring standard protocols.

Medicolegal Implications

- Malpractice is a civil or criminal offense, depending on the intent and severity. In India, claims can be filed under: Consumer Protection Act (for compensation), and Indian Penal Code (IPC) for criminal negligence (e.g. IPC Section 304A).
- *Burden of proof:* Patients (plaintiffs) must establish: duty of care existed, there was a breach, and the breach caused injury, damage: Physical, emotional, or financial harm.
- ***Compensation and legal penalties:*** Courts can award **monetary compensation**, revoke licenses, or impose **imprisonment** in severe cases.

Ethical Issues

- Malpractice undermines ethical principles such as nonmaleficence, beneficence (act in the patient's best interest), autonomy (violated when informed consent is missing, justice (patients are denied fair, safe treatment).
- *Lack of transparency*: Failing to disclose errors or attempting to conceal malpractice violates honesty and integrity.

- *Exploitation and overtreatment*: Performing unnecessary procedures for financial gain (e.g. induced demand) is an ethical breach and malpractice.

Professional Issues

- *Erosion of trust*: Malpractice incidents reduce public trust in the profession and increase defensive medicine.
- *Disciplinary action*: Medical councils (like NMC) may impose suspensions, censures, or license revocation for malpractice.
- *Duty to improve*: Professionals must engage in continued education to avoid malpractice due to outdated knowledge or skills.
- *Team responsibility*: Poor teamwork and communication can contribute to malpractice, especially in surgical and emergency settings.

Sociocultural Issues

- *Public reaction and doctor-patient dynamics*: In societies like India, malpractice often triggers mistrust, legal suits, or even violence against doctors. The belief that doctors are infallible contributes to unrealistic expectations, escalating blame when outcomes are poor.
- *Media sensationalism:* News reports often sensationalize malpractice claims, damaging the image of doctors, even before due legal process.
- *Healthcare inequity*: Resource-limited settings may push doctors to take shortcuts, increasing malpractice risk—but society may still hold individual doctors solely responsible.
- *Cultural variations*: What is considered acceptable practice may vary culturally. This can create conflicts in expectations, particularly with end-of-life care, childbirth practices, or gender-sensitive issues.

Q. Discuss the medicolegal, sociocultural, professional and ethical issues in dealing with impaired physicians.

- The impaired physician is a medical doctor who suffers from alcoholism, drug addiction, physical, or mental illness. Impairment affects the physician's life both personally and professionally. The physician's personal life is usually affected first, then his professional interactions with colleagues, and the last area to be affected is the physician's patient care skills.
- Physicians have a higher prevalence of impairment. The high rate of impairment is generally attributed to two sources—the high stress inherent in medical practice and the access to chemical substances.
- Physician impairment raises several medicolegal, sociocultural, professional, and ethical challenges. Below is a detailed discussion and defense of these issues from various perspectives:

Medicolegal Issues

- ***Duty to protect patients:*** Legal responsibility exists to prevent patient harm. Healthcare institutions and regulators (e.g. Medical Council of India/NMC or international equivalents) are legally bound to investigate and act upon reports of impairment.
- ***Mandatory reporting:*** In many jurisdictions, colleagues are legally required to report impaired practitioners to the regulatory body. Failure to report may result in professional liability or civil litigation if patient harm occurs.
- ***Licensure and fitness to practice:*** Impairment can lead to temporary suspension, mandated rehabilitation, or permanent revocation of medical licenses. There must be a balance between public safety and due process.
- ***Confidentiality vs public interest*:** Medical records of the impaired physician must be handled carefully. Exceptions to confidentiality are legally justified when the physician poses a clear risk to patient safety.

Sociocultural Issues

- Many physicians do not reveal or seek treatment for their impairment because of many reasons. Fear of being looked down upon and loss of respect prevent the physician from revealing and seeking help for his impairment. In addition, fear of losing practice, and disciplinary actions by law enforcing agencies, and fear of losing license to practice are all reasons behind impaired physician not seeking help.

Professional Issues

- ***Impairment vs incompetence*:** It is crucial to distinguish temporary impairment (e.g. grief, burnout) from permanent incompetence. Requires systematic assessment by peer review or health boards.
- ***Role of medical institutions:*** Hospitals and medical boards must implement early intervention programs, peer support systems, and confidential reporting mechanisms.
- ***Rehabilitation and reintegration:*** A nonpunitive, supportive approach facilitates safe return to practice after recovery (e.g. drug rehab, psychiatric treatment). Monitored re-entry protects both the physician and the public.
- ***Duty to peers*:** Professionalism demands compassion and accountability toward impaired colleagues. Silence or collusion violates the ethical and professional obligation to maintain standards.

Ethical Issues

- In the framework of physician impairment, the patient's autonomy and the physician's autonomy come into conflict. Patient autonomy takes priority over physician autonomy. The physician may have the autonomy to self-destruct, namely to leave addiction untreated, but this right cannot be extended to be a right to damage a patient.
- The application of the principle of nonmaleficence in case of physician impairment implies the need to protect the patient from the impaired physician who would likely do harm.

- The principle of justice places the needs of the patients above the physician's needs, resulting in regulation of medical practice while impaired. Policy resulting from the principle of justice would emphasize its primary focus on removal of the impaired physician from practice, and secondarily address the treatment programs to benefit physicians.

Identification of the Impaired Physician

- An impaired physician can be identified if his addiction leads to an interaction with law enforcement authorities. For physicians still in training, a supervisor may identify their impairment based on work performance.
- In most cases, the first people to become aware of the physician's impairment are family and close friends.

Intervention and Treatment of the Impaired Physician

- It is important to identify and treat the impaired physician earlier in the course of their impairment. Early identification and intervention result in the best outcome.
- The professionals who intervene and treat the impaired physician must exude hope and potential for recovery or the impaired physician may view continued substance abuse or suicide as better options.
- Confidentiality is another key element to successful intervention and treatment. The impaired physician is likely to fear exposure to colleagues and thus deny addiction or refuse treatment. In general, the impaired physician does best when treated in an in-patient unit particularly if the unit is dedicated specifically to the treatment of medical professionals so that the impaired physician is not being treated alongside nonmedical professionals.

Q. Discuss the medicolegal, sociocultural and ethical issues as they pertain to refusal of medical care.

- A patient's right to the refusal of care is founded upon one of the basic ethical principles of medicine, autonomy. Competent patients have a right to refuse treatment. Competent adults can refuse care even if the care would likely save or prolong the patient's life. However, this respect for patient autonomy may sometimes conflict with other ethical principles of beneficence and nonmaleficence, because patient may wrongly refuse treatment and harm himself. In such situations whether the doctor should respect the patient's decision of refusing treatment (as per the principle of autonomy) or force the patient to undergo treatment for patients benefit becomes a dilemma.

Procedure to follow when Patient Refuses Treatment

- Explain the patient in detail about the benefits of treatment and the risks of no treatment.
- Try to discover the patient's reasons for refusing care and discuss these with the patient to see if there are ways to overcome these so that the patient can receive care that is in his or her best interests.
- With the patient's permission, speak with family, clergy or another mediator if you think this might help the patient reconsider his or her refusal.
- Determine the patient's capacity to refuse. Capacity is defined as a person's ability to process information and make an informed decision about their care in a way that is in line with their beliefs, values, and preferences. If the patient does not have the capacity to make right decisions because of influence of alcohol, drugs, or mental illness, then the physician needs to identify another person who can decide on behalf of patient, or if no one is available, then physician himself can decide about treatment in the best interest of patient.
- Consider a mental health referral if the patient has overwhelming anxieties about receiving care or shows psychiatric comorbidities and is willing to be evaluated.
- Document your efforts to educate the patient, the rationale for your recommended treatment, and the patient's refusal of care.
- Ask the patient to sign a refusal of care form.

Exceptions to the Rule of Autonomy When Patient Refuses Treatment

- *Emergency situation*: Informed consent may be bypassed if immediate treatment is necessary for the patient's life or safety.
- *Altered mental status*: Patients may not have the right to refuse treatment if they have an altered mental status due to alcohol and drugs, brain injury, or psychiatric illness.
- *Children:* A parent or guardian cannot refuse life-sustaining treatment or deny medical care from a child. This includes those with religious beliefs that discourage certain medical treatments. Parents cannot invoke their right to religious freedom to refuse treatment for a child.
- *Threat to the community*: If a patient is a threat to the community (e.g. communicable diseases, violent mentally ill patient), then informed consent is not necessary for treatment as the safety of public takes priority here.

Q. Do not resuscitate (DNR) order and do not intubate order (DNI).

- These two are often part of advance care planning for patients with terminal illnesses, advanced age, or poor prognosis.
- Used to respect patient autonomy and prevent unwanted aggressive interventions at end of life.

Do not Resuscitate (DNR) Order

- In the event of a cardiopulmonary arrest, cardiopulmonary resuscitation is done for every patient unless a do not attempt resuscitation (DNAR) also known as do not resuscitate (DNR) order has been requested by the patient or is written in the medical record by the physician. DNR order may be in the form of advanced directive by the patient.

- If the doctor feels that CPR is futile, then he can write a DNR order, but this should be after discussion with the patient and family members.

Do Not Intubate (DNI) Order

- A DNI order indicates that if the patient stops breathing or experiences respiratory failure, no endotracheal intubation or mechanical ventilation should be performed. It does not preclude other supportive care, such as supplemental oxygen or medication.
- It may accompany a DNR or be issued separately.

Ethical and Legal Considerations

- DNR/DNI orders are legally binding in most jurisdictions and must be respected. Requires informed consent from the patient or their legally authorized representative. If patient wants a DNR order in spite him knowing that CPR may benefit him, patient's decision should be respected and honored. This is respecting patient's autonomy and is supported by law in most countries that recognize a competent patient's right to refuse treatment. Consent of the family is not necessary if the decision is made by the patient—family disagreement is not sufficient to override the patient's choice. If the patient is mentally incompetent, decisions not covered by advance directives are taken after discussion with family members or appropriate surrogate decision makers. If conflict or dilemmas arise, the Ethics Committee assists in clarifying available options and improving communications.
- Nurses and the entire medical team should be aware of this DNR order. When a DNR is written on the medical record no resuscitative treatment is done such as CPR or ACLS.
- Must be clearly documented and communicated to the healthcare team.
- DNR does not mean "do not treat"—patients may still receive all other forms of medical care, including antibiotics, fluids, and pain relief.

Q. Withdrawal of treatment.

- Modern medicine has progressed so much that patients can often be kept alive almost indefinitely with the aid of mechanical ventilators, artificial feeds and organ support strategies. However, in terminally ill patients and permanently unconscious patients, it is futile to do so. In such situations, end of life decisions become important.
- End-of-life decisions are of two types: withdrawal of therapy and withholding of therapy. Withdrawal is removal of a therapy that has been started in an attempt to sustain life but is not, or is no longer effective. Examples are stopping mechanical ventilation and inotropic agents. Withholding means not to make any further therapeutic interventions. Examples are do not resuscitate (DNR) order, withholding dialysis in renal failure, etc.
- Although these two actions are considered ethically equivalent, withdrawing life-sustaining therapy may be preferable to withholding.

Why the Decision on Withdrawal of Therapy is Important?

- If withdrawal of therapy were not permitted, then ICUs would be full of hopelessly ill patients receiving (often expensive) therapies that no longer benefit them and only prolongs suffering. Such futile therapy also puts lot of burden to patient's relatives.
- By continuing ineffective therapy, an ICU bed may be blocked and not available for another patient who may benefit from ICU care. In addition, the costs of the futile care could be better employed elsewhere.

When is Withdrawal Considered Appropriate?

- Treatment is futile or prolongs the dying process.
- Patient has a terminal illness or is in a persistent vegetative state.
- Patient has an advance directive, DNR/DNI, or expresses a wish to stop treatment.
- The burden outweighs the benefit, such as severe suffering or poor quality of life.

Withdrawal may be Better than Withholding

- In case of withholding a therapy, where a treatment is not started in the first place deprives the patient from possible benefit from that therapy. For example, consider an elderly, frail patient who develops severe pneumonia. The prognosis in this case is not sure. Should the patient be put on mechanical ventilation and put on antibiotics or should he be left alone without mechanical ventilation. In this case it is better to put him on mechanical ventilation and later withdraw it if not helping. Hence in many places withdrawal of therapy is more common than withholding.

Legal Aspects

- Legal in many countries, including India, when done with patient consent or proxy decision-making.
- Requires adherence to Supreme Court guidelines in India regarding passive euthanasia and advance directives.
- Must be well-documented, transparent, and ethically justified.
- Not equivalent to euthanasia: Withdrawal lets nature take its course without actively causing death.
- Does not mean abandonment: Patients continue to receive palliative and supportive care.

Essentials when Withdrawing Therapy

- End-of-life decisions should be made in advance whenever possible. This is particularly true for decisions to withhold therapy because there is often less time to think in emergencies.

- It is also important that end-of-life decisions are made by consensus, after open discussion involving patient, relatives and doctor. However, such decisions should not be left to the relatives alone because it is difficult for them to decide, and ultimately it is the physician who is responsible for administering or discontinuing any treatment. Any such discussions and decisions should be documented clearly in the patient notes.

Problems

- Problems arising from decisions to withdraw treatment can be divided into four types.

Referring Team Request Continued Futile Therapy

- This can usually be resolved by explaining the rationale and offering a second opinion. If conflict still remains, treatment cannot be withdrawn.

Patient's Family Requests Continued Futile Therapy

- Guilt usually plays a part in the family's request to continue treatment. Agreement can usually be obtained by explaining the rationale again and offering a second opinion from within or outside the intensive care team. It is best not to withdraw treatment if there is conflict. However, the final decision rests with the intensive care team. This underlines the need for good communication.

Family Requests Inappropriate Discontinuation of Therapy

- The rationale behind the therapy and the reasons why continuing treatment is thought appropriate should be explained. The duty of care is to the patient, not the family. Again, a second opinion can be offered.

Patient Requests Discontinuation of Therapy

- Explain to the patient the rationale for the treatment and that, in the opinion of the intensive care team, a chance of recovery exists. It may be appropriate to offer a short-term contract for treatment (for example, 48 hours then review). Ultimately, the competent patient has the right to refuse treatment even if that treatment is lifesaving.

Chapter 20

Geriatrics

Q. What is geriatrics? Describe the key aspects of geriatrics.

- Geriatrics is the branch of medicine that focuses on the health care of geriatric age group (older adults). The geriatric age group typically refers to individuals who are **65 years of age and older**.
- It aims to promote healthy aging by preventing, diagnosing, and managing diseases and conditions commonly affecting elderly people.

Key Aspects of Geriatrics

- Holistic care: Addresses physical, psychological, social, and functional aspects of aging.
- Multimorbidity management: Older adults often have multiple chronic conditions (e.g. diabetes, hypertension, arthritis).
- Polypharmacy management: Avoids harmful drug interactions due to multiple medications.
- Functional status evaluation: Assesses ability to perform activities of daily living (ADLs) and instrumental ADLs.
- Cognitive and mental health: Deals with conditions like dementia, delirium, and depression.
- Fall and frailty prevention.
- End-of-life care and advance directives.
- Geriatrics is often interdisciplinary, involving physicians, nurses, social workers, physiotherapists, and others to provide comprehensive care tailored to the elderly population.

Q. Describe the epidemiology, pathogenesis, clinical evolution, presentation and course of common diseases in the elderly.

- As people age, they are more prone to certain chronic and degenerative diseases due to physiological changes, declining organ function, and cumulative exposure to risk factors.

Epidemiology of Diseases in the Elderly

- The elderly population (≥65 years) is rapidly increasing worldwide due to rising life expectancy.
- Noncommunicable diseases (NCDs) are the leading cause of morbidity and mortality in this age group.
- Common diseases in the elderly include:
  - Cardiovascular diseases: Hypertension, ischemic heart disease, heart failure
  - Diabetes mellitus
  - Chronic respiratory diseases: COPD, asthma
  - Neurodegenerative diseases: Alzheimer's disease, Parkinson's disease
  - Osteoarthritis and osteoporosis
  - Malignancies: Colorectal, prostate, breast, and lung cancers
  - Depression, dementia, and delirium
  - Urinary incontinence and BPH
  - Sensory deficits: Hearing and vision loss
  - Falls and fractures.

Pathogenesis

Aging-related Physiological Changes

- Reduced organ reserve and adaptability
- Altered immune response (immunosenescence)
- Increased oxidative stress and cellular senescence
- Impaired homeostatic mechanisms.

These Changes Increase Vulnerability to

- Multisystem diseases
- Polypharmacy effects
- Atypical presentations
- Poor recovery after illness.

Clinical Evolution and Presentation

- Diseases often have atypical or subtle symptoms in the elderly.
- Infections may present without fever but with confusion or falls.
- Myocardial infarction may present as fatigue or breathlessness instead of chest pain.
- Depression may mimic dementia ("pseudodementia").
- Thyroid dysfunction may present as cognitive decline.
- Urinary tract infection may present with delirium.

- Symptoms often overlap and may be masked by comorbidities.

Course of Common Diseases

- Chronic and progressive in nature
- Slower onset, but with higher risk of complications
- Higher rates of hospitalizations, disability, and institutionalization
- Recovery is often prolonged and may be incomplete.
- High prevalence of frailty, sarcopenia, and functional decline
- Often complicated by: Polypharmacy, falls, nutritional deficiencies, and cognitive impairment.

Examples of Specific Conditions in Elderly

(Table 20.1)

TABLE 20.1: Common diseases affecting elderly

Disease	Presentation	Course
Hypertension	Often asymptomatic or presents with headaches/dizziness	Increases risk of stroke, heart failure, renal failure
Diabetes	Fatigue, weight loss, recurrent infections	Risk of neuropathy, nephropathy, retinopathy; needs individualised targets
Osteoporosis	Silent in early stages (diagnosed only by bone mineral density test). Symptomatic patients may present with back pain and fractures.	Progressive functional decline: Difficulty in ambulation, activities of daily living (ADLs). Many elderly with hip fractures require long-term care. Recurrent fractures likely if untreated.
Osteoarthritis	Joint pain, stiffness	Progressive; leads to mobility issues
Dementia	Memory loss, disorientation, personality change	Gradual decline in cognitive and functional abilities
COPD	Chronic cough, dyspnea	Progressive, with exacerbations; often coexists with heart disease
Benign prostatic hyperplasia (BPH)	Weak urine stream (poor stream), straining to urinate, hesitancy (delay in starting urination), dribbling at the end of urination, increased frequency of urination (day and night), nocturia (waking up at night to urinate), urgency (sudden need to urinate), urge incontinence (leakage)	Symptoms gradually worsen. If untreated can lead to acute urinary retention, recurrent urinary tract infections, bladder stones, hydronephrosis (back pressure on kidneys), and chronic kidney disease
Depression	Sadness, withdrawal, sleep issues, somatic complaints	May be underdiagnosed; affects quality of life and recovery from illness

Q. Describe the multidimensional geriatric assessments that includes medical, psychosocial and functional components.

- Multidimensional geriatric assessment (MGA) also known as comprehensive geriatric assessment (CGA), is a structured, interdisciplinary process used to evaluate the overall health status of elderly individuals, especially those who are frail, chronically ill, or functionally impaired.
- It includes medical, psychological, social, and functional domains to identify problems, develop a coordinated care plan, and improve outcomes.

Goal of Multidimensional Geriatric Assessment

- Identify reversible problems.
- Maintain independence.
- Improve quality of life.
- Prevent hospitalizations and institutionalization.
- Guide individualized and multidisciplinary care planning.

Medical Assessment

- Medical assessment focuses on identifying and managing diseases, medications, and nutritional status.

Chronic Disease Review

- *Common illnesses:* Hypertension, diabetes, COPD, heart failure, arthritis, osteoporosis, BPH, cognitive dysfunction, malignancy, risk of falls, incontinence, pressure ulcers, frailty, sensory deficits.

Medication Review (Polypharmacy)

- Identify potentially inappropriate medications (e.g. using Beers criteria).
- Assess for adverse drug reactions, drug interactions, and compliance.

Nutritional Assessment

- Unintentional weight loss
- Appetite changes
- Tools: Mini-nutritional assessment (MNA)

Psychological Assessment

Evaluates Cognitive and Emotional Health

- *Cognitive function*: Detects dementia, delirium, and mild cognitive impairment. Can be assessed by using mini-mental state examination (MMSE) or montreal cognitive assessment (MoCA).
- *Mood and mental health*: Depression and anxiety are common and often underdiagnosed. Can be assessed by geriatric depression scale (GDS) hospital anxiety and depression scale (HADS).

Functional Assessment

Assesses the Person's Ability to Perform Daily Activities Independently

- Activities of daily living (ADLs): Bathing, dressing, eating, toileting, transferring, continence.

- Instrumental activities of daily living (IADLs): Managing finances, cooking, using the phone, transportation, shopping.
- Mobility and fall risk: Gait, balance, and strength.
- There are tools to assess these functions.

Social Assessment

Looks at the Support System, Living Conditions, and Socioeconomic Factors

- Living arrangement (alone, with family, in a care home)
- Caregiver availability and burden
- Financial resources and insurance status
- Risk of neglect, elder abuse, or social isolation.

Environmental Assessment

Evaluates the Home Environment and Safety Risks

- Hazards: Slippery floors, poor lighting, stairs
- Need for assistive devices (grab bars, walkers)
- Accessibility and suitability for the elderly.

Q. Beers criteria.

- Beers criteria is a guideline developed by the American Geriatrics Society (AGS) that lists potentially inappropriate medications (PIMs) for use in older adults (usually ≥65 years). It is used to improve medication safety, reduce adverse drug events, and support clinical decision-making in geriatric care.

Purpose of Beers Criteria

- Identify drugs with high risk of side effects in the elderly.
- Prevent polypharmacy and drug interactions.
- Guide safe prescribing practices.

Why Older Adults are at Risk

- Age-related changes in pharmacokinetics and pharmacodynamics
- Decreased renal and hepatic function
- Increased sensitivity to CNS drugs
- More likely to have multiple comorbidities.

Key Categories in Beers Criteria (Table 20.2)

TABLE 20.2: Beers criteria

Category	Description
1. Medications to avoid in older adults	High risk of adverse effects outweighs potential benefits
2. Medications to avoid in certain diseases or conditions	May worsen underlying conditions (e.g. dementia, heart failure)
3. Medications to use with caution	Use only if benefits clearly outweigh risks
4. Drug-drug interactions	Combinations to avoid due to harmful interactions
5. Dose adjustments based on kidney function	Drugs that require renal dose adjustments in elderly

Examples of Drugs in Beers Criteria

Drugs to Avoid in Most Older Adults

Drug/Class	Risk
Anticholinergics (e.g. diphenhydramine)	Confusion, constipation, dry mouth, falls
Benzodiazepines (e.g. diazepam, lorazepam)	Sedation, falls, cognitive impairment
Nonbenzodiazepine hypnotics (e.g. zolpidem)	Delirium, falls, fractures
NSAIDs (e.g. ibuprofen, diclofenac)	GI bleeding, kidney injury, hypertension
Sliding scale insulin	Risk of hypoglycemia
Digoxin (>0.125 mg/day)	Increased toxicity in renal impairment

Drugs to Avoid in Certain Conditions

Condition	Avoid
Dementia	Anticholinergics, benzodiazepines
Heart failure	NSAIDs, certain calcium channel blockers (e.g. diltiazem)
History of falls/fractures	Sedatives, antipsychotics, opioids

Use with Caution

Drug/Class	Concern
Aspirin for primary prevention	Increased bleeding risk
Tricyclic antidepressants	Anticholinergic side effects, orthostatic hypotension
Diuretics	Electrolyte imbalance, dehydration

Drug Combinations to Avoid in Elderly

Combination	Risk
Anticholinergic + Anticholinergic	Delirium, cognitive decline
Opioids + Benzodiazepines	Respiratory depression, death
Warfarin + NSAIDs/Antibiotics	Major bleeding
ACEI/ARB + Potassium sparing diuretics	Hyperkalemia
Digoxin + Loop Diuretic	Arrhythmia from hypokalemia
CNS depressants (≥3)	Falls, sedation, cognitive impairment

Dose Adjustments Based on Kidney Function

- Renal function commonly declines due to aging—even in the absence of overt kidney disease. This makes renal dose adjustment critical for many drugs to avoid toxicity, especially in medications that are renally excreted.
- Many elderly patients may have normal creatinine levels due to low muscle mass, but reduced renal function.

Q. Describe the etiopathogenesis, clinical presentation, identification, functional changes, acute care, stabilization, management and rehabilitation of acute confusional states.

- Acute confusional state (delirium) is a transient, fluctuating disturbance of consciousness, attention, and cognition, with an acute onset, often reversible.
- Delirium and confusional states are among the most common mental disorders encountered in patients with medical illness, particularly among those who are older.

Etiopathogenesis

- Preexisting dementia or cognitive impairment
- Electrolyte imbalance: Hypernatremia, hyponatremia
- Metabolic causes: Hypoglycemia, hypoxia
- Infection
- Severe medical illness
- Sensory deprivation (visual/hearing impairment)
- Drugs: Anticholinergics, opioids, benzodiazepines, corticosteroids, polypharmacy
- Intracranial pathology: Stroke, hemorrhage, trauma, tumor
- Urinary/fecal retention
- Substance use or withdrawal.

Clinical Presentation

- Acute onset and fluctuating course
- Inattention (hallmark feature)
- Disorganized thinking or altered level of consciousness
- Disorientation (time/place), memory deficits
- Perceptual disturbances (hallucinations)
- Sleep-wake disturbances.

Subtypes

- Hyperactive: Agitation, hallucinations, restlessness.
- Hypoactive: Apathy, reduced alertness (often missed).
- Mixed: Fluctuates between hyperactive and hypoactive.

Identification/Diagnosis

- Clinical features
- Mini-mental state examination (MMSE).

Investigations

- CBC, electrolytes, LFTs, RFTs, blood glucose
- Urine analysis (UTI common cause)
- Chest X-ray, ECG
- CT/MRI brain (if focal signs or trauma)
- Blood cultures, if sepsis suspected.

Functional changes

- Impairment in attention, orientation, memory
- Impaired ADLs (Activities of Daily Living)
- Increased fall risk, poor nutritional intake
- Social withdrawal, sleep disturbances
- Impacts long-term cognitive and physical recovery.

Management

Acute Care and Stabilization

- Ensure patient safety (prevent falls, remove restraints if possible)
- Address life-threatening conditions (e.g. hypoxia, sepsis, hypoglycemia)
- Create a calm, well-lit environment
- Reorient frequently (clock, calendar, family)
- Hydration, nutrition
- Encourage mobility if possible
- Optimize vision and hearing (use aids)
- Avoid or minimize catheterization, restraints.

Treatment of Underlying Cause

- Antibiotics for infections
- Correct metabolic imbalances
- Stop/adjust offending medications
- Pharmacological treatment (only if severely agitated): Haloperidol (0.5–1 mg orally or IM)—preferred first-line in most cases. Olanzapine or risperidone (atypical antipsychotics). Avoid benzodiazepines (except in alcohol/sedative withdrawal delirium).

Rehabilitation

- Monitor for persistent cognitive impairment
- Address nutrition, mobility, psychosocial needs
- Involve multidisciplinary team: Geriatrician, physiotherapist, occupational therapist, psychiatrist/psychologist, social worker
- Cognitive exercises
- Re-establish routines
- Reduce environmental triggers
- Gradual reintroduction to social interaction.

Q. Describe the etiopathogenesis, clinical features, diagnosis, functional changes, management, and rehabilitation of vascular events in the elderly.

- Vascular events in the elderly are common, multifactorial in etiology, and often disabling. Prompt recognition, timely intervention, and coordinated rehabilitation can significantly improve outcomes and quality of life.

Etiopathogenesis of Vascular Events in the Elderly

Age-related Vascular Changes

- Atherosclerosis: Progressive narrowing and hardening of arteries
- Endothelial dysfunction
- Reduced cerebral autoregulation
- Arterial stiffness and calcification.

Risk Factors

- Hypertension
- Diabetes mellitus
- Hyperlipidemia
- Atrial fibrillation and other arrhythmias
- Smoking and alcohol use.

- Sedentary lifestyle
- Prior TIA or stroke
- Carotid artery disease.

Clinical Features

Symptoms vary by vascular territory involved, commonly:
- Sudden-onset weakness or paralysis (hemiparesis/hemiplegia)
- Speech disturbances (aphasia or dysarthria)
- Vision loss (amaurosis fugax, hemianopia)
- Facial asymmetry
- Gait disturbances
- Loss of coordination or balance (ataxia)
- Altered consciousness in severe strokes
- Cognitive decline (vascular dementia)
- Atypical presentations in elderly: Confusion, repeated falls, urinary incontinence, isolated dizziness.

Diagnosis

- Based on clinical features
- Imaging: CT/MRI brain/CT/MR angiography
- Cardiovascular evaluation: ECG, Holter monitoring—to detect atrial fibrillation, echocardiography—for cardioembolic sources, carotid doppler USG—to detect carotid stenosis.

Lab Investigations

- CBC, blood glucose, HbA1c
- Lipid profile
- Renal function tests
- Coagulation profile.

Functional Changes

- Motor deficits: Hemiplegia/hemiparesis, spasticity
- Speech and language impairments: Aphasia, dysarthria
- Swallowing difficulty: Risk of aspiration
- Cognitive decline: Executive dysfunction, vascular dementia
- Emotional disturbances: Depression, pseudobulbar affect
- Loss of independence: Impaired ADLs and IADLs
- Bowel/bladder dysfunction.

Management

Ischemic Stroke

- IV thrombolysis (Alteplase) if within 4.5 hours and no contraindications
- Mechanical thrombectomy in selected large vessel occlusions (up to 24 hours in some cases)
- Antiplatelets (aspirin, clopidogrel) after excluding hemorrhage.

Hemorrhagic Stroke

- Blood pressure control (target SBP <140 mm Hg).
- Neurosurgical evaluation (e.g. for hematoma evacuation).
- Reverse anticoagulation, if applicable.

Secondary Prevention

- Antiplatelets or anticoagulants (for AF or embolic strokes)
- Statins
- Blood pressure control
- Glycemic control
- Lifestyle modifications: Diet, exercise, smoking cessation.

Rehabilitation

- Multidisciplinary approach is started as early as possible, ideally within 24–48 hours after stabilization
- *Physiotherapy:* Improve strength, balance, mobility, prevent contractures and pressure sores
- *Occupational therapy*: Focus on activities of daily living, adaptive techniques, home modifications
- *Speech and swallow therapy*: For aphasia, dysphagia, communication training
- *Neuropsychological support*: Cognitive rehabilitation, behavior therapy, depression screening and management
- *Social and family support*: Involvement in care planning, vocational therapy if applicable
- *Assistive devices*: Wheelchairs, walkers, communication aids.

Q. Discuss the etiopathogenesis, clinical presentation, identification, functional changes, acute care, stabilization, management and rehabilitation of depression in the elderly.

- Depression in the elderly is a common but under-recognized condition with atypical presentations. Early diagnosis and management can significantly improve prognosis, quality of life, and functional independence in the elderly.

Etiopathogenesis of Depression in the Elderly

- Depression in older adults is **multifactorial**, involving **biological, psychosocial** components.

Biological Factors

- **Neurotransmitter imbalance:** ↓ serotonin, norepinephrine, dopamine.
- **Structural brain changes:** White matter lesions, frontal lobe atrophy.
- **Neuroendocrine dysregulation:** ↑ cortisol (HPA axis overactivity).
- **Chronic medical conditions:** Stroke, Parkinson's, dementia, hypothyroidism, chronic pain, cancer.
- **Polypharmacy:** Some drugs (e.g. corticosteroids, beta-blockers, benzodiazepines) may contribute.

Psychosocial Factors

- Bereavement
- Loneliness, social isolation
- Financial dependency or insecurity
- Retirement, loss of status/role
- Institutionalization.

Clinical Presentation

- May be **atypical** in the elderly and often misdiagnosed as cognitive decline ("pseudodementia").
- **Core symptoms:** Persistent sadness, low mood, anhedonia (loss of interest/pleasure), fatigue, low energy.
- **Other symptoms:** Poor concentration, memory complaints, appetite and weight changes, sleep disturbances (early morning awakening), psychomotor retardation or agitation, feelings of worthlessness, excessive guilt, suicidal ideation (elderly have highest suicide rates), somatic complaints (pain, constipation) common.

Identification and Diagnosis

- Detailed history (including recent bereavement, social factors)
- Mental status examination
- Rule out delirium and dementia
- Screening tools: Geriatric depression scale.

Investigations

To rule out reversible causes:

- CBC, TSH, B_{12}, folate.
- ECG, LFTs, RFTs (if on medications).
- Neuroimaging (MRI/CT brain) if atypical features or cognitive decline.

Functional Changes in Elderly with Depression

- Impaired ADLs (activities of daily living)
- Loss of motivation → neglect of self-care
- Cognitive slowing and memory loss (may mimic dementia)
- Social withdrawal
- Falls and physical deconditioning
- Reduced medication adherence and increased healthcare utilization.

Management

Risk Assessment

- Suicide risk (ask directly; elderly have high risk)
- Safety–home hazards, neglect, nutrition
- Admission to hospital if there is suicidal ideation or attempts, severe psychomotor retardation, refusal of food/water, psychotic features, coexisting medical instability.

Pharmacological Therapy

- **SSRIs (first-line):** e.g. sertraline, escitalopram (start low, go slow)
- **SNRIs:** Duloxetine (if also pain), venlafaxine
- **Mirtazapine:** Good for insomnia, weight loss
- **Avoid:** TCAs and MAOIs (anticholinergic side effects, cardiac risks).

Psychotherapy

- Cognitive behavioral therapy (CBT)
- Interpersonal therapy (IPT)
- Problem-solving therapy.

Social Interventions

- Family education and involvement
- Day care programs
- Community and senior support groups.

Rehabilitation

Goals of Rehabilitation

- Functional recovery
- Reintegration into community
- Prevent relapse.

Approach

- Multidisciplinary team: Physician, psychiatrist, psychologist, physiotherapist, social worker
- Occupational therapy: Reinforce independence in ADLs
- Social support: Enhance social networks
- Regular follow-up: Monitor recurrence or cognitive decline
- Home care services: If physical or cognitive limitations persist.

Q. Describe the etiopathogenesis, clinical features, management and rehabilitation of dementia in elderly.

- Dementia is a chronic, progressive decline in cognitive function severe enough to interfere with daily life and independence. It primarily affects memory, executive function, language, and behavior.

Etiopathogenesis of Dementia in the Elderly

Alzheimer's disease

- Accumulation of β-amyloid plaques and tau tangles
- Neuronal loss and cortical atrophy

Vascular dementia

- Chronic cerebral ischemia/infarcts
- Associated with hypertension, diabetes, stroke, atherosclerosis

Lewy body dementia

- Accumulation of alpha-synuclein (Lewy bodies) in cortex and brainstem

Other risk factors

- Advanced age
- Family history
- Traumatic brain injury
- Depression
- Low educational attainment

Clinical Features

Cognitive Symptoms

- Memory loss (especially short-term memory)
- Disorientation to time/place
- Language difficulties (anomia, aphasia)
- Impaired judgment and reasoning
- Visuospatial disorientation
- Apraxia, agnosia.

Neuropsychiatric Symptoms

- Depression, apathy
- Delusions, hallucinations (common in Lewy body dementia)
- Personality changes, disinhibition (especially in FTD)
- Anxiety, agitation, aggression.

Functional Impairment

- Difficulty with activities of daily living (ADLs)
- Poor self-care, safety issues (wandering, forgetting stove).
- Falls, incontinence in later stages.

Management

General Principles

- No cure; Focus is on symptom control, functional support, and safety.
- Address reversible or treatable causes
- Involve multidisciplinary team and caregivers.

Pharmacological Management

- Cognitive enhancers: Cholinesterase inhibitors (donepezil, Rivastigmine, Galantamine) are indicated in mild–moderate Alzheimer's disease. NMDA antagonist memantine is helpful in moderate to severe Alzheimer's disease.
- Psychiatric Symptoms: SSRIs for depression and anxiety (e.g. sertraline). Atypical antipsychotics (e.g. quetiapine, risperidone) for severe agitation, psychosis.
- Treatment of comorbidities: Control of BP, glucose, lipids
- Avoid sedatives, anticholinergics.

Rehabilitation and Supportive Care

- ***Cognitive rehabilitation***: Memory aids (calendars, clocks, notes), routine-based training, reality orientation and reminiscence therapy.
- ***Occupational therapy***: Training in ADLs, environmental modifications to reduce fall risk.
- ***Speech and language therapy***: For aphasia or communication deficits.
- ***Physical therapy***: Balance and gait training, fall prevention strategies.
- ***Caregiver support and education***: Stress management and respite care, training on handling behavioral issues.
- ***Safety measures:*** Simplify home layout, remove tripping hazards, use of identification bracelets.
- ***Advanced planning***: Discuss advance directives, legal guardianship. Plan for end-of-life care and nursing home placement if needed.

Q. Describe the etiopathogenesis, clinical presentation, identification, functional changes, acute care, stabilization, management and rehabilitation of personality changes in the elderly.

- Personality changes in the elderly are often under-recognized but highly impactful, signaling underlying neurological or psychiatric pathology.
- A careful evaluation, prompt identification of treatable causes, and a comprehensive, interdisciplinary management approach are essential to minimize disability, preserve dignity, and enhance the elderly person's overall well-being.

Etiopathogenesis

- Personality changes in the elderly can result from a complex interplay of biological, psychological, and social factors.

Biological Factors

- Neurodegenerative diseases: Alzheimer's disease, frontotemporal dementia (especially behavioral variant FTD), Parkinson's disease, and Lewy body dementia.
- Cerebrovascular disease: Multi-infarct dementia and silent strokes affecting the frontal lobes.
- Frontal lobe lesions: Tumors, trauma, or infections can alter executive functioning and personality traits.
- Delirium and metabolic encephalopathy: Acute confusional states may present with abrupt personality changes.
- Medication effects: Psychotropic drugs, corticosteroids, anticholinergics, and polypharmacy.

Psychological Factors

- Depression, anxiety, grief reactions
- Chronic stress or adjustment disorders
- Preexisting personality traits may become exaggerated with aging.

Social and Environmental Factors

- Loss of spouse, friends, retirement, social isolation
- Institutionalization or abuse/neglect
- Role changes and lack of purpose.

Clinical Presentation

Personality changes may be gradual or abrupt, and include:

- Apathy or withdrawal
- Irritability or aggression
- Disinhibition (e.g. inappropriate jokes, sexual behavior)
- Paranoia or suspiciousness (belief that others are stealing or harming them)
- Emotional lability (rapid mood swings, crying or laughing without clear cause)
- Compulsiveness or ritualistic behavior
- Lack of empathy (seen in frontotemporal dementia)
- Rigid or stubborn behavior
- Social withdrawal or fearfulness.

Identification and Diagnosis

- *History:* Family or caregiver input is essential. Onset, duration, progression, and associated symptoms.
- *Clinical examination*: Look for focal deficits, gait abnormalities, extrapyramidal signs.
- *Mental status and psychological Assessment*: Mini-mental state examination (MMSE), Montreal cognitive assessment (MoCA)'
- *Investigations:* CBC, electrolytes, thyroid function, B_{12}, folate, LFTs, RFTs. CT or MRI brain to assess for stroke, atrophy, or lesions.

Differential Diagnosis

- Dementias (especially frontotemporal)
- Depression ("pseudodementia")
- Delirium
- Normal pressure hydrocephalus
- Primary psychiatric disorders (late-onset schizophrenia, bipolar).

Functional Changes

- Decline in activities of daily living (ADLs)
- Social dysfunction: Isolation, relationship difficulties
- Loss of executive functioning: Impaired judgment, planning
- Impaired work/leisure capabilities
- Increased caregiver burden and potential for elder abuse.

Management

Acute Care and Stabilization

- Identify and treat reversible causes: e.g. infections, metabolic derangements, drug toxicity
- Safety assessment: Prevent self-harm, manage aggression or wandering
- Hospitalization: If there is risk of harm or severe behavioral dysregulation
- Environmental modifications: Calm, well-lit, structured setting.

Pharmacological

- Antidepressants: SSRIs for depression or irritability
- Antipsychotics: Only if severe agitation or psychosis; use lowest dose and shortest duration (e.g. risperidone)
- Mood stabilizers: Valproate for mood lability in dementia
- Cholinesterase inhibitors: Donepezil or rivastigmine for Alzheimer's disease
- Avoid benzodiazepines and anticholinergic drugs.

Nonpharmacological

- Psychoeducation for patient and family
- Cognitive-behavioral therapy (CBT) or supportive psychotherapy
- Behavioral interventions: Reinforcement strategies, activity scheduling.
- Environmental adjustments: Reduce overstimulation, use memory aids.
- Occupational therapy: To promote routine and independence.

Rehabilitation

- *Multidisciplinary approach:* Geriatrician, neurologist, psychiatrist, psychologist, social worker, physiotherapist. Goal is to maximize independence, enhance quality of life, and support caregivers.
- *Strategies:*
  - Cognitive rehabilitation and stimulation
  - Structured activities: Art, music, reminiscence therapy
  - Social engagement: Day-care centers, senior clubs
  - Caregiver support and training
  - Advance care planning and legal counseling, if progressive condition.

Q. Describe the etiopathogenesis, clinical presentation, diagnosis, and management of osteoporosis in the elderly.

- Osteoporosis is a systemic skeletal disorder characterized by reduced bone mass and microarchitectural deterioration of bone tissue, leading to increased bone fragility and fracture risk.

Etiology

Primary Osteoporosis

- Type I (Postmenopausal): Due to estrogen deficiency, seen in women aged 50–70 years.
- Type II (Senile): Due to age-related bone loss, seen in both sexes, especially after age 70.

Secondary Osteoporosis

Due to underlying medical conditions or medications, e.g.:

- Calcium/vitamin D deficiency: Impairs bone mineralization
- Endocrine disorders: Hyperthyroidism, hyperparathyroidism, diabetes
- GI disorders: Malabsorption, chronic liver disease
- Renal disease: Chronic kidney disease (CKD), renal tubular acidosis
- Medications: Glucocorticoids, heparin, anticonvulsants, proton-pump inhibitors.

Pathophysiological Mechanisms

- Decreased bone formation due to reduced osteoblast activity and increased bone resorption due to increased osteoclast activity. These changes may be age related which is a normal physiological phenomenon or due to some underlying cause as in secondary osteoporosis.

Clinical Presentation

- Osteoporosis is often asymptomatic until a fracture occurs. When symptomatic, features include:

Fragility Fractures

- Vertebral compression fractures (most common). Other sites include Colles' fracture (distal radius), neck of femur fracture, humerus, pelvis, and rib fractures.

Symptoms

- Back pain (due to vertebral collapse)
- Loss of height due to vertebral compression fracture
- Kyphosis ("Dowager's hump")
- Functional impairment, reduced mobility.

Complications

- Chronic pain
- Disability
- Increased morbidity and mortality post-fracture.

Diagnosis

- History of fractures, risk factors, dietary habits, medications
- Physical exam: Height loss, kyphosis, tenderness over vertebrae.
- Investigations (*see* below).

Investigations

- Bone mineral density (BMD): DEXA scan (dual-energy X-ray absorptiometry). This is the gold standard test to diagnose osteoporosis.
  - WHO criteria (T-score):
    - Normal: ≥–1
    - Osteopenia: –1 to –2.5
    - Osteoporosis: ≤–2.5
- Serum calcium, phosphate, alkaline phosphatase
- Serum vitamin D level
- PTH, TSH
- Renal and liver function tests
- X-rays: May show vertebral fractures, but poor sensitivity for early bone loss.

Management

Lifestyle Modifications

- Diet rich in calcium and vitamin D
- Exercise: Weight-bearing and muscle-strengthening exercises
- Fall prevention: Home safety, vision correction, balance training
- Avoid smoking, alcohol, and excessive caffeine.

Pharmacological Treatment

- Antiresorptive agents: Bisphosphonates (1st line, e.g. alendronate, risedronate, zoledronate). Denosumab (monoclonal antibody, esp. in renal impairment).
- Anabolic agents: Teriparatide (PTH analog), abaloparatide, Romosozumab (for severe osteoporosis).
- Hormonal therapy: Estrogen replacement therapy in postmenopausal women (with caution), raloxifene).
- Calcium and vitamin D supplementation: Adjunct to all therapies.

Management of Fractures

- Orthopedic intervention (surgery or conservative), rehabilitation and pain control, post-fracture osteoporosis therapy initiation.

Q. Describe the etiology, clinical presentation, investigations, functional changes, management and rehabilitation of CVA in the elderly.

- Cerebrovascular accident (CVA), or stroke, refers to the sudden loss of brain function due to disturbance in blood supply.
- It is classified as ischemic (85%) or hemorrhagic (15%).

Etiology of CVA in the Elderly

Ischemic Stroke (most common in elderly)

- Thrombotic: Due to atherosclerotic plaque rupture in cerebral arteries.
- Embolic: Often from atrial fibrillation, valvular heart disease, or mural thrombus.
- Lacunar infarcts: Small vessel occlusion due to chronic hypertension or diabetes.

Hemorrhagic Stroke

- Intracerebral hemorrhage (ICH): From chronic hypertension, amyloid angiopathy.
- Subarachnoid hemorrhage (SAH): Rupture of aneurysm or AV malformation (less common in elderly).

Risk Factors

- Age
- Hypertension
- Atrial fibrillation
- Diabetes mellitus
- Dyslipidemia
- Smoking, alcohol
- Carotid artery stenosis
- Prior TIA or stroke

Clinical Presentation

- Hemiparesis or hemiplegia.
- Aphasia (expressive/receptive).
- Facial droop.
- Visual disturbances (e.g. hemianopia).
- Ataxia or vertigo.
- Loss of coordination or balance.
- Sudden headache (more in hemorrhagic).
- Altered consciousness.
- Hemi-neglect (usually right hemispheric stroke).

Investigations

- Noncontrast CT head: Rule out hemorrhage (done first).
- MRI brain: More sensitive for early ischemia.
- CT/MR angiography: To detect large vessel occlusion.
- Carotid Doppler: For carotid stenosis.
- Echocardiography: To identify cardiac embolic sources.

- ECG and Holter: Detect atrial fibrillation
- CBC, PT/INR, aPTT
- Blood glucose
- Lipid profile
- Renal and liver function tests.

Functional Changes

- Motor impairment: Weakness, spasticity, contractures
- Sensory deficits
- Speech/language disorders: Aphasia, dysarthria
- Swallowing difficulty (dysphagia)
- Cognitive impairment: Memory, attention deficits
- Emotional changes: Depression, apathy
- Visual-spatial deficits
- Bladder/bowel dysfunction
- Loss of independence in activities of daily living.

Management

Ischemic Stroke

- IV thrombolysis with alteplase (tPA): Within 4.5 hours of symptom onset. Contraindications must be ruled out.
- Mechanical thrombectomy: Within 6–24 hours for large vessel occlusion.

Hemorrhagic Stroke

- Blood pressure control
- Surgical evacuation in selected cases
- Neurocritical care.

Supportive Measures

- Oxygen, fluid-electrolyte balance
- Control of blood glucose and blood pressure
- Seizure control (if needed)
- DVT prophylaxis
- Manage comorbidities (HTN, diabetes, AF)
- Prevent complications (e.g. aspiration pneumonia, pressure sores).

Long-term Management

Secondary prevention:

- Antiplatelets: Aspirin, clopidogrel (if noncardioembolic)
- Anticoagulation: In atrial fibrillation (e.g. warfarin)
- Statins: For atherosclerotic stroke
- Blood pressure control
- Glycemic control
- Lifestyle changes: Smoking cessation, diet, exercise.

Rehabilitation

Multidisciplinary Approach

- Physiotherapy: Motor recovery, gait training
- Occupational therapy: ADL training, assistive devices
- Speech therapy: For aphasia and dysphagia
- Cognitive rehabilitation: Memory, attention training
- Psychological support: Depression screening and treatment.

Goals of Rehabilitation

- Maximize functional independence
- Improve quality of life
- Prevent complications (e.g. contractures, depression)
- Reintegration into community.

Q. Discuss the functional changes, pre and post-op management and rehabilitation of the elderly undergoing surgery.

- Elderly patients undergoing surgery are at increased risk of complications due to age-related physiological changes, comorbidities, and reduced physiological reserve. A comprehensive, multidisciplinary approach is essential for optimal outcomes.

Functional Changes in the Elderly Affecting Surgery

Cardiovascular System

- Decreased cardiac output, compliance
- Increased arterial stiffness and afterload
- Increased risk of ischemia, arrhythmias, heart failure.

Respiratory System

- Reduced lung elasticity and chest wall compliance
- Decreased cough reflex and mucociliary clearance
- Higher risk of atelectasis, pneumonia, hypoxia.

Renal Function

- Reduced glomerular filtration rate (GFR)
- Impaired drug clearance
- Increased risk of fluid and electrolyte imbalance.

Hepatic Function

- Decreased metabolic capacity
- Altered drug metabolism (especially phase I reactions).

Nervous System

- Increased sensitivity to anesthetics and opioids
- Risk of postoperative cognitive dysfunction (POCD) and delirium.

Musculoskeletal System

- Sarcopenia and osteoporosis increase risk of immobility, falls, and fractures.

Immune Function

- Immunosenescence leads to poor wound healing and increased infection risk.

Nutritional and Functional Status

- Malnutrition is common.
- Baseline frailty affects postoperative recovery.

Preoperative Assessment

- Comprehensive geriatric assessment (CGA): Functional, cognitive, nutritional, psychosocial.
- Optimization of comorbidities: e.g. diabetes, hypertension, cardiac disease.

- Medication review: Discontinue or adjust nephrotoxic or sedating drugs
- Nutritional supplementation
- Risk stratification: ASA score, frailty index, cardiac clearance.
- Anesthesia considerations: Prefer regional anesthesia when feasible. Lower doses of anesthetics due to increased sensitivity. Avoid long-acting sedatives and anticholinergics

Postoperative Care

- Close monitoring in postoperative ICU/ICU, if indicated.
- Respiratory support to prevent hypoxia and pneumonia.
- Cardiac monitoring for arrhythmias or ischemia.
- Adequate pain Control: Minimize opioids; consider acetaminophen, NSAIDs (cautiously), regional blocks.
- Avoid sedatives, ensure orientation, maintain sleep-wake cycle.
- Early Mobilization: Prevent deconditioning, DVT, and pulmonary complications.
- Nutrition: Early enteral feeding when possible. High-protein, high-calorie diet.
- Infections: Early recognition of surgical site infections, UTI, pneumonia.
- Wound care: Meticulous and frequent inspection.
- Pressure ulcer prevention.
- Minimize use of restraints and catheters.
- Prevention of falls.

Rehabilitation

Goals

- Restore preoperative functional status
- Promote independence in activities of daily living (ADLs)
- Prevent readmission or institutionalization.

Multidisciplinary Team Involvement

- Physiotherapy: Strength, balance, mobility
- Occupational therapy: ADL training
- Speech therapy: If dysphagia or cognitive issues present
- Geriatrician and nursing care: Overall management and monitoring.

Psychosocial Support

- Address depression, anxiety, and social isolation.
- Family and caregiver involvement.

Q. Discuss the etiopathogenesis, clinical presentation, identification, functional changes, management and rehabilitation of degenerative joint disease in the elderly.

- Degenerative joint diseases (DJDs) are a group of conditions characterized by the progressive degeneration of joints, particularly affecting the articular cartilage, subchondral bone, and supporting structures.
- They are highly prevalent in the elderly and a leading cause of pain, disability, and reduced quality of life.

Common Degenerative Joint Diseases in the Elderly

Osteoarthritis (OA): Most Common Joint Disease in Elderly

- Primary OA: Age-related, idiopathic
- Secondary OA: Follows trauma, obesity, metabolic disease, etc.
- Commonly affects knees, hips, spine, hands
- Features: Joint pain, stiffness (<30 min), crepitus, deformities (e.g. Heberden's nodes)
- Highly disabling
- Major cause of gait instability, falls, and dependence
- Often leads to total joint replacement surgery in advanced cases.

Degenerative Disc Disease

- Affects the intervertebral discs in the spine
- Leads to disc herniation, spinal stenosis, and radiculopathy
- Common in cervical and lumbar spine
- Symptoms: Back/neck pain, radiating limb pain, numbness, weakness.

Cervical and Lumbar Spondylosis

- DJD of the facet joints and vertebral bodies
- Can cause nerve root compression and myelopathy
- Features: Neck/back pain, stiffness, limited mobility, neurological symptoms.

Facet Joint Arthropathy

- Involves degeneration of zygapophyseal (facet) joints
- Common in the lumbar spine
- Pain worsens with extension and improves with flexion.

Erosive Osteoarthritis

- Inflammatory variant, more aggressive
- Common in elderly women, especially in hand joints
- Features: Joint pain, swelling, central erosions.

Risk Factors in the Elderly

- Aging (↓ cartilage repair, ↓ bone quality)
- Female sex (especially post-menopausal)
- Obesity
- Joint overuse or trauma
- Genetics and family history
- Vitamin D deficiency or osteoporosis.

Functional Consequences

- Chronic pain
- Impaired mobility
- Difficulty in activities of daily living (ADLs)
- Muscle wasting and joint deformity
- Increased fall risk and fractures
- Psychosocial issues: Depression, isolation.

Diagnosis

- Clinical evaluation: Pain pattern, stiffness, deformities.
- Imaging: X-ray (osteophytes, joint space narrowing, sclerosis), MRI (for discs, soft tissue).
- Rule out inflammatory arthritis (e.g. RA, gout).

Management

Nonpharmacological

- Exercise therapy (focus in range of motion, strengthening). Exercises improve pain, function, and quality of life without the side effects of medication. Exercise therapy is individualized based on joint involved, pain level, comorbidities. Always start low and go slow. Avoid high-impact or pain-provoking movements. Include warm-up and cool-down. Supervision by physiotherapist may be needed initially.
- Weight reduction to reduce joint load.
- Physical aids: walkers, orthotics.
- Patient education on activity pacing and ergonomics and lifestyle modification.

Pharmacological

- Paracetamol, topical NSAIDs, for pain control.
- Oral NSAIDs for moderate to severe pain (with caution due to GI, renal, CV risks).
- Intra-articular injections (corticosteroids, hyaluronic acid). They provide short-term pain relief in severe cases.
- Supplements (glucosamine, chondroitin—evidence mixed).

Surgical

- Considered when conservative measures fail and quality of life is severely affected.
- Total joint replacement (arthroplasty), especially hip or knee.
- Osteotomy or arthrodesis in selected cases.
- Spinal decompression or fusion (for severe spondylosis).

Rehabilitation

- Multidisciplinary care: Geriatrician, physiotherapist, occupational therapist, pain specialist
- Customized rehab plans to restore independence
- Physical rehabilitation: Regular supervised exercises (ROM, strengthening, balance training)
- Gait training. With assistive devices if needed
- Fall prevention strategies
- Psychological support for chronic pain management.

Q. Discuss the etiology, clinical presentation, functional changes, management, and rehabilitation of falls in the elderly.

Q. Falls prevention in elderly.

- Falls are a common and serious problem in the elderly, often leading to injury, loss of independence, and even death. Around 30–40% of people >65 years fall at least once per year. Falls are a geriatric syndrome—multifactorial, with physical, psychological, and environmental contributors.

Etiology

Intrinsic Factors (Patient-related)

- Age-related changes: Impaired balance, slower reflexes, visual and auditory decline
- Neurological disorders: Parkinson's disease, dementia, stroke
- Musculoskeletal conditions: Osteoarthritis, sarcopenia (low muscle mass), foot disorders
- Cardiovascular causes: Orthostatic hypotension, arrhythmias, syncope
- Sensory deficits: Vision or vestibular impairment
- Cognitive impairment: Inattention, poor judgment
- Medication side effects: Benzodiazepines, antipsychotics, antihypertensives, hypoglycemics, diuretics.

Extrinsic Factors (Environment-related)

- Poor lighting
- Slippery floors
- Uneven surfaces
- Inappropriate footwear
- Lack of assistive devices.

Pathogenesis

- Falls occur when an individual's postural control mechanisms fail to respond to a challenge or hazard. The combination of age-related decline + acute triggers (e.g. hypotension, medication, trip hazard) leads to instability and falls.

Clinical Presentation

- Reported or witnessed fall
- Unexplained injuries: bruises, lacerations, fractures
- Fear of falling (post-fall syndrome)
- Loss of consciousness (if syncope or stroke involved)
- Functional decline after recurrent falls
- Head injury or altered mental status (if severe).

Identification and Assessment

History

- Circumstances of the fall (where, how, when)
- Symptoms before the fall (dizziness, palpitations, weakness)
- Medication review
- Fall history and frequency
- Functional and cognitive status.

Physical Examination

- Vital signs including orthostatic BP
- Neurological exam: balance, gait, strength, coordination
- Cardiovascular exam
- Visual acuity, hearing
- Foot and footwear inspection.

Investigations

- ECG, Holter monitor (if cardiac cause suspected)
- Blood tests: Glucose, CBC, electrolytes
- Brain imaging (if head injury or neurological signs)
- X-rays (if fracture suspected)
- Comprehensive geriatric assessment (CGA).

Functional Changes Following Falls

- Reduced mobility
- Dependency in activities of daily living (ADLs)
- Fear of falling → decreased physical activity → deconditioning
- Depression, anxiety
- Institutionalization in severe cases.

Management

- ABCs (airway, breathing, circulation)
- Hemodynamic stabilization: Manage hypotension or arrhythmia
- Correct reversible causes: Hypoglycemia, electrolyte imbalance
- Temporary immobilization (splints, traction) if needed
- Treat fractures and head injury, if any
- Investigate the cause: Was it due to syncope, stroke, infection, or environmental hazard?

Rehabilitation

Goals

- Restore physical function
- Prevent recurrence
- Promote independence and confidence.

Components

- Physiotherapy: Strength, ROM, balance retraining
- Occupational therapy: ADL training, home safety
- Psychological support: Treat depression, fear of falling
- Social support: Community programs, caregiver education
- Nutritional support: Address malnutrition and sarcopenia.

Prevention of Falls

- Preventing falls in older adults is crucial to reduce injury, maintain independence, and enhance quality of life. Since falls are multifactorial, prevention strategies must be comprehensive and individualized, addressing both intrinsic (health-related) and extrinsic (environmental) risk factors.
- *Review medications and deprescribe high risk medications*: Sedatives/hypnotics (e.g. benzodiazepines), antihypertensives causing orthostatic hypotension, antipsychotics, antidepressants, and anticholinergics. Use Beers criteria to identify inappropriate medications.
- *Correct sensory deficits*: Regular eye and hearing exams. Correct refractive errors, treat cataracts, provide hearing aids, if needed.
- *Address cognitive impairment:* Screen for and manage dementia or delirium. Supervise patients with impaired judgment.
- *Treat medical conditions:* Parkinson's, diabetes, cardiac issues (e.g. syncope, arrhythmias), osteoporosis
- *Exercise programs*: Balance training, muscle strengthening (especially lower limb), gait training, flexibility and endurance.
- *Nutritional and bone health support*: Vitamin D and calcium supplementation (if deficient). Screen and treat osteoporosis to prevent fractures. Prevent malnutrition and dehydration.
- *Environmental modifications:*
  - Install grab bars in bathrooms and near toilets
  - Use non-slip mats in showers and on floors
  - Secure or remove loose rugs and cords
  - Ensure stable furniture and handrails on stairs

o Keep walkways clear and clutter-free grab bars, non-slip mats, adequate lighting.

- *Assistive devices*: Canes, walkers, hip protectors (in high-risk patients), well-fitted, non-slip, low-heeled shoes.

Q. Discuss the etiology, clinical presentation, identification, functional changes, management and rehabilitation of common fractures in the elderly.

- Fractures in the elderly are common and often result from low-energy trauma, such as falls from standing height, due to underlying osteoporosis, frailty, and age-related changes in balance, coordination, and bone strength. These fractures can lead to loss of independence, prolonged hospitalization, and increased morbidity and mortality.

Etiology

Predisposing factors for falls and fractures:

- Osteoporosis (most important risk factor for fracture)
- Sarcopenia (loss of muscle mass and strength)
- Poor vision or hearing
- Balance and gait disturbances
- Neurological disorders: Parkinson's disease, stroke, dementia
- Medications: Sedatives, antihypertensives, psychotropics
- Comorbidities: Diabetes, cardiovascular disease
- Poor lighting, slippery floors, clutter
- Minor trauma (even a sudden twist or strain)
- Syncopal episodes or seizures.

Common Fractures in the Elderly

Fracture site	Mechanism
Hip (Femoral neck/ intertrochanteric)	Fall on side
Distal radius (Colles' fracture)	Fall on outstretched hand
Vertebral compression fracture	Spontaneous or minor trauma
Proximal humerus	Fall on outstretched arm
Pelvic fractures	Low-energy trauma in osteoporotic bone

Clinical Presentation

- Pain at the site of injury
- Swelling, deformity, or bruising
- Inability to bear weight or use the limb
- Shortening and external rotation of leg (hip fracture)
- Loss of function in affected area
- Neurological deficits (in spinal or severe limb fractures)
- Vertebral fractures: May present with height loss or kyphosis.

Identification (diagnosis)

History

- Mechanism of injury (fall, trauma)
- Past history of osteoporosis, fractures
- Comorbidities and medication history

Physical Examination

- Inspect for deformity, swelling, bruising
- Palpation for tenderness
- Assess neurovascular status
- Gait and mobility assessment (if ambulatory).

Investigations

- X rays: First-line for suspected fractures
- CT/MRI: For complex, occult, or vertebral fractures
- DEXA scan: To assess bone mineral density
- Blood tests: To evaluate secondary causes of osteoporosis (calcium, vitamin D, PTH, TSH).

Functional Changes

- Reduced mobility or complete immobility
- Loss of independence in activities of daily living (ADLs)
- Deconditioning and muscle atrophy
- Psychological effects: Depression, fear of falling
- Increased risk of complications: pressure ulcers, deep vein thrombosis, pneumonia, delirium.

Management

- Pain control: Paracetamol, opioids, nerve blocks
- Immobilization: Splints, casts, traction as appropriate
- Surgical intervention:
    - Hip fracture: Internal fixation or arthroplasty
    - Vertebral fracture: Conservative or vertebroplasty/kyphoplasty
    - Wrist fracture: Closed reduction + casting or ORIF
- DVT prophylaxis: Especially in immobile patients
- Early mobilization: To prevent complications
- Treat osteoporosis: Bisphosphonates, calcium, vitamin D, denosumab
- Correct underlying disorders: Vision, balance, nutrition, medications.

Rehabilitation

Goals

- Restore function
- Prevent complications
- Promote independence
- Reduce risk of future falls and fractures.

Components

- Physiotherapy: ROM (range of motion) exercises, muscle strengthening, gait training
- Occupational therapy: ADL training, use of assistive devices
- Fall prevention: Environmental modification, balance training, medication review
- Nutritional support: Protein, calcium, vitamin D
- Social support: Family education, community resources.

Q. Vision abnormalities and visual loss in the elderly and its management.

- Vision abnormalities and visual loss are common in the elderly and can significantly impact independence, safety, cognitive function, and quality of life. Aging affects all components of the visual system—from the cornea to the visual cortex—leading to multiple potential causes of visual impairment.

Etiology

- Age-related eye diseases: Cataract, macular degeneration, glaucoma, presbyopia
- Diabetic retinopathy
- Hypertensive retinopathy
- Posterior vitreous detachment
- Retinal detachment
- Optic neuritis
- Neurological causes: Stroke (occipital cortex or optic tract involvement), brain tumors
- Drug side effects (e.g. steroids causing cataracts/glaucoma)
- Nutritional deficiencies (vitamin A)
- Trauma.

Clinical Presentation

Symptoms

- Blurred or cloudy vision
- Decreased visual acuity (near/far)
- Glare sensitivity (e.g. with cataracts)
- Loss of central vision (ARMD)
- Peripheral vision loss (glaucoma)
- Difficulty with night vision
- Visual field defects (e.g. hemianopia in stroke)
- Visual hallucinations (Charles Bonnet syndrome in severe vision loss).

Signs

- Abnormal visual acuity test results
- Abnormal pupillary responses
- Fundus abnormalities on ophthalmoscopy
- Changes in intraocular pressure.

Investigations

- Visual acuity test (Snellen chart)
- Fundoscopic examination
- Intraocular pressure measurement (tonometry)
- Visual field testing (confrontation or automated perimetry)
- Slit lamp examination (for cataracts, cornea, anterior chamber)
- Optical coherence tomography (OCT): Macular and retinal analysis
- Fluorescein angiography: Retinal vasculature in ARMD/diabetic retinopathy
- MRI/CT brain: If neurological causes suspected.

Functional Changes as a Consequence of Visual Abnormalities

- Impaired reading, driving, recognizing faces
- Increased risk of falls, accidents, and social isolation
- Dependency in daily activities
- Depression and anxiety
- Cognitive decline may be worsened by visual impairment.

Management

General Measures

- *Optimize systemic conditions*: BP, glucose control
- *Medication review*: Avoid drugs causing ocular side effects
- *Protective eyewear* for trauma prevention.

Disease-specific Treatment

- *Refractory error:* Corrective glasses
- *Cataract:* Surgical removal with intraocular lens implant
- *Glaucoma*: Topical agents (latanoprost, timolol), surgery
- *Diabetic retinopathy*: Glycemic control, laser therapy, anti-VEGF
- *Dry eyes*: Artificial tears, humidifiers.

Rehabilitation

Low Vision Aids and Assistive Devices

- Magnifiers, large-print books
- High-contrast materials
- Audio books, screen readers
- Talking watches, tactile keyboards.

Environmental Modifications

- Improved lighting
- Contrasting colors for steps and doorways
- Elimination of tripping hazards.

Psychological Support

- Counseling for coping with vision loss
- Address depression and anxiety
- Support groups.

Occupational Therapy

- Training in using assistive devices
- Strategies for ADL adaptation.

Multidisciplinary Care

- Ophthalmologist, optometrist, geriatrician, occupational therapist, social worker.

Q. Describe the principles of physical and social rehabilitation, functional assessment, role of physiotherapy and occupational therapy in the management of disability in the elderly.

- Disability in the elderly arises from chronic diseases, frailty, falls, sensory deficits, and cognitive decline. Rehabilitation aims to restore or maintain physical function, independence, and social participation, thus improving quality of life. A comprehensive, multidisciplinary approach is essential.

Principles of Physical Rehabilitation

- *Holistic and individualized approach*: Tailored to the person's physical condition, cognitive status, social support, and goals.
- *Early mobilization*: Prevents deconditioning and complications of immobility (e.g. pressure ulcers, pneumonia).
- *Restoration of function*: Enhance strength, endurance, balance, and coordination through structured exercise programs.
- *Maintenance of independence*: Focus on regaining ability to perform activities of daily living (ADLs).
- *Compensation for irreversible deficits*: Use of assistive devices, environmental modifications.
- *Continuity of care*: Smooth transition from hospital to home or community-based rehabilitation.
- *Patient and family education:* Empower the elderly and caregivers to participate in care and goal-setting.

Principles of Social Rehabilitation

- *Community reintegration*: Encourage social participation and prevent isolation.
- *Vocational and recreational support*: Enable engagement in meaningful activities, hobbies, or even part-time work.
- *Psychosocial support*: Address depression, anxiety, and cognitive impairment.
- *Environmental adaptation*: Ensure home safety (grab bars, ramps, lighting).
- *Support services*: Link with NGOs, senior centers, or government schemes for elder care.

Functional Assessment

- This is a key step in planning rehabilitation.

Components

- *Physical function*: Mobility, strength, endurance
- *ADLs (activities of daily living)*: Bathing, dressing, eating, toileting
- IADLs (*instrumental activities of daily living*): Cooking, shopping, managing finances
- *Cognitive function*: Memory, judgment, executive function.

- *Sensory function*: Vision, hearing
- *Emotional and social status*: Depression, isolation, support systems.

Tools Used

- Barthel Index–Basic ADL scoring
- Lawton IADL scale
- Timed up and go (TUG) test: Mobility and fall risk
- Mini-mental state sxamination (MMSE): Cognitive assessment
- Geriatric depression scale (GDS)
- Functional independence measure (FIM).

Role of Physiotherapy in Elderly Disability

- *Restores mobility and strength*: Through gait training, resistance exercises, and aerobic conditioning
- *Prevents falls*: Balance and coordination training
- *Pain management*: Modalities such as TENS (transcutaneous electrical nerve stimulation), ultrasound, hot/cold therapy
- *Post-surgical or fracture rehabilitation*: Especially after hip/knee replacements or strokes
- *Pulmonary and cardiac rehab*: In COPD or post-MI patients
- *Assistive device training*: Proper use of canes, walkers, wheelchairs.

Role of Occupational Therapy in Elderly Disability

- *Enhances functional independence*: Through retraining in ADLs and IADLs
- *Environmental modification*: Adapting the home/workplace to accommodate limitations
- *Cognitive rehabilitation*: For dementia or post-stroke patients
- *Hand therapy and fine motor skills*: Useful in arthritis, Parkinson's disease, stroke recovery
- *Energy conservation techniques*: For elderly with fatigue or chronic illnesses
- *Adaptive equipment training*: Use of reachers, special utensils, dressing aids.

Q. Describe the etiology, functional impact, management, and rehabilitation of hearing loss in the elderly.

- Hearing loss in the elderly, known as presbycusis, is a common sensory impairment that affects communication, social interaction, and quality of life. It is usually progressive, bilateral, and sensorineural, and is associated with aging-related degeneration of the auditory system.

Etiology

- *Age-related (presbycusis):* Most common cause of hearing loss in older adults. Involves degeneration of hair cells in the cochlea, auditory nerve fibers, and central auditory pathways.
- *Noise-induced hearing loss*: Cumulative exposure to loud noise over a lifetime damages cochlear hair cells.
- *Ototoxic drugs*: Medications like aminoglycosides, loop diuretics, chemotherapeutic agents (cisplatin)
- *Vascular and metabolic disorders*: Diabetes, hypertension, and atherosclerosis affecting cochlear blood supply
- *Ear diseases*: Chronic otitis media, otosclerosis, impacted cerumen (wax), tympanic membrane perforation
- *Neurological disorders*: Tumors (e.g. acoustic neuroma), stroke affecting auditory centers.

Functional Impact

- Communication difficulties: Trouble understanding speech, especially in noisy environments
- Social isolation: Avoidance of conversations or group activities
- Cognitive decline: Hearing loss is associated with increased risk of dementia
- Depression and anxiety
- Reduced safety: Difficulty hearing alarms, traffic, or verbal warnings
- Reduced independence and confidence.

Management

- Identification of cause
- Audiometric testing
- Referral to ENT or audiologist when needed.

Medical and Surgical Treatment

- Remove impacted cerumen (wax)
- Treat infections (otitis media, external otitis)
- Surgery: Tympanoplasty, stapedectomy (if indicated for conductive causes)
- Discontinue or adjust ototoxic drugs.

Hearing Aids and Devices

- Most effective for sensorineural hearing loss (presbycusis)
- Bone conduction devices (for conductive/mixed hearing loss)
- Cochlear implants for severe/profound bilateral sensorineural loss.

Rehabilitation

Auditory Rehabilitation

- Speech therapy and auditory training
- Lip reading and communication strategies
- Assistive listening devices (ALDs): amplified phones, TV listening devices, FM systems.

Environmental and Social Modifications

- Quiet surroundings during conversations
- Good lighting to aid lip reading
- Face-to-face communication
- Written instructions and visual aids.

Psychological and Social Support

- Counseling for the individual and family
- Support groups.

- Addressing depression or anxiety related to hearing loss.

Education and Advocacy

- Educate about hearing hygiene, hearing aid care, and regular screening.
- Encourage social engagement to prevent isolation.

Q. Describe the Impact of the demographic changes in aging on the population.

- Demographic changes in aging, marked by an increase in the proportion of elderly individuals in the population, have profound implications for society, healthcare, the economy, and social systems. These changes are primarily driven by declining fertility rates, increased life expectancy, and improved healthcare.

Healthcare System Impact

- *Increased demand for healthcare services:* Elderly populations require more frequent and prolonged medical attention due to chronic diseases like diabetes, hypertension, dementia, osteoarthritis, and cardiovascular diseases.
- *Rise in geriatric and long-term care needs*: There is a growing need for specialized geriatric care, home-based services, palliative care, and rehabilitation facilities.
- *Healthcare costs*: Ageing populations significantly increase healthcare expenditures, both at the individual and governmental levels.

Economic Impact

- *Shrinking workforce*: As the working-age population declines and more people retire, labor shortages may occur, potentially reducing economic productivity.
- *Increased pension and social security burden*: Governments must allocate more resources to pensions and social welfare programs, creating fiscal pressures.
- *Changes in consumption patterns*: The elderly tend to spend more on healthcare and less on durable goods, shifting economic demand and affecting market dynamics.

Social Impact

- *Changing family structures*: Smaller family sizes and nuclear families lead to decreased availability of informal caregivers, increasing reliance on institutional care.
- *Intergenerational tensions*: Economic dependency of a larger elderly population on a smaller working population may lead to intergenerational equity issues.
- *Elder abuse and neglect*: Social isolation and dependency can make elderly individuals more vulnerable to abuse or neglect.

Urban Planning and Infrastructure

- *Need for age-friendly infrastructure*: Demand rises for accessible housing, public transport, healthcare facilities, and public spaces designed for elderly mobility and safety.
- *Increased demand for assisted living facilities*: More elderly people living alone or with disabilities increases the need for residential care institutions.

Political and Policy Implications

- *Shift in policy priorities*: Governments may need to redirect policies toward aged care, social security reform, and age-friendly employment practices.
- *Political influence of the elderly*: A growing elderly demographic may influence election outcomes and policy preferences, focusing on healthcare and pension benefits.

Impact on Education and Youth Services

- *Resource reallocation*: Budget priorities may shift away from education and child services to aged care, affecting opportunities for younger generations.

Q. Enumerate and describe the social problems in the elderly including isolation, abuse, change in family structure and their impact on health.

- The elderly population is vulnerable to a range of social problems that can significantly affect their physical, mental, and emotional well-being. These issues often arise due to retirement, bereavement, declining health, and changing family and societal structures.

Social Isolation and Loneliness

- *Description*: A state in which elderly individuals have limited social interaction, often living alone or lacking meaningful relationships.

Causes

- Loss of spouse or peers
- Migration of children
- Reduced mobility or disability
- Retirement from work.

Impact on Health

- Increased risk of depression and anxiety
- Higher incidence of dementia
- Poor immune function and increased mortality
- Risk of malnutrition due to neglect of self-care.

Elder Abuse

- *Description*: Physical, emotional, financial, or sexual abuse or neglect of elderly individuals, often by caregivers or family members.

Types

- Physical: Hitting, restraining
- Emotional: Insults, threats, humiliation
- Financial: Misuse of money or property
- Neglect: Withholding food, medication, or care.

Impact on Health

- Physical injuries, fractures
- Chronic stress, PTSD
- Increased risk of suicide
- Delay in seeking or receiving healthcare.

Changes in Family Structure

- *Description*: Transition from joint families to nuclear families, urban migration, and reduced intergenerational co-residence.

Consequences

- Loss of traditional caregiver roles
- Reduced family support and emotional bonding
- Dependency on institutions or hired caregivers.

Impact on Health

- Feelings of abandonment, leading to depression
- Poor adherence to treatment and self-care
- Increased risk of institutionalization.

Financial Insecurity

- *Description*: Limited income post-retirement, absence of pension, or financial exploitation.

Sources

- Lack of savings or insurance
- Rising healthcare costs
- Economic dependency on children.

Impact on Health

- Inability to afford medications, nutritious food, or healthcare
- Delay in seeking treatment
- Increased mental stress and anxiety.

Bereavement and Grief

- *Description*: Loss of spouse, friends, or siblings is common in older age.

Impact on Health

- Depression and insomnia
- Increased risk of cardiovascular events (widowhood effect)
- Social withdrawal.

Inadequate Access to Social Support Services

- *Description*: Elderly may not have access to government schemes, disability aids, or home-based care.

Impact on Health

- Increased burden of disease
- Unmanaged disabilities and reduced independence
- Higher hospitalization rates.

Ageism and Social Discrimination

- *Description*: Negative attitudes or prejudices toward older adults.

Manifestations

- Disregard in decision-making
- Stereotyping as "nonproductive".

Impact on Health

- Lower self-esteem and social participation
- Diminished quality of life.

Q. Enumerate and describe social interventions in the care of elderly including domiciliary services, rehabilitation facilities, old age homes and state interventions.

- Social interventions play a critical role in promoting the health, independence, and dignity of elderly individuals. These interventions address the social, economic, and functional needs of the ageing population and aim to prevent isolation, neglect, and institutionalization.

Domiciliary Services (home-based care)

- *Description*: Provision of medical and nonmedical support services at the elderly person's home.

Components

- Home visits by doctors, nurses, physiotherapists
- Assistance with activities of daily living (ADLs) such as bathing, dressing, feeding
- Delivery of meals, medications, and assistive devices.

Advantages

- Promotes independence and comfort in familiar surroundings
- Reduces burden on hospital infrastructure
- Cost-effective and prevents unnecessary hospitalization.

Rehabilitation Facilities

- *Description*: Institutions providing comprehensive services for physical, psychological, and social rehabilitation of the elderly.

Types

- Physiotherapy centers for mobility restoration
- Occupational therapy units for promoting functional independence
- Geriatric psychiatric units for managing depression, dementia, and anxiety.

Benefits

- Improves quality of life and functional capacity
- Facilitates reintegration into the community
- Reduces caregiver burden.

Old Age Homes (residential care facilities)

- *Description*: Institutions offering shelter, food, health care, and companionship to elderly individuals who are homeless, abandoned, or unable to live independently.

Types

- Free homes for the destitute
- Paid homes for those who can afford it
- Day-care centers for day-time engagement and support.

Services Provided

- Accommodation, food, medical care, recreational activities
- Emotional support and social interaction.

Challenges

- May lead to emotional distress due to separation from family
- Quality of care varies between institutions.

State Interventions and Government Schemes

- *Description*: Government-led programs aimed at supporting the elderly through financial, medical, and legal means.

Key Initiatives in India

- Maintenance and Welfare of Parents and Senior Citizens Act: Legal provision for maintenance of elderly by children/relatives.
- National Programme for Health Care of the Elderly (NPHCE): Focuses on geriatric healthcare at primary, secondary, and tertiary levels.
- Indira Gandhi National Old Age Pension Scheme (IGNOAPS): Monthly pension to elderly below poverty line.
- Senior Citizens' Helpline (14567): Toll-free number for emergency support.
- Concessions in rail and air travel, income tax benefits, priority in government schemes

Impact

- Enhances financial security and healthcare access.
- Reduces neglect and promotes ageing with dignity.

Community-based and NGO Interventions

Examples

- Self-help groups, senior citizen clubs.
- NGOs like HelpAge India, which provide mobile health clinics, counselling, and advocacy.

Role

- Foster community participation and social inclusion.
- Create awareness about elderly rights and health issues.

Legal and Policy Framework

Purpose

- Protection from abuse, exploitation, and neglect.
- Ensure right to maintenance, shelter, and healthcare.

Implementation Needs

- Stronger enforcement mechanisms.
- Greater awareness and access to legal aid.

Q. Enumerate and describe ethical issues in the care of the elderly.

- The care of elderly individuals presents several ethical challenges, owing to age-related decline, chronic illness, dependency, and vulnerability. Ethical issues arise in medical decisions, social care, legal matters, and resource allocation, and require a careful balance between autonomy, beneficence, nonmaleficence, and justice.
- **Autonomy and decision-making:** Respecting elderly individuals' right to make informed choices is crucial, though cognitive decline may limit their capacity.
- **Informed consent:** Ethical care demands clear communication of treatment options, acknowledging the risks of cognitive impairment and undue influence from others.
- **End-of-life care:** Decisions on life-sustaining treatments and palliative care should prioritize patient dignity and respect for advance directives.
- **Agism and discrimination:** Bias against the elderly in healthcare access or treatment violates the principle of justice and must be addressed.
- **Elder abuse and neglect:** Protecting elders from harm while maintaining confidentiality and respecting their wishes presents ethical dilemmas.
- **Resource allocation:** Fair distribution of limited healthcare resources, especially during crises, must balance individual needs with societal good.
- **Institutionalization *vs* home care:** Ethical decisions should weigh the elder's autonomy and quality of life against family burden and safety.
- **Confidentiality and privacy:** Maintaining respect for personal health information while involving caregivers requires careful ethical navigation.
- **Participation in research:** Inclusion of elders in research must be based on valid informed consent and protection from exploitation.
- **Cultural and religious sensitivities:** Honoring individual beliefs in care delivery is essential to providing respectful and dignified elder care.

Q. Discuss the etiopathogenesis, clinical presentation, complications, assessment and management of nutritional disorders in the elderly.

- Nutritional disorders in the elderly are common and often underdiagnosed, yet they significantly affect morbidity, functional status, and quality of life. A multidisciplinary, individualized approach involving dietary modifications, medical treatment, psychosocial support, and regular monitoring is essential to ensure optimal nutrition and healthy aging.

Etiopathogenesis

- Nutritional disorders in the elderly are multifactorial and arise due to physiological, psychological, medical, and social factors.

Physiological Factors

- Decreased basal metabolic rate
- Loss of appetite (anorexia of aging) due to altered taste, smell, and delayed gastric emptying
- Poor dentition or ill-fitting dentures affecting chewing
- Impaired absorption of nutrients (e.g. B_{12}, calcium, iron).

Medical Causes

- Chronic diseases like diabetes mellitus, chronic kidney disease, chronic infections or malignancies.
- Medications causing anorexia, nausea, or altered metabolism (e.g. diuretics, laxatives, antidepressants).
- Depression, dementia, or dysphagia post-stroke.

Socioeconomic and Psychological Factors

- Social isolation, widowhood
- Poverty or limited access to nutritious food
- Cognitive decline leading to poor meal preparation.
- Alcohol abuse.

Clinical Presentation

General Symptoms

- Weight loss or cachexia
- Fatigue, lethargy
- Muscle wasting or sarcopenia
- Poor wound healing
- Dehydration or dry skin.

Specific Deficiency Symptoms

- Protein-energy malnutrition (PEM): Muscle weakness, edema, hypoalbuminemia
- Iron deficiency: Pallor, fatigue, angular stomatitis
- Vitamin B_{12} deficiency: Paresthesia, ataxia, confusion
- Vitamin D deficiency: Bone pain, fractures, osteomalacia
- Calcium deficiency: Muscle cramps, tetany.

Complications of Nutritional Disorders in the Elderly

- Immunosuppression → increased infections
- Delayed wound healing
- Pressure ulcers
- Increased risk of falls and fractures
- Cognitive decline and dementia
- Sarcopenia and frailty syndrome
- Hospitalization and institutionalization
- Increased mortality

Assessment of nutritional status

- A comprehensive assessment includes clinical, anthropometric, and biochemical evaluations.

Clinical Assessment

- Diet history (appetite, meal frequency, dietary intake)
- Weight changes over past 6 months
- Functional assessment (ADLs, mobility)
- Look for signs of deficiencies.

Anthropometry

- Body Mass Index (BMI)
- Mid-upper arm circumference
- Skinfold thickness
- Grip strength (sarcopenia).

Biochemical Parameters

- Serum albumin, prealbumin (visceral protein stores)
- Hemoglobin, ferritin (iron status)
- Vitamin D, B_{12} levels
- Electrolytes, creatinine.

Nutritional Screening Tools

- Mini nutritional assessment (MNA).
- Malnutrition universal screening tool (MUST).

Management

- Management involves correcting deficiencies, restoring nutritional balance, and addressing underlying causes.

Dietary Intervention

- Caloric and protein-rich diets
- Small, frequent meals
- Use of nutritional supplements (oral or enteral)
- Texture-modified diets in dysphagia
- Ensure adequate hydration
- Micronutrient supplementation: Vitamin D and calcium, iron, folic acid, B_{12}, other vitamins as needed.

Treat Underlying Conditions

- Manage chronic diseases (e.g. diabetes, heart failure)
- Treat dental issues or oral infections
- Adjust medications causing anorexia or GI upset.

Rehabilitation and Functional Support

- Physiotherapy for muscle strength
- Occupational therapy for meal preparation support
- Swallowing therapy in dysphagia.

Psychosocial Support

- Counseling for depression or anxiety
- Encouraging communal meals to reduce isolation
- Social services for food delivery (e.g. meals-on-wheels).

Monitoring

- Regular weight and nutritional status checks
- Laboratory monitoring of deficiencies
- Adjustments based on disease progression or improvement.

Chapter 21

Case Scenario-based Discussions

Case scenario-based discussions are very helpful to sharpen your diagnostic and interpreting skills. They are an excellent way of learning medicine. Recently, many UG and PG medical examinations include one or two case scenario-based questions. In the following pages, there are many case scenarios which we commonly encounter in our daily clinical practice.

Q. A 30-year-old man presents with 5 days history of fever, headache and vomiting. Headache is diffuse and severe. Examination shows neck stiffness and Kernig's sign is positive. Discuss about the most likely diagnosis in this patient.

- Because of presence of fever, headache and neck stiffness, the most likely diagnosis in this patient is acute meningitis most probably pyogenic. Differential diagnosis includes migraine headache, subarachnoid hemorrhage, and encephalitis. In case of migraine similar episodes of headache are usually present previously with spontaneous recovery and fever is absent. Subarachnoid hemorrhage is usually characterized by abrupt onset of severe diffuse headache and fever is usually absent. Encephalitis is also a differential diagnosis, but neck stiffness is usually absent and altered sensorium is usually present. Other differential diagnosis are brain abscess and cortical venous sinus thrombosis.
- CSF analysis will confirm the diagnosis in this patient.
- Acute meningitis is a medical emergency. Empiric antibiotic therapy should be started as early as possible. The empirical drug of choice is a combination of third generation cephalosporin (such as ceftriaxone or cefotaxime) plus vancomycin. Ceftriaxone covers *Streptococcus pneumoniae* (the most common organism causing meningitis in adults) whereas vancomycin covers penicillin resistant *Streptococcus pneumoniae*. Vancomycin can be stopped if *Streptococcus pneumoniae* penicillin sensitive as per culture sensitivity report.
- Complications of this condition include hearing loss, cortical blindness, cranial nerve palsies, stroke, seizures, mental retardation, subdural effusions, hydrocephalus, cerebral atrophy and sepsis.
- Refer 'acute pyogenic meningitis' for more detailed discussion.

Q. A middle aged farmer presents with 4 days h/o fever and generalized bodyache. He has also noticed yellowish discoloration of eyes and oliguria. Examination reveals muscle tenderness.

1. **What is your diagnosis?**
2. **What investigation will you do to confirm the diagnosis?**
3. **How do you treat this patient?**

- The most likely diagnosis is leptospirosis because it presents with prominent myalgia due to muscle involvement, jaundice due to liver involvement and oliguria due to kidney involvement. Leptospirosis is common in certain occupations such as farmers, sewage workers and abattoir workers. This patient is a farmer. Patients may also present with meningo-encephalitis and ARDS. Leptospirosis is transmitted via direct contact with the body fluid of an acutely infected animal or by exposure to soil or fresh water contaminated with the urine of an animal (usually rats) that is a chronic carrier.
- Differential diagnosis includes dengue, acute viral hepatitis, brucellosis, malaria, and other infectious diseases with sepsis.
- Serum IgM leptospira antibody will be positive in the blood. Creatine kinase (CK) levels will be elevated in the blood due to muscle damage. LFT and RFT will also be abnormal in this case. Darkfield microscopy can demonstrate leptospira, but not available in all the labs.
- Oral doxycycline can be used in stable patients. For seriously ill patients intravenous penicillin G is the treatment of choice. Third-generation cephalosporins (cefotaxime, ceftriaxone) are as effective as doxycycline and penicillin.
- Refer 'leptospirosis' in 'infectious diseases' chapter for detailed discussion.

Q. A 30-year-old lady presents with h/o breathlessness and wheezing of 2 days duration. She also gives

h/o similar episodes since childhood usually during spring season. She is not a smoker. Her mother also has similar complaints.

What is your diagnosis? Discuss the etiology, pathogenesis, clinical features and treatment of the same.

- Most likely diagnosis is acute exacerbation of asthma because of similar episodes in the past with seasonal exacerbation, positive family history and onset since childhood. She is also a non-smoker (COPD has to be considered in chronic smokers). All these points favor the diagnosis of asthma.
- Other possibilities to be considered when a patient presents with acute onset breathlessness with wheezing are acute pulmonary edema due to left ventricular failure, acute exacerbation of COPD, allergic reactions causing bronchospasm, tropical pulmonary eosinophilia, eosinophilic pneumonias etc. Acute bronchitis needs to be considered for a single isolated episode of wheezing. But this patient has recurrent episodes.
- Treatment involves bronchodilators preferably given via nebulizer, i.e. salbutamol nebulization plus ipratropium bromide nebulization 4th–6th hourly. Nebulized steroids also help in decreasing the severity of attack (e.g. budesonide nebulization every 12th hourly). Oral steroids or parenteral steroids can be given in acute severe asthma. Antibiotics can be given if the cause of asthma exacerbation is respiratory tract infection.
- For a detailed discussion refer asthma under respiratory system.

Q. A 55-year-old man, who has been smoking for the last 25 years presents with dyspnea on exertion of 8 years duration. Dyspnea has progressed from grade 1 to grade 2 for the last 3 years. He also gives h/o recurrent episodes of cough with scanty mucoid sputum associated with wheezing. He does not report any chest pain, orthopnea or paroxysmal nocturnal dyspnea (PND).

1. **What is your diagnosis?**
2. **What findings are you likely to get on examination?**
3. **How do you treat this patient?**

- Most likely diagnosis is COPD, predominantly chronic bronchitis because of chronic cough with wheezing. Other points favoring a diagnosis of COPD are smoking history and progressive breathlessness. It is unlikely to be asthma because asthma does not lead to progressive worsening of breathlessness over the years. It is unlikely to be IHD or heart failure because of the absence of chest pain, orthopnea and PND.
- Other differentials for progressive breathlessness are heart disease (IHD, rheumatic heart disease, cardiac failure), interstitial lung diseases, etc.
- Examination may show barrel-shaped chest, bilateral lung crepitations, and bilateral rhonchi. In advanced COPD, cyanosis, signs of pulmonary HTN such as loud P2, right ventricular hypertrophy (suggested by parasternal heave, shift of apex beat laterally) may be present. Corpulmonale may develop in advanced cases with significant pulmonary HTN which produces raised JVP with peripheral edema.
- Refer COPD in respiratory system for detailed discussion.

Q. A 40-year-old lady presents with h/o recurrent episodes of cough with copious amount of sputum for the past 10 years. She had suffered from pulmonary tuberculosis 15 years ago. Examination reveals presence of clubbing and bilateral basal coarse crepitations.

1. **What is the most likely diagnosis? Discuss the etiology, clinical features, investigations and management of the same.**
2. **How do you prevent recurrent chest infections in her?**

- The most likely diagnosis is bronchiectasis which has developed as a sequelae of past pulmonary tuberculosis. Recurrent episodes of cough with sputum are due to recurrent lower respiratory tract infections.
- Differential diagnosis of chronic cough with bilateral crepitations include extrinsic allergic alveolitis, heart failure, interstitial lung disease, pneumonia and tuberculosis.
- Diagnosis can be confirmed by high-resolution CT (HRCT) of chest which will show dilated bronchi. Bronchography can also be done but not commonly done nowadays due to the availability of CT scan.
- Treatment involves antibiotics and chest physiotherapy. Surgery is an option for selected patients with advanced or complicated disease. Antibiotic choices include amoxicillin, doxycycline, trimethoprim-sulfamethoxazole, a newer macrolide (e.g. azithromycin or clarithromycin), cephalosporins or a fluoroquinolone.
- Recurrent infections can be prevented to some extent by smoking cessation, avoidance of second-hand smoke, good nutrition and immunizations for influenza and pneumococcal pneumonia.
- Refer bronchiectasis in respiratory system for more detailed discussion.

Q. A 50-year-old man presents with cough with expectoration of 2 weeks duration. He says his sputum is of large quantity and foul smelling. Patient says cough and sputum quantity are more on lying in left lateral position. He also gives h/o fever.

1. **What is your diagnosis?**
2. **What are the causes of this condition?**
3. **What investigation will you do to confirm the diagnosis?**
4. **How do you treat this patient?**

- Diagnosis is lung abscess in view of large quantity of foul smelling sputum, postural variation of cough and sputum and high-grade fever. The abscess is probably in the right lung since the patient gets more cough in left lateral position. In left lateral position right lung is in the upper position and due to gravity the abscess drains into central airways producing more cough and sputum.

- Causes of lung abscess include necrotizing pneumonias due to staphylococcus aureus and *Klebsiella pneumoniae*, tuberculosis, and aspiration pneumonia. Other organisms causing lung abscess are anaerobes such as Peptostreptococcus species, Bacteroides species, Fusobacterium species, and microaerophilic streptococci. Aerobic bacteria that may infrequently cause lung abscess include *Streptococcus pyogenes, Streptococcus pneumoniae* (rarely), *Haemophilus influenzae,* Actinomyces species, Nocardia species, and gram-negative bacilli. A malignant lesion can cavitate and produce lung abscess. Nonbacterial pathogens may also cause lung abscesses in the in the immunocompromised host. These include parasites (e.g. Paragonimus and Entamoeba species), and fungi (e.g. Aspergillus, Cryptococcus, Histoplasma, Blastomyces, and Coccidioides species).
- A chest X-ray will show a cavity with air fluid level. HRCT chest can clearly show the size and extent of an abscess. Microbiological studies of the sputum will identify the microorganism.
- Treatment depends on the presumed infecting organism. For Infections caused by anaerobic bacteria, clindamycin (600 mg four times daily IV initially followed by oral dosage of 300 mg four times daily once the patient becomes afebrile and improves clinically) is the drug of choice. Other options are any beta-lactam/beta-lactamase inhibitor combination (example amoxicillin/clavulanate) or carbapenems (e.g. meropenem). Lung abscess due to *S. aureus* is usually treated with vancomycin. Duration of therapy is usually 4–6 weeks.
- Refer 'lung abscess' for a detailed discussion.

Q. A 25-year-old man who is a known case of rheumatic heart disease (RHD) presents with fever of three weeks duration. Examination shows petechial hemorrhages, subungual (splinter) hemorrhages, and tender subcutaneous nodules on the digits.

1. **What is the most likely diagnosis?**
2. **What investigation will you do to confirm the diagnosis?**
3. **How do you treat this patient?**

- The most likely diagnosis is infective endocarditis because the patient is a known case of RHD. Tender subcutaneous nodules are Osler nodes. Other signs suggestive of endocarditis should be looked for in this patient such as Janeway lesions (nontender maculae on the palms and soles) and Roth's spots (retinal hemorrhages with small, clear centers). Infective endocarditis can be acute or subacute. Acute infective endocarditis is caused by Staphylococcus and Pseudomonas whereas subacute infective endocarditis is caused by *Streptococcus viridans*.
- Though, the obvious possibility is infective endocarditis, simultaneous work up to rule out other causes of fever such as tuberculosis, HIV infection, etc. should be done.
- Duke criteria are used in the diagnosis of infective endocarditis. Presence of two major criteria, or one major and three minor criteria, or five minor criteria is required to make a clinical diagnosis of definite endocarditis. Blood culture and echocardiogram are the most important investigations used to confirm the diagnosis of infective endocarditis and form the major Duke criteria. At least three blood culture sets, ideally with the first separated from the last by at least 1 hour, should be sent from different venipuncture sites over 24 hours.
- Treatment involves empirical antibiotic therapy started as soon as possible after obtaining blood cultures. Empirical therapy should be targeted at the most likely pathogens. Initial choices of antibiotics include benzyl penicillin plus gentamicin. If MRSA is suspected vancomycin should be added. Antibiotics should be given parenteraly.

Q. A 50-year-old chronic smoker presents with retrosternal chest pain on exertion which lasts few minutes and subsides on taking rest. Pain radiates to left shoulder. He also gives h/o excessive sweating during episodes of pain.

Discuss the etiology, pathogenesis, clinical features, investigations and management of the most likely diagnosis?

- The most likely diagnosis is stable angina.
- Investigations to confirm the diagnosis include ECG, treadmill testing and coronary angiogram (CAG). Resting ECG can be normal, hence all patients with suspected angina should undergo treadmill testing even if the ECG is normal. CAG can identify which and how much of the coronary artery is blocked.
- Treatment involves nitrates (glyceryl trinitrate, isosorbide dinitrate and mononitrate), beta blockers, antiplatelet agents (aspirin or clopidogrel) and statins (atorvastatin, rosuvastatin). Other useful drugs are ACE inhibitors, nondihydropyridine calcium channel blockers (diltiazem, verapamil) and nicorandil (potassium-channel activator with a nitrate component). Percutaneous transluminal coronary angioplasty (PTCA) with stenting and coronary artery bypass grafting (CABG) can be used to relieve or bypass the stenotic area. Transmyocardial laser revascularization (TMR) is another new technique where laser is used to make channels (small holes) in the myocardium to allow direct perfusion of the myocardium from blood within the ventricular cavity.
- *See* 'stable angina' for a detailed discussion.

Q. A 55-year-old diabetic and hypertensive develops severe left sided chest pain while working. Pain has been present for the last

30 minutes. He also has dyspnea and fatigue. Examination shows diaphoresis, pale cool skin, tachycardia, presence of S3 and bilateral basal lung crepitations.

1. **What is your diagnosis?**
2. **What investigation will you do to confirm the diagnosis?**
3. **How do you treat this patient?**

- Most likely diagnosis is acute myocardial infarction with left ventricular failure (LVF). Chest pain of MI is more severe than angina and lasts for more than 20 minutes (this patient has severe pain and pain is present for 30 minutes). Diaphoresis and tachycardia are due to sympathetic stimulation. Pale cool skin is due to peripheral vasoconstriction due to heart failure and sympathetic stimulation. Presence of S3 and bibasal lung crepitations is due to left ventricular failure and pulmonary edema respectively.
- Investigations to confirm the diagnosis of MI include ECG, CK-MB, troponins and echocardiogram. ECG usually shows ST elevation and formation of pathological Q waves. However, ST elevation may not be present in non-ST elevation MI. cardiac enzymes such as CK-MB and troponins get elevated after MI. Echocardiogram may show dilated heart and hypokinesia or akinesia of the affected myocardium. Coronary angiogram (CAG) can identify which and how much of the coronary artery is blocked.
- Treatment involves nitrates (glyceryl trinitrate, isosorbide dinitrate and mononitrate), beta blockers, antiplatelet agents (aspirin or clopidogrel) and statins (atorvastatin, rosuvastatin). Other useful drugs are ACE inhibitors, nondihydropyridine calcium channel blockers (diltiazem, verapamil) and nicorandil (potassium-channel activator with a nitrate) component. Percutaneous transluminal coronary angioplasty (PTCA) with stenting and coronary artery bypass grafting (CABG) can be used to relieve or bypass the stenotic coronary arteries. Thrombolysis (using streptokinase or urokinase) can be considered if facility for percutaneous coronary interventions is not available. Transmyocardial laser revascularization (TMR) is another new technique here laser is used to make channels (small holes) in the myocardium to allow direct perfusion of the myocardium from blood within the ventricular cavity.
- *See* 'myocardial infarction' under CVS chapter for detailed discussion.

Q. A 35-year-old lady presents with easy fatigability and dyspnea on exertion of 4 years duration. She also gives h/o recurrent respiratory tract infections. Examination shows hyperdynamic precordium, signs of pulmonary hypertension, widely split and fixed second heart sound.

1. **What is your diagnosis?**
2. **What investigation will you do to confirm the diagnosis?**
3. **How do you treat this patient?**

- Most likely diagnosis is atrial septal defect (ASD). In ASD there is shunting of blood from high pressure left atrium to low pressure right atrium. Consequently, there is increased blood flow into pulmonary circulation. Increased pulmonary blood flow leads to development of pulmonary HTN. This usually happens above the age of 30 years. Dyspnea and easy fatigability are due to development of pulmonary hypertension. Recurrent respiratory infections are due to increased pulmonary blood flow leading to congestion of pulmonary circulation.
- Differential diagnosis includes total anomalous pulmonary venous connection (TAPVC), ventricular septal defect (VSD), pulmonary stenosis, truncus arteriosus, and tricuspid atresia. All these conditions can produce split second sound.
- Echocardiogram and cardiac catheterization can be used to confirm the diagnosis. Echocardiogram shows right ventricular hypertrophy, dilated pulmonary artery, and presence of ASD. Abnormal shunt and blood flow can be assessed by color Doppler. Cardiac catheterization can confirm the presence of ASD but usually Echo is enough for confirmation. Cardiac catheterization shows increased oxygen content of right atrial blood due to blood flow from left atrium.
- Surgical closure should be done between 3 and 6 years of age or as soon as possible in significant ASD (i.e. pulmonary flow more than 50% increased compared with systemic flow). Closure should not be carried out in patients with small defects and trivial left-to-right shunts or in those with severe pulmonary hypertension. Angiographic closure is now possible by using a transcatheter device. Infective endocarditis prophylaxis is not required for uncorrected ASDs unless there is another accompanying valvular lesion.
- *See* 'Atrial Septal Defect' under CVS chapter for detailed discussion.

Q. A 55-year-old man with h/o hypertension presents with sudden onset retrosternal chest pain which is tearing in nature. Examination shows blood pressure of 200/120 and asymmetric peripheral pulses.

Discuss the etiology, pathogenesis, clinical features, investigations and management of the most likely diagnosis.

- This is a case of aortic dissection. Most patients with aortic dissection have h/o hypertension. Pain is usually tearing in nature, but it can also be sharp or stabbing in nature. Asymmetry of pulses is a common finding. The DeBakey classification divides the dissection into 3 types. Type 1 involves the ascending aorta, aortic arch, and descending aorta. Type II is confined to the ascending aorta. Type III is confined to the descending aorta distal to the left subclavian artery.
- Differential diagnosis includes myocardial infarction, aortic aneurysm rupture, cardiac tamponade, esophageal rupture (Boerhaave syndrome), spontaneous pneumothorax, and pulmonary embolism.

- Chest X-ray may show mediastinal widening. Echocardiography can identify proximal dissections but not very useful for confirmation of diagnosis. CT or MRI of chest is required for the confirmation of diagnosis.
- See 'Aortic dissection' under CVS chapter for detailed discussion.

Q. A 25-year-old man presents with 2 months h/o of diarrhea, low-grade fever, and pain abdomen. Stools are watery and contain blood and mucus. Patient has had similar episodes in the past and has recovered without treatment. Examination is normal.

1. **What could be the diagnosis in this case? What are the differential diagnoses?**
2. **How do you confirm the diagnosis?**
3. **How do you treat this patient?**

- The diagnosis in this case could be inflammatory bowel disease (IBD, ulcerative colitis) because of chronic diarrhea, presence of blood and mucus in the stool and recurrent exacerbations and remissions. IBD is of two types; ulcerative colitis and Crohn's disease.
- Other possibilities can be chronic amebiasis, intestinal tuberculosis and AIDS-related infections (*Mycobacterium avium* complex, Microsporida, Cryptosporidium, *Isospora belli*). Irritable bowel syndrome (IBS) is unlikely because there will not be weight loss and blood in the stool. In addition, IBS will not be associated with fever. Malabsorption syndromes are unlikely again because there will not be fever in these conditions and blood will not be present in the stool.
- Diagnosis can be confirmed by colonoscopy and mucosal biopsy.
- The mainstay of therapy for IBD is 5-ASA (amino salicylic acid) agents. Example is sulfasalazine. Sulfasalazine is not broken down in small intestine and the intact molecule reaches colon where it is broken down by colonic bacteria into sulfa and 5-ASA moieties. 5-ASA acts as local anti-inflammatory agent in the colon. Newer sulfa-free agents such as mesalamine, olsalazine and balsalazide have less of side effects. Glucocorticoids (prednisolone) can be tried in patients with moderate to severe UC and CD. Immunosuppressive agents (azathioprine, 6-mercaptopurine, methotrexate and cyclosporine) are useful as steroid sparing agents in the management of glucocorticoid-dependent IBD. Tacrolimus and mycophenolate mofetil are newer immunosuppressive agents.

Q. A 30-year-old man who is a chronic alcoholic presents with epigastric pain of 2 days duration after a binge of alcohol intake. Epigastric pain radiates to the back between the scapulae and is associated with nausea and vomiting. Pain worsens on taking food and on lying down. Pain is relieved partially on sitting and bending forward. There is no h/o of fever or diarrhea.

Discuss the etiology, pathogenesis, clinical features, investigations and management of the most likely diagnosis in this case.

- Diagnosis is acute pancreatitis. It presents with epigastric pain which radiates to back between the scapulae. Pain also worsens with food intake and in supine position. Pain reduces on sitting and bending forward. It is common in alcoholics and alcohol binge often triggers an attack. Other causes of acute pancreatitis are gallstones, post-ERCP, post-surgical (abdominal, cardiopulmonary bypass), trauma (blunt or penetrating abdominal injury), drugs (azathioprine, thiazides, sulphasalazine, valproate), hypercalcemia, hypertriglyceridemia, infection (mumps, coxsackievirus, HIV, Leptospira, Ascaris), and idiopathic.
- Diagnosis can be confirmed by measuring serum amylase and lipase which will be elevated. Other useful tests are ultrasound abdomen and CT abdomen which can show inflamed and bulky pancreas.
- *Treatment*: Patient should be kept NPO (nil per oral). Ryle's tube aspiration is also required if there is recurrent vomiting. Intravenous fluids are given to maintain intravascular volume. Analgesics are given for to control abdominal pain. Proton-pump inhibitors are used to decrease the acid output. The role of somatostatin or octreotide infusion is controversial.
- Complications of acute pancreatitis include abscess and pseudocyst formation, splenic or portal vein thrombosis, systemic inflammatory response syndrome (SIRS) and multiorgan failure, ARDS, and hypocalcemia (due to sequestration of calcium in fat necrosis).
- See pancreatitis for detailed discussion.

Q. A 20-year-old girl presents with pain abdomen and vomiting of 2 days duration. Initially pain was in the periumbilical region, but later on pain has shifted to right iliac fossa. Examination reveals tachycardia and rebound tenderness in the right iliac fossa at the McBurney's point.

Discuss the clinical features, investigations and management of the most likely diagnosis in this case.

- Diagnosis is acute appendicitis. In acute appendicitis pain is initially felt in the umbilical area (referred pain), but later, it shifts to right iliac fossa due to involvement of peritoneum surrounding the inflamed appendix. Other differential diagnoses are pelvic inflammatory disease (PID) or tubo-ovarian abscess, endometriosis, ovarian cyst or torsion, ureteric colic, diverticulitis, ectopic pregnancy, Crohn's disease, and urinary tract infection (UTI).
- Diagnosis can be confirmed by ultrasound abdomen and if required CT abdomen.
- Patient should undergo emergency appendicectomy. Supportive measures include intravenous antibiotics

(ceftriaxone and metronidazole), intravenous fluids and analgesics.

- Complications are bowel obstruction, abdominal/pelvic abscess, and, rarely, death.

Q. A 35-year-old man presents with painless, profuse diarrhea of 2 days duration. There is no h/o fever or pain abdomen. Stool is watery and appears like rice water. Examination shows moderate dehydration and no other abnormal findings.

1. **What is the possible diagnosis?**
2. **What investigations are helpful to confirm the diagnosis?**
3. **How do you treat this patient?**

- Diagnosis is cholera. Cholera commonly presents as sudden onset, painless diarrhea. Since the causative organism vibrio cholera does not invade the intestinal mucosa, there is no fever or pain abdomen. Stool appears like 'rice water' because of mucus flecks floating in the watery stools (resemblance to the water in which rice has been washed).
- Other causes of noninvasive watery diarrhea are ETEC (enterotoxigenic *E. coli*), rotavirus, Cryptosporidum, and Girardia.
- Diagnosis of cholera can be confirmed by hanging drop preparation of stool sample (shows rapidly motile organisms) and also by stool culture.
- Mainstay of therapy is oral rehydration salt (ORS). ORS takes advantage of a cotransport mechanism not affected by cholera toxin wherein sodium (Na^+) moves across the gut mucosa along with actively transported glucose. Intravenous fluids may be required if the patient is severely dehydrated or has vomiting. Ringer's lactate is the fluid of choice since it contains almost all the electrolytes lost in the stools. Antibiotics can diminish the duration and volume of fluid loss and hasten clearance of the organism from the stool. Single-dose doxycycline (300 mg) is effective in adults but is not recommended for children <8 years of age because of possible deposition in bone and developing teeth.

Q. About 15 people have been brought to emergency department with h/o nausea, vomiting, and abdominal cramps. Five of them also have fever and diarrhea. All of them had food at a function 30 minutes prior to the onset of the above symptoms.

1. **What is the possible diagnosis?**
2. **What investigations would you do?**
3. **How do you treat them?**

- The diagnosis is food poisoning probably due to a preformed toxin produced by Staphylococcus or *Bacillus cereus* since the onset of symptoms after the food intake is within 1–6 hours and many are affected at the same time after having the same food.
- Suspected food can be tested for the presence of enterotoxin and Staphylococcus, but usually not necessary.
- Most cases of food poisoning are self-limiting. Intravenous fluids and anti-emetics should be given to patients with severe vomiting and diarrhea.
- *See* 'Food poisoning' in 'infectious diseases' chapter for more details.

Q. A 20-year-old lady complains of recurrent episodes of headache since 5 years. She gets 1–2 attacks of headache per week lasting 4–12 hours. Headache is unilateral and throbbing type and interferes with routine activity. She also reports nausea and vomiting during attacks. Headache worsens on exposure to bright light. There are no other symptoms before or during the headache. Her mother also has similar h/o headache.

1. **What is the diagnosis?**
2. **How do you treat her?**

- Diagnosis is migraine without aura (also known as common migraine). Migraine with aura is less common and the headache is preceded by transient neurological symptoms such as visual aura (fortification spectra, scotomas), vertigo, speech difficulty, motor weakness, etc. the lady in this case scenario does not have any aura symptoms, hence, it is a case of migraine without aura.
- Migraine is three times more common in females than males and young females are commonly affected. It tends to run in families. Migraine headache is usually unilateral and commonly associated with nausea and/or vomiting. Photophobia (sensitivity to light) and phonophobia (sensitivity to sound) are also common in migraine.
- For an acute attack, paracetamol or any other analgesic can be given along with an antiemetic such as metoclopramide. Triptans (sumatriptan, zolmitriptan) can also abort an attack. Attacks can be prevented by prophylactic drug therapy such as beta-blockers (propranolol, atenolol, metoprolol), amitriptyline, verapamil, sodium valproate and topiramate. Precipitating factors such as certain foods and scents should be avoided.

Q. A 35-year-old man presents with 4 days h/o fever, headache, altered mental status, siezures and aphasia. Neck stiffness is absent on examination.

1. **What is the likely diagnosis?**
2. **What are the differential diagnoses?**
3. **What investigations would you do to confirm the diagnosis?**
4. **How do you treat him?**

- Likely diagnosis is acute encephalitis probably due to herpes virus. Acute encephalitis typically presents with the above symptoms and speech deficits are common in herpes encephalitis because of involvement of temporal lobe. Absence of neck stiffness argues against meningitis.

- Encephalitis should be differentiated from other causes of altered sensorium such as: fever with delirium, meningitis with cerebral edema, metabolic encephalopathy, stroke, cerebral venous thrombosis, cerebral abscess, acute disseminated encephalomyelitis (ADEM), and cerebral malaria.
- Diagnosis can be confirmed by CSF analysis which shows a raised WBC count with predominant lymphocytes, normal sugar and mildly elevated protein. CSF PCR for herpes simplex and other viral serology is helpful to identify the virus. CT and MRI scan may show areas of cerebral edema, often in the temporal lobes. EEG often shows characteristic slow waves.
- Treatment of herpes simplex encephalitis is with intravenous acyclovir (10 mg/kg IV Q8h) for 10–14 days. There is no specific treatment for other viral encephalitis. Supportive treatment involves anticonvulsants, antiedema measures, bedsore prevention, and attention to nutrition through Ryle's tube.

Q. A 40-year-old man presents with 2 days h/o progressive bilateral lower limb weakness. Patient says he first noticed weakness in the proximal muscles of lower limbs which has then progressed to involve trunk and upper limbs also. There are no sensory symptoms and there is no h/o bowel bladder involvement. Examination shows absent deep tendon reflexes in all 4 limbs and there are no sensory deficits. He also gives h/o upper respiratory tract infection 1 week prior to the onset of weakness.

1. **What is the diagnosis?**
2. **What are the differential diagnoses?**
3. **What investigations would you do to confirm the diagnosis?**
4. **How do you treat him?**

- Diagnosis is acute inflammatory demyelinating polyneuropathy (AIDP) also known as Guillain-Barré syndrome (GBS). The cardinal features of GBS are progressive, symmetric muscle weakness and absent or depressed deep tendon reflexes. Weakness usually starts in the proximal legs, and then ascends up to involve trunk and upper limbs (ascending paralysis). However, in some patients weakness can begin in the arms or facial muscles and then descend down to involve trunk and lower limbs (descending paralysis). Sensory symptoms such as paresthesias occur in the hands and feet in most of the patients, but usually there are no objective sensory deficits. There is often prominent severe pain in the lower back.
- Differential diagnosis includes other causes of symmetric flaccid paralysis such as hypokalemic and hyperkalemic periodic paralysis, tick paralysis and toxin induced neuropathies. Neurotoxic snake bite and botulism can mimic GB syndrome of descending type where the weakness first starts in bulbar muscles.
- Investigations to confirm the diagnosis are nerve conduction studies (NCS) and electromyography (EMG) which show decreased nerve conduction velocity due to demyelination and decreased amplitude of nerve action potentials due to axonal injury. CSF analysis shows elevated protein with normal WBC count which is known as albuminocytologic dissociation.
- Treatment is by plasmapheresis or intravenous immune globulin (IVIG). Plasmapheresis removes the circulating antibodies and helps in fast recovery. Four sittings of plasmapheresis are recommended. Intravenous immune globulin (IVIG) acts by neutralizing circulating antibodies and immunomodulation. IVIG is given in a dose of 0.4 g/kg daily for 5 days. Both plasmapheresis and IV immunoglobulins have equal efficacy and combining both of them is not better than anyone given alone. Steroids are not effective in GBS.
- *See* 'Guillain-Barré syndrome' in neurology chapter for detailed discussion.

Q. A 30-year-old man presents with 3 days h/o bilateral lower limb weakness which developed over few hours. He says he has decreased sensation below the level of umbilicus. He also has urinary retention for which he has undergone bladder catheterization in a local hospital. He had suffered from an acute febrile illness 1 week prior to the onset of lower limb weakness. Examination reveals a sensory level at the level of umbilicus, increased tone in lower limbs, exaggerated deep tendon reflexes and bilateral extensor plantar response.

1. **What is the likely diagnosis?**
2. **What are the differential diagnoses?**
3. **What investigations would you do to confirm the diagnosis?**
4. **How do you treat him?**

- Likely diagnosis is transverse myelitis. The term myelitis is a nonspecific term for inflammation of the spinal cord; transverse refers to involvement of complete width of spinal cord. In this case the lesion seems to be at the level of T10, since below this level (level of umbilicus) there is both sensory and motor weakness. Transverse myelitis produces UMN type weakness below the level of lesion which this patient has (as evidenced by exaggerated reflexes, extensor plantars and increased tone in lower limbs). Definite sensory level and bladder involvement also support a diagnosis of transverse myelitis. Causes of transverse myelitis include idiopathic, para-infectious (occurring in association with an acute infection), post-vaccinial (rabies, cowpox), autoimmune diseases (e.g. SLE, sarcoidosis), multiple sclerosis, paraneoplastic syndrome and thrombosis of spinal arteries.
- Differential diagnosis include other causes of paraparesis/paraplegia such as GB syndrome (LMN type paralysis, absent reflexes, absent sensory level, and no objective sensory deficits), compression of

spinal cord (due to tumor, disc prolapse, trauma, epidural abscess), and unpaired ACA territory infarct (absent sensory level, and sensory deficits).
- MRI of spinal cord should be done to rule out any alternate pathology (abscess, mass, etc.).
- Treatment of idiopathic transverse myelitis is by intravenous steroids (methylprednisolone). Any underlying cause should also be treated.

Q. A 65-year-old man is brought with h/o episodes of motionless stare with altered consciousness followed by lip smacking. Each episode lasts 1–2 minutes.

1. **What is the diagnosis?**
2. **What investigations would you do to confirm the diagnosis?**
3. **How do you treat him?**

- Diagnosis is focal (partial) seizure with impaired awareness. A motionless stare with altered consciousness followed by automatism (e.g. lip smacking, chewing, swallowing) is the usual pattern. This type of seizure commonly arise from the temporal lobe.
- EEG usually shows abnormal spikes in the temporal area if done during an attack. MRI brain can pick up any lesion responsible for the seizure.
- Almost all the antiepileptic drugs (AEDs), except ethosuximide are effective in complex focal seizures. Some examples are carbamazepine, phenytoin, sodium valproate, and gabapentin.

Q. A 70-year-old man, who is a known diabetic for the past 30 years is brought with h/o recurrent episodes of right-sided hemiparesis which recovers fully within one hour. He also gives h/o episodes of transient loss of vision in the left eye.

Discuss the clinical features, investigations and management of the most likely diagnosis in this case.

- Diagnosis is transient ischemic attack (TIA). TIA is defined as a transient episode of neurological dysfunction caused by focal brain, spinal cord, or retinal ischemia, without acute infarction (this is the new definition from American Heart Association and American Stroke Association (AHA/ASA)) which has eliminated the earlier time limit of 24 hours). This man also has episodes of transient loss of vision in the left eye (amaurosis fugax) indicating left carotid artery disease causing emboli into retinal artery as well as into the brain.
- As per definition, brain imaging should not show any infarct. Hence, we expect a normal CT or MRI brain. Cardiac source of emboli should be ruled out by echocardiogram. Four vessel Doppler study of neck (2 vertebral and 2 carotid arteries) can show any stenosis in these vessels which can be further confirmed by angiogram.
- Treatment involves antiplatelet agents (aspirin or clopidogrel) daily lifelong along with lipid lowering agents (statins; atorvastatin, rosuvastatin etc.). These agents reduce the risk of stroke. Internal carotid endarterectomy is recommended if internal carotid artery stenosis is greater than 70%. Percutaneous transluminal angioplasty (stenting) is an alternative procedure which is being commonly done now-a-days.

Q. A 24-year-old man c/o fever, nausea and vomiting of 1 week duration. For the past 2 days, fever has come down but the patient has noticed yellowish discoloration of eyes. There is no h/o alcohol or any drug intake. There is no h/o clay colored stools or pain abdomen. His brother also had similar complaints 2 weeks before. Examination shows moderate icterus and tender hepatomegaly.

1. **How do you approach this patient?**
2. **What is the likely diagnosis?**
2. **What investigations are helpful to confirm the diagnosis?**
3. **How do you treat him?**

- Basically this patient has fever with jaundice. Some important causes of fever with jaundice are acute viral hepatitis, liver abscess, cholecystitis, cholangitis, sepsis, malaria, leptospirosis, dengue, ricketsial fever, etc.
- First possibility to be considered in this patient is acute viral hepatitis. Other causes of acute hepatitis are alcoholic hepatitis, ischemic hepatitis, drug induced hepatitis, autoimmune hepatitis, and Wilson's disease. This patient does not have h/o alcohol or drug ingestion; hence, these are ruled out. Fever is unusual in autoimmune hepatitis and Wilson's disease. Malaria, dengue and leptospirosis produce multi-organ involvement and fever is a prominent feature. Fever continues along with jaundice. In viral hepatitis, jaundice becomes prominent as the fever subsides. Hence, this patient most likely has viral hepatitis, though other causes described above have to be ruled out with appropriate investigations.
- Acute viral hepatitis typically presents with fever, nausea and vomiting. Tender hepatomegaly also supports the diagnosis of acute hepatitis. Jaundice appears when fever starts coming down. Absence of clay colored stool and abdominal pain goes against the diagnosis of obstructive jaundice. Hemolytic anemia typically has mild jaundice and pallor also will be present which is not the case here (this patient has moderate icterus). Hemolytic anemia is usually not associated with fever (this patient has fever). Hepatitis A and hepatitis E spreads through food and water and may affect multiple family members. The fact that this patient's brother also had jaundice supports the diagnosis of hepatitis A or E. However, hepatitis B and C also may spread among family members through close contact and have to be ruled out.

- Diagnosis can be confirmed by liver function tests and viral serology. AST and ALT will be usually elevated to above thousand IU. Viral markers such as IgM anti HAV, HBsAg, anti-HCV, anti-HEV should be sent to identify the specific virus. Appropriate test are done to rule out malaria, dengue, and leptospirosis. Ultrasound abdomen usually shows hepatomegaly and can rule out other causes of jaundice such as cholecystitis, obstruction to biliary tree, liver abscess etc.
- Acute viral hepatitis is usually self-limited, and treatment is mainly supportive with hydration, vitamins and antipyretics. Hepatoprotective agents such as silymarin and vitamin C are particularly useful. Liver transplantation should be considered for patients who develop fulminant liver failure.

Q. A 35-year-old man who is a known case of cholelithiasis presents with 5 days h/o of jaundice, right hypochondrial pain, generalized pruritus, and passing clay colored stool.

1. **What is the likely diagnosis?**
2. **What investigations are helpful to confirm the diagnosis?**
3. **How do you treat him?**

- Diagnosis is obstructive jaundice probably due to a gallstone blocking the common bile duct. Right hypochondrial pain, clay-colored stools and generalized itching all support the diagnosis of obstructive jaundice.
- Ultrasound abdomen is useful to confirm the diagnosis. It may visualize the stone and also show dilated common bile duct. CT abdomen is even more sensitive in picking up the common bile duct stone.
- Endoscopic retrograde cholangiopancreatography (ERCP) can be used to remove stone from common bile duct. If ERCP is not possible, laparotomy and direct removal of stone can be attempted.

Q. A 55-year-old man who is a chronic alcoholic for the past 25 years presents with 10 days h/o passing black colored stools and abdominal distension. Examination shows presence of dilated veins over the abdomen, ascites and moderate splenomegaly.

Discuss the pathogenesis, clinical features, investigations and treatment of the most likely diagnosis in this patient.

- Diagnosis is cirrhosis of liver with portal hypertension. Black colored stool indicates melena due to esophageal varices due to portal hypertension. Presence of ascites, dilated veins over the abdomen and splenomegaly also support the diagnosis of portal hypertension due to cirrhosis. Portal hypertension can also occur without liver disease such as extrahepatic portal hypertension due to portal vein thrombosis, portal vein fibrosis, etc. Here, in this case scenario, there is no mention of features suggestive of liver parenchymal involvement such as jaundice, bleeding tendency, gynecomastia, testicular atrophy, spider nevi, hepatic encephalopathy, etc. These features should be looked for in this patient. Since there is chronic alcohol consumption, probably there is cirrhosis causing portal hypertension.
- Refer 'Cirrhosis' in the chapter 'Diseases of Liver and Biliary System' for detailed discussion.

Q. A 52-year-old man who is a known case of cirrhosis of liver presents with 15 days h/o jaundice, abdominal distension and right hypochondrial pain. Examination shows irregularly enlarged and tender liver.

1. **What is the most likely diagnosis?**
2. **What investigations are helpful to confirm the diagnosis?**
3. **How do you treat him?**

- Diagnosis is hepatocellular carcinoma which can develop as a complication of cirrhosis of liver. Worsening of liver function, painful irregular enlargement of liver point towards the diagnosis of hepatocellular carcinoma. Other possibility is acute hepatitis developing in a previously diseased liver due to alcohol binge or viral hepatitis.
- Diagnosis can be confirmed by ultrasound abdomen, serum alpha-fetoprotein (AFP) level and biopsy of the lesion. Additional imaging such as CT abdomen may also be required.
- Surgical resection and liver transplantation offers the only chance of cure but is limited by the availability of donors. Local therapies (chemoembolization, ethanol ablation, radiofrequency ablation, cryoablation, and radiotherapy) can be used to reduce the tumor burden. For advanced disease systemic chemotherapy can be tried but response is poor.

Q. A 30-year-old lady presents with 5 months h/o easy fatigability and palpitation. She also has h/o geophagia and craving for ice. Examination shows presence of pallor, glossitis, angular stomatitis and koilonychia.

Discuss the etiology, clinical features, investigations and treatment of the most likely diagnosis.

- Diagnosis is iron deficiency anemia because all the above features are typically seen in iron deficiency.
- Serum iron profile (iron, ferritin, TIBC) is helpful in confirming the diagnosis. Iron and ferritin will be low and TIBC will be elevated. Peripheral smear shows microcytic hypochromic RBCs.
- She should be treated with oral iron supplements. Hemoglobin level will normalize in about 6–8 weeks of iron therapy. However, iron therapy has to be continued for a total of 6 months to ensure repletion of the body iron stores. In addition, any underlying cause of iron deficiency (such as menorrhagia, hemorrhoids, worm infestation, peptic ulcer) should be diagnosed and treated.
- For detailed discussion refer 'Iron Deficiency Anemia' under the chapter 'Diseases of Blood'.

Q. A 35-year-old lady presents with 5 months h/o easy fatigability, tingling and numbness of both feet. She is a pure vegetarian and there is no h/o HTN/DM/IHD/asthma or COPD. Examination shows pallor and signs of peripheral neuropathy.

Discuss the etiology, clinical features, investigations and treatment of the most likely diagnosis.

- Diagnosis is anemia due to vitamin B_{12} deficiency because she has both anemia and peripheral neuropathy. Fatigability and pallor are due to anemia. Tingling and numbness is due to peripheral neuropathy due to vitamin B_{12} deficiency. Pure vegetarians like this patient are prone to develop vitamin B_{12} deficiency because vitamin B_{12} is found only in foods of animal origin. Vegetarians get their vitamin B_{12} mainly from milk and milk products.
- Diagnosis can be confirmed by measuring serum vitamin B_{12} levels. B_{12} level <200 pg/ml is suggestive of deficiency. Peripheral smear shows macrocytic RBCs and hyper-segmented neutrophils.
- Vitamin B_{12} should be replaced by parenteral route since malabsorption is the cause most of the time. 1000 µg should be given intramuscularly per week for 8 weeks, followed by 1000 µg every month for the rest of the patient's life. Oral replacement therapy with 2 mg vitamin B_{12} per day is also effective if malabsorption is not a problem. Any underlying cause of vit-B12 deficiency should be treated (e.g. antibiotics for intestinal bacterial overgrowth, deworming for tape worm infestation).
- Refer 'vitamin B_{12} deficiency' under the chapter 'Diseases of Blood' for detailed discussion.

Q. A 25-year-old lady presents with h/o feeling tired even with routine physical activity for the last 2 months. She also gives h/o passing red-brown urine. Her relatives have noticed yellowish discoloration of her eyes. Examination shows pallor, mild icterus and mild splenomegaly.

1. **What is the most likely diagnosis?**
2. **What investigations are helpful to confirm the diagnosis?**
3. **How do you treat her?**

- Most likely diagnosis is hemolytic anemia in view of presence of tiredness, pallor and jaundice. Red brown urine is due to hemoglobinuria. There are many causes of hemolytic anemia such as hereditary spherocytosis, G6PD deficiency, thalassemias, sickle cell anemia, autoimmune hemolytic anemia, drugs, etc.
- Diagnosis can be confirmed by peripheral blood smear (may show spherocytes, sickle cells, polychromasia, nucleated RBCs), reticulocyte count (increased), Coombs' test (to identify autoimmune hemolytic anemia), and bone marrow examination (shows erythroid hyperplasia). In addition, there will be indirect hyperbilirubinemia and decreased serum haptoglobin levels. Shortened RBC survival as demonstrated by chromium-51 labeled RBCs.
- Treatment depends on the underlying cause—steroids for autoimmune hemolytic anemia, splenectomy in hereditary spherocytosis and sickle cell anemia, withdrawal of offending drug, etc.
- For detailed discussion refer hemolytic anemia in the chapter 'Diseases of Blood'.

Q. A 50-year-old man presents with h/o easy fatigability and left hypochondrial pain. Examination shows pallor and massive splenomegaly. His complete blood count shows Hb of 5 g/dl, WBC count of 1,50,000/mm^3 and platelet count of 2,25000/mm^3.

1. **What is the most likely diagnosis?**
2. **What further investigations would you like to do?**
3. **How do you treat him?**

- Most likely diagnosis is chronic myeloid leukemia in view of very high leukocyte count and massive splenomegaly.
- Other causes of massive splenomegaly such as hairy cell leukemia, kala-azar, tropical splenomegaly, etc. should also be considered in this case and ruled out by appropriate investigations. But the presence very high leukocyte count argues against kala-azar, and tropical splenomegaly.
- Peripheral blood smear shows presence of myelocytes and metamyelocytes. Bone marrow aspiration and biopsy shows myeloid hyperplasia, increase in reticulin fibers and vascularity. There is increase in the myeloid-to-erythroid ratio in the bone marrow. Diagnosis of CML can be confirmed by the demonstration of the Philadelphia chromosome or the BCR-ABL fusion gene. BCR-ABL can be detected in the peripheral blood by polymerase chain reaction (PCR) test, which has now supplanted cytogenetics.
- Conventional treatment of CML in chronic phase has been single agent therapy with busulphan or hydroxyurea. Alpha interferon is also helpful. Introduction of imatinib mesylate which inhibits the tyrosine kinase activity of the BCR/ABL oncogene has revolutionized the treatment of CML.

Q. A 36-year-old lady c/o multiple joint pain involving bilateral ankle, knee, small joints of hands, wrist, elbow and shoulder since 6 months. Joint pain is worse in the morning and is associated with early morning stiffness.

1. **What is the most likely diagnosis?**
2. **What are the differential diagnoses?**
3. **What further investigations would you like to do?**
4. **How do you treat her?**

- This is a case of chronic symmetric inflammatory polyarthritis. Most likely diagnosis is rheumatoid arthritis (RA). Characteristic clinical features of RA are as follows:
  - Morning stiffness of at least 1 hour and present for at least 6 weeks.
  - Swelling of three or more joints for at least 6 weeks.

- Arthritis of hand joints.
- Symmetrical arthritis.
- Presence of rheumatoid subcutaneous nodules.
- Positive rheumatoid factors or anti-cyclic citrullinated peptide (anti-CCP) antibodies.
- Elevated acute phase reactants (erythrocyte sedimentation rate or C-reactive protein).
- Radiological changes (erosions or unequivocal bony decalcification adjacent to the involved joints.

- **Differential diagnoses include other diseases which can present with polyarthritis as follows:**
  - Acute viral polyarthritis (such as chickungunya, associated with acute onset polyarthritis, usually transient, subsides without any residual deformities)
  - Systemic rheumatic diseases such as SLE, systemic sclerosis.
  - Reactive arthritis (usually oligoarthritis involving large joints such as knee, ankle, etc.)
  - Lyme arthritis
  - Psoriatic arthritis (usually oligoarthritis)
  - Polymyalgia rheumatic (frank arthritis is unusual).
  - Crystalline arthritis (e.g. gout. Usually monoarthritis)
  - Infectious arthritis (such as tuberculous arthritis, gonococcal arthritis: Usually oligoarthritis involving large joints)
  - Osteoarthritis (usually involves large weight bearing joints such as knee, hip, etc. pain worse in the evening, seen in elderly)
- Further investigations which are helpful are rheumatoid factor, anti-CCP antibody, CRP, ESR, ANA (a negative ANA helps to rule out SLE and other systemic rheumatic diseases), hand X-rays to look for joint erosions.
- Refer rheumatoid arthritis for detailed discussion.

Q. A 30-year-old lady presents with malar rash, photosensitivity, and polyarthralgia of 5 years duration. She also gives h/o recurrent abortions and Raynaud phenomenon.

Discuss the etiology, clinical features, investigations and treatment of the most likely diagnosis.

- Most likely diagnosis is systemic lupus erythematosus (SLE). SLE frequently affects women in their 20s and 30s. It affects almost all the organs and usually begins with one or several of the following features such as: fever, fatigue, malar rash (butterfly rash), arthralgia or arthritis, Raynaud phenomenon, serositis (pleuritis, pericarditis, peritonitis), nephritis or nephrotic syndrome, seizures, alopecia, recurrent abortions, and anemia.
- Complete blood count shows anemia or pancytopenia. ESR, CRP are elevated and complement levels (C3, and C4) are decreased. Antinuclear antibodies (ANA), antiphospholipid antibodies, antibodies to double-stranded DNA and anti-Smith (Sm) antibodies may be positive. Anti dsDNA and anti Sm antibodies are highly specific for the diagnosis of SLE.
- Mainstay of treatment is steroids. Immunosuppressive drugs (azathioprine, methotrexate, ciclosporin, tacrolimus, mycophenolate mofetil) are useful either alone or in combination with steroids for severe manifestations. Hydroxychloroquine also is useful for cutaneous and joint symptoms. Lifelong anticoagulation is required for patients with the antiphospholipid antibody syndrome with thrombotic events.
- For detailed discussion refer 'SLE' in Chapter 10 'Diseases of Immune system, Connective tissue and Joints'.

Q. A 25-year-old man presents with insidious onset of low back pain and stiffness of 6 months duration. He also has pain in the ankle, knee and hip joints. Examination shows restricted spinal mobility and sacroiliac joint tenderness.

1. **What is the most likely diagnosis?**
2. **What investigations are helpful to confirm the diagnosis?**
3. **How do you treat him?**

- Most likely diagnosis is ankylosing spondylitis. It is a type of seronegative spondyloarthropathy. It mainly affects males and the peak incidence is between 20 and 30 years. Most important feature is involvement of lumbosacral spine with restriction of mobility in all directions. Note that rheumatoid arthritis also involves spine but usually cervical spine. In addition, restriction of spine mobility is unusual in rheumatoid arthritis. Degenerative spine diseases such as spondylosis also involve spine and cause restricted mobility, but occur in old age and also do not affect peripheral joints. Extra-articular features are also common in seronegative spondyloarthropathies and include enthesitis (inflammation at tendon insertion sites), scleritis, uveitis, mucosal ulcers, etc.
- ESR and CRP are elevated. Rheumatoid factor is usually negative. HLA-B27 is usually positive. X-ray of sacroiliac joint shows irregularity and loss of cortical margins, sclerosis, narrowing and fusion. In advanced cases, there will be fusion of vertebras which produces bamboo spine appearance on X-ray.
- Treatment involves both nonpharmacological and pharmacological therapy. Nonpharmacological therapy involves smoking cessation and exercise. Pharmacological therapy involves NSAIDs, DMARDs (sulfasalazine, methotrexate), and TNF-alpha antagonists (infliximab, etanercept, adalimumab). However, methotrexate has been shown to be of little use in ankylosing spondylitis.

Q. A 60-year-old lady presents with right temporal headache of 5 days duration. She also has blurring of vision in the right eye. Routine investigations showed that her ESR is 100 mm/hour.

Discuss the etiology, clinical features, investigations and treatment of the most likely diagnosis.

- The diagnosis is temporal arteritis. Temporal arteritis is common in elderly (above 50 years of age). It is more common in females. Typical presentation is temporal headache with blurring of vision. There will be tenderness over the temporal artery. ESR is usually high.

- Diagnosis can be confirmed by temporal artery biopsy. Biopsy will show infiltration of temporal artery with lymphocytes, fragmentation of internal elastic lamina and destruction of tunica media.
- Treatment is with steroids. Steroids should be started immediately on suspicion without waiting for confirmation of diagnosis. Dose of prednisolone is 40–60 mg per day for 1–2 months initially, followed by slow tapering. Typical duration of therapy is 9–12 months. Low dose aspirin is also useful to reduce the risk of visual loss, TIA and stroke.
- For detailed discussion refer 'temporal arteritis' in Chapter 10 'Diseases of Immune system, Connective tissue and Joints'.

Q. A 50-year-old man who is a chronic alcoholic presents with confusion and disorientation. Examination shows nystagmus, ophthalmoplegia and ataxia. There are no motor or sensory deficits. CT brain is essentially normal. Discuss the etiology, clinical features, and treatment of the most likely diagnosis.

- Most likely diagnosis is Wernicke's encephalopathy (WE). WE typically occurs in chronic alcoholics due to thiamine deficiency. It should be suspected in any alcoholic presenting with the triad of encephalopathy, ataxia and ophthalmoplegia.
- WE is mainly a clinical diagnosis. Imaging (CT or MRI brain) is useful to rule out alternative diagnosis). Measurement of erythrocyte transketolase activity after adding thiamine pyrophosphate can be used to diagnose thiamine deficiency.
- Patients suspected to have WE should be treated with intravenous thiamine immediately, without waiting for confirmation of diagnosis. Thiamine 500 mg should be given as IV infusion three times daily for 2 days followed by 500 mg once daily IV or IM once daily for 5 days. This is followed by 100 mg daily orally as long as the patient is at risk of developing deficiency. Administration of glucose in the presence of thiamine deficiency can precipitate thiamine deficiency, because thiamine is an important co-enzyme in glucose metabolism (conversion of pyruvate to acetyl CoA). Hence, thiamine should be given before giving glucose.

Q. A 50-year-old chronic alcoholic presents with confusion and memory loss. He also gives h/o diarrhea of 3 months duration. Examination shows dark, dry and scaly skin lesions around the neck, hands and legs.

1. **What is the most likely diagnosis?**
2. **What investigations are helpful to confirm the diagnosis?**
3. **How do you treat this patient?**

- Most likely diagnosis is pellagra due to niacin deficiency. Niacin deficiency is common in alcoholics, malabsorption disorders and anorexia nervosa. Niacin deficiency can occur in Hartnup's disease which is characterized by defective absorption of several amino acids. Similarly niacin deficiency can also occur in carcinoid syndrome where tryptophan is converted to 5-HT and serotonin rather than niacin. Pellagra is characterized by 3 D's, diarrhea, dementia and dermatitis. This patient has all these features.
- Pellagra is treated by niacin supplements 100 mg 3 times daily orally or parenterally for 5 days.
- Refer 'pellagra for more details.

Q. A 30-year-old lady presents with, easy fatigability, cold intolerance, and amenorrhea after the last child birth. She had suffered severe postpartum hemorrhage and also lactation failure after last child birth. Examination is otherwise normal except dry skin.

1. **What is the most likely diagnosis?**
2. **What investigations are helpful to confirm the diagnosis?**
3. **How do you treat this patient?**

- Most likely diagnosis is hypopituitarism due to Sheehan's syndrome. Hypopituitarsim due to infarction of the pituitary gland after postpartum hemorrhage is called Sheehan syndrome. The pituitary gland is physiologically enlarged in pregnancy and is therefore very sensitive to the decreased blood flow caused by massive hemorrhage and hypovolemic shock.
- Failure to lactate or difficulty with lactation are common initial symptoms of Sheehan syndrome (due to prolactin deficiency). Many women also report amenorrhea or oligomenorrhea after delivery (due to FSH and LH deficiency). Other features include fatigue, anorexia, weight loss (due to decreased ACTH), and features of hypothyroidism (due to decreased TSH).
- There is deficiency of all the hormones, i.e. growth hormone, prolactin, gonadotropins, TSH and ACTH. CT scan or MRI shows a small pituitary within a sella of normal size, sometimes referred to as "empty sella".
- Treatment of hypopituitarism involves the treatment of each individual target gland hormone deficiencies. ACTH deficiency is treated by giving hydrocortisone or other glucocorticoid. TSH deficiency, which results in thyroxine deficiency, is treated with L-thyroxine.

Q. A 30-year-old woman c/o weight loss, increased appetite, heat intolerance and palpitations since 2 months. Examination shows a pulse rate of 105/minute and fine tremors of hands.

1. **What is your diagnosis?**
2. **How do you confirm the diagnosis?**
3. **How do you treat this patient?**

- Diagnosis is thyrotoxicosis.
- Diagnosis can be confirmed by thyroid function tests. In primary hyperthyroidism, T3, T4 will be

elevated and TSH will be suppressed. In central hyperthyroidism, all three will be elevated.

- Treatment involves antithyroid drugs. Methimazole is started at 5–10 mg OD and can be increased to 30–40 mg per day. Propyl thiouracil (PTU) is given at a dose of 100–150 mg every 8 hours. Radioactive iodine (^{131}I) is used to treat hyperthyroidism in older patients but is contraindicated in pregnant ladies. Subtotal thyroidectomy is another option for patients with thyroid enlargement causing obstructive symptoms.
- For more details refer 'hyperthyroidism' in the chapter 'Endocrinology and Diabetes Mellitus'.

Q. A 35-year-old patient presents with weight gain, cold intolerance and hoarseness of voice since 2 months. Examination shows dry skin and bilateral nonpitting pedal edema.

1. **What is your diagnosis?**
2. **How do you confirm the diagnosis?**
3. **How do you treat this patient?**

- Diagnosis is hypothyroidism.
- Diagnosis can be confirmed by thyroid function tests. In primary hypothyroidism, T3, T4 will be low and TSH will be elevated. In central hypothyroidism, all three will be low.
- Treatment involves thyroxine supplementation. Thyroxine should be started at a low dose and increased every 6–8 weeks till thyroid function is normalized. Initial dose should be low especially in patients with IHD, because high initial dose of thyroxine can precipitate angina and heart failure by increasing BMR.
- For more details refer 'hypothyroidism' in the chapter 'Endocrinology and Diabetes Mellitus'.

Q. A 40-year-old man presents with weight loss, easy fatigability, and darkening (hyperpigmentation) of skin of few months duration. Examination shows BP of 90/60 mm Hg. Investigations show Na^+ of 130, K^+ of 5.6 and his random blood sugar is 70 mg/dl.

1. **What could be the diagnosis?**
2. **How do you confirm the diagnosis?**
3. **How do you treat this patient?**

- Diagnosis is adrenal insufficiency (Addison's disease). Adrenal insufficiency is of two types: primary (inability of the adrenals to produce hormones), secondary (due to pituitary or hypothalamic disease leading to ACTH and CRH deficiency). Symptoms and signs are due to low glucocorticoid, low mineralocorticoid, low adrenal androgen levels and secondary increase in ACTH. Glucocorticoid deficiency causes malaise, fatigue, generalized weakness, nausea, vomiting, anorexia, weight loss, postural hypotension with postural drop and hypoglycemia. Mineralocorticoid deficiency causes hyponatremia and hyperkalemia. ACTH excess in primary adrenal deficiency causes hyperpigmentation. Hyperpigmentation is not seen in secondary adrenal insufficiency as ACTH is low.
- Refer Addison disease for detailed discussion.

Q. A 50-year-old patient presents with polyuria, excessive thirst and increased appetite. He also has weight loss since last 3 months and recurrent skin infections.

1. **What is your diagnosis?**
2. **How do you confirm the diagnosis?**
3. **How do you treat this patient?**

- Diagnosis is diabetes mellitus in v/o of polyuria, polydipsia, polyphagia and recurrent skin infections. The type of diabetes is probably type 2 DM, because the patient is 50 years old. Type 1 DM is unlikely because it usually occurs in children and young adults. Secondary diabetes due to pancreatic disease is possible and should be ruled out by appropriate investigations. Patients with chronic pancreatitis usually c/o epigastric pain worsened by food intake, and bulky foul smelling stools (steatorrhea).
- Polyuria occurs due to the osmotic diuresis caused by sugar in the urine. Polydipsia occurs secondary to excess loss of fluid in the urine and also due to increased osmolality of blood due to excess sugar. Polyphagia is due to loss of calories in the urine (as glucose) and also the inability of the body to use glucose due to lack of insulin or insulin resistance.
- Diagnosis can be confirmed by doing FBS and PPBS. An FBS of more than 110 mg/dl and PPBS of more than 200 mg/dl confirms diabetes mellitus.
- Treatment involves diet control, exercise, antidiabetic drugs and insulin. Antidiabetic drugs include sulphonylureas, biguanides, glitazones, alpha-glucosidase inhibitors, meglitinides, PPP-4 inhibitors.

Q. A 34-year-old lady who has undergone total thyroidectomy for papillary carcinoma thyroid 2 months ago presents with h/o episodes of paresthesias involving fingertips, toes, perioral area and muscle cramps involving low back, legs and feet.

1. **What is your diagnosis?**
2. **How do you confirm the diagnosis?**
3. **How do you treat this patient?**

- Diagnosis is hypoparathyroidism. This patient has undergone total thyroidectomy, hence even the parathyroid glands which are very close to the thyroid glands must have been removed leading to hypoparathyroidism. Paresthesias and muscle cramps are due to hypocalcemia. Other causes of hypoparathyroidism are irradiation of the neck, Type 1 autoimmune polyglandular syndrome, and congenital agenesis or hypoplasia of the parathyroid gland.
- Diagnosis can be confirmed by measuring serum calcium which will be low and serum parathormone (PTH) level which also will be low. Measurement

of 25-hydroxy vitamin D is important to exclude vitamin D deficiency as a cause of hypocalcemia. Serum magnesium level should also me measured as low magnesium also causes symptoms similar to hypocalcemia. In addition, hypomagnesemia may cause PTH deficiency and subsequent hypocalcemia.

- Treatment involves supplementation of vitamin D and calcium. Currently parathormone use is approved for use only in patients with osteoporosis.

Q. A 30-year-old man is brought with 1 month h/o altered behavior. He is socially withdrawn, appears depressed, has difficulty in taking care of himself, reports hearing voices, and believes that people are inserting thoughts into his mind. His routine blood tests are normal.

1. **What is your diagnosis?**
2. **How do you treat this patient?**

- Diagnosis is schizophrenia.
- Treatment is by antipsychotics such as clozapine, risperidone, olanzapine, and quetiapine.
- For detailed discussion refer 'schizophrenia' in the chapter 'psychiatric disorders'.

Q. A 25-year-old man is found unconscious at his house. Examination shows kerosene smell in his breath. Patient is tachypneic with a pulse rate of 35/min and BP of 90/60 mm Hg. There is excess salivation and excess sweating. His pupils are constricted and there are fasciculations also.

Discuss the etiology, clinical features, investigations and treatment of the most likely diagnosis in this patient.

- Diagnosis is organophosphorus poisoning. Usually organophosphorus compounds have the smell of kerosene. Clinical features can be divided into 3 phases: acute cholinergic phase, intermediate syndrome, and organophosphate-induced delayed polyneuropathy (OPIDN). Acute cholinergic phase is characterized by bradycardia, constricted pupils, increased body secretions and fasciculations. Intermediate syndrome starts 1–3 days after exposure to poison. It occurs due to receptor dysfunction at the neuromuscular junction and is characterized by weakness of neck muscles, decreased deep tendon reflexes, cranial nerve abnormalities, proximal and respiratory muscle weakness or paralysis. OPIDN occurs about 1–3 weeks after acute OP exposure and is characterized by transient, painful "stocking-glove" paresthesias followed by a symmetrical motor polyneuropathy
- Diagnosis can be confirmed by history and by measuring plasma cholinesterase levels which will be reduced to less than 50% of normal.
- Treatment involves gastric lavage, activated charcoal and IV fluids. Antidote is atropine which antagonizes the muscarinic effects of acetylcholine. Atropine does not reverse nicotinic effects such as muscle fasciculation. Initially 2–5 mg is given IV. If no effect is noted, the dose is doubled every three to five minutes until the muscarinic signs and symptoms are reversed. Atropine infusion is usually required for several days after the exposure. Intravenous glycopyrrolate is an alternative and does not have many CNS side effects of atropine. Oximes such as pralidoxime (PAM) and obidoxime are cholinesterase reactivating agents and are effective in treating both muscarinic and nicotinic effects of OP compound. Dose of PAM is 2 g IV infusion over 30 minutes. Intermediate syndrome is treated by ventilator support. There is no specific therapy for OPIDN. Regular physiotherapy may reduce deformities and muscle-wasting.
- Refer organophosphorus poisoning for more details.

Q. A 22-year-old student is found unconscious in his room. Examination shows low respiratory rate (10 breaths per minute), pulse rate of 55/min, normal BP, decreased chest movements, decreased bowel sounds and miotic pupils. Discuss the etiology, clinical features, investigations and treatment of the most likely diagnosis in this patient.

- The diagnosis is opioid intoxication. The classic signs of opioid intoxication include depressed mental status, decreased respiratory rate, decreased tidal volume, decreased bowel sounds, and constricted pupils. Rarely normal sized pupils can be seen if the patient has taken meperidine or propoxyphene or presence of sympathomimetic or anticholinergic co-ingestants. Constricted pupils can also be seen in organosphosphorus poisoning and pontine hemorrhage. However, absence of kerosene smell, decreased bowel sounds argue against OP poisoning. Pontine hemorrhage can present with similar picture and should be ruled out by CT or MRI brain.
- Diagnosis of opioid poisoning is made clinically. However diagnosis can be confirmed by response to naloxone which is an opioid antagonist.
- Initial management involves support of patient's airway and breathing. Naloxone (opioid antagonist) is given intravenously. Activated charcoal and gastric emptying are usually not necessary and may increase the chances of aspiration in an unconscious patient.

Q. A 44-year-old man presents with h/o ingestion of illicit liquor followed by nausea, vomiting, abdominal pain, and severe watery diarrhea. There is garlic odor of the breath and stool. Discuss about the most likely diagnosis in this patient.

- The diagnosis is acute arsenic poisoning. Arsenic poisoning can occur in people working in industries dealing with semiconductors (gallium arsenide), smelting/refining, mining, metallurgy, and decorative glass-making. It can also occur after ingestion of arsenic-containing pesticides, herbicides and some "moonshine" (illegally distilled alcohol). Symptoms start in the gastrointestinal system and include nausea, vomiting, abdominal pain, and watery diarrhea which can lead to dehydration and hypotension. Garlic odor of breath and stool is typically found in severe poisoning. Other features are cardiac arrhythmias, shock, ARDS, acute encephalopathy, and sometimes death.

- Another consideration is methanol poisoning. But it is associated with blurring of vision or blindness, features of metabolic acidosis, etc.
- Diagnosis of arsenic poisoning can be established by taking an X-ray of the abdomen which may show radiopaque material soon after ingestion. ECG may show QT prolongation. Blood arsenic level are usually raised but since blood arsenic is cleared rapidly, measurement of urine arsenic levels can confirm the diagnosis. In acute poisoning, urine arsenic levels are usually in the thousands of micrograms per liter.
- Refer arsenic poisoning for more details.

Q. A 35-year-old man who works in a battery manufacturing unit has come with colicky abdominal pain, constipation, joint pains, decreased libido, and difficulty concentrating. Examination shows impaired short-term memory, anemia, a bluish pigmentation at the gum-tooth line, and bilateral weakness of extensors of ankle and wrist.

Discuss about the most likely diagnosis in this patient.

- Diagnosis is lead poisoning. Lead exposure can occur in places involved in manufacturing or use of batteries, pigments, solder, ammunitions, paint, car radiators, cable and wires, and some cosmetics. Leaded fuel was another source of lead exposure, but now lead is not being added to fuels.
- Diagnosis can be confirmed by measuring blood lead levels. Chelation is indicated for individuals with blood lead levels greater than 80 µg/dl. Other useful tests are free erythrocyte protoporphyrin (FEP) or zinc protoporphyrin (ZPP). These two tests measure the effect of lead on hemoglobin synthesis, and can be used as an indicator of lead exposure.

Q. A 25-year-old lady presents with h/o fever, increased frequency and burning micturition of 2 days duration. Discuss briefly the most likely diagnosis in this patient.

- This patient has urinary tract infection (UTI). Fever, increased frequency and burning micturition are all pointing towards urinary tract infection. Usually females are more likely to get UTI than males because of short urethra (4 cm) and *E. coli* is the common organism causing UTI. More than 5 WBCs in the urine per high power field will confirm the diagnosis of UTI.
- Other helpful investigations in this patient are urine culture and sensitivity. Rarely ultrasound abdomen may be required in cases of recurrent UTI to rule out any urinary tract abnormality.
- A 5-day course of antibiotics should be given to this patient. Antibiotic choices include quinolones (ciprofloxacin or levofloxacin), amoxicillin-clavulinic acid, co-trimoxazole, azithromycin or cephalosporins. Reccurent UTI can be prevented by maintaining good hygiene in the perinial and genitourinary area, passing urine after sexual intercourse. Cranberry juice has been shown to reduce the incidence of UTI by preventing the attachment of *E. coli* fimbriae to urothelium.

Q. A 30-year-old lady has presented with facial puffiness, leg swelling and passing frothy urine. BP is 130/80 mm Hg. Her LFT and RFT reports are normal. Her urine analysis report shows 4+ proteinuria.

Discuss the etiology, clinical features, investigations and treatment of the most likely diagnosis in this patient.

- Diagnosis is nephrotic syndrome. Nephrotic syndrome is defined as proteinuria of more than 3.5 g/day accompanied by hypoalbuminemia, edema, and hyperlipidemia. Normal BP also goes in favor of nephrotic syndrome as hypertension is a feature of nephritic syndrome. Etiology includes minimal change disease (in children), focal segmental glomerulosclerosis (FSGS), membranous nephropathy, diabetes mellitus, SLE and other collagen diseases, amyloidosis, vasculitis, infections (post-streptococcal, hepatitis B, hepatitis C, HIV), and drugs (penicillamine, NSAIDs).
- Other useful investigations are measurement of 24 hour urinary protein excretion, lipid profile and investigations to find out the cause of nephrotic syndrome (such as blood sugar, ANA, cANCA, hepatitis-B and C serology, ASO titer, HIV ELISA, etc.). Renal biopsy is required if the cause is not clear especially in an adult patient.
- *Management:* Edema is managed by dietary salt restriction and diuretics. Hyperlipidemia is treated by dietary modification and statins. Minimal change disease responds to steroids. Membranous nephropathy responds to alternating monthly corticosteroids and monthly oral chlorambucil over 6 months. Membranous nephropathy with progressive renal failure may benefit from cyclophosphamide plus corticosteroids. Underlying cause should also be addressed. Anticoagulation may be required if there is evidence of thrombosis because nephrotic syndrome is a hypercoagulable state due to loss of antithrombin-III in urine.

Q. A 20-year-old boy presents with hematuria, oliguria and generalized edema. His BP is 160/100 mm Hg. His urine analysis shows presence of 1+ poteinuria, WBCs, RBCs and RBC casts. Urea and creatinine are elevated.

- Diagnosis is acute glomerulonephritis. Glomerulonephritis typically presents with hypertension, hematuria, RBC casts, pyuria (WBCs) and mild-to-moderate proteinuria. Causes of acute glomerulonephritis include primary glomerular diseases (diffuse proliferative glomerulonephritis, focal segmental glomerulosclerosis, membranous glomerulonephritis, crescentic glomerulonephritis, IgA nephropathy), systemic diseases (SLE, Wegener's granulomatosis, polyarteritis, Goodpasture's syndrome), infections (post-streptococcal, syphilis, hepatitis B and C), and serum sickness, etc.

- Treatment usually requires high-dose steroids and cytotoxic agents such as cyclophosphamide. Plasmapheresis can be used in Goodpasture's disease. Underlying disease requires specific treatment.
- Refer 'acute glomerulonephritis' for detailed discussion.

Q. A 30-year-old man who is a known case of type 1 diabetes mellitus has come to emergency with fatigue, diffuse abdominal pain, vomiting and drowsiness. He was taking insulin daily (total 60 units per day), but has skipped the insulin for the past 4 days. On examination he is tachypneic, has pulse rate of 110 beats per minute, respiratory rate of 28 breaths per minute (deep and sighing type breaths), blood pressure of 100/70 mm Hg. He also has dry mucous membranes, poor skin turgor and is slightly confused. His blood sugar is 450 mg/dl. An ABG done at the bedside shows arterial pH of 6.9, PO_2 95 mm Hg, PCO_2 28 mm Hg, and HCO of 9 mEq/L. Urine shows presence of large amount of ketone bodies.

Discuss in detail the most likely diagnosis in this patient.

- Diagnosis is diabetic ketoacidosis (DKA). DKA is common in type 1 DM. it is precipitated by acute illness or skipping of insulin. Blood sugar is usually more than 250 mg/dl. Patients present with fatigue, diffuse abdominal pain due to acidosis and altered sensorium. Patients usually have severe dehydration due to osmotic diuresis caused by hyperglycemia. This patient has dry mucus membranes, poor skin turgor and low normal BP, all of which suggest dehydration. Tachypnea and deep sighing breathing is due to metabolic acidosis. ABG shows metabolic acidosis (low pH and low bicarbonate) and urine shows large amount of ketone bodies confirming the diagnosis of DKA.
- For detailed discussion refer 'DKA' in 'Endocrinology and Diabetes Mellitus' chapter.

Q. A 52-year-old male presents with increasing fatigue and weakness for the past few days. He is a known case of type 2 diabetes mellitus on glimepiride and insulin. He also c/o excessive thirst and passing large amount of urine for the past few days. Examination shows BP of 70/40 mm Hg; pulse 115/min; respiratory rate, 22/min; and temperature of 36.9°C. The patient is awake and responsive but disoriented. Mucus membranes are dry and skin turgor is poor. Lab data show blood sugar of 950 mg/dl, and negative ketone bodies in the urine. ABG shows normal pH and normal PO_2 and CO_2.

Discuss the most likely diagnosis in this patient.

- Most likely diagnosis in this patient is hyperglycemic hyperosmolar state (HHS). It is common in type 2 DM. In type 2 DM, there is some residual insulin secretion in the body which prevents formation of ketone bodies. If DKA develops due to ketone bodies, patient become sick and seeks medical attention early. However, in type 2 DM residual insulin prevents ketone body formation and there is rise of blood glucose to very high level (>800 mg/dl) which causes hyperosmolality of blood. Hyperosmolality leads to dehydration of neurons producing altered sensorium and sometimes seizures. Severe hyperglycemia also leads to osmotic diuresis, dehydration and excessive thirst. Low BP and increased pulse rate in this patient are due to dehydration. Another consideration in a patient presenting with hyperglycemia, weakness and dehydration is DKA. But absence of ketone bodies in the urine and normal pH in this patient suggest that it is not DKA.
- For detailed discussion refer 'HHS' in 'Endocrinology and Diabetes Mellitus' chapter.

Q. A 55-year-old man presents with fever, breathlessness, cough with purulent sputum and right sided chest pain of 3 days duration. Chest pain is sharp, stabbing type and increases on deep breathing and coughing. Examination shows pulse rate of 110/min, respiratory rate of 30/min and BP of 130/80 mm Hg. Chest examination shows crepitations and bronchial breath sounds in right infrascapular area.

Discuss the most likely diagnosis in this patient.

- The most likely diagnosis is lobar pneumonia. Lobar pneumonia usually produces pleuritic type chest pain which this patient has. Bronchopneumonia usually affects both lung and there will be findings in both the lungs which is not the case here. Another consideration is lung abscess, but it presents with significant amount of foul smelling sputum. In addition, pleuritic type chest pain is unusual in lung abscess unless it is closer to the periphery of the lung.
- For detailed discussion refer 'pneumonia' in 'Diseases of Respiratory System' chapter.

Index

A

Abdominal tuberculosis 331
Achalasia 313
Acne vulgaris 761
Acoustic neuroma 453
Acromegaly/gigantism 592
Actinomycosis 37
Acute abdomen 341
Acute adrenal insufficiency 616
Acute bronchitis 130
Acute cholangitis 558
Acute confusional state—elderly 825
Acute confusional state (delirium) 450, 451
Acute cor pulmonale 210
Acute diarrhea 301
Acute inflammatory demyelinating polyneuropathy (AIDP) 440
Acute kidney injury (AKI) 565
Acute lung injury (ALI) 803
Acute lymphoid leukemia (ALL) 481
Acute mountain sickness 796
Acute myeloid leukemia (AML) 480
Acute myocardial infarction (STEMI) 236
Acute peritonitis 342
Acute pulmonary edema 211
Acute pyelonephritis 582
Acute respiratory distress syndrome (ARDS) 803
Acute rheumatic fever 246
Acute severe asthma (status asthmaticus) 136
Addisonian crisis 616
Adrenal insufficiency 615
Advanced directives 813
African trypanosomiasis (sleeping sickness) 91
Agglutination test 3
Agranulocytosis 471
Air embolism 284
Alcohol use disorder 705
Alcohol withdrawal syndrome (delirium tremens) 706
Alcoholic liver disease (ALD) 536
Alopecia (baldness) 768
Alpha thalassemias 476
Alpha-fetoprotein 553
Aluminum phosphide poisoning 777
Alzheimer's disease 448
Amaurosis fugax 404
Amebiasis 88
Amebic liver abscess 554
American Diabetes Association (ADA) criteria for diabetes 628
American trypanosomiasis (Chagas' disease) 93
Amniotic fluid embolism 284
Amyotrophic lateral sclerosis (ALS) 438
Anemia 457
Anemia in CKD 572
Anemia of chronic disease 464
Angina 230
Angina equivalents 230
Angina-treatment 232
Angioedema 760
Anion gap 722
Ankylosing spondylitis (AS) 652
Anomic aphasia 370
Anorexia nervosa 703
Anthrax 20
Antiarrhythmic drugs 276
Anticancer drugs 730
Anticoagulants (coagulation inhibitors) 505
Anticyclic citruillinated peptide (anti-CCP) antibody 651
Antiepileptic drugs 413
Antigenic drift 54
Antigenic shift 54
Antileprosy drugs 41
Antineutrophil cytoplasmic antibodies (ANCA) 672
Antinuclear antibodies (ANA) 673
Antioxidants 746
Antiphospholipid antibody syndrome (APLA) 673
Antiplatelet agents in stroke patients 397
Antiretroviral drugs 75
Antithyroid drugs 597, 605
Antituberculous drugs 158
Anuria 562
Anxiety disorders 695
Aortic aneurysm 293
Aortic dissection 294
Aortic regurgitation (AR)-peripheral signs 257
Aortic regurgitation (AR) 256
Aortic sclerosis 256
Aortic stenosis 254
Aphasia 369
Aphthous ulcers 306
Aplastic anemia 469
Aplastic crisis 475
Approach to a case of cough 119
Approach to a case of FUO 6
Approach to a case of hematuria 564
Approach to a case of jaundice 522
Approach to a case of joint pain 657
Approach to a case of motor weakness 356
Approach to a case of vertigo 382
Approach to a case of vomiting 299
Apraxia 369
Argyll Robertson pupil (ARP) 367
Arrhythmia 265
Arsenic poisoning 783
Arthralgia *vs* arthritis 658, 659
Arthrocentesis 645
Asbestosis 170
Ascaris lumbricoides (Ascariasis) 102
Aschoff nodule 247
Ascites 547
Aseptic meningitis 387
Aspergillosis 113
Asthma 131
Asthma-COPD overlap (ACO) 140
Asthma–treatment 134
Atherosclerosis–risk factors 229
Athetosis 422
Atrial fibrillation (AF) 269
Atrial flutter 271
Atrial septal defect (ASD) 226
Atrioventricular blocks (heart blocks) 265, 266
Attention-deficit hyperactivity disorder (ADHD) 699
Atypical pneumonia 145
Austin flint murmur 259, 264
Autism spectrum disorder 700
Autoantibodies in SLE 661
Autoimmune hemolytic anemias 466
Autonomic neuropathy 442
Autonomic neuropathy 640
Autonomy and shared responsibility 810
Autosomal dominant disorders 740
Autosomal recessive disorders 740

B

Babesiosis 94
Bacteremia 1, 802
Bariatric surgery 682
Barrett's esophagus 309
Basal cell carcinoma (BCC) (rodent ulcer) 770
Becker muscular dystrophy 446
Bee sting 789
Beers criteria 824
Behçet disease 671
Bell's palsy 381
Beneficence in patient care 811
Beriberi 686
Beryllium disease 170
Beta thalassemias 476
Bilirubin metabolism 520
Binasal hemianopia 366
Biomarkers in acute myocardial infarction 240

Bioterrorism 797
Bipolar disorder 699
Blackwater fever 87
Bladder dysfunction 433
Blast crisis in CML 484
Bleeding and clotting disorders 499
Blood loss anemia 464
Blood supply of the heart 180
Blood transfusion 511
Blood transfusion reactions 513
Body mass index (BMI) 675, 676
Bone marrow aspiration and biopsy 514
Bone pain 646
Botulism 17
Bradycardia 189
Brain abscess 407
Brain death 362
Brain natriuretic peptide (BNP) 198
Brain tumors 452
Breast cancer 732
Bronchiectasis 149
Bronchogenic carcinoma (lung cancer) 176
Brown-Séquard syndrome 430
Brucellosis 35
Brudginski's sign 386
Brugada syndrome 275
Bubonic plague 33
Budd-Chiari syndrome 551
Bulimia nervosa 703
Bullous pemphigoid 757
Bundle branch blocks 266
Burkitt's lymphoma 494
Byssinosis (Monday fever) 171

C

CABG contraindications 243
CABG indications 243
Calorie requirements of normal person 676
Cancer chemotherapy 730
Cancer–genetic factors 725
Cancer epidemiology 724
Cancer screening 726
Cancer–palliative care 733
Cancer–radiotherapy 731
Cancer–risk factors/etiology 724
Cancer–treatment 729
Candidiasis 112
Cannabis abuse 708
Carcinoid syndrome 344
Cardiac biomarkers 197
Cardiac catheterization 200, 201
Cardiac cirrhosis 542
Cardiac rehabilitation 240
Cardiac remodeling 208
Cardiac tamponade 297
Cardiogenic shock 242
Cardiomyopathies 289
Cardiopulmonary resuscitation (CPR) 244
Cardioversion and defibrillation 245
Carey-Coombs murmur 264
Carpal tunnel syndrome 442
Case scenario-based discussions 842–858
Cat-scratch disease 34
Causes of loud S1 194
Causes of unresolving pneumonia 145
Celiac sprue 328
Central sleep apnea 173
Cerebellopontine angle tumors 453
Cerebral malaria 86
Cerebrovascular accident 392
Chancroid 22
Charcot's joint (neuropathic arthropathy) 436
Charcot's triad 550
Chemoprophylaxis 8
Chest pain 181
Chickenpox 56
Chikungunya fever 72
Chilblains (pernio) 793
Child-Turcotte-Pugh scoring system 540
Cholangitis 550
Cholecystitis 557
Cholera-clinical features 30
Cholera—pathogenesis 29
Cholera 28
Cholinergic crisis 445
Chorea 421
Chromosomal disorders 741
Chronic bronchitis 137
Chronic cor pulmonale 210
Chronic diarrhea 304
Chronic fatigue syndrome 58
Chronic hepatitis 532
Chronic hepatitis B 528
Chronic hepatitis B carrier 530
Chronic hepatitis C 530
Chronic kidney disease (CKD) 567
Chronic lymphocytic leukemia (CLL) 485
Chronic myeloid leukemia (CML) 482, 483
Chronic obstructive pulmonary disease (COPD) 137
Chronic pancreatitis 349
Churg-Strauss syndrome) 670
Chvostek sign 610
Circle of Willis 392
Cirrhosis of liver 537
Classification of epilepsy 409
Clubbing 122
Cluster headache 375
CML–accelerated phase 484
Coagulation cascade 497, 498
Coal worker's pneumoconiosis (CWP) 169
Coarctation of aorta 227
Cold hemagglutinin disease (cold AIHA) 466
Collapsing pulse 190
Colonization 1
Coma 359, 360
Common cold 130
Common diseases in the elderly 822
Common fractures in the elderly 834
Community-acquired pneumonia 142
Complement fixation test 3
Complete blood count—CBC 455
Complications of blood transfusion 512
Complications of diabetes 632
Complications of insulin therapy 632
Complications of smoking 708
Compressive myelopathy 428
Computed tomography (CT scan) 353
Conduction system of the heart 181
Confidentiality in patient care 813
Congenital adrenal hyperplasia 618
Congenital heart diseases 221
Congenital hyperbilrubinemic disorders 524
Congenital syphilis 45
Conn's syndrome 614
Constipation 304
Constrictive pericarditis 296
Contact dermatitis 753
Continuous murmurs 264
Conversion disorder 704
Coombs' test (antiglobulin test) 468
Cor pulmonale 210
Coronary angiography (CAG) 201
Coronary artery bypass grafting (CABG) 242
Coronavirus infection 78
Corrosives ingestion 784
Cortical (frontal) bladder 435, 436
Corticosteroids in tuberculosis treatment 165
COVID-19 infection 79
COVID-19 vaccines 81
Creatine kinase-MB (CK-MB) 198
Creutzfeldt-Jakob disease (CJD) 449
Crohn's disease 333
Crystal induced arthropathies 655
CSF findings in meningitis 386
Cullen's sign 347
CURB-65 scoring 144
Cushing's syndrome 611, 612
Cutaneous leishmaniasis 92
CVA in the elderly 830
Cyanide poisoning 779
Cyanosis 185
Cystic fibrosis 151
Cysticercosis 98

D

Datura poisoning 782
Dawn phenomenon 638
Decision-making in emergency care 814
Decompression sickness (Caisson's disease) 796
Deep vein thrombosis (DVT) 278
Deep vein thrombosis (DVT)–prophylaxis 280
Degenerative joint disease in the elderly 833
Dementia 447
Dementia in elderly 827
Demyelinating neurological disorders 426
Dengue fever 67
Dengue hemorrhagic fever 67

Dengue shock syndrome 68
Depression 698
Depression in the elderly 826
Dermatitis (eczema) 752
Dermatitis herpetiformis 329
Dermatomyositis 665
Dermatophytoses 751
Diabetes insipidus (DI) 594
Diabetes mellitus 619
Diabetic foot 640
Diabetic ketoacidosis (DKA) 633
Diabetic nephropathy 638
Diabetic neuropathy 639
Diabetic retinopathy 638, 639
Dialysis disequilibrium syndrome 584, 585
Diarrhea 300
Dicrotic pulse/twice beating pulse 191
Differences between hemoptysis and hematemesis 130
Differences between stable angina, unstable angina, and MI 241
Differential cyanosis 186
Diffuse abdominal pain 351
Diffuse esophageal spasm 314
Digoxin 209
Dilated cardiomyopathy 291
Diphtheria 14
Diphyllobothriasis 99
Diplopia 368
Direct agglutination test (DAT) 3
Direct Coombs' test 468
Direct immunofluorescence 3
Disseminated intravascular coagulation (DIC) 508
Disseminated tuberculosis 163
Dissociated sensory loss 431
DKA diagnostic criteria 634
DKA management 634
Do not resuscitate (DNR) order 819
DOTS (Directly Observed Treatment-short Course) 162
DOTS-Plus 159
Down syndrome (mongolism) 742
Dracunculiasis (guinea worm disease) 110
Drowning 793
Drug-induced liver injury (hepatitis) 532
Duchenne muscular dystrophy 445
Duke criteria 213
Dyspepsia 312
Dysphagia 309
Dyspnea 124
Dystonia 420

E

Early diastolic murmur (EDM) 262
Eaton-Lambert myasthenic syndrome 445
Ebola virus disease 69
ECG changes in MI 237
Echinococcosis (dog tape worm) 100
Echocardiography (Echo) 200
Eisenmenger's syndrome 228
Ejection systolic murmur (ESM) 261
Electric shock/lightening injury 794
Electrocardiography (ECG) 198
Electroconvulsive therapy 712
Electroencephalography (EEG) 355
Emphysema 137
Empyema 176
Endobronchial tuberculosis 156
Endocrine glands 589
End-of-life care 736, 737
Endoscopic retrograde cholangiopancreatography (ERCP) 519
Endoscopic ultrasound (EUS) 520
Enteric fever 24
Enzyme-linked immunosorbent assay (ELISA) 1
Eosinophilia 472
Eosinophilic lung diseases (ELD) 171
Epidemic typhus fever 50
Epigenetics 740
Erysipelas 13
Erythema marginatum 248
Erythema migrans 49
Erythema multiforme 759
Erythema nodosum 766
Erythroderma (exfoliative dermatitis) 758
Erythropoietin 471
Essential thrombocytosis 489
Essential tremor 424, 425
Ethical issues in the care of the elderly 840
Ethylene glycol poisoning 780
Extradural hematoma (epidural hematoma) 415
Extrapulmonary tuberculosis (EPTB) 164

F

Facial nerve – course 378
Facial pain 375
Facial palsy—bilateral 381
Facial palsy—LMN 379
Facial palsy—UMN 379
Factor VIII (antihemophilic factor) 505
Fall and rise phenomenon in tuberculosis (TB) 164
Falls in the elderly 833
Falls prevention in elderly 833
Fanconi anemia 470
Farmer's lung (hypersensitivity pneumonitis) 167
Fat embolism 284
Fatty liver 535
Felty syndrome 650
Fever in pregnancy 52
Fever of unknown origin (FUO) 5
Fibrinolysis-for MI 238
Fibromyalgia 671
Filariasis 106
First heart sound 193
First-degree AV block 266
Fixed drug eruption (FDE) 758
Flaccid (LMN) bladder 435
Fluid volume depletion 713
Fluorosis 688
Folic acid deficiency 463
Food poisoning 11
Forced vital capacity 118
Fourth heart sound (S4) 197
Fractional excretion of sodium (FENA) 567
Frostbite (freezing cold injury) 792
Fulminant hepatic failure 533
Functional anatomy of the brain 389
Functional dyspepsia 313
Functions of liver 516
Functions of respiratory system 115
Functions of the kidneys 561

G

Galactorrhea 594
Gallstone disease (cholelithiasis) 558
Gardner's syndrome (familial adenomatous polyposis) 346
Gas gangrene 19
Gastroesophageal reflux disease (GERD) 307
Gene therapy 744
General paralysis of the insane 436
Generalized anxiety disorder 696
Generalized edema 714
Generalized lymphadenopathy 510
Generalized tonic clonic seizures (GTCS) 409
Genetic basis of heart failure 207
Genetic basis/pathophysiology of autoimmune disease 644
Genetic counseling 739
Genetic diseases–prevention 739
Genetics 738
Geriatrics 822
Gestational diabetes mellitus (GDM) 641
Giant cell arteritis (temporal arteritis) 668
Giardiasis 90
Glasgow Coma Scale (GCS) 361
Global aphasia 369
Glomerular filtration rate (GFR) 562
Glomerulonephritis (nephritic syndrome) 575
Glossopharyngeal neuralgia 377
Glucose-6-phosphate dehydrogenase deficiency 478
Glycated hemoglobin (HbA1c) 629
Gonococcal urethritis 21
Gonorrhea 21
Gout 655
Graft-versus-host disease (GVHD) 495
Granuloma inguinale (donovanosis) 36
Grattage test (scraping test) 755
Graves' disease 598
Grey-Turner's sign 347
Growth hormone deficiency 593
Guillain-Barre syndrome 440
Gynecomastia 618

H

H1N1 influenza 55
Hairy cell leukemia 486
Hanging 794
Hashimoto's thyroiditis 604
HbSag 529
Headache 370
Hearing loss in the elderly 837
Heart failure–classification 203
Heart failure–treatment 205
Heart failure 202
Heat cramps 790
Heat exhaustion 790
Heat stroke 790
Heat syncope 790
Helicobacter pylori 318
Hematemesis 320
Hematopoietic stem cell transplantation 494
Hematuria 563
Hemiballismus 423
Hemochromatosis 555
Hemodialysis 583
Hemoglobin structure 473
Hemoglobinopathies 474
Hemoglobin-S (Hb-S) 474
Hemolytic anemias 465
Hemolytic transfusion reactions 513
Hemolytic-uremic syndrome (HUS) 503
Hemophilia B (Christmas disease) 505
Hemophilia-A (classic hemophilia) 504
Hemoptysis 128
Hemoptysis in pulmonary tuberculosis 163
Hemorrhagic stroke 399
Henoch-Schönlein purpura (HSP) 670
Heparin-induced thrombocytopenia (HIT) 500
Hepatic encephalopathy 545
Hepatitis A 525
Hepatitis B 526
Hepatitis B-vaccination 528
Hepatitis C 530
Hepatitis D (delta hepatitis) 531
Hepatitis E 532
Hepatocellular carcinoma (hepatoma) 552
Hepatojugular reflux (abdominaojugular reflux) 193
Hepatorenal syndrome 547
Hereditary spherocytosis 477
Herpes labialis (cold sores) 763
Herpes zoster (shingles) 57
Hiatus hernia 306
Hiccups 311
High altitude illness 796
Hill's sign 259
Hirsutism 619
HIV transmission 74
HIV treatment 75
HIV virus 72, 73
Hodgkin's lymphoma (HL) 490
Holter monitoring 199
Homonymous hemianopia 366
Hook worm infestation 104
Hormones secreted by pituitary 590
Horner syndrome 367
Hospital-acquired pneumonia (HAP) 147
Human genome project 738
Human leukocyte antigen (HLA) system 745
Human metapneumovirus (HMPV) 82
Human papillomavirus (HPV) infection 59
Huntington's chorea 423
Hydatid cyst 100
Hydrocephalus 449
Hymenolepis nana (dwarf tapeworm) 100
Hypercalcemia 608
Hypercalcemic crisis 608, 609
Hyperkalemia 719
Hyperkalemia-ECG changes 719
Hypermagnesemia 720
Hypernatremia 717
Hyperosmolar hyperglycemic state (HHS) 635
Hyperparathyroidism 607
Hyperprolactinemia 594
Hypersplenism 510
Hypertension 284
Hypertensive emergency 288, 289
Hypertensive urgency 289
Hyperthermia (hyperpyrexia) 789
Hyperthyroidism (thyrotoxicosis) 596
Hypertrophic obstructive cardiomyopathy (HOCM) 289
Hypertrophic osteoarthropathy 124
Hypervitaminosis A 686
Hypervitamiosis D 692
Hypocalcemia 609
Hypoglycemia 636
Hypokalemia 718
Hypomagnesemia 720
Hyponatremia 714
Hypoparathyroidism 609
Hypopituitarism (panhypopituitarism) 590
Hypothalamic-pituitary-thyroid (HPT) axis 606
Hypothermia 791, 792
Hypothyroidism 600
Hypoxia 805

I

IBD-associated arthritis 655
Idiopathic intracranial hypertension 378
IgA nephropathy 577
Ileus (paralytic ileus) 343
Immune deficiency disorders 746
Immune reconstitution inflammatory syndrome (IRIS) 78
Immune thrombocytopenic purpura (ITP) 501
Immunoelectrophoresis 4
Immunofluorescence applications 3
Immunofluorescence test 3
Impaired fasting glucose (IFG) 629
Impaired glucose tolerance (IGT) 629
Impaired physicians 818
Implantable cardioverter-defibrillator (ICD) 276
Inclusion body myositis 666
Indications for colonoscopy in GI bleed 323
Indications for endoscopy in UGI bleed 322
Indications of anticoagulation 505
Indirect (passive) agglutination test 4
Indirect Coombs' test 468
Indirect immunofluorescence 3
Infection 1
Infection and cancers 731
Infectious mononucleosis (glandular fever) 58
Infective endocarditis 213
Infective endocarditis prophylaxis 219, 220
Infective endocarditis-treatment 218
Infestation 1
Inflammatory bowel diseases (IBD) 332
Influenza 53
Inhalant abuse 709
Initial management of poison ingestion/ drug overdose 772
Insomnia 709
Insulin analogues 631
Insulin preparations 629
Intellectual disability disorder (mental retardation) 711
Intention tremor 425
Intermediate syndrome (IMS) 775
Internal capsule 392
Interstitial lung disease (ILD) 166
Intestinal obstruction 343
Intracranial pressure 384
Intracranial space-occupying lesions 451, 452
Intravascular ultrasound (IVUS) 202
Iodization programs of India 606
Iron deficiency anemia 458
Iron metabolism 457
Irritable bowel syndrome (IBS) 339
Ischemic heart disease (IHD) 229
Ischemic stroke–clinical features 395
Ischemic stroke–treatment 396
Ischemic stroke 393

J

Janeway leisons 220
Japanese encephalitis 70
Jones criteria 248
Jugular venous pulse 192

K

Keratoconjuctivitis sicca 667
Kernicterus 479
Kernig's sign 386
Kidney biopsy 565
Killip classification of acute MI 241
Klebsiella pneumonia 148
Klinefelter's syndrome 743
Koplik's spots 60

Korsakoff psychosis 447
Kussmaul sign 193
Kyasanur forest disease (KFD) 71

L

Lactic acidosis 636
Lactose intolerance 330
Lacunar infarcts (lacunar stroke) 398
Latent autoimmune diabetes in adults (LADA) 627
Latent TB 161
Lead poisoning (plumbism) 782
Left ventricular hypertrophy (LVH) 245, 246
Legal aspects of poisoning 798
Legionnaires' disease 149
Leishmaniasis 91
Lepra reactions 42
Leprosy-lepromatous (LL) 40
Leprosy – tuberculoid (TT) 39
Leprosy (Hansen's disease) 39
Leprosy treatment 41
Leptrospirosis 47
Leukemia–acute 480
Levine's sign 231
LFTs in acute hepatitis 518
LFTs in obstructive jaundice 519
LGBTQA+ community 702
Libman-Sacks endocarditis 221
Lichen planus 764
Life cycle of malaria life cycle 83
Lifelong learning 810
Light's criteria 174
Listeriosis 13
Liver abscess 553
Liver biopsy 520
Liver function tests (LFT) 516
Liver transplantation 554, 555
Locked-in syndrome 362
Low backache 673
Lower abdominal pain 351
Low-molecular weight heparins (LMWHs) 506
Lown-Ganong-Levine syndrome 267
Lucio's phenomenon 43
Lumbar puncture 354
Lung abscess 153
Lung defense mechanisms 115
Lupus anticoagulant 673
Lyme disease (Lyme borreliosis) 49
Lymphogranuloma venereum (LGV) 53

M

Macrocytic anemia 460
Macrocytosis 460
Magnetic resonance angiography (MRA) 354
Magnetic resonance cholangiopancreatography (MRCP) 519
Magnetic resonance imaging (MRI) 353
Malabsorption syndrome 325
Malaria 83
Malignant melanoma 770, 771
Mammography 733
Management of cardiac arrest 244
Management of disability in the elderly 836
Mania 699
Marfan's syndrome 666
Massive splenomegaly 508
MDR tuberculosis 160
Measles (rubeola) 59
Mechanical ventilation 807
Mechanism of vomiting 299
Medical malpractice 817
Medical negligence 816, 817
Medical nutrition therapy (MNT) 642
Melanocytic nevi (moles) 768
Melioidosis 34
Meningitis 385
Meningovascular syphilis 435
Meralgia paresthetica 443
Mesenteric ischemia 338
Metabolic acidosis 721
Metabolic alkalosis 722
Metabolic syndrome 642
Methanol (methyl alcohol) poisoning 780
Methemoglobinemia 478, 479
Mid diastolic murmur (MDM) 263
Migraine headache 371
Migraine precipitants 372
Migraine–prophylaxis 373, 374
Migraine–treatment 373
Miliaria (heat rash) 762
Miliary mottling in chest X-ray 179
Miliary tuberculosis 163
Minimal change disease 574
Mitral regurgitation (MR) 252
Mitral stenosis 249
Mitral valve prolapse (MVP) 253
Mitral valve replacement 252
Modified Duke criteria 216
Molluscum contagiosum 764
Monoarthritis 645
Mood disorders 698
Motor aphasia 369
Motor neurone diseases (MND) 438
Movement disorders 417
Mucocutaneous leishmaniasis (ML) 92
Mucormycosis 114
Multidimensional geriatric assessments 823
Multinodular goiter 603
Multiple myeloma 496
Multiple sclerosis 426
Mumps 61
Munchausen syndrome 705
Muscular dystrophies 445
Mutation 738
Myasthenia gravis 443
Myasthenic crisis 445
Mycetoma (Madura foot or Maduromycosis) 38
Mycosis fungoides 494
Myelodysplastic syndrome 489, 490
Myelofibrosis 488
Myeloproliferative disorders 486
Myocardial infarction-treatment 237
Myocarditis 292
Myoclonus 423
Myopathy 445
Myxedema coma 601
Myxedema madness 602

N

Narcolepsy 710
National programs for anemia prevention 470
Necrotizing pneumonia 148
Negri bodies 65
Nelson's syndrome 614
Nephrotic syndrome 573
Nerve conduction velocity (NCV) studies 356
Nerve supply of the heart 181
Nerve supply of urinary bladder 433
Neurocysticercosis (NCC) 408
Neurocysticercosis 98
Neuroleptic malignant syndrome (NMS) 791
Neurosyphilis 435
Neurosyphilis 44
Neurotic *vs* psychotic disorders 693
Newer methods of diagnosis of tuberculosis 157
Newer oral anticoagulants (NOACs) 506
Niacin deficiency (pellagra) 687
Nicotine abuse 707
Nikolsky's sign 756
Nocardiosis 37
Nonalcoholic fatty liver disease (NAFLD) 535
Nonalcoholic steatohepatitis (NASH) 535
Noncardiogenic pulmonary edema 212
Non-Hodgkin's lymphomas (NHL) 492
Nonmaleficence in patient care 810
Non-ST elevation myocardial infarction (NSTEMI) 235
Nonthrombotic pulmonary embolism 204
Normal and abnormal functions of the brain lobes 390
Normal pressure hydrocephalus (NPH) 450
Northern blotting 5
Nosocomial infections (hospital-acquired infections) 10
N-Terminal pro-BNP 198
Nutcracker Esophagus 315
Nutritional assessment in adults 675
Nutritional disorders in the elderly 840
Nutritional requirement during illness 677
NYHA classification of heart failure 204
Nystagmus 383

O

Obesity 680
Obesity hypoventilation syndrome 172
Obesity–environmental factors 683

Obesity–natural history 684
Obesity–onogenic forms 683
Obesity–prevention 684
Obsessive-compulsive disorder (OCD) 697
Obstructive sleep apnea 173
Occult blood in the stool 305
Octreotide 324
Oleander poisoning 782
Oligoarthritis 645
Onchocerciasis (river blindness) 109
Oncogene 725
Opioid abuse 708
Opioid/morphine poisoning 781
Opportunistic infections 9
Opportunistic infections in AIDS 76
Optic atrophy 365
Optic neuritis 365
Oral glucose tolerance test (OGTT) 628
Oral iron therapy 459
Oral rehydration salt (ORS) 30
Organ donation 812
Organic *vs* functional disorders 693
Organophosphate-induced delayed neuropathy (OPIDN) 776
Organophosphorus poisoning 775
Osler's nodes 220
Osteoarthritis 646
Osteomalacia 689
Osteoporosis 691
Osteoporosis in the elderly 829
Oxygen therapy 806

P

Pain in cancer 734, 735
Pain relief in acute coronary syndrome 240
Palpitations 187
Pancreas or islet cell transplantation 627
Pancreatitis 347
Pancytopenia 472
Panic attack 697
Pansystolic murmur (holosystolic murmur) 262
Papilledema 364
Paracetamol (acetaminophen) poisoning 777
Paraesophageal or rolling hernia 306
Paraneoplastic syndrome 176
Paraneoplastic syndromes 728
Paraplegia 432
Paratyphoid fever 26
Parenteral iron therapy 459
Parenteral nutrition 678
Parkinsonism 417
Paroxysmal cold hemoglobinuria (PCH) 467
Paroxysmal nocturnal hemoglobinuria (PNH) 467
Paroxysmal supraventricular tachycardia (PSVT) 268
Patent ductus arteriosus (PDA) 226
Patient rights in health care 813
Peak expiratory flow rate (PEFR) 117
Pediculosis 750
Pemphigus 756
Peptic ulcer disease 315
Percutaneous balloon mitral valvotomy (PBMV) 251
Percutaneous transhepatic cholangiography (PTC) 520
Pericardial effusion 297
Pericarditis 295
Peripheral blood smear 455, 456
Peripheral neuropathy 439
Peritoneal dialysis 584
Pernicious anemia 463
Persistent vegetative state 362
Personality changes in the elderly 828
Pertussis 23
Peutz-Jeghers syndrome 346
Pheochromocytoma 614
Physician's role and responsibility to society 815
Physician-industry relationships 816
Pica 458
Pickwickian syndrome 172
Pinpoint pupils 367
Pinta 46
Pinworm infestation (enterobiasis, oxyuriasis) 106
Pituitary gland 590
Pituitary infarction (Sheehan's syndrome) 591
Pityriasis rosea 756
Plague 31
Plague-clinical features 32
Plague-treatment 33
Plantar reflex (Babinski sign) 359
Plasma cell disorders 496
Pleural effusion 174
Plummer-Vinson syndrome 311, 459
Pneumoconioses 168
Pneumocystis jiroveci pneumonia 95
Pneumonia 141
Pneumonic plague 33
Poison center 799
Polyarteritis nodosa (PAN) 669
Polyarthritis 646
Polycystic kidney disease (PKD) 579
Polycythemia 486
Polycythemia vera 487
Polygenic (multifactorial) disorders 741
Polymerase chain reaction (PCR) 4
Polymyalgia rheumatica (PMR) 672
Polymyositis 665
Polyuria 563
Portal hypertension 542
Post exposure prophylaxis (PEP) for HIV 76, 77
Posterior columns – diseases 437
Postherpetic neuralgia 378
Post-MI drug therapy 239
Poststreptococcal glomerulonephritis (PSGN) 577
Posttraumatic stress disorder (PTSD) 698
Prebiotics 344
Pre-excitation syndromes 267
Prenatal diagnosis 738, 739
Prevention of HIV transmission 76
Pre-XDR TB 161
Primary biliary cirrhosis 541
Primary hyperaldosteronism 614
Primary tuberculosis 156
Prinzmetal's angina (variant angina) 234
Probiotics 344
Professional qualities of a physician 809
Prolactinoma 594
Prophylaxis for opportunistic infections in HIV 77
Protein energy malnutrition (PEM) 679
Protein-calorie malnutrition in the hospital 676, 677
Protein-losing enteropathy 330
Proteinuria 563
Proteome 739
Proteomics 739
Proto-oncogene 725
Pseudo-clubbing 124
Pseudodiarrhea (false diarrhea) 300
Pseudogout 656
Pseudomembranous colitis 19, 337
Pseudotumor cerebri 378
Pseuodcyanosis 187
Psittacosis (parrot fever) 52
Psoriasis 753
Psoriatic arthritis 654
Psychiatric consultation in poisoning 798
Psychiatric disorders-classification 693
Psychosexual disorders 701
Psychosis 694
Ptosis (blepharoptosis) 363
Puddle sign 548
Pulmonary embolism 280
Pulmonary function tests (PFT) 116
Pulmonary hypertension 277
Pulmonary regurgitation (PR) 260
Pulmonary stenosis 260
Pulmonary tuberculosis 154
Pulsus alternans 191
Pulsus bigeminy 192
Pulsus bisferiens 191
Pulsus paradoxus 190
Pulsus parvus et tardus 191
Pyoderma 769
Pyramidal tract (corticospinal tract) 359

Q

Q fever 51

R

Rabies-antemortem diagnosis 64
Rabies-post-exposure prophylaxis of rabies 65
Rabies-pre-exposure prophylaxis 64
Rabies-prevention 64

Rabies 62
Rabies clinical features 63
Radial pulse 189
Radioiodine therapy 605
Radionuclide thyroid scanning 596
Ramsay-Hunt syndrome (herpes zoster oticus) 381
Ranson criteria 348
Rapid immunochromatographic test 2
Rapidly progressive glomerulonephritis (crescentic glomerulonephritis) 578
Raynaud's phenomenon 662
Reactive arthritis 653
Reed-Sternberg cells 492
Refractory ascites 549
Refusal of medical care 819
Rehabilitation of patients with a CVA 402
Reiter syndrome 653
Relapsing fever 48
Renal artery stenosis (RAS) 857, 588
Renal cell carcinoma (RCC) 588
Renal diet 571
Renal osteodystrophy 572
Renal replacement therapy 583
Renal transplantation 585
Renal tuberculosis 587
Renal tubular acidosis 586
Reperfusion therapy – MI 238
Research on human subjects 815
Respiratory acidosis 722
Respiratory alkalosis 723
Respiratory failure 804
Restrictive cardiomyopathy 291
Retrobulbar neuritis 365
Reye's syndrome 534
Rheumatic chorea (Sydenham's chorea; St. Vitus dance) 248
Rheumatic diseases 641
Rheumatic fever prophylaxis 249
Rheumatoid arthritis 647
Rheumatoid factor (RF) 651
Rickets 690
Right heart failure (RHF) 212
Role of a physician in healthcare system 809, 810
Romberg sign 437
Rome IV criteria for the diagnosis of IBS 339
Rose spots 25
Roth's spots 221
Rubella (German measles) 60

S

Salicylate (aspirin) poisoning 778
Sarcoidosis 664
Scabies 749
Scarlet fever 13
Schilling test (vitamin B_{12} absorption test) 463
Schilling test 327
Schistosomiasis (bilharziasis) 110
Schizophrenia 694
Schizophrenia-negative symptoms 695
Schizophrenia-positive symptoms 695
Scorpion stings 788
Scrub typhus 51
Scurvy 687
Second heart sound (S2) 195
Secondary (reactivation or post primary) TB 156
Secondary biliary cirrhosis 542
Secondary HTN 285
Second-degree AV block 266
Sedative-hypnotic (benzodiazepines, barbiturates) overdose 776
Sedative-hypnotic abuse 709
Seizure episode – acute management 411
Sensory aphasia 369
Sepsis 1, 802
Septic shock 1
Septicemic plague 33
Sequelae of pulmonary tuberculosis 160
Seronegative spondyloarthropathies 651
Shigellosis 27
Shock 800
Short stature 592
SIADH 716
Sick sinus syndrome 265
Sickle cell anemia 474
Sickle cell crisis 474
Sideroblastic anemias 472, 473
Silicosis 168
Simple goiter 602
Sinus arrhythmia 265
Sinus bradycardia 265
Sinus tachycardia 267
Sjögren's syndrome 667
Skin manifestations of internal disease 771
Sleep apnea 173
Sleep disorders 709
Sleepwalking (somnambulism) 710
Sliding hiatus hernia 306
Smoking cessation 708
Snake bite – management 787
Snake bite 785
Social interventions in the care of elderly 839
Solitary pulmonary nodule (SPN) 125
Somatic symptom disorders 704
Somogyi phenomenon 637
Southern blotting 5
Spastic (UMN) bladder 435
Spirometry 116
Splenic sequestration syndrome 475
Splenomegaly 508
Spondyloarthritis 651
Spontaneous bacterial peritonitis (SBP) 550
Sporotrichosis (rose gardener's disease) 114
Squamous cell carcinoma (SCC) 770
Staphylococcal food poisoning 12
Staphylococcal pneumonia 148
Status epilepticus 414
Stepwise treatment of asthma 135
Sterile pyuria 581
Steroid therapy 617
Stevens-Johnson syndrome 757
Stress ulcers 317
Stroke in young 402, 403
Strongyloidiasis 104, 105
Structure of a nephron 561
Subacute combined degeneration 437
Subarachnoid hemorrhage 400
Subclinical hypothyroidism 601
Subdural hematoma (SDH) 416
Sudden cardiac arrest (SCA) 243
Sudden cardiac death (SCD) 243
Supraventricular ectopics 274
Supraventricular tachycardias (svts) 267
Surgery in hemorrhagic stroke 401
Surgical intervention in GI Bleeding 322
Surrogate decision making 814
Sydenham chorea (St Vitus dance) 422
Syncope 183
Syphilis 43
Syphilis-latent 44
Syphilis-primary 43
Syphilis-secondary 44
Syphilis-tertiary 44
Syringomyelia 431
Systemic inflammatory response syndrome (SIRS) 801
Systemic lupus erythematosus (SLE) 659
Systemic sclerosis (scleroderma) 663

T

Tabes dorsalis 436
Tachycardia 189
Taenia saginata (beef tapeworm) 98
Taenia solium (pork tapeworm) 98
Takayasu arteritis 669
Tamm-Horsfall protein 564
Targeted therapy-in cancer 729
Tender hepatomegaly 522
Tetanus 15
Tetany 610
Tetralogy of Fallot (TOF) 223
Thalassemia major (Cooley's anemia) 476
Thalassemias 476
Third heart sound (S3) 196
Third-degree AV block (complete AV block) 266
Thrombocytopenia 500
Thrombolytic therapy in ischemic stroke 397
Thrombotic thrombocytopenic purpura (TTP) 502
Thyroid dermopathy (pretibial myxedema) 599
Thyroid function tests 595
Thyroiditis 603
Thyrotoxic crisis (thyroid storm) 599
Thyroxine (levothyroxine sodium) 604
Tinea versicolor (pityriasis versicolor) 751
Torsades de pointes 272

Tourniquet test (Hess test) 500
Toxic epidermal necrolysis 757
Toxic megacolon 336
Toxic shock syndrome (TSS) 12
Toxidromes 774
Toxoplasmosis 95
Transfusion-related acute lung injury (TRALI) 514
Transient ischemic attack (TIA) 403
Transjugular intrahepatic portosystemic stent (TIPS) 544
Transposition of the great arteries (TGA) 223, 224
Transverse myelitis 429
Traveler's diarrhea 302
Treadmill test (TMT) or exercise stress test 199
Treatment of opportunistic infections of HIV 77
Treatment of tuberculosis (TB) 158, 159
Tremor 424
Trench fever 35
Trench or immersion foot 793
Trichomonas vaginalis (trichomoniasis) 91
Trichuriasis (whipworm) 105
Tricuspid regurgitation 260
Tricuspid stenosis (TS) 259
Trigeminal neuralgia 376, 377
Tropical pulmonary eosinophilia 108
Tropical splenomegaly 88
Tropical sprue 329
Troponins (troponin I and troponin T) 197
Trousseau sign 610
Trypanosomiasis 93
Tuberculin skin test (Montoux test) 162
Tuberculous meningitis (TBM) 388
Tuberculous pericarditis 296
Tubulointerstitial nephritis (interstitial nephritis) 579
Tumor lysis syndrome 727
Tumor markers 726
Tumor suppression genes 726
Tumors of the mediastinum 79
Turner's syndrome 744
Type 1 diabetes 621
Type 2 diabetes 623
Type 2 diabetes-treatment 624
Type 2 lepra reaction (erythema nodosum leprosum) 42
Type I lepra reaction (reversal reaction) 42
Typhoid carrier 27
Typhoid fever 24
Typhoid fever-complications 25
Typhoid vaccines 26

U

Ulcerative colitis 335
Unstable angina 234
Upper abdominal pain 350
Uremia 571
Urinary tract infection (UTI) 580
Urticaria 759

V

Van den Bergh reaction 522
Variceal bleeding 544
Varicella-zoster virus infection 56
Vascular anatomy of the brain 389
Vascular events in the elderly 825
Vasculitis 667
Vasovagal syncope 184
Vena caval filters 283
Venereal disease research laboratory (VDRL) test 46
Ventilator associated pneumonia (VAP) 147
Ventricular ectopics/ventricular premature complexes 275
Ventricular fibrillation (VF) 273
Ventricular septal defect (VSD) 224
Ventricular tachycardia (VT) 271
Vertigo 382
Vesicoureteral reflux 582
Viral encephalitis 406, 407
Visceral leishmaniasis (kala-azar) 92
Vision abnormalities in the elderly 835
Visual pathway 366
Vital capacity 118
Vitamin A (retinol) deficiency 685
Vitamin B_1 (thiamine) deficiency 686
Vitamin B_{12} (cyanocobalamin) deficiency 460
Vitamin C (ascorbic acid) deficiency 687
Vitamin D deficiency 688
Vitamin K deficiency 692
Vitiligo 766
Vomiting 299
Von-Willebrand's disease 503

W

Wallenberg's syndrome (lateral medullary syndrome) 405
Warts 765
Wasting of small muscles of hand 446
Water hammer pulse 190
Waterhouse-Friderichsen syndrome 617
Wegener's granulomatosis 670
Weight loss 306
Weight loss 680
Weil's syndrome 48
Wells scoring system 281
Wernicke's encephalopathy 446
Wernicke-Korsakoff syndrome 686
Western blot (immunoblot) test 2
Whipple's disease 329
Whooping cough 23
Wide fixed split S2 195
Wilson disease 556
Withdrawal of treatment 820
Wolff-Parkinson-White (WPW) syndrome 267
Wuchereria bancrofti 107

X

XDR tuberculosis161
X-linked dominant diseases 741
X-linked recessive diseases 741

Y

Yaws 46
Yellow fever 66

Z

Zinc phosphide poisoning 777
Zollinger-Ellison syndrome (gastrinoma) 345